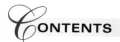ONTENTS

CONGRATULATIONS

You now have access to Mosby's "Get Smart" Bonus Package!

Here's what's included to help you "Get Smart"

sign on at:

http://www.mosby.com/MERLIN/matern_lowdermilk

A Web site just for you as you learn maternity nursing with the new 5th edition of *Maternity Nursing*

what you will receive:

Whether you're a student, an instructor, or a clinician, you'll find information just for you. Things like:
- Content Updates ● Links to Related Products
- Author Information . . . and more

plus:

 WebLinks

An exciting new program that allows you to directly access hundreds of active Web sites keyed specifically to the content of this book. The WebLinks are continually updated, with new ones added as they develop. **Simply peel off the sticker on this page and register with the listed passcode.**

LIFT HERE

PASSCODE INSIDE

If passcode sticker is removed, this textbook cannot be returned to Mosby, Inc.

Free CD-ROM Companion
with every copy of *Maternity Nursing*, 5th Edition

With Strong Emphasis on Clinical and Functional Relevance, this Valuable CD-ROM Features:

Critical Thinking Case Studies
Matching and Fill-in-the-Blank Questions
NCLEX - Style Review Questions
Vocabulary Review with Sound Pronunciations

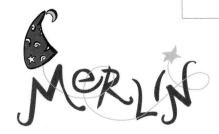

Mosby's **E**lectronic **R**esource **L**inks & **I**nformation **N**etwork

M Mosby

Maternity Nursing

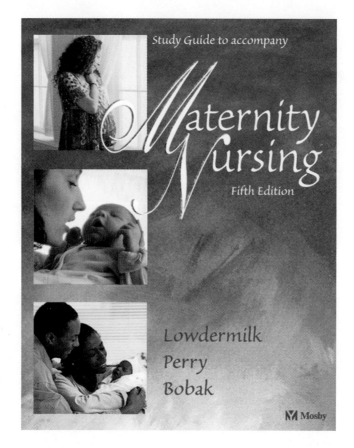
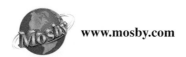

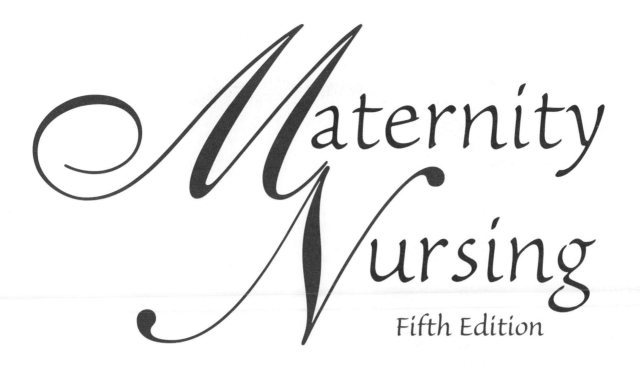

Maternity Nursing

Fifth Edition

Deitra Leonard Lowdermilk, RNC, PhD, FAAN
Clinical Professor, School of Nursing
University of North Carolina
Chapel Hill, North Carolina

Shannon E. Perry, RN, PhD, FAAN
Professor and Director, School of Nursing
San Francisco State University
San Francisco, California

Irene M. Bobak, RN, PhD, FAAN
Professor Emerita
San Francisco State University
San Francisco, California

with 640 illustrations

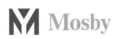 Mosby

St. Louis   Baltimore   Boston   Carlsbad   Chicago   Naples   New York   Philadelphia   Portland
London   Madrid   Mexico City   Singapore   Sydney   Tokyo   Toronto   Wiesbaden

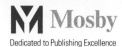
Mosby
Dedicated to Publishing Excellence

Publisher: **Sally Schrefer**
Editor: **Michael S. Ledbetter**
Developmental Editor: **Laurie K. Muench**
Project Manager: **Dana Peick**
Senior Production Editor: **Dottie Martin**
Designer: **Amy Buxton**
Manufacturing Supervisor: **Karen Boehme**
Cover Photos: **The Stock Market**

A NOTE TO THE READER:
The authors and publisher have made every attempt to check dosages and nursing content for accuracy. Because the science of pharmacology is continually advancing, our knowledge base continues to expand. Therefore we recommend that the reader always check the product information for changes in dosage or administration before administering any medication. This is particularly important with new or rarely used drugs.

FIFTH EDITION

Composition by Carlisle Communications
Printing by Von Hoffmann Press

Mosby, Inc.
11830 Westline Industrial Drive
St. Louis, Missouri 63146

Library of Congress Cataloging-in-Publication Data

Maternity nursing/[edited by] Deitra Leonard Lowdermilk, Shannon E.
    Perry, Irene M. Bobak.–5th ed.
            p.   cm.
    Includes bibliographic references and index.
    ISBN 0-323-00215-3
    1. Maternity nursing.   2. Pediatric nursing.   I. Lowdermilk,
    Deitra Leonard.   II. Perry, Shannon E.   III. Bobak, Irene M.
    [DNLM: 1. Maternal-Child Nursing.   2. Obstetric Nursing.   WY
157.3M4266 1999]
RG951.B66   1999
610.73'678–dc21
DNLM/DLC
for Library of Congress   98-33732
                                                 CIP

98 99 00 01 02 / 9 8 7 6 5 4 3 2 1

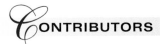
Kathryn Rhodes Alden, MSN, RN, IBCLC
Clinical Assistant Professor
University of North Carolina
Chapel Hill, North Carolina;
Lactation Consultant
Rex Healthcare
Raleigh, North Carolina

Debbie Fraser Askin, MN, RNC
Neonatal Nurse Practitioner
St. Boniface General Hospital;
Adjunct Professor
University of Manitoba
Winnipeg, Manitoba, Canada

Jean A. Bachman, RN, BSN, MSN, DSN
Associate Professor
Barnes College of Nursing
University of Missouri
St. Louis, Missouri

Kitty Cashion, RNC, MSN
Clinical Nurse Specialist
Department of Obstetrics & Gynecology
Division of Maternal-Fetal Medicine
University of Tennessee College of Medicine
Memphis, Tennessee

Jane G. Conner, MSN, WHCNP, RNC
Assistant Professor
Department of Nursing
California State University
Los Angeles, California

Carol Fowler Durham, RN, MSN
Clinical Assistant Professor
School of Nursing
University of North Carolina
Chapel Hill, North Carolina

Lienne D. Edwards, RN, PhD
Assistant Professor and Director
Office of Continuing Education
College of Nursing and Health Professions
University of North Carolina at Charlotte
Charlotte, North Carolina

Lisa B. Fikac, RN, BSN, MSN
Clinical Nurse I
Neonatal Intensive Care Unit
University of North Carolina Hospitals
Chapel Hill, North Carolina

Anne H. Fishel, PhD, RN, CS
Professor
School of Nursing
University of North Carolina
Chapel Hill, North Carolina

Catherine Ingram Fogel, RNC (WHNP), PhD, FAAN
Professor
University of North Carolina
Chapel Hill, North Carolina

Cynthia Garrett, RNC, BSN, MSN
Women's Health Clinical Nurse Specialist
University of North Carolina Hospitals
Chapel Hill, North Carolina

Bette B. Hammond, RN, BSN, MSN
Former Assistant Professor
St. Charles County Community College
St. Peters, Missouri

Sharon E. Lock, PhD, RNC, FNP
Assistant Professor
College of Nursing
University of Kentucky
Lexington, Kentucky

Mary Courtney Moore, RN, RD, PhD
Research Assistant Professor
Vanderbilt University
Nashville, Tennessee

Karen Piotrowski, RNC, MSN
Assistant Professor of Nursing
D'Youville College
Buffalo, New York

Rebecca Burdette Saunders, PhD, RNC
Associate Professor
School of Nursing
University of North Carolina at Greensboro
Greensboro, North Carolina

Barbara Peterson Sinclair, MN, RNC, OGNP, FAAN
Professor of Nursing;
Director, Institute of Nursing
California State University
Los Angeles, California

Betsy Stetson, EdD, RN, FACCE
Associate Professor
School of Nursing
University of San Francisco
San Francisco, California

Cecilia Tiller, RNC, DSN, WHNP
Professor and Dean
Abilene Intercollegiate School of Nursing
Abilene, Texas

Susan M. Tucker, MSN, RN, PHN, CNAA
Healthcare Consultant
Roseville, California

Rhea P. Williams, RN, MN, PhD
Professor
Department of Nursing
California State University
Los Angeles, California

Jan Lamarche Zdanuk, RNC, MSN, CNS, CFNP
Certified Family Nurse Practitioner
Health Partners Medical Group
Fort Worth, Texas

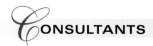

Carol M. Arnold, RN, MS, ACCE
Assistant Clinical Professor
Texas Woman's University
Dallas, Texas

Natalie Cloutman Arnold, RN,
MSN, PNP, CBE
Assistant Professor
Nursing Division
Tulsa Community College
Tulsa, Oklahoma

Nancy C. Barnum, MSN, RNC
Instructor
University of Kentucky College of
Nursing
Lexington, Kentucky

Jane Hoppe Berg, MSN, RNC,
FNP
Family Nurse Practitioner
Family Health Care Center
Pueblo West, Colorado

Bernadette Butler, EdD, MSN,
BSN, RNC
Associate Professor and Learning
Facilitator
University of Toledo/Medical
College of Ohio
Toledo, Ohio

Darlene Nebel Cantu, BSN,
MSN, RNC
Assistant Director
Baptist Health System School of
Professional Nursing
San Antonio, Texas

Joyce Cirrito, RNC, MS
Instructor
St. Joseph's Hospital Health Center
Syracuse, New York

Dorothy S. Crowder, RN, BSN,
MS, CCE
Professor Emeritus
Medical College of Virginia Campus
Virginia Commonwealth University
School of Nursing
Richmond, Virginia

Kathleen Didominicis, RN,
BSN, MSN
Professor of Nursing
Moraine Valley Community College
Palos Hills, Illinois

Dusty Dix, RN, MSN
Clinical Instructor
University of North Carolina
Chapel Hill, North Carolina

Lisa A. Dreyer, MSN, CNS, RNC
Senior Consultant
Fairfield, Ohio;
Phillips & Fenwick
Scotts Valley, California

Denise D. Estridge, RN, BSN,
MPH
Nursing Instructor
Guilford Technical Community
College
Jamestown, North Carolina

Polly D. Fehler, RN, AS, BSN,
MSN
Head of the Department of Nursing
Tri-County Technical College
Pendleton, South Carolina

Kathy Goodwin, RN, BSN,
MSN, CNM
SDBD
St. Louis, Missouri

Lynn Grommet, RNC, BSN,
MNSc
Course Coordinator for Nursing
Childbearing Family
East Arkansas Community College
Forrest City, Arkansas

Lois Hamel, RN, MS
Assistant Professor of Nursing
University of New England
Portland, Maine

Bette B. Hammond, RN, BSN,
MSN
Former Assistant Professor
St. Charles County Community
College
St. Peters, Missouri

Judith Johnson Hilton, BSN,
MSN, RNC
Assistant Professor of Nursing
Lenoir-Rhyne College
Hickory, North Carolina

Diane B. Longobucco, APRN,
NNP
Clinical Nurse Specialist
St. Francis Hospital and Medical
Center
Hartford, Connecticut

Anna Romig Nickels, RNC,
BSN
Perinatal Consultant
Herndon, Virginia

Patti F. Nicks, RN, MSN
Nursing Faculty
Angelina College
Lufkin, Texas

Karen Polansky, RN, MSN
Assistant Professor of Nursing
Indiana University of Pennsylvania
Indiana, Pennsylvania

Melissa Powell, BSN, MSN, RN
Assistant Professor
Eastern Kentucky University
Richmond, Kentucky

Sharon Rose, RN, MS
Professor of Nursing
Illinois Central College
Peoria, Illinois

Sara Alicia Peña Rounder, RN,
BA
Spanish Directives
Wilson, North Carolina

Shirley Schantz, RN, EdD
Assistant Professor
Barry University School of Nursing
Miami Shores, Florida

Colleen Tracy Snell, RN, BSN,
MS
Nursing Instructor
Anoka-Ramsey Community College
Coon Rapids, Minnesota

Sue A. Tedford, MNSc, APN,
CNS
Level III Coordinator
Jefferson School of Nursing
Pine Bluff, Arkansas

Sue G. Thacker, RNC, AS,
BSN, MS, PhD
Professor
Wytheville Community College
Wytheville, Virginia

Celesta L. Warner, RN, BSN,
MS
Clinical Instructor
Wright State University-Miami
Valley College of Nursing and Health
Dayton, Ohio

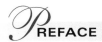

This fifth edition of *Maternity Nursing* focuses on the care of women during their reproductive years. Childbearing issues and concerns, including neonatal care, are the primary focus, but the promotion of wellness and the management of common women's health problems are also addressed.

Many exciting changes will be noted throughout the book; they demonstrate the different dimensions of women's health care. However, we have retained the underlying philosophy of the previous editions: we believe pregnancy and childbirth and developmental changes in a woman's life are natural processes. Our goal continues to be one of helping students understand and recognize normal processes before asking them to identify any complications and comprehend their implications for care.

The specialty of maternity and women's health nursing offers both challenges and opportunities. Nurses are challenged to assimilate knowledge and to develop the technical and critical thinking skills needed to apply that knowledge to practice. Each woman presents a new challenge because her individual needs must be identified and met. However, the opportunities are sufficiently extraordinary to make this one of the most fulfilling specialties of nursing practice.

The goal of nursing education is to prepare today's student to meet the challenges of tomorrow. This preparation must extend beyond the mastery of facts and skills. Nurses must be able to combine competence with caring and critical thinking. They must address both the physiologic and the psychosocial needs of patients. Above all, they must look beyond the condition and see the woman as an individual with distinctive needs but in the context of her family.

Maternity Nursing was developed to provide students with the knowledge and skills they need to become competent, think critically, and attain the sensitivity needed to become caring nurses. This fifth edition has been revised and refined in response to comments and suggestions from educators, clinicians, and students. It includes the most accurate, current, and clinically relevant information available.

▌ APPROACH

Professional nursing practice continues to evolve and adapt to society's changing health priorities. The rapidly changing health care delivery system offers new opportunities for nurses to alter the practice of maternity and women's health nursing and to improve the way care is given. Consumers of maternity and women's health care vary in age, ethnicity, culture, language, social status, marital status, and sexual preference. They seek care from obstetricians, gynecologists, family practice physicians, nurse midwives, nurse practitioners, and other health care providers in a variety of health care settings, including the home.

Nursing education must reflect these changes. Clinical education must be planned to offer students a variety of maternity and women's health care experiences in settings that include hospitals and birth centers, homes, clinics and private physicians' offices, shelters for the homeless or women in need of protection, and other community-based settings. The changing needs of nursing students must also be addressed. Today's nursing students are challenged to learn more than ever before—often in less time than their predecessors. Students are diverse. They may be high school graduates, college students, or older adults with families. They may be men or women. They may have college degrees in other fields and be interested in switching to a nursing career. They may represent various cultures; English may not be their primary language.

As we move into the twenty-first century, this fifth edition of *Maternity Nursing* is designed to meet the changing needs of women during their childbearing years and students in all types of nursing programs. This edition presents content in a clearly written and easy-to-read manner, but it retains the comprehensiveness of the previous editions.

To ensure a logical and consistent presentation of material, *Care Management* has been used as an organizing framework for discussion in the nursing care chapters. This approach incorporates the nursing process and collaborative care approach to demonstrate how nursing care is combined with care from other health care providers to give the most comprehensive care to women and newborns. Assessments, nursing diagnoses, expected outcomes, nursing and collaborative interventions, and evaluations of care are highlighted throughout the chapters for emphasis. Nursing plans of care reinforce the problem-solving approach to patient care. In chapters that focus on complications of childbearing and reproductive conditions, medical care is often the priority for patient care. Therefore, in these discussions, the specific condition and medical therapy are discussed first, followed by the nursing care management.

Health care today emphasizes *wellness*. This focus is an integral part of our philosophy. Likewise, the developmental changes a woman experiences throughout her life are considered to be natural and normal. In women's health care the goal is promotion of wellness for the woman through knowledge of her body and its normal functions throughout her reproductive years; health care also helps her develop an awareness of conditions that require professional intervention. The unit on women's health care has been expanded to emphasize the wellness aspect of care. This unit has been placed before the units on pregnancy because many of the aspects of assessment and care can be applied to later chapters. Pregnancy and childbirth are also part of a natural developmental process. We believe that students need to thoroughly understand and recognize the normal processes before they can identify complications and comprehend their implications for care. Therefore we present the entire normal childbearing cycle before discussing potential complications.

Teaching for self-care is an essential component of nursing care for women and newborns. The chapter on women's health promotion and screening emphasizes teaching for self-care to promote wellness and to encourage preventive care. A new chapter on adaptation to parenthood focuses on teaching for new mothers and infants at home. Special boxed features highlight teaching guidelines, patient self-care, and home care throughout the text.

To implement *preventive care,* perinatal and women's health nurses must be able to recognize signs and symptoms of emergent problems. Throughout the discussion of assessment and care, we alert the nurse to signs of potential problems and provide boxed information highlighting warning signs and emergency situations.

The family chapter includes a discussion of cultural implications and focuses on specific customs related to childbearing and women's health. This chapter also stresses the importance of assessing both the nurse's and the patient's cultural beliefs. Cultural implications are integrated throughout the text to emphasize the wide range of ethnic diversity and its effects on maternity and women's health. Boxes throughout the text highlight cultural aspects of care. A new chapter on care in the community and home has been added to prepare the student to provide maternity and women's health care in a variety of settings.

To truly meet the specific needs of each woman, the nurse must include family members and significant others in the plan of care. *Family dynamics* are rarely more prominent than in pregnancy and childbirth. The nurse is often the family's primary advocate. A separate chapter on the family, as well as integrated family considerations throughout the chapters on pregnancy, labor and birth, postpartum, and newborn care, demonstrate the importance of the entire family. Issues concerning grandparents, siblings, and different family constellations are addressed.

Nursing research is an integral part of nursing education and practice. Nursing research has been incorporated throughout the text to demonstrate the effect of research utilization on the practice of maternity and women's health nursing. In addition, boxed research highlights throughout the text describe selected studies and discuss clinical implications.

Maternity and women's health nurses confront ethical and legal challenges daily. Nurses need to develop a reflec-

tive stance that assesses the new reproductive and women's health technologies and policies in light of their potential to influence human well being. Information on legal tips are integrated throughout the text to emphasize these issues as they relate to maternal and women's health nursing.

▌FEATURES

The fifth edition features a contemporary design and spacious presentation. Students will find that the logical, easy-to-follow headings and attractive four-color design highlight important content and increase visual appeal. Hundreds of color photographs and drawings throughout the text illustrate important concepts and techniques to further enhance comprehension.

Each chapter begins with a list of *Key Terms* that alert students to new vocabulary; these terms are then boldfaced within the chapter. *Learning Objectives* focus students' attention on the important content to be mastered.

The organizing framework, *Care Management,* is used consistently to discuss nursing care. The five steps of the *Nursing Process* are incorporated into this framework. *Plans of Care* are included to help students apply the nursing process in the clinical setting. The *Plans of Care* use only NANDA-approved nursing diagnoses, describe expected outcomes for patient care, provide rationales for interventions, and include evaluations of care. *Care Paths, Protocols,* and *Procedures* for care are included to provide students with examples of various approaches to the implementation of care.

Special boxed features are integrated throughout for quick access of information and visual appeal. *Teaching Guidelines* supplement the narrative and emphasize the information needed by the nurse in teaching the patient. **NEW** for the fifth edition are *English-Spanish Guidelines* boxes that provide common English-to-Spanish phrases for patient instructions during care. *Home Care: Patient Instructions for Self-Care* boxes emphasize guidelines for the patient to practice self-care and provide information to help students transfer learning from the hospital to the home setting. *Emergency* boxes alert students to the signs and symptoms of various emergency situations and provide interventions for immediate implementation. **NEW** *Nurse Alert* boxes highlight critical information for the student. *Research* boxes include a brief summary of the study and a discussion of application to practice.

Although childbearing is a normal process, complications may occur. During assessment the nurse must be alert for *Signs of Potential Complications;* therefore we have included these signs as boxes in chapters that cover uncomplicated pregnancy and childbirth. Other features include *Cultural Considerations* boxes, which describe beliefs and practices about pregnancy, childbirth, parenting, and women's health concerns. *Legal Tip* boxes are integrated throughout to provide students with relevant information to deal with important legal areas in the context of maternity and women's health nursing.

At the end of each chapter, *Key Points* summarize important content. *Critical Thinking Exercises* guide students in applying their knowledge and in increasing their ability to think critically about maternity and women's health care issues.

ORGANIZATION

The fifth edition of *Maternity Nursing* comprises seven units organized to enhance understanding and learning and to facilitate easy retrieval of information.

Unit I, *Introduction to Maternity Nursing,* begins with an overview of contemporary maternity and women's health nursing practice. It then addresses the family as a unit of care, incorporating cultural aspects of care. The unit concludes with a **NEW** chapter on community and home care that provides understanding of these practice settings in relation to maternity and women's health nursing.

Unit II, *Reproductive Years,* is a revised and expanded unit on women's health. Four chapters discuss health promotion and screening, including a **NEW** chapter on the assessment of women and the presentation of common reproductive concerns.

Unit III, *Pregnancy,* describes nursing care of the woman and her family from conception through preparation for childbirth. A separate chapter on maternal and fetal nutrition emphasizes the important aspects of care, highlights cultural variations on diet, and stresses the importance of early recognition and management of nutritional problems.

Unit IV, *Childbirth,* focuses on collaborative care among physicians, nurse midwives, nurses, and women and their families during the processes of labor and birth. Separate chapters deal with the nurse's role in management of discomfort during labor and childbirth and fetal monitoring. These chapters familiarize students with current childbirth practices and focus on interventions to support and educate the woman and her family.

Unit V, *Postpartum Period,* deals with a time of significant change for the entire family. The mother requires both physical and emotional support as she adjusts to her new role. A **NEW** chapter on assessment and care during the fourth trimester focuses on these needs. A **NEW** chapter on adaptation to parenthood discusses family dynamics in response to the birth of a child and describes ways nurses can facilitate parent-infant adjustment, including anticipatory guidance for the first few days at home and with home follow-up care.

Unit VI, *The Newborn,* addresses the immediate assessment and care of the newborn. Information on the nutritional needs of the newborn and nursing care associated with breastfeeding and formula feeding are highlighted in a separate chapter.

Unit VII, *Complications of Childbearing,* discusses the conditions that place the woman, fetus, infant, and family at risk. This unit has been extensively reorganized and includes a chapter on high risk assessment of pregnancy complications, two **NEW** chapters on pregnancy at risk: preexisting and gestational conditions, and labor and birth complications; a **NEW** chapter on postpartum complications; and two chapters on newborn complications. Care management focuses on achieving the best possible outcomes as well as supporting the woman and family when expectations are not met. Loss and grief issues of the family experiencing a fetal, neonatal, or maternal loss are integrated throughout this unit.

The text concludes with a glossary of important terms, appendixes that provide valuable resource information, and a detailed, cross-referenced index.

TEACHING AND LEARNING PACKAGE

A number of ancillaries to this text have been developed to assist instructors and students in the teaching and learning process. For the instructor, these include an *Instructor's Resource Manual* and *Test Bank,* a CD-ROM version of the test bank, and a **NEW** CD-ROM product, *Mosby's Electronic Image Collection.* For the student, the fifth edition includes a *Study Guide* and a **NEW** interactive CD-ROM product, *Mosby's Maternal-Newborn CD-ROM.* Also **NEW** for the instructor and student is *Mosby's Electronic Resource Links and Information Network* (MERLIN).

The *Instructor's Resource Manual* and *Test Bank* are keyed chapter by chapter to the text to help coordinate course objectives to chapter content. Each chapter includes an outline of content with course guidelines, suggested learning activities, and a summary of key concepts. A sample syllabus that includes a proposed class schedule and reading assignments for 6- to 7-week courses or 14- to 16-week courses is provided. This gives educators suggestions for using the text in the most essential manner or in a more comprehensive way. New additions to the manual are the case study presentations, which can be used by educators to foster critical thinking skills. The test bank portion includes approximately 500 new questions that parallel the NCLEX format. The answer key provides page references and coding of questions according to the NCLEX test plan categories of nursing process and patient needs.

NEW to the fifth edition is *Mosby's Electronic Image Collection* CD-ROM. This valuable tool for instructors provides easy access to electronic images from the main textbook. Each image can easily be imported to a slide presentation program to enhance lecture materials.

A separate *Study Guide* includes *Chapter Review Activities* and *Critical Thinking Exercises* to reinforce learning and evaluate comprehension. The *Study Guide* can be used for homework assignments or for remedial practice. The exercises in the guide were developed to assist students in synthesizing knowledge of maternity and women's health care and to foster critical thinking.

NEW to the fifth edition is *Mosby's Maternal-Newborn CD-ROM*. This exciting, interactive program provides the students with a resource to solve critical thinking case studies, review questions, study questions, and review vocabulary. The vocabulary review will include a sound card so the student can easily hear and practice the correct pronunciations.

Also **NEW** for both the instructor and student is *Mosby's Electronic Resource Links and Information Network* (MERLIN). This exciting new resource is provided through Mosby's web page at www.mosby.com/MERLIN/matern_lowdermilk and allows access to information and resources based on topics covered in *Maternity Nursing*, fifth edition.

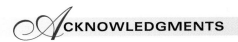
ACKNOWLEDGMENTS

Maternity Nursing would not have been possible without the contributions of many people. First, we want to thank the many nurse educators, clinicians, and nursing students in the United States, Canada, Australia, and Taiwan whose comments and suggestions about the manuscript led to this collaborative effort by an outstanding group of contributors. A special thanks goes to these contributors whose names are listed in the contributors list; their expertise and knowledge of current clinical practice and research has added to the relevancy and accuracy of the materials presented. We are also appreciative of the critiques given by the consultants, especially in their attention to validating the accuracy of the content and their challenge to present content differently and include new ideas. These combined efforts have resulted in a revision that incorporates the most recent research and current information about the practice of maternity and women's health care.

We offer thanks for shared expertise and photographs to the staffs of Lactation Consultants of North Carolina, University of North Carolina Hospitals, and University of North Carolina School of Nursing.

We would also like to thank the following photographers: Marjorie Pyle, RNC, Lifecircle, Costa Mesa, California; Kim Molloy, San Jose, California; Jonas N. McCoy, Raleigh, North Carolina; and Michael S. Clement, MD, Mesa, Arizona.

This edition also contains artwork by George Wassilchenko, Broken Arrow, Oklahoma; and Julie Perry, Burlingame, California. Their talent is evident in the precise detailed illustrations throughout the text.

Special words of gratitude are extended to Michael Ledbetter, editor; Laurie Muench, developmental editor; Dana Peick, project manager; Dottie Martin, production editor; and Amy Buxton, designer, for their encouragement, inspiration, and assistance in the preparation and production of this text. These talented and hardworking people helped change our manuscript into a beautiful book by editing the manuscript, designing an attractive format for our special features, and overseeing the production of the book from start to finish. We are especially thankful to Laurie Muench who always had time to answer our questions and to reassure us that we were doing a great job and were going to finish on time. A special thank you to Karen A. Piotrowski, RNC, MSN, for all her hard work in developing the *Instructor's Resource Manual and Test Bank*, the *Study Guide,* and *Mosby's Maternal-Newborn CD-ROM.* We also thank Sally Schrefer, publisher, for her support and encouragement throughout the project.

Finally, we thank Irene Bobak for her continued support and encouragement as we took on the responsibility for this fifth edition. We hope that we have continued her tradition of excellence.

Deitra Leonard Lowdermilk
Shannon E. Perry

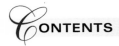
CONTENTS

unit four
CHILDBIRTH

unit five
POSTPARTUM PERIOD

unit six
THE NEWBORN

unit seven
COMPLICATIONS OF CHILDBEARING

Maternity Nursing

CHAPTER

1

Contemporary Maternity Nursing

SHANNON E. PERRY

LEARNING OBJECTIVES

- *Define the key terms.*
- *Describe the scope of maternity nursing.*
- *Evaluate contemporary issues and trends in maternity nursing.*
- *Describe sociopolitical issues affecting the care of mothers and infants.*
- *Compare selected biostatistical data among races.*
- *Describe social concerns in maternity nursing.*
- *Relate legal issues to standards of practice.*
- *Debate ethical issues in perinatal nursing.*

KEY TERMS

AWHONN
birthrate
evidence-based practice
fertility rate
infant mortality rate
low-birth-weight
managed care
maternal mortality rate
maternity nursing
outcomes-oriented care
preterm infants
self-care
standard of care
telemedicine

Maternity nursing focuses on the care of childbearing women and their families through all stages of pregnancy and childbirth, as well as the first 4 weeks after birth. Throughout the prenatal period, nurses, nurse-practitioners, and nurse-midwives provide care for women in clinics and doctor's offices and teach classes to help families prepare for childbirth. They also care for childbearing families during labor and birth in hospitals, in birthing centers, and in the home. Nurses with special training may provide intensive care for high-risk neonates in special care units and for high-risk mothers in antepartal units, critical care obstetric units, or at home. Maternity nurses teach about pregnancy; the process of labor, birth, and recovery; and parenting skills. Investment in health promotion during childbearing can make a significant difference not only in the health of individual women and their infants but also in society.

The strength of a society rests on the health of its mothers and infants. In the United States serious problems related to the health and health care of mothers and infants exist. Access to prepregnancy and pregnancy-related care for all women and the lack of reproductive health services for adolescents are major concerns. Nurses can influence health policy by their active participation in education of the public and of state and federal legislators (Hastings, 1995).

This chapter presents a general overview of issues and trends related to the health and health care of women and infants during the maternity cycle.

I CONTEMPORARY ISSUES AND TRENDS

Changing Health Care Delivery Structure

In 1995 health care consumed 13.6% of the gross domestic product. To control costs, managed care links providers and insurers; health maintenance organizations (HMOs) were the prototype for this system (Barter et al., 1995). The consolidation, merger, and integration of hospitals occurred; these systems were designed for provision of services throughout the continuum of care (Barter et al., 1995). The number of nurses in hospitals has declined and unlicensed assistive personnel and multiskilled workers have been substituted. The role of the nurse is evolving from primary caregiver to leader of the interdisciplinary care team. Documentation of patient outcomes has become essential (Barter et al., 1995). Advanced practice roles will increase as nurses assume more responsibility for care of patients.

Changing Childbirth Practices

Maternity care has changed dramatically. Women can choose either a physician or a nurse-midwife as their primary

1

care provider. In 1993 physicians attended 93.6% of all births in hospitals and nurse-midwives attended 4.8% of all births in hospitals; 1% were out-of-hospital births (Guyer et al., 1995). Home births comprised 0.6% of all births (Ventura et al., 1994). Women can give birth in a hospital labor room (rather than a delivery room), in a birthing room, a free-standing birthing center (Ernst, 1994), or at home.

Certified nurse midwives provide safe, quality care (Fischler & Harvey, 1995). Women who choose nurse-midwives as their primary providers participate actively in childbirth decisions and receive fewer interventions, such as epidural anesthesia for labor (Callister, 1995).

No longer are laboring mothers and their support persons separated. With family-centered care, fathers, partners, grandparents, siblings, and friends may be present for labor and birth. Fathers or partners may be present for cesarean births. Newborn infants remain with the mother and may breastfeed immediately after birth. Parents participate in caring for their infants in nurseries and neonatal intensive care units.

Nursing care is changing to single-room maternity care in which a woman labors, gives birth, and recovers in the same room (Labor-Delivery-Recovery [LDR]). In some settings, the entire hospital stay for a birth may occur in the same room (Labor-Delivery-Recovery-Postpartum [LDRP]). Instead of having one nurse care for the baby and another nurse care for the mother, some hospitals have one nurse caring for the mother and baby as a unit (couplet or mother-baby care). In some hospitals, central nurseries have been eliminated and babies "room-in" with their mothers. Many hospitals employ lactation consultants to assist mothers with breastfeeding.

Discharge of a mother and baby in 24 to 48 hours after birth is a common practice, resulting in a growing need for follow-up or home care. In some settings when mutually agreed upon by the primary provider and the mother, discharge may occur as early as 6 hours after birth. Legislation now ensures that mothers and babies are permitted to stay in the hospital at least 48 hours. Early discharge creates a need for focused and efficient teaching to enable parents and infant to have a safe transition to home. Nurses may establish "warm lines" or incorporate follow-up telephone calls or home visits into their practice as they assist families needing information and reassurance.

Neonatal security in the hospital setting is receiving increasing attention. A number of cases of "baby-napping" and sending home the wrong baby have been reported. Parents have expressed concerns for their infant's safety. Security systems are being placed in nurseries and nurses required to wear a photo identification or some other security badge.

Changing Views of Women

Women must be viewed holistically and in the context in which they live. Their physical, mental, and social needs must be considered because these areas are interdependent and influence women's health and illness (Breslin, 1995). Even the language health care providers use to describe women and their problems needs to be examined (Freda, 1995). For example, providers describe women who have an "incompetent cervix," who "fail to progress," or who have an "arrest" of labor, or they describe a fetus with intrauterine growth "retardation"; providers "allow" women a "trial" of labor. Caregivers might better describe a woman who has recurrent premature dilatation of the cervix or the fetus whose intrauterine growth has been restricted (Freda, 1995). In communications with women, health care providers must move away from punitive terms associated with confinement and prison (Peterson & Cefalo, 1990).

Violence is a major factor affecting pregnant women. Violence includes battery (which may increase during pregnancy), rape or other sexual assaults, and attacks with various weapons. It is estimated that 8.3% of pregnant women are battered (Loring & Smith, 1994). Sexual abuse survivors may have "body memories" that interfere with the process of childbirth.

Human immunodeficiency virus (HIV) and acquired immunodeficiency syndrome (AIDS) are increasingly affecting women and children. Approximately 30% of infants born to women with HIV will be infected with HIV (Kass, 1994). By the year 2000, AIDS will be among the top five causes of death in women of childbearing age (Covington & Collins, 1994). Limitation of reproductive choice of women infected with HIV is being discussed (Kass, 1994), and mass screening of infants and mothers is occurring (Grady, 1994).

Trends in Fertility and Birthrate

Fertility trends and birthrates reflect women's needs for health care. (See Box 1-1 for an explanation of biostatistical terminology useful in analyzing maternity health care.) In 1996 the **fertility rate,** the number of births to women of childbearing age (15 to 44), was 65.6 live births per 1,000 women. The highest birthrates were for women between the ages of 20 and 29 (Table 1-1). **Birthrate,** the number of live births per 1,000 population in 1 year, was 14.8 in 1996, the same as in 1995. Almost one third of all births in the United States in 1996 were to unmarried women with wide variation in rate among racial groups: African-American, 70.8 per 1,000; Hispanic, 104.4 per 1,000; and Caucasian 64.7 per 1,000 (Guyer et al., 1997). Births to unmarried women are commonly related to less favorable outcomes because there are typically a large number of teenagers in the unmarried group (32% in 1995). The rates of pregnancy (54.7 per 1,000) and abortion among adolescents is higher in the United States than in any other industrialized country (Burnhill, 1994; Guyer et al., 1997).

BOX 1-1 Maternal-Infant Biostatistical Terminology

Abortus: An embryo/fetus that is removed or expelled from the uterus at 20 weeks' gestation or less, or weighing 500 g or less, or measuring 25 cm or less.

Birthrate: Number of live births in 1 year per 1,000 population.

Fertility rate: Number of births per 1,000 women between ages 15 and 44 (inclusive), calculated on a yearly basis.

Infant mortality rate: Number of deaths of infants under 1 year of age per 1,000 live births.

Maternal mortality rate: Number of maternal deaths from births and complications of pregnancy, childbirth, and puerperium (the first 42 days after termination of the pregnancy) per 100,000 live births.

Neonatal mortality rate: Number of deaths of infants under 28 days of age per 1,000 live births.

Perinatal mortality rate: Number of stillbirths and the number of neonatal deaths per 1,000 live births.

Stillbirth: An infant who, at birth, demonstrates *no* signs of life, such as breathing, heartbeat, or voluntary muscle movements.

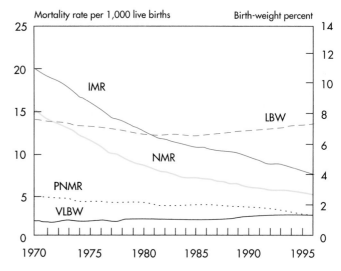

Fig. **1-1** Infant, neonatal, postnatal mortality and low-birth-weight and very low-birth-weight, United States, 1970 to 1995. *IMR,* infant mortality rate; *LBW,* low-birth-weight (<2,500 g); *NMR,* neonatal mortality rate; *PNMR,* perinatal mortality rate; *VLBW,* very low-birth-weight (<1,500 g). (Guyer B et al: Annual summary of vital statistics–1996, *Pediatrics* 100(6):905, 1997.)

TABLE 1-1 Birthrate According to Age—1996

AGE	RATE (/1,000 WOMEN)
15 to 17	36
18 to 19	89.1
20 to 24	109.8
25 to 29	112.2
30 to 34	82.5
35 to 39	34.3
40 to 44	6.6

Data from Guyer B et al.: Annual summary of vital statistics—1996, *Pediatrics* 100(6):905, 1997.

Number of low-birth-weight infants

Babies born weighing less than 2,500 grams are classified as **low-birth-weight (LBW),** and their risks for morbidity and mortality increase. By reducing the number of LBW infants, the health of infants improves. In 1996 the incidence of LBW infants reached 7.4%, the highest level since 1975 (Guyer et al., 1997). African-American babies are more than twice as likely as Caucasian babies to be LBW and to die in the first year of life. For African-American births, the incidence of LBW was 13.0% while the rate for Caucasian births was 6.3%. Cigarette smoking is associated with LBW, prematurity, and intrauterine growth restriction (Shu et al., 1995). In 1995, 13.9% of pregnant women smoked; this proportion represented a decline from 1993 (Guyer et al., 1997).

The proportion of **preterm infants,** those born before 38 weeks of gestation, was 10.7% in 1993, a slight decline attributed to the decline in African-American preterm births from 18.9% to 18.4%. The rate of Caucasian preterm births remained at 9.1% (Ventura et al., 1994). The number of multiple births increased in 1995; most of the increase is attributed to delay in childbearing and use of fertility drugs (Guyer et al., 1997).

Infant mortality in the United States

A common indicator of the adequacy of prenatal care and the health of a nation as a whole is the **infant mortality rate** (deaths per 1,000 live births). The infant mortality rate for 1996 was 7.2, the lowest ever recorded in the United States (Guyer et al., 1997). The infant mortality rate continues to be higher for African-American babies than for Caucasian babies, a gap that has widened since the mid-1970s (Kochanek & Hudson, 1995). Figure 1-1 illustrates the trend in infant mortality over the years. Limited maternal education, young maternal age, unmarried status, poverty, and lack of prenatal care appear to be associated with higher infant mortality rates. Poor nutrition, smoking and alcohol use, as well as maternal conditions such as poor health or hypertension, are also important contributors to infant mortality. A shift from the current emphasis on high-technology medical interventions to a focus on improving access to preventive care for low-income families is necessary.

International infant mortality trends

In comparing the infant mortality rates of Canada and the United States with other industrialized nations, it is significant to note that in 1995 Canada ranked fifteenth and the United States had the twentieth lowest rate (Guyer et al., 1997). Even though infant mortality decreased some in the United States, the United States did not keep pace with other industrialized countries. Some suggest that the problem in the United States is rooted in economic barriers and inadequate access to prenatal care, as well as poor financial and social benefits for childbearing women (National Commission, 1990).

Maternal mortality trends

Maternal mortality rate is defined as the number of maternal deaths per 100,000 live births. In 1994, 270 women in the United States died from complications of pregnancy, childbirth, and the puerperium (National Center for Health Statistics, 1995). African-American women were 4 times more likely to die from these complications than were Caucasian women, at a rate of 20.5 for African-American women compared with 4.8 for Caucasian women (Mortality Patterns–1993, 1996).

Trends Toward Consumer Involvement and Self-Care

In the 1960s patients began to demand information about medical technology and their medical care. A movement toward self-help and assuming responsibility for wellness also occurred. No longer do patients passively accept and follow the advice of health care providers. Patients demand information and take active roles in their health care. They make changes in health behaviors to improve pregnancy outcome (Higgins, Frank & Brown, 1994). Consumers are demanding a choice of health plans and providers but choice based on knowledge. In efforts to influence choice, increasing numbers of agencies, health plans, and employers are issuing report cards, that is, reports that contain ratings or scores that indicate quality or measure performance (Grimaldi, 1997). Consumers can use these ratings to judge quality or safety and make selections of providers or care delivery systems based on this information.

Self-care has been appealing to both patients and the health care system because of its potential to reduce health care costs. Maternity care is especially suited to self-care because childbearing is essentially health focused, patients are usually well when they enter the system, and visits to health care providers can present the opportunity for health and illness interventions. Measures to improve health and reduce risks associated with poor pregnancy outcomes and illness can be addressed. Visits to health care providers provide opportunities to address topics such as nutrition education, stress management, smoking cessation, alcohol and drug treatment, improvement of social supports, and parenting education.

High-Risk Pregnancies Escalate

High-risk pregnancies have increased, which means that a greater number of pregnant women are at risk for poor pregnancy outcomes. Escalating drug use (11% to 27% of pregnant women, depending on the geographic location) has contributed to higher incidences of prematurity, LBW, congenital defects, learning disabilities, and withdrawal symptoms in infants. Alcohol use in pregnancy has been associated with miscarriages (spontaneous abortions), mental retardation, LBW, and fetal alcohol syndrome.

Trend to High-Technology Care

Advances in scientific knowledge and the large number of high-risk pregnancies have contributed to a health care system that emphasizes high-technology care. Obstetrics has branched out to preconception counseling, more and better scientific techniques to monitor the mother and fetus, more definitive tests for hypoxia and acidosis, and neonatal intensive care units. Strides are being made in identifying genetic codes; genetic engineering is occurring in laboratories. In general, high-technology care has flourished while "health" care has been relatively neglected. These technologic advances have also contributed to higher health care costs.

Trends and Issues of High Costs

Health care is one of the fastest growing sectors of the U.S. economy. National health expenditures are 14.3% of the gross domestic product or one seventh of the U.S. economy (Vincenzino, 1994). Perinatal care cost $27.8 billion in 1989, representing $6,850 for each mother-infant pair (Long, Marquis & Harrison, 1994). A shift in demographics, an increased emphasis on high-cost technology, and liability costs of a litigious society contribute to the high cost of care. Most researchers agree that the costs of caring for the increased number of LBW infants in intensive care units has also contributed significantly to overall health care costs, especially because 19% of all uninsured women gave birth to an infant of LBW (National Commission, 1990).

In 1991 Medicaid funded 32% of all births in states reporting the data (Singh, Gold & Frost, 1994). Nursing is making some impact on cost-containment by providing midwifery care to pregnant women, but the lack of direct access to reimbursement for nurse practitioners and clinical nurse specialist services as direct care providers continues to be a problem (Ernst, 1994).

Managed Care Expands

Managed care continues to expand. Stahl (1997) predicted that enrollment in health maintenance organizations (HMOs) would increase 16% by 1997 and by the year 2000, there would be 100 million people enrolled in HMOs. **Managed care** focuses on meeting the patients' needs while promoting efficiency and cost-effectiveness. The drive to contain costs may compromise quality of services. Access to services and quality outcomes are hallmarks of success in managed care. The concept of care management is applied to maternity nursing in this text. Approaches such as protocols and critical paths are used where applicable.

Access to Care Problems

Access to prenatal care continues to be an issue through the 1990s. The proportion of women in 1994 who began prenatal care in the first trimester was 80.2%, the highest level ever reported; 4.4% or fewer delayed care until the third trimester or had no care (Guyer et al., 1997). Older mothers (86%) seek care earlier than those under 20 years of age (59%) (Ventura et al., 1994). However, many women with access to prenatal care entered the health care system late or came only sporadically. Minority women were less likely than Caucasian women to receive early prenatal care; 82% of Caucasian women, 67% of Hispanic women, and 66% of African-American women had prenatal care in the first trimester (Ventura et al., 1995). African-American women had fewer prenatal visits than Caucasian women (LaVeist, Keith & Gutierrez, 1995). Homelessness inhibits access to care.

Barriers to access need to be removed so pregnancy outcomes can be improved. The most significant barrier to access is the inability to pay. Lack of transportation and dependent child care are other barriers. When barriers are removed, low-income women seek care earlier and more often (Piper, Mitchel & Ray, 1994). Simple incentives to increase participation in prenatal care do not work (Laken & Ager, 1995). In addition to a lack of insurance and high costs, there is a shortage of providers for low-income women because many physicians either refuse to take Medicaid patients or take only a few such patients. This presents a significant problem because one in six births is to a mother who receives Medicaid.

Home Health Care Flourishes

A shift in settings from acute care institutions to the home has been occurring. Even high-risk childbearing women are increasingly cared for in the home. Technology previously available only in the hospital is now found in the home. This has affected the organizational structure of care, the skills required in providing such care, and the costs to consumers (deLissovoy & Feustle, 1991). Home health also has a community focus. Nurses are involved in providing care for women and infants in homeless shelters; school-based care for adolescents; and health promotion and prevention activities in community sites, such as schools, churches, and shopping malls. Nursing education curricula are increasingly community based.

TRENDS IN NURSING PRACTICE

The increasing complexity of care for maternity patients has contributed to specialization of nurses working with these patients. This specialized knowledge is being gained through experience, advanced degrees, and certification programs. Nurses in advanced practice—nurse-practitioners and nurse-midwives—may provide primary care throughout a woman's life, including during the pregnancy cycle. Lactation consultants provide services in the postpartum unit or on an outpatient basis.

Nursing Interventions Classification

When the National Institutes of Medicine proposed that all patient records be computerized by the year 2000, a need for a common language to describe the contributions of nurses to patient care became evident (Eganhouse, McCloskey & Bulachek, 1996). Nurses from the University of Iowa developed a comprehensive standardized language that describes interventions that are performed by generalist or specialist nurses. This language is included in the Nursing Interventions Classification (NIC). Interventions commonly used by maternal-child nurses include those in Box 1-2.

Evidence-Based Practice

There is increasing emphasis on providing **evidence-based practice** gained through research and clinical trials. As much as possible, nursing practice should be based on such evidence. Although not all practice can be based on evidence, practitioners must use the best available information upon which to base their interventions. Health care providers may write practice guidelines based on findings of research. The American College of Obstetricians and Gynecologists (ACOG) issues *Practice Patterns* based on evidence that has been evaluated and graded (Zinberg, 1997). The first consensus initiative of the Coalition for Improving Maternity Services, the *Mother-Friendly Childbirth Initiative*, is an evidence-based model that focuses on prevention and wellness as alternatives to costly programs of screening, diagnosis, and treatment (The Mother-Friendly Childbirth Initiative, 1997). AWHONN's 1998 edition of *Standards and Guidelines for Professional Nursing Practice in the Care of Women and Newborns* includes an evidence-based approach to practice.

Outcomes Orientation

Outcomes of care, that is, the effectiveness of interventions and quality of care, are receiving increased emphasis. **Outcomes-oriented care** measures effectiveness of care against benchmarks or standards based on results achieved by others. Quality indicators include cost, length of stay, and patient satisfaction. This focus requires nurses to take more responsibility for their actions and monitor the effects of their interventions.

BOX 1-2   *Childbearing Care Interventions*

LEVEL 1 DOMAIN: FAMILY
Care that supports the family unit

LEVEL 2 CLASS: CHILDBEARING CARE
Interventions to assist in understanding and coping with the psychologic and physiologic changes during the childbearing period

LEVEL 3: INTERVENTIONS
Amnioinfusion
Anticipatory guidance
Attachment promotion
Birthing
Bleeding reduction: antepartum uterus
Bleeding reduction: postpartum uterus
Bottle feeding
Breastfeeding assistance
Cesarean-section care
Childbirth preparation
Electronic fetal monitoring: antepartum
Electronic fetal monitoring: intrapartum
Environmental management: attachment process
Family integrity promotion: childbearing family
Family planning: contraception
Family planning: infertility
Family planning: unplanned pregnancy
Genetic counseling

Grief work facilitation: perinatal death
High-risk pregnancy care
Infant care
Intrapartal care
Kangaroo care
Labor induction
Labor suppression
Lactation counseling
Lactation suppression
Newborn care
Newborn monitoring
Nonnutritive sucking
Parent education: childbearing family
Phototherapy: neonate
Postpartal care
Preconception counseling
Pregnancy termination care
Prenatal care
Reproductive technology management
Resuscitation: fetus
Resuscitation: neonate
Risk identification: childbearing family
Surveillance: late pregnancy
Teaching: infant care
Tube care: umbilical line
Ultrasonography: limited obstetric

From Iowa Intervention Project: *Nursing interventions classification (NIC)*, ed 2, St Louis, 1996, Mosby.

Telemedicine

Telemedicine is an umbrella term for the use of communication technologies and electronic information to provide or support health care when the participants are separated by distance (Field, 1996; Fishman, 1997). Nurses can interact with patients and physicians using live, real-time, two-way audiovisual interaction. It is estimated that this technology will save billions of dollars annually for health care (Fishman, 1997). There are two types of telenursing: teletriage nursing and home health nursing (see also Chapter 3). Teletriage nursing is conducted over the telephone and involves timely referral of patients to appropriate health care resources. Nurses use protocols or guidelines to assess needs and symptoms and prioritize the urgency of the needs of the patient. In home health nursing, nurses use interactive video-based applications in the home. Patients can be monitored and reminded to take medications or vital signs. When telephone outreach crosses state lines, regulatory issues such as license to practice in more than one state cause concern. The National Council of State Boards of Nursing is addressing the issue of multistate regulation and licensing.

A Global Perspective

Advances in medicine and nursing have resulted in increased knowledge and understanding in the care of mothers and infants and reduced perinatal morbidity and mortality. However, these advances have affected predominantly the industrialized nations. As the world becomes smaller because of travel and communication technologies, nurses and other health care providers are gaining a global perspective and participating in activities to improve the health and health care of peoples worldwide. Nurses participate in medical outreach, providing obstetric, surgical, ophthalmologic, orthopedic, or other services; attend international meetings; conduct research; and provide international consultation. International student and faculty exchanges occur. More articles about health care in various countries are appearing in nursing journals. Several schools of nursing in the United States are World Health Organization (WHO) Collaborating Centers.

▌ STANDARDS OF PRACTICE AND LEGAL ISSUES IN DELIVERY OF CARE

Nursing standards of practice in perinatal and women's health nursing have been described by several organizations, including the American Nurses Association (ANA), which publishes standards for maternal-child health nursing; The Association of Women's Health, Obstetric, and Neonatal Nurses **(AWHONN),** which publishes standards and guidelines of

BOX 1-3 *Standards of Care for Women and Newborns*

STANDARDS THAT DEFINE THE NURSE'S RESPONSIBILITY TO THE PATIENT

Assessment
Collection of health data of the woman or newborn

Diagnosis
Analysis of data to determine nursing diagnosis

Outcome identification
Identification of expected outcomes that are individualized

Planning
Development of a plan of care

Implementation
Performance of interventions for the plan of care

Evaluation
Evaluation of the effectiveness of interventions in relation to expected outcomes

STANDARDS OF PROFESSIONAL PERFORMANCE THAT DELINEATE ROLES AND BEHAVIORS FOR WHICH THE PROFESSIONAL NURSE IS ACCOUNTABLE

Quality of care
Systemic evaluation of nursing practice

Performance appraisal
Self-evaluation in relation to professional practice standards and other regulations

Education
Participation in ongoing educational activities to maintain knowledge for practice

Collegiality
Contribution to the development of peers, students, and others

Ethics
Use of Code for Nurses to guide practice

Collaboration
Involvement of patient, significant others, and other health care providers in the provision of patient care

Research
Use of research findings in practice

Resource utilization
Consideration of factors related to safety, effectiveness, and costs in planning and delivering patient care

Practice environment
Contribution to the environment of care delivery

Accountability
Legal and professional responsibility for practice

Source: Association of Women's Health, Obstetric, and Neonatal Nurses (AWHONN): *Standards and guidelines for professional nursing practice in the care of women and newborns,* ed 5, Washington, DC, 1998, AWHONN.

practice and education; and the National Association of Neonatal Nurses (NANN), which publishes standards of practice for neonatal nurses. These standards reflect current knowledge and represent levels of practice agreed upon by leaders in the specialty (AWHONN, 1998) (Box 1-3). Because nursing practice, society, and the health care system are dynamic rather than static, guidelines may change while standards are intended to remain the same over time.

In addition to these more formalized standards, agencies often have their own policy and procedure books that outline standards to be followed in that setting. In determining legal negligence, the care given is compared to the standards of care. If the standard was not met and harm resulted, then negligence occurred. The number of legal suits in the perinatal area has typically been high. As a consequence, malpractice insurance costs are high for physicians, nurse-midwives, and nurses in labor and delivery.

LEGAL TIP **Standard of Care**
When you are uncertain about how to perform a procedure, consult the agency procedure book and follow the guidelines printed therein. These guidelines are the standard of care for that agency.

ETHICAL ISSUES IN PERINATAL NURSING

Ethical concerns and debates have multiplied with the increased use of technology and scientific advances. For example, with reproductive technology, pregnancy is now possible in women who thought they would never bear children, including some who are menopausal or postmenopausal. With induced ovulation and in vitro fertilization, multiple pregnancies occur and multifetal pregnancy reduction (selectively terminating one or more fetuses) may be considered (Lipitz, Mashiach & Seidman, 1994). Innovations such as intrauterine fetal surgery, therapeutic insemination, genetic engineering, surrogate childbearing, surgery for infertility, "test-tube" babies, fetal research, and treatment of very low-birth-weight (VLBW) babies have resulted in questions about informed consent and allocation of resources. The introduction of long-acting contraceptives has created moral choices and policy dilemmas for health care providers and legislators; that is, should some women (substance abusers, women with low incomes, or women who are HIV positive) be required to take the contraceptives

(Moskowitz, Jennings & Callahan, 1995)? With the potential for great good that can come from fetal tissue transplantation, what research is ethical? What are the rights of the embryo (Robertson, 1995)? Discussion and debate about these issues will continue for many years; nurses and patients, as well as scientists, physicians, attorneys and clergy, must be involved in the discussions.

RESEARCH INTO PRACTICE

The incorporation of research findings into practice is essential in developing a science-based practice. Practicing nurses can identify problems and read research literature to identify studies that address their clinical concerns. Research use must increase (Gennaro, 1994). AWHONN has conducted four research utilization (RU) projects: Transition of an Infant from an Incubator to an Open Crib, Management of Second-Stage Labor, Urinary Continence in Women, and Neonatal Skin Care. These projects were multistate and staff nurses were involved in data collection. Nurses can develop protocols and procedures based on published research. Health care providers need to support researchers in their endeavors.

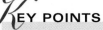
KEY POINTS

- Maternity nursing focuses on women and their infants and families during the childbearing cycle.
- Nurses caring for women can play an active role in shaping health care systems to be responsive to the needs of contemporary families.
- Childbirth practices have changed to become more family focused and to allow alternatives in care.
- Home care is an increasing and cost-effective alternative locus of care.
- The United States ranks twentieth among industrialized nations in infant mortality.
- Nursing is changing to include evidence-based and outcomes-oriented practice.
- Ethical concerns have multiplied with the increased use of technology and scientific advances.

CRITICAL THINKING EXERCISES

1 Consult the "yellow pages" of the telephone directory. What kind of and how many pregnancy-related services are you able to identify? Select one of the services and call to inquire if there is a bus stop close to the service and who can use the services. What does this information say about access to services?

2 Select five issues of a newspaper at random. Are there any articles that have relevance for mothers, infants, and families? Is there a theme to the articles? What "slant" do you perceive in the articles (e. g., welfare mothers need to work; teenage pregnancy is a problem). As a regular reader of that newspaper, would your view of women, infants, and families be influenced?

References

Association of Women's Health, Obstetric, and Neonatal Nurses (AWHONN): *Standards and guidelines for professional nursing practice in the care of women and newborns,* ed 5, Washington, DC, 1998, AWHONN.

Barter M et al.: The changing health care delivery structure: opportunities for nursing practice and administration, *Nurs Admin Q* 19(3):74, 1995.

Breslin E: Integrating women's health concepts in a nursing course, *Nurs Educ* 20(1):30, 1995.

Burnhill M: Adolescent pregnancy rates in the US, *Contemp Obstet Gynecol* 39(2):26, 1994.

Callister L: Beliefs and perceptions of childbearing women choosing different primary health care providers, *Clin Nurse Res* 4(2):168, 1995.

Covington C & Collins J: Back to the future of women's health and perinatal nursing in the 21st century, *J Obstet Gynecol Neonatal Nurs* 23(2):183, 1994.

deLissovoy G & Feustle J: Advanced home health care, *Health Policy* 17:227, 1991.

Eganhouse D, McCloskey J & Bulachek G: How NIC describes MCH nursing, *MCN Am J Matern Child Nurs* 21(5):247, 1996.

Ernst E: Health care reform as an ongoing process, *J Obstet Gynecol Neonatal Nurs* 23(2):129, 1994.

Field M, editor: *Telemedicine: a guide to assessing telecommunications in health care,* IOM, Washington, DC, 1996, National Academy Press, p 1.

Fischler N & Harvey S: Setting and provider of prenatal care: association with pregnancy outcomes among low-income women, *Health Care for Women Int* 16(4):309, 1995.

Fishman D: Telemedicine: bringing the specialist to the patient, *Nurs Manage* 28(7):30, 1997.

Freda M: Arrest, trial, and failure, *J Obstet Gynecol Neonatal Nurs* 24(5):393, 1995.

Gennaro S: Research utilization: an overview, *J Obstet Gynecol Neonatal Nurs* 23(4):313, 1994.

Grady G: HIV mass screening of infants and mothers: historical, technical, and practical issues, *Acta Paediatr Suppl* 400:39, 1994.

Grimaldi P: Report cards can improve choice, *Nurs Manage* 28(5):26, 1997.

Guyer B et al.: Annual summary of vital statistics—1994, *Pediatrics* 96(6):1029, 1995.

Guyer B et al.: Annual summary of vital statistics—1995, *Pediatrics* 98(6):1007, 1996.

Guyer B et al.: Annual summary of vital statistics—1996, *Pediatrics* 100(6):905, 1997.

Hastings K: Health care reform: we need it, but do we have the national will to shape our future? *Nurse Pract* 20(1):52, 1995.

Higgins P, Frank B & Brown M: Changes in health behaviors made by pregnant women, *Health Care Women Int* 15(2):149, 1994.

Kass N: Policy, ethics, and reproductive choice: pregnancy and childbearing among HIV-infected women, *Acta Paediatr Suppl* 400:95, 1994.

Kochanek K & Hudson B: Advance report of final mortality statistics, 1992, *Monthly Vital Stat Rep* 43 (suppl 6):1, 1995.

Laken M & Ager J: Using incentives to increase participation in prenatal care, *Obstet Gynecol* 85(3):326, 1995.

LaVeist T, Keith V & Gutierrez M: Black/white differences in prenatal care utilization: an assessment of predisposing and enabling factors, *Health Serv Res* 30(1):43, 1995.

Lipitz S, Mashiach S & Seidman D: Multifetal pregnancy reduction: the case for non-directive patient counseling, *Hum Reprod* 9(11):1978, 1994.

Long S, Marquis M & Harrison E: The costs and financing of perinatal care in the United States, *Am J Public Health* 84(9):1473, 1994.

Loring M & Smith R: Health care barriers and interventions for battered women, US Department of Health and Human Services, *Public Health Reports* 109(3):328, 1994.

Mortality Patterns—1993: *MMWR* 45(8):1, 1996.

Moskowitz E, Jennings B & Callahan D: Long-acting contraceptives: ethical guidance for policymakers and health care providers, *Hastings Center Report* 25(1):S1, 1995.

The Mother-Friendly Childbirth Initiative: The first consensus initiative of the coalition for improving maternity services, *J Nurs Midwifery* 42(1):59, 1997.

National Center for Health Statistics: Births, marriages, divorces, and deaths for 1994, *Monthly Vital Stat Rep* 43(12):1, 1995.

National Commission to Prevent Infant Mortality: *Troubling trends: the health of America's next generation*, Washington, DC, 1990.

Peterson R & Cefalo R: Terms of confinement, *Obstet Gynecol* 76(2):308, 1990.

Piper J, Mitchel E & Ray W: Presumptive eligibility for pregnant Medicaid enrollees: its effects on prenatal care and perinatal outcome, *Am J Public Health* 84(10):1626, 1994.

Robertson J: Symbolic issues in embryo research, *Hastings Center Report* 25(1):37, 1995.

Shu X, Hatch M & Mills J: Maternal smoking, alcohol drinking, caffeine consumption, and fetal growth: results from a prospective study, *Epidemiology* 6(2):115, 1995.

Singh S, Gold R & Frost J: Impact of the Medicaid eligibility expansions on coverage of deliveries, *Fam Plann Perspect* 26(1):31, 1994.

Stahl D: Managed care trends: the effect on subacute care, *Nurse Manage* 28(3):17, 1997.

Ventura S et al.: Advance report of final natality statistics, 1992, *Monthly Vital Stat Rep* 43(suppl 5):1, 1994.

Ventura S et al.: Advance report of final natality statistics, 1993, *Monthly Vital Stat Rep* 44(suppl 3):1, 1995.

Vincenzino J: Development in health care costs—an update, *Stat Bull* 75(1):30, 1994.

Zinberg S: A guest editorial: evidence-based practice guidelines: a current perspective, *Obstet Gynecol Surv* 52(5):265, 1997.

CHAPTER

The Family and Culture

RHEA P. WILLIAMS

LEARNING OBJECTIVES

- *Define the key terms.*
- *Identify key factors in determining the quality of family health.*
- *Identify and describe the key characteristics of various family forms.*
- *Explain the functions carried out by a family for the well-being of its members and society.*
- *Explain components of family dynamics and how these contribute to accomplishing family functions.*
- *Explain three theoretic approaches (family systems theory, family developmental theory, and family stress theory) for working with childbearing families. Describe the nursing implications of each theory.*
- *Relate the role and impact of culture on childbearing families.*

KEY TERMS

binuclear family
cultural competence
cultural context
extended family
family
family developmental theory
family dynamics
family functions
family stress theory
family systems theory
homosexual (lesbian and gay) family
nuclear family
reconstituted family
single-parent family

Maternity nurses have a unique privilege and opportunity to affect the future through their work with families. In traditional or nontraditional settings, whether in hospitals, homes, or communities, they are among the first health care practitioners to touch the lives of families. Thus the nurse acknowledges the family unit as the focus of care.

The **family,** one of society's most important institutions, represents a primary social group that influences and is influenced by other people and institutions. The family is recognized as the fundamental social unit because most people have more continuous contact with this social group than with any other. The family assumes most of the responsibility for the introduction and socialization of people. A family transmits its fundamental cultural background to its members. Despite modern stresses and strains, the family forms a social network that acts as a potent support system for its members.

To deliver safe, comprehensive, and holistic care, nurses working with childbearing families in hospitals and in the community need a clear understanding of the family as an institution in our society.

▌ DEFINING THE FAMILY

Families are defined in many ways. Definitions of the family usually involve explaining family *structure, functions, composition,* and *affectional ties.*

Friedman (1998) offers a broad definition of family, emphasizing the importance of emotional involvement as a necessary characteristic. She says, the family is "two or more persons who are joined together by bonds of sharing and emotional closeness and who identify themselves as part of the family." Wright and Leahey (1994) offer an even broader interpretation saying "The family is who they say they are." These definitions include a variety of family forms such as the nuclear family, the extended family, the binuclear family, and the reconstituted family.

Nuclear Family

The **nuclear family** consists of parents and their dependent children. The family lives apart from either the husband's or wife's family of origin, and is usually economically independent.

The nuclear family has long represented the "traditional" American family. In this family group, parents of different genders once played complementary roles of husband-wife and father-mother in giving emotional and physical support to each other and their children. Recent trends in contemporary society, however, have caused many variations in the "ideal" family structure. The "idealized" two-parent, two-child nuclear family, in which the father is the sole provider and the mother is the homemaker (Fig. 2-1), represents a small number of modern American families; this type of family constitutes fewer than 8% of all households (Walsh, 1993).

Extended Family

The **extended family** includes the nuclear family and other people related by blood. Called *kin,* these people include grandparents, aunts, uncles, and cousins (Fig. 2-2) (Friedman, 1998). Through its kinship network, the extended family provides role models and support to all members.

Alternative family forms

Variations of the traditional nuclear and extended families have always existed. Until recently, most of these alternative family forms have been considered deviations from the norm. Today, society recognizes and generally accepts these forms.

Single-Parent Family

The **single-parent family** is becoming an increasingly recognized structure in our society. The single-parent family may result from the loss of a spouse by death, divorce, separation, or desertion; from the out-of-wedlock birth of a child; or from the adoption of a child. Today almost 4 out of every 10 children in the United States are either currently living with a single parent or have lived with one in the past (Bianchi, 1994). Of all children 17 years old or younger, approximately 26% live in a family with a single parent, another relative, or a nonrelative. Fewer than 4% live with fathers in a single-parent household (Evolving American Family, 1993).

The single-parent family tends to be vulnerable economically and socially. Many single-mother households are poor, with the most disadvantaged being children living with mothers who were never married (Bianchi, 1994). Unless buttressed by a concerned society, single-parent families may create an unstable and deprived environment for the growth potential of children.

For other adults, the single-parent family is a chosen lifestyle that provides a free and open system for development of parents and children. In these families decision making and communication are seen as joint commitments between parent and child, and the parent-child relationship is considered a major source of life fulfillment.

Binuclear Family

Binuclear family refers to the family after divorce in which the child is a member of both their maternal and paternal nuclear households (Ahron & Perlmuller, 1982 as cited in

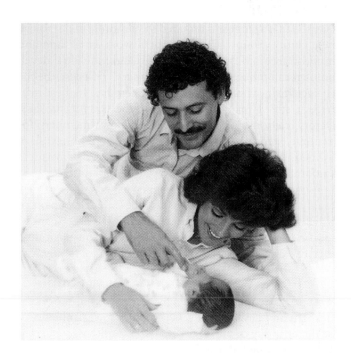

Fig. **2-1** Nuclear family. (Courtesy Ross Laboratories, Columbus, Ohio.)

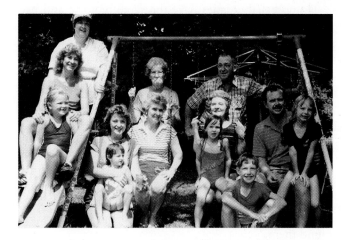

Fig. **2-2** Extended family. (From Lowdermilk D, Perry S & Bobak I: *Maternity & women's health care,* ed 6, St Louis, 1997, Mosby.)

Friedman, 1998). In these families, the degree of cooperation between the parents varies.

Reconstituted Family

The **reconstituted family,** also called a *blended, combined,* or *remarried family,* includes stepparents and stepchildren. Separation, divorce, and remarriage commonly take place in the United States, where approximately 50% of marriages end in divorce. Divorce and remarriage may occur at any time in the family life cycle and affect family function differently, depending on when they occur in the cycle. Whatever the timing, effort is required to constitute and stabilize new family groups. This emotional work takes time and must be accomplished before family and individual development can proceed. Visher and Visher (1993) describe the characteristics of successful remarried families. In these marriages a strong relationship between the couple and satisfactory relationships among unrelated family members (for example, stepparents, stepchildren, and stepsiblings) have formed. The separate households cooperate to provide a smooth transition as children move back and forth between households. The family has realistic expectations of new family relationships, and they provide an environment in which losses (for example, death and divorce) can be mourned. In addition, through creativity and flexibility, they can establish satisfying rituals for the new family.

Homosexual (Lesbian and Gay) Family

Western society has increasingly recognized **homosexual (lesbian and gay) families.** Children in such families may be the offspring of previous heterosexual unions, conceived by one member of a lesbian couple through therapeutic insemination, or adopted. Laird (1993) estimates that the number of children in lesbian and gay families ranges from 6 to 14 million.

Homosexual couples have the same biologic and psychologic needs as heterosexual couples. They too desire quality health care for themselves and for their children. The attitude toward lesbians and gays and their experiences when seeking health care, however, suggests much room for improvement. Homosexuals often encounter humiliation, disregard, and intimidation. Partners are often not allowed in the examining room or in pediatric care. Because of negative experiences within the health care system, lesbians may delay seeking health care for important symptoms (Quimby, 1994). Despite this, Laird (1993) points out that "children of gay and lesbian parents appear to grow and thrive as well as children in heterosexual families in spite of the prejudice and discrimination that can and does surround them."

Family Unit

Although society finds it difficult to precisely define the family, the members of a family can readily describe its composition. Family members know who is kin and who is not, how the family has affected their lives, and in what family style they believe.

However the family is defined, the lack of an adult makes the family unit incomplete. From an adult's perspective, the family can be composed of people of any age or gender who are bound by a blood or love relationship. From the child's perspective, the family involves relationships between the child's dependent self and one or more protective adults.

Regardless of the form that a family assumes or the society in which it lives, the family possesses enduring characteristics that have far-reaching personal and societal effects.

What then are the functions that families must perform, and how can nurses best support families facing economic and social pressures?

I FAMILY FUNCTIONS

Although family functions have evolved and changed over time (Friedman, 1998; Hanson & Boyd, 1996) in response to social and economic changes, the family progresses through its life cycle (Table 2-1) and continues to carry out certain functions for the well-being of family members and the wider society.

Friedman (1998) describes the **family functions** as the affective, socialization, reproductive, economic, and health care functions. The affective function focuses on meeting family members' needs for affection and understanding. It is seen as one of the most vital functions of families. The socialization function refers to the learning experiences provided within the family to teach children their culture and how to function and assume adult social roles. It is a lifelong process that includes internalizing norms and values appropriate for each developmental milestone. The reproductive function serves to ensure family continuity over the generations and the survival of society. Economic functions involve the family's provision and allocation of sufficient resources. Health care functions are met by provision of physical necessities including food, clothing, shelter, and health care. The health care function of families has expanded in recent years. Cox (1997) maintains that: "As the U.S. health care system shifts its focus from illness to wellness and health promotion, health professionals must empower families to be responsible for their own health and offer them access to do so."

Although certain functions are relegated to or emphasized more in one phase of the family's life cycle than another (e.g., the care and socialization of children are part of the childbearing and childrearing phase of the cycle), many of the functions are continuous for the family's survival and progress. Because families reflect societal changes, many functions that were previously performed almost exclusively by one gender (e.g., child care, financial support) are now shared by both genders.

I FAMILY DYNAMICS

Families work cooperatively to accomplish family functions. Through **family dynamics,** (interactions and communication), family members assume appropriate social roles. Social roles are learned in the family and in pairs (e.g., mother-father, parent-child, and brother-sister). Role pairing enables social interactions to take place in an orderly, predictable manner—the roles are said to be complementary. Some families maintain a traditional pairing of roles, whereas other families change behavior patterns to suit a change in family lifestyle. Rather than mother-father, brother-sister, the roles

	TABLE 2-1	*Stages of the Family Life Cycle*

FAMILY LIFE CYCLE STAGE	EMOTIONAL PROCESS OF TRANSITION: KEY PRINCIPLES	SECOND-ORDER CHANGES IN FAMILY STATUS REQUIRED TO PROCEED DEVELOPMENTALLY
Leaving home: single young adults	Accepting emotional and financial responsibility for self	Differentiation of self in relation to family of origin Development of intimate peer relationships Establishment of self regarding work and financial independence
The joining of families through marriage: the new couple	Commitment to new system	Formation of marital system Realignment of relationships with extended families and friends to include spouse
Families with young children	Accepting new members into the system	Adjusting marital system to make space for child(ren) Joining in child-rearing, financial, and household tasks Realignment of relationships with extended family to include parenting and grandparenting roles
Families with adolescents	Increasing flexibility of family boundaries to include children's independence and grandparents' frailties	Shifting of parent-child relationships to permit adolescent to move in and out of system Refocus on midlife marital and career issues Beginning shift toward joint caring for older generation
Launching children and moving on	Accepting a multitude of exits from and entries into the family system	Renegotiation of marital system as a dyad Development of adult-to-adult relationships between grown children and their parents Realignment of relationships to include in-laws and grandchildren Dealing with disabilities and death of parents (grandparents)
Families in later life	Accepting the shifting of generational roles	Maintaining own and/or couple functioning and interests in face of physiologic decline; exploration of new familial and social role options Support for a more central role of middle generation Making room in the system for the wisdom and experience of the elderly, supporting the older generation without overfunctioning for them Dealing with loss of spouse, siblings, and other peers and preparation for own death; life review and integration

From Carter B & McGoldrick M: *The changing family life cycle: a framework for family therapy,* ed 2, New York, 1998, Allyn & Bacon.

may be mother-daughter, mother-son. *Negotiation* brings these pair roles into a new alignment. Negotiation is essential to maintain family equilibrium.

Each family sets up *boundaries* between itself and society. Each member is extremely conscious of the difference between "family members" and "outsiders," people without kinship status. Some families isolate themselves from the outside community. Others have a wide community network to help in times of stress. Although boundaries exist for every family, family members set up *channels* through which they interact with society. These channels also ensure that the family receives its share of social resources.

Ideally the family uses its resources to provide a safe, intimate environment for the biopsychosocial development of the family members. The family nurtures the newborn and teaches gradual *socialization* of the growing child. Children form their earliest and closest relationships with their parents or guardians; these affiliations continue throughout their lifetime. For better or worse, parent-child relationships influence self-worth and the ability to form later relationships. The family also influences the child's perceptions of the outside world. The family provides the growing child with an identity that possesses both a past and a sense of the future. Cultural values and rituals are passed from one generation to the next through the family (Friedman, 1998).

Through everyday interactions, the family develops and uses its own patterns of verbal and nonverbal *communication.* These patterns give insight into the emotional exchange within a family and act as reliable indicators of interpersonal functioning. Family members not only react to the communication or actions of other family members, but also interpret and define them.

Over time the family develops protocols for *problem solving,* particularly regarding important decisions such as having a baby, buying a house, or sending children to college. The criteria used in making decisions are based on *family values* and *attitudes* concerning the appropriateness of the behavior and the moral, social, political, and economic events of society. The *power* to make critical decisions is given to a family member through tradition or negotiation. This power is not always stated. Power reflects the family's concepts of male or female dominance and the cultural practices, social customs, and community norms. As a result, family members attain certain *statuses* or *hierarchies.* They play out these statuses by assuming various *roles.* Most families have a member who "takes charge" or "is supportive" or "can't be expected to do anything."

I FAMILY THEORIES

Many academic disciplines study the family and have developed theories that provide differing perspectives for assessment and interventions. By knowing these theories, nurses can understand family functioning and dynamics. The theories provide a basis for planning and intervening in the day-to-day care of families and help predict events that may necessitate a modification of care.

Family Systems Theory

Wright and Leahey (1994) define *system* as a complex of elements in mutual interaction. When applied to families, the systems theory allows nurses to "view the family as a unit and thus focus on observing the interaction among family members rather than studying family members individually"

(Wright & Leahey, 1994). The individual maintains uniqueness and importance as an individual system. However, as a family member, the individual remains a part of a larger system (the family) and also a subsystem.

Wright and Leahey outline the key characteristics of the **family systems theory:**

1. A family system is part of a larger suprasystem and comprises many subsystems. The target or focal system (the family) must relate to a suprasystem (e.g., community, cultural group, church, or health care system) and its subsystem (e.g., spousal or parent-child subsystem). As with all systems, the family has boundaries that identify its members. These boundaries have various degrees of permeability, which determine the extent of influence by those outside the system.
2. The family as a whole is greater than the sum of its individual members. Viewing the interaction of the whole family helps nurses more fully understand the functioning of individual family members.
3. A change in one family member affects all family members.
4. The family is able to create a balance between change and stability. This balance allows the family to remain flexible and adapt to changes.
5. Family members' behaviors are best understood from a view of circular rather than linear causality. With circular causality, an individual's behavior affects and is affected by the behavior of others; with the linear view, one behavior simply causes another.

Implications for maternity nursing

The family systems theory encourages nurses to view individual family members as part of a larger family system influenced by and influencing others. Application of these concepts can guide assessment and interventions for the family. For example, the childbearing family as a system interacts with many elements in the environmental suprasystem, including the health care community. The extent to which this suprasystem influences the family in matters such as prenatal care, childbirth education, and infant care depends on the family's boundary permeability. A relatively closed family may only want instructions from others within the family, whereas a relatively open family may be more receptive to instruction from health care providers.

Family Developmental Theory

The **family developmental theory** focuses on the family as it moves in time. Family members pass through phases of growth, from dependence through active independence to interdependence. The family's structure and function also varies over time. Together, these stages constitute the family life cycle. Carter and McGoldrick (1988) outline the tasks of the family life cycle in Table 2-1.

Mercer (1989) summarizes the essence of the developmental approach in family nursing:

> Developmental concepts include movement to a higher level of functioning. This implies continuous, unidirectional progression. However, during transitional periods from one stage or phase to the next, disequilibrium occurs, during which time the individual may revert to an earlier level of developmental responses. Families face normative and unexpected transitions that also create a period of disorganization, during which the family functions at a lower level than usual. Resolution of the disequilibrium or crisis has potential to lead to a higher level of family functioning.

Implications for maternity nursing

The developmental perspective provides many useful insights into family functioning. Knowing about the phases of the life cycle can assist nurses in providing anticipatory guidance for families. For example, helping childbearing families prepare for the birth of a newborn may minimize the development of crises.

The family as a group and as individuals simultaneously engages in developmental tasks (Duvall, 1977; Erikson, 1968). If the developmental task of the family does not correspond with that of the person, disharmony occurs. Two examples include the adolescent father who is grappling with the need to break from his own family ties but is also expected to establish monetary and other support for his new family and a toddler learning socially acceptable behaviors who may revert to infantile behavior when introduced to a new sibling. Using this knowledge, the nurse helps the family develop appropriate coping mechanisms.

The developmental approach presents a realistic, constantly evolving concept of family. The phases of the life cycle are easier to plot in the nuclear family than in an extended family because the extended family may involve many generations (Fig. 2-3). Sometimes it may be difficult to document the life cycle of a family, because it often changes or disintegrates before the nurse can grasp its significance.

Family Stress Theory

Hill originally developed the **family stress theory** in 1949. Known as the *ABCX theory*, it describes how families adapt differently to the same stressor. Researchers use three factors to explain the outcome (X): the stressor itself (A), the family's existing resources (B), and the family's perception of the stressor (C). Other researchers, including Boss (1996), modified and expanded Hill's theory. Boss views this linear approach to understanding family stress as no longer valid. She believes that family stress must be studied within the internal and external contexts in which the family is living. The internal context involves elements that a family can change or control, such as family structure (i.e., boundaries and roles), psychologic defenses (i.e., perception of the

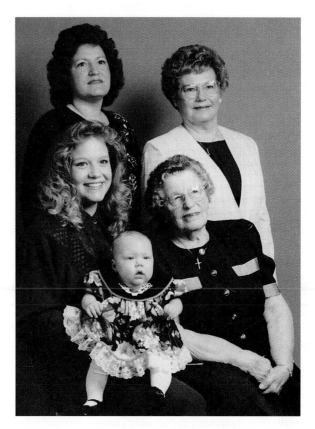

Fig. **2-3** Five generations of a family. (From Lowdermilk D, Perry S & Bobak I: *Maternity & women's health care*, ed 6, St Louis, 1997, Mosby.)

event), and philosophic values and beliefs. On the other hand, the external context consists of the time and place in which a particular family finds itself. A family has no control over these elements, which include the culture of the larger society, time in history in which the events happen to the family, economic state of society, maturity of the individuals involved, success of the family in coping with stressors, and genetic inheritance. According to Boss, the nurse should ascertain a family's internal context before helping its members manage stress.

Implications for maternity nursing

Nurses working with childbearing families may find the family stress theory particularly useful because of its realistic and practical approach. As expressed by Boss (1996), because today's families experience a great deal of pressure, they need to develop stress-management strategies. Maternity nurses usually care for healthy but highly stressed families. Nurses who understand the components of the family stress theory and stress management can intervene to reduce the stress level.

Boss considers birth one of the expected developmental (maturational) stressor events. Although a birth is expected and normal, its occurrence causes family dynamics to shift, thus having the potential to change the family's stress level. Boss says that families "experience increased levels of stress at each transition point, at least until the process of reorganization is accomplished after each addition or loss of a family member."

Maternity nurses work with families experiencing nonnormative (unexpected or situational) stressor events such as complicated pregnancies. These highly stressful events require the interventions of nurses who understand family stress management.

Nurses can assist families in changing their stress levels by helping families control internal context factors. For example, if a family's perception of a stressful event is based on incorrect or incomplete information, the nurse intervenes through educational strategies. Nurses can also explain various dimensions of the external context. For example, explaining normal infant growth and development (maturation) may reduce the stress of parenting.

▌KEY FACTORS IN FAMILY HEALTH

With childbearing families, family dynamics, family socioeconomics, and family response to stress and culture are important in determining the quality of family health. For example, family dynamics (see previous discussion) encompass the coordination of intrafamilial roles, distribution of power within the family, and decision-making process. Family dynamics also affect the use of health services.

Family socioeconomic characteristics influence the family's ability to access and use health care services. Socioeconomic factors govern expectations, obligations, and rewards, all of which influence the use of health services. In addition, the family acts as the primary economic unit in which incomes may be pooled, expenditure decisions made jointly, and services rendered internally.

Friedman (1998) considers a family's social class as the prime molder of its lifestyle. She says that socioeconomic factors and cultural background "exert the greatest overall influence on family life, influencing family values and practices, family behavior patterns, socialization, and world experiences families have." The interplay among stress, perception, and resources affects the level of support given to family members. The family's response to stress influences its members' physiologic and psychologic well-being. Cultural responses to childbearing and the use of related health care services also play central roles in family health.

▌CULTURAL FACTORS

Cultural Context of the Family

The **cultural context** of the family should concern nurses, especially when they provide care to the childbearing family. A critical life experience, such as childbearing, often involves traditional beliefs and practices. A culture's economic, religious, kinship, and political structures pervade its beliefs and practices regarding childbearing. All cultures maintain behavioral norms and expectations for each stage of the perinatal cycle. These norms and expectations evolve from a culture's view of how people stay healthy and prevent illness. To practice with **cultural competence**, nurses must focus on the way people of different cultures perceive life events and the health care system. Patients have a right to expect that their physiologic and psychologic health care needs will be met and that their cultural beliefs will be respected.

Culture has many definitions. Helman (1990) views culture as a set of guidelines, which individuals inherit as members of a particular society, that tell people how to view the world and how to relate to other people, supernatural forces, and the natural environment. Cultural knowledge includes beliefs and values about each facet of life. These guidelines have been tested over time. They relate to food, language, religion, art, health and healing practices, kinship relationships, and all other systems of behavior.

Many subcultures may be found within each culture. *Subculture* refers to a group existing within a larger cultural system that retains its own characteristics. A subculture may be an ethnic group or a group organized in other ways. For example, in the United States, many ethnic subcultures such as African-Americans, Asians, and Mexican-Americans exist, as do subcultures within these groups. Nurses should also remember that the Caucasian population in America has diverse and multiple subcultures. Although the recent literature in the area of ethnicity and health has focused on people of color, little has been written about Caucasian ethnic communities (e.g., Italian-, Polish-, and German-Americans) (Spector, 1996). In issues of health, illness, and major life transitions, there may be greater differences among Caucasian groups than has generally been acknowledged.

Each subculture holds rich and complex traditions, including health practices. These traditions vary from group to group. In a multicultural society, many groups can influence these traditions and practices. As cultural groups come in contact with each other, acculturation and assimilation may occur.

Acculturation refers to changes that take place in one or both groups when people from different cultures come in contact with one another. People may retain some of their own culture while adopting some of the cultural practices of the dominant society. This familiarization among cultural groups results in much overt behavioral similarity, especially in mannerisms, styles, and practices. Dress, language patterns, food choices, and health practices especially reveal differences among cultural groups within a society. In the United States, acculturation is generally thought to take three generations. The adult grandchild of the immigrant is usually fully Americanized (Spector, 1996). An example of acculturation would be the adoption of ethnic food practices in the United States. It is important to note that even when individuals have become acculturated, during times of childbearing, childrearing, crisis, and illness, a person may rely on old cultural patterns (Ramer, 1992).

Assimilation, on the other hand, refers to when a cultural group loses its identity and becomes a part of the dominant culture. According to Friedman (1998), "assimilation denotes the more complete and one-way process of one culture being absorbed into the other." Assimilation is the process by which groups "melt" into the mainstream, thus accounting for the notion of a "melting pot," a phenomenon that has been said to occur in the United States. In contrast, Spector (1996) asserts that in the United States, the melting pot, with its dream of a common culture, "has proved to be a myth and faded; it is now time to identify the mosaic phenomenon and both accept and appreciate the differences among people."

A wide range of cultural diversity exists within society. The health care provider striving to provide culturally appropriate health care must assess the beliefs and practices of the patient. Nurses must also be aware of factors that may prevent some health care practitioners from providing optimal care. Understanding the concepts of ethnocentrism and cultural relativism may help nurses care for families in a multicultural society.

Ethnocentrism refers to "the view that one's culture's way of doing things is the right and natural way" (Galanti, 1991). Essentially, ethnocentrism supports the notion "my group is best." Although the United States is a culturally diverse nation, the prevailing practice of health care is based on the beliefs and practices held by members of the dominant culture, primarily Caucasians. This practice is based on the biomedical model that represents pregnancy and childbirth as phenomena with inherent risk most appropriately managed through specific knowledge and technology. When encountering behavior in women unfamiliar with this model, the nurse may become frustrated and impatient. The nurse may label the women's behavior inappropriate and believe that it conflicts with "good" health practices. If this system, the Western health care system, provides the nurse's only standard for judgment, the behavior of the nurse is called *ethnocentric.*

Cultural relativism, the opposite of ethnocentrism, refers to learning about and applying the standards of another person's culture to activities within that culture. To be culturally relativistic, the nurse recognizes that people from different cultural backgrounds comprehend the same objects and situations differently. In other words, culture determines a person's viewpoints.

Cultural relativism does not require nurses to *accept* the beliefs and values of another culture; rather nurses recognize that others' behavior may be based on a system of logic different from their own. Cultural relativism affirms the uniqueness and value of every culture. Spector (1996) states that "because health care providers learn from their culture the way and the how of being healthy or ill, it behooves them to treat each patient with deference to his own cultural background."

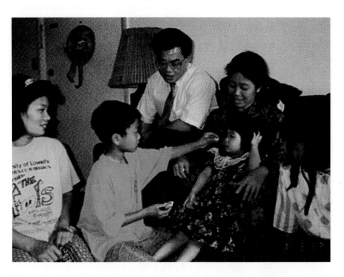

Fig. 2-4 Southeast Asian families may be large and closely spaced. They are often a closely knit group. (From Dickason E, Silverman B & Kaplan J: *Maternal-infant nursing care,* ed 3, St Louis, 1998, Mosby.)

Childbearing Beliefs and Practices

Nurses working with childbearing families in the United States and Canada care for families from different cultures and ethnic groups (Fig. 2-4). To provide culturally competent care, the nurse should be aware of the cultural beliefs and practices important to individual families. Countless beliefs and practices stem from a religious or an ethnic origin and may be observed by families with differing cultural backgrounds. Spector (1995) observed that people who have maintained a strong sense of their heritage may hold onto traditional health beliefs.

A nurse should consider the products of culture, including communication, space, time, and family roles, when working with childbearing families (Giger & Davidhizar, 1995). Communication often creates the most difficult problem for nurses working with patients from diverse cultural groups. Communication includes understanding not only the individual's language, varied dialect, and style, but also volume of speech and meaning of touch and gestures. Whenever the patient, family, or both do not speak the same language as the nurse, the nurse can use an interpreter to address the family's health care needs in a culturally competent manner. When using an interpreter, the nurse respects the family by addressing questions to them and not the interpreter (Box 2-1).

Personal space needs and feelings of territoriality develop in a cultural setting. Although personal space varies from person to person and with the situation, the dimensions of comfort zones differ from culture to culture. Actions such as touching, placing the patient in proximity to others, taking away personal possessions, and making decisions for the patient can decrease personal security and heighten anxiety. On the other hand, if the nurses respect the need for

---

| BOX 2-1 | *Working with a Translator* |

STEP 1: BEFORE THE INTERVIEW

A. Outline your statements and questions. List the key pieces of information you want/need to know.

B. Learn something about the culture so that you can converse informally with the translator.

STEP 2: MEETING WITH THE TRANSLATOR

A. Introduce yourself to the translator and converse informally. This is the time to find out how well he or she speaks English. No matter how proficient or what age the translator is, be respectful. Some ways to show respect are to ask a cultural question to acknowledge that you can learn from the translator, or you could learn one word or phrase from the translator.

B. Emphasize that you *do* want the patient to ask questions because some cultures consider this inappropriate behavior.

C. Make sure the translator is comfortable with the technical terms you need to use. If not, take some time to explain them.

STEP 3: DURING THE INTERVIEW

A. Ask your questions and explain your statements (see Step 1 above)

B. Make sure that the translator understands which parts of the interview are most important. You usually have limited time with the translator and you want to have adequate time at the end for patient questions.

C. Try to get a "feel" for how much is "getting through." No matter what the language is, if in relating information to the patient the translator uses far fewer or far more words than you do, "something else" is going on.

D. Stop every now and then and ask the translator, "How is it going?" You may not get a totally accurate answer,

but you will have emphasized to the translator your strong desire to focus on the task at hand. If there are language problems: (1) speak *slowly*; (2) use gestures (e.g., fingers to count or point to body parts); and (3) use pictures.

E. Ask the translator to elicit questions. This may be difficult, but it is worth the effort.

F. Identify cultural issues that may conflict with your requests or instructions.

G. Use the translator to help problem solve, or at least give insight into possibilities for solutions.

STEP 4: AFTER THE INTERVIEW

A. Speak to the translator and try to get an idea of what went well and what could be improved. This will help you to be more effective with this or another translator.

B. Make notes on what you learned for your future reference or to help a colleague.

Remember:

Your interview is a *collaboration* between you and the translator. *Listen* as well as speak.

Notes:

1. The translator may be a child, grandchild, or sibling of the patient. Be sensitive to the fact that the child is playing an adult role.

2. Be sensitive to cultural and situational differences (e.g., an interview with someone from urban Germany will likely be different from an interview with someone from a transitional refugee camp).

3. Younger females telling older males what to do may be a problem for both a female nurse and for a female translator. This is not the time to pioneer new gender relations. Be aware that in some cultures it is difficult for a woman to talk about some topics with a husband or a father present.

Courtesy Elizabeth Whalley, PhD, San Francisco State University.

---

distance, they allow the patient to maintain control over personal space and support the patient's autonomy, thereby increasing the patient's sense of security. For example, since Chinese-Americans have traditionally been a noncontact group, some may consider closeness, increased eye contact, and touch offensive or impolite. Nurses can avoid misunderstandings by providing explanations whenever performing tasks that require close contact (Chang, 1995). Nurses often use touch, especially in areas such as labor and delivery. The acceptance and effectiveness of these approaches must be considered in a cultural context.

Nurses must also understand time as it pertains to culture. People in cultural groups may be oriented to the past, present, or future. People who focus on the past strive to maintain tradition and have little motivation for formulating future goals.

Some individuals who focus on the present neither save for the future nor appreciate the past; these individuals do not necessarily adhere to strict schedules. Individuals oriented to the future use the present to achieve future goals.

The time orientation of the childbearing family may affect nursing care. For example, talking to a family about bringing the infant to the clinic for follow-up examinations (events in the future) may be difficult for the family that focuses on the present. On the other hand, a family with a future-oriented sense of time, in which events are planned, may be more likely to return as scheduled for follow-up visits. Despite the differences in time orientation, each family may be equally concerned for the well-being of its newborn.

Family roles involve the expectations and behaviors associated with a member's position in the family (e.g., mother,

CULTURAL CONSIDERATIONS

Questions to Obtain Cultural Explanations about Childbearing

1. What do you and your family think you should do to remain healthy during pregnancy?
2. What are the things you can do or not do to improve your health and the health of your infant?
3. Who do you want with you during your labor?
4. What things or actions are important to you and your family after the infant's birth?
5. What do you and your family expect from the nurse or nurses caring for you?
6. How will family members participate in your pregnancy, childbirth, and parenting?

father, or grandparent). Social class and cultural norms also affect these roles; distinct roles for men and women may be stressed. For example, culture may influence whether a man actively participates in the pregnancy and childbirth. The way that health care practitioners manage this family's care in turn molds its experience in and perception of the Western health care system. Maternity care practitioners expect fathers to be involved, but this role expectation may conflict with that of Mexican- and Arab-Americans, who usually view the birthing experience as a female affair (see Cultural Considerations box).

The nurse must be familiar with each woman as an individual and validate her cultural beliefs. The nurse supports and nurtures the beliefs that promote physical or emotional adaptation to childbearing. However, if certain beliefs might be harmful, the nurse should carefully explore them with the woman and use them in the reeducation and modification process.

Table 2-2 provides examples of some cultural beliefs and practices regarding childbearing among European-Americans (Caucasians), Hispanics, Asians, African-Americans, and Native Americans. Most of these cultural beliefs and customs reflect the traditional culture and are not universally practiced by all members of the cultural group in every part of the country. Callister (1995) states that "stereotypical assumptions should not be made based on identified sociocultural-spiritual affiliations; rather, there is a need for sensitivity to the individual family, who may uniquely apply cultural background to their lives." Variables such as an individual subculture within the primary group, degree of acculturation, educational and income levels, and amount of contact with the older generations influence the extent to which people practice these customs. Women from these cultural and ethnic groups may adhere to some, all, or none of the practices listed.

In planning the care of a family or an individual family member the nurse may find it useful to view the family at a developmental phase in the life cycle, facing stressful life events, and operating as a system. No one family member has a problem; if a problem exists, the whole family has a problem. The best solutions evolve through family participation when the nurse uses knowledge of family dynamics and culture and works with the family as a unit.

KEY POINTS

- The family forms a social network that acts as an important support system for its members.
- Ideally, the family provides a safe, intimate environment for the biopsychosocial development of its children and adult members.
- The family systems, developmental, and stress theories provide nurses with useful guidelines for understanding family function.
- A family's life cycle may be difficult to document.
- The reproductive beliefs and practices of a culture are embedded in its economic, religious, kinship, and political structures.
- The expression of parental roles and the way that children are viewed reflect cultural differences.
- Many ethnic, religious, and cultural groups coexist in the United States; therefore, varying family forms are recognized and accepted in differing degrees.

CRITICAL THINKING EXERCISES

1 *Using one of the family theories discussed in this chapter (family systems theory, developmental theory, family stress theory) explain how you would assess family function and dynamics for families representing various family structures.*

2 *Select families representing various cultural groups in your community (include both recently immigrated and acculturated families). Discuss strategies and possible interventions for providing culturally competent care to these families during the childbearing cycle.*

TABLE 2-2 *Traditional* Cultural Beliefs and Practices*

PREGNANCY	CHILDBIRTH	PARENTING

HISPANIC

(Members of the Hispanic community have their origins in Spain, Cuba, Central and South America, Mexico, Puerto Rico, and other Spanish-speaking countries. These beliefs are based primarily on knowledge of Mexican-Americans.)

PREGNANCY	CHILDBIRTH	PARENTING
Pregnancy is desired soon after marriage. Prenatal care is sought late.	**Labor**	**Newborn**
Expectant mother is influenced strongly by mother or mother-in-law.	Use of "partera" or lay midwife is preferred in some places; expectant mother may prefer presence of mother rather than husband.	Breastfeeding begins after third day; colostrum may be considered "filthy" or "spoiled;" belief that there is no milk.
Cool air in motion is considered dangerous during pregnancy.	After birth of infant, mother's legs are brought together to prevent air from entering the uterus.	Olive or castor oil is given to stimulate passage of meconium.
Unsatisfied food cravings cause birthmarks.	Loud behavior occurs during labor.	Male infant is not circumcised.
Some pica is observed in eating ashes or dirt (not common).		Female infant's ears are pierced.
Milk is avoided because it causes large infants and difficult births.	**Postpartum period**	Belly band is used to prevent umbilical hernia.
Many predictions are made about sex of the infant.	Diet may be restricted after birth; for first 2 days, only boiled milk and toasted tortillas are permitted. (These are special foods to restore warmth to the body.)	Religious medal worn by mother during pregnancy is placed around the infant's neck.
It may be unacceptable and frightening to have pelvic examination by a male health care provider.	Mother has bed rest for 3 days after birth.	Infant is protected from "evil eye."
Women use herbs to treat common complaints of pregnancy.	Mother is to keep warm and delay bathing.	Various remedies are used to treat "mal ojo" and fallen fontanel (depressed fontanel).
Drinking chamomile tea is thought to ensure effective labor.	Mother's head and feet are protected from cold air; bathing is permitted after 14 days.	
	Mother is often cared for by her own mother.	
	There is 40-day restriction on sexual intercourse.	

AFRICAN-AMERICAN

(Members of the African-American culture have their origins in Africa, many of whom are descendants of slaves. Today a number of blacks have immigrated from Africa, the West Indian Islands, the Dominican Republic, Haiti, and Jamaica. These beliefs are based primarily on knowledge of southern, rural African-Americans.)

PREGNANCY	CHILDBIRTH	PARENTING
Acceptance of pregnancy depends on economic status.	**Labor**	**Newborn**
Pregnancy is thought to be state of "wellness," which is often reason for delay in seeking prenatal care, especially by lower-income African-Americans.	Use of "Granny midwife" occurs in certain parts of the United States.	Feeding is very important: "Good" infant eats well. Early introduction of solid foods occurs. Mother may breastfeed or bottle feed; breastfeeding may be considered embarrassing.
Old wives tales include the following: having picture taken during pregnancy will cause stillbirth and reaching up will cause cord to strangle baby.	Varied emotional responses occur: some cry out, whereas some display stoic behavior to avoid calling attention to themselves.	Parents fear spoiling infant.
Mother may crave certain foods, including chicken, greens, clay, starch, and dirt.	Emotional support is often provided by other women, especially own mother.	Patient may arrive at hospital in far-advanced labor.
Pregnancy may be viewed by men as sign of virility.	**Postpartum period**	Parents commonly call infant by nicknames.
Self-treatment occurs for various discomforts of pregnancy, including constipation, nausea, vomiting, headache, and heartburn.	Vaginal bleeding may be seen as sign of sickness; tub baths and shampooing of hair are prohibited.	Parents may use excessive clothing to keep infant warm.
	Sassafras tea is thought to have healing power.	Belly band is used to prevent umbilical hernia.
	Eating liver is thought to cause heavier vaginal bleeding because of its high "blood" content.	Large amounts of oil are used on infant's scalp and skin.
		Strong feeling of family, community, and religion exists.

Data compiled from Amaro, 1994; Bar-Yam, 1994; Galanti, 1991; Geissler, 1994; Mattson, 1995; Spector, 1996; Williams, 1989 (see p. 22 for full citations).
*Variations exist in some beliefs and practices within subcultures. Most of these cultural beliefs and customs reflect the traditional culture and are not universally practiced. These lists are not intended to stereotype patients; rather they serve as guidelines while discussing meaningful cultural beliefs with a patient and her family. Examples of other cultural beliefs and practices are found throughout this text.

TABLE 2-2 *Traditional* Cultural Beliefs and Practices—cont'd*

PREGNANCY	CHILDBIRTH	PARENTING

ASIAN

(The term *Asian* commonly refers to groups from China; Korea; the Philippines; Japan; and Southeast Asia, particularly Thailand, Indochina, and Vietnam.)

PREGNANCY	CHILDBIRTH	PARENTING
Pregnancy is considered time when mother "has happiness in her body." Pregnancy is seen as natural process. Strong preference for female health care provider exists. Mother believes in theory of hot and cold. Mother may omit soy sauce in diet to prevent dark-skinned baby. Mother prefers soup made with ginseng root as general strength tonic. Milk is usually excluded from diet; is thought to cause stomach distress. Inactivity or sleeping late is thought to cause difficult birth.	**Labor** Mother is attended by other women, especially her own mother. Father does not actively participate. Labor occurs in silence. Cesarean birth is not welcome. **Postpartum period** Mother must protect herself from yin (cold forces) for 30 days. Ambulation is limited. Shower and bathing are prohibited. Warm environment to restore warmth to body. Diet: Warm fluids. Some patients are vegetarians. Korean mother is served seaweed soup with rice.	Chinese diet is high in hot foods. Chinese mother avoids fruits and vegetables. Concept of family is important and valued. Father is head of household; wife plays subordinate role. **Newborn** Birth of boy is preferred. Parents may delay naming child. Some groups (e.g., Vietnamese) believe colostrum is dirty; therefore, they may delay breastfeeding until milk comes in; belief that there is no milk.

CAUCASIAN/EUROPEAN-AMERICANS

(These beliefs are based primarily on knowledge of European-Americans.)

PREGNANCY	CHILDBIRTH	PARENTING
Pregnancy is viewed as condition that requires medical attention to ensure health. Emphasis is placed on early prenatal care. Variety of childbirth education programs are available, and participation is encouraged. Technology driven. Emphasis is placed on nutritional science. Involvement of the father is valued. Written information is valued.	**Labor** Birth is public concern. Technology dominated. Birthing process in institutional setting is valued. Varied emotional response; stoic or cry out. Involvement of the father is expected. Physician is seen as head of team. **Postpartum period** Emphasis or focus on early bonding occurs. Medical interventions for dealing with discomfort are valued. Early ambulation and activity are emphasized. Self-care is valued.	**Newborn** Breastfeeding has increased in popularity. Breastfeeding begins as soon as possible after childbirth. **Parenting** Motherhood and transition to parenting are seen as stressful times. Nuclear family is valued, although single parenting and other forms of parenting are more acceptable than in past. Women often deal with multiple roles. Early return to prepregnancy activities occurs.

NATIVE AMERICAN

(There are many different tribes within the Native American culture; viewpoints vary according to tribal customs and beliefs.)

PREGNANCY	CHILDBIRTH	PARENTING
Pregnancy is considered as normal, natural process. Prenatal care is late. Mother avoids heavy lifting. Herb teas are encouraged.	**Labor** Mother prefers female attendant, although husband, mother, or father may assist with birth. Birth may be attended by whole family. Herbs may be used to promote uterine activity. Birth may occur in squatting position.	**Postpartum period** Herb teas are used to stop bleeding. **Newborn** Infant is not fed colostrum. Use of herbs increases flow of milk. Cradle boards are used for infant. Babies are not handled often.

References

Amaro H: Women in the Mexican-American community: religion, culture, and reproductive attitudes and experiences, *J Comm Psych* 16(1):6, 1994.

Bar-Yam N: Learning about culture: a guide for birth practitioners, *Int J Childbirth Educ* 9(2):8, 1994.

Bianchi S: The changing demographics and socioeconomic characteristics of single-parent families, *Marriage and Family Review* 20(1):71, 1994.

Boss P: *Family stress management,* ed 2, Newbury Park, Calif, 1996, Sage.

Callister L: Cultural meanings of childbirth, *J Obstet Gynecol Neonatal Nurs* 24(4):327, 1995.

Carter B & McGoldrick M: *The changing family life cycle: a framework for family therapy,* ed 2, New York, 1988, Allyn & Bacon.

Chang K: Chinese Americans. In Giger J & Davidhizar R, editors: *Transcultural nursing assessment and interventions,* ed 2, St Louis, 1995, Mosby.

Cox R: Family health care delivery for the 21st century, *J Obstet Gynecol Neonatal Nurs* 21(1):109, 1997.

Duvall E: *Marriage and family development,* ed 5, Philadelphia, 1997, JB Lippincott.

Erikson E: *Identity: youth and crisis,* New York, 1968, WW Norton.

Evolving American family, *Stat Bull* 74:2, 1993.

Friedman M: *Family nursing theory and assessment,* ed 4, New York, 1998, Appleton-Century-Crofts.

Galanti G: *Caring for patients from different cultures: case studies from American hospitals,* Philadelphia, 1991, University of Pennsylvania.

Geissler E: *Pocket guide to cultural assessment,* St Louis, 1994, Mosby.

Giger J & Davidhizar R, editors: *Transcultural nursing assessment and interventions,* ed 2, St Louis, 1995, Mosby.

Hanson S & Boyd S: *Family health care nursing: theory, practice and research,* Philadelphia, 1996, FA Davis.

Helman C: *Culture, health and illness,* London, 1990, Wright.

Hill R: *Families under stress,* New York, 1949, Harper & Row.

Laird J: Lesbian and gay families. In Walsh F, editor: *Normal family processes,* ed 2, New York, 1993, Guilford.

Mattson S: Culturally sensitive prenatal care for Southeastern Asians, *J Obstet Gynecol Neonatal Nurs* 24(4):335, 1995.

Mercer R: Theoretical perspective on the family. In Gillis C et al., editors: *Toward a science of family nursing,* Menlo Park, Calif, 1989, Addison-Wesley.

Quimby S: Women and the family of the future, *J Obstet Gynecol Neonatal Nurs* 23(2):113,1994.

Ramer L: *Culturally sensitive caregiving and childbearing families,* White Plains, NY, 1992, March of Dimes Birth Defects Foundation.

Spector R: Cultural concepts of women's health and health promoting behaviors, *J Obstet Gynecol Neonatal Nurs,* 24(3):241, 1995.

Spector R: *Cultural diversity in health and illness,* ed 4, New York, 1996, Appleton-Century-Crofts.

Visher E & Visher J: Remarried families and stepparenting. In Walsh F, editor: *Normal family processes,* ed 2, New York, 1993, Guilford.

Walsh F: Conceptualization of normal family processes. In Walsh F, editor: *Normal family processes,* ed 2, New York, 1993, Guilford.

Williams R: Issues in women's health care. In Johnson B, editor: *Psychiatric mental health nursing: adaptation and growth,* Philadelphia, 1989, JB Lippincott.

Wright L & Leahey M: *Nurses and families,* ed 2, Philadelphia, 1994, FA Davis.

CHAPTER

Community and Home Care

JANE G. CONNER

LEARNING OBJECTIVES

- Define the key terms.
- Compare community-based health care and community health (population or aggregate focused) care.
- Select appropriate methods of community assessment for specific situations.
- List health indicators of community health status and their relevance to perinatal health care.
- Explain how age, gender, socioeconomic status, health status, and life experiences can predispose people to vulnerability.
- Discuss perinatal concerns and related nursing interventions for selected vulnerable populations: homeless, migrant laborers, and refugees.
- List the potential advantages and disadvantages of home visits.
- Describe the way home care fits into the maternity continuum of care.
- Define common perinatal conditions amenable to home care.
- Discuss safety and infection control principles as they apply to the care of patients in their homes.
- Describe the nurse's role in perinatal home care.

KEY TERMS

aggregates
census data
clinical integration
community
community-as-partner
home health care
homeless
key informants
levels of prevention
Medicaid
migrant laborers
participant observation

KEY TERMS—cont'd

proprietary agencies
refugees
surveys
third-party payers
vulnerable populations
windshield or walking survey

In the past most nurses have been employed in hospitals, and textbooks have reflected that. However, most health care actually occurs outside of secondary and tertiary institutions, in primary care facilities or patients' homes. It is anticipated that in the future hospitals will assume a smaller role, limiting their services to technologically complex care for the acutely ill. The movement to reduce health care costs has shortened hospitalization time and led to exploration of home- and community-based options for the provision of care (Henry, 1997). Attention to the role of health care providers in community-oriented health promotion and disease prevention activities is increasing (Expert Panel on Women's Health, 1997; Zyzanski, Williams & Flocke, 1996). Managed care organizations have a vested interest in maintaining the health of all of their members, not just those who present themselves for care. Publication of the U.S. national health objectives in *Healthy People 2000* and *Healthy Communities 2000* focused attention on the unequal distribution of disease and disability and the need to reach out to vulnerable populations not being adequately served by the current health system. Hospital-based nurses are increasingly involved in follow-up of patients and families after discharge (Fowler et al., 1997). Professional organizations cite the need for all nurses to be prepared to function in community settings and hospitals (Zotti, Brown & Stotts, 1996). Chapter 2 provided an overview of family and cultural theory and assessment. In this chapter we discuss the larger system of which the family is a part—the community. Methods of community assessment and the special perinatal health needs of vulnerable aggregates in the population are identified. Guidelines and issues related to the provision of home care for patients across the perinatal continuum are included.

ASSESSING LEVELS OF COMMUNITY WELLNESS

Definitions of Community

There are many definitions of **community,** but most share three characteristics: people, place and interaction, or function. We are all simultaneously part of several communities, such as an ethnic or religious group or a professional organization, but this discussion is limited to geographically based communities. The people are the residents of the community; place refers to geographic dimensions; function refers to the activities of the community that meet the needs of the residents (Schuster & Goeppinger, 1996). Figure 3-1 shows the core of the community surrounded by the multiple systems that serve to meet their collective needs. The people who reside there make up the core of the community. Significant characteristics include the demographics of the population and their values, beliefs, and culture. As residents of the community, the people affect, and are influenced by, the subsystems of the com-

munity. Economics, education, public safety, environmental factors, and availability of health and social services all have significant impact on community health and well-being. The broken lines between the segments emphasize the interaction and interdependence among the subsystems of the community (Anderson & McFarlane, 1996).

Methods of Community Assessment

Perinatal Health: Strategies for the 21st Century (1992), a plan produced by a federally funded expert panel, has as one of its basic principles that the organization and focus of perinatal care at the community level must be responsive to the unique characteristics of the populations and their special needs.

Multiple sources of data about communities are available. The extent and nature of the assessment to be performed depends on the time and resources available and the way the information is to be used. A nurse who is providing family-focused home care may be primarily interested in becoming familiar with the neighborhoods and

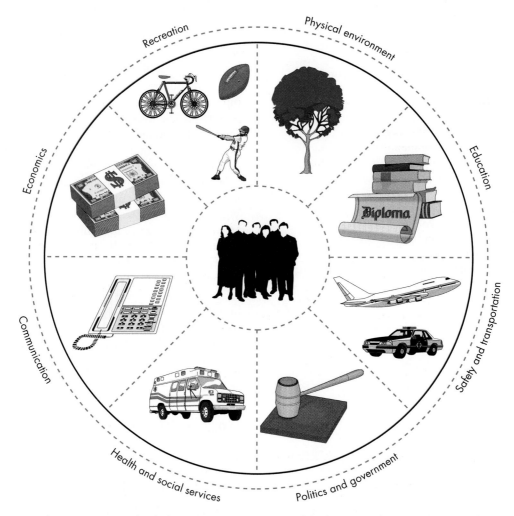

Fig. 3-1 The community assessment wheel, the assessment segment of the community-as-partner model. (From Anderson E & McFarlane J: *Community-as-partner: theory and practice in nursing,* Philadelphia, 1996, JB Lippincott.)

resources with which her patients interact. A community health agency must conduct a comprehensive needs assessment in order to plan and evaluate health services for the community as a whole. A variety of methods may be used to obtain both the community's perceptions of its strengths and problems and quantitative analyses of health and well-being, which can be compared with state and national statistics. Methods of data collection include windshield survey, participant observation, interviews, focus groups, analysis of existing data, and surveys.

Using one's senses while traveling through a community is the essence of the **windshield (or walking) survey** (Table 3-1). By focusing skills of observation during a trip through a community, a nurse can obtain significant information about its sociocultural characteristics and the environment, housing, transportation, and local community

TABLE 3-1 *Windshield Survey Components*

ELEMENT	DESCRIPTION
Housing and zoning	What is the age of the houses, their architecture, of what materials are they constructed? Are all the neighborhood houses similar in age, architecture? How would you characterize the differences? Are they detached from or connected to others? Do they have space in front and behind? What is their general condition? Are there signs of disrepair—broken doors, windows, leaks, locks missing? Is there central heating, modern plumbing, air conditioning?
Open space	How much open space is there? What is the quality of the space—green parks or rubble-filled lots? What is the lot size of the houses? Lawns? Flower boxes? Do you see trees on the pavements, a green island in the center of the streets? Is the open space public or private? Used by whom?
Boundaries	What signs are there of where this neighborhood begins and ends? Are the boundaries natural—a river, a different terrain? Physical— a highway, railroad? Economic—difference, in real estate or presence of industrial, commercial units along with residential? The neighborhood has an identity, a name? Do you see it displayed? Are there unofficial names?
"Commons"	What are the neighborhood hangouts? For what groups, at what hours? (e.g., schoolyard, candy store, bar, restaurant, park, 24-hour drugstore?) Does the "commons" have a sense of "territoriality" or is it open to the stranger?
Transportation	How do people get in and out of the neighborhood? Car, bus, bike, walk, etc.? Are the streets and roads conducive to good transportation and also to community life? Is there a major highway near the neighborhood? Whom does it serve? How frequent is public transportation available?
Service centers	Do you see social agencies, patients , recreation centers, signs of activity at the schools? Are there offices of doctors, dentists? Palmists, spiritualists, etc.? Parks? Are they in use?
Stores	Where do residents shop? Shopping centers, neighborhood stores? How do they travel to shop?
Street people	If you are traveling during the day, who do you see on the street? An occasional housewife, a mother with a baby? Do you see anyone you would not expect? Teenagers, unemployed males? Can you spot a welfare worker, an insurance collector, a door-to-door salesman? Is the dress of those you see representative or unexpected? Along with people, what animals do you see? Stray cats, dogs, pedigreed pets, "watchdogs"?
Signs of decay	Is this neighborhood on the way up or down? Is it "alive"? How would you decide? Trash, abandoned cars, political posters, neighborhood meeting posters, real estate signs, abandoned houses, mixed-zoning usage?
Race	Are the residents white, black, or is the area integrated?
Ethnicity	Are there indices of ethnicity—food stores, churches, private schools, information in a language other than English?
Religion	Of what religion are the residents? Do you see evidence of heterogeneity or homogeneity? What denomination are the churches? Do you see evidence of their use other than on Sunday mornings?
Health and morbidity	Do you see evidence of acute or of chronic diseases or conditions? Of accidents, communicable diseases, alcoholism, drug addiction, mental illness, etc.? How far is it to the nearest hospital? Clinic?
Politics	Do you see any political campaign posters? Is there a headquarters present? Do you see any evidence of a predominant party affiliation?
Media	Do you see outdoor TV antennas? What magazines, newspapers do residents read? Do you see *Forward Times, Hampton Post, Enquirer, Readers' Digest* in the stores? What media seem most important to the residents? Radio? TV?

From Anderson E & McFarlane J: *Community as partner: application of the nursing process*, Philadelphia, 1996, Lippincott.

agencies. Using **participant observation,** in which nurses are part of the situation they wish to learn about, it is possible to more fully understand the people and processes involved and to validate perceptions and inferences.

Every 10 years the U.S. government conducts a national census. **Census data** offer a broad range of information that is extremely helpful to nurses and other health care providers who wish to become familiar with a community. Data include population size, age, sex and ethnic distribution, socioeconomic status, educational level, employment, and housing characteristics. Reports are available in libraries, in print, on CD-ROM, and through the Internet. Summaries are prepared for municipalities; large metropolitan areas; zip codes; and the smallest unit, a census tract. A census tract is a portion of a larger urban area, usually consisting of 3,000 to 6,000 persons and often corresponding to a neighborhood. Depending on the density of the population, this can be a few square blocks or several square miles. Looking at individual census tracts helps to identify subpopulations, or **aggregates,** with differing needs that would be obscured by the statistics gathered on the entire community. Census tract–level data on socioeconomic status and environmental stressors have been used to identify women at risk for delivery of a low-birth-weight (LBW) infant. Based on this information, outreach activities can be appropriately targeted (O'Campo et al., 1997).

Vital statistics and other sources of health data

Official records of births and deaths are reported annually for the preceding year by city, county, and state health departments. In addition to the number of births and deaths, certificates include the type of birth and any complications, as well as causes of death. Local health departments compile extensive statistics about the incidence of communicable and other diseases within their jurisdictions. The National Center for Health Statistics publishes annual National Health Survey data, which describe health trends on a national sample. Many state and local government reports from health and planning agencies provide data that assist the nurse in assessing the community. Hospitals and voluntary agencies may conduct detailed assessments focused on a particular health area. The March of Dimes Birth Defects Foundation, for example, has supported perinatal needs assessments in many communities across the United States. Other local sources of information include the Chamber of Commerce, newspapers, community center newsletters, libraries, public safety agencies, school districts, and the American Red Cross.

Interviews with selected individuals in positions of leadership, **key informants,** allow input from many different perspectives. Persons such as health care providers or administrators; religious leaders; government officials; representatives of voluntary health organizations; service clubs; and cultural groups can provide an "insider's" viewpoint not available in published documents. Similarly, focus groups can be conducted with potential patients or collaborators to discuss needs and services important to the community. Using structured open-ended questions, exploration of community strengths and needs can be facilitated. Formal **surveys,** either by mail, telephone, or face-to-face, are expensive and time consuming but can be sources of information not available from secondary sources. Knowledge of support groups, educational programs, and social service agencies allows the nurse to make appropriate referrals for perinatal patients. Information about community resources may be obtained from many of the sources listed above, as well as the local United Way organization, telephone directory, or community services directory.

▌ HEALTH AND WELLNESS IN THE COMMUNITY

Community Health Status Indicators

Just as norms have been developed for individual health assessment, the data collected about communities can be compared with state or national standards to assess the well-being of the population as a whole. What percentage of the population has income below the poverty level? What is the unemployment rate? Do most women begin prenatal care in the first trimester? What are the fetal and infant mortality rates?

Box 3-1 displays a set of community health status indicators developed by a committee of experts from many community health-related organizations. Infant mortality, because it is affected by the preconceptional health, prenatal, and intrapartal care of the mother, as well as living conditions for the infant after birth, is a statistic widely used to compare the health status of different populations. Three of the five indicators of risk—incidence of low birth rate, adolescent pregnancy, and early prenatal care—refer to maternal-infant health. Poverty and a high percentage of young children in a community are strongly associated with significant community health needs (Zyzanski, Williams & Flocke, 1996). *Healthy People 2000* has set national goals for maternal-child health. One of the overall goals is to reduce disparities in health between groups within the population. Infant mortality in the African-American population remains twice that of the nation as a whole in spite of efforts to address this concern. The rate of pregnancy in young adolescents is still higher than the targeted goal. Reported child abuse and neglect continue to increase. These and many other health problems require intervention at the community level in addition to assisting individuals to improve their personal health behaviors.

| BOX 3-1 | *Consensus Set of Indicators* for Assessing Community Health Status* |

INDICATORS OF HEALTH STATUS OUTCOME

1. Race/ethnicity-specific infant mortality, as measured by the rate (per 1,000 live births) of deaths among infants <1 year of age

Death rates (per 100,000 population)[†] for:

2. Motor vehicle crashes
3. Work-related injury
4. Suicide
5. Lung cancer
6. Breast cancer
7. Cardiovascular disease
8. Homicide
9. All causes

Reported incidence (per 100,000 population) of:

10. Acquired immunodeficiency syndrome
11. Measles
12. Tuberculosis
13. Primary and secondary syphilis

INDICATORS OF RISK FACTORS

14. Incidence of LBW, as measured by percentage of total number of live-born infants weighing <2,500 g at birth
15. Births to adolescents (females aged 10 to 17 years) as a percentage of total live births
16. Prenatal care, as measured by percentage of mothers delivering live infants who did not receive prenatal care during first trimester.
17. Childhood poverty, as measured by the proportion of children <15 years of age living in families at or below the poverty level
18. Proportion of persons living in counties exceeding U.S. Environmental Protection Agency standards for air quality during previous year

From Consensus set of indicators for assessing community health status, *MMWR* 40(27):449, 1991.
*Position or number of the indicator does not imply priority.
†Age-adjusted to the 1940 standard population

Population- or Aggregate-Focused Care

Levels of prevention

Population-focused health care uses a framework of **levels of prevention.**

- Primary prevention includes efforts made before the development of illness to promote general health and well-being. It also includes the use of specific protection, such as immunizations or approved infant car seats.
- Secondary prevention involves early detection of health problems so that treatment can begin before significant disability occurs. This includes various methods of health screening.
- Tertiary prevention is the treatment and rehabilitation of persons who have developed disease. Because most women are healthy during pregnancy, maternal-newborn nursing emphasizes primary and secondary prevention activities regardless of where care is provided. However, in general, the ill, hospitalized patient is the focus of tertiary prevention.

Health promotion in group settings

The use of established groups for health promotion activities has many advantages. Members are used to meeting on a regular basis and are comfortable with each other. Their shared experience may help them focus on a new goal and provide support to each other in initiating new health behaviors. Settings for community health promotion may include day care centers and schools; work sites; religious, service, or social organizations; community nursing centers; and the community at large (Pender, 1996). School-based programs can address many of the needs of adolescents regarding sexual and reproductive health. Employers are concerned about rising health insurance costs and absenteeism and are increasingly willing to sponsor prevention and health promotion programs for employees (Lassiter, 1996; Pender, 1996). The March of Dimes Birth Defects Foundation (1991) developed and supports "Babies + You," a campaign using volunteers to bring prenatal health education to women at work. In the growing parish nursing movement, coalitions of religious groups sponsor community health nursing activities for the areas they serve (Bergquist & King, 1994; Dixon, 1996). With **community-as-partner,** nurses can function as members, leaders, advisors, or consultants. Community nursing centers have been established in many areas to provide primary care, health promotion, and home care. Two such centers, based in low-income housing projects and cosponsored by the University of Pennsylvania School of Nursing, in collaboration with other health care organizations, were able to reduce the incidence of LBW infants born to residents from 13.6% to only 2% in just 3 years. They offer a comprehensive range of services, staffed by nurse practitioners who provide primary care, prenatal care, home visits, group health education, parenting and grandparenting support and education, mental health services, violence prevention education, and drug and alcohol treatment (USDHHS, 1997).

High Risk Aggregates or Vulnerable Populations

Definition of vulnerability

The health care system is moving toward managed care rather than fee-for-service. Providers recognize the need to target health education and outreach programs toward vulnerable populations. **Vulnerable populations** are groups who are at higher risk of developing physical, mental, or social health problems or who are more likely to have worse outcomes from these health problems than the population as a whole (Aday, 1997; Sebastian, 1996). People often have problems along more than one of these dimensions. Increasingly the need for multidisciplinary approaches to the needs of vulnerable populations has been recognized (Pew Health Professions Commission, 1995).

Many special population groups are more vulnerable to reproductive health risks, including pregnant adolescents, substance abusers, violence-prone families, the mentally ill, those with sexually transmitted or other communicable diseases, and those with malnutrition. These groups are often served by community health nurses who participate in community outreach (i.e., seeking underserved individuals, families, and groups and facilitating their entry into the health care system) and family- and community-based health promotion interventions. In the following section, selected vulnerable populations who may have some or all of these problems are discussed: homeless families, immigrants and refugees, and migrant laborers. These groups, living in poverty and marginalized by mainstream society, have many common characteristics and needs.

Homeless

The term **homeless** as defined by the U.S. Department of Housing and Urban Development includes those who are homeless (i.e., living on the streets or in shelters) and those who are at risk of being homeless, such as those sharing housing and transients. Each year an estimated 2.5 to 3 million people lack access to a conventional dwelling; families are the fastest growing segment of that population. Families with children account for 33% to 43% of the homeless. Young, single women head 53% of homeless families. Many of these women have a history of physical or sexual abuse as children and have also abused alcohol or drugs (American Academy of Pediatrics, 1996; Stanhope & Lancaster, 1996). It is estimated that as many as 2 million homeless adolescents may be living on the streets of major cities. Many engage in "survival sex," exchanging sexual favors for food, clothing, and shelter, making them vulnerable to sexually transmitted diseases and unintended pregnancies. They seldom appear at agencies serving the adult homeless population (Rew, 1996).

Homeless people have fewer resources than other poor families. Preexisting health problems are complicated by homelessness, and other health problems are caused by homelessness. Living conditions contribute to higher levels of infectious disease, including respiratory infections, especially antibiotic-resistant tuberculosis and enteric infections. Anemia and other nutritional deficits are common. Obesity is often present because of lack of storage and cooking facilities and reliance on fast foods and convenience stores. Family members are at higher risk for injury because of accidents, violence, or environmental exposure. Access to health care, especially preventive care, is limited because of the energy required for the daily struggle to meet needs for food and shelter and by frequent moves and reliance on emergency rooms for the most acute needs (American Academy of Pediatrics, 1996; Burg, 1994).

Killion (1995) followed 15 homeless pregnant women living in several different shelters in southern California for periods of several weeks to more than 1 year. Conception among this group of women was rarely planned and usually occurred during the period of homelessness as a result of factors such as victimization, economic survival, lack of access to contraceptives, need for closeness and intimacy, and doubt of fertility. None had consistent prenatal care. Some did not admit to being homeless when seen in clinics or emergency rooms for fear of having children removed by protective services. They reported difficulty in dealing with the normal discomforts of pregnancy such as fatigue and nausea and vomiting. Some addicted women found the stress of pregnancy increased their reliance on drugs, while for others the pregnancy was an impetus to help them work toward reestablished stability in their lives.

Although most research has focused on urban homeless families, Wagner, Menke, and Ciccone (1995) studied the needs of rural homeless families. These families were similar to those in cities, but as a group had been homeless for longer periods because fewer resources were available in their communities.

Many homeless women are covered by **Medicaid** and may present in private offices and hospitals for care. Because of distrust of the system, they may try to hide their status. Nurses working with homeless women and families agree that treating patients with dignity and respect is basic to establishing a therapeutic relationship. Case management is recommended to coordinate the various agencies and disciplines that may be involved in meeting the multiple needs of these families. Time for appointments must be flexible and patients should not be penalized if they fail to appear when scheduled. Health is of lower priority than food and shelter, except in emergencies. Whenever possible, the service must be provided when the patient presents herself. Each interaction should be purposeful and offered with the awareness that this may be the only encounter possible with the woman. Health information and strategies that are feasible within the context of her living situation are offered. The health care provider builds on existing coping strategies and strengths. The woman is allowed to do as much as possible for herself to reduce her feelings of powerlessness. The woman (and her family) is helped to reconnect with her social support system. At the local, state, and federal levels, health care providers can advocate for adequate funding for homeless prevention programs and comprehensive health care for all homeless people, with a focus on continuity of preventive care (Acquaviva & Lancaster, 1996; American Academy of Pediatrics, 1996; Burg, 1994: Killion, 1995).

Migrants

An estimated 3 to 5 million people are classified as migrant farm workers, 16% of whom are women (Maternal and Child Health Bureau, 1997). **Migrant laborers** are those who must establish temporary residence in various areas on a seasonal basis in order to obtain employment. Most live in temporary housing for at least 6 months out of the year; others move continuously throughout the year. They may be thought of as episodically homeless because their shelter is often dependent on employment, and as the seasons change, they become homeless until the next job is obtained. Ethnic groups among migrants include African-Americans, European-Americans, Hispanics, Haitians, and some Southeast Asians. Those in the western and central states are predominantly Mexican, while the population in the east, traveling north from Florida, is more varied. (Lambert, 1995; Rodriguez, 1996).

Migrant laborers and their families face many problems, including financial instability, child labor, poor housing, lack of education, language and cultural barriers, and limited access to health and social services (Clemen-Stone, Eigsti & McGuire, 1998). Migrant farm work is one of the most hazardous occupations in the United States because of heavy physical demands, fatigue, operation of potentially dangerous machinery, exposure to pesticides and naturally occurring irritants, and limited enforcement of Occupational Safety and Health Administration (OSHA) standards. Housing is often substandard and overcrowded because of lack of availability and/or cost (Jones & Schenk, 1996). Although comprehensive studies of migrant health have not been reported, analyses of records of patients seen at Migrant Health Centers indicate that there are high rates of poor dental health, diabetes, hypertension, malnutrition, tuberculosis, substance abuse, and parasitic infections. The average life expectancy for migrant laborers is 49 years as compared with 75 years for the population as a whole. Substance abuse and domestic violence are significant problems. Most farm workers do not view illness as a problem unless the condition prevents working. Health promotion and disease prevention are not values to those with orientation to the present, limited education, and lack of access to health care (Jones & Schenk, 1996).

A typical day for the mother of a migrant family may begin at 4 or 5 AM when she arises to prepare food for the family. She works in the fields until 5 or 6 PM and then continues her workday with housework and child care (Rodriguez, 1996). Higher rates of spontaneous abortion, inadequate prenatal care, and infant mortality are reported. There is concern about the reproductive effects of exposure to toxic chemicals. Less consistent use of contraception and increased rates of sexually transmitted diseases, including human immunodeficiency virus (HIV) and inflammatory conditions of the cervix, vagina, and vulva are reported (Lambert, 1995). Compared with other poor women attending public nutrition clinics, migrants are more likely to have late initiation of prenatal care and inadequate pregnancy weight gain. The incidence of preterm birth and the birth of a LBW infant was similar for both groups and higher than the *Healthy 2000* objective targets (Maternal and Child Health Bureau, 1997).

Although a system of 100 federally funded Migrant Health Centers has been established in the United States and Puerto Rico, they see less than 15% of the 3 to 5 million farm workers, and the gap is not closed by the various voluntary agencies that also serve this community. Many migrants seek help at local community hospitals and clinics in the areas in which they are working. Lack of time is a major barrier to obtaining health care. Even if services are free, the loss of wages incurred in leaving the fields is a deterrent to preventive care. To ensure access, offices should be open after the migrants' usual working hours. Lack of trust (i.e., reluctance to share personal problems with a stranger or fear of being reported to the Immigration and Naturalization Services if they are undocumented) prevents many from obtaining care. Domestic violence is a significant problem, and men's control over women's activities limits women's ability to seek help (Rodriguez, 1996).

Providing culturally competent care to a multiethnic population is a challenge for health care workers (Jones & Schenk, 1996; Lambert, 1995). (See Chapter 2 for discussion of cultural competence.) One approach that has been successful is the use of lay camp aides to assist in outreach and health education. Among Hispanic women the use of camp volunteers, known as "promotoras," who assist families in obtaining prenatal, postpartum, and infant care and meeting other health needs, has been effective. This partnership with the community provides a link between the formal health care system and traditional practices (Rodriguez, 1996). Guidance and information about other resources are available to health care providers through the National Migrant Resource Program and the Migrant Clinicians Network (Lambert, 1995).

Refugees and immigrants

From 1975 through 1993, 1.85 million refugees were admitted to the United States, with 1 of every 140 persons of the U.S. population being of refugee origin (U.S. Committee on Refugees, 1995). The surge in refugee immigration began with Southeast Asians after the Vietnam War, and continued with those from Ethiopia, Cuba, Eastern Europe, and the Kurds from Iraq. Other countries whose emigrants are not always officially recognized as refugees include Haiti, China, and uncounted numbers from Central America. Governmental agencies make a distinction between those who voluntarily immigrate for economic reasons and **refugees,** who are forced to flee for political reasons. Refugees are automatically eligible for permanent resident status and additional services and support. However, the differences are not always clear, and many voluntary immigrants come from countries in political turmoil (Bollini & Siem, 1995).

Although most immigrants find adaptation to a new language and culture stressful, refugees share common characteristics that significantly increase the difficulties families experience. These include the following:

- Leaving their homeland without hope of return
- Surviving the trauma of war and/or refugee camps—women are commonly raped while in transit or in refugee camps
- Grief related to deaths of family members and loss of home
- Multiple health problems, including malnutrition, infectious disease, and stress-related mental health disorders (e.g., posttraumatic stress disorder)
- Lack of previous experience with the Western health care system, in particular no previous experience with prenatal care and family planning
- Unique cultural beliefs that are unfamiliar to most U.S. health workers (Kemp, 1996).

In addressing the needs of refugee women, the World Health Organization recommends that reproductive health programs include a minimum package of care related to issues of family planning; maternal mortality; unwanted pregnancy; sexually transmitted diseases, including HIV and acquired immunodeficiency syndrome (AIDS); and physical and sexual violence. If they have lost children during the exodus from their country, women may want to rebuild their families soon after resettlement. A participatory approach is needed to bring together the many agencies and groups working with refugees and to allow for input into decision making by the refugees themselves (Djeddah, 1995). Foss (1996) explored the difficulty of experiencing the overlapping transitions of adjustment to a new country and parenthood while grieving for the many losses experienced as refugees. Health workers with immigrant and refugee groups have found that most are receptive to new health education but prefer to receive it in their own language from someone who is part of their culture. Bicultural professionals and trained community workers from the refugee group have successfully reached women and families who were reluctant to interact with the health system of the new country (Ganguly, 1995; Lipson & Omidian, 1997). When refugee and other immigrant women are hospitalized, a cultural liaison who can interpret not only language but also differing cultural expectations is invaluable. Understanding reproductive health needs through the eyes of refugee communities is an essential step towards providing appropriate and culturally sensitive services and information (Djeddah, 1995; Gany & Bocanegra, 1996). Many immigrants who have strong ties to traditional medical practices from their homeland also respect Western or scientific practices. This pluralistic view allows them to combine both modalities without conflict (Rodriguez, 1996).

HOME CARE ALONG THE PERINATAL CONTINUUM OF CARE

A continuum of care is defined as a range of clinical services provided for an individual or group that reflects care given during a single hospitalization or care for multiple conditions over a lifetime (United HealthCare Corporation, 1994). Home care is one delivery component available along the perinatal continuum of care (Fig. 3-2). This continuum begins with family planning and continues with preconception, prenatal care, intrapartum care, postpartum, newborn care, interconceptional, and infant care until the infant is 1 year old. Independent self-care, ambulatory care, home care, low-risk hospitalization or specialized intensive care may be appropriate at different points along this continuum.

Current Trends and Historical Perspectives

A priority for future decades will be the development of innovative, cost-effective methods of health care delivery. Large health care organizations are developing clinically integrated health care delivery networks. The goals of **clinical integration** are improved coordination of care and care outcomes; better communication among health care providers; increased patient, payer, and provider satisfaction; and reduced cost. With clinical integration the focus changes from illness to health, from the individual to the population, and from care provided in one setting to care across the continuum (Porter et al., 1996). The following several factors make home care a growth area in perinatal services:

- Increased interest in family birthing alternatives
- Shortened hospital stays
- Availability of new technologies that allow sophisticated assessments and treatments to be performed in the home setting
- Increasing reimbursement by third-party payers.

Fig. **3-2** Perinatal continuum of care. (From Lowdermilk D, Perry S & Bobak I: *Maternity & women's health care,* ed 6, St Louis, 1997, Mosby.)

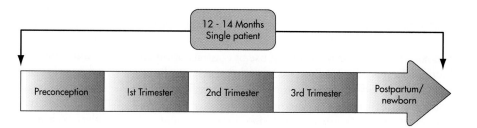

In 1877 the Women's Branch of the New York City Mission provided the first training program for home health care nursing. These home care nurses focused on caring for the sick within their homes. In 1893 Lillian Wald established the Henry Street Settlement House and expanded this visitation to include some preventive care. Modern home care nursing has its foundation in public health nursing, which provided comprehensive care to sick and well patients within their own homes.

Specialized maternity home care nursing services began in the 1980s when public health maternity nursing services were limited and services had not kept pace with the changing practices of high-risk obstetrics and emerging technology. Lengthy antepartal hospitalizations for such conditions as preterm labor and pregnancy-induced hypertension created nursing care challenges for staff members on inpatient units. Many women expressed their concern for the negative effect of antepartal hospitalizations on the family. Although clinical indications showed that a new nursing care approach was needed, home health care did not become a viable alternative until **third-party payers** (i.e., public/private organizations or employer groups that pay for health care expenses) pushed for cost containment in maternity services.

Communication to Bridge the Continuum

As maternity care continues to consist of frequent and brief contacts with health care providers throughout the prenatal and postpartum periods, nurses need to develop innovative nursing delivery methods, as well as innovative ways to communicate that care is provided. Bakewell-Sachs and Persily (1995) and Brooten (1995) discuss the need for the development of services that link maternity patients throughout the perinatal continuum of care, including critical pathways, telephonic nursing assessments, discharge planning, specialized education programs, parent support groups, home visiting programs, nurse advice lines, and perinatal home care. Some hospitals have provided cross-training for hospital-based nurses to make postpartum home visits (Fowler et al., 1997). Another has developed an outpatient follow-up center staffed by nurses from the maternity unit (Blystad-Keppler, 1995).

Telephonic nursing care

Telephonic nursing care through services such as warm lines, nurse advice lines, and telephonic nursing assessments are emerging as valuable services to manage health care problems and bridge the gaps among acute, outpatient, and home care services. This type of nursing care occurs by telephone and is very interactive and responsive to the immediate health care questions consumers have about particular health care needs. Warm lines are telephone lines that are offered as a community service to provide new parents with support,

encouragement, and basic parenting education (Jones, Maestri & McCoy, 1993). Nurse advice lines, or toll-free nurse consultation services, provide answers to medical questions, guide callers through urgent health care situations, suggest treatment options, and provide health education (Barnett, 1995). Telephonic nursing assessments, or nurse consultation, assessment, and health education that take place during a telephone conversation, can be added to the plan of care in conjunction with skilled nursing visits or may be a separate nursing contact for the woman. Telephonic nursing assessments are commonly used after a postpartum home care visit to reassess a woman's knowledge about the signs and symptoms of adequate hydration in breastfeeding, or, after initiating home phototherapy, to assess the caregiver's knowledge regarding equipment complications. In the new health care environment with limited resources, warm lines, nurse advice lines, and telephonic nursing assessments can influence patients' health care decisions by empowering them with knowledge to make wiser and more cost-efficient health care decisions. Some hypothesize that most future health care will be provided in patients' homes by two-way telecommunication systems (Jones, 1996).

Guidelines for Nursing Practice

Although the home care industry continues to grow rapidly, perinatal home care nursing practice is still emerging. As a specialist nursing practice area, perinatal home care has only approximately 15 years of experience. Clarifying the role of the perinatal home care nurse and the ways this role differs from other health care providers is still being molded by clinical practice and regulatory and accreditation organizations.

Until the Association of Women's Health, Obstetric, and Neonatal Nurses (AWHONN) published a document describing perinatal home care nursing practice in 1994, no specific guidelines for perinatal home care existed. These practices are directed toward the following:
- Assisting women in optimizing their state of health before conception
- Assessing and managing actual or potential problems of pregnancy that can be managed safely outside the inpatient setting
- Facilitating postpartum physical restoration and adaptation to parenthood
- Promoting the achievement of maximum health for the newborn and family

The guidelines in this document identified specific knowledge and clinical skills needed, and criteria for the verification of this knowledge and skills were suggested (AWHONN, 1994).

According to the Health Care Financing Administration (HCFA), a patient who meets the following criteria may receive home health care services: homebound status, need for intermittent skilled care, medically reasonable and necessary need for treatment, and has a plan of care authorized by the health care provider (HCFA, 1990).

A wide range of professional health care services and health products can be delivered or used in the home. The primary difference between health care in a hospital and home care is the absence of the continuous presence of professional health care providers in a patient's home. Most **home health care** is given as intermittent care with the professional staff visiting in the patient's home or providing care on site for fewer than 4 hours at a time. The home health care agency maintains on-call professional staff to assist home care patients who have questions about their care and for emergencies, such as equipment failure.

Perinatal Services

Home care perinatal services may be provided by hospital-based programs, independent **proprietary** (for profit) **agencies** or nonprofit home care agencies, and official or tax-supported agencies. Innovative programs may be supported by research grants for a period of years, but ultimately must be sponsored by an agency with long-term funding. Home visits have both advantages and disadvantages. The mother is able to maintain bed rest if indicated, and vulnerable neonates are not exposed to the weather or external sources of infection. The nurse can observe and interact with family members in their most natural and secure environment. Adequacy of resources and safety factors can be assessed. Teaching can be tailored to the actual home conditions and other family members included. A home visit is less expensive than a day's hospitalization, but a 60- to 90-minute visit requires 2½ to 3 hours of nursing time, including travel and documentation. It is more cost effective to see patients in an office setting where professional time is not spent in travel. Availability of nurses with expertise in maternity care may be limited, and concerns about the nurse's physical safety in some communities may limit visits.

Visits for outreach and health promotion are an integral part of community (or public) health nursing. In countries with national health systems, a nurse may see all women during pregnancy and after birth. In the United States visits of this sort have been provided mainly to low-income families without health insurance who use the clinics provided by local health departments (Olds, Kitzman & Cole, 1995; Zotti & Zahner, 1995). Until recently, private insurers did not reimburse for health promotion visits. Managed care organizations now recognize that anticipatory guidance is cost effective, but home visit programs are still targeted to specific high-risk populations, such as young adolescents or women at risk for preterm labor.

Home care agencies are subject to regulation by governmental and professional organizations and provide interdisciplinary services including social work, nutrition, and occupational and physical therapy. Increasingly their caseloads are made up of patients who require high-technologic care, such as infusions or home monitoring. Although the home health nurse develops the care plan, all care must be ordered by a physician. Interventions must meet the insurer's criteria for reimbursement, and services are limited to the registered patients. Preconception care and low-risk antepartum care can usually be provided more efficiently in office settings and are not currently reimbursable. High-risk antepartum care is often provided by home care agencies. Women with hyperemesis gravidarum who require parenteral nutrition may be treated at home. Conditions requiring bed rest, such as preterm labor and hypertension, are common indications for home care. Other conditions may include cardiac disease and substance abuse (Kemp & Hatmaker, 1996) and diabetes in pregnancy (Persily, Brown & York, 1996).

Postpartum home care is a growing area of perinatal services. Some insurers reimburse for at least one visit to families after early discharge or in the presence of high risk factors. Home phototherapy is used for treatment of neonatal hyperbilirubinemia and to avoid separation of mother and infant. Many other neonates who require long-term high technology care are also managed with home care. Consumer demand and education of insurers by case managers is increasing the availability of home care options (Women's Health Center Management, 1997).

Patient selection and referral

The office- or hospital-based nurse is often the key person in making effective referrals to home care. When considering a referral to home care the following factors need to be evaluated:
- Health status of mother and fetus or infant: Is condition serious enough to warrant home care and is it stable enough for intermittent observation to be sufficient?
- Availability of professionals to provide the needed services within the patient's community
- Family resources, including psychosocial, social, and economic resources: Will the family be able to provide care between nursing visits? Are relationships supportive? Is third-party reimbursement available or can it be negotiated with the insurer? Is there a voluntary or tax-supported community agency that could provide needed care without payment?
- Cost-effectiveness: Is it more reasonable for the patient to receive these services at home or to go to a local outpatient facility to receive them?

Standardized referral forms simplify the referral process and ensure that all needed information will be forwarded to the home health agency.

The nursing assessment should include the woman's physical and psychologic status, her level of knowledge about self-care activities, her willingness to learn, the availability of caregivers and social support in the home, and her level of comfort with home care. If the referral is for a mother and infant home care visit, then the nursing assessment should include newborn data.

High-technology home care requires additional information to be collected from the chart and consultation with the referring physician and other members of the health care team before making a home care referral. These additional data include the medical diagnosis, medical prognosis, prescribed therapies, medication history, drug dosing information, potential ancillary supplies, and type of infusion access device. The nursing assessment and therapies data provide baseline information for the home care nurse and pharmacist.

Whenever a referral is called into a home health care agency, a member of the nursing or admission staff determines the agency's ability to accept the patient for service. The use of fax machines to transmit information has eliminated delays in initiating home care services.

Admission to home care

Once the patient is admitted to the agency, the determination of staffing is addressed by nursing management. Patient assignments are generally determined according to diagnosis, geographic location, potential length of service, and skill level of the home care nurse. An agency may have a number of nurses with various clinical backgrounds and certifications. Clinical nurse specialists are assuming leadership roles in many perinatal home care agencies (Broussard, 1996; Christian, 1996).

Preparing for the home visit

The home care nurse reviews the available clinical data, demographic information, and completed plan of care form, and consults with the home care pharmacist or other health care team members who have previously contacted the patient to determine the goals of the visit. At this point the nurse uses the medical diagnosis and stage on the perinatal continuum as a starting point to organize the patient's care. The nurse reviews agency policies and procedures, professional literature about diagnosis, and community resources as part of the previsit preparation work (Box 3-2).

Before going on a home visit, the nurse should contact the patient to make necessary arrangements. Contact by telephone has several goals besides establishing a convenient visit date and time and obtaining directions to the patient's home. Setting the stage for the first home care visit is essential. The nurse should identify himself/herself by name, title, and agency. The nurse should explain who referred the patient to the agency for home care and the purpose of the home care visits. The patient should be encouraged to verbalize an understanding of her home care needs. Then the nurse should briefly explain what will occur during the visit and approximately how long the visit will last. Patients should be requested to restrain their pets during the visit. Lastly, the nurse should ask about health supplies that may be needed for the patient's care.

Before going out on the first visit, the home care nurse collects the patient's clinical record, patient education materials, medical supplies, and equipment necessary for the visit. Medications and specialized equipment should be ordered before the visit and delivered at the time of the scheduled visit.

CARE MANAGEMENT

First Home Care Visit

Making the first home care visit can be stressful for the nurse and patient. The home care nurse is faced with an unknown environment controlled by the patient and her family. The woman and her family also experience feelings of the unknown, such as anxiety about the way the nurse will treat them or what the nurse will do during the visit. The challenge for the home care nurse is to establish a nurse-patient relationship and provide the prescribed home care services within the time provided for the initial home visit.

Introductions generally begin the visit; the nurse identifies self and home care agency (Fig. 3-3). The patient introduces herself and the other family members who are present. Sometimes, the patient may feel uncertain of her role or be uncomfortable in taking the lead in introductions, so other people in the home may not be introduced to the nurse. In these situations the nurse can politely ask about other people in the home and their relationship to the woman.

Before performing any services, the home care nurse must obtain written agreement and consent for the home health care services. This consent-for-care serves two major purposes: agreement for care and authorization to release medical information. Many third-party payers require written documentation of the services provided, therefore the

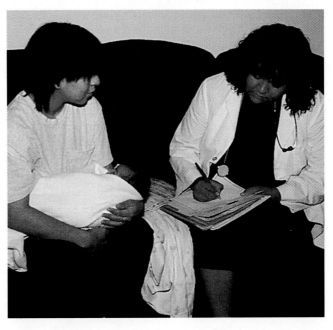

Fig. **3-3** Home care nurse visiting with woman and her infant. (Courtesy Michael S. Clement, MD, Mesa, Ariz.)

BOX 3-2   *Protocol for Perinatal Home Visits*

PREVISIT INTERVENTIONS

1. Contact family to arrange details for home visit.
   a. Identify self, credentials, and agency role.
   b. Review purpose of home visit follow-up.
   c. Schedule convenient time for visit.
   d. Confirm address and route to family home.
2. Review and clarify appropriate data.
   a. All available assessment data for mother and fetus or infant (i.e., referral forms, hospital discharge summaries, family identified learning needs).
   b. Review records of any previous nursing contacts.
   c. Contact other professional caregivers as necessary to clarify data (i.e., obstetrician, nurse-midwife, pediatrician, referring nurse).
3. Identify community resources and teaching materials appropriate to meet needs already identified.
4. Plan the visit, and prepare bag with equipment, supplies, and materials necessary for assessments of mother and fetus or infant, actual care anticipated, and teaching.

IN-HOME INTERVENTIONS: ESTABLISHING A RELATIONSHIP

1. Reintroduce self and establish purpose of visit for mother, infant, and family; offer family opportunity to clarify their expectations of contact.
2. Spend brief time socially interacting with family to become acquainted and establish trusting relationship.

IN-HOME INTERVENTIONS: WORKING WITH FAMILY

1. Conduct systematic assessment of mother and fetus or newborn to determine physiologic adjustment and any existing complications.
2. Throughout visit, collect data to assess the emotional adjustment of individual family members to pregnancy or birth and lifestyle changes. Note evidence of family-newborn bonding and sibling rivalry; note relationships among mother, father, children, and grandparents.
3. Determine adequacy of support system.
   a. To what extent does someone help with cooking, cleaning, and other home management tasks?
   b. To what extent is help being provided in caring for the newborn and any other children?
   c. Are support persons encouraging the new mother to care for herself and get adequate rest?
   d. Who is providing helpful information? Emotional support?
4. Throughout the visit, observe home environment for adequacy of resources:
   a. Space: privacy, safe play of children, sleeping.
   b. Overall cleanliness and state of repair.
   c. Number of steps pregnant woman/new mother must climb.
   d. Adequacy of cooking arrangements.
   e. Adequacy of refrigeration and other food storage areas.
   f. Adequacy of bathing, toilet, and laundry facilities.
   g. Arrangements in home for newborn: sleeping, bathing, formula preparation (if needed), layette items, and diapers.
5. Throughout the visit, observe home environment for overall state of repair and existence of safety hazards:
   a. Storage of medications, household cleaners, and other substances hazardous to children.
   b. Presence of peeling paint on furniture, walls, or pipes.
   c. Factors that contribute to falls, such as dim lighting, broken steps, scatter rugs.
   d. Presence of vermin.
   e. Use of crib or playpen that fails to meet safety guidelines.
   f. Existence of emergency plan in case of fire; fire alarm or extinguisher.
6. Provide care to mother and/or newborn as prescribed by their respective primary care provider or in accord with agency protocol.
7. Provide teaching on basis of previously identified needs.
8. Refer family to appropriate community agencies or resources, such as warm lines and support groups.
9. Ascertain that woman knows potential problems to watch for and whom to call if they occur.
10. Ensure that used disposable items have been handled appropriately and that reusable items are cleaned and repacked appropriately in the nurse's bag.

IN-HOME INTERVENTIONS: ENDING THE VISIT

1. Summarize the activities and main points of the visit.
2. Clarify future expectations, including schedule of next visit.
3. Review teaching plan and provide major points in writing.
4. Provide information about reaching the nurse or agency if needed before the next scheduled visit.

POSTVISIT INTERVENTIONS

1. Document the visit thoroughly, using the necessary agency forms to serve as a legal record of the visit and to allow third-party reimbursement, as possible.
2. Initiate the plan of care on which the next encounter with the patient/family will be based.
3. Communicate appropriately (by telephone, letter, progress notes, or referral form) with primary care provider, other health professionals, or referral agencies on behalf of patient/family.

agency obtains authorization from the patient to give information to her physician and any individual or company involved in payment for the services. Agencies that bill third-party payers for the rendered services will include agreement language for assignment of benefits and financial remuneration. By agreeing to assign insurance benefits to the agency, the patient allows her insurance company to pay the home health care agency directly.

All patients have the right to actively participate in their home care plan of care. These patient rights and responsibilities should begin the discussion about the nurse-patient roles during this initial visit.

Assessment and nursing diagnoses

The primary goals of the assessment phase are to develop a trusting relationship and collect data by various methods to obtain a comprehensive patient profile. It may not be feasible or appropriate to collect in-depth information about all areas of assessment during the first visit (Clemen-Stone, Eigsti & McGuire, 1998). However, in many instances the nurse may be limited to one visit and must obtain information pertinent to the current situation in that hour.

The establishment of a trusting relationship began with the previsit telephone call. An interview style that reflects sensitivity, a nonjudgmental, accepting attitude, and a respect for the patient's rights facilitates the development of that trusting relationship. A skillful interviewer avoids barriers to communication such as false reassurance, advice-giving, excessive talking, and the showing of approval or disapproval (Clemen-Stone, Eigsti & McGuire, 1998). This nurse-patient relationship continues to develop over the course of home visits.

The nurse is a guest in the woman's home and should show respect for her and her belongings. Some adaptation of the home visit schedule may need to occur if there are numerous distractions during a visit, such as caring for the needs of small children. The nurse may need to ask to have the volume of the television lowered or to suggest moving to another room where it is more quiet and private.

The major areas of the assessment are demographics, medical history, general health history, medication history, social/cultural assessment, home and community environment, and physical assessment. Some of this information can be obtained from patient records sent to the home care agency at the time of referral or from the previsit interview. These data will be used to develop the nursing care plan and complete the plan of care, which is required for many licensed home health care agencies. Two areas requiring further discussion are the social assessment and the home environment assessment.

Social assessment includes information regarding the number and roles of each household member, which family members or individuals have taken on the role of caregiver,

and the woman's social support network. Identifying the roles of each member is helpful for developing the nursing care plan (Box 3-3).

Physical assessment of the home environment is an essential element of the home care assessment. The major areas of the home environment assessment include physical features of the home, access to the home, sanitary conditions, the presence of utilities (for example, telephone, electricity), safety features, and access to transportation and emergency support. Although some of this information can be collected during an interview, physically inspecting many areas of the home essential to care is a critical part of developing an accurate nursing care plan. Before any physical inspection, the home care nurse should ask the patient or caregiver for permission and assistance in identifying areas

---

BOX 3-3 | *Psychosocial Assessment*

LANGUAGE

Identify the primary language spoken in the home
Assess whether there are any language barriers to receiving support

COMMUNITY RESOURCES/ACCESS TO CARE

Identify primary and secondary means of transportation
Identify community agencies family currently uses for health care and support
Assess cultural and psychosocial barriers to receiving care

SOCIAL SUPPORT

Determine the people living with the pregnant woman
Identify who assists with household chores
Identify who assists with child care/parenting activities
Identify who the pregnant woman turns to for problems or during a crisis

INTERPERSONAL RELATIONSHIP

Identify the way decisions are made in the family
Identify the family's perception of the need for home care
Identify roles of adults in caring for family members

CAREGIVER

Identify the primary caregiver for home care treatments
Identify other caregivers and their roles
Assess the caregiver's knowledge of treatments and care process
Identify potential strain from the caregiver role
Identify the level of satisfaction with the caregiver role

STRESS AND COPING

Identify what the woman perceives as lifestyle changes and their impact on her and her family
Identify the changes she and her family have made to adjust to her health condition and home health care treatments

in the home that will be involved in the caregiving activities. During the physical inspection, careful consideration should be taken to avoid moving personal belongings that are not affected by the care.

Each specific plan of care has a different emphasis in the home environment. For example, patients on infusion therapy for hyperemesis gravidarum need a safe place to store medications and infusion supplies that are out of reach of small children living in the home. The home care nurse should incorporate the agency policies and procedures for the storage and handling of infusion supplies into her walk-through inspection. During the walk through, the home care nurse looks at the potential storage areas for supplies that are dry, clean, and where the temperature can be maintained. The home care nurse should include an inspection of the work areas, such as counter tops, table tops, sink and trash areas, that the patient or caregiver may use for mixing medications, changing infusion tubing, handling supplies, or disposing of used equipment and supplies.

Patients using electronic home health care equipment, such as phototherapy equipment or infusion pumps, require physical inspection of electrical outlets, electrical cords, and extension cords that will be used. Homes with faulty electrical wiring may place the patient at risk for being involved in an electrical fire; faulty wiring may require inspection and repair by a professional electrician before electronic devices are used. Findings from the assessment are incorporated into the plan of care.

Nursing diagnoses are derived from the data collected at the first home visit. Examples of nursing diagnoses for perinatal home health care patients are contained in the box below.

I Nursing Diagnoses

Perinatal Home Visits
Knowledge deficit related to
- Lack of understanding of management of vomiting
- Importance of bed rest for preterm labor
- Newborn care and feeding

Anxiety related to
- Performing blood glucose monitoring at home

Caregiver role strain, risk for, related to
- Providing care to a pregnant woman while working full-time

Coping, ineffective family: compromised, related to
- Care of newborn on oxygen therapy
- Lack of child care while woman is on bed rest for preterm labor

Sleep pattern disturbance related to
- Performing treatment at night

Impaired physical mobility related to
- Prescribed bed rest for preeclampsia, preterm labor

Expected outcomes of care

The home care nurse formulates patient-centered expected outcomes. Many of the interventions will be carried out by the patient or the designated caregiver; therefore, their participation in the planning process is critical to achieving positive outcomes. Examples of expected outcomes for perinatal patients include the following:
- The woman will verbalize understanding of treatments.
- The woman will report decreased anxiety about performing procedures (e.g., blood glucose monitoring).
- The woman will use support systems to cope effectively with problems (e.g., pregnancy complications, newborn complications/treatments).
- The woman and/or caregiver will return to demonstrate procedures.
- The caregiver will verbalize decreased role strain.

Plan of care and interventions

The nursing care plan is developed based on the individual health care needs of the patient. The care plan describes the nursing diagnoses and interventions needed to meet the patient's health care needs.

Home care nurses working in HCFA-regulated home health care agencies use a plan of care (POC) that includes patient demographics, the health care provider's orders, home care goals, and the level of functioning as a basis for nursing care plans. This document is initiated at the time of referral to the home care agency and must be updated every 60 days or as specified by state regulations.

The frequency of the skilled nursing visit may vary with the individual POC, nursing care plan, and reimbursement criteria established by the third-party payers.

Nurse safety and infection control are two important aspects specific to home care.

Safety issues for the home care nurse. The nurse should be fully aware of the home environment and neighborhood in which the home care is being provided. Unlike hospitals, in which the environment is more predictable and controlled, the patient's neighborhood and home have the potential for uncertainty. Home care nurses should take necessary safety precautions and avoid dangerous areas.

Agencies that serve patients in high-crime areas may conduct a violence-potential assessment by telephone before the visit and enlist the patient's cooperation in minimizing risk (Hunter, 1997). Others have hired full-time security personnel to accompany nurses on their visits. Personal strategies recommended for nurses visiting families with a history of violence or substance abuse include: (1) self-awareness; (2) environmental assessment; (3) using listening and observation skills with patients to be aware of behavioral changes indicating aggression or lack of impulse control; (4) planning for dealing with aggressive behavior (i.e., allowing personal space and taking a nonaggressive stance (Whitley, Jacobson & Gowrys, 1996); (5) making visits in pairs; and (6) having access to a cellular phone at all times.

Personal safety. The home care nurse needs to be aware of personal safety behaviors before going on a home visit. Dress should be casual but professional in appearance with a name-identification tag. Limited jewelry should be worn. Valuable personal items, such as an expensive purse or coat, should not be worn on a visit. Carrying an extra set of car keys in the nursing home care bag saves time and frustration if the nurse becomes locked out of the automobile. Automobile keys spread between the fingers with sharp ends outward can be used as a weapon if necessary. The same common sense behaviors and precautions that guide a person's behavior when alone in any setting should be followed by home care nurses.

The agency should have a copy of the nurse's home care itinerary, including contact telephone numbers if a patient does not have a telephone, and information on the nurse's car, the make, model, and color, as well as the license plate number. Many home care nurses carry agency-provided pagers or cellular telephones that allow the agency to contact the nurse throughout the day to give information about patient updates, changes in orders or services, schedule changes, and new patients who require an initial visit. The telephone is also useful to notify patients when the nurse is delayed.

The automobile used for the home care visits, whether a personal or agency-owned vehicle, should have regular preventive maintenance checks, an adequate fuel level, and road safety items stored in the trunk. Items to carry in the vehicle include change for telephone calls and tolls, maps, emergency telephone numbers, a flashlight, a first aid kit, flares, and equipment for inclement weather conditions.

Home care nurses should park and lock their cars in a safe place that is visible from the street and patient's home and away from hidden alleys. While driving to the patient's home, the nurse should assess the neighborhood for safety, especially if the neighborhood is unfamiliar. All valuable items should be stored out of sight before leaving the office. While walking to the patient's home, nurses should not walk near groups of strangers hanging out in doorways or alleys, enter into vacant buildings, or enter a yard that has an unrestrained dog. The home or building should not be entered if the nurse has any safety concerns. All home care agencies should have policies to follow for such situations (OSHA, 1996).

Patient's home. Once inside the patient's home, the nurse may encounter unsafe situations such as the presence of weapons, abusive behavior, or health hazards. Each potentially hazardous situation must be dealt with according to agency policies and procedures. If abuse or neglect is reasonably suspected, the home care nurse should follow home care agency and state and federal regulations for reporting and documenting the situation. Nurses should maintain their own safety first and act accordingly throughout the visit.

Infection control. The nurse carries the necessary supplies and equipment to provide nursing care to the patient. Home care bags should contain infection control supplies, such as personal protection equipment; disposable non-sterile, sterile, and utility gloves; disinfectants; disposable cardiopulmonary resuscitation (CPR) masks; gowns; shoe covers; caps; leakproof and puncture-resistant specimen containers; sharps container; dry-hand disinfectants; and leakproof barriers. Proper infection control techniques should be used in stocking, storing, handling, and transporting this bag. When a procedure is to be performed, the nurse should set up a clean area for necessary supplies. A dirty area is designated with a trash bag for the collection of soiled equipment and supplies. Hands are washed before all supplies and equipment for the visit are removed from the bag and placed in a clean area.

The importance of infection control does not diminish because nursing care is provided in the patient's home rather than in a hospital. Patients are not likely to become infected because of their home environment, but the nurse may become exposed to a communicable disease.

The Centers for Disease Control and Prevention (CDC) has recommended standard precaution guidelines for the protection of health care workers from blood-borne pathogens. These guidelines recommend that standard precautions should be used whenever a treatment is performed because it is difficult to determine which patients have a communicable disease.

Handwashing remains the single most important infection control procedure. Hands should be washed before and after each patient contact. Wearing gloves does not eliminate the necessity for handwashing. If running water or clean facilities are unavailable, the hands can be cleaned with an antiseptic foam.

Using gloves reduces the incidence of exposure to blood-borne pathogens. Gloves should be selected according to the nursing activity to be performed. Nonsterile latex or vinyl gloves should be worn with each procedure that has the potential for contact with bodily substances (e.g., performing venipunctures, heelsticks on the newborn, and perineal care). Sterile gloves should be worn with clinical procedures requiring sterile technique, such as insertion of peripherally inserted central lines and certain dressing changes. General-purpose utility gloves should be used for housekeeping activities, such as cleaning equipment or spills. Nonsterile and sterile gloves should be discarded after each use in a leak-resistant waste receptacle. Utility gloves may be disinfected and reused.

Disposable personal protection equipment should be removed after each use and discarded in a plastic trash container. Safety glasses or goggles can be cleaned with soap and water after each use.

Whenever specimens are collected, standard precautions should be used. Any specimen of bodily fluids should be placed in a leakproof bag and secured in a puncture-proof container. The outside of the container is washed off, if it was soiled, before transporting it. Specimens should be labeled with the patient's name and additional identifying information according to the home health care agency or laboratory policies. If specimens are being transported, they should be placed in a container on a flat surface in the vehicle. An insulated container may be used to keep specimens cool in transit.

Sharps containers are puncture-proof and leakproof containers that are labeled with a biohazard sign on the outside and should be used to collect needles and sharp objects. Patients are instructed to fill containers between two thirds and three fourths full to prevent spillage of their contents. As part of the patient-teaching process, information about storage and handling is covered by the home care nurse. When the container reaches its maximum capacity, it should be returned to the home health care agency and replaced. Medical-waste material, such as urine and secretions, can be discarded via the sewer or septic system.

Contaminated dressings and disposable supplies should be placed in a leakproof, plastic bag and securely fastened for disposal at the patient's home. The patient should be instructed regarding the proper disposal of medical waste in the home. Agency policies and procedures and local waste-management ordinances should be consulted before the patient is instructed.

Documentation of care. The home care nurse continually reassesses the patient's condition and response to the interventions during every home visit and revises the nursing diagnoses and care plan. Nursing documentation should reflect an objective description of the nursing assessment data collected at each visit. Statements such as "no change" or "same as last visit" do not accurately reflect the monitoring of the patient condition that occurred during the skilled nursing visit. Once the home care outcomes are achieved, and the patient is discharged from the home care agency, documentation should include information about the patient status at the time of discharge, progress toward attaining health care goals, and plans for follow-up care.

The role of the clinical record in home care has been affected by social, economic, and legal health care changes. The clinical record serves as the only written documentation of the home care nursing visits and is required to qualify for reimbursement for services from most third-party payers. Appropriate care should be taken to accurately and in a timely manner complete the necessary home health care records. Documentation guidelines include writing or dictating notes or using a laptop computer at the patient's home or shortly after the visit.

Evaluation

Evaluation is based on the expected outcomes of care. The plan is revised as necessary.

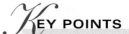 **EY POINTS**

- A community is defined as a locality-based entity, composed of systems of societal institutions, informal groups, and aggregates that are interdependent and whose function is to meet a wide variety of collective needs.
- Community-oriented practice is targeted to the community, the population group in which healthful change is sought.
- Of necessity, most changes aimed at improving community health involve partnerships among community residents and health workers.
- Assessing community health requires gathering and interpreting data.
- Methods of collecting data useful to the nurse working in the community include windshield surveys, analysis of existing data, informant interviews, and participant observation.
- The health care system is giving increasing attention to health promotion and disease prevention for populations or aggregates.
- Knowledge of the community in which patients live helps in the planning and organization of care that is responsive to their unique characteristics and needs.
- Vulnerable populations are groups who are at higher risk of developing physical, mental, or social health problems.
- Perinatal home care is a unique nursing practice that incorporates knowledge from community health nursing, acute care nursing, family therapy, health promotion, and patient education.
- Social and economic factors affect the scope of perinatal nursing practice.
- External organizations, such as federal and state government, professional organizations, and health care accrediting agencies, influence the standards of perinatal home health care practice.
- Perinatal home care can be provided for women and infants throughout the perinatal period beginning with preconception and ending in the postpartum period.
- Perinatal home care nurses should incorporate personal safety and infection control practices into the nursing care plan.
- Telephonic nurse advice lines, telephonic nursing assessments, and warm lines are low-cost health care services that facilitate continuous patient education, support, and health care decision making even though health care is delivered in multiple sites.
- Communication protocols among members of the home health care team are critical to diminish fragmentation and duplication of health care services.

CRITICAL THINKING EXERCISES

1 *With a classmate, complete a windshield survey of a neighborhood in which many of your hospital's maternity patients live. How might knowledge of the patient's community affect your discharge teaching?*

2 *Read your local newspaper and identify articles illustrating community partnerships to meet health needs of vulnerable populations. Were these needs identified by providers or consumers? What needs are unmet?*

3 *Prepare education materials that could be used for teaching patients self-care for preterm labor. Describe the difference between hospital teaching and home care teaching. What follow-up is necessary?*

References

Acquaviva T & Lancaster J: Poverty and homelessness. In Stanhope M & Lancaster J, editors: *Community health nursing: promoting the health of aggregates, families and individuals*, ed 4, St Louis, 1996, Mosby.

Aday L: Vulnerable populations: a community-oriented perspective, *Fam Comm Health* 19(4):1, 1997.

American Academy of Pediatrics Committee on Community Health Services: Health needs of homeless children and families, *Pediatrics* 98(4 pt 1):789, 1996.

Anderson E & McFarlane J: *Community as partner: theory and practice in nursing*, ed 2, Philadelphia, 1996, Lippincott-Raven.

Association of Women's Health, Obstetric, and Neonatal Nurses (AWHONN): *Didactic content and clinical skills verification for professional nurse providers of perinatal home care*, Washington, DC, 1994, AWHONN.

Bakewell-Sachs S & Persily C: Perinatal partnerships in practice: a conceptual framework for giving care across the childbearing continuum, *J Perinat Neonatal Nurs* 9(1):31, 1995.

Barnett A: Is knowledge really power for patients? *Business & Health* 13(5):29, 1995.

Bergquist S & King J: Parish nursing—a conceptual framework, *J Holist Nurs* 12(2):155, 1994.

Blystad-Keppler A: Postpartum care center: follow-up care in a hospital-based clinic, *J Obstet Gynecol Neonatal Nurs* 24(1): 17, 1995.

Bollini P & Siem H: Health needs of migrants, *World Health* 48(6):20, 1995.

Brooten D: Perinatal care across the continuum: early discharge and nursing home follow-up, *J Perinat Neonatal Nurs* 9(1):38, 1995.

Broussard B: The role of the perinatal home care clinical specialist, *Home Healthc Nurse* 14(11):855, 1996.

Burg M: Health problems of sheltered homeless women and their dependent children, *Health Soc Work* 19(2):125, 1994.

Christian A: Clinical nurse specialists: creating new programs for neonatal home care, *J Perinatal Neonatal Nurs* 10(1):54, 1996.

Clemen-Stone S, Eigsti D & McGuire S: *Comprehensive community health nursing: family, aggregate, and community practice*, ed 5, St Louis, 1998, Mosby.

Consensus set of indicators for assessing community health status, *MMWR* 40(27):449, 1991.

Dixon S: Parish nurse ministry improves health outcomes of low-income community, *Aspens Advis Nurse Exec* 11(11):7, 1996.

Djeddah C: Refugee families, *World Health* 48(6):10, 1995.

Expert Panel on Women's Health: Women's health and women's health care: recommendations of the 1996 AAN expert panel on women's health, *Nurs Outlook* 45(1):7, 1997.

Foss G: A conceptual model for studying parenting behaviors in immigrant populations, *Adv Nurs Sci* 19(2):74, 1996.

Fowler B et al.: Cross-training to develop a home visit program: a rural experience, *Mother Baby J* 2(2):30, 1997.

Ganguly I: Promoting the health of women of non-English-speaking backgrounds in Australia, *World Health Forum* 16(2):157, 1995.

Gany F & Bocanegra H: Maternal-child immigrant health training: changing knowledge and attitudes to improve health care delivery, *Patient Educ Couns* 27(1):23, 1996.

Health Care Financing Administration: *Homehealth insurance manual* Pub No 11-Rev 229, Washington, DC, 1990, USDHHS.

Henry J: Community nursing centers: models of nurse managed care, *J Obstet Gynecol Neonatal Nurs* 26(2):224, 1997.

Hunter E: Violence prevention in the home health setting, *Home Healthc Nurse* 15(6):403, 1997.

Jones K & Schenk C: Migrant health issues. In Stanhope M & Lancaster J, editors: *Community health nursing: promoting the health of aggregates, families and individuals*, ed 4, St Louis, 1996, Mosby.

Jones L, Maestri B & McCoy K: Why parents use the warm line, *MCN Am J Matern Child Nurs* 18(5):258, 1993.

Jones M: *Electronic house calls: 21st century options*, Washington, DC, 1996, Consumer Interest Research Institute.

Kemp C: Refugee health and community nursing—Dallas, Texas. In Anderson E & McFarlane J, editors: *Community as partner: theory and practice in nursing*, Philadelphia, 1996, Lippincott-Raven.

Kemp V & Hatmaker D: Perinatal home care: issues in family and community health, *Family Comm Health* 18(4):40, 1996.

Killion C: Special health care needs of homeless pregnant women, *Adv Nurs Science* 18(2):44, 1995.

Lambert M: Migrant and seasonal farm worker women, *J Obstet Gynecol Neonatal Nurs* 24(3):66, 1995.

Lassiter P: Group approaches in community health. In Stanhope M & Lancaster J, editors: *Community health nursing: promoting the health of aggregates, families and individuals*, ed 4, St Louis, 1996, Mosby.

Lipson J & Omidian P: Afghan refugee issues in the U.S. social environment, *Western J Nurs Res* 19(1):110, 1997.

March of Dimes Birth Defects Foundation: *Babies + you: a prenatal health promotion program*, White Plains, New York, 1991, March of Dimes Birth Defects Foundation.

Maternal and Child Health Bureau: Pregnancy-related behaviors among migrant farm workers—four states, 1989-1993, *MMWR* 46 (13): 283, 1997.

O'Campo P et al.: Neighborhood risk factors for low birthweight in Baltimore: a multilevel analysis, *Am J Public Health* 87(7):1113, 1997.

Occupational Safety and Health Administration: *Guidelines for preventing workplace violence for health care and social service workers-OSHA 3148-1996*, Washington, DC, 1996, United States Department of Labor.

Olds D, Kitzman H & Cole R: Effect of home visitation by nurses on caregiving and maternal life-course, *Arch Pediatr Adolesc Med* 149:76, 1995.

Pender N: *Health promotion in nursing practice*, ed 3, Stamford, Conn, 1996, Appleton & Lange.

Perinatal health: strategies for the 21st century, Providence, RI, 1992, National Perinatal Information Center.

Persily C, Brown L & York R: A model of home care for high-risk childbearing families: women with diabetes in pregnancy, *Nurs Clin North Am* 31(2):327, 1996.

Pew Health Professions Commission: *Critical challenges: revitalizing the health professions for the 21st century,* San Francisco, 1995, Pew Charitable Trust.

Porter A et al.: Clinical integration: an interdisciplinary approach to a system priority; corporatization of health care, *Nurs Adm Q* 20(2):65, 1996.

Rew L: Health risks of homeless adolescents. Implications for holistic nursing, *J Holist Nurs* 14(4): 348, 1996.

Rodriguez R: Promoting healthy partnerships with migrant farm workers–Colorado. In Anderson E & McFarlane J, editors: *Community as partner: theory and practice in nursing,* Philadelphia, 1996, Lippincott-Raven.

Sebastian J: Vulnerability and vulnerable populations: an introduction. In Stanhope M & Lancaster J, editors: *Community health nursing: promoting the health of aggregates, families, and individuals,* ed 4, St Louis, 1996, Mosby.

Shuster G & Goeppinger J: Community as client: using the nursing process to promote health. In Stanhope M & Lancaster J, editors*: Community health nursing: promoting the health of aggregates, families and individuals,* ed 4, St Louis, 1996, Mosby.

Stanhope M & Lancaster J, editors: *Community health nursing: promoting the health of aggregates, families, and individuals,* ed 4, St Louis, 1996, Mosby.

United HealthCare Corporation*: A glossary of terms: the language of managed care and organized health care systems,* Minnetonka, Minn, 1994, United HealthCare Corporation.

U.S. Committee on Refugees: *World refugee survey,* Washington, DC, 1995, Immigration and Refugee Services of America.

U.S. Department of Health and Human Services: CHCs staffed by nurses win "models that work" award, *Public Health Rep* 112(2):94, 1997.

Wagner J, Menke E & Ciccone J: What is known about the health of rural homeless families? *Public Health Nursing* 12(6):400, 1995.

Whitley G, Jacobson G & Gawrys M: The impact of violence in the health care setting upon nursing education, *J Nurs Educ* 35(5):211, 1996.

Women's Health Center Management: Making insurers want to pay for home care, *Women's Health Care Management* 5(1):2, 1997.

Zotti M, Brown P & Stotts R: Community-based nursing versus community health nursing: what does it all mean? *Nurs Outlook* 44(2):211, 1996.

Zotti M & Zahner S: Evaluation of public health nursing home visits to pregnant women on WIC, *Public Health Nurs* 12(5):294, 1995.

Zyzanski S, Williams R & Flocke S: Selection of key community descriptors for community-oriented primary care, *Family Practice* 13(3):280, 1996.

CHAPTER

Health Promotion and Prevention

BARBARA PETERSON SINCLAIR

BARBARA PETERSON SINCLAIR

LEARNING OBJECTIVES

- *Define the key terms.*
- *List factors influencing a woman's contact with the health care system.*
- *Identify reasons for women to enter the health care delivery system.*
- *Discuss financial, cultural, and gender barriers to seeking health care.*
- *Explain conditions and characteristics that increase health risks.*
- *Review programs of anticipatory guidance that promote health and prevention.*
- *Suggest community resources to combat violence against women.*
- *Outline health screening schedules for women in the childbearing years.*

KEY TERMS

cycle of violence
health promotion
human chorionic gonadotropin (hCG)
infertility
Kegel exercises
menopause
osteoporosis
perimenopause
preconception counseling
prevention
rape

REASONS FOR ENTERING THE HEALTH CARE SYSTEM

In addition to regular human health care needs, women have unique and special health circumstances related to their reproductive capacity. As a result, many women initially enter the health care system because of some reproductive system–related situation such as pregnancy; irregular menses; desire for contraception; or episodic illness, such as vaginal infection. Once in the system, however, it is incumbent on health care providers to recognize the need for health promotion and preventive health maintenance and to provide these services as part of lifelong care for women. It has been demonstrated repeatedly that lifestyle and health habits influence the development of illness, both chronic and acute. In fact, the leading five causes of death in women are to some degree preventable, or at least modifiable, if individuals eat well, are not exposed to tobacco or environmental hazards, engage in physical activity, are immunized, and maintain appropriate health screening and follow-up (U.S. Preventive Services Task Force, 1996).

One cannot generalize among all women, but rather must view the individual woman within the context of her particular age, family, culture, religion, society, and physical being. Also, women cannot be viewed in the same way as men because women may respond differently physiologically, emotionally, and cognitively. Women's roles in society have changed dramatically during recent decades, and as a result, women's attitudes in regard to health care have changed. In addition to quality health services for themselves and their families, women want information and the opportunity to be involved in decision making and self-care. Nurses have the responsibility to provide health education and health promotion and to show compassion for and understanding of the woman's circumstances while doing so (Sinclair, 1997).

Preconception Counseling

Preconception health promotion provides women and their partners with information that is needed to make decisions about their reproductive future. **Preconception counseling** guides couples on how to avoid unintended pregnancies, stresses risk management, and identifies healthy behaviors that promote the well-being of the woman and her potential fetus. Some couples are simply desirous of information pertaining to normal physiology or the timing of coitus to achieve pregnancy or to have myths or beliefs confirmed or denied.

The initiation of activities that promote healthy mothers and babies must occur before the period of critical fetal organ development, which is between 17 and 56 days following fertilization. By the end of the eighth week after conception and certainly by the end of the first trimester, any major structural anomalies in the fetus are already present.

BOX 4-1	*Components of Preconception Care*

HEALTH PROMOTION: GENERAL TEACHING

Nutrition
  Healthy diet, including folic acid
  Optimum weight
Exercise and rest
Avoidance of substance abuse (tobacco, alcohol, "recreational" drugs)
Use of safer sex practices
Attending to family and social needs

RISK FACTOR ASSESSMENT

Medical history
  Immune status (e.g., rubella, hepatitis B)
  Family history (e.g., genetic disorders)
  Illnesses (e.g., infections)
  Current use of medication (prescription, nonprescription)
Reproductive history
  Contraceptive
  Obstetric
Psychosocial history
  Spouse/partner and family situation, including domestic violence
  Availability of family or other support systems
  Readiness for pregnancy (e.g., age, life goals, stress)
Financial resources
Environmental (home, workplace) conditions
  Safety hazards
  Toxic chemicals
  Radiation

INTERVENTIONS

Anticipatory guidance/teaching
Treatment of medical conditions and results
  Medications
  Cessation/reduction in substance use/abuse
  Immunizations (e.g., rubella, tuberculosis, hepatitis)
Nutrition, diet, and weight management
Exercise
Referral for genetic counseling
Referral to and use of
  Family planning services
  Family and social needs management

Because many women do not realize that they are pregnant and do not seek prenatal care until well into the first trimester, the rapidly growing fetus may be exposed to many types of intrauterine environmental hazards during this most vulnerable developmental phase. Thus preconception health care should occur well in advance of an actual pregnancy.

Every woman of childbearing age should be viewed as a potential mother. Therefore, identifying and treating risk factors and providing anticipatory guidance with emphasis on healthy lifestyles may be the keys to improving the health of the next generation (Frede, 1993). The components of preconception care, such as health promotion, risk assessment, and interventions, are outlined in Box 4-1.

Preconception care is important for women who have had a problem with a previous pregnancy (e.g., spontaneous abortion or preterm birth). Although causes are not always identifiable, in many cases, problems can be identified and treated and may not recur in subsequent pregnancies. Preconception care is also important to minimize fetal malformations. For example, research has consistently shown that offspring of women who have type 1 diabetes mellitus have significantly more congenital anomalies than do children of mothers without diabetes. Furthermore, it has been shown that the rate of malformation is greatly reduced when the insulin-dependent diabetic woman has excellent blood glucose control when she becomes pregnant and maintains euglycemia (normal blood sugar) throughout the period of organ development in the fetus. Therefore, education and glucose control must begin before conception to benefit from this knowledge.

There are many examples illustrating effects of maternal age or illnesses, conditions that produce anomalies in the fetus (teratogenic agents), such as drugs, viruses, chemicals, genetically inherited diseases, or conditions that might be harmful to the woman should a pregnancy occur. In many instances, counseling can allow for behavior modification before damage is done or a woman can make an informed decision about her willingness to accept potential hazards. There is no doubt that the concept of counseling bears out the adage that risk reduction before conception may offer greater benefits than risk reduction during a pregnancy (Moos, 1994).

Pregnancy

A woman's entry into health care is often associated with pregnancy, either for diagnosis or for actual care. Suspicion of pregnancy occurs most commonly when a woman is late with her menses. However, other presumptive symptoms such as breast tenderness, nausea, or urinary frequency may also encourage her to seek confirmation. Pregnancy testing is often the first diagnostic tool to be used and can be performed at home or in the health care provider's clinic, office, or laboratory. **Human chorionic gonadotropin (hCG)** is the biologic marker on which both serum and urine pregnancy tests are based. Earlier and more accurate results occur from testing the blood but a first-voided morning urine sample can yield valid findings approximately 1 week after the missed period.

Pregnancy is divided into three, 3-month segments called trimesters. It is highly desirous for a woman to enter prenatal care within the first 12 weeks, the first trimester. This allows for early pregnancy counseling especially for the woman who has had no preconception care. Subjective information is obtained by history taking and objective findings are gathered by physical examination, laboratory tests, and diagnostic analysis. Major goals of prenatal care are found in Box 4-2 and should be initiated at the first visit.

BOX 4-2 — *Major Goals of Prenatal Care*

- Define health status of mother and fetus.
- Determine the gestational age of the fetus and monitor fetal development.
- Identify the woman at risk for complications and minimize the risk whenever possible.
- Anticipate and try to prevent problems before they occur.
- Provide appropriate education and counseling.

Gestational age of the fetus and estimated date of birth (EDB) are often predicated on menstrual history. If there is a question about gestational age, ultrasonography during early pregnancy is helpful in accurate dating.

Education and counseling for women in the first trimester include discussion and self-care concepts in the areas of nutrition, exercise, sexual relations, employment, travel, rest, social habits (tobacco, alcohol, drugs), genetic counseling, avoidance of environmental insult to the fetus, physical changes, management of common complaints, prenatal classes, other resources, and what to expect for follow-up (Fahey & Sinclair, 1996). Women should be encouraged to ask questions and to share concerns or fears. It is preferable that husbands/partners are invited to attend prenatal visits and are provided the opportunity to ask questions and share their concerns. Extensive discussion of pregnancy is found in Unit Three.

Well-Woman Care

Current trends in the health care of women have expanded beyond a reproductive focus. A holistic approach to women's health care includes a woman's health needs throughout her lifetime. This view is one that goes beyond simply her reproductive needs. This restructuring places women's health within the primary health care delivery system. Women's health assessment and screening focus on a multisystem evaluation emphasizing the maintenance and enhancement of wellness (Allen & Phillips, 1997). Support and reassurance begin with the woman's first contact with the health care team. It is often the nurse's responsibility in health promotion to coordinate the woman's care. A nurse often takes the history, orders diagnostic tests, interprets test results, makes referrals, and directs attention to the problems that require medical intervention and referral. Nurses who function in the expanded role as advanced practice nurses can also perform complete physical assessments, including the gynecologic examination.

Many women first enter the health care delivery system for a Papanicolaou (Pap) smear or contraception. Visits to the nurse may be their only contact with the system unless they become ill. Some women postpone examination until a specific need arises, such as pregnancy, pain, abnormal bleeding, or vaginal discharge. Embarrassing signs and symptoms, such as urinary incontinence, dyspareunia (painful intercourse), and annoying vaginal discharge, are often elicited only by sensitive interviewing and careful examination. Some women report a minor symptom as a way of entering the health care system when stronger motives for seeking care, either conscious or unconscious, underlie their primary complaint. It is not uncommon that serious concerns, such as fear of pregnancy, sexually transmitted disease, cancer, or sexual dysfunctioning, begin to surface during the interview.

Health care needs vary with culture, religion, age, and personal differences. The changing responsibilities and roles of women, their socioeconomic status, and their personal lifestyles also contribute to differences in the health and behavior of women. Employment outside of the home, physical disability, inadequate or lack of health insurance, divorce, single parenthood, and sexual orientation also can affect women's ability to seek and receive health care in clinical settings (Bartman, 1996). As women age, many continue to address their primary health care needs within their established gynecologic care setting. Therefore, well-women's health care should include a complete history, physical examination, and age-appropriate screening. In addition, health promotion must be included because it increases the levels of health and well-being and actualizes or maximizes the health potential of all women.

Fertility Control and Infertility

As women become more informed about themselves and their health care, they are more willing to seek counseling and techniques of contraception appropriate to their varied and specific needs. Some women first enter the health care system to obtain such advice. Over half of the pregnancies in the United States each year are unintended, and the majority of these occur in the 10% of women who do not use birth control. Education is the key to encouraging women to make family planning choices based on preference and actual benefit-to-risk ratios. Providers can influence the user's motivation and ability to use the method correctly (Hatcher et al., 1998).

Many types of birth control or contraceptives have a high degree of safety and effectiveness. Included are (1) hormonal methods such as combined oral contraceptives (OCs), pills that contain both estrogen and progestin, and progestin-only systems delivered via injectables, subdermals, or orals; (2) barrier methods with physical deterrents such as latex in diaphragms or condoms and chemical deterrents such as nonoxynol-9, a spermicide found in foams and creams; and (3) natural family planning, which involves a combination of calendar, basal body temperature, and cervical mucus/ovulation record keeping as a basis for periodic abstinence. Information on the specifics of these methods plus intrauterine devices, sterilization, and postcoital options can be found in Chapter 7.

The concept of health promotion applies to contraception as can be seen in Box 4-3. The nurse is in a prime

BOX 4-3	*Contraceptive Health Promotion*

- Childspacing and quality maternity care improve perinatal outcomes and health in general of mother and children.
- Achieving desired family size infers a better sharing of all resources with attendant increases in education, health care, and other positive societal parameters.
- Contraceptives themselves may positively affect future health. For example, use of condoms may prevent acquisition of HIV infection; combined OCs may provide some protection against later development of cancer of ovary and endometrium; barrier methods decrease transmission of STDs, which can develop into pelvic inflammatory disease (PID) with resultant infertility or sterility and thus affect future childbearing capacity.

situation to influence women positively regarding the need for child spacing, methods of family planning that are consistent with religious and personal preferences, noncontraceptive benefits of certain methods, the appropriate use of methods selected, and the protection of future fertility when so desired.

Women also enter the health care system because of their desire to achieve a pregnancy. Approximately 15% of couples in the United States have some degree of **infertility** as defined by not becoming pregnant after 1 year of unprotected intercourse or not being able to carry a pregnancy to viability. Infertility can cause emotional pain for many couples and the inability to produce an offspring sometimes results in feelings of failure and inordinate stress on the relationship. Significant amounts of time, money, and emotional investment can be spent on testing and treatment in efforts to build a family (Epps & Stewart, 1995).

Infertility appears to be an ever-increasing problem. Not only is it addressed more often in the media, but also we may be seeing more couples trying to have babies because America's largest population group, the baby boomers, are well into their reproductive years. Many couples have delayed starting their families until they are in their 30s or 40s, which allows for more time to be exposed to situations negatively affecting fertility (including age-related infertility for the female). In addition, sexually transmitted diseases (STDs), which can predispose to decreased fertility, are on the rise, and many women and men are in workplaces and home settings where they may be exposed to reproductive environmental hazards.

Approximately 30% to 40% of all couples treated for infertility conceive at some point. However, steps toward prevention of infertility should be undertaken as part of on-going routine health care, and such information is especially appropriate in preconception counseling (Lemcke et al., 1995). Primary care providers can undertake initial evaluation and counseling before couples are referred to specialists. For additional information about infertility, see Chapter 7.

Menstrual Problems

Under the influence of hormones, the initiation of menstruation, called the menarche, heralds the beginning of the ability to reproduce and occurs at a mean age of 13 years. Reproductive capacity extends until menstruation ceases at **menopause** at a mean age of 51 years. Irregularities or problems with the menstrual period are among the most common concerns of women and often cause them to seek help within the health care system. Common menstrual disorders include the following:

- Amenorrhea (absence of menses), which is most often but not always caused by pregnancy
- Dysmenorrhea (cramps or painful menstruation), which is perhaps the most common of all gynecologic problems
- Premenstrual syndrome, which represents a constellation of recurrent physical and psychologic discomforts that occur only during the time period preceding menstruation
- Endometriosis (endometrial tissue outside of the uterus that responds to monthly hormonal changes that cause it to thicken and bleed), which possibly causes discomfort or decreased fertility
- Menorrhagia (excessive bleeding) or metrorrhagia (irregular bleeding), which can be due to a variety of causes and should be investigated to allow for appropriate management

Simple explanation and counseling may handle the concern; however, history and examination must be completed, as well as laboratory or diagnostic tests, if indicated. Questions should never be considered inconsequential and age-specific reading materials are recommended, especially for teenagers. The reader is referred to Chapter 6 for an in-depth discussion of menstrual problems.

Perimenopause

Although menopause or the last menstrual period occurs at an average age of 51 years, it is preceded by a period known as the **perimenopause,** or climacteric, during which ovarian function declines. Ova slowly diminish, menstrual cycles are anovulatory, resulting in irregular bleeding; the ovary stops producing estrogen, and eventually menses no longer occurs. The body responds to this natural transition in a number of ways, most of which are due to the decrease in estrogen (Box 4-4). Although fertility is greatly reduced during the climacteric, women are urged to maintain some method of birth control because pregnancies still can occur. Most women seeking health care at this time do so because of irregular bleeding that may accompany the perimenopause. Others are concerned about vasomotor symptoms (hot flashes and flushes). All women need to have

BOX 4-4 **Effects from Decreased Estrogen in Perimenopausal Women**

- Hot flashes and flushes may occur. These are periodic feelings of warmth that spread over the body and occasionally interfere with sleep.
- Urogenital tissues become dry and less flexible, possibly resulting in painful intercourse, atrophic vaginitis, and urinary problems.
- Accelerated bone loss occurs (**osteoporosis**), eventually causing bones to be brittle and at risk for fracture.
- Cardiovascular risk increases and continues to rise with aging.
- Mood swings and irritability are occasionally reported but are probably due to poor sleep patterns caused by hot flashes at night.

factual information, the dispelling of myths, a thorough examination, and periodic health screenings thereafter.

Not all women have the same symptoms, nor do symptoms have the same intensity or duration. Hormone replacement therapy (HRT), a combination of estrogen and progestin, relieves many symptoms and also reduces the risk of osteoporosis and heart disease. However, the risk of breast cancer may be increased. Perimenopausal and postmenopausal women are encouraged to maintain a well-balanced diet, physical activity, and adequate calcium and vitamin D intake (supplementation is recommended), and to have regular mammograms, pelvic examinations, Papanicolaou tests, and diagnostic tests to evaluate bone density, cholesterol levels, and presence of occult blood in stools.

I BARRIERS TO SEEKING HEALTH CARE

Financial Issues

The United States spends almost 15% of its gross domestic product on health, far more than any other industrialized nation in the world, yet major problems still exist (*Failure of Health Care Reform*, 1995). Employment-based financing of health insurance has resulted in a system in which one's health insurance is linked to a job, and the system is working well for fewer and fewer people, especially women. Fourteen million young women have no health insurance and 5 million more have coverage so inadequate that it does not even include maternity care (Rosenfeld, 1997).

In the United States disparity occurs among races and socioeconomic classes affecting many facets of life, including health. With limited money and awareness, there is a lack of access to care, delay in seeking care, few prevention activities, and little accurate information about health and the health care system. Women use health services more often than men but are more likely than men to have difficulty in financing them; they are twice as often underinsured (i.e., have limited coverage with high cost copayments

or deductibles). Women make up the majority of Medicaid recipients; however, only 42% of poor women are eligible. Medicaid has been expanded to include special benefits for pregnant women but they are limited to treatment of pregnancy-related conditions and terminate 60 days after birth (Lemcke et al., 1995). Current questions abound regarding possible changes in the Medicaid coverage related to care for mother and child during the maternity cycle. More and more states are requiring their Medicaid recipients to enroll in managed care programs; whether this improves access and outcomes is yet to be determined.

Insurance coverage varies significantly by age, marital status, race, and ethnicity (Horton, 1995). Caucasians of all ages are more likely than African-Americans and other racial or ethnic groups to have private insurance. Caucasians possess insurance 2.5 times more often than Hispanics and 1.8 times more often than African-Americans. Single, separated, or divorced individuals are less likely to have insurance. Often unmarried teenagers who are usually covered by their parent's medical insurance do not have maternity coverage because policies have inclusion statements for only the employee or spouse.

Midwifery care has helped contain some health care costs, but not all insurance carriers reimburse nurse-practitioners and clinical nurse-specialists as direct care providers, a situation that continues to be a problem (Ernst, 1994). Nursing data need to be identified and placed in a database to be included in public policy decisions; nursing variables such as education and supportive care must become part of the national data-gathering system. Nurses should deal with the politics involved in cost-containment health care policies, since they, as knowledgeable experts, can provide solutions to many of the health care problems at a relatively low cost (Hastings, 1995).

Cultural Issues

Although they are most significant, financial considerations are not the only barriers to obtaining quality health care. As our nation becomes more racially, ethnically, and culturally diverse, the health of minority groups becomes a major issue. The National Center for Health Statistics reports 1996 data that reflect racial differences in health. For example, life expectancy for Caucasian women was 79.6 years while for African-American women it was 74.2 years. The proportion of mothers who began receiving prenatal care during the first trimester of pregnancy was 84% for Caucasians, 71% for African-Americans and 72% for Latinas (National Center for Health Statistics, 1997). According to the 1990 census, one of every four persons in the United States is a person of color; however, it is expected that this ratio will become even greater after the census in 2000. The United States is truly a multicultural, pluralistic society. Cox (1997) suggests that differences for all racial/ethnic groups will be more significant than their aggregate numbers indicate and health care workers will need to deal with even more distinct racially and ethnically diverse populations—obviously presenting another health care challenge.

A variety of reasons converge to explain some of the differences in accessing care when financial barriers are adjusted. Insufficient numbers of providers willing to see low-income women was a powerful disincentive; however, with more of the Medicaid population being admitted into managed care programs, this barrier may be modified. Transportation problems and availability of clinic hours prohibit many women from seeking care. A lack of cross-cultural communication also presents problems. Desired health outcomes are best achieved when the health care provider has knowledge and understanding about the culture, language, values, priorities, and health beliefs of those in minority groups. Conversely, members of the group should understand the health goals to be achieved and the methods proposed to do so. Language differences can produce profound barriers between women patients and those in the health care system. Even when using a translator, information may be skewed in either direction. It is particularly difficult to use a family member to translate when personal information is being requested because cultural mores and personal biases may interfere with accurate interpretations (see Chapter 2).

Providers must consider culturally based differences that could affect the treatment of diverse groups of women, and the women themselves must share practices and beliefs that could influence their management responses or willingness to comply. For example, women in some cultures value privacy to such an extent that they are reluctant to disrobe and as a result avoid physical examination unless absolutely necessary. Other women rely on their husbands to make major decisions, including those affecting the woman's health. Religious beliefs may dictate a plan of care as with birth control measures or blood transfusions. Some cultural groups prefer folk medicine, homeopathy, or prayer to traditional western medicine, and yet others attempt combinations of some or all practices. Even the perceived effectiveness of medications may be tempered by route of administration or color of the pill. In any event, it is incumbent on health care providers to value and appreciate their own and their patient's various sources of information and beliefs about sickness and health.

Gender Issues

Gender influences provider-patient communication and may influence access to health care in general. The most obvious gender consideration is that between men and women. Researchers have reported significant male-female differences in receipt of major diagnostic and therapeutic interventions, especially with cardiac and kidney problems. Women tend to use primary care services more often than men, and some believe, more effectively. The sex of the provider plays a role because studies have shown that female patients have Pap smears and mammograms more consistently if they are seen by female providers. Also, women providers generally engage in greater positive, partnership-building communication that is vital to facilitating patients' lifestyle changes (Lemcke et al., 1995).

Gender issues also pervade the manner in which scientific knowledge is generated. Although women may respond uniquely to treatment, the scientific research used as a basis for the development of treatment modalities was conducted on men and then applied to women. It was not until 1993, when the National Institutes of Health (NIH) launched the Women's Health Initiative, that scientifically appropriate research was undertaken on selected conditions of concern to women (e.g., cardiovascular disease; cancers, especially breast and colorectal; and osteoporosis). At about the same time, The Food and Drug Administration changed its guidelines to allow potentially fertile women to be included in clinical drug trials. Although future findings may not be directly responsible for producing better access for women, they may indirectly allow for the focus of care to be based on what constitutes optimal health for a woman throughout her entire life span.

Sexual orientation may produce another barrier. Lesbian women have primary erotic attractions and relations with other women. Some lesbians may not disclose their orientation to health care providers because they may be at risk for hostility, inadequate health care, or breach of confidentiality. To offset stereotypes, it is necessary for providers to develop an approach that does not assume that all patients are heterosexual (Roberts & Sorensen, 1995). Primary care of lesbians is not different from caring for any other group of women, and lesbian couples have basic physical and psychologic needs similar to those of any couple. Finding supportive providers to provide quality care may be difficult and, as a result, lesbians may have poor access to care.

| CONDITIONS AND CHARACTERISTICS THAT INCREASE HEALTH RISKS IN THE CHILDBEARING YEARS

Maintaining optimum health is a goal for all women. Essential components of health maintenance are identification of unrecognized problems and potential risks and the education/promotion needed to reduce them. This is especially important for women in their childbearing years because conditions that increase a woman's health risks are of concern not only to her well-being but also are potentially associated with negative outcomes for both mother and baby in the event of a pregnancy. Prenatal care is the prime example of prevention that is practiced after conception. However, prevention and health maintenance are needed before pregnancy because many of the mother's risks can be identified and then eliminated or at least modified. An overview of conditions and circumstances that increase health risks in the childbearing years is presented below.

DEMOGRAPHICS

Age

Adolescents

As a female progresses through developmental ages and stages, she is faced with conditions that are age-related. All teens undergo progressive growth of sexual characteristics and also undertake developmental tasks of adolescence, such as establishing identity, developing sexual preference, emancipating from family, and establishing career goals. Some of these situations can produce great stress for the adolescent, and the health care provider should treat her very carefully. Female teenagers who enter the health care system usually do so for screening (Pap smears start at age 18 or when sexually active), or because of a problem such as episodic illness or accidents. Gynecologic problems are often associated with menses (either bleeding irregularities or dysmenorrhea), vaginitis or leukorrhea, STDs, contraception, or pregnancy.

Teenage pregnancy. Pregnancy in the teenager who is 16 years of age or younger often introduces additional stress on an already stressful developmental period. The emotional level of such teens is commonly characterized by impulsiveness and self-centered behavior, and they often place primary importance on the beliefs and actions of their peers. In attempts to establish a personal and independent identity, many teens do not realize the consequences of their behavior, and planning for the future is not part of their thinking processes.

Unless very young, teens are sufficiently mature to physically support the pregnancy, but they may be non-compliant in many areas of prenatal instruction, especially nutrition and continuing care. Studies have shown that when adolescents maintain access to regular prenatal care, their outcomes are similar to those of adults; conversely, when prenatal care is lacking, there is higher risk for preterm birth, intrauterine growth restriction, and pregnancy-induced hypertension (Lubarsky et al., 1994; Scholl, Hediger & Belsky, 1994). However, other risks are present such as the psychosocial implications of unwed status, high divorce rates of those who do marry, and single parent families; education that is disrupted, delayed or ended; and socioeconomic hardships of women raising children alone without much economic support and with few skills for the job market. Children of teen mothers may be at risk for abuse or neglect because of the teen's inadequate knowledge of growth, development, and parenting. Implementation of specialized adolescent programs in schools, communities, and health care systems are demonstrating continued success in lowering the birth rate in teens as evidenced by an overall 12% decline in teenage pregnancy between 1991 and 1996 (National Center for Health Statistics, 1997).

Young and middle adulthood

Because women ages 20 to 40 have need for contraception, pelvic and breast screening, and pregnancy care, they may prefer to use their gynecologic or obstetric provider as their primary care provider also. During these years, the woman may be "juggling" family, home, and career responsibilities with resulting increases in stress-related conditions. Health maintenance includes not only pelvic and breast screening, but also promotion of a healthy lifestyle, that is, good nutrition, regular exercise, no smoking, moderate alcohol consumption, sufficient rest, stress reduction, and referral for medical conditions and other specific problems. Common conditions in well-woman care include vaginitis, urinary tract infections, menstrual variations, obesity, sexual and relationship issues, and pregnancy.

Late reproductive age

Women of later reproductive age are often experiencing change and reordering personal priorities. Generally, the goals of education, career, marriage, and family have been achieved, and now the woman has increased time and opportunity for new interests and activities. Conversely, divorce rates are high at this age, and children leaving home may produce an "empty nest syndrome," resulting in levels of depression. Chronic diseases also become more apparent. Most problems for the well woman are associated with perimenopause (e.g., bleeding irregularities and vasomotor symptoms). Health maintenance screening continues to be of importance because some conditions such as breast disease or ovarian cancer occur more often during this stage.

Parenthood after age 35. The woman over 35 does not have a different physical response to a pregnancy, per se, but rather has had health status changes as a result of time and the aging process. These changes may be responsible for age-related pregnancy conditions. For example, a woman with type 2 diabetes may not have had expression of her diabetes at age 22 but may have full-blown disease at age 38. Other chronic or debilitating diseases or conditions increase in severity with time and these, in turn, may predispose to increased risks during pregnancy. Of significance to women in this age group is the risk for certain genetic anomalies (e.g., Down Syndrome), and the opportunity for genetic counseling should be available to all (see Chapter 8).

Social/Cultural

Differences exist among people from different socioeconomic levels and ethnic groups with respect to risk for illness and distribution of disease and death. Some diseases are more common among people of selected ethnicity, for example, sickle cell anemia in African-Americans, Tay-Sachs disease in Ashkenazi Jews, adult lactase deficiency in Chinese, beta thalassemia in Mediterranean peoples, and cystic fibrosis in northern Europeans. Cultural and religious influences also increase health risks because the woman and her family may have life and societal values and a view of health and illness that dictate practices different from those expected in the Judeo-Christian Western model. These may include food taboos or frequencies, methods of hygiene, effects of climate, care-seeking behaviors, willingness to undergo screening and diagnostic procedures, and value conflicts. Culturally induced belief in magic can cause illness and death (Murray & Zentner, 1997).

Socioeconomic contrasts result in major health differences as exemplified in birth outcomes. The rates of perinatal and maternal deaths, preterm births, and low-birth-weight babies are considerably higher in disadvantaged populations (National Center for Health Statistics, 1997). Social consequences for poor women as single parents are great because many mothers with few skills are caught in the bind of insufficient income to afford child care. These families generate fewer and fewer resources and increase their risks for health problems. Multiple roles for women in general produce overload, conflict, and stress, resulting in higher risks for psychosocial health care (Cox, 1997).

Health Behaviors

Smoking

Cigarette smoking is a major preventable cause of death and illness. Smoking is linked to cardiovascular heart disease, various types of cancers (especially lung and cervical), chronic lung disease, and negative pregnancy outcomes. Tobacco contains nicotine, which is an addictive substance that creates a physical and a psychologic dependence. Tobacco smoke contains known carcinogens. An average cigarette smoker shortens life by 6 to 8 years.

Between 1990 and 1994 the incidence of smoking among persons 18 years of age and over remained stable at 25.5%. Among adolescents and young adults, more women than men smoke. Smoking in persons over the age of 25 ranges from 12% for college graduates to 38% for those with less than a high school education.

Cigarette smoking impairs fertility in both women and men, may reduce the age for menopause, and increases the risk for osteoporosis after menopause. Passive or second-hand smoke contains similar hazards and presents additional problems for the smoker, as well as harm for the non-smoker.

Smoking in pregnancy is known to cause a decrease in placental perfusion and is the cause of low birth weight in 21% to 39% of all such infants (Creasy & Resnik, 1994). The harmful effects of smoking are numerous because the oxygen-carrying capacity of hemoglobin is decreased when carbon monoxide passes through the placenta. Furthermore, nicotine causes vasoconstriction and decreased uterine

BOX 4-5	*Maternal Complications of Pregnancy Associated with Smoking*

Ectopic pregnancy
Spontaneous abortion
Premature rupture of membranes
Preterm birth
Placenta previa
Abruptio placentae
Chorioamnionitis

perfusion. In addition, smokers generally have a nutrient-poor diet. Finally, smoking interferes with the body's ability to process essential vitamins and minerals, resulting in calcium loss from the bones, a decreased intestinal synthesis of vitamin B12, and increased usage of vitamin C. The woman who smokes during pregnancy is at risk for a variety of complications (Box 4-5).

Substance use and abuse

The inappropriate use of illicit and prescription drugs continues to increase and is found in all ages, races, ethnic groups, and socioeconomic strata. When abused, psychoactive (mind-altering) drugs can disturb relationships, cause psychologic and physical dependency, and create serious health problems. Such substances interfere with the brain's neurotransmitters and normal chemistry, which in turn affects an individual's mood. They particularly affect the part of the brain that produces euphoria, pleasure, or pain release and, as a result, lead easily to abuse. There are four types of mind-altering drugs: sedatives (e.g., sleeping pills, tranquilizers, and street drugs such as red devils, yellow jackets, and downers); narcotics (e.g., codeine, Darvon, Lomotil, morphine, Percodan, and street drugs such as heroin and methadone); stimulants (e.g., caffeine, nicotine, dexedrine, Preludin, Ritalin, and street drugs such as cocaine, bennies, and speed); and hallucinogens (e.g., street drugs such as marijuana, LSD, and PCP). Risk increases with the strength, amount, frequency, and route of administration.

Addiction to substances is seen as a biopsychosocial disease with several factors leading to risk. These include biogenetic predisposition, lack of resilience to stressful life experiences, and poor social support (Jessup, 1997). Women are less likely than men to abuse drugs but the rate in women is increasing significantly. Substance-abusing pregnant women create severe problems for themselves and their offspring, including interference with optimal growth and development and addiction.

Alcohol. Women ages 35 to 49 have the highest rates of chronic alcoholism, but women ages 21 to 34 have the highest rates of specific alcohol-related problems (Jessup, 1997). About one third of alcoholics are women, and many relate onset of their drinking problem to stressful events. Women who are problem drinkers are often depressed, have more motor vehicle injuries, and have a higher incidence of attempted suicide than women in the general population. Also, they are at particular risk for alcohol-related liver damage. Early case finding and early treatment are important in alcoholism for both the ill individual and for family members.

Alcohol abuse during pregnancy is the leading cause of mental retardation in the United States (Lewis & Woods, 1994). In addition, alcohol abuse during pregnancy has been associated with fetal growth restriction, altered facies, and developmental problems. For this reason, abstinence from alcohol consumption during pregnancy is recommended (Cefalo & Moos, 1995).

Illicit Drugs

Cocaine. Cocaine is a powerful central nervous system stimulant that is addictive because of the tremendous sense of pleasure or feeling good that it creates. It can be snorted, smoked, or injected. Crack, or rock, is a form of cocaine that is exceedingly potent and even more highly addictive (some say that an individual is "hooked" after the first use or, at the least, after two or three "hits"). After ingestion of cocaine, an intensely pleasurable high results that is followed by an uncomfortable low, which increases the urge to repeat the drug.

Cocaine affects all of the major body systems. Among other complications, it produces cardiovascular stress that can lead to heart attack or stroke, liver disease, central nervous system stimulation that can cause seizures, and even perforation of the nasal septum. Users are often poorly nourished and commonly have STDs. If the user is pregnant, there is an increased incidence of spontaneous abortion, preterm labor, small-for-dates babies, abruption of placenta, and stillbirth. Anomalies have also been reported (Fox, 1994).

Heroin. Heroin is an opiate that is usually injected but can be smoked or snorted. It produces euphoria, relaxation, relief from pain, and "nodding out" (apathy, detachment from reality, impaired judgment, and drowsiness). Signs and symptoms are constricted pupils, nausea, constipation, slurred speech and respiratory depression (Stuart & Sundeen, 1998). Users are at increased risk for HIV and hepatitis B, C, and D, primarily because of sharing needles that contain contaminated blood. Perinatal effects include interference with fetal growth, premature rupture of membranes, preterm labor, and prematurity. Newborns can be born addicted to heroin and may need to undergo a withdrawal process.

Marijuana. Marijuana is a substance derived from the cannabis plant. It is usually rolled into cigarettes and smoked. But it may also be mixed into food and eaten. It produces an intoxicating and sensory-distorting high. Marijuana smoke has the same characteristics as tobacco smoke and, for this reason, has similar dangers (Cook, Peterson & Moore, 1994). Both readily cross the placenta and have the effect of increasing carbon monoxide levels in the mother's blood, which reduces the oxygen supply to the fetus.

Research findings regarding the effects of marijuana on pregnancy are inconsistent, however. That is, maternal use has not been consistently found to be associated with an increased incidence of spontaneous abortion or stillbirths (Cook, Peterson & Moore, 1994).

Other illicit drugs. A number of other street drugs pose risk to users. A few are derived from organic materials, but more and more are synthetically produced in various laboratories. Variations of stimulants, such as speed, meth, and ice, produce signs and symptoms similar to cocaine, although fewer maternal and fetal complications have been attributed to them. Sedatives such as downers, yellow jackets, or red devils are used to come off of "highs." Hallucinogens alter perception and body function. PCP (angel dust) and LSD produce vivid changes in sensation, often with agitation, euphoria, paranoia, and a tendency toward antisocial behavior. Their use may lead to flashbacks, chronic psychosis, and violent behavior. Hallucinogens taken during pregnancy may have a negative neurobehavioral effect on the newborn.

Prescription drugs

Psychotherapeutic drugs. Stimulants, sleeping pills, tranquilizers, and pain relievers are used by an estimated 2% of American women (Epps & Stewart, 1995). Such drugs can bring relief from undesirable conditions such as insomnia, anxiety, and pain, but because the drugs have mind-altering capacity, misuse can produce psychologic and physical dependency in the same manner as illicit drugs. Risk-to-benefit ratios should be considered when such drugs are used for more than very short periods of time. All of these categories of drugs have some effect on the fetus when taken during pregnancy and should be very carefully monitored.

Stimulants. These drugs increase energy and reduce appetite. In the past, they were occasionally used for weight loss but because of their tendency to create dependence, they are no longer sanctioned for this purpose. They may be prescribed for narcolepsy or attention deficit disorder.

Sleeping pills. Barbiturates and hypnotics are used to relieve insomnia but with long-term use, tolerance develops and larger amounts are needed for the same effect. Larger amounts of the drugs can result in poor concentration, mood swings, anxiety, and depression. Again, dependency occurs. Withdrawal symptoms can include emotional distress, anxiety, headache, gastrointestinal disturbances, and restlessness.

Narcotics. The use of opiate narcotics is of great benefit in many circumstances because they act on the brain and nervous system to decrease sensitivity to pain and produce a sense of well-being. Yet, they are highly addictive over time and can produce severe physical and mental symptoms when withdrawn.

Tranquilizers. Tranquilizers provide short-term relief from anxiety and stress caused by unexpected emotional conflict or trauma. Their effect is similar to that of alcohol; low doses produce relaxation and buoyancy, and higher doses produce intoxication. Tranquilizers are not appropriate for long-term therapy. Withdrawal effects are similar to those of sleeping pills but less severe.

Psychotropic drugs. Depression is the most common mental health problem in women. Everyone has a case of the "blues" periodically, but true depression impairs the ability to live a normal life and involves symptoms of pervasive sadness, isolation, fatigue, changes in eating and sleeping patterns, and general negativity. Severely depressed people are at risk for suicide. Typical drugs used to treat depression are tricyclic antidepressants (e.g., imipramine [Tofranil] and amitriptyline [Elavil], monoamine oxidase (MAO) inhibitors (e.g., phenelzine [Nardil]), selective serotonin reuptake inhibitors (SSRIs) (e.g., fluoxetine [Prozac] or sertraline [Zoloft]), and lithium. Tricyclic antidepressants relieve symptoms of depression without artificial mood enhancement seen with stimulants.

Caffeine. Caffeine is found in society's most popular drinks: coffee, tea, and soft drinks. It is a stimulant that can affect mood and interrupt body functions by producing anxiety and sleep interruptions. Heart arrhythmias may be made worse by caffeine, and there can be interactions with certain medications such as lithium. Birth defects have not been related to caffeine consumption; however, high intake has been related to a slight decrease in birth weight. The U.S. Food and Drug Administration recommends that pregnant women eliminate or limit their consumption of caffeine to less than 300 mg per day (3 cups of coffee or cola).

Nutrition

Essential to good health is good nutrition. A well-balanced diet helps prevent illness and also is used to treat certain health problems. Conversely, poor eating habits, eating disorders, and obesity are linked to disease and discomfort.

Nutritional deficiencies. Overt disease caused by lack of certain nutrients is rarely seen in the United States. However, insufficient amounts or imbalances of nutrients do pose problems for individuals and families. Overweight or underweight status, listlessness, fatigue, frequent colds and other minor infections, constipation, dull hair and nails, and dental caries are examples of problems that could be nutritionally related and indicate the need for further nutritional assessment. Poor nutrition, especially related to obesity and high fat/cholesterol intake, may lead to more serious conditions and is said to contribute to 6 of the 10 leading causes of death in the United States: heart disease, cancer, stroke and hypertension, arteriosclerosis, cirrhosis of the liver, and diabetes (Williams, 1995).

Obesity. Obesity is the accumulation of excess poundage caused by extra body fat. In addition to the risks previously mentioned, obesity is also a factor in other disorders such as gallbladder disease, gout, breathing problems, varicose veins, and osteoarthritis. Extreme obesity contributes to a shortened life span. Obesity is occurring at earlier ages and is disproportionately high among women (Rosenfeld, 1997). Because it is a chronic disease, short-term approaches to weight loss rarely succeed. Management of obesity requires a lifelong commitment to changes in lifestyle, behaviors, and attitudes toward food and eating (Edwards, 1993). Pregnant women who are morbidly obese are at increased risk for hypertension, diabetes, gallbladder disease, postterm pregnancy, and musculoskeletal problems (Lachat, Owen & Ebel, 1995).

Other considerations. Other dietary extremes can also produce risk. For example, insufficient amounts of calcium can lead to osteoporosis, too much sodium contributes to hypertension, and megadoses of vitamins can create adverse effects in several body systems. Fad weight loss programs and yo-yo dieting (repeated weight gain and weight loss) result in nutritional inequality and, in some instances, medical problems. Such diets and programs are not appropriate for weight maintenance. Adolescent pregnancy produces a special nutritional circumstance because the metabolic needs of pregnancy are superimposed on the teen's own needs for growth and maturation and eating habits, which are often less than nutritious.

Eating disorders

Anorexia nervosa. Some women have a distorted view of their bodies and, no matter what their weight, perceive themselves to be much too heavy. As a result, they undertake strict and severe diets and rigorous extreme exercise. This chronic and rarest of eating disorders is known as anorexia nervosa. A coexisting depression usually accompanies anorexia. Women can carry this condition to the point of starvation, with resulting endocrine and metabolic abnormalities. If not corrected, significant complications of arrhythmias, cardiomyopathy, and congestive heart failure occur and, in the extreme, can lead to death. The condition commonly begins during adolescence in young women who have some degree of personality disorder. They gradually lose weight over several months, have amenorrhea, and are abnormally concerned with body image. The condition requires both psychiatric and medical interventions.

Bulimia nervosa. Bulimia refers to secret, uncontrolled binge eating alternating with methods to prevent weight gain: self-induced vomiting, laxatives or diuretics, strict diets, fasting, and rigorous exercise. During a binge episode, large numbers of calories are consumed usually consisting of sweets and "junk foods." Binges occur at least two times per week. Bulimia usually begins in early adulthood (18 to 25) and is found primarily in females. Complications can include dehydration and electrolyte imbalance, gastrointestinal abnormalities, and cardiac arrhythmias. Bulimia is somewhat similar to anorexia in that it is an eating disorder and usually involves some degree of depression. Unlike anorexia, individuals may feel shame or disgust about their disorder and tend to seek help earlier.

Physical fitness and exercise. Exercise contributes to good health by lowering risks for a variety of conditions that are influenced by obesity and a sedentary lifestyle. It is effective in the prevention of cardiovascular disease and in the management of chronic conditions such as hypertension, arthritis, diabetes, respiratory disorders, and osteoporosis. Exercise also contributes to stress reduction and weight maintenance. Women report that engaging in regular exercise improves their body image and self-esteem and acts as a mood enhancer. Aerobic exercise produces cardiovascular involvement because increasing amounts of oxygen are delivered to working muscles. Anaerobic exercise, such as weight training, improves individual muscle mass without stress on the cardiovascular system. Because women are concerned about both cardiovascular and bone health, weight-bearing aerobic exercises such as walking, running, racket sports, and dancing are preferred. Excessive or strenuous exercise can lead to hormonal imbalances, resulting in amenorrhea and its consequences. Physical injury is also a potential risk.

Stress

The modern woman faces increasing levels of stress and as a result is prone to a variety of stress-induced complaints and illness. Stress often occurs because of multiple roles in which coping with job and financial responsibilities conflict with parenting and home. To add to this burden, women are socialized to be caretakers, which is emotionally draining by itself. Also, they find themselves in positions of minimal power that do not allow them to have control over their everyday environments (Epps & Stewart, 1995). Some stress is normal and, in fact, contributes to positive outcomes. Many women thrive in busy surroundings. However, excessive or high levels of on-going stress trigger physical reactions in the body, such as rapid heart rate, elevated blood pressure, slowed digestion, release of additional neurotransmitters and hormones, muscle tenseness, and weakened immune system. Consequently, constant stress can contribute to clinical illnesses such as flareups of arthritis or asthma, frequent colds or infections, gastrointestinal upsets, cardiovascular problems, and infertility. Box 4-6 lists physical symptoms that may be related to chronic or extreme stress. Psychologic signs such as anxiety, irritability, eating disorders, depression, insomnia and substance abuse also have been associated with stress.

Sexual Practices

Potential risks related to sexual activity are undesired pregnancy and STDs. The risks are particularly high for

BOX 4-6	*Physical Symptoms of Stress*
Headache	Nausea, vomiting
Dizziness or feeling faint	Diarrhea
Muscle tension	Constipation
Backache	Loss of appetite
Grinding of teeth	Shortness of breath
Skin rash or hives	Pounding heart
Sweaty palms	Nonradiating chest pain
Indigestion	Frequent colds

Modified from Epps R & Stewart S: *The women's complete healthbook,* New York, 1995, The Philip Lief Group, Inc.

adolescents and young adults who engage in sexual intercourse at earlier and earlier ages. Adolescents report many reasons for wanting to be sexually active, among which are peer pressure, to love and be loved, experimentation, to enhance self-esteem, and to have fun (Murray & Zentner, 1997). However, many teens do not have the decision-making or values-clarification skills needed to take this important step at a young age and are also lacking the knowledge base regarding contraception and STDs. They also do not believe that becoming pregnant or getting an STD will happen to them. Pregnancy raises further issues of continuing the pregnancy versus abortion, adoption versus childrearing, continuing with education and career goals versus quitting school, and accepting jobs that require little skill.

Although some STDs can be cured with antibiotics, many can cause significant problems. Possible sequelae include infertility, ectopic pregnancy, neonatal morbidity and mortality, genital cancers, acquired immunodeficiency syndrome, and even death (Hatcher et al., 1998). Sexually transmitted diseases are increasing rapidly and are in epidemic proportion. Choice of contraception has an impact on the risk of contracting an STD. Natural family planning, hormones, and intrauterine devices offer no protection. Diaphragms offer some cervical protection. Condoms combined with nonoxynol-9 (a spermicide) offer the most protection. No method of contraception offers complete protection.

Medical Conditions

Most women of reproductive age are relatively healthy. However, certain medical conditions present during pregnancy can have deleterious effects on both mother and fetus. Of particular concern are risks from all forms of diabetes, urinary tract disorders, thyroid disease, hypertensive disorders of pregnancy, cardiac disease, and seizure disorders. Effects on the fetus vary and include intrauterine growth restriction, macrosomia, anemia, prematurity, immaturity, and stillbirth. Effects on the mother can also be quite severe. Refer to Chapter 23 for information on specific conditions.

Gynecologic Conditions Affecting Pregnancy

Gynecologic conditions that may contribute negatively to pregnancy include the following:

- *Pelvic inflammatory disease (PID)* can cause stricture or occlusion of uterine (fallopian) tubes, resulting in infertility or ectopic pregnancy.
- *Endometriosis* occurs when endometrial tissue grows outside of the uterus; it responds to hormonal influences and causes scarring and adhesions in the tubes.
- Some *STDs* can be vertically transmitted to the fetus (e.g., HIV, syphilis) or cause damage during the birth process (e.g., *Chlamydia, Neisseria gonorrhoeae,* herpes simplex virus [HSV], or group B streptococci).
- *Fibroids,* benign fibrous growths from the uterine muscle that are under the influence of estrogen, can press on the lining of the uterus causing infertility, or occasionally, impinge on the space needed by the growing fetus or require a cesarean delivery for a pregnancy occurring after surgical removal of the growth.
- *Uterine deformities* (bicornuate uterus) can cause spontaneous abortion, preterm labor, and fetal growth problems.
- *Vaginal infection* caused by *Trichomonas* or *Candida* or bacterial vaginosis can result in uncomfortable vaginal discharge and be confused with normal leukorrhea (*Candida* has a propensity for the glycogen-laden vaginal epithelium found during pregnancy, and reinfections can occur.)
- *Reproductive or breast cancer treatments* (radiation, surgery, and chemotherapy) can cause fetal anomalies, spontaneous abortion, and preterm labor.

Risks for gynecologic cancers

Women are also at risk for gynecologic cancer. Risk factors differ, depending on the type of cancer.

Cervical cancer

Risks for cervical cancer include the following:

- *Early age of first sexual intercourse:* This introduces foreign bodies to young teen's rapidly changing cells at the junction of columnar tissue from the endometrium and squamous tissue from the vagina.
- *Cigarette smoking:* Organic residues from tobacco are preferentially deposited in the cervix.
- *HIV infection:* HIV-positive women have an increased rate of dysplastic cervical cells.
- *Human papillomavirus (HPV) infection:* A few particular strains of HPV, such as types 16, 18, 45, and 56, are associated with cervical cancer.
- *Multiple sexual partners:* This exposes the cervix to many microorganisms.

In the United States, Vietnamese women have the highest rate of cervical cancer, followed by Hispanic women.

Abnormal spotting or vaginal bleeding is the primary symptom (ACS, 1997b).

Endometrial cancer

The most common malignancy of the reproductive system is endometrial cancer. Estrogen-related exposures such as nulliparity, unopposed estrogen therapy, infertility, and early or late menopause are the most significant risk factors. Other risk factors include obesity, hypertension, diabetes, gallbladder disease, and family history of breast or ovarian cancer. Use of birth control pills and pregnancy appears to provide some protection against endometrial cancer. It occurs most frequently in Caucasian women and after menopause. Abnormal uterine bleeding is the cardinal sign (ACS, 1997b).

Ovarian cancer

Ovarian cancer is the most malignant of all gynecologic cancers, accounting for the most deaths from these cancers. Risk factors include family history of ovarian or breast cancer and having no children or having them late in life. Native American women have the highest rates of ovarian cancer in the United States. There are usually no early warning symptoms (ACS, 1997b).

Other gynecologic cancers

Cancer of the vulva, vagina, and uterine tubes accounts for less than 6% of all female reproductive cancers. Cancer of the vulva and vagina have been linked to HPV and HSV. The cause of uterine tube cancer is unknown. These cancers occur most often in postmenopausal women. Lesions are often the first sign of vulvar cancer. Women with vaginal or uterine tube cancer may be asymptomatic or have vaginal bleeding (DiSaia & Creasman, 1997).

Environmental and Workplace Hazards

Environmental hazards in the home, workplace, and community can contribute to poor health at all ages. Categories and examples of health-damaging hazards include: (1) pathogenic agents (viruses, bacteria, fungi, parasites), (2) natural and synthetic chemicals, (natural toxins from animals, insects, and plants; consumer and industrial products such as pesticides and hydrocarbon gases; medical and diagnostic devices; tobacco; fuels; and drug and alcohol abuse), (3) radiation (radon, heatwaves, sound waves), (4) food substances (added components that are not necessary for nutrition), and (5) physical objects (moving vehicles, machinery, weapons, water, building materials) (Pender, 1996).

Environmental hazards can affect fertility, fetal development, live birth, and the child's future mental and physical development. Children are at special risk for poisoning from lead found in paint and soil. Everyone is at risk from air pollutants, such as tobacco smoke, carbon monoxide, smog, suspended particles, (dust, ash, and asbestos), and cleaning solvents; noise pollution; pesticides; chemical additives; and poor preparation of food. Workers also face safety and health risks caused by ergonomically poor work stations and stress. The lists could go on and on. It is important that risk assessments continue to be in effect to identify and understand environmental public health problems.

Violence Against Women

Violence against women is a major health care problem in the United States, affecting 2 to 4 million women each year and costing $44 million annually in medical costs (Bash & Jones, 1994). Forty-two percent of women who are murdered die at the hands of an intimate partner (*Day One,* 1995). Women of all races and of all ethnic, educational, religious, and socioeconomic backgrounds are affected (Gelles, 1993). The magnitude of the problem is far greater than the statistics indicate, since violent crimes against women are the most underreported data because of fear, lack of understanding, and stigma surrounding violent situations.

Maternity and women's health nurses, by the very nature of their practice, are in a unique position to conduct case finding, provide sensitive care to women experiencing abusive situations, engage in prevention activities, and influence health care and public policy toward decreasing the violence.

Battered women

Wife battering, spouse abuse, and *domestic* or *family violence* are all terms applied to a pattern of assaultive and coercive behaviors that includes physical, sexual, and psychologic attacks, as well as economic coercion inflicted by a male partner in a marriage or other heterosexual, significant, intimate relationships. The terms *domestic violence* and *spouse abuse* connote that abuse can occur by either partner against the other and do not address that women are the victims of abuse at a rate much greater than men.

Relationship violence rarely consists of a single episode, but rather is a pattern that may start with intimidation or threats (Fig. 4-1) and progress to more aggressive physical and sexual acts, resulting in injury to the woman. Common elements of battering are economic

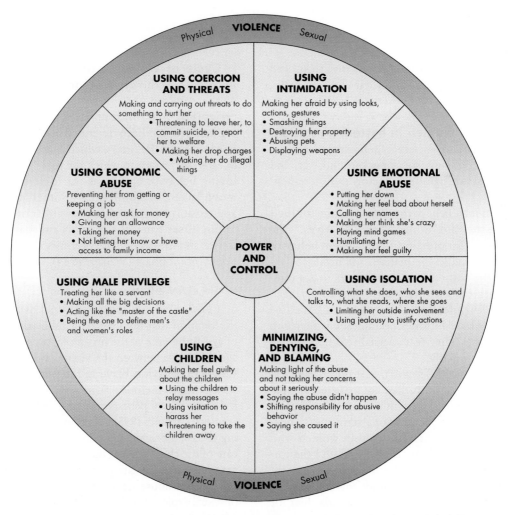

Fig. **4-1** Model of how power and control issues perpetuate battering. (From Duluth Domestic Abuse Intervention Project: *Power and control tactics of men who batter,* Duluth, Minn.)

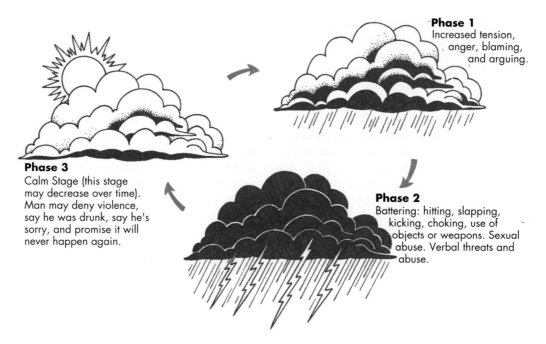

Phase 1
Increased tension, anger, blaming, and arguing.

Phase 3
Calm Stage (this stage may decrease over time). Man may deny violence, say he was drunk, say he's sorry, and promise it will never happen again.

Phase 2
Battering: hitting, slapping, kicking, choking, use of objects or weapons. Sexual abuse. Verbal threats and abuse.

Fig. 4-2 Cycle of violence. (From Helton A: *A protocol of care for the battered woman,* White Plains, NY, 1987, March of Dimes Birth Defects Foundation.)

deprivation, sexual abuse, intimidation, isolation, and stalking and terrorizing victims and their children (Yllo, 1993). Pregnancy is often a time when violence begins or escalates (see Chapter 10).

Characteristics of women in battering relationships. Every segment of society is represented among abused women; race, religion, social background, age, and educational level are not significant factors in differentiating women at risk.

Battered women may believe they are to blame for their situations because they are "not good enough wives." The woman blames herself for bringing on the violent behavior in her relationship because she believes she needs to "try harder" to please the abuser. In many cases there is a traumatic bonding with the man that hinges on loyalty, fear, terror, and learned helplessness. Many women have low self-esteem and may have histories of domestic violence in their families of origin. They fear societal rejection if they discuss their problem openly.

Warren and Lanning (1992) found that strong, traditional feminine characteristics of nurturing, compassion, sympathy, and yielding were more apparent in women in abusive relationships, in contrast to the traits of assertiveness, independence, and willingness to take a stand in women who were in nonviolent relationships. They also found the former group to be more willing to tolerate control from others. Social isolation seems to be another characteristic of battered women, which may result from stigma, fear, or restrictions placed on them by their partners.

Cycle of violence: the dynamics of battering. According to the **cycle of violence** concept, battering is neither random nor constant; rather, it occurs in repeated cycles (Fig. 4-2). A three-phase cyclic pattern to the battering behavior has been described as a period of *increasing tension* leading to the *battery*, which is then followed by a period of *calm and remorse* in which the male partner displays kind, loving behavior and pleas for forgiveness. This "honeymoon" phase lasts until stress or other factors cause conflict and tension to mount again toward another episode of battering. Over time, the tension and battering phases last longer and the calm phase becomes shorter until there is no honeymoon phase (Walker, 1984).

Sexual abuse

Childhood sexual abuse is defined as any type of sexual exploitation that involves (1) a child younger than 18 years of age at the time of the first molestation, (2) at least a 3-year age difference between the victim and perpetrator, and (3) a variety of behaviors between the victim and the perpetrator, which may include disrobing; nudity; masturbation; fondling; digital penetration; and anal, oral, or vaginal penetration (Urbanic, 1993). Childhood sexual abuse acts, according to law, are acts perpetrated by someone responsible for care of the child, such as the parents, boyfriends, stepfathers, grandparents, day-care provider, or baby-sitter. These childhood sexual abuse acts may include incest, which is any type of sexual exploitation between blood relatives or surrogate relatives before the victim reaches 18 years of age. If a stranger commits sexual abuse, it is considered *sexual assault*. Childhood sexual abuse continues over time and gradually escalates. The child is pressured by the adult to cooperate and maintain the relationship. This continuing victimization and accompanying feeling of helplessness, together with lack of confiding, lead to the long-term behavioral and relationship consequences seen in adult survivors of sexual abuse. Hulme and Grove (1994) have identified the following, most prominent long-term symptoms found in some incest survivors:

- *Physical:* insomnia, sexual dysfunction, overeating, drug and alcohol abuse, severe headaches, and two or more major surgeries
- *Psychosocial:* depression, guilt, low self-esteem, inability to trust others, mood swings, suicidal thoughts, difficulty in relationships, confusion, extreme anger, and memory lapse.
- Women may also exhibit feelings of self-blame, shame, body rejection, anxiety, fear, mistrust, and hatred.

Rape

Rape is an act of violence rather than a sexual act. Rape is a legal and not a medical entity and in its strictest sense is the penile penetration of the female sex organ or labia without her consent. *Sexual assault,* a term used interchangeably with rape, is also an act of force and has a much broader definition to include unwanted or uncomfortable touches, kisses, hugs, petting, intercourse, or other sexual acts. States may also use different legal definitions of rape.

Hymenal penetration or ejaculation does not have to occur to qualify as rape. The key feature to establish rape is the absence of consent: threat or coercion implies the lack of consent. The victim who is mentally retarded, who is unconscious or otherwise physically unable to move, who has been drugged without her knowledge, or who is a minor (statutory rape) is not capable of giving consent. The court must prove absence of consent; thus the term *alleged rape* or *alleged sexual assault* is used in medical records.

It is vital that nurses understand the definition of rape because many people (possibly including the victim of rape) believe that the woman "invited" the rape through either seductive dress or seductive behavior (Campbell & Landenburger, 1995). The fact is that no woman deserves to be forced into any sexual behavior.

The types of rape are reported as date or acquaintance rape, marital rape, gang rape, stranger rape, and psychic rape. *Acquaintance rape* involves persons who know one another, such as a classmate, neighbor, family member, or date, and is sexual assault that occurs when the trust of a relationship is violated and one person is forced by another into sexual activity (Stuart & Sundeen, 1998). Victims of date and acquaintance rape are most often between 15 and 19 years of age.

Marital rape occurs partly because men may believe it is their right to engage in sex whenever they desire, regardless of the partner's desire or condition. It commonly occurs whenever there is physical abuse of the woman.

Gang rape occurs when one woman is raped by two or more men. *Stranger rape* is when an unknown attacker actively seeks a woman who is vulnerable. This is the type of rape most feared by women (Aguilera, 1994).

Psychic rape occurs when one's personal dignity and self-respect are assaulted (Stuart & Sundeen, 1998). *Sexual harassment,* although not classified as rape, is another form of using power and control tactics to victimize women sexually, particularly in the workplace. The anticipatory fear of rape in women, the trauma experienced during an attack, and the terror that persists after the attack are all damaging to women's lives.

ANTICIPATORY GUIDANCE FOR HEALTH PROMOTION AND PREVENTION

Over the last several decades, women have made tremendous strides in education, careers, policy making, and overall participation in today's complex society. There have been costs for these advances, and although women are living longer, they may not be living better. As a result, the health care system needs to pay greater attention to the health consequences for women. In addition, women need to be active participants in their own health promotion and illness prevention. Pender (1996) describes **health promotion** as the motivation to increase well-being and actualize health potential. **Prevention** is the desire to avoid illness, detect it early, or maintain optimal functioning when illness is present.

Nurses have a major opportunity and responsibility to help women understand risk factors and to motivate them to adopt healthy lifestyles that prevent disease. Lifestyle factors that affect health over which the woman has some control include diet; tobacco, alcohol, and substance use; exercise; sunlight exposure; stress management; and sexual practices. Other influences, such as genetic and environmental factors, may be beyond the woman's control, although some opportunities for prevention exist (e.g., through environmental legislation activism or genetic counseling services).

Knowledge alone is not enough to bring about healthy behaviors. The woman must be convinced that she has some control over her life and that healthy life habits, including periodic health examinations, are a sound investment. She must believe in the efficacy of prevention, early detection, and therapy and in her ability to perform self-care practices, such as breast self-examination. Many people believe that they have little control over their health, or they become immobilized by fear and anxiety in the face of life-threatening illnesses, such as cancer, so that they delay seeking treatment. The nurse must explore the reality of each woman's perceptions about health behaviors

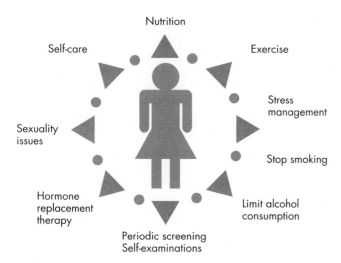

Nutrition

Self-care   Exercise

Stress management

Sexuality issues

Stop smoking

Hormone replacement therapy

Limit alcohol consumption

Periodic screening Self-examinations

Fig. 4-3 Nursing care model for counseling women about self-care. (Courtesy Design Center, University of North Carolina at Chapel Hill School of Nursing, Chapel Hill, NC.)

and individualize teaching if it is to be effective. The model illustrated in Fig. 4-3 incorporates the major aspects to be included when counseling women.

Nutrition

To maintain good nutrition, women should be counseled to include recommended servings from the major food categories of the Food Guide Pyramid (see Fig. 11-6). Complex carbohydrates should make up 45% to 60% of daily intake, including grains, breads, fruits, and vegetables. Moderate amounts of proteins, sugars, and salt should be ingested, and diets should be low in total fat (no more than 30% of total calories), saturated fat (no more than 10%), and cholesterol (up to 300 mg per day). Recommended servings from the food groups also provide for adequate vitamins, minerals, iron, and fiber. Fluid intake is not included in the Food Guide Pyramid, but individuals should be encouraged to drink at least four to six glasses of water every day in addition to other fluids such as juices. Coffee, tea, soft drinks, and alcoholic beverages should be used in moderation.

The technique of basic nutrition counseling does not differ significantly between pregnant and nonpregnant women. The diet can be assessed using a standard assessment form—a 24-hour recall is adequate and quick—and then food likes and dislikes, including cultural variations and typical food portions and dietary habits, should be discussed and incorporated into counseling. The woman should be actively involved in evaluating her intake with the nurse, using a standard food group guide, and should suggest modifications in the diet where needed. Many women have a fair knowledge of food groups and their importance for various nutrients; with guidance they can critique their own intake and suggest changes to improve nutrition. Cultural background and age have a major influence

on eating behaviors. A nonjudgmental approach is important, since many women, especially if they are obese or know they are not eating as they should, are sensitive about diet. Unless the motivation to change food habits is intrinsic, efforts to change the diet will fail. If the nurse is supportive, this approach can increase the woman's self-esteem and reinforce good practices while motivating change where needed.

The nurse can provide information about the risks associated with high fat intake and ways to reduce dietary fat intake. Although many people are aware of the association between high fat and cholesterol and disease, they may be ignorant of the major sources of saturated fat and need help in changing eating patterns established during childhood. Because there are more than twice as many calories in fat as there are in protein and carbohydrate, gram for gram, weight control can be facilitated by encouraging women to choose foods relatively low in fat and calories. Fiber-rich foods can be substituted for foods high in fat; they delay digestion and absorption and increase the feeling of satiety.

Most women do not recognize the importance of calcium to health, and their diets are insufficient in calcium. If an adequate bone mass is not achieved at skeletal maturity (usually by about age 20), the woman is at increased risk of developing osteoporosis in later life. Osteoporosis is a disabling, life-threatening disease of epidemic proportions in the United States. The ideal daily calcium intake is unknown, but it is agreed that most women, especially adolescents, should increase their intake. Women under age 50 need 1,000 mg of calcium per day and postmenopausal women over age 50 need 1,500 mg. Pregnant and lactating women also need 1,500 mg.

Women who are unlikely to get enough calcium in the diet may need calcium supplements in the form of calcium carbonate, which contains more elemental calcium than other preparations.

Long-standing dietary habits are difficult to modify, but given the potential health benefits and positive influence a woman can have on the nutrition of other family members, she may respond to the nurse's encouragement and reinforcement of her good intentions. Chances of success may be enhanced if she becomes involved in a support group or enlists significant others in goal setting.

Exercise

Physical activity/exercise counseling for persons of all ages should be undertaken at schools, worksites, and primary care settings. It is characterized as integrating short bouts of exercise into daily living (Pender, 1996). Specific recommendations include 20 to 30 minutes of moderate activity at least three times per week. Unfortunately, few Americans exercise this often, and physical inactivity increases with age, especially during adolescence and early adulthood.

Nurses are respected care providers who can influence patients to become more active and help them to develop

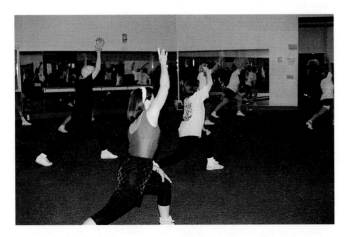

Fig. 4-4 Weight-bearing exercise may delay bone loss and increase bone mass. (Courtesy Jonas McCoy, Raleigh, NC.)

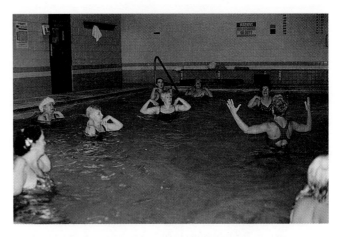

Fig. 4-5 Water aerobics improves cardiovascular function. (Courtesy Jonas McCoy, Raleigh, NC.)

an exercise program geared to their age and personal fitness and goals. Even small increases in activity can be beneficial. The nurse should stress the importance of daily exercise throughout life for weight management and health promotion, suggesting exercises that are enjoyable to the individual. (Fig. 4-4).

Walking, as part of the daily routine, if more vigorous activities cannot be performed, is feasible for most women. Swimming is good for cardiorespiratory fitness but will not prevent osteoporosis, since it is not a weight-bearing exercise (Fig. 4-5). Many women who are sedentary during leisure time can profit from gradually increasing their physical activity. They may be encouraged to exercise with their children or in groups. Worksite fitness programs or community-based programs are increasing. Young women can be involved in physical education activities, games and group sports, and more active pursuits. Home maintenance, yard work, and gardening are other activities that promote health and a sense of well-being, especially for older adults. Attention to safety factors and clothing and shoes appropriate to each activity are advised. Care should be taken not to aggravate existing conditions or create muscle and joint discomfort by an overly aggressive approach to exercise.

During pregnancy, an on-going exercise regimen can be continued but should be decreased in intensity and duration. Sedentary women should obtain medical clearance to initiate exercise during pregnancy and should begin with low-intensity and low-impact workouts.

Kegel exercises

Kegel exercises, or pelvic muscle exercises, were developed to strengthen the supportive pelvic floor muscles to control or reduce incontinent urine loss. These exercises are also beneficial during pregnancy and postpartum. They strengthen the muscles of the pelvic floor, providing support for the pelvic organs and control of the muscles surrounding the vagina and urethra.

The Association of Women's Health, Obstetric, and Neonatal Nurses is conducting a research utilization project focused on continence for women (Sampselle et al., 1997). Educational strategies for teaching women how to perform Kegel exercises that were compiled by nurse researchers involved in the project are described in the Teaching Guidelines box.

Stress Management

Because it is neither possible nor desirable to avoid all stress, women need to learn how to manage stress. The nurse should assess each woman for signs of stress, using therapeutic communication skills to determine risk factors and the woman's ability to function.

Some women must be referred for counseling or other mental health therapy. Women are twice as likely as men to suffer from depression, anxiety, or panic attacks (Japenga, 1998). Nurses need to be alert to the symptoms of serious mental disorders, such as depression and anxiety, and make referrals to mental health practitioners when necessary. Women experiencing major life changes, such as divorce and separation, bereavement, serious illness, and unemployment, also need special attention.

For many women the nurse is able to provide comfort, reassurance, and advice concerning helping resources, such as support groups. Many centers offer support groups to help women prevent or manage stress. The nurse can help them become more aware of the relationship between good nutrition, rest, relaxation and exercise/diversion and their ability to deal with stress. In the case of role overload, determining what needs immediate attention and what can wait are important. Practical advice includes regular breaks, taking time for friends, developing interests outside of work or the home, setting realistic goals, and learning self-acceptance. Discussing how women can maintain meaningful relationships is very important. Social support and good coping skills can improve a woman's self-esteem and give

TEACHING GUIDELINES

Kegel Exercises

DESCRIPTION AND RATIONALE

Kegel exercise, or pelvic muscle exercise, is a technique used to strengthen the muscles that support the pelvic floor. This exercise involves regularly tightening (contracting) and relaxing the muscles that support the bladder and urethra. By strengthening these pelvic muscles, a woman can prevent or reduce accidental urine loss.

TECHNIQUE

The woman needs to learn how to target the muscles for training and how to contract them correctly. One suggestion for teaching is to have the woman pretend she is trying to prevent the passage of intestinal gas. Have her use this tightening motion on the muscles around her vagina and the upper pelvis. She should feel these muscles drawing inward and upward. Other suggested techniques are to have the woman pretend she is trying to stop the flow of urine in midstream or to have her think about how her vagina is able to contract around and move up the length of the penis during intercourse.

The woman should avoid straining or bearing-down motions while performing the exercise. She should be taught how bearing down feels by having her take a breath, hold it, and push down with her abdominal muscles as though she were trying to have a bowel movement. Then the woman can be taught how to avoid straining down by exhaling gently and keeping her mouth open each time she contracts her pelvic muscles.

SPECIFIC INSTRUCTIONS

1. Each contraction should be as intense as possible without contracting the abdomen, thighs, or buttocks.
2. Contractions should be held for at least 10 seconds. The woman may have to start with as little as 2 seconds per contraction until her muscles get stronger.
3. The woman should rest for 10 seconds or more between contractions so that the muscles have time to recover and each contraction can be as strong as the woman can make it.
4. The woman should feel the pulling up and over the three muscle layers so that the contraction reaches the highest level of her pelvis.

OTHER SUGGESTIONS FOR IMPLEMENTATION

1. At first the woman should set aside about 15 minutes a day to do the Kegel exercises.
2. The woman may want to put up reminders, such as notes on her bathroom mirror, her refrigerator, her TV, or on a calendar, to do the exercises.
3. Guidelines for practicing Kegel exercises suggest performing between 30 and 80 contractions a day; however, positive results can be achieved with only 30 a day.
4. The best position for learning how to do Kegel exercises is to lie supine with the knees bent. Another position to use is on the hands and knees. Once the woman learns the proper technique, she can perform the exercises in other positions such as standing or sitting.

From Breeding D: You don't have to live with incontinence, *Female Patient* 53:29, 1996; Sampselle C & Miller J: Pelvic muscle exercise: effective patient teaching, *Female Patient* 21:29, 1996; Sampselle C et al.: Continence in women: evidence-based practice, *J Obstet Gynecol Neonatal Nurs* 26(4):375, 1997.

her a sense of mastery. Anticipatory guidance for developmental or expected situational crises can help her plan strategies for dealing with potentially stressful events.

There is a great deal of literature on stress management interventions. Role-playing, relaxation techniques, biofeedback, meditation, desensitization, imagery, assertiveness training, yoga, diet, exercise, and weight control are techniques nurses can include in their repertoire of helping skills. Insufficient time prevents one-on-one assistance in many situations, but the more nurses know about these resources, the better able they are to intervene, counsel, and direct women to appropriate resources. Careful follow-up of all women experiencing difficulty in dealing with stress is important.

Substance Use

All women at all ages will receive substantial and immediate benefits from smoking cessation. However, this is not easy and most people stop several times before they accomplish their goal. Many are never able to do so.

New approaches to increase cessation among smokers and to discourage smoking among young women—especially in adolescence and during pregnancy—are needed. Health care providers can have an impact on smoking behavior and should attempt to motivate smokers to stop. Raising questions about social consequences—stained teeth, foul-smelling breath and clothes—is sometimes effective with young people.

Those who wish to stop smoking can be referred to a smoking cessation program where individualized methods can be implemented. At the very least, individuals should be guided to self-help materials available from The March of Dimes Birth Defects Foundation, American Lung Association, and the American Cancer Society. During pregnancy, women seem to be highly motivated to stop or at least to limit smoking to 10 or fewer cigarettes a day. Insult to the fetus can be reduced or even avoided if this is done by the end of the first trimester.

Alcohol and other drugs exact a staggering toll on society, not only in terms of personal health, but also in their association with poverty and homelessness, family disorganization, violence, crime, motor vehicle injuries, reduced productivity, and economic costs. The abuse of alcohol and other drugs increases the risk of victimization and date rape and of acquiring HIV through shared needles or sexual contact. Alcohol use and drug use are the leading preventable causes of birth defects.

A national awareness of the seriousness of problems associated with substance abuse has led to raising the legal drinking age to 21 in all states and tighter controls on advertising. Stronger regulation of advertising and tougher laws and law enforcement for alcohol- and drug-related offenses are being implemented. There is still much that must be done to increase the accessibility to care for low-income people, minorities, and young people. Women have special needs that must be addressed, especially mothers of young children and pregnant women.

All primary care providers should screen for alcohol and other drug use problems, with an understanding of the obvious problems in relying on self-reporting of these behaviors. The use of over-the-counter drugs by women should also be explored. Counseling women who appear to be drinking excessively or using drugs may include strategies to increase self-esteem and teaching new coping skills to resist and maintain resistance to alcohol abuse and drug use. Appropriate referrals should be made, with the health care provider arranging the contact and then following up to be sure that appointments are kept. General referral to sources of support should also be provided. National groups that provide information and support for those who are chemically dependent are listed in Box 4-7. Many of these organizations have local branches or contacts that are listed in the telephone book.

Anticipatory guidance includes teaching about the health and safety risks of alcohol and mind-altering substances and discouraging drug experimentation among preteen and high school students, since the use of drugs at an early age tends to predict greater involvement later.

Safer Sexual Practices

Prevention of STDs is predicated on the reduction of high-risk behaviors by educating toward a behavioral change. Behaviors of concern include multiple and casual sexual partners and unsafe sexual practices. Specific self-care measures for "safer sex" can be reviewed in Box 4-8. The abuse of alcohol and drugs is also a high risk behavior resulting in impaired judgment and thoughtless acts.

Behavioral changes must come from within, and therefore the nurse must provide sufficient information for the individual or group to "buy into" the need for change. Education for STDs includes the following: (1) verbal desensitizing (e.g., talking about sex and sexual practices); (2) offering specific information (e.g., the signs and symptoms of diseases and their complications and specifically how to

---

BOX 4-7	National Groups Providing Information and/or Support for Chemical Dependency

Alcoholics Anonymous (for individuals who are alcohol
  dependent) 212-686-1100*
  Al-Anon (for families of alcoholics)
  Al-Ateen (for teenage children of alcoholics)
COCAINE Hotline 1-800-COCAINE
National Alcohol and Drug Abuse Hotline
  1-800-252-6465
Narcotics Anonymous (for drug abusers)
  1-888-336-4066*

*Also check your telephone book for local listing.

BOX 4-8	"Safer" Sex

"Safer" sex is possible only if there is no oral, genital,
  or rectal exchange of body fluids.
Correct use of condoms, although greatly reducing risk,
  is not exclusively protective.
Use of spermicides containing nonoxynol-9 may offer
  additional protection.
Select sexual partners with extreme care.
Ask partner about history of STDs.

---

prevent disease); (3) endorsing use of condoms (although not 100% effective, condoms are our best form of protection and should be used each and every time unless abstinence or mutual monogamy is ensured); (4) providing behavioral scripts (e.g., suggest ways to discuss sexual situations before they actually occur); (5) providing referrals for screening (even in the absence of symptoms), additional information, or treatment.

In addition to the prevention of STDs, women of childbearing years need information and behavioral considerations regarding contraception and family planning (see Chapter 7). Education is a powerful tool in health promotion and prevention of sexually associated diseases or pregnancy. However, it works best when delivered in the language or parlance of the intended listener and takes into account the culture and lifestyle of the individual or group to whom it is intended.

Health Screening Schedule

Periodic health screening includes history, physical examination, education, counseling, and selected diagnostic and laboratory tests. This regimen provides the basis for overall health promotion, prevention of illness, early diagnosis of problems, and referral for appropriate management. Such screening should be customized according to a woman's age and risk factors. In most instances, it is completed in health care offices, clinics, or hospitals; however, portions of the screening are now being carried out at events such as

Community Health Fairs. An overview of health screening recommendations for women over 18 years of age is found in Table 4-1. Consistent with information provided earlier in this chapter, it is important for the nurse to continually educate and counsel on diet, exercise, cessation of smoking, alcohol moderation, help for drug abuse, and stress management.

Health Risk Prevention

Often, simple safety factors are forgotten or perceived not to be important; yet injuries continue to have major impact on health status of all ages. Being aware of hazards and implementing safety guidelines will reduce risks. The nurse should frequently reinforce the following common sense concepts that will protect the individual:

- Wear seat belts at all times in a moving vehicle.
- Wear safety helmets when riding a motorcycle or bicycle.
- Follow driving "rules of the road."
- Place smoke alarms throughout the home and workplace.

TABLE 4-1   *Health Screening Recommendations for Women 18+ Years of Age*

INTERVENTION	RECOMMENDATION*
PHYSICAL EXAMINATION	
Blood pressure	Every visit, but at least every 2 years
Height and weight	
Pelvic examination	
Breast examination	
Self-examination	Initiated/taught at time of first pelvic examination; done monthly at end of menses.
Clinical breast examination[†]	Every 1 to 3 years starting at age 30; annually over age 40
High risk	Annually over 18 with history of premenopausal breast cancer in first-degree relative
Risk groups	At least annually:
Skin examination	Family history of skin cancer or increased exposure to sunlight
Oral cavity examination	Mouth lesion or exposure to tobacco or excessive alcohol
LABORATORY/DIAGNOSTIC TESTS	
Blood cholesterol[†]	Every 5 years
High Risk	More often per clinical judgment with potential for cardiac or lipid abnormalities
Papanicolaou smear[†]	Initially at age 18 or when sexually active; after three normal consecutive annual examinations, Pap can be per risk, but at least every 3 years
Mammography[‡]	Annually over age 50[†]
	Annually over age 40[§],
	Every 1 to 2 years, ages 40 to 49 and annually thereafter[‖]
Risk groups	
Fasting blood sugar	Annually with family history of diabetes, gestational diabetes, or significantly obese
Hearing	Annually with exposure to excessive noise
STD screen	As needed with multiple sexual partners
Tuberculin skin test	Annually with exposure to persons with TB or in risk categories for close contact with the disease
IMMUNIZATIONS	
Tetanus-diphtheria	Booster is given every 10 years after primary series
Measles, mumps, rubella	Once if born after 1956 and no evidence of immunity
Hepatitis B	Primary series of three for all who are in risk categories
Influenza	Annually after age 65 or in risk categories, such as chronic diseases, immunosuppression, renal dysfunction

From the United States Preventive Services Task Force, 1996.
*Unless otherwise noted, the recommended intervention should be performed routinely every 1 to 3 years.
†U.S. Preventive Service Task Force, 1996.
‡Note: There is no consensus regarding mammograms for women between 40 and 49, thus various recommendations are listed. Women are urged to discuss circumstances with their health care provider.
§American College of Obstetricians and Gynecologists, 1997.
‖American Cancer Society, 1997a.(See pp. 62-63 for full citations.)

- Avoid second-hand smoke.
- Reduce noise pollution or safeguard against hearing loss.
- Protect skin from ultraviolet light via sunscreen and clothing.
- Handle and store firearms appropriately.
- Practice water safety.

Taking necessary precautions and avoiding dangerous situations are imperative.

Health Protection

Nurses can make a difference in stopping the violence and preventing further injury. Educating women that abuse is a violation of their rights and facilitating their access to protective and legal services constitute a first step. Other helpful measures for women to discourage their fall into abusive relationships are promoting assertiveness and self-defense courses; suggesting support and self-help groups that encourage positive self-regard, confidence, and empowerment; and recommending educational and skills development classes that will enhance independence or at least the ability to take care of oneself (Hadley et al., 1995).

Numerous national and local organizations provide information and assistance for women experiencing abusive situations. Nurses and victims may find these resources helpful. Box 4-9 lists national resources and hotlines. All nurses who work in women's health care should become familiar with local services and legal options.

BOX 4-9   *Resources for Violence Against Women*

Center for Women Policy Studies
2000 P St. NW, Suite 580
Washington, DC 20036
(202) 872-1770
(Publications and current federal legislation information)

National Child Abuse Hotline
(800) 422-4453

National Coalition Against Domestic Violence
PO Box 34103
Washington, DC 20043-4301
(202) 638-8638
Hotline (800) 333-SAFE (7223)
(Many states have local coalition against domestic violence.)

National Coalition Against Sexual Assault
912 North 2nd St.
Harrisburg, PA 17102
(717) 232-6771

National Organization for Women (NOW)
Legal Defense and Education Fund
99 Hudson St.
New York, NY 10013-2871
(212) 925-6635

The National Center on Women and Family Law
799 Broadway, Room 402
New York, NY 10003
(212) 674-8200
(Legal Information)

RESEARCH

Women's Sense of Well-Being Before and After Hysterectomy

Hysterectomy is among the most frequently performed surgeries in the United States. Most research in the area of hysterectomies has focused on the medical necessity of this procedure. Few studies have looked at the broader implications of hysterectomy for women. Specifically, few studies have examined how symptoms that lead to the surgery affect the various domains of women's lives and whether the impact is positive or negative. The purpose of this prospective, descriptive study was to describe women's perceived sense of well-being before and after hysterectomy by examining a broad array of outcomes experienced by women undergoing the surgery for benign conditions. A total of 178 women needing hysterectomies for nononcologic reasons were chosen from a regional tertiary care facility. Sense of well-being was measured by women's responses on three measurements on the SF-36 Health Survey and a questionnaire assessing information pertinent to current gynecologic health at three times during the study: before surgery, 4 months after surgery, and 11 months after surgery. The women also completed the Zung Self-Rating Depression Scale preoperatively and at 4 months postoperatively. In the initial period after surgery, the patients experienced an improved health status. In addition, the women reported an improvement in their psychologic well-being, including less depression and improved sexual functioning. Outcomes for these women undergoing hysterectomy for nononcologic reasons were generally positive.

CLINICAL APPLICATION OF THE STUDY

The findings from this study can be valuable in counseling women considering or awaiting hysterectomy. Myths continue regarding body changes after hysterectomy related to the women's loss of femininity and sense of personal value. These myths can be challenged with current research findings.

Source: Lambden M et al.: Women's sense of well-being before and after hysterectomy, *J Obstet Gynecol Neonatal Nurs* 26(5):540, 1997.

KEY POINTS

- Culture, religion, socioeconomic status, personal circumstances, the uniqueness of the individual, and stage of development are among the factors that influence a person's recognition of need for care and response to the health care system and therapy.
- The changing status and roles of women affect their health, needs, and ability to cope with problems.
- Assessment is more comprehensive and learning is best in a safe environment in which the atmosphere is nonjudgmental and sensitive, and the interaction is strictly confidential.
- Every woman is entitled to be respected and fully involved in the assessment and educational processes.
- Preconception counseling allows identification and possible remediation of potentially harmful personal and social conditions, medical and psychologic conditions, environmental conditions, and barriers to care before the advent of pregnancy.
- Conditions that increase a woman's health risks also increase risks for her offspring.
- Periodic health screening, including history, physical examination, and diagnostic and laboratory tests, provides the basis for overall health promotion, prevention of illness, early diagnosis of problems, and referral for management.
- Health promotion and prevention assist women to actualize health potential by increasing motivation, providing information, and suggesting how to access specific resources.

CRITICAL THINKING EXERCISES

1 *Interview at least two women of different cultures.*
  a *Ask them about their beliefs in relation to seeking health care.*
  b *Identify reasons for differences and how these would influence planning to teach about preventive health care and health promotion.*
2 *Prepare a consultation plan for a 32-year-old, never-married, nulliparous woman needing general anticipatory guidance for health promotion and prevention.*
  a *Ascertain her view regarding her health risk status.*

CRITICAL THINKING EXERCISES—cont'd

  b *Obtain overview information about need for counseling regarding nutrition, exercise, stress management, and safer sexual practices.*
  c *Suggest recommendations for screening, based on information obtained.*
3 *Identify and visit resources in your community appropriate for referring the following women. Then evaluate the resource in terms of access, costs, and follow-up service.*
  a *one who wants to stop smoking*
  b *one who is battered by her husband*
  c *one who is requesting a mammogram*
  d *one whose mother is an alcoholic.*
4 *Interview a woman to determine her risk for cervical cancer.*
  a *What are her perceptions about cervical cancer?*
  b *Ask her about her age of first sexual intercourse and her experience with multiple partners.*
  c *Ask about the sexual history of her partner(s)*
  d *Determine her cigarette smoking history.*
  e *Formulate a plan of care.*
5 *Interview nursing and other students regarding knowledge of screening methods for cancer.*
  a *Analyze your findings to determine the degree of awareness among nonnursing students and nursing students.*
  b *Examine reasons for the differences and similarities.*
  c *Propose an educational strategy to increase awareness of resources for cancer detection and prevention.*

References

Aguilera D: *Crisis intervention: theory and methodology,* ed 7, St Louis, 1994, Mosby.

Allen K & Phillips J: *Women's health across the lifespan: a contemporary perspective,* Philadelphia, 1997, Lippincott.

American Cancer Society: Breast cancer ACS checkup guidelines, announcement posted on World Wide Web, retrieved September 3, 1997a, from http://www.cancer.org/guide/quickchec.html

American Cancer Society: *Cancer facts and figures 1997,* New York, 1997b, American Cancer Society.

American College of Obstetricians and Gynecologists: *Committee opinion: routine cancer screening,* Washington, DC, 1997, ACOG.

Bartman B: Women's access to appropriate providers within managed care: implications for the quality of primary care, *Women's Health Issues* 6(1):45, 1996.

Bash K & Jones F: Domestic violence in America, *NC Med J* 455(9):400, 1994.

Breeding D: You don't have to live with incontinence, *Female Patient* 53:29, 1996.

Campbell J & Landenburger K: Violence against women. In Fogel C & Woods N, editors: *Women's health care,* Thousand Oaks, Calif, 1995, Sage.

Cefalo R & Moos M: *Preconceptional health care,* St Louis, 1995, Mosby.

Cook P, Peterson R & Moore D: *Alcohol, tobacco, and other drugs may harm the unborn,* Rockville, Md, 1994, US DHHS.

Cox R: Family health care delivery for 21st century, *J Obstet Gynecol Neonatal Nurs* 26(1):109, 1997.

Creasy R & Resnick R: *Maternal fetal medicine: principles and practice,* ed 3, Philadelphia, 1994, Saunders.

Day One, *ABC News Magazine* June 22, 1995.

DiSaia P & Creasman W: *Clinical gynecologic oncology,* ed 5, St Louis, 1997, Mosby.

Edwards K: Obesity, anorexia, and bulimia (review), *Med Clin North Am* 77(4):899, 1993.

Epps R & Stewart S: *The women's complete healthbook,* New York, 1995, The Philip Lief Group, Inc.

Ernst E: Health care reform as an ongoing process, *J Obstet Gynecol Neonatal Nurs* 23(2):129, 1994.

Fahey L & Sinclair B: *Nurse practitioner, certified nurse midwife, physician assistant protocols,* ed 2, Pasadena, 1996, Kaiser Permanente.

Failure of health care reform (special section), *J Health Politics, Policy and Law* 20(2):271, 1995.

Fox C: Cocaine use in pregnancy, *J Am Board Fam Pract* 7(3):225, 1994.

Frede D: Preconceptional education, *AWHONN Clin Issues Perinat Women Health Nurs* 4(1):60, 1993.

Gelles R: Through a sociological lens: social structure and family violence. In Gelles R & Loseke D, editors: *Current controversies on family violence,* Newbury Park, Calif, 1993, Sage.

Hadley S et al.: Womankind: an innovative model of health care response to domestic abuse, *Women's Health Issues* 5(4):189, 1995.

Hastings K: Health care reform: we need it, but do we have the national will to shape our future? *Nurse Pract* 20(1):52, 1995.

Hatcher R et al.: *Contraceptive technology,* ed 17, New York, 1998, Irvington Publishers, Inc.

Helton A: *A protocol of care for the battered woman,* White Plains, NY, 1987, March of Dimes Birth Defects Foundation.

Horton J: *The women's health data book,* ed 2, New York, 1995, Elsevier.

Hulme P & Grove S: Symptoms of female survivors of child sexual abuse, *Issues Ment Health Nurs* 15(5):519, 1994.

Japenga A: Depression: are men hiding? *USA Weekend* Jan 2 1998, p 20.

Jessup M: Addiction in women: Prevalence, profiles, and meaning, *J Obstet Gynecol Neonatal Nurs* 26(4):449, 1997.

Lachat M, Owen J & Ebel M: Caring for the morbidly obese pregnant woman, *MCN Am J Matern Child Nurs* 20(2): 101, 1995.

Lemcke D et al.: *Primary care of women,* East Norwalk, Conn, 1995, Appleton & Lange.

Lewis D & Woods S: Fetal alcohol syndrome, *Am Fam Physician* 50(5):1025, 1994.

Lubarsky S et al.: Obstetric characteristics among nulliparas under age 15, *Obstet Gynecol* 84(3):365, 1994.

Moos M: *Preconceptional health promotion,* White Plains, NY, 1994, March of Dimes Birth Defects Foundation.

Murray R & Zentner J: *Health assessment promotion strategies through the life span,* ed 6, Stamford, Conn, 1997, Appleton & Lange.

National Center for Health Statistics: *Health, United States, 1996-1997,* Atlanta, 1997, Centers for Disease Control and Prevention.

Pender N: *Health promotion in nursing practice,* ed 3, Stamford, Conn, 1996, Appleton & Lange.

Roberts S & Sorensen L: Lesbian health care: A review and recommendations for health promotion in primary care settings, *J Obstet Gynecol Neonatal Nurs* 20(6):42, 1995.

Rosenfeld J, editor: *Women's health in primary care,* Baltimore, 1997, Williams & Wilkins.

Sampselle C & Miller J: Pelvic muscle exercise: effective patient teaching, *Female Patient* 21:29, 1996.

Sampselle C et al.: Continence for women: evidence-based practice, *J Obstet Gynecol Neonatal Nurs* 26(4):375, 1997.

Scholl T, Hediger M & Belsky D: Prenatal care and maternal health during adolescent pregnancy: a review and meta-analysis, *J Adolesc Health* 15(6):444, 1994.

Sinclair B: Advanced practice nurses in integrated health care systems, *J Obstet Gynecol Neonatal Nurs* 26(2):217, 1997.

Stuart G & Sundeen S: *Principles and practices of psychiatric nursing,* ed 6, St Louis, 1998, Mosby.

United States Preventive Services Task Force: *Guide to clinical preventive services,* ed 2, Baltimore, 1996, Williams & Wilkins.

Urbanic J: Intrafamilial sexual abuse. In Campbell J & Humphreys J, editors: *Nursing care of survivors of family violence,* St Louis, 1993, Mosby.

Walker L: *The battered woman syndrome,* vol 6, New York, 1984, Springer.

Warren J & Lanning W: Sex role beliefs, control, and social isolation of battered women, *J Fam Violence* 7(1):1, 1992.

Williams S: *Nutrition and diet therapy,* ed 10, St Louis, 1995, Mosby.

Yllo K: Through a feminist lens: gender, power, and violence. In Gelles R & Loseke D, editors: *Current controversies on family violence,* Newbury Park, Calif, 1993, Sage.

CHAPTER

5

Health Assessment

JAN LAMARCHE ZDANUK

LEARNING OBJECTIVES

- Define the key terms.
- Identify the structures and functions of the female reproductive system.
- Summarize the menstrual cycle in relation to hormonal, ovarian, and endometrial response.
- Identify the four phases of the sexual response cycle.
- Compare natural and acquired immunity.
- Discuss the effects of age, lifestyle, environment and nutrition on the immune system.
- Identify cultural and communication variations that may affect a woman's decision to seek and follow through with health care.
- Discuss how assessment and physical examination can be adapted for women with special needs.
- List strategies for teaching safety and injury prevention during routine health examinations.
- Identify indications of abuse, appropriate screening, and referral to community agencies.
- Define components of taking a woman's history and performing a physical examination.
- Identify the correct procedure for assisting with and collecting Pap smear specimens.

KEY TERMS

acquired or adaptive immunity
active immunity
breast self-examination (BSE)
climacteric
endometrial cycle
hypothalamic-pituitary cycle
immunocompetent
immunology
menarche
menopause
menstruation

KEY TERMS—cont'd

natural immunity
ovarian cycle
ovulation
Papanicolaou (Pap) smear
passive immunity
perineum
prostaglandins (PGs)
puberty
sexual response cycle
vaccination
vulvar self-examination (VSE)

The purpose of this chapter is to review female anatomy and physiology, the menstrual cycle, immunology, and gynecologic health assessment. Knowledge of the anatomy and physiology of female structures involved in reproduction is necessary in order to assess, plan, implement, and evaluate nursing care of women. Each structure has a vital role in expression of human sexuality, generating and maintaining secondary sexual characteristics, and in reproduction. The breasts, genitals, and pelvis develop the unique adaptations necessary for childbearing through hormonal influences and organ maturation. The female reproductive system consists of the following four principal components:

1. External genitals
2. Primary sex glands
3. Ducts leading from the gonads to the body's exterior
4. Secondary sex glands

FEMALE REPRODUCTIVE SYSTEM

The female reproductive system consists of external structures visible from the pubis to the perineum and internal structures located in the pelvic cavity. The external and internal female reproductive structures develop and mature in response to estrogen and progesterone starting in fetal life and continuing through puberty and the childbearing years. Reproductive structures atrophy with age or in response to a decrease in ovarian hormone production. A complex nerve and blood supply supports the functions of these structures. The appearance of the external genitals varies greatly among women. Heredity, age, race, and the number of children a woman has borne determine the size, shape, and color of her external organs.

External Structures

The external genital organs, or *vulva,* include all structures visible externally from the pubis to the perineum: the mons pubis, labia majora, labia minora, clitoris, vestibular glands, vaginal vestibule, vaginal orifice, and urethral opening. The external genital organs are illustrated in Fig. 5-1. The *mons pubis* is a fatty pad that lies over the anterior surface of the symphysis pubis. In the postpubertal female, the mons is covered with coarse curly hair. The *labia majora* are two rounded folds of fatty tissue covered with skin that extend downward and backward from the mons pubis. The labia are highly vascular structures that develop hair on the outer surfaces after puberty. They protect the inner vulvar structures. The *labia minora* are two flat, reddish folds of tissue visible when the labia majora are separated. No hair follicles are in the labia minora, but many sebaceous follicles and a few sweat glands are present. The interior of the labia minora is composed of connective tissue and smooth muscle, which are supplied with nerve endings that are extremely sensitive. Anteriorly, the labia minora fuse to form the *prepuce* (hoodlike covering of the clitoris) and the *frenulum* (fold of tissue under the clitoris). The labia minora join to form a thin flat tissue called the *fourchette* underneath the vaginal opening at midline. The *clitoris* is located underneath the prepuce. It is a small structure composed of erectile tissue with numerous sensory nerve endings. During sexual arousal the clitoris increases in size.

The vaginal *vestibule* is an almond-shaped area enclosed by the labia minora that contains openings to the urethra, Skene's glands, vagina, and Bartholin glands. The urethra is not a reproductive organ but is considered here because of its location. It usually is found about 2.5 cm below the clitoris. The Skene's glands are located on each side of the urethra and produce mucus, which aids in lubrication of the vagina. The vaginal opening is in the lower portion of the vestibule and varies in shape and size. The hymen, a connective tissue membrane, surrounds the vaginal opening. It can be perforated during strenuous exercise, insertion of tampons, masturbation, and vaginal intercourse. Bartholin glands (see Fig. 5-1) lie under the constrictor muscles of the vagina and are located posteriorly on the sides of the vaginal opening, although the ductal openings are usually not visible. During sexual arousal the glands secrete a clear mucus to lubricate the vaginal introitus.

The area between the fourchette and the anus is the **perineum,** a skin-covered muscular area that covers the pelvic structures. The perineum forms the base of the perineal body, a wedged-shaped mass that serves as an anchor for the muscles, fascia, and ligaments of the pelvis. The pelvic organs are supported by muscles and ligaments that form a sling.

Internal Structures

The internal structures include the vagina, uterus, uterine tubes, and ovaries.

The *vagina* is a fibromuscular, collapsible tubular structure that extends from the vulva to the uterus and lies between the bladder and rectum. During the reproductive years the mucosal lining is arranged in transverse folds called *rugae.* These rugae allow the vagina to expand during childbirth. Estrogen deprivation that occurs after childbirth, during lactation, and at menopause causes dryness and thinness of the vaginal walls and the rugae to become smooth. The vagina, particularly the lower segment, has few sensory nerve endings. Vaginal secretions are slightly acidic (pH 4 to 5) so that the vagina's susceptibility to infections is reduced. The vagina serves as a passageway for menstrual flow, a female organ of copulation, and as a part of the birth canal for vaginal childbirth. The uterine cervix projects into a blind vault at the upper end of the vagina. There are anterior, posterior, and lateral pockets called *fornices* that surround the cervix. The internal pelvic organs can be palpated through the thin walls of these fornices.

Fig. **5-1** External female genitals.

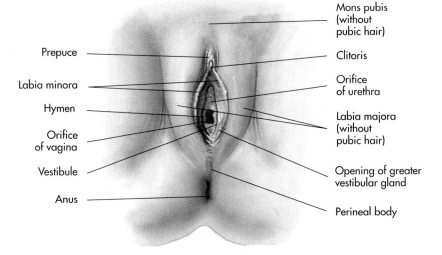

Prepuce

Labia minora

Hymen

Orifice of vagina

Vestibule

Anus

Mons pubis (without pubic hair)

Clitoris

Orifice of urethra

Labia majora (without pubic hair)

Opening of greater vestibular gland

Perineal body

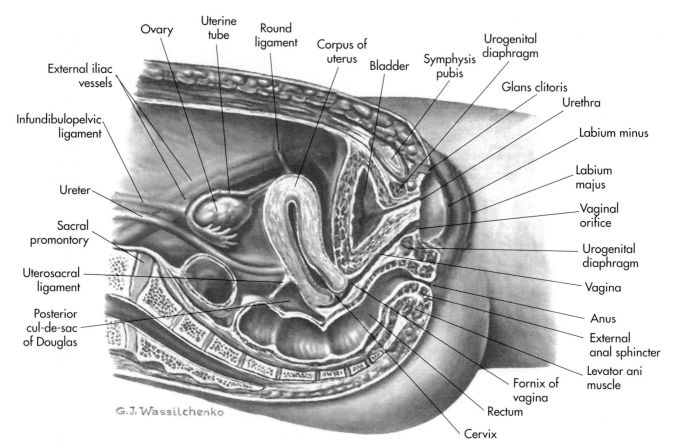

Fig. 5-2 Midsagittal view of female pelvic organs, with woman lying supine.

The *uterus* is a muscular organ shaped like an upside-down pear that sits midline in the pelvic cavity between the bladder and rectum above the vagina. Four pairs of ligaments support the uterus: the cardinal, uterosacral, round, and broad. Single anterior and posterior ligaments also support the uterus. The cul-de-sac of Douglas is a deep pouch, or recess, posterior to the cervix formed by the posterior ligament.

The uterus is divided into two major parts, an upper triangular portion called the corpus and a lower cylindrical portion called the cervix (Fig. 5-2). The fundus is the dome-shaped top of the uterus and is the site the uterine tubes enter the uterus. The isthmus (lower uterine segment) is a short, constricted portion that separates the corpus from the cervix.

The uterus serves for reception, implantation, retention, and nutrition of the fertilized ovum and later the fetus during pregnancy and expulsion of the fetus during childbirth. It also is responsible for cyclic menstruation.

The uterine wall comprises three layers: the endometrium, the myometrium, and part of the peritoneum. The *endometrium* is a highly vascular lining made up of three layers, the outer two of which are shed during menstruation. The *myometrium* is made up of layers of smooth muscles that extend in three different directions (longitudinal, transverse, and oblique) (Fig. 5-3). Longitudinal fibers of the outer myometrial layer are found mostly in the fundus, and this arrangement assists in expelling the fetus during the birth process. The middle layer contains fibers from all three directions, which form a figure-eight pattern encircling large blood vessels. This arrangement assists in ligating blood vessels after childbirth and controls blood loss. Most of the circular fibers of the inner myometrial layer are around the site where the uterine tubes enter the uterus and around the internal cervical os (opening). These fibers help to keep the cervix closed during pregnancy and prevent menstrual blood from flowing back into the uterine tubes during menstruation.

The *cervix* is made up of mostly fibrous connective tissues and elastic tissue, making it possible for the cervix to stretch during vaginal childbirth. The opening between the uterine cavity and the canal that connects the uterine cavity to the vagina (endocervical canal) is the internal os. The narrowed opening between the endocervix and the vagina is the external os, a small circular opening in women who have never been pregnant. The cervix feels firm (like the end of a nose) with a dimple in the center, which marks the external os.

Fig. **5-3** Schematic arrangement of directions of muscle fibers. Note that uterine muscle fibers are continuous with supportive ligaments of uterus.

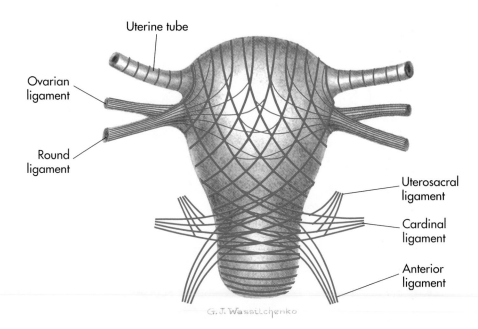

The outer cervix is covered with a layer of squamous epithelium. The mucosa of the cervical canal is covered with columnar epithelium and contains numerous glands that secrete mucus in response to ovarian hormones. The *squamocolumnar junction,* where the two types of cells meet, is usually located just inside the cervical os. This junction is the most common site for neoplastic changes, and cells from this site are scraped for the Papanicolaou test (see p. 86).

The *uterine tubes* (fallopian tubes) attach to the uterine fundus. The tubes are supported by the broad ligaments and range from 8 to 14 cm in length. The tubes are divided into four sections: the interstitial portion is closest to the uterus; the isthmus and the ampulla are the middle portions; and the infundibulum is closest to the ovary. The uterine tubes provide a passage between the ovaries and the uterus for the passage of the ovum. The infundibulum has fimbriated ends, which pull the ovum into the tube. The ovum is pulled along the tubes to the uterus by rhythmic contractions of the muscles of the tubes and by the current that is produced by the movement of the cilia that line the tubes. The ovum is usually fertilized by the sperm in the ampulla portion of one of the tubes.

The *ovaries* are almond-shaped organs located on each side of the uterus below and behind the uterine tubes. During the reproductive years, they are approximately 3 cm long, 2 cm wide, and 1 cm thick; they diminish in size after menopause. Before menarche, each ovary has a smooth surface; after menarche they become nodular because of repeated ruptures of follicles at ovulation. The two functions of the ovaries are ovulation and hormone production. **Ovulation** is the release of a mature ovum from the ovary at intervals (usually monthly). Estrogen, progesterone, and androgen are the hormones produced by the ovaries.

The Bony Pelvis

The bony pelvis serves three primary purposes: protection of the pelvic structures; accommodation of the growing fetus during pregnancy; and anchorage of the pelvic support structures. Two innominate (hip) bones (consisting of ilium, ischium, and pubis), the sacrum, and the coccyx make up the four bones of the pelvis (Fig. 5-4). Cartilage and ligaments form the symphysis pubis, sacrococcygeal, and two sacroiliac joints that separate the pelvic bones. The pelvis is divided into two parts: the false pelvis and the true pelvis (Fig. 5-5). The false pelvis is the upper portion above the pelvic brim or inlet. The true pelvis is the lower curved bony canal, which includes the inlet, the cavity, and the outlet through which the fetus passes during vaginal birth. The upper portion of the outlet is at the level of the ischial spines and the lower portion is at the level of the ischial tuberosities and the pubic arch (see Fig. 5-4). Variations that occur in the size and shape of the pelvis are usually due to age and race. Pelvic ossification is complete at about 20 years of age.

Breasts

The breasts are paired mammary glands located between the second and sixth ribs (Fig. 5-6). About two thirds of the breast overlies the pectoralis major muscle, between the sternum and midaxillary line, with an extension to the axilla referred to as the tail of Spence. The lower one third of the breast overlies the serratus anterior muscle. The breasts are attached to the muscles by connective tissue or fascia.

The breasts of healthy mature women are approximately equal in size and shape, but are often not absolutely symmetric. The size and shape vary depending on the woman's age, heredity, and nutrition. However, the contour should be smooth with no retractions, dimpling, or masses.

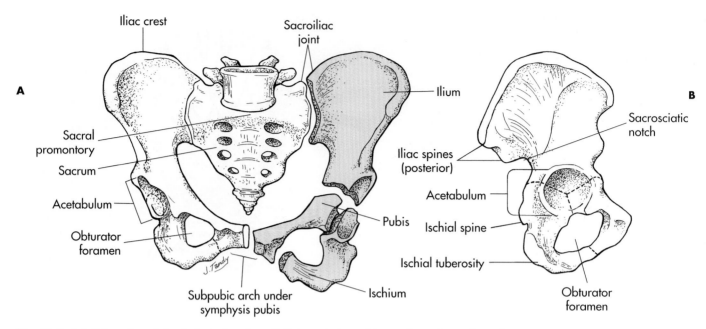

Fig. **5-4** Adult female pelvis. **A,** Anterior view. **B,** External view of innominate bone (fused).

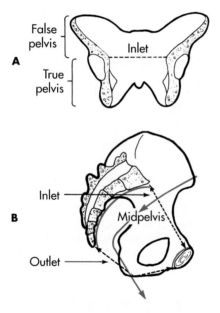

Fig. **5-5** Female pelvis. **A,** Cavity of false pelvis is shallow. **B,** Cavity of true pelvis is an irregularly curved canal *(arrows).*

Estrogen stimulates growth of the breast by inducing fat deposition in the breasts, development of stromal tissue (i.e., increase in its amount and elasticity), and growth of the extensive ductile system. Estrogen also increases the vascularity of breast tissue.

Once ovulation begins in puberty, progesterone levels increase. The increase in progesterone causes maturation of

mammary gland tissue, specifically the lobules and acinar structures. During adolescence, fat deposition and growth of fibrous tissue contribute to the increase in the gland's size. Full development of the breasts is not achieved until after the end of the first pregnancy or in the early period of lactation.

Each mammary gland is made of 15 to 20 lobes, which are divided into lobules. Lobules are clusters of acini. An acinus is a saclike terminal part of a compound gland emptying through a narrow lumen or duct. In discussions of mammary glands, the correct anatomic term (*acinus*) is often used interchangeably with *alveolus*. The acini are lined with epithelial cells that secrete colostrum and milk. Just below the epithelium is the myoepithelium (*myo,* or muscle), which contracts to expel milk from the acini.

The ducts from the clusters of acini that form the lobules merge to form larger ducts draining the lobes. Ducts from the lobes converge in a single nipple (mammary papilla) surrounded by an areola. Just as the ducts converge, they dilate to form common lactiferous sinuses, which are also called ampullae. The lactiferous sinuses serve as milk reservoirs. Many tiny lactiferous ducts drain the ampullae and exit in the nipple.

The glandular structures and ducts are surrounded by protective fatty tissue and are separated and supported by fibrous suspensory *Cooper's ligaments.* Cooper's ligaments provide support to the mammary glands while permitting their mobility on the chest wall (see Fig. 5-6). The round nipple is usually slightly elevated above the breast. On each breast the nipple projects slightly upward and laterally. It contains 15 to 20 openings from lactiferous ducts.

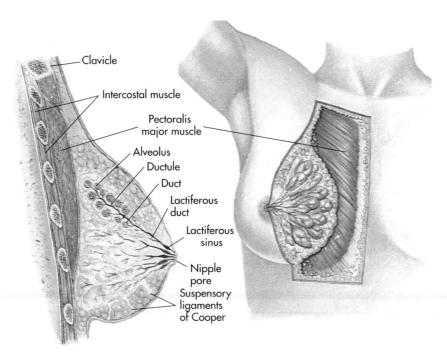

Fig. 5-6 Anatomy of the breast, showing position and major structures. (From Seidel H et al.: *Mosby's guide to physical examination*, ed 4, St Louis, 1998, Mosby.)

The nipple is surrounded by fibromuscular tissue and covered by wrinkled skin. Except during pregnancy and lactation, there is usually no discharge from the nipple.

The nipple and surrounding areola are usually more deeply pigmented than the skin of the breast. The rough appearance of the areola is caused by sebaceous glands, *Montgomery tubercles* (see Fig. 5-6), directly beneath the skin. These glands secrete a fatty substance, thought to lubricate the nipple. Smooth muscle fibers in the areola contract to stiffen the nipple to make it easier for the breastfeeding infant to grasp.

The vascular supply to the mammary gland is abundant. In the nonpregnant state the skin does not have an obvious vascular pattern. The normal skin is smooth without tightness or shininess. The skin covering the breasts contains an extensive superficial lymphatic network that serves the entire chest wall and is continuous with the superficial lymphatics of the neck and abdomen. In the deeper portions of the breasts, the lymphatics form a rich network as well. The primary deep lymphatic pathway drains laterally toward the axillae.

Besides their function of lactation, breasts function as organs for sexual arousal in the mature adult.

The breasts change in size and nodularity in response to cyclic ovarian changes throughout reproductive life. Increasing levels of both estrogen and progesterone in the 3 to 4 days before menstruation increase vascularity of the breasts, induce growth of the ducts and acini, and promote water retention. The epithelial cells lining the ducts proliferate in number, the ducts dilate, and the lobules distend. The acini become enlarged and secretory, and lipid (fat) is deposited within their epithelial cell lining. As a result, breast swelling, tenderness, and discomfort are common symptoms just before the onset of menstruation. After menstruation, cellular proliferation begins to regress, acini begin to decrease in size, and retained water is lost. After breasts have undergone changes numerous times in response to the ovarian cycle, the proliferation and involution (regression) are not uniform throughout the breast. In time, after repeated hormonal stimulation, small persistent areas of nodulations may develop. This normal physiologic change must be remembered when breast tissue is examined. Nodules may develop just before and during menstruation, when the breast is most active. The physiologic alterations in breast size and activity reach their minimum level about 5 to 7 days after menstruation stops. Therefore **breast self-examination (BSE)** (systematic palpation of breasts to detect signs of breast cancer or other changes) is best carried out during this phase of the menstrual cycle (see Home Care box). Table 5-1 compares the variations in physical assessment related to age differences in women.

MENSTRUATION

Knowledge of menstruation is important for nurses providing care to women across the life span. Nurses should be

HOME CARE *Patient Instructions for Self-Care*
Breast Self-Examination

1. The best time to do breast self-examination is after your period, when breasts are not tender or swollen. If you do not have regular periods or sometimes skip a month, do it on the same day every month.
2. Lie down and put a pillow under your right shoulder. Place your right arm behind your head (Fig. 1).
3. Use the finger pads of your three middle fingers on your left hand to feel for lumps or thickening. Your finger pads are the top third of each finger.
4. Press firmly enough to know how your breast feels. If you're not sure how hard to press, ask your health care provider, or try to copy the way your health care provider uses the finger pads during a breast examination. Learn what your breast feels like most of the time. A firm ridge in the lower curve of each breast is normal.
5. Move around the breast in a set way. You can choose either circles (Fig. 2, *A*), vertical lines (Fig. 2, *B*), or wedges (Fig. 2, *C*). Do it the same way every time. It will help you to make sure that you've gone over the entire breast area and to remember how your breast feels.
6. Gently compress the nipple between your thumb and forefinger and look for discharge.
7. Now examine your left breast using the finger pads of your right hand.
8. If you find any changes, see your health care provider right away.

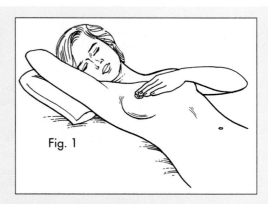
Fig. 1

9. You may want to check your breasts while standing in front of a mirror right after you do your breast self-examination each month. See if there are any changes in the way your breasts look: dimpling of the skin, changes in the nipple, or redness or swelling.
10. You may also want to do an extra breast self-examination while you're in the shower (Fig. 3). Your soapy hands will glide over the wet skin, making it easy to check how your breasts feel.
11. It is important to check the area between the breast and the underarm and the underarm itself. Also examine the area above the breast to the collarbone and to the shoulder.

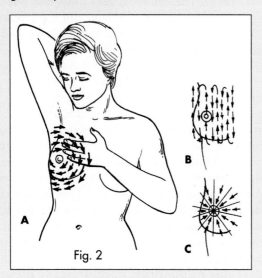
Fig. 2

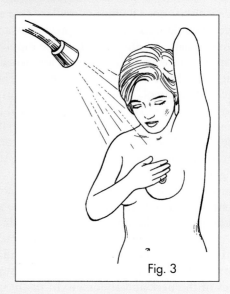
Fig. 3

knowledgeable about menarche, the endometrial cycle, the hypothalamic-pituitary cycle, the ovarian cycle, other cyclic changes, and the climacteric.

Menarche and Puberty
Although young girls secrete small, rather constant amounts of estrogen, a marked increase occurs between 8 and 11 years of age. The term **menarche** denotes first menstruation. **Puberty** is a broader term that denotes the entire transitional stage between childhood and sexual maturity. Increasing amounts and variations in gonadotropin and estrogen secretion develop into a cyclic pattern at least a year before menarche. In North America this occurs in most girls at about 13 years of age.

TABLE 5-1	*Female Reproductive Physical Assessment Across the Life Cycle*		
	ADOLESCENT	**ADULT**	**POSTMENOPAUSAL**
Breasts	Tender when developing; buds appear; small, firm, one side may grow faster; areola diameter increases; nipples more erect	Grow to full shape in early adulthood; nipples and areolae become pinker and darker	Become stringy, irregular, pendulous and nodular; borders less well delineated; may shrink, become flatter, elongated, and less elastic; ligaments weaken; nipples are positioned lower
Vagina	Vagina lengthens; epithelial layers thicken; secretions become acidic	Growth complete by age 20	Introitus constricts; vagina narrows, shortens, loses rugation; mucosa is pale, thin, and dry; walls may lose structural integrity
Uterus	Musculature and vasculature increase; lining thickens	Growth complete by age 20	Size decreases; endometrial lining thins
Ovaries	Increase in size and weight; menarche occurs between 8 to16 years of age; ovulation occurs monthly	Growth complete by age 20	Size decreases to 1 to 2 cm; follicles disappear; surface convolutes; ovarian function ceases between 40 and 55 years of age
Labia majora	Become more prominent; hair develops	Growth complete by age 20	Labia become smaller and flatter; pubic hair sparse and gray
Labia minora	Become more vascular	Growth complete by age 20	Become shinier and dryer
Uterine tubes	Increase in size	Growth complete by age 20	Decrease in size

Initially, periods are irregular, unpredictable, painless, and anovulatory. After 1 or more years, a hypothalamic-pituitary rhythm develops, and the ovary produces adequate cyclic estrogen to make a mature ova. Ovulatory periods tend to be regular, monitored by progesterone.

Although pregnancy can occur in exceptional cases of true precocious puberty, most pregnancies in young girls occur after the normally timed menarche. *All girls would benefit from knowing pregnancy can occur at any time after the onset of menses.*

Menstrual Cycle

Menstruation is the periodic uterine bleeding that begins approximately 14 days after ovulation. It is controlled by a feedback system of three cycles: endometrial, hypothalamic-pituitary, and ovarian. The average length of a menstrual cycle is 28 days, but variations are normal. The first day of bleeding is designated as day 1 of the menstrual cycle or *menses* (Fig. 5-7). The average duration of menstrual flow is 5 days (range of 3 to 6 days), and the average blood loss is 50 ml (range of 20 to 80 ml), but these vary greatly.

For about 50% of women, menstrual blood does not appear to clot. The menstrual blood clots within the uterus, but the clot usually liquefies before being discharged from the uterus. Uterine discharge includes mucus and epithelial cells in addition to blood.

The menstrual cycle is a complex interplay of events that occur simultaneously in the endometrium, hypothalamus and pituitary glands, and ovaries. The menstrual cycle prepares the uterus for pregnancy. When pregnancy does not occur, menstruation follows. The woman's age, physical and emotional status, and environment influence the regularity of her menstrual cycles.

Endometrial cycle

The four phases of the **endometrial cycle** are (1) the menstrual phase, (2) the proliferative phase, (3) the secretory phase, and (4) the ischemic phase (see Fig. 5-7). During the *menstrual phase,* shedding of the functional two thirds of the endometrium (the compact and spongy layers) is initiated by periodic vasoconstriction in the upper layers of the endometrium. The basal layer is always retained, and regeneration begins near the end of the cycle from cells derived from the remaining glandular remnants or stromal cells in the basalis.

The *proliferative phase* is a period of rapid growth lasting from about the fifth day to the time of ovulation. The endometrial surface is completely restored in approximately 4 days, or slightly before bleeding ceases. From this point on an eightfold to tenfold thickening occurs with a leveling off of growth at ovulation. The proliferative phase depends on estrogen stimulation derived from ovarian follicles.

The *secretory phase* extends from the day of ovulation to about 3 days before the next menstrual period. After ovulation, larger amounts of progesterone are produced. An edematous, vascular, functional endometrium is now apparent.

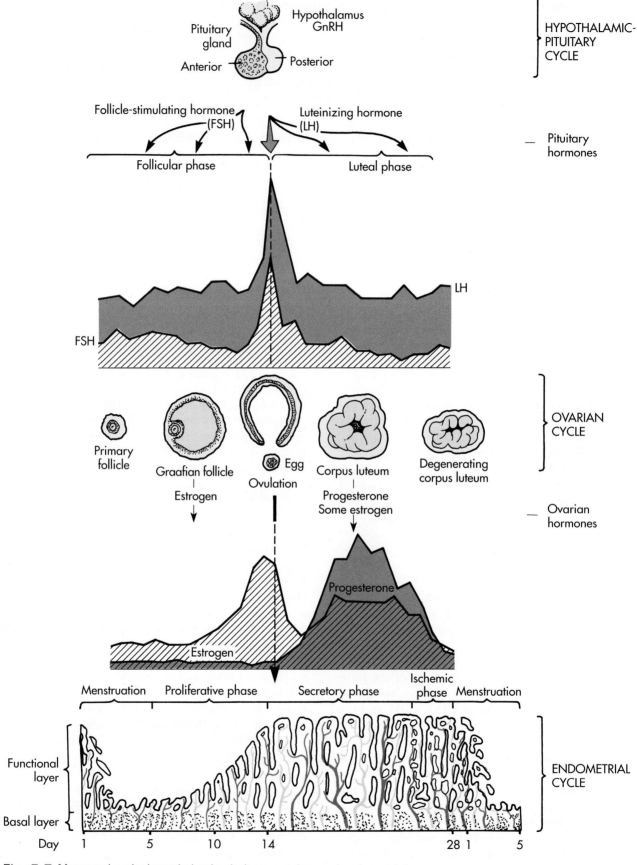

Fig. **5-7** Menstrual cycle: hypothalamic-pituitary, ovarian, and endometrial.

At the end of the secretory phase the fully matured secretory endometrium reaches the thickness of heavy, soft velvet. It becomes luxuriant with blood and glandular secretions, a suitable protective and nutritive bed for a fertilized ovum.

Implantation of the fertilized ovum generally occurs about 7 to 10 days after ovulation. If fertilization and implantation do not occur, the corpus luteum, which secretes estrogen and progesterone, regresses. With the rapid fall in progesterone and estrogen levels, the spiral arteries go into a spasm. During the *ischemic phase,* the blood supply to the functional endometrium is blocked and necrosis develops. The functional layer separates from the basal layer, and menstrual bleeding begins, marking day 1 of the next cycle (see Fig. 5-7).

Hypothalamic-pituitary cycle

Toward the end of the normal menstrual cycle, blood levels of estrogen and progesterone fall. Low blood levels of these ovarian hormones stimulate the hypothalamus to secrete gonadotropin-releasing hormone (Gn-RH). In turn, Gn-RH stimulates anterior pituitary secretion of follicle stimulating hormone (FSH). FSH stimulates development of ovarian graafian follicles and their production of estrogen. Estrogen levels begin to fall, and hypothalamic Gn-RH triggers the anterior pituitary release of luteinizing hormone (LH). A marked surge of LH and a smaller peak of estrogen (day 12; see Fig. 5-7) precede the expulsion of the ovum from the graafian follicle by about 24 to 36 hours. LH peaks about the thirteenth or fourteenth day of a 28-day cycle. If fertilization and implantation of the ovum have not occurred by this time, regression of the corpus luteum follows. Levels of progesterone and estrogen decline, menstruation occurs, and the hypothalamus is once again stimulated to secrete Gn-RH. This process is called the **hypothalamic-pituitary cycle.**

Ovarian cycle

The primitive graafian follicles contain immature oocytes (primordial ova). Before ovulation, from 1 to 30 follicles begin to mature in each ovary under the influence of FSH and estrogen. The preovulatory surge of LH affects a selected follicle. The oocyte matures, ovulation occurs, and the empty follicle begins its transformation into the corpus luteum. This *follicular phase* (preovulatory phase) (see Fig. 5-7) of the **ovarian cycle** varies in length from woman to woman. *Almost all variations in ovarian cycle length are the result of variations in the length of the follicular phase.* On rare occasions (i.e., 1 in 100 menstrual cycles), more than one follicle is selected, and more than one oocyte matures and undergoes ovulation.

After ovulation, estrogen levels drop. For 90% of women, only a small amount of *withdrawal bleeding* occurs so that it goes unnoticed. In 10% of women, there is sufficient bleeding for it to be visible, resulting in what is known as *midcycle bleeding.*

The *luteal phase* begins immediately after ovulation and ends with the start of menstruation. This postovulatory phase of the ovarian cycle usually requires *14* days (range of 13 to 15 days). The corpus luteum reaches its peak of functional activity 8 days after ovulation, secreting both of the steroids estrogen and progesterone. Coincident with this time of peak luteal functioning, the fertilized ovum is implanted in the endometrium. If no implantation occurs, the corpus luteum regresses, and steroid levels drop. Two weeks after ovulation, if fertilization and implantation do not occur, the functional layer of the uterine endometrium is shed through menstruation.

Other cyclic changes

When the hypothalamic-pituitary-ovarian axis functions properly, other tissues undergo predictable responses. Before ovulation the woman's basal body temperature (BBT) is often below 37° C; after ovulation, with rising progesterone levels, her BBT rises. Changes in the cervix and cervical mucus follow a generally predictable pattern. Preovulatory and postovulatory mucus is viscous (thick) so that sperm penetration is discouraged. At the time of ovulation, cervical mucus is thin and clear. It looks, feels, and stretches like egg white. This stretchable quality is termed *spinnbarkheit.* Some women experience localized lower abdominal pain called *mittelschmerz* that coincides with ovulation.

Prostaglandins

Prostaglandins (PGs) are oxygenated fatty acids classified as hormones. The different kinds of PGs are distinguished by letters (PGE, PGF), numbers (PGE_2), and letters of the Greek alphabet ($PGF_{2\alpha}$).

PGs are produced in most organs of the body, but most notably by the endometrium. Menstrual blood is a potent prostaglandin source. PGs are metabolized quickly by most tissues. They are biologically active in minute amounts in the cardiovascular, gastrointestinal, respiratory, urogenital, and nervous systems. They also exert a marked effect on metabolism, particularly on glycolysis. Prostaglandins play an important role in many physiologic, pathologic, and pharmacologic reactions. $PGF_{2\alpha}$, PGE_4, and PGE_2 are most commonly used in reproductive medicine.

Prostaglandins affect smooth muscle contractility and modulation of hormonal activity. Indirect evidence supports PGs' effects on: ovulation, fertility, changes in the cervix and cervical mucus that affect receptivity to sperm, tubal and uterine motility, sloughing of endometrium (menstruation), onset of abortion (spontaneous and induced), and onset of labor (term and preterm).

After exerting their biologic actions, newly synthesized PGs are rapidly metabolized by tissues in such organs as the lungs, kidneys, and liver.

PGs may play a key role in ovulation. If PG levels do not rise along with the surge of LH, the ovum remains trapped within the graafian follicle. After ovulation, PGs may influence production of estrogen and progesterone by the corpus luteum.

The introduction of PGs into the vagina or into the uterine cavity (from ejaculated semen) increases the motility of uterine musculature, which may assist the transport of sperm through the uterus and into the oviduct.

PGs produced by the woman cause regression of the corpus luteum, regression of the endometrium, and sloughing of the endometrium, resulting in menstruation. PGs increase myometrial response to oxytocic stimulation, enhance uterine contractions, and cause cervical dilatation. They may be one factor in the initiation or maintenance of labor, or both. They may also be involved in the following pathologic states: dysmenorrhea, hypertensive states, preeclampsia-eclampsia, and anaphylactic shock.

Climacteric

The *climacteric* is a transitional phase during which ovarian function and hormone production decline. This phase spans the years from the onset of premenopausal ovarian decline to the postmenopausal time when symptoms stop. **Menopause** (from the Latin *mensis*, month, and Greek *pausis*, to cease) refers only to the last menstrual period. Unlike menarche, however, menopause can be dated only with certainty 1 year after menstruation ceases. The average age at natural menopause is 51.4 years, with an age range of 35 to 60 years.

Sexual Response

The hypothalamus and anterior pituitary gland in females regulate the production of FSH and LH. The target tissue for these hormones is the ovary, which produces ova and secretes estrogen and progesterone. A *feedback mechanism* between hormone secretion from the ovaries, hypothalamus, and anterior pituitary aids in the control of the production of sex cells and steroid sex hormone secretion.

Physiologic response to sexual stimulation

Although the first outward appearance of maturing sexual development occurs at an earlier age in females, both females and males achieve physical maturity at approximately 17 years of age. However, individual development varies greatly. Anatomic and reproductive differences notwithstanding, women and men are more alike than different in their physiologic response to sexual excitement and orgasm. For example, the glans clitoris and the glans penis are embryonic homologues. Not only is there little difference between female and male sexual response, but the physical response is essentially the same whether stimulated by coitus, fantasy, or masturbation. Physiologically, according to Masters (1992), sexual response can be analyzed in terms of two processes: vasocongestion and myotonia.

Sexual stimulation results in circumvaginal blood vessels (lubrication in the female), causing engorgement and distention of the genitals. Venous congestion is localized primarily in the genitals, but also occurs to a lesser degree in the breasts and other parts of the body. Arousal is characterized by *myotonia* (increased muscular tension), resulting in voluntary and involuntary rhythmic contractions. Examples of sexually stimulated myotonia are pelvic thrusting, facial grimacing, and spasms of the hands and feet (carpopedal spasms).

The **sexual response cycle** is divided into four phases: excitement phase, plateau phase, orgasmic phase, and resolution phase. The four phases occur progressively with no sharp dividing line between any two phases. Specific body changes take place in sequence. The time, intensity, and duration for cyclic completion also vary for individuals and situations. Table 5-2 compares male and female body changes during each of the four phases of the sexual response cycle.

▌IMMUNOLOGY

Immunology is the study of the molecules, cells, organs, and systems responsible for the recognition and disposal of foreign material, and how the human body defends itself against this material. The human immune system is necessary for survival. Foreign substances can be as diverse as life-threatening infectious microorganisms or a lifesaving organ transplant. The desirable consequences of immunity include natural resistance, recovery, and acquired resistance to infectious diseases.

Body Defenses

The first barrier to infection is unbroken skin and mucous membranes. These surfaces form a physical barrier against many microorganisms. Secretions, such as mucus or those produced in the process of eliminating liquid and solid wastes (i.e., the urinary and gastrointestinal processes), are also important as nonspecific mechanisms for removing potential pathogens from the body. The acidity and alkalinity of the fluids of the stomach and intestinal tract, and the acidity of the vagina, can destroy many potentially infectious microorganisms. These fluids can also have chemical properties that defend the body. For example, lysozyme is an enzyme found in tears and saliva that attacks the cell wall of susceptible bacteria.

The body has a wide variety of barrier-assisting defenses that initially protect the body against disease. Although these barriers vary among individuals, they do assist in the general resistance to infectious organisms. When barrier-assisting defenses break down, the potential for disease increases. For instance, when the new mother's skin integrity is impaired (e.g., through episiotomy or lacerations) or when she has cracking of the nipples, she is at increased risk for infection. In older women, the pH and amount of vaginal

TABLE 5-2 *Four Phases of Sexual Response*

REACTIONS COMMON TO BOTH SEXES	FEMALE REACTIONS	MALE REACTIONS
EXCITEMENT PHASE		
Heart rate and blood pressure increase. Nipples become erect. Myotonia begins.	Clitoris increases in diameter and swells. External genitals become congested and darken. Vaginal lubrication occurs; upper two thirds of vagina lengthen and extend. Cervix and uterus pull upward. Breast size increases.	Erection of the penis begins; penis increases in length and diameter. Scrotal skin becomes congested and thickens. Testes begin to increase in size and elevate toward the body.
PLATEAU PHASE		
Heart rate and blood pressure continue to increase. Respirations increase. Myotonia becomes pronounced; grimacing occurs.	Clitoral head retracts under the clitoral hood. Lower one third of vagina becomes engorged. Skin color changes occur—red flush may be observed across breasts, abdomen, or other surfaces.	Head of penis may enlarge slightly. Scrotum continues to grow tense and thicken. Testes continue to elevate and enlarge. Preorgasmic emission of 2 or 3 drops of fluid appears on the head of the penis.
ORGASMIC PHASE		
Heart rate, blood pressure, and respirations increase to maximum levels. Involuntary muscle spasms occur. External rectal sphincter contracts.	Strong rhythmic contractions are felt in the clitoris, vagina, and uterus. Sensations of warmth spread through the pelvic area.	Testes elevate to maximum level. Point of "inevitability" occurs just before ejaculation and an awareness of fluid in the urethra. Rhythmic contractions occur in the penis. Ejaculation of semen occurs.
RESOLUTION PHASE		
Heart rate, blood pressure, and respirations return to normal. Nipple erection subsides. Myotonia subsides.	Engorgement in external genitalia and vagina resolves. Uterus descends to normal position. Cervix dips into seminal pool. Breast size decreases. Skin flush disappears.	Fifty percent of erection is lost immediately with ejaculation; penis gradually returns to normal size. Testes and scrotum return to normal size. Refractory period (time needed for erection to occur again) varies according to age and general physical condition.

fluid is altered, resulting in the increased risk of yeast infection (i.e., *Candida albicans*).

Types of Immunity

Natural immunity

Natural (innate or inborn) resistance is one of two ways the body resists infection after microorganisms have penetrated the first line of resistance. The second form, acquired or adaptive resistance, specifically recognizes and selectively eliminates exogenous (or endogenous) agents.

Natural immunity is characterized as a nonspecific mechanism. If a microorganism penetrates the skin or mucous membranes, cellular and humoral defense mechanisms become operational. The elements of natural resistance are phagocytic cells, complement, and the acute inflammatory reaction. Despite their relative lack of specificity, these components are essential, because they are largely responsible for natural immunity to many environmental microorganisms.

Acquired immunity

If a microorganism overwhelms the body's natural resistance, another form of defensive resistance, **acquired** or **adaptive immunity,** allows the body to recognize, remember, and respond to a specific stimulus—an antigen.

Acquired immunity can eliminate microorganisms and commonly leaves the host with antigen-specific immunologic memory. This condition of memory or recall, *acquired resistance,* allows the host to respond more effectively if reinfection with the same microorganism occurs. Acquired immunity, like natural immunity, is composed of cellular and humoral components.

The major cellular component of this mechanism is the lymphocyte; the major humoral component is the antibody.

Lymphocytes selectively respond to foreign materials, antigens, which leads to immune memory and a permanently altered pattern of response or adaptation to the environment. The two categories of the adaptive response are antibody-mediated and cell-mediated immunity. Antibody-mediated immunity is the primary defense against bacterial infection. Cell-mediated immunity is the primary defense against viral and fungal infections, intracellular organisms, tumor antigens, and graft rejections.

Antibody-mediated immunity

If specific antibodies have been formed to antigen stimulation, they are available to protect the body against foreign substances. The recognition of foreign substances and subsequent production of antibodies to these substances is the specific meaning of immunity. Antibody-mediated immunity to infection occurs when the antibodies are formed by the host or received from another source. These two types of immunity are called *active* and *passive* immunity.

Active immunity can be acquired by natural exposure in response to an infection or acquired by injection of an antigen. This injection of antigen, called **vaccination,** effectively stimulates antibody production and memory (acquired resistance) without suffering from the disease. The selected antigenic agent should produce the antibodies without the clinical signs and symptoms of the disease in an **immunocompetent** host (a person whose immune system is able to recognize a foreign antigen and build specific antigen-directed antibodies) and produce permanent antigenic memory. Booster vaccinations may be needed to expand the pool of memory cells.

Artificial **passive immunity** is achieved by infusion of serum or plasma containing high concentrations of antibody. This provides immediate antibody protection against microorganisms such as hepatitis A or antigens such as Rh-positive (fetal) red blood cells. The antibodies have been produced by another person or animal that has been actively immunized, not by the ultimate recipient. As long as the antibodies persist in the circulation, recipients will benefit from passive immunity. Passive immunity can also be acquired naturally by the fetus through the transfer of antibodies through maternal circulation in utero. Maternal antibodies are also transferred to the newborn after birth in the prelactation fluid called *colostrum.* For the newborn to have lasting protection, active immunity must occur.

Cell-mediated immunity

Cell-mediated immunity consists of immune activities that differ from those of antibody-mediated immunity. Cell-mediated immunity is moderated by the link between T-lymphocytes and phagocytic cells (i.e., monocyte-macrophage cells). Lymphocytes (T-cells) do not directly recognize the antigens of microorganisms or other living cells, such as an *allograft* (a graft of tissue from a genetically different member of the same species [e.g., a human kidney], but do so when the antigen is present on the surface of an antigen-presenting cell—the macrophage. Lymphocytes are immunologically active through various types of direct cell-to-cell contact and by the production of soluble factors, such as *lymphokines,* for specific immunologic functions. These include the recruitment of phagocytic cells to the site of inflammation. The term *delayed hypersensitivity* is often used synonymously with the term *cell-mediated immunity.* Delayed hypersensitivity refers to the slow appearance of a secondary response in the skin. The term dates back to when antibody responses were detected by immediate hypersensitivity and reflected the difference in the length of time that it took for a delayed response to occur (e.g., tuberculin skin test).

Under some conditions, the activities of cell-mediated immunity may not be beneficial. Suppression of the normal adaptive immune response (*immunosuppression*) by drugs or other means is necessary in conditions such as organ transplantation, hypersensitivity, and autoimmune disorders.

Factors Associated with Immunologic Disease

Factors such as general health and the age of an individual are important considerations in the functioning of the immune system in defense against infectious disease. In the case of noninfectious diseases or disorders, however, additional factors may be important. In caring for women and their families, nurses must consider the effects of the environment, nutritional status, and lifestyle on the developing immune system. Standard precautions should be practiced at all times whether caring for women in the hospital, community, or home (see Box 6-3).

I HEALTH ASSESSMENT

Profound changes in society and the family and in roles and expectations of women make maternity nursing and women's health care a challenging field. Current women's health trends have expanded beyond a reproductive focus to include a holistic approach to health care across the life span. This restructuring deemphasizes tertiary care and places women's health within the scope of primary care. Women's health assessment and screening focus on a systems evaluation beginning with a careful history and physical examination. During the assessment and evaluation, the responsibility for self-care, health promotion, and enhancement of wellness are emphasized. Nursing is an interactive process that begins with establishing trust and a caring relationship with the broader goal of enhancing and maintaining wellness. The nurse provides care that includes assessment, planning, education, counseling, and referral as needed, as well as commendations of good self-care that the woman has practiced. This enables women to make informed decisions about their own health care.

It is the nurse's responsibility to coordinate the woman's care in accordance with established guidelines and protocols (US Department of Health and Human Services, 1997).

In a market-driven system such as managed care, there may be specific guidelines provided for health screening by the insurer or managed care organization. A nurse often takes the history, orders diagnostic tests, interprets test results, makes referrals, coordinates care, and directs attention to problems requiring medical intervention. Advance practice nurses who have specialized in women's health, such as nurse practitioners, clinical nurse specialists, and nurse midwives, perform complete physical assessments, including gynecologic examinations.

Culturally competent nursing care should be delivered with an awareness of cultural diversity while respecting the unique qualities of each woman. Such care cannot be provided in the absence of self-awareness. Nurses need to acknowledge their own values, beliefs, and communication styles in order to understand what they contribute to cross-cultural communication (Lipson et al., 1996).

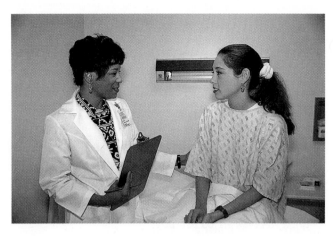

Fig. 5-8 Nurse interviews patient as part of annual physical examination. (From Potter P & Perry A: *Fundamentals of nursing: concepts, process, and practice,* ed 4, St Louis, 1997, Mosby.)

Interview

The interview should be conducted in a private, comfortable, and relaxed setting and in an unhurried manner. (Fig. 5-8). The nurse is seated and makes sure the woman is comfortable. The woman is addressed by her title and name (e.g., Mrs. Miller), and the nurse introduces herself or himself using name and title. It is important to phrase questions in a sensitive and nonjudgmental manner. Body language should match verbal communication. The nurse is cognizant of a woman's vulnerability and assures her of strict confidentiality. For many women, fear, anxiety, and modesty make the examination a dreaded and stressful experience. Many women are uninformed, misguided by myths, or afraid they will appear ignorant by asking questions about sexual or reproductive functioning. The woman is assured that no question is irrelevant. The history begins with an open-ended question such as, "What brings you in to the office/clinic/hospital today? Anything else? Tell me about it." Additional ways to get women to share information include:

- **Facilitation:** Using a word or posture that communicates interest; leaning forward; making eye contact; or saying "Mm-hmmm" or "Go on."
- **Reflection:** Repeating a word or phrase that a woman has used.
- **Clarification:** Asking the woman what is meant by a word or phrase.
- **Empathic responses:** Acknowledging the feelings of a woman by statements such as, "That must have been frightening."

- **Confrontation:** Identifying something about the woman's behavior or feelings not expressed verbally or apparently inconsistent with her history.
- **Interpretation:** Putting into words what you infer about the woman's feelings or about the meaning of her symptoms, events, or other matters.

Direct questions may be necessary to get specific details. This should be worded in language that is understandable to the woman and expressed neutrally so that the woman will not be led into a specific response. The nurse asks about one item at a time and proceeds from the general to the specific (Bates, 1991).

Biographic Information

At a woman's first visit, she is often expected to fill out a form with biographic and historical data before meeting with the examiner. The nurse is usually responsible for ensuring that the woman's name, age, marital status, race, ethnicity, address, phone numbers, occupation, and date of visit are recorded. The name should be recorded on all pages of the record. Common patient names should also have additional identifying patient information such as date of birth or social security number on each page.

Old records are considered a reliable source of patient information. The nurse records a subjective judgment about the reliability of the person giving the history—the woman, parent, spouse, or other historian.

Cultural and Communication Variations

Recognition of signs and symptoms of disease and deciding when to seek treatment are influenced by cultural perceptions. Culture evolves over time and is a system of symbols that are learned, shared, and passed on through generations of a social group. Cultural competence in nursing is a complex combination of knowledge, attitudes, and

GUIDELINES/GUÍAS

Take off all your clothes.
Quítese toda la ropa.

Put on the gown.
Póngase la bata.

I'm going to examine you.
Le voy a hacer un examen.

You will feel less discomfort if you relax.
Se sentirá mejor si relaja su cuerpo.

Lie down, please.
Acuéstese, por favor.

Put your feet in the stirrups.
Ponga sus pies en los estribos.

Open your legs.
Separa las piernas, por favor.

I'm going to take a sample from the lining of the cervix (Pap smear).
Voy a tomarle una muestra del cuello de la matriz para una prueba del cáncer; se llama la prueba "el pap."

We will test this sample for cancer.
Se le hara la prueba de cáncer.

It won't hurt.
Esto no le va a doler.

Everything looks fine.
Todo está bien.

You may get dressed.
Puede vestirse.

skills mixed with personal attributes of flexibility, empathy, and language facility. It is more than simply acquiring knowledge about another ethnic group. It is essential that a nurse have respect for the rich and unique qualities that cultural diversity brings to individuals. In recognizing the value of these differences, the nurse can modify the plan of care to meet the needs of each woman. Trust that the woman is the expert on her life, culture, and experiences. If the nurse asks with respect and a genuine desire to learn, the patient will tell the nurse how to care for her (Lipson et al., 1996). The nurse communicates in an even-toned and nonjudgmental manner, keeping a calm facial expression, and recognizes that modifications may be necessary for the physical examination. In some cultures, it may be considered inappropriate for the woman to completely disrobe for the physical examination. In many cultures, a woman examiner is preferred.

Communication may be hindered by different beliefs even when the nurse and patient speak the same language. Communication variations include the following (modified from Lipson et al., 1996):

- **Conversational style and pacing:** Silence may show respect or acknowledgment that the listener has heard. In cultures in which a direct "no" is considered rude, silence may mean no. Repetition or loudness may mean emphasis or anger.
- **Personal space:** Cultural conceptions of personal space differ, based on one's culture. Someone may be perceived as distant for backing off when approached or aggressive for standing too close.
- **Eye contact:** Eye contact varies among cultures from intense to fleeting. In an effort to refrain from invading personal space, avoiding direct eye contact may be a sign of respect.
- **Touch:** The norms about how people should touch each other vary among cultures. In some cultures physical contact with the same sex (embracing, walking hand in hand) is more appropriate than with an unrelated person of the opposite sex.
- **Time orientation:** In some cultures involvement with people is more valued than being "on time." In other cultures, life is scheduled and paced according to clock time, which is valued over personal time.

Women with Special Needs

Women with emotional or physical disorders have special needs. Women who are visually, auditorily, emotionally, or physically disabled should be respected and involved in the assessment and physical examination to the full extent of their abilities. The nurse should communicate openly and directly with sensitivity. It is often helpful to learn about the disability directly from the woman while maintaining eye contact. Family and significant others should be relied on only when absolutely necessary. The assessment and physical examination can be adapted to each woman's individual needs.

Communication with a woman who is hearing impaired can be accomplished without difficulty. Most of these women read lips and/or write; thus, an interviewer who speaks and enunciates each word slowly and in full view may be easily understood. If a woman is not comfortable with lip reading, she may use an interpreter. In this case, it is important to continue to address the woman directly, avoiding the temptation to speak directly with the interpreter. The visually impaired woman needs to be oriented to the examination room and may have her guide dog with her. As with all patients, the visually impaired woman needs a full explanation of what the examination entails before proceeding. Before touching her, the nurse explains, "Now I am going to take your blood pressure. I am going to place the cuff on your right arm." The woman can be asked if she would like to touch each of the items that will be used in the examination to reduce her anxiety.

Many physically disabled women cannot comfortably lie in the lithotomy position for the pelvic examination. Several alternative positions may be used, including a lateral (side-lying) position, a V-shaped position, a diamond-shaped position, and an M-shaped position (Fig. 5-9). The woman

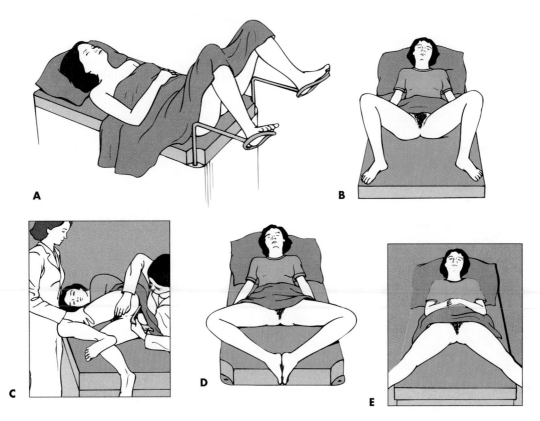

Fig. **5-9** Lithotomy and variable positions for women who have a disability. **A,** Lithotomy position. **B,** M-shaped position. **C,** Knee-chest position. **D,** Diamond-shaped position. **E,** V-shaped position. (From Lowdermilk D, Perry S & Bobak I: *Maternity & women's health care,* ed 6, St Louis, 1997, Mosby.)

can be asked what has worked best for her previously. If she has not had a pelvic or a comfortable examination in the past, the nurse proceeds slowly by showing her a picture of various positions and asking her which one she prefers. The nurse's support and reassurance can help the woman to relax, which will make the examination go more smoothly. The woman is informed that she is in charge, and if the examination needs to stop for whatever reason, it can be scheduled again at a later date.

Abused Women

Nurses should screen all women entering the health care system for potential abuse. It is important to keep in mind the possibility that violence against this woman may have occurred. Abuse is a life-threatening public health problem that affects millions of women and their children. Abuse of women knows no socioeconomic, racial, ethnic, religious, or age barriers. The risk for domestic violence increases during pregnancy and after separation or divorce. Many health care providers avoid questions about family violence because they are unaware of the extent of the problem, or they find it difficult to ask about violence. Help for the woman may depend on the sensitivity with which the nurse screens for abuse, the discovery of abuse, and subsequent

intervention. The nurse must be familiar with the laws governing abuse in the state in which she or he practices and inform the woman of these laws before eliciting this information. Awareness of the law can ensure the woman's confidentiality and trust.

Pocket cards listing emergency numbers (abuse counseling, legal protection, and emergency shelter) may be available by calling the local police department, women's shelter, or going to an emergency room or 24-hour clinic. It is helpful to have these on hand in the setting where screening is done. The National Family Violence Helpline is 1-800-222-2000. An abuse assessment screen (Fig. 5-10) can be used as part of the interview or written history (Parker & McFarlane, 1991). Reports show an increase in identification of victims of domestic violence when screening takes place at each visit. If a male partner is present, he should be asked to leave the room because the woman may not disclose experiences of abuse in his presence, or he may try to answer questions for her to protect himself. The same procedure would apply for partners of lesbians or adult children of older women.

Fear, guilt, and embarrassment may keep many women from giving information about family violence. Clues in the history and evidence of injuries on physical examination

ABUSE ASSESSMENT SCREEN

1. Have you ever been emotionally or physically abused by your partner or someone important to you?

YES ☐

NO ☐

2. Within the last year, have you been hit, slapped, kicked, or otherwise physically hurt by someone?

YES ☐

NO ☐

If YES, by whom _____

Number of times _____

Mark the area of injury on body map.

3. Within the last year, has anyone forced you to have sexual activities?

If YES, who _____

Number of times _____

4. Are you afraid of your partner or anyone you listed above?

YES ☐

NO ☐

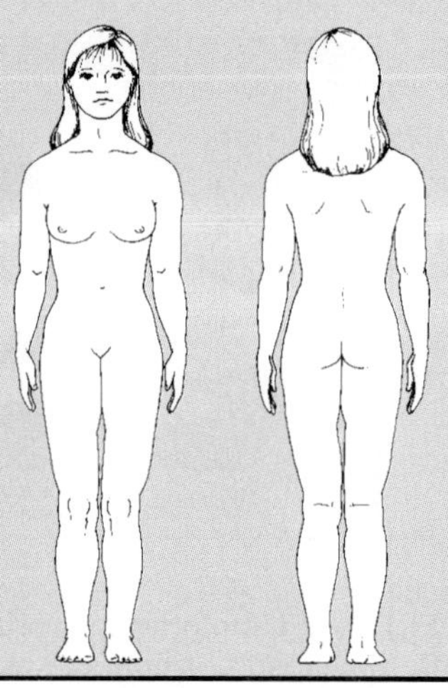

Fig. **5-10** Abuse assessment screen. (Modified from the Nursing Research Consortium on Violence and Abuse, 1991.)

BOX 5-1   *Indications of Possible Abuse*

1. Change in appointment pattern, either increased appointments with somatic, vague complaints or frequently missed appointments
2. Self-directed abuse, depression, attempted suicide
3. Severe anxiety, insomnia or violent nightmares
4. Alcohol or drug abuse; overuse or abuse of prescription medications
5. Bruises

Data from Edge V & Miller M: *Women's health care,* St Louis, 1994, Mosby.

---

should give a high index of suspicion (Box 5-1). The areas most commonly injured in women are the head, neck, chest, abdomen, breasts, and upper extremities. Burns and bruises in patterns resembling hands, belts, cords, or other weapons and multiple traumatic injuries may be seen. Attention should be given to women who present repeatedly with somatic complaints such as headaches, insomnia, choking sensation, hyperventilation, gastrointestinal symptoms, and pain in the chest, back, and pelvis. During pregnancy, the nurse should assess for injuries to the breasts, abdomen, and genitals. Assessment requires a detailed history of the woman's abuse and her living arrangements.

If a woman discloses battering as a problem, this disclosure is acknowledged and affirmed that it is unacceptable. The woman is told that she is at risk for recurrence. She also needs to know that battering is a common problem because she may think she is alone in experiencing violence perpetrated by a family member or loved one. She needs to be told that help is available and that she does not even deserve to be abused. The nurse's goal is to empower the woman. She needs to gain a feeling of control over her life, set her own goals, and make her own decisions. It is vital for the nurse to communicate two messages: (1) the nurse is deeply concerned for her welfare, and (2) the woman does not deserve to be abused (US Department of Health and Human Services, 1997).

The nurse can help the woman formulate a plan: What referrals (shelters, agencies, and legal aid) can help her? Where can she go if she needs to leave immediately? What necessary documents and personal items should be packaged that can be easily accessed?

Age-related Considerations

Age 13 to 19 years

As a young woman matures, she should be asked the same questions that are included in any history. Particular attention should be paid to hints about risky behaviors, eating disorders, and depression. Do not assume that a teenager is not sexually active. After rapport has been established it is best to talk to a teen with the parent (partners or friend) out of the room. Questions should be asked with sensitivity and in a gentle and nonjudgmental manner (Seidel et al., 1998).

A teen's first speculum examination is the most important because she will develop perceptions that will remain with her for future examinations. What the examination entails should be discussed with the teen while she is dressed. Models or illustrations can be used to show exactly what will happen. All of the necessary equipment should be assembled so that there are no interruptions. Pediatric specula that are 1 to 1.5 cm wide can be inserted with minimal discomfort. If the teen is sexually active, a small adult speculum may be used.

Injury prevention should be a part of the counseling at routine health examinations with special attention to seat belts, helmets, firearms, recreational hazards, and sports involvement. The use of drugs and alcohol and nonuse of seat belts contribute to motor vehicle injuries, accounting for the greatest proportion of accidental deaths in women (Fogel & Woods, 1995). Contraceptive options including safety should be addressed during visits.

To provide developmentally appropriate care, it is important to review the major tasks for women in this stage of life. Major tasks for teens include value assessment; education and work goal setting; formation of peer relationships that focus on love, commitment, and sex; and separation from parents. Individuality may be reflected in areas such as sexuality, politics, and career choices. Conflict exists between making and keeping commitments in order to keep options open. The teen is egocentric as she progresses rapidly through emotional and physical change. Her feelings of invulnerability may lead to misconceptions, such as unprotected sexual intercourse will not lead to pregnancy (Youngkin & Davis, 1994).

Age 50 years and older

The assessment of women age 50 and over presents unique challenges. Women may be experiencing major lifestyle changes such as children leaving home, caretaking for their aging parents, job retirement, or divorce or death of a partner, as well as aging changes and health problems. The nurse has an opportunity to use reflection and empathy while listening and ensuring open and caring communication. It may be necessary to schedule a longer appointment time because older women have longer histories or have a need to talk. Some women may fail to report symptoms because they fear their complaints will be attributed to old age or they feel that they have lived with a chronic condition (e.g., incontinence, dyspareunia) for so long that nothing can be done. Women may choose to ignore a problem if they have symptoms that are life threatening (e.g., chest pain or a breast lump) because they traditionally put the needs of others first. As a result, the nurse needs to encourage the woman to express her concerns and fears and reassure her that her problems are important and will be addressed. Hormone replacement therapy, diet, vitamin and calcium supplementation, daily aspirin, breast self-examination, mammogram, sigmoidoscopy/colonoscopy, updating immunizations, and need for exercise should be discussed.

Sexual assessment is important in women age 50 and over. Unless directly asked, women may omit mention of sexual concerns. Questions asked with sensitivity may invite responses regarding changes in sexual desire/response or physical issues that challenge her sexual enjoyment. Open and reflective questions also affirm a woman's right to sexual enjoyment throughout the life span.

Women over 50 commonly experience menopause (cessation of menses) and have physical changes associated with decreased estrogen. A decrease in estrogen causes thinning of the mucosal tissue layers, resulting in a narrowing and a decrease in lubrication of the vagina. Estrogen also plays a role in the formation of bone matrix, and a decrease may lead to osteoporosis. Decreases in estrogen cause a relaxation of the ligaments and connective tissue, which affects the support of the bladder and uterus. Decreases in estrogen also affect the hypothalamus, causing hot flashes, which are disturbing to most women (Edge & Miller, 1994).

Physical changes can result in increased discomfort during the pelvic examination. It is important to be both gentle and thorough during the examination. A small adult speculum may be used to view the cervix. The uterus in a menopausal woman is small and firm and the ovaries are nonpalpable. A woman with palpable adnexal masses or vaginal bleeding after menopause needs immediate gynecologic referral.

A respectful and reassuring approach toward caring for women age 50 and older will ensure their continued participation in seeking health care. Because the risk of breast, ovarian, uterine, cervical, and colon cancer increases with age, the nurse has the opportunity to educate women about the importance of preventive screening. It is the nurse's responsibility to ensure a positive health care experience that encourages future visits for preventive health, chronic, and acute care.

Advance Directives can be introduced on any entry into a health care system. It is a good idea to have a formal statement in the medical record regarding a woman's wishes in the event of accident or illness regarding life maintenance measures or organ donation. Most states have laws formalizing such statements in writing. The Durable Power of

Attorney for Health Care can be used by a patient to delegate decision-making authority to a trusted relative or friend.

Functional assessment is included as part of the history in women over 70 and those with disabilities. In the review of systems, the nurse needs to ask about self-care activities such as walking, getting to the bathroom, bathing, hair combing, dressing, and eating. Questions about driving, using public transportation or the telephone, hanging up clothes, buying groceries, taking medications, and meal preparation should be included.

History

A medical history usually includes the following:

1. **Identifying Data:** Name, age, race, living household preference, occupation, religion, culture, and ethnicity are obtained.
2. **Chief Complaint(s):** A verbatim response to the question, "What problem or symptom brought you here today?" If a lengthy list is recited and the nurse's schedule is slotted for one or two complaints, it may be necessary to tell the woman that her two complaints with the highest priority will be addressed today. Then in order to give all of her problems the full attention they deserve, a follow-up appointment in 1 to 2 weeks will be scheduled. Women are usually appreciative that the nurse is taking extra time and are agreeable to this.
3. **History of Present Illness:** A chronologic narrative that includes onset of the problem, the setting in which it developed, its manifestations, and any treatments received are noted. The woman's state of health before the onset of the present problem is determined. If the problem is long standing, the reason for seeking attention at this time is elicited. The principal symptoms should be described as to:
   • Location
   • Quality
   • Quantity or severity
   • Timing (onset, duration, frequency)
   • Setting
   • Factors that aggravate or relieve
   • Associated manifestations
4. **Past Medical History:** Determine general state of health and strength:
   • Infectious diseases: measles, mumps, rubella, whooping cough, chicken pox, rheumatic fever, scarlet fever, diphtheria, polio, tuberculosis (TB), hepatitis
   • Chronic disease and system disorders: arthritis, cancer, diabetes, heart, lung, kidney, seizures, stroke, or ulcers
   • Adult injuries, accidents, illnesses, disabilities, hospitalizations, or blood transfusions. Note if the injury occurred on the job (Workmen's Compensation) or if potential litigation is being considered.

5. **Present Health Status:**
   • Allergies: medications, previous transfusion reactions, or environmental allergies
   • Immunizations: diphtheria, pertussis, tetanus, polio, measles, mumps, rubella (MMR), hepatitis B, varicella, influenza, and pneumococcal vaccine; last TB skin test
   • Screening tests: Pap smear, mammogram, stool for occult blood, sigmoidoscopy/colonoscopy, chest x-ray, hematocrit, hemoglobin, rubella titer, urinalysis and cholesterol test; blood type/Rh; last eye examination; last dental examination
   • Environmental/chemical hazards: home, school, work, and leisure setting; exposure to extreme heat/cold, noise, industrial toxins such as asbestos or lead, pesticides, diethylstilbestrol (DES), radiation exposure, cat feces, or cigarette smoke
   • Use of safety measures: seat belts, bicycle helmets, designated driver
   • Exercise and leisure activities
   • Sleep patterns: length and quality
   • Sexuality: Is she sexually active? With men, women, or both?
   • Diet, including beverages: 24-hour dietary recall
   • Medications: name, dose, frequency, duration, reason for taking, and compliance with prescription medications; home remedies, over-the-counter drugs, vitamin and mineral supplements used over a 24-hour period
   • Nicotine, alcohol, illicit or recreational drugs: type, amount, frequency, duration, and reactions
   • Caffeine: coffee, tea, cola, or chocolate intake
6. **Past Surgical History:** Type, date, reason, outcome, and any complications should be noted.
7. **Family History:** Information about age and health of family members may be presented in narrative or genogram: age, health/death of parents, siblings, spouse, children. Check for history of diabetes, heart disease, hypertension, stroke, respiratory, renal, thyroid, cancer, bleeding disorders, hepatitis, allergies, asthma, arthritis, TB, epilepsy, mental illness, human immunodeficiency virus (HIV), or other disorders.
8. **Social History:** Note birthplace, education, employment, marital status, living accommodations, children, persons at home, and hobbies. Does she enjoy what she is doing?
   • Screen for abuse: Has she ever been hit, kicked, slapped or forced to have sex against her wishes? Verbally or emotionally abused? History of childhood sexual abuse? If yes, has she received counseling or does she need referral (Seng & Petersen, 1995)?
9. **Review of Systems:** It is probable that all questions in each system will not be included every time a history is taken. Some questions regarding each

system should be included in every history. The essential areas to be explored are listed in the following head-to-toe sequence. If a woman gives a positive response to a question about an essential area, more detailed questions should be asked.

- **General:** weight change, fatigue, weakness, fever, chills, or night sweats
- **Skin:** skin, hair and nail changes, itching, bruising, bleeding, rashes, sores, lumps, or moles
- **Lymph nodes:** enlargement, inflammation, pain, suppuration (pus), or drainage
- **Head, Eyes, Ears, Nose, and Throat (HEENT):**
  - **Head:** trauma, vertigo (dizziness), convulsive disorder, syncope (fainting), headache location, frequency, pain type, nausea/vomiting, or visual symptoms
  - **Eyes:** glasses, contact lenses, blurriness, tearing, itching, photophobia, diplopia, inflammation, trauma, cataracts, glaucoma, or acute visual loss
  - **Ears:** hearing loss, tinnitus (ringing), vertigo, discharge, pain, fullness, recurrent infections, or mastoiditis
  - **Nose/Sinuses:** trauma, rhinitis, nasal discharge, epistaxis, obstruction, sneezing, itching, allergy, or smelling impairment
  - **Mouth/Throat/Neck:** hoarseness, voice changes, soreness, ulcers, bleeding gums, goiter, swelling, or enlarged nodes
- **Breasts:** masses, pain, lumps, dimpling, nipple discharge, fibrocystic changes or implants; breast self-examination (BSE)
- **Respiratory:** shortness of breath, wheezing, cough, sputum, hemoptysis, pneumonia, pleurisy, asthma, bronchitis, emphysema, or TB; last chest x-ray (CXR)
- **Cardiac:** hypertension, rheumatic fever, murmurs, angina, palpitations, dyspnea, tachycardia, orthopnea, edema, chest pain, cough, cyanosis, cold extremities, ascites, intermittent claudication (calf pain), phlebitis, or skin color changes
- **Gastrointestinal (GI):** appetite, nausea, vomiting, indigestion, dysphagia, abdominal pain, ulcers, hematochezia (bleeding with stools), melena (black, tarry stools), bowel habit changes, diarrhea, constipation, bowel movement frequency, food intolerance, hemorrhoids, jaundice, or hepatitis; sigmoidoscopy/colonoscopy/barium enema/ or ultrasound
- **Genitourinary (GU):** frequency, hesitancy, urgency, polyuria, dysuria, hematuria, nocturia, incontinence, stones, infection, or urethral discharge; dysmenorrhea, intermenstrual bleeding, dyspareunia, discharge, sores, itching, sexually transmitted diseases (STD), gravidity (G), parity (P), problems in pregnancy, contraception, menopause, hot flashes, or sweats (may be included here or as part of endocrine)

- **Vascular:** leg edema, claudication, varicose veins, thromboses, or emboli
- **Endocrine:** heat/cold intolerance, dry skin, excessive sweating, polyuria, polydipsia, polyphagia, thyroid problems, diabetes, or secondary sex characteristic changes; age at menarche, length/flow of menses, last menstrual period (LMP), age at menopause, libido, or sexual concerns
- **Hematologic:** anemia, easy bruising, bleeding, petechiae, purpura, or transfusions
- **Musculoskeletal:** muscle weakness, pain, joint stiffness, scoliosis, lordosis, kyphosis, range of motion instability, redness, swelling, arthritis, or gout
- **Neurologic:** loss of sensation, numbness, tingling, tremors, weakness, vertigo, paralysis, fainting, twitching, blackouts, seizures, convulsions, loss of consciousness or memory
- **Psychiatric:** moodiness, depression, anxiety, obsessions, delusions, illusions, or hallucinations
- **Functional Assessment:** should be done on women with disabilities and age 70 and over; see Age-Related Considerations Age 50 and Over in this chapter.

Physical Examination

Objective data are recorded by system or location. A general statement of overall health status is a good way to start. Findings are described in detail.

- **General Appearance:** age, race, sex, state of health, stature, development, dress, hygiene, affect, alertness, orientation, cooperativeness, and communication skills
- **Vital Signs:** temperature, pulse, respiration, blood pressure, height and weight
- **Skin:** color; integrity; texture; hydration; temperature; edema; excessive perspiration; unusual odor; presence and description of lesions; hair texture and distribution; nail configuration; color, texture, condition, or presence of nail clubbing
- **Head:** size, shape, trauma, masses, scars, rashes or scaling; facial symmetry; presence of edema or puffiness
- **Eyes:** pupil size, shape, reactivity, conjunctival injection, scleral icterus, fundal papilledema, hemorrhage, lids, extraocular movements, visual fields and acuity
- **Ears:** shape/symmetry, tenderness, discharge, external canal, and tympanic membranes; hearing: Weber should be midline (loudness of sound equal in both ears) and Rinne negative (no conductive or sensorineural hearing loss); should be able to hear whisper at 3 feet
- **Nose:** symmetry, tenderness, discharge, mucosa, turbinate inflammation, frontal/maxillary sinus tenderness; discrimination of odors
- **Mouth, Throat:** hygiene, condition of teeth, dentures, appearance of lips, tongue buccal and oral mucosa, erythema, edema, exudate, tonsillar enlargement, palate, uvula, gag reflex, or ulcers

- **Neck:** mobility, masses, range of motion, trachea deviation, thyroid size, carotid bruits
- **Lymphatic:** cervical, intraclavicular, axillary, trochlear, or inguinal adenopathy; size, shape, tenderness, and consistency
- **Breasts:** skin changes, dimpling, symmetry, scars, tenderness, discharge or masses; characteristics of nipples and areolae
- **Heart:** rate, rhythm, murmurs, rubs, gallops, clicks, heaves, or precordial movements
- **Peripheral Vascular:** jugular vein distention (JVD), bruits, edema, swelling, vein distention, Homans' sign, or tenderness of extremities
- **Lungs:** chest symmetry with respirations, wheezes, crackles, rhonchi, vocal fremitus, whispered pectoriloquy, percussion, and diaphragmatic excursion; breath sounds equal and clear bilaterally
- **Abdomen:** shape, scars, bowel sounds, consistency, tenderness, rebound, masses, guarding, organomegaly, liverspan, percussion (tympany, shifting, dullness), costovertebral angle (CVA) tenderness
- **Extremities:** edema, ulceration, tenderness, varicosities, erythema, tremor, or deformity
- **Genitourinary:** external genitalia, perineum, vaginal mucosa, cervix, inflammation, tenderness, discharge, bleeding, ulcers, nodules, masses, internal vaginal support, bimanual, and rectovaginal; palpation of cervix, uterus, and adnexae
- **Rectal:** sphincter tone, masses, hemorrhoids, rectal wall contour, tenderness, and stool for occult blood
- **Musculoskeletal:** posture, symmetry of muscle mass, muscle atrophy, weakness, appearance of joints, tenderness or crepitus, joint range of motion, instability, redness, swelling, or spine deviation
- **Neurologic:** mental status, orientation, memory, mood, speech clarity and comprehension, cranial nerves II to XII, sensation, strength, deep tendon and superficial reflexes, gait, balance, and coordination with rapid alternating motions.

Pelvic examination

Many women are intimidated by the gynecologic portion of the physical examination. The nurse in this instance can take an advocacy approach that supports a partnership relationship between the woman and the care provider.

The woman is assisted into the lithotomy position (see Fig. 5-9, *A*) for the pelvic examination. When she is in the lithotomy position, the woman's hips and knees are flexed with the buttocks at the edge of the table, and her feet are supported by heel or knee stirrups.

Some women prefer to keep their shoes or socks on, especially if the stirrups are not padded. Many women express feelings of vulnerability and strangeness when in the lithotomy position. During the procedure the nurse assists the woman with relaxation techniques.

One method of helping the woman relax is to have her place her hands on her chest at about the level of the diaphragm, breathe deeply and slowly (in through her nose and out through her O-shaped mouth), concentrate on the rhythm of breathing, and relax all body muscles with each exhalation (Barkauskas et al., 1994). This breathing technique is particularly helpful for the adolescent or the woman whose introitus may be especially tight or for whom the experience may be new or may provoke tension. Some women relax when they are encouraged to become involved with the examination with a mirror placed so that they can view the area being examined. This type of participation helps with health teaching as well. Distraction is another technique that can be used effectively (e.g., placement of interesting pictures on the ceiling over the head of the table).

Many women find it distressing to attempt to converse in the lithotomy position. Most women appreciate an explanation of the procedure as it unfolds, as well as coaching for the type of sensations they may expect. Generally, however, women prefer not to have to respond to questions until they are again upright and at eye level with the examiner. Questioning during the procedure, especially if they cannot see their questioner's eyes, may make women tense.

External inspection. The examiner sits at the foot of the table for the inspection of the external genitals and for the speculum examination. To facilitate open communication and to help the woman relax, the woman's head is raised on a pillow and the drape is arranged so that eye-to-eye contact can be maintained. In good lighting, external genitals are inspected for sexual maturity, clitoris, labia, and perineum. After childbirth or other trauma there may be healed scars.

External palpation. The examiner proceeds with the examination using palpation and inspection. The examiner wears gloves for this portion of the assessment. Before touching the woman, the examiner explains what is going to be done and what the woman should expect to feel (e.g., pressure). The examiner may touch the woman in a less sensitive area such as the inner thigh to alert her that the genital examination is beginning. This gesture may put the woman more at ease. The labia are spread apart to expose the structures in the vestibule: urinary meatus, Skene's glands, vaginal orifice, and Bartholin's glands (Fig. 5-11). To assess the Skene's glands, the examiner inserts one finger into the vagina and "milks" the area of the urethra. Any exudate from the urethra or the Skene's glands is cultured. Masses and erythema of either structure are assessed further. Ordinarily the openings to the Skene's glands are not visible; prominent openings may be seen if the glands are infected (e.g., with gonorrhea). During the examination, the examiner keeps in mind the data from the review of systems, such as history of burning on urination.

The vaginal orifice is examined. Hymenal tags are normal findings. With one finger still in the vagina, the examiner repositions the index finger near the posterior part of the

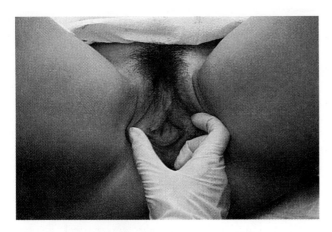

Fig. **5-11** External examination. Separation of the labia. (From Edge V & Miller M: *Women's health care,* St Louis, 1994, Mosby.)

Assisting with Pelvic Examination

Wash hands. Assemble equipment (Fig. 5-13).

Ask woman to empty her bladder before the examination (obtain clean-catch urine specimen as needed).

Assist with relaxation techniques. Have the woman place her hands on her chest at about the level of the diaphragm, breathe deeply and slowly (in through her nose and out through an O-shaped mouth), concentrate on the rhythm of breathing, and relax all body muscles with each exhalation (Barkauskas et al., 1994).

Encourage the woman to become involved with the examination if she shows interest. For example, a mirror can be placed so that she can see the area being examined.

Assess for and treat signs of problems such as supine hypotension.

Warm the speculum in warm water if a prewarmed one is not available.

Instruct the woman to bear down when the speculum is being inserted.

Apply gloves and assist the examiner with collection of specimens for cytologic examination, such as a Pap test. After handling specimens, remove gloves and wash hands.

Lubricate the examiner's fingers with water or water-soluble lubricant before bimanual examination.

Assist the woman at completion of the examination to a sitting position and then a standing position.

Provide tissues to wipe lubricant from perineum.

Provide privacy for the woman while she is dressing.

orifice. With the thumb outside the posterior part of the labia majora, the examiner compresses the area of Bartholin's glands located at the 8 o'clock and 4 o'clock positions and looks for swelling, discharge, and pain.

The support of the anterior and posterior vaginal wall is assessed. The examiner spreads the labia with the index and middle finger and asks the woman to strain down. Any bulge from the anterior wall (urethrocele or cystocele) or posterior wall (rectocele) is noted and compared with the history, such as difficulty to start the stream of urine or constipation.

The perineum (area between the vagina and anus) is assessed for scars from old lacerations or episiotomies, thinning, fistulas, masses, lesions, and inflammation. The anus is assessed for hemorrhoids, hemorrhoidal tags, and integrity of the anal sphincter. The anal area is also assessed for lesions, masses, abscesses, and tumors. If there is a history of sexually transmitted disease, the examiner may want to obtain a culture specimen from the anal canal at this time. Throughout the genital examination, the examiner notes the odor. Odor may indicate infection or poor hygiene.

Vulvar self-examination. The pelvic examination provides a good opportunity for the practitioner to emphasize the need for regular **vulvar self-examination (VSE)** and to teach this procedure. Because there has been a dramatic increase in cancerous and precancerous conditions of the vulva in recent years, a VSE should be performed as an integral part of preventive health care by all women who are sexually active or 18 years of age or older, monthly between menses or more frequently if there are symptoms or a history of serious vulvar disease. Most lesions, including malignancy, condyloma acuminatum (wartlike growth), and Bartholin's cysts, can be seen or palpated and are easily treated if diagnosed early.

The examination can be performed by the practitioner and woman together, using a mirror. A simple diagram of the anatomy of the vulva can be given to the woman, with instructions to perform the examination herself that evening to reinforce what she has learned. She does the examination in a sitting position with adequate lighting, holding a mirror in one hand and using the other hand to expose the tissues surrounding the vaginal introitus. She then systematically examines the mons pubis, clitoris, urethra, labia majora, perineum, and perianal area and palpates the vulva, noting any changes in appearance of abnormalities, such as ulcers, lumps, warts, and changes in pigmentation.

Internal examination. A vaginal speculum consists of two blades and a handle. Speculums come in a variety of types and styles. A vaginal speculum is used to view the vaginal vault and cervix (see Procedure box). The speculum is gently placed into the vagina and inserted to the back of the vaginal vault. The blades are opened to reveal the cervix and are locked into the open position. The cervix is inspected for position and appearance of the os: color, lesions, bleeding, and discharge (Fig. 5-12). Cervical findings that are not within normal limits include ulcerations, masses, inflammation, and excessive protrusion into the vaginal vault. Anomalies, such as a cockscomb (a protrusion over the cervix that looks like a rooster's comb), a hooded or collared cervix (seen in DES daughters), or polyps are noted.

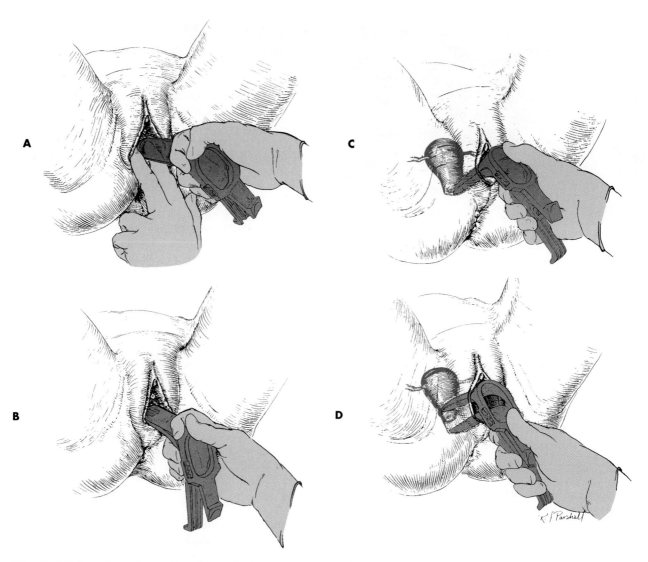

Fig. **5-12** Insertion of speculum for vaginal examination. **A,** Opening of the introitus. **B,** Oblique insertion of the speculum. **C,** Final insertion of the speculum. **D,** Opening of the speculum blades. (From Barkauskas
V et al.: *Health and physical assessment,* St Louis, 1994, Mosby.)

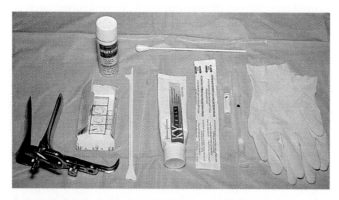

Fig. **5-13** Equipment used for pelvic examination. (Courtesy
Michael S. Clement, MD, Mesa, Ariz.)

Collection of specimens. The collection of specimens
for cytologic examination is an important part of the gynecologic examination. Infection can be diagnosed through
examination of specimens collected during the pelvic examination. These infections include *Candida albicans, Trichomonas vaginalis,* bacterial vaginosis, β-hemolytic streptococci, *Neisseria gonorrhoeae, Chlamydia trachomatis,* and
herpes simplex virus. Once the diagnoses have been made,
treatment can be instituted.

Papanicolaou (Pap) smear. Carcinogenic conditions,
potential or actual, can be determined by examination of
cells from the cervix **(Papanicolaou smear)** collected during the pelvic examination (see Procedure Box) (Fig. 5-14).

PROCEDURE
Papanicolaou Smear

In preparation, make sure the woman has not douched, used vaginal medications, or had sexual intercourse for at least 24 hours before the procedure. Reschedule the test if the woman is menstruating.

The woman is assisted into a lithotomy position. A speculum is inserted into the vagina.

Explain to the woman the purpose of the test and what sensations she will feel as the specimen is obtained (e.g., pressure but not pain).

The cytologic specimen is obtained before any digital examination of the vagina is made or endocervical bacteriologic specimens are taken with cotton swabbing of the cervix.

The Pap smear is obtained by using an endocervical sampling device (Cytobrush, Cervex-Brush, papette, or broom) (see Fig. 5-14). If the two-sample method of obtaining cells is used, the cytobrush is inserted into the canal and rotated 90 to 180 degrees, followed by a gentle smear of the entire transformation zone using a spatula. Broom devices are inserted and rotated 360 degrees five times. They obtain endocervical and ectocervical samples at the same time. If the patient has had a hysterectomy, the vaginal cuff is sampled. Areas that appear abnormal on visualization will require colposcopy and biopsy. If using a one-slide technique, the spatula sample is smeared first. This is followed by applying the cytobrush sample (rolling the brush in the opposite direction from which it was obtained), which is less subject to drying artifact, and then the slide is sprayed with preservative within 5 seconds.

The ThinPrep Pap Test is an improved method of preserving cells that reduces blood, mucus, and inflammation. The Pap specimen is obtained in the manner described above and the collection device (brush, spatula, or broom) is simply rinsed in a vial of preserving solution that is provided by the lab. The sealed vial with solution is sent off to the appropriate lab. A special processing device filters the contents and a thin layer of cervical cells is deposited on a slide, which is then examined microscopically. Initial reports state that specimen adequacy is improved by 50% and improved detection of low-grade and more severe lesions by 65%.

Label the slides with the woman's name and site. Include on the form to accompany the slides the woman's name, age, parity, and chief complaint or reason for taking the cytologic specimens.

Send specimens to the pathology laboratory promptly for staining, evaluation, and a written report, with special reference to abnormal elements, including cancer cells.

Advise the woman that repeat smears may be necessary if the specimen is not adequate.

Instruct the woman concerning routine checkups for cervical and vaginal cancer. The American Cancer Society advises that women over 18 years of age and those under 18 who are sexually active have the test at least every 3 years, *but only after they have had three negative Pap tests a year apart.* A pelvic examination is recommended every 3 years from age 20 to 40 and every 1 to 3 years thereafter.

Record the examination date on the woman's record.

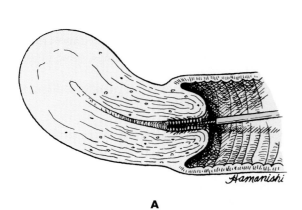
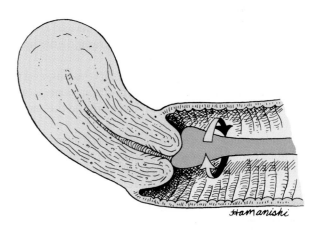

A **B**

Fig. **5-14** Pap smear. **A,** Collecting cells from endocervix using a cytobrush. **B,** Obtaining cells from the transformation zone using a wooden spatula. (From Mishell D et al.: *Comprehensive gynecology,* ed 3, St Louis, 1997, Mosby.)

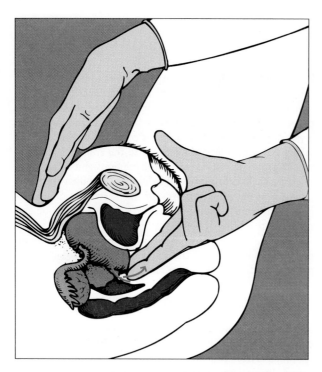

Fig. **5-15** Bimanual palpation of the uterus. (From Lowdermilk D, Perry S & Bobak I: *Maternity & women's health care*, ed 6, St Louis, 1997, Mosby.)

Vaginal examination. After the specimens are obtained, the vagina is viewed when the speculum is rotated. The speculum blades are unlocked and partially closed. As the speculum is withdrawn, it is rotated and the vaginal walls are inspected for color, lesions, rugae, fistulas, and bulging.

Bimanual palpation. The examiner stands for this part of the examination. A small amount of lubricant is placed on the first and second fingers of the gloved hand for the internal examination. To avoid tissue trauma and contamination, the thumb is abducted and the ring and little fingers are flexed into the palm (Fig. 5-15).

The vagina is palpated for distensibility, lesions, and tenderness. The cervix is examined for position, shape, consistency, motility, and lesions. The fornix around the cervix is palpated.

The other hand is placed on the abdomen halfway between the umbilicus and symphysis pubis and exerts pressure downward toward the pelvic hand. Upward pressure from the pelvic hand traps reproductive structures for assessment by palpation. The uterus is assessed for position, size, shape, consistency, regularity, motility, masses, and tenderness.

With the abdominal hand moving to the right lower quadrant and the fingers of the pelvic hand in the right lateral fornix, the adnexa is assessed for position, size, tenderness, and masses. The examination is repeated on the woman's left side.

Just before the intravaginal fingers are withdrawn, the woman is asked to tighten her vagina around the fingers as

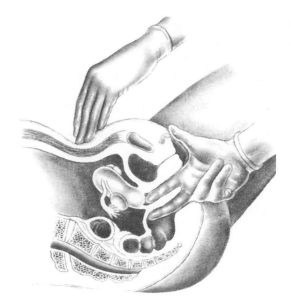

Fig. **5-16** Rectovaginal examination. (From Seidel H et al: *Mosby's guide to physical examination*, ed 4, St Louis, 1998, Mosby.)

much as she can. If the muscle response is weak, the woman is assessed for her knowledge about Kegel exercises.

Rectovaginal palpation. To prevent contamination of the rectum from organisms in the vagina (such as *Neisseria gonorrhoeae*) it is necessary to change gloves, add fresh lubricant, and then reinsert the index finger into the vagina and the middle finger into the rectum (Fig. 5-16). Insertion is facilitated if the woman strains down. The maneuvers of the abdominovaginal examination are repeated. The rectovaginal examination permits assessment of the rectovaginal septum, the posterior surface of the uterus, and the region behind the cervix and the adnexa. The vaginal finger is removed and folded into the palm, leaving the middle finger free to rotate 360 degrees. The rectum is palpated for rectal tenderness and masses.

After the rectal examination, the woman is assisted into a sitting position, given tissues or wipes to cleanse herself, and privacy to dress. The woman often returns to the examiner's office for a discussion of findings, prescriptions for therapy, and counseling.

Pelvic examination during pregnancy is discussed in Chapter 10.

Laboratory and diagnostic procedures

The following laboratory and diagnostic procedures are ordered at the discretion of the clinician: hemoglobin, total blood cholesterol, fasting plasma glucose, urinalysis for bacteria, syphilis serology (VDRL or RPR) and other screening tests for sexually transmitted diseases, Papanicolaou smear, mammogram, tuberculin skin test, hearing, electrocardiogram, chest x-ray, fecal occult blood, and bone mineral density. HIV and drug screening may be offered or encouraged with informed consent, especially in high-risk populations.

KEY POINTS

- Normal feedback regulation of the menstrual cycle depends on an intact hypothalamic-pituitary-gonadal mechanism.
- The female's reproductive tract structures and breasts respond predictably to changing levels of sex steroids across her life span.
- The myometrium of the uterus is uniquely designed to expel the fetus and promote hemostasis after birth.
- Prostaglandins play an important role in reproductive functions by their effect on smooth muscle contractility and modulation of hormones.
- Nurses need to be aware of their own feelings and values regarding sexuality before they can competently help patients meet their information needs or refer them for further counseling.
- The desirable consequences of immunity include natural resistance, recovery, and acquired resistance to infectious diseases.
- Vaccination is an effective method of stimulating antibody production and memory.
- Culture, religion, socioeconomic status, personal circumstances, the uniqueness of the individual, and stage of development are among the factors that influence a person's recognition of need for care and responses to the health care system and therapy.
- Profound changes in society and in roles and expectations of women have affected their health, needs, and ability to cope with problems.
- Assessment is more comprehensive and learning is best in a safe environment in which the atmosphere is nonjudgmental and sensitive, and the interaction is strictly confidential.
- Every woman is entitled to be respected and fully involved in the assessment process to the fullness of her capacity.
- Nurses in all specialties must respond with sensitivity and caring toward women who experience abuse and victimization.
- Well-women's health care includes a complete history, physical examination, and age-appropriate screening.
- Monthly breast self-examination, routine screening mammography, and yearly breast examinations by practitioners are recommended for early detection of breast cancer.

CRITICAL THINKING EXERCISES

1 *A young woman who has had one leg amputated above the knee arrives at the clinic for a yearly physical examination and Pap smear.*
   a *What alterations in the assessment procedure need to be considered?*
   b *Are there any impediments in your clinical site that would prevent women with disabilities from receiving adequate care? What needs to be changed and how would you make those changes?*

2 *You are assigned to teach breast self-examination (BSE) at a clinic for non–English-speaking migrant women from Mexico. The clinic provides you with an aide who is bilingual.*
   a *Compare the migrant women's perceptions and beliefs about health and BSE to your own.*
   b *Analyze how these factors may affect the health-seeking behaviors of these women.*
   c *How would you incorporate this knowledge into your teaching plan?*

References

Barkauskas V et al.: *Health and physical assessment,* St Louis, 1994, Mosby.

Bates B: *A pocket guide to physical examination and history taking,* Philadelphia, 1991, JB Lippincott.

Edge V & Miller M: *Women's health care,* St Louis, 1994, Mosby.

Fogel C & Woods N: *Women's health care, a comprehensive handbook,* Thousand Oaks, Calif, 1995, Sage.

Lipson J et al.: *Culture & nursing care: a pocket guide,* San Francisco, 1996, UCSF Nursing Press.

Lowdermilk D, Perry S & Bobak I: *Maternity & women's health care,* ed 6, St Louis, 1997, Mosby.

Masters W: *Human sexuality,* ed 4, New York, 1992, Harper Collins.

Mishell D et al.: *Comprehensive gynecology,* ed 3, St Louis, 1997, Mosby.

Parker B & McFarlane J: Identifying and helping battered pregnant women, *MCN Am J Maternal Child Nurs* 16(3):161, 1991.

Potter P & Perry A: *Fundamentals of nursing: concepts, process, and practice,* ed 4, St Louis, 1997, Mosby.

Seidel H et al.: *Mosby's guide to physical examination,* ed 4, St Louis, 1998, Mosby.

Seng J & Petersen B: Incorporating routine screening for history of childhood sexual abuse in well-women and maternity care, *J Nurse Midwifery* 40(1):26, 1995.

US Department of Health and Human Services, Public Health Service: Clinician's handbook of preventive services, Washington, DC, 1997, US Government Printing Office.

Youngkin E & Davis M: *Women's health, a primary care clinical guide,* Norwalk, Conn, 1994, Appleton & Lange.

CHAPTER

6

Common Health Problems

CATHERINE INGRAM FOGEL

LEARNING OBJECTIVES

- *Define the key terms.*
- *Develop a nursing care plan for the woman with primary dysmenorrhea.*
- *Outline patient teaching about premenstrual syndrome.*
- *Relate the pathophysiology of endometriosis to associated symptoms.*
- *Describe prevention of sexually transmitted infections in women.*
- *Differentiate signs, symptoms, diagnosis, and management of women with sexually transmitted infections.*
- *Summarize the care of women with selected viral infections (HIV, hepatitis B).*
- *Differentiate signs, symptoms, and management of selected vaginal infections.*
- *Review principles of infection control, including Standard Precautions and precautions for invasive procedures.*
- *Discuss the pathophysiology of selected benign breast conditions and malignant neoplasms of the breasts found in women.*
- *Discuss the emotional effects of benign and malignant neoplasms.*
- *Develop a plan of care for the woman with a lump in her breast.*

KEY TERMS

amenorrhea
dysfunctional uterine bleeding (DUB)
dysmenorrhea
endometriosis
fibroadenoma
fibrocystic change
human immunodeficiency virus (HIV)
human papillomavirus (HPV)
hypogonadotropic amenorrhea
intraductal papilloma
leiomyoma
lumpectomy
mammary duct ectasia
mammography
menorrhagia (hypermenorrhea)
metrorrhagia
modified radical mastectomy
oligomenorrhea (hypomenorrhea)
pelvic inflammatory disease (PID)
premenstrual syndrome (PMS)
primary dysmenorrhea
radical mastectomy
secondary dysmenorrhea
sexually transmitted infections (STI) or sexually
  transmitted diseases (STDs)
simple mastectomy
Standard Precautions
vulvovaginitis

Throughout her life, the average woman is likely to have some concerns related to her menstrual and gynecologic health and will experience bleeding, pain, or discharge associated with her reproductive organs or functions. In addition, during a woman's lifespan, she may experience infections associated with her reproductive or sexual life. Many women will seek out nurses as advisors, counselors, and health care providers for these concerns. If they are to meet their patients' needs, nurses must have accurate, up-to-date information. This chapter provides information on common menstrual problems, sexually transmitted infections, and selected other infections that can affect reproductive func-

tions, and benign breast conditions. Breast cancer is also included as the most common reproductive cancer occurring in women.

MENSTRUAL PROBLEMS

Women typically have menstrual cycles for about 40 years. Once the irregular nature of menses in the first 2 to 3 years following menarche subsides and a cyclic, predictable pattern of monthly bleeding is established, women may worry about any deviation from that pattern, or what they have been told is normal for all menstruating women. A woman may be concerned about her ability to conceive and bear children, or she may believe that she is not really a woman without monthly evidence. A sign such as amenorrhea or excess menstrual bleeding can be a source of severe distress and a concern for a woman as she wonders what is wrong. Sexual issues often are expressed and must be examined.

Amenorrhea

Amenorrhea, the absence or cessation of menstrual flow, is a clinical sign of a variety of disorders. Although the criteria used to determine when amenorrhea is a clinical problem are not universal, the following circumstances should generally be evaluated: (1) the absence of both menarche and secondary sexual characteristics by age 14; (2) the absence of menses by age 16, regardless of presence of normal growth and development (primary amenorrhea); or (3) a 6-month cessation of menses after a period of menstruation (secondary amenorrhea) (Fogel, 1997).

Although amenorrhea is not a disease, it is often the sign of one. It is most commonly a result of pregnancy. Amenorrhea may occur from any defect or interruption in the hypothalamic-pituitary-ovarian-uterine axis (see Chapter 4). It may also result from anatomic abnormalities; other endocrine disorders, such as hypothyroidism or hyperthyroidism; chronic diseases, such as type 1 diabetes; medications, such as dilantin; eating disorders; strenuous exercise; and emotional stress. Finally, amenorrhea can result from oral contraceptive use.

Assessment of amenorrhea begins with a thorough history and physical examination. An important but often overlooked initial step is to confirm that the woman is not pregnant. Specific components of the assessment process depend on a woman's age—adolescent, young adult, or perimenopausal—and whether or not she has previously menstruated.

Hypogonadotropic amenorrhea

Hypogonadotropic amenorrhea reflects a problem in the central hypothalamic-pituitary axis. In rare instances, a pituitary lesion or genetic inability to produce follicle-stimulating hormone (FSH) and luteinizing hormone (LH) is at fault. Once pregnancy has been ruled out, a diagnostic workup, including thyroid-stimulating hormone (TSH) and prolactin levels, x-rays or CT scan of the sella turcica, and a progestational challenge, is done to determine the cause (Kiningham, Apgar & Schwenk, 1996).

Hypogonadotropic amenorrhea often results from hypothalamic suppression as a result of two principal influences: stress (in the home, school, or workplace) or a body fat-to-lean ratio that is inappropriate for an individual woman, especially during a normal growth period. Current research on the interaction between nervous system or neurotransmitter functions and hormonal regulation throughout the body has demonstrated a biologic basis for the relation of stress to physiologic processes. Exercise-associated amenorrhea can occur in women undergoing vigorous physical and athletic training (Castiglia, 1996) and is thought to be associated with many factors, including body composition (height, weight, and percentage of body fat); type, intensity, and frequency of exercise; nutritional status; and presence of emotional or physical stressors. Amenorrhea is one of the classic signs of anorexia nervosa, and the interrelatedness of disordered eating, amenorrhea, and premature osteoporosis has been described (Golden & Shenker, 1994). Calcium loss from the bone, comparable to that seen in postmenopausal women, may occur with this type of amenorrhea.

Management. When amenorrhea is caused by hypothalamic disturbances, the nurse is an ideal health professional to assist women because many of the causes are potentially reversible (e.g., stress, weight loss for nonorganic reasons). Counseling and education are primary interventions. When a stressor known to predispose a woman to hypothalamic amenorrhea is identified, initial management involves addressing the stressor. Together the woman and nurse plan how to decrease or discontinue medications known to affect menstruation, correct weight loss, deal more effectively with psychologic stress, and eliminate substance abuse, including, for example, alcohol and marijuana.

The nurse and woman working together can identify, cope with, and possibly resolve sources of stress in the patient's life. Teaching the woman deep breathing exercises and relaxation techniques are simple, yet effective stress-reduction measures. Referral for biofeedback or massage therapy also may be useful. In some instances, referrals for psychotherapy may be indicated.

If a woman's exercise program is thought to contribute to her amenorrhea, several options exist for management. She may decide to decrease the intensity or duration of her training, if possible, or to gain some weight, if appropriate. Accepting this alternative may be difficult for one who is committed to a strenuous exercise regimen, and the nurse and patient may have several sessions before the woman elects to try exercise reduction. Many young women athletes may not understand the consequences of low bone density or osteoporosis; nurses can point out the connection between low bone density and stress fractures. The nurse and patient also should investigate other factors that may be contributing to the amenorrhea and develop plans for altering lifestyle and decreasing stress.

If amenorrhea continues after a patient has decreased her exercise level and/or gained weight and altered her lifestyle, hormonal therapy may be indicated to prevent additional problems. Because estrogen therapy in postmenopausal women has been shown to protect from bone loss that normally occurs, estrogen therapy also is used in exercise-associated amenorrhea (EAA) (Castiglia, 1996). Oral contraceptive pills (OCPs) and calcium are commonly used to treat extremely low levels of estrogen seen in EAA. OCPs have the additional advantage of providing pregnancy protection in sexually active women. Further, the few side effects of OCPs often yield higher compliance than other forms of hormonal supplementation.

Dysmenorrhea

Dysmenorrhea, or painful menstruation, is one of the most common gynecologic problems in women of all ages. Between 50% and 80% of women report some level of discomfort associated with menses and 10% to 18% report severe dysmenorrhea (Fankenauser, 1996; Fogel, 1995a); however, the amount of disruption in women's lives is difficult to determine. It has been estimated that up to 10% of women have severe enough pain to interfere with their functioning for 1 to 3 days a month (Fankenauser, 1996). Traditionally dysmenorrhea is differentiated as primary or secondary. Symptoms usually begin with menstruation, although some women experience discomfort several hours before onset of flow. The range and severity of symptoms are different from woman to woman and from cycle to cycle in the same woman. Symptoms of dysmenorrhea may last several hours or several days.

Pain is usually located in the suprapubic area or lower abdomen. Women describe the pain as sharp, cramping, or gripping or as a steady dull ache; pain may radiate to the lower back or upper thighs.

Primary dysmenorrhea

Traditionally **primary dysmenorrhea** has been defined as dysmenorrhea that occurs in the absence of anatomic abnormalities or pelvic pathology. This definition is no longer accurate because research has shown that primary dysmenorrhea has a biochemical basis and arises from the release of prostaglandins with menses. During the luteal phase and subsequent menstrual flow, prostaglandin F2 alpha ($PGF_{2\alpha}$) is secreted. Excessive release of $PGF_{2\alpha}$ increases the amplitude and frequency of uterine contractions and causes vasospasm of the uterine arterioles, resulting in ischemia and cyclic lower abdominal cramps. The degree of discomfort is related to duration of menstrual flow but not to cycle length. Systemic responses to $PGF_{2\alpha}$ include backache, weakness, sweats, gastrointestinal symptoms (anorexia, nausea, vomiting, and diarrhea), and central nervous system symptoms (dizziness, syncope, headache, and poor concentration).

Although primary dysmenorrhea is not a normal condition, it is not caused by underlying pathology; rather, it is the occurrence of a physiologic alteration in some women. Primary dysmenorrhea usually appears in 6 to 12 months after menarche when ovulation is established. Anovulatory bleeding, common in the few months or years after menarche, is painless. Because both estrogen and progesterone are necessary for primary dysmenorrhea to occur, it is experienced only with ovulatory cycles. This problem is most commonly experienced by women in their late teens and early twenties; the incidence declines with age. Contrary to what was once thought, pregnancy and parity have a variable effect. Psychogenic factors may influence symptoms, but symptoms are definitely related to ovulation and do not occur when ovulation is suppressed.

Management. Management of primary dysmenorrhea depends on the severity of the problem and the individual woman's response to various treatments. Important components of nursing care are information and support. Because menstruation is so closely linked to reproduction and sexuality, menstrual problems such as dysmenorrhea can have a negative influence on sexuality and self-worth. Nurses can do a lot to correct myths and misinformation about menstruation and dysmenorrhea by providing facts about what is normal. Nurses must support their patients' feelings of positive sexuality and self-worth.

Often more than one alternative for alleviating menstrual discomfort and dysmenorrhea can be offered, giving women options to try and decide which works best for them. Heat (heating pad or hot bath) minimizes cramping by increasing vasodilation and muscle relaxation and minimizing uterine ischemia. Massaging the lower back can reduce pain by relaxing paravertebral muscles and increasing pelvic blood supply. Soft, rhythmic rubbing of the abdomen (effleurage) may be useful because it provides distraction and an alternative focal point. Biofeedback, progressive relaxation, Hatha Yoga, and meditation also have been used successfully to decrease menstrual discomfort.

Exercise has been found to help relieve menstrual discomfort through increased vasodilation and subsequent decreased ischemia; release of endogenous opiates, specifically beta-endorphins; suppression of prostaglandins; and/or shunting of blood flow away from the viscera, resulting in less pelvic congestion. Specific exercises that nurses can suggest include pelvic rock and heels-over-the-head yoga position.

In addition to maintaining good nutrition at all times, specific dietary changes may be helpful in decreasing some of the systemic symptoms associated with dysmenorrhea. Decreased salt and refined sugar intake 7 to 10 days before expected menses may reduce fluid retention. Natural diuretics, such as asparagus, cranberry juice, peaches, parsley, or watermelon may help reduce edema and related discomforts. Decreasing red meat intake may also help to minimize dysmenorrheal symptoms. Some women with primary dysmenorrhea have reported a decrease in symptoms when they switched from a high-fat to a low-fat diet.

Medications used to treat primary dysmenorrhea include prostaglandin synthesis inhibitors, primarily nonsteroidal antiinflammatory drugs (NSAIDs) (Apgar, 1997) (Table 6-1). They are most effective if started several days before menses. All NSAIDs have potential gastrointestinal side effects, including nausea, vomiting, and indigestion. All women taking NSAIDs should be warned to report dark colored stools because this may be an indication of gastrointestinal bleeding. Women with a history of aspirin sensitivity or allergy should avoid all NSAIDs. Often if one NSAID is

TABLE 6-1	*Medications Used to Treat Dysmenorrhea (NSAIDs)*			
DRUG	**DOSAGE***	**SIDE EFFECTS†**	**COMMENTS**	**CONTRAINDICATIONS**
Aspirin‡	650-975 mg qid	Gastrointestinal irritation; tinnitus with excess dose	Not as potent a prostaglandin synthesis inhibitor as NSAIDs Do not take with NSAIDs	Hemophilia, hemorrhagic states, bleeding ulcers
Fenoprofen (Nalfon)‡	300-600 mg qid to 2,400 mg/day	Diarrhea, abdominal distention, nausea and vomiting, dyspepsia, constipation	For mild-to-moderate pain Take with meals Avoid alcohol	See aspirin
Ibuprofen (Motrin, Advil, Nuprin)	400-800 mg qid to 3,200 mg/day	Nausea, dyspepsia, rash, pruritus	Most commonly used Take with meals Do not take with aspirin Avoid alcohol Side effects more likely	See aspirin
Indomethacin (Indocin)‡	25-50 mg tid to 200 mg/day	Nausea, dyspepsia		See aspirin
Mefenamic acid (Ponstel)	500 mg initially, then 250 mg qid	Diarrhea, nausea, abdominal distention	Very potent and effective prostaglandin synthesis inhibitor Antagonizes already formed prostaglandins Increased incidence of adverse GI side effects	See aspirin
Naproxen sodium (Anaprox, Aleve)	275-550 mg bid	Nausea, abdominal distress, dyspepsia, rash, pruritus	See ibuprofen	See aspirin

Adapted from Fogel C: Common symptoms. In Fogel C & Woods N, editors: *Women's health care,* Thousand Oaks, Calif, 1995a, Sage; Facts and Comparisons: Loose-leaf drug information service, St Louis, 1995, Facts and Comparisons.
qid, Four times a day; *tid,* three times a day; *GI,* gastrointestinal; *bid,* two times a day.
*Dosages are current recommendations and should be verified before use. Recommended dosage for over-the-counter preparations are generally less than recommendations for therapeutic dosage.
†Risk with all NSAIDs is gastrointestinal ulceration, possible bleeding, and prolonged bleeding time. Incidence of side effects is dose related. Reported incidence 3% to 9%.
‡Unlabeled indications for use in treating dysmenorrhea.

ineffective, a different one may be effective. If the second drug is unsuccessful after a 4-month trial, OCPs may be used. OCPs inhibit ovulation and thus decrease menstrual cramps and bleeding (see Chapter 7).

OCPs prevent ovulation and can decrease the amount of menstrual flow, which can decrease the amount of prostaglandin, thus decreasing dysmenorrhea. OCPs may be used in place of NSAIDs if the woman wants oral contraception and has primary dysmenorrhea. It should be remembered that OCPs have side effects and women who do not need them or want them may not wish to use them for dysmenorrhea. OCPs also may be contraindicated for some women.

Before the development of NSAIDs, numerous medications were used to treat dysmenorrhea, including narcotics, antispasmodics, tranquilizers, amphetamines, and diuretics. Because of their potential harmful effects or undocumented effectiveness, these should no longer be used for the treatment of dysmenorrhea.

Over-the-counter (OTC) preparations that are indicated for primary dysmenorrhea include the same active ingredients (e.g., ibuprofen, naproxen sodium) as prescription preparations. However, the labeled recommended dose may be subtherapeutic. Preparations containing acetaminophen are even less effective because acetaminophen does not have the antiprostaglandin properties of NSAIDs.

Secondary dysmenorrhea

Secondary dysmenorrhea is acquired menstrual pain that developed later in life than primary dysmenorrhea, typically after age 25. It is associated with pelvic pathology such as adenomyosis, endometriosis, pelvic inflammatory disease (PID), endometrial polyps, submucous or interstitial myomas (fibroids), or use of intrauterine devices (IUD). Pain often begins a few days before menses, but it can be present at ovulation and continue through the first days of menses or start after menstrual flow has begun. In contrast to primary dysmenorrhea, the pain of secondary dysmenorrhea is often characterized by dull, lower abdominal aching radiating to back or thighs. Often women experience feelings of bloating or pelvic fullness. Treatment is directed toward removal of the underlying pathology. Many of the measures described for pain relief of primary dysmenorrhea are also helpful for women with secondary dysmenorrhea.

Premenstrual Syndrome

Although almost all women experience minor physical and emotional changes preceding menstruation, a much smaller percentage (estimated at about 5%) experience physical or psychologic symptoms that become severe or temporarily disabling during the premenstrual phase. These experiences have been categorized as premenstrual syndrome (PMS).

Premenstrual syndrome is a constellation of physical and psychologic symptoms beginning in the luteal phase of the menstrual cycle (ACOG, 1995). Symptoms associated include: fluid retention (abdominal bloating, pelvic fullness, edema of the lower extremities, breast tenderness, and weight gain); behavioral or emotional changes (depression, crying spells, irritability, panic attacks, and impaired ability to concentrate); premenstrual cravings (sweets, salt, increased appetite, and food binges); and headache, fatigue, and backache. In contrast, some women experience a heightened sense of creativity and increased mental and physical energy. A diagnosis of PMS is made only if the following criteria are met:

- Symptoms occur in the luteal phase and resolve within a few days of menses onset.
- Symptom-free period occurs in follicular phase.
- Symptoms are recurrent.

The cause of PMS is unknown. Theories include serotonin system dysfunction, estrogen and progesterone changes, circadian rhythm abnormalities, and vitamin (vitamin B_6) and mineral (e.g., magnesium, calcium, and zinc) deficiencies (Fankenauser, 1996).

There is much controversy regarding PMS. Its existence, diagnosis, and etiology are hotly and widely debated. Readers are encouraged to explore current feminist, medical, and social science literature for more information on these topics.

Management

There is little agreement on management. A careful, detailed history and daily log of symptoms and mood fluctuations spanning several cycles may give direction to a plan of management. Diet and exercise changes are a useful way to begin and may provide symptom relief for some women. Nurses can suggest that women limit consumption of refined sugar (<5 tbs/day), salt (<3 g/day), red meat (up to 3 oz/day), alcohol (less than 1 oz/day), and caffeinated beverages. Women can be encouraged to include whole grains, legumes, seeds, nuts, vegetables, fruits, and vegetable oils in

their diet. Use of natural diuretics may help reduce fluid retention as well. Nutritional supplements may assist in symptom relief. Calcium, magnesium, and vitamin E have been shown to be moderately effective in relieving symptoms, to have few side effects, and to be safe. However, Vitamin B_6, once widely recommended, is not an effective form of PMS treatment (Carter & Verhoef, 1994). Daily supplements of evening primrose oil are thought to be useful in relieving breast symptoms with minimal side effects. Exercise has been recommended widely for relief of PMS symptoms. Women who exercise regularly seem to have less premenstrual anxiety than nonathletic women do. It is thought that aerobic exercise increases beta-endorphin levels to offset symptoms of depression and elevate mood. Exercise programs should be at least 30 minutes long for at least 4 times a week. A monthly program that varies in intensity and type of exercise according to PMS symptoms is recommended.

Counseling, in the form of support groups or individual/couple counseling, may be helpful. Stress-reduction techniques may also assist with symptoms management (Baker, 1998).

If these strategies do not provide significant symptom relief in 1 to 2 months, medication is often begun. Many medications have been used in treating PMS. At present no one medication alleviates all PMS symptoms. Medications often used in the treatment of PMS include diuretics, prostaglandin inhibitors (NSAIDs), progesterone, and OCPs. Selective serotonin reuptake inhibitors (SSRIs) (e.g., fluoxetine [Prozac] and clomipramine [Anafranil]) are often used for PMS with a resultant decrease in emotional symptoms, especially depression (Baker, 1998; Chandraiah, 1996). Melfenamic acid (250 mg daily during the luteal phase of the menstrual cycle) may relieve or resolve many symptoms, specifically fatigue, headaches, general aches and pains, and mood swings (Chuong, Pearsall-Otley & Rosenfeld, 1995). Bromocriptine (5 mg daily at night from days 10 to 26 of the cycle) helps reduce breast tenderness and swelling.

Endometriosis

Endometriosis is characterized by the presence and growth of endometrial tissue outside of the uterus. The tissue may be implanted on the ovaries, cul-de-sac, uterine ligaments, rectovaginal septum, sigmoid colon, pelvic peritoneum, cervix, and/or inguinal area (Fig. 6-1). Endometrial lesions have been found in the vagina and surgical scars; on the vulva, perineum, and bladder; and in sites far from the pelvic area such as the thoracic cavity, gallbladder, and heart. A chocolate cyst is a cystic area of endometriosis in the ovary. The dark coloring of the cyst's contents is caused by old blood.

Endometrial tissue contains glands and stoma and responds to cyclic hormonal stimulation in the same way that the uterine endometrium does but often out of phase with it. During the proliferative and secretory phases of the

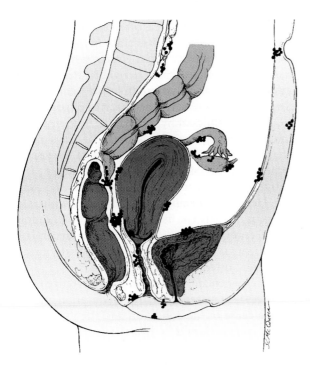

Fig. **6-1** Common sites of endometriosis. (From Mishell D et al.: *Comprehensive gynecology*, ed 3, St Louis, 1997, Mosby.)

cycle, the endometrial tissue grows. During or immediately after menstruation, the tissue bleeds, resulting in an inflammatory response with subsequent fibrosis and adhesions to adjacent organs.

Endometriosis is a common gynecologic problem affecting between 1.7 and 5.6 million American women and accounting for about 40,000 hysterectomies each year (Ryan & Taylor, 1997). While the condition usually develops in the third or fourth decade of life, endometriosis has been found in adolescents with disabling pelvic pain or abnormal vaginal bleeding. The condition occurs across all socioeconomic levels (Sangi-Haghpeykar & Poindexter, 1995). The condition is found equally in Caucasian and African-American women and is slightly more prevalent in Asian women. Endometriosis may worsen with repeated cycles, or it may remain asymptomatic and undiagnosed, eventually disappearing after menopause.

Several theories to account for the cause of endometriosis have been suggested, yet the etiology and pathology of this condition continue to be poorly understood. One of the most widely accepted, long-debated theories is transtubal migration or retrograde menstruation. According to this theory, endometrial tissue is regurgitated or mechanically transported from the uterus during menstruation to the uterine tubes and into the peritoneal cavity, where it implants on the ovaries and other organs. Recent assisted reproductive technology (ART) data suggest that patients with endometriosis also have ovulatory dysfunction (Ryan & Taylor, 1997).

Symptoms vary among women and change over time. The major symptom is dysmenorrhea. Women also experience chronic noncyclic pelvic pain, pelvic heaviness, or pain radiating into the thighs. Many women report bowel symptoms such as diarrhea, pain with defecation, and constipation secondary to avoiding defecation because of the pain. Less common symptoms include pain on exercise or during intercourse (dyspareunia) as a result of adhesions, and intermenstrual bleeding. Impaired fertility may result from adhesions around the uterus that pull the uterus into a fixed, retroverted position. Adhesions around the uterine tubes may block the fimbriated ends or prevent the spontaneous movement that carries the ovum to the uterus.

Management

Treatment is based on the severity of symptoms and the goals of the woman or couple. Women without pain who do not want to become pregnant need no treatment. Women with mild pain who may desire a future pregnancy may require analgesics. Those who have severe pain and can postpone pregnancy may be treated with combined oral contraceptives to shrink endometrial tissue. Often the daily dosage has to be increased to 2 to 3 pills to maintain amenorrhea. Side effects such as nausea, edema, and breakthrough bleeding often lead to discontinuation of therapy. Because of the increased risk of deep vein thrombosis with this therapy, patients should be warned of possible side effects and danger signs, (e.g., abdominal pain, severe headache, and leg pain) (Lu & Ory, 1995). When this therapy is stopped, women often experience high rates of recurrence of pain and other symptoms.

Hormonal antagonists that suppress ovulation and reduce endogenous estrogen production and subsequent endometrial lesion growth have been used to treat mild-to-severe endometriosis in women who wish to become pregnant. Gonadotropin-releasing hormone (Gn-RH) agonist therapy (Leuprolide, Synarel, Zoladex) acts by suppressing pituitary gonadotropin secretion. FSH/LH stimulation to the ovary declines notably, and ovarian function decreases significantly. The hypoestrogenism results in hot flashes in almost all women. In addition, there may be minor bone loss, most of which is reversible within 12 to 18 months after the medication is stopped. Leuprolide (3.75 mg intramuscular injection given once a month) or nafarelin (200 mg administered twice daily by nasal spray) are both effective and well tolerated. Both medications reduce endometrial lesions and pelvic pain associated with endometriosis and have posttreatment pregnancy rates similar to that of danazol therapy (Garner, 1994). Common side effects of these drugs are those of natural menopause—hot flashes and vaginal dryness. Occasionally women report headaches and muscle aches.

Danazol (Danocrine), a mildly androgenic synthetic steroid, suppresses FSH and LH secretion, thus producing anovulation and hypogonadotropinism with resulting decreased secretion of estrogen and progesterone and regression of endometrial tissue. This medication was widely used to treat endometriosis in the 1970s and 1980s. Danazol can produce side effects that may cause a woman to discontinue using the drug. Side effects include masculinizing traits in the woman—weight gain, edema, decreased breast size, oily skin, hirsutism, and deepening of the voice—all of which often disappear when treatment is discontinued. Other side effects are amenorrhea, hot flashes, vaginal dryness, insomnia, and decreased libido. Migraine headaches, dizziness, fatigue, and depression are also reported. Further, decreases in bone density have been noted that may be only partially reversible. Danazol should never be prescribed when pregnancy is suspected, and contraception should be used with it because ovulation may not be suppressed. Danazol can produce pseudohermaphroditism in female fetuses. The drug is contraindicated in women with liver disease and should be used with caution in women with cardiac and renal disease. Because it is an expensive drug, danazol may not be available to all women.

Surgical intervention is often needed for severe, acute, or incapacitating symptoms. Decisions regarding the extent and type of surgery are influenced by a woman's age, desire for children, and location of the disease. For women who do not want to preserve their ability to have children, the only definite cure is hysterectomy and bilateral salpingo-oophorectomy (total abdominal hysterectomy [TAH] with BSO). For those women in their childbearing years who want children and in whom the disease does not prevent it, reproductive capacity should be retained through careful removal of all endometrial tissue possible by surgery or laser therapy, with retention of ovarian function (Garner, 1995).

Short of TAH with BSO, endometriosis recurs in approximately 40% of women, regardless of the form of treatment. Thus for many women, endometriosis is a chronic disease with conditions such as chronic pain or infertility. Counseling and education are critical components of nursing care of women with endometriosis. Women need an honest discussion of treatment options with potential risks and benefits of each option reviewed. Because pelvic pain is a subjective, personal experience that can be frightening, support is very important. Sexual dysfunction resulting from painful intercourse (dyspareunia) may be present and may necessitate referral for counseling. Support groups for women with endometriosis may be found in some locations. The nursing care measures discussed in the section on dysmenorrhea are appropriate for managing chronic pelvic pain associated with endometriosis.

Alterations in Cyclic Bleeding

Women often experience changes in amount, duration, interval, or regularity of menstrual cycle bleeding. Often women worry about menstruation that is short, of a small amount, or occurs too frequently.

The term **oligomenorrhea** often is used to describe decreased menstruation, either in amount or time, or both. However, oligomenorrhea more correctly refers to infrequent menstrual periods characterized by intervals of 40 to 45 days or longer, and **hypomenorrhea** refers to scanty bleeding at normal intervals. The causes of oligomenorrhea are often abnormalities of hypothalamic, pituitary, or ovarian function. Oligomenorrhea also can be physiologic or part of a woman's normal pattern for the first few years after menarche or for several years before menopause.

Treatment is aimed at reversing the underlying cause, if possible. Hormonal therapy using progestins, with or without estrogens, may also be used to prevent complications of unopposed estrogen production (endometrial hyperplasia or carcinoma) or of absent estrogen (vaginal dryness, hot flashes/flushes, osteoporosis).

Women experiencing menstruation characterized by prolonged intervals between cycles need education and counseling. The cause of the condition and the rationale for a specific treatment should be discussed, as should advantages and disadvantages of hormonal therapy. If a woman chooses medical intervention, she should be provided with written instructions, taught how to take the medications, and made aware of side effects of any drugs. Teaching and counseling should emphasize the importance of the woman keeping careful records of her vaginal bleeding.

One of the most common causes of scanty menstrual flow is OCPs. If a woman is considering OCPs for contraception, it is important that the nurse explain in advance that the use of OCPs can decrease menstrual flow by as much as two thirds. This effect is caused by the continuous action of the progestin component, which produces a decidualized endometrium with atrophic glands.

Hypomenorrhea also may be caused by structural abnormalities of the endometrium or uterus that result in partial destruction of the endometrium. These conditions include Asherman's syndrome, in which adhesions resulting from curettage or infection obliterate the endometrial cavity, and congenital partial obstruction of the vagina.

Metrorrhagia or intermenstrual bleeding refers to any episode of bleeding, whether spotting, menses, or hemorrhage, that occurs at a time other than the normal menses. *Mittlestaining*, a small amount of bleeding or spotting that occurs at the time of ovulation (14 days before onset of next menses), is considered normal. The cause of mittlestaining is not known; however, it is a common occurrence that can be documented by its repetition in the menstrual cycle. Women taking OCPs may experience midcycle bleeding or spotting. (See Chapter 7.) If the contraceptive pill does not sufficiently maintain a hypoplastic endometrium, it will begin to shed, usually in small amounts at a time, a process called "breakthrough bleeding." Breakthrough bleeding is most common in the first three cycles of OCPs. The lowered potency of OCPs (resulting in increased safety) has decreased the amount of available hormones, making it more important that blood levels be kept constant. Suggesting that women take their pill at exactly the same time each day may alleviate the problem. If the spotting continues, a different formulation of OCP that increases either the estrogen or progestin component of the pill can be tried.

Contraceptive implants, such as Norplant, that are filled with synthetic progestin also may cause midcycle bleeding, especially in the first several cycles after implantation. Women should be advised of this and counseled to report continuation of breakthrough bleeding after the first three to six cycles to their health care provider. Women with an intrauterine device (IUD) may experience spotting between their periods and heavier menstrual flow.

The causes of intermenstrual bleeding are varied. It is important that the nurse always consider the possibility that a woman is, or recently has been, pregnant when a woman seeks care for intermenstrual bleeding.

Treatment of intermenstrual bleeding depends on the cause and may include reassurance and education concerning mittlestaining through observation of three menstrual cycles for presumed functional ovarian cyst, adjustment of an oral contraceptive, removal of IUDs, and treatment for vaginal infections. More complex treatment may consist of removal of polyps; evaluation and treatment of abnormal Pap smear, including colposcopy, biopsy, cautery, cryosurgery, and/or conization; and finally surgery, chemotherapy, and radiation treatment for malignancy. Important nursing roles include reassurance, counseling, education, and support.

Menorrhagia (hypermenorrhea) is defined as excessive menstrual bleeding, either in duration or amount. The causes of heavy menstrual bleeding are many, including hormonal disturbances, systemic disease, benign and malignant neoplasms, infection, and contraception (IUDs). A single episode of heavy bleeding may occur, or a woman may experience regular flooding as a pattern in which she changes tampons or pads every few hours for several days. If the woman herself considers the amount or duration of bleeding to be excessive, the problem should be investigated. Hemoglobin and hematocrit are objective indicators of actual blood loss and should always be assessed.

A single episode of heavy bleeding may signal an early pregnancy loss such as a spontaneous abortion or ectopic pregnancy. This type of bleeding is often thought to be a period that is heavier than usual, perhaps delayed, and is associated with abdominal pain or pelvic discomfort. When early pregnancy loss is suspected, a hematocrit and pregnancy test should be done.

Infectious and inflammatory processes such as acute or chronic endometritis and salpingitis may cause heavy menstrual bleeding. Although rare, systemic diseases of nonreproductive origin such as blood dyscrasias, cirrhosis of the liver, and renal disease also can cause hypermenorrhea. Medications also may cause abnormal bleeding. Chemotherapy, anticoagulants, neuroleptics, major tranquilizers, and steroid hormone therapy all have been associated with excessive menstrual flow.

Uterine **leiomyoma** (fibroids or myomas) are a common cause of menorrhagia. Fibroids are benign tumors of the smooth muscle of the uterus whose etiology is unknown. Fibroids occur in a quarter of women of reproductive age; the incidence of fibroids is three to nine times higher in African-American women (Speroff, Glass & Kase, 1994). Other uterine growths ranging from endometrial polyps to adenocarcinoma and endometrial cancer are common causes of heavy menstrual bleeding, as well as intermenstrual bleeding.

Nonsteroidal antiinflammatory drugs (NSAIDs) are often used to treat menorrhagia because they increase vasoconstriction and improve platelet aggregation (Rosenfeld, 1996). The cause of the bleeding also determines treatment. If the bleeding is related to contraceptive method, the nurse provides factual information and reassurance and discusses other contraceptive options. The degree of disability and discomfort associated with fibroids and the woman's plans for childbearing will influence treatment decisions. Most fibroids can be followed by frequent examinations to judge growth, if any, and correction of anemia, if present. Women with menorrhagia should be warned not to use aspirin because of its tendency to increase bleeding. Hormonal therapy may be tried in an effort to reduce the size of the tumors. If the woman wishes to have children, a myomectomy may be done. Myomectomy, or removal of the tumors only, is particularly difficult if multiple myomas must be removed. If the woman does not want to preserve her childbearing function or if she has severe symptoms (severe anemia, severe pain, considerable disruption of lifestyle), hysterectomy or endometrial ablation (laser surgery or electrocoagulation used to destroy endometrial tissue) may be done.

Dysfunctional uterine bleeding

Dysfunctional uterine bleeding (DUB) refers to a wide variety of menstrual irregularities, but most often is associated with excessive bleeding of some type: flow that is too frequent, too heavy, too prolonged, or irregular. DUB is most commonly caused by anovulation. When there is no surge of LH or if insufficient progesterone is produced by the corpus luteum to support the endometrium, it will begin to involute and shed. This most often occurs at the extremes of a woman's reproductive years—when the menstrual cycle is just becoming established at menarche or when it draws to a close at menopause (Mehring, 1997). DUB can also be found with any condition that gives rise to chronic anovulation associated with continuous estrogen production. Such conditions include obesity, hyperthyroidism and hypothyroidism, polycystic ovarian syndrome, and any of the endocrine conditions discussed in the sections on amenorrhea and oligomenorrhea. A diagnosis of DUB is made only after all other causes of abnormal menstrual bleeding have been ruled out (Rosenfeld, 1996).

When uterine bleeding is severe, the woman may be hospitalized and given conjugated estrogens (Premarin) 25 mg intravenously, every 4 hours until bleeding stops or slows significantly (up to 3 doses) (Speroff, Glass & Kase, 1994). Following this, oral conjugated estrogen 2.5 mg to 3.75 mg is given for 21 days. During the last 7 to 10 days of the estrogen regimen, progesterone (e.g., medroxyprogesterone [Provera] 10 mg po) is added. Alternatively, a combined OCP is given for 21 days after intravenous therapy (Starr, Lommel & Shanon, 1995). Once the acute phase has passed, the woman is maintained on cyclic, low-dose oral contraceptives for at least 3 months. If she wants contraception, she should continue to take OCPs. If she has no need for contraception, the treatment may be stopped in order to assess the woman's bleeding pattern. If her menses does not resume, a progestin regimen (e.g., Provera, 10 mg each day, for 10 days before the expected date of her menstrual period) may be prescribed after ruling out pregnancy. This is done to prevent persistent anovulation (Mehring, 1997) with chronic unopposed endogenous estrogen hyperstimulation of the endometrium, which can result in eventual atypical tissue changes. Such long-term treatment also helps prevent recurrence of the pattern of DUB and hemorrhage.

If the recurrent, heavy bleeding is not controlled by hormonal therapy, ablation of the endometrium through laser treatment may be performed. Nursing roles include informing patients of their options, counseling and education as indicated, and referring to the appropriate specialists and health care services.

I CARE MANAGEMENT

Assessment and Nursing Diagnoses

In addition to taking a careful menstrual, obstetric, sexual, and contraceptive history, the nurse should explore the woman's perceptions of her condition, cultural or ethnic influences, experiences with other caregivers, lifestyle, and patterns of coping. The amount of pain and/or bleeding experienced and its effect on daily activities should be evaluated. Home remedies and prescriptions to relieve discomfort are noted. A symptom diary, in which the woman records emotions, behaviors, physical symptoms, diet, and exercise and rest patterns, is a useful diagnostic tool. Nursing diagnoses for the woman experiencing menstrual disorders are listed in the accompanying box.

I Nursing Diagnoses

Women Experiencing Menstrual Disorders
Risk for ineffective individual or family coping related to:
* Insufficient knowledge of the cause of the disorder
* Emotional and physiologic effects of the disorder

Knowledge deficit related to:
* Self-care
* Available therapy for the disorder
Risk for body image disturbance related to:
* Menstrual disorder
* Sexual dysfunction
Risk for low self-esteem related to:
* Others' perception of her discomfort
* Inability to conceive
Pain related to:
* Menstrual disorder

Expected Outcomes of Care

After data collection and review, mutual expected outcomes are established and a plan of care is developed. Expected outcomes for the woman are that she will:
* Verbalize her understanding of reproductive anatomy, etiology of her disorder, medication regimen, and diary use.
* Verbalize understanding and accept her emotional and physical responses to her menstrual cycle.
* Develop personal goals that benefit her emotionally and physically.
* Choose appropriate therapeutic measures for her menstrual problems.
* Adapt successfully to the condition, if cure is not possible.

Plan of Care and Interventions

During the history and diagnostic workup, the clinician's concern and acceptance of the woman's symptoms as valid are in themselves therapeutic. Data from the daily diary of emotional status, subjective feelings, and physical state are correlated with physiologic changes. If the woman has a partner, both the woman and her partner keep separate diaries that include how each perceives the other's responses day by day. Through the diaries, feelings are vented, problems are identified and clarified, insights occur, and possible solutions begin to develop. The clinician facilitates insights and suggests therapeutic options. The woman (couple) makes choices considered best for her (them). Nurses need to discuss the options available to women with menstrual disorders. They must understand basic information about the anatomy and physiology, pathophysiology, psychologic impact, and treatment for the condition.

Support groups are an important resource. Nurses can use a local women's center or clinic to bring together women who want to learn more about their condition and support each other.

Evaluation

The nurse can be assured that care has been effective when the woman reports improvement in the quality of her life, skill in self-care, and a positive self-concept and body image.

| INFECTIONS

Infections of the reproductive tract can occur throughout a woman's life and are often the cause of significant morbidity and mortality. The direct economic costs of these infections can be substantial and the indirect cost equally overwhelming. Some consequences of maternal infection such as infertility last a lifetime. The emotional costs may include damaged relationships and lowered self-esteem.

Sexually Transmitted Diseases

Sexually transmitted diseases (STDs) or **sexually transmitted infections (STIs)** are infections or infectious disease syndromes primarily transmitted by sexual contact (Box 6-1). Caused by a wide spectrum of bacteria, viruses, protozoa, and ectoparasites (organisms that live on the outside of the body such as a louse), STDs are a direct cause of tremendous human suffering, place heavy demands on health care services, and cost hundreds of millions of dollars to treat (Fogel, 1995b). The term "STD" is not specific for any one disease; rather, the term includes more than 25 infectious organisms that are transmitted through sexual activity and the dozens of clinical syndromes that they cause (Eng & Butler, 1997). Despite the U.S. Surgeon General targeting STDs as a priority for prevention and control efforts, STDs are among the most common health problems in the United States today (Eng & Butler, 1997). The CDC estimates that more than 12 million Americans are infected with STDs every year (CDC, DSTD/HIVP, 1995). The most common STDs in women, chlamydia, human papilloma virus, gonorrhea, herpes simplex virus type-2, syphilis, and human immunodeficiency virus (HIV) infection, are discussed in this chapter. Effects on pregnancy and the fetus are discussed in Chapter 24. Neonatal effects are discussed in Chapter 28.

Prevention of STDs

Preventing infection (primary prevention) is the most effective way of reducing the adverse consequences of STDs for women. With the advent of serious and potentially lethal STDs that are not readily cured or are incurable, primary prevention becomes critical. Prompt diagnosis and treatment of current infections (secondary prevention) also can prevent personal complications and transmission to others.

Primary preventive measures are individual activities aimed at deterring infection. Risk-free options include complete abstinence from sexual activities that transmit semen, blood, or other body fluids, or that allow for skin-to-skin contact. Alternatively, involvement in a mutually monogamous relationship with an uninfected partner also eliminates risk of contracting an STD. When neither of these options is realistic for a woman, however, the nurse must focus on other, more feasible measures.

To be motivated to take preventive actions, a woman must believe that catching a disease will be serious for her and that she is at risk for infection. Unfortunately most

| BOX 6-1 | *STDs* |

BACTERIA
Chlamydia
Gonorrhea
Syphilis
Chancroid
Lymphogranuloma venereum
Genital mycoplasmas
Group B streptococci

VIRUSES
Human immunodeficiency virus
Herpes simplex virus, types 1 and 2
Cytomegalovirus
Viral hepatitis A and B
Human papillomavirus

PROTOZOA
Trichomoniasis

PARASITES
Pediculosis*
Scabies*

*This may or may not be sexually transmitted.

individuals tend to underestimate their personal risk of infection in a given situation. Thus many women may not perceive themselves as at risk for contracting an STD, and telling them that they need to carry condoms may not be well received. Though levels of awareness of STDs are generally high, widespread misconceptions or specific gaps in knowledge also exist. Therefore nurses have a responsibility to ensure that their patients have accurate, complete knowledge about transmission and symptoms of STDs and behaviors that place them at risk for contracting an infection.

Safer sex practices. An essential component of primary prevention is counseling women regarding safer sex practices, including knowledge of her partner, reduction of number of partners, low-risk sex, and avoiding the exchange of body fluids.

No aspect of prevention is more important than knowing one's partner. Reducing the number of partners and avoiding partners who have had many previous sexual partners decreases a woman's chance of contracting an STD. Deciding not to have sexual contact with casual acquaintances also may be helpful. Discussing each new partner's previous sexual history and exposure to STDs will augment other efforts to reduce risk. Critically important is whether or not male partners resist wearing condoms. This is crucial when women are not sure about their partner's history. Counseling on ways to negotiate with the partner about condom use may be helpful. The nurse may also suggest that women carefully examine a partner for lesions, sores, ulcerations, rashes, redness, discharge, swelling, and odor before initiating sexual activity.

TABLE 6-2   *Safer Sex Guidelines*

SAFEST	LOW RISK	POSSIBLY RISKY (POSSIBLE EXPOSURE)	HIGH-RISK (UNSAFE)
Behavior: Abstinence Self-masturbation Monogamous (both partners and no high-risk activities) Hugging,* massage,* touching* Dry kissing Mutual masturbation Drug abstinence	*Behavior:* Wet kissing Vaginal intercourse with condom Anal intercourse with condom Fellatio interruptus Urine contact with intact skin	*Behavior:* Cunnilingus[†] Fellatio[‡] Mutual masturbation with skin breaks Vaginal intercourse after anal contact without new condom	*Behavior:* Unprotected anal intercourse Unprotected vaginal intercourse Oral-anal contact Fisting Multiple sexual partners Sharing sex toys, douche equipment Sharing needles
Prevention: Avoid high-risk behaviors	*Prevention:* Avoid exposure to potentially infected body fluids Consistent use of condom and spermicide Avoid anal intercourse	*Prevention:* Use dental dam or female condom with cunnilingus Use condom with fellatio Use latex gloves	*Prevention:* Avoid exposure to potentially infected body fluids Use condom and spermicide consistently Avoid anal penetration If anal penetration occurs, use condom with intercourse, latex glove with hand penetration Avoid oral-anal contact Do not share sex toys, needles, douching equipment If sharing needles, clean with bleach before and after use.

Adapted from Fogel C: Common Symptoms. In Fogel C & Woods N, editors: *Women's health care,* Thousand Oaks, Calif, 1995b, Sage.
*Assumes no breaks in skin.
[†]Cunnilingus: oral stimulation of the female genitalia.
[‡]Fellatio: oral stimulation of the male genitalia.

Women should be taught low-risk sexual practices and which sexual practices to avoid (Table 6-2). Mutual masturbation is low risk as long as bodily fluids only come in contact with intact skin. Caressing, hugging, body rubbing, massage, and hand-to-genital touching are low-risk behaviors. Currently, the sole physical barrier promoted for the prevention of sexual transmission of HIV and other STD infection is the condom. Nurses can encourage women to use condoms by first discussing the subject with them. Such a discussion gives women permission to discuss any concerns, misconceptions or hesitations they may have about using condoms. Women need to know how to purchase and use condoms. Information to be discussed includes importance of using latex rather than natural skin condoms and using only condoms with a reservoir that are lubricated with nonoxynol-9. The nurse should remind women to use only condoms with a current expiration date and to store them away from high heat. Contrary to popular myth, studies have found no increase in breakage after carrying condoms in a wallet for a lengthy period of time. Though not ideal, women may choose to safely carry condoms in wallets, shoes, or inside a bra. Women can be taught the differences among condoms, price ranges, sizes, and where they can be purchased. Instructions for how to apply a condom are found in Chapter 7. Women should be reminded to use a condom only one time and with every sexual encounter.

Women should be counseled to watch out for situations that make it hard to talk about and practice safer sex. These include romantic times when condoms are not available and when alcohol or drugs make it difficult to make wise decisions about safer sex.

Certain sexual practices should be avoided in order to reduce one's risk of infection. Abstinence from any sexual activities that could result in exchange of infective body fluids will help decrease risk. Anal-genital intercourse, anal-oral contact, and anal digital activity are high-risk sexual behaviors and should be avoided.

Bacterial STDs

Chlamydial infection

Chlamydia trachomatis is the most common and fastest spreading STD in American women with an estimated 2.6 million new cases each year (Eng & Butler, 1997). These infections are often silent and very destructive; their sequelae and complications can be very serious. In women, chlamydial infections are difficult to diagnose; the symptoms, if present, are nonspecific and the organism expensive to culture.

Acute salpingitis or PID is the most serious complication of chlamydial infections. Past chlamydial infections are associated with an increased risk of ectopic pregnancy and tubal factor infertility. Further, chlamydial infection of the cervix causes inflammation, resulting in microscopic cervical ulcerations that may increase risk of acquiring HIV infection.

Sexually active women younger than 20 years are two to three times more likely to become infected with chlamydia than women between 20 and 29 years. Women over age 30 have the lowest rate of infection. Risky behaviors, including multiple partners and not using barrier methods of birth control, increase a woman's risk of chlamydial infection. Lower socioeconomic status may be a risk factor, especially with respect to treatment-seeking behaviors.

Diagnosis. In addition to obtaining information regarding the presence of risk factors, the nurse should inquire about the presence of any symptoms. Centers for Disease Control and Prevention (CDC, 1998) strongly urges screening of sexually active adolescents, women between the ages of 20 and 34 years, women who do not use barrier contraceptives, and women with new or multiple partners.

Although usually asymptomatic, some women may experience spotting or postcoital bleeding, mucoid or purulent cervical discharge, or dysuria. Bleeding results from inflammation and erosion of the cervical columnar epithelium.

Diagnosis of chlamydia is by culture, which is expensive, requires special transport and storage, and up to 10 days for results. Special culture media and proper handling of specimens are important, so the nurse should always know what is required in her individual practice site.

Management. Treatment recommendations for chlamydia include azithromycin, doxycycline or erythromycin (CDC, 1998). Because chlamydia is often asymptomatic, the patient should be cautioned to take all medication prescribed. All exposed sexual partners should be treated. Women treated with doxycycline or azithromycin do not need to be retested unless symptoms continue. Women treated with erythromycin may be retested 3 weeks after completing the medication.

Gonorrhea

Gonorrhea is probably the oldest communicable disease in the United States. An estimated 600,000 American men and women contract gonorrhea each year. Gonorrhea is caused by the aerobic, gram-negative diplococci *Neisseria gonorrhoeae*. Gonorrhea is almost exclusively transmitted by the contact of sexual activity. The principal means of communication is genital-to-genital contact; however, it is also spread by oral-to-genital and anal-to-genital contact. Gonorrhea also can be transmitted to the newborn in the form of ophthalmia neonatorum during birth by direct contact with gonococcal organisms in the cervix. Although the organism has been recovered from inanimate objects artificially inoculated with the bacteria, there is no evidence that natural transmission occurs this way (Schaffer, 1998).

Age is probably the most important risk factor associated with gonorrhea. The majority of those contracting gonorrhea are under age 20 years. Other risk factors include early onset of sexual activity and multiple sexual partners.

Women are often asymptomatic, but when symptomatic, they may have a greenish-yellow purulent endocervical discharge or may experience menstrual irregularities. Women may complain of pain, chronic or acute severe pelvic or lower abdominal pain, or longer, more painful menses. Gonococcal rectal infection may occur in women following anal intercourse. Individuals with rectal gonorrhea may be completely asymptomatic or, conversely, experience severe symptoms with profuse purulent anal discharge, rectal pain, and blood in the stool. Rectal itching, fullness, pressure, or pain also are common symptoms, as is diarrhea. A diffuse vaginitis with vulvitis is the most common form of gonococcal infection in prepubertal girls. There may be few signs of infection; or vaginal discharge, dysuria, and swollen, reddened labia may be present.

Diagnosis. Gonococcal infection cannot be diagnosed reliably by clinical signs and symptoms alone. Individuals may present with "classic" symptoms, with vague symptoms that may be attributed to a number of conditions, or with no symptoms at all. Cultures are considered the "gold standard" for diagnosis of gonorrhea. Cultures should be obtained from the endocervix, rectum, and when indicated, the pharynx. Thayer-Martin cultures are recommended to diagnose gonorrhea in women. Because STDs tend to coexist, any woman suspected of having gonorrhea should have a chlamydial culture and serologic test for syphilis if one has not been done in the past 2 months.

Management. Management of gonorrhea is straightforward, and the cure is usually rapid with appropriate antibiotic therapy. Single-dose efficacy is a major consideration in selecting an antibiotic regimen for women with gonorrhea. Another important consideration is the high percentage (45%) of women with coexisting chlamydial infections. The recommended treatment is ceftriaxone and azithromycin or doxycycline (CDC, 1998). The CDC also suggests concomitant treatment for chlamydia because coinfection is common. All patients with gonorrhea should be offered confidential counseling and testing for HIV-infection.

Gonorrhea is a highly communicable disease. Recent (past 30 days) sexual partners should be examined, cultured, and treated with appropriate regimens. Most treatment failures result from reinfection: the woman needs to be informed of this, as well as of the consequences of reinfection in terms of chronicity, complications, and potential infertility. Women are counseled to have their partners use condoms.

Gonorrhea is a reportable communicable disease. Health care providers are legally responsible for reporting all cases to the health authorities, usually the local health department in the woman's county of residence. Women should be informed that the case will be reported, told why, and informed of the possibility of being contacted by a health department epidemiologist.

Syphilis

Syphilis, one of the earliest described STDs, is caused by *Treponema pallidum,* a motile spirochete. Transmission is thought to be by entry in the subcutaneous tissue through microscopic abrasions that can occur during sexual intercourse. The disease can also be transmitted through kissing, biting, or oral-genital sex. Transplacental transmission may occur at any time during pregnancy; the degree of risk is related to the quantity of spirochetes in the maternal bloodstream.

There are more than 100,000 new cases of syphilis in the United States each year (Eng & Butler, 1997). Rates are highest among young adult African-Americans in urban areas and in southern states. Much of the rise in cases seen since 1990 is directly attributable to illicit drug use—particularly crack cocaine—and the exchange of sex for drugs and money.

Syphilis is a complex disease that can lead to serious systemic disease and even death if untreated. Infection manifests itself in distinct stages with different symptoms and clinical manifestations. *Primary* syphilis is characterized by a primary lesion, the chancre, that appears 5 to 90 days after infection; this lesion often begins as a painless papule at the site of inoculation and then erodes to form a nontender, shallow, indurated, clean ulcer several millimeters to centimeters in size (Fig. 6-2, *A*). *Secondary* syphilis occurring 6 weeks to 6 months after the appearance of the chancre is characterized by a widespread, symmetrical maculopapular rash on the palms and soles and generalized lymphadenopathy. The infected individual also may experience fever, headache, and malaise. Condyloma lata (wartlike infectious lesions) may develop on the vulva, perineum, or anus (Fig. 6-2, *B*). If the patient is untreated, she enters a latent phase that is asymptomatic for most individuals. If left untreated, about one third of patients will develop tertiary syphilis. Neurologic/cardiovascular, musculoskeletal, or multiorgan system complications can develop in this third stage.

Diagnosis. Diagnosis is dependent on microscopic examination of primary and secondary lesion tissue and serology during latency and late infection. Any test for anti-

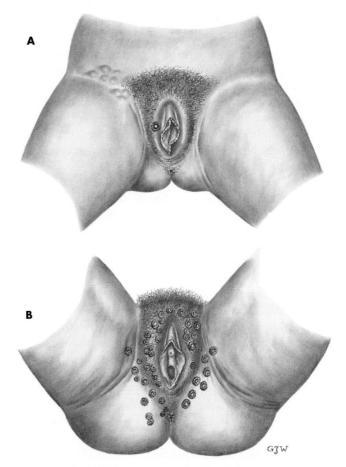

Fig. **6-2** Syphilis. **A,** Primary stage: chancre with inguinal adenopathy. **B,** Secondary stage: condyloma lata.

bodies may not be reactive in the presence of active infection because it takes time for the body's immune system to develop antibodies to any antigens. Two types of serologic tests are used: nontreponemal and treponemal. Nontreponemal antibody tests such as the Venereal Disease Research Laboratory (VDRL) or rapid plasma reagin (RPR) are used as screening tests. False-positive results are not unusual, particularly when conditions such as acute infection, autoimmune disorders, malignancy, pregnancy, and drug addiction exist and after immunization or vaccination. The treponemal tests, fluorescent treponemal antibody absorbed (FTA-ABS) and microhemagglutination assays for antibody to *T. pallidum* (MHA-TP), are used to confirm positive results. Test results in patients with early primary or incubating syphilis may be negative. Seroconversion usually takes place 6 to 8 weeks after exposure so testing should be repeated in 1 to 2 months when a suspicious genital lesion exists. Most patients with positive treponemal antibody tests will remain positive for life, regardless of treatment or disease activity; more than 15% to 20% of patients treated during the primary stage might return to nonreactivity after 2 to 3 years (CDC, 1998).

TABLE 6-3	*Wet Smear Tests for Vaginal Infections*	
INFECTION	**TEST**	**POSITIVE FINDINGS**
Trichomoniasis	Saline wet smear (vaginal secretions mixed with normal saline on a glass slide)	Presence of many white blood cell protozoa
Candidiasis	Potassium hydroxide (KOH) prep (vaginal secretions mixed with KOH on a glass slide)	Presence of hyphae and pseudohyphae (buds and branches of yeast cells)
Bacterial vaginosis	Normal saline smear	Presence of clue cells (vaginal epithelial cells coated with bacteria)
	Whiff test (vaginal secretions mixed with KOH)	Release of fishy odor

Tests for chlamydia and gonorrhea should be done, HIV testing offered, and, if indicated, wet smears to detect vaginosis carried out (Table 6-3).

Management. Penicillin is the preferred medication for treating patients with syphilis (CDC, 1998). It is the only proven therapy that has been widely used for patients with neurosyphilis, congenital syphilis, or syphilis during pregnancy. Patients treated for syphilis may experience a Jarisch-Herxheimer reaction, an acute febrile reaction often accompanied by headache, myalgias, and arthralgias that develop within hours of treatment (Fogel, 1995b).

Monthly follow-up is mandatory so that retreatment may be given if needed. The nurse should emphasize the necessity of long-term serologic testing even in the absence of symptoms. The patient should be advised to practice sexual abstinence until treatment is completed, all evidence of primary and secondary syphilis is gone, and serologic evidence of a cure is demonstrated. Women should be told to notify all partners who may have been exposed. They should be informed that the disease is reportable. Preventive measures should be discussed.

Pelvic inflammatory disease

Pelvic inflammatory disease (PID) is an infectious process that most commonly involves the uterine tubes (salpingitis), uterus (endometritis), and, more rarely, the ovaries and peritoneal surfaces. Multiple organisms have been found to cause PID and most cases are associated with more than one organism. *Chlamydia trachomatis* is estimated to cause one half of all cases of PID. In addition to gonorrhea and chlamydia, a wide variety of anaerobic and aerobic bacteria are recognized to cause PID. Because PID may be caused by a wide variety of infectious agents and encompasses a wide variety of pathologic processes, the infection can be acute, subacute, or chronic, and has a wide range of symptoms.

Most PID results from ascending spread of microorganisms from the vagina and endocervix to the upper genital tract. This spread most frequently happens at the end of or just after menses following reception of an infectious agent. PID also may develop following an abortion, pelvic surgery, or childbirth.

Each year more than 1 million women in the United States will have an episode of symptomatic PID (Eng & Butler, 1997). Risk factors for acquiring PID are those associated with the risk of contracting an STD–a history of PID or STDs, intercourse with a partner who has untreated urethritis, recent intrauterine device (IUD) insertion, and nulliparity.

Women who have had PID are at increased risk for ectopic pregnancy, infertility, and chronic pelvic pain. After a single episode of PID, a woman's risk for ectopic pregnancy increases sevenfold compared with the risk for women who have never had PID. Other problems associated with PID include dyspareunia (painful intercourse), pyosalpinx (pus in the uterine tubes), tubo-ovarian abscess, and pelvic adhesions.

The symptoms of PID vary, depending on whether the infection is acute, subacute, or chronic; however, pain is common to all types of infection. It may be dull, cramping, and intermittent (subacute) or severe, persistent, and incapacitating (acute). Women may also report one or more of the following: fever, chills, nausea and vomiting, increased vaginal discharge, symptoms of a urinary tract infection, and irregular bleeding. Abdominal pain is usually present; upper abdominal pain may be due to liver capsule inflammation (Fitz-Hugh-Curtis Syndrome) (Forrest, 1998).

Diagnosis. PID is difficult to diagnose because of the accompanying wide variety of symptoms. CDC (1998) recommends treatment for PID in all sexually active young women and others at risk for STDs, if the following criteria are present and no other causes(s) of the illness can be found: lower abdominal tenderness, bilateral adnexal tenderness, and cervical motion tenderness. Other criteria for diagnosing PID include oral temperature > 38.3° C, abnormal cervical or vaginal discharge, elevated erythrocyte sedimentation rate, elevated C-reactive protein, and laboratory documentation of cervical infection with *N. gonorrhoeae* or *C. trachomatis*.

Management. Perhaps the most important nursing intervention is prevention. Primary prevention would be education in avoiding acquisition of STDs, whereas secondary prevention involves preventing a lower-genital tract infection from ascending to the upper-genital tract.

Instructing women in self-protective behaviors such as practicing safer sex and using barrier methods is critical. Also important is the detection of asymptomatic gonorrheal and chlamydial infections through routine screening of women with risky behaviors and/or specific risk factors such as age. Partner notification and treatment when an STD is diagnosed is essential to prevent reinfection.

Although treatment regimens vary with the infecting organism, a broad-spectrum antibiotic generally is used (ofloxacin plus metronidazole or ceftriaxone plus doxycycline) (CDC, 1998). Several antimicrobial regimens have proved to be effective and no single therapeutic regimen of choice exists. The woman with acute PID should be on bedrest in a semi-Fowler's position. Comfort measures include analgesics for pain and all other nursing measures applicable to a patient confined to bed. As few pelvic examinations as possible should be done during the acute phase of the disease. During the recovery phase, the woman should restrict her activity and make every effort to get adequate rest and a nutritionally sound diet. Follow-up laboratory work after treatment should include endocervical cultures for a test of cure.

Health education is central to effective management of PID. Nurses should explain to women the nature of their disease and should encourage them to comply with all therapy and prevention recommendations, emphasizing the necessity of taking all medication, even if symptoms disappear. Any potential problems such as lack of money for prescriptions or lack of transportation to return to clinic for follow-up appointments that would prevent a woman from completing a course of treatment should be identified and the importance of follow-up visits stressed. Women should be counseled to refrain from sexual intercourse until their treatment is completed. Contraceptive counseling should be provided. The nurse can suggest the woman select barrier methods such as condoms or a diaphragm. A woman with a history of PID should not choose an IUD as her contraceptive method.

The woman who suffers from PID may be acutely ill or experience long-term discomfort. Either or both take an emotional toll. Pain in itself is debilitating and is compounded by the infectious process. The potential or actual loss of reproductive capabilities can be devastating and can adversely affect a woman's self-concept. Part of the nurse's role is to help the woman adjust her self-concept to fit reality and to accept alterations in a way that promotes health. Because PID is so closely tied to sexuality, body image, and self-concept, the woman diagnosed with it will need supportive care. Her feelings need to be discussed and her partner(s) included when appropriate.

Viral STDs

Human papillomavirus infections

Human papillomavirus (HPV) infections, also known as condyloma acuminata, or genital warts, is an STD that

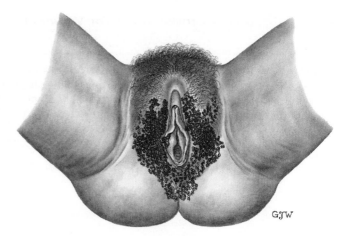

Fig. 6-3 HPV infection. Condyloma acuminata.

was first described in 25 AD and is now one of the most common STDs seen in ambulatory health care settings. An estimated 24 million Americans are infected with HPV and as many as 1 million new infections occur every year (CDC, 1998). HPV, a double-stranded DNA virus, has over 40 known serotypes, five of which are known to cause genital wart formation and eight of which are currently thought to have oncogenic potential (CDC, 1998). HPV types 6 and 11 are responsible for most benign anal-genital disease.

Genital warts in women are most commonly seen in the posterior part of the introitus (Fig. 6-3); however, lesions also are found on the buttocks, vulva, vagina, anus, and cervix. Typically warts are small, 2 to 3 mm in diameter and 10 to 15 mm in height, soft, papillary swellings occurring singularly or in clusters on the genital and anal-rectal region. Infections of long duration may appear as a cauliflower-like mass. In moist areas such as the vaginal introitus, the lesions may appear to have multiple, fine, finger-like projections. Vaginal lesions are often multiple. Flat-topped papules, 1 to 4 mm in diameter, are seen most often on the cervix. Often these lesions are visualized only under magnification. Warts are usually flesh-colored or slightly darker on Caucasian women, black on African-American women, and brownish on Asian women. Condyloma acuminata are often painless, but may also be uncomfortable, particularly when very large. They can become inflamed and ulcerated.

Diagnosis. Viral screening and typing for HPV is not standard practice yet. History, evaluation of signs and symptoms, Pap smear, and physical examination are used in making a diagnosis. The only definitive diagnostic test for presence of HPV is by histologic evaluation of a biopsy specimen.

Management. Treatment of genital warts is with topical application of podofilox 0.5% solution or gel (CDC, 1998). Cryotherapy, electrocautery, and laser therapy may also be used. No therapy has been shown to eradicate HPV.

The goal of treatment is removal of warts and relief of signs and symptoms, not the eradication of HPV. The woman often must make multiple office visits; frequently, many different treatments will be tried.

Women who are experiencing discomfort associated with genital warts may find that bathing with an oatmeal solution and drying the area with a cool hair dryer will provide some relief. Keeping the area clean and dry will also decrease growth of the warts. Cotton underwear and loose fitting clothes that decrease friction and irritation also may decrease discomfort. Women should be advised to maintain a healthy lifestyle to aid the immune system; women can be counseled regarding diet, rest, stress reduction, and exercise.

Patient counseling is essential. Women must understand the virus, how it is transmitted, that no immunity is conferred with infection, and that reinfection is likely with repeated contact. Women need to know that their partners should be checked, even if they are asymptomatic. All sexually active women with multiple partners or a history of HPV should be encouraged to use latex condoms and a vaginal spermicide for intercourse to decrease acquisition or transmission of the infection. Semiannual or annual health examinations are recommended to assess disease recurrence and screening for cervical cancer. At least annual Pap smears should be done on women who have been treated for HPV infections.

Genital herpes simplex virus

Unknown until the middle of the twentieth century, genital herpes simplex virus (HSV) is now one of the most common STDs in the United States, especially in women. HSV is a painful vesicular eruption of the skin and mucosa of the genitals caused by two different antigen subtypes of herpes simplex virus: herpes simplex virus I (HSV-1) and herpes simplex virus II (HSV-2). HSV-2 is usually transmitted sexually and HSV-1, nonsexually. Although HSV-1 is more commonly associated with gingivostomatitis and oral labial ulcers (fever blisters) and HSV-2 with genital lesions, neither type is exclusively associated with the respective sites.

It is estimated that at least one in every four women in the United States will become infected with herpes in her lifetime (Eng & Butler, 1997). Between 200,000 and 500,000 persons contract an initial (or primary) infection each year; recurrent HSV infections are much more common. Prevalence is higher in women with multiple sex partners. The greatest number of new cases occur in individuals between the ages of 15 and 34.

An initial herpetic infection characteristically has both systemic and local symptoms and lasts about 3 weeks. Women generally have a more severe clinical course than do men. Often the first symptoms following incubation are genital discomfort and neuralgic pain. Systemic symptoms appear early, peak about 3 to 4 days after lesions appear, and then subside over 3 to 4 days (Fig. 6-4). Ulcerative lesions last

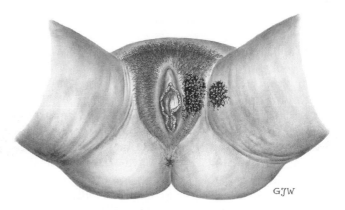

Fig. **6-4** Herpes genitalis.

4 to 15 days before crusting over. New lesions may develop up to the tenth day of the course of the infection. Viral shedding and thus infectivity may last 6 or 8 weeks.

Common systemic symptoms with the primary infection include fever, malaise, headache, and photophobia. Women with primary genital herpes have many lesions that progress from macules to papules, then vesicles, pustules, and ulcers that crust and heal without scarring. These ulcers are extremely tender, and primary infections may be bilateral. Women also may have itching, inguinal tenderness, and lymphadenopathy. Severe vulvular edema may develop and women may have difficulty sitting. Cervicitis also is common with initial infections and a heavy, watery to purulent vaginal discharge is common. Extragenital lesions may be present because of autoinoculation. Urinary retention and dysuria may occur secondary to autonomic involvement of the sacral nerve root.

Women experiencing recurrent episodes of HSV infections commonly will have only local symptoms, which are usually less severe than those associated with the initial infection. Systemic symptoms are usually absent, although the characteristic prodromal genital tingling is common. Recurrent lesions are unilateral, less severe, and usually last 7 to 10 days without prolonged viral shedding. Lesions begin as vesicles and progress rapidly to ulcers. Very few women with recurrent disease have cervicitis.

Diagnosis. Although a diagnosis of herpes infection may be suspected from the history and physical, it is confirmed by laboratory studies. A viral tissue culture is taken during the vesicular stage by swabbing exudate from a lesion and placing it in a viral medium. Preliminary results are available in 48 hours and final results in 1 to 2 weeks (Youngkin, 1995).

Management. Genital herpes is a chronic and recurring disease for which there is no known cure. Medications used for treating HSV infections include acyclovir, famciclovir, and valacyclovir (CDC, 1998). Management is directed toward specific treatment during primary and recurrent infections, prevention, self-help measures, and psychologic support.

Cleaning lesions twice a day with saline will help prevent secondary infection. Bacterial infection must be treated with appropriate antibiotics. Measures that may increase comfort for women when lesions are active include warm sitz baths with baking soda; keeping lesions warm and dry by blowing area dry using a hair dryer set on cool or patting dry with soft towel; wearing cotton underwear and loose clothing; using drying aids such as hydrogen peroxide, Burrow's solution, or oatmeal baths; applying cool, wet black tea bags to lesions and applying compresses with an infusion of cloves or peppermint oil and clove oil to lesions.

Analgesics such as aspirin or ibuprofen may be used to relieve pain and systemic symptoms associated with initial infections. Because the mucous membranes affected by herpes are very sensitive, any topical agents should be used with caution. Nonantiviral ointments, especially those containing cortisone, should be avoided. A thin layer of lidocaine ointment or an antiseptic spray may be applied to decrease discomfort, especially if walking is difficult.

Counseling and education are critical components of the nursing care of women with herpes infections. Information regarding the etiology, signs and symptoms, transmission, and treatment should be provided. Women should be helped to understand when viral shedding and thus transmission to a partner is most likely, and that they should refrain from sexual contact from the onset of prodrome until complete healing of lesions. Condoms may not prevent transmission, particularly male-to-female transmission: This does not mean however that the partners should avoid all intimacy. Women can be encouraged to maintain close contact with their partners while avoiding contact with lesions. Women should be taught how to look for herpetic lesions using a mirror and good light source to aid vision and a wet cloth or finger covered with a finger cot to rub lightly over the labia. The nurse should ensure that patients understand that when lesions are active, sharing intimate articles (e.g., washcloth, wet towel) that come into contact with the lesions should be avoided. Plain soap and water are all that is needed to clean hands that have come in contact with herpetic lesions; isolation is neither necessary nor appropriate.

The nurse should explain the role of precipitating factors in the reactivation of the latent virus and recurrent episodes. Stress, menstruation, trauma, febrile illnesses, chronic illness, and ultraviolet light have all been found to trigger genital herpes. Women may wish to keep a diary to identify which stressors seem to be associated with recurrent herpes attacks so that they can then avoid those stressors when possible. Referral for stress reduction therapy, yoga, or meditation classes may be done when indicated. The role of exercise in reducing stress can be discussed. Avoiding excessive heat and sun and hot baths and using a lubricant during sexual intercourse to reduce friction also may be helpful.

The emotional impact of contracting herpes is considerable. No cure is available and most women will experience recurrences. At diagnosis many emotions may surface—helplessness, anger, denial, guilt, anxiety, shame, or inadequacy. Women need the opportunity to discuss their feelings and help in learning to live with the disease. A woman can be encouraged to think of herself as a person who is not diseased but rather healthy and inconvenienced from time to time. Herpes can affect a woman's sexuality, her sexual practices, and her current and future relationships. She may need help in raising the issue with her partner or with future partners.

Hepatitis B

Hepatitis B virus (HBV), a common STD, is much more contagious than HIV, and is the virus most threatening to the fetus and neonate. Rates have been increasing steadily in the United States since the early 1980s. It is caused by a large DNA virus and is associated with three antigens and their antibodies: hepatitis B surface antigen (HBsAG), HBV antigen (HBeAG), HBV core antigen (HBcAG), antibody to HBsAG (anti-HBs), antibody to HBeAG (anti-HBe), and antibody to HBcAG (anti-HBc). Screening for active or chronic disease or disease immunity is based on testing for these antigens and their antibodies.

Populations at risk include women of Asian, Pacific Islander (Polynesian, Micronesian, Melanesian) or Alaskan Eskimo descent and women born in Haiti or sub-Saharan Africa. Women with a history of acute or chronic liver disease, who work or receive treatment in a dialysis unit, or who have household or sexual contact with a hemodialysis patient are at greater risk. Women who work or live in institutions for the mentally retarded are considered to be at risk as are women with a history of multiple blood transfusions. Health care workers and public safety workers exposed to blood in the workplace are at risk. Behaviors such as multiple sexual partners and a history of intravenous drug use increase risk of contracting HBV infections.

HBsAG has been found in blood, saliva, sweat, tears, vaginal secretions, and semen. Drug abusers who share needles are at risk as are health care workers who are exposed to blood and needle sticks. Perinatal transmission most often occurs in mothers who have acute hepatitis infection late in the third trimester or during the intrapartum or postpartum periods from exposure to HBsAG-positive vaginal secretions, blood, amniotic fluid, saliva, and breast milk. HBV has also been transmitted by artificial insemination. Although HBV can be transmitted via blood transfusion, the incidence of such infections has decreased significantly since testing of blood for HBsAG became routine.

Hepatitis B (HB) is a disease of the liver and is often a silent infection. In the adult, the course of the infection can be fulminating and the outcome fatal. Early symptoms include skin eruptions, urticaria, arthralgias, arthritis, lassitude, anorexia, nausea, vomiting, headache, fever, and mild abdominal pain. Later the patient may have clay-colored stools, dark urine, increased abdominal pain, and jaundice. Between 5% and 10% of individuals with HB have persistence of HBsAg and become chronic hepatitis B carriers.

Diagnosis. All women at high-risk for contracting hepatitis B should be screened on a regular basis. The HbsAg screening test is usually done as a rise in HbsAg occurs at the onset of clinical symptoms and usually indicates an active infection. If HbsAg persists in the blood, the women is identified as a carrier. If the HBsAG is positive, further laboratory studies may be ordered: anti-Hbe, anti-Hbc, SGOT, alkaline phosphatase, and liver panel.

Management. There is no specific treatment for hepatitis B. Recovery is usually spontaneous in 3 to 16 weeks. Women should be advised to increase bedrest, eat a high protein, low-fat diet, and increase their fluid intake. They should avoid drugs and alcohol and medications metabolized in the liver. Women with a definite exposure to hepatitis B should be given hepatitis B immune globulin (HBIG) and begin the hepatitis B vaccine series within 14 days of the most recent contact to prevent infection (CDC, 1998). Vaccination during pregnancy is not thought to pose risks to the fetus.

Hepatitis B vaccination is the most effective means of preventing HBV infections. High-risk adolescents who have not been previously vaccinated should be vaccinated (CDC, 1998). Vaccination is also recommended for all nonimmune women who have had multiple sex partners within the past 6 months, IV-drug users, residents of correctional or long-term-care facilities, persons seeking care for an STD, sex workers, women whose partners are IV-drug users or bisexual, and women who work in high-risk occupations. The vaccine is given in a series of three (some authorities recommend four) doses over a 6-month period, with the first two doses given at least 1 month apart and the first and third doses at least 4 months apart (CDC, 1998). The vaccine may be given in the deltoid muscle or gluteal muscle in adults.

Patient education includes explaining the meaning of hepatitis B infection, including transmission, state of infectivity, and sequelae. The nurse should also explain the need for immunoprophylaxis for household members and sexual contacts. In order to decrease transmission of the virus, women with hepatitis B or who test positive for HBV should be advised to maintain a high level of personal hygiene: wash hands after using the toilet; carefully dispose of tampons, pads, and Band-Aids in plastic bags; do not share razor blades, toothbrushes, needles, and manicure implements; have male partner use a condom if unvaccinated and without hepatitis; avoid sharing saliva through kissing, or sharing of silverware or dishes; wipe up blood spills immediately with soap and water. They should inform all health care providers of their carrier state.

Human immunodeficiency virus infection

Although human immunodeficiency virus (HIV) has traditionally been thought to be a homosexual or gay disease, heterosexual transmission is now the most common means of transmission in women. Women are the fastest-growing population of individuals with HIV infection and acquired immunodeficiency syndrome (AIDS) (Wortley & Flemming, 1997). An estimated 8 million women are infected with HIV worldwide (CDC, 1995). Between 1991 and 1995, the number of American women diagnosed as having AIDS increased by 63%. In 1993, AIDS became the fourth leading cause of death in women 25 to 44 years of age; in many of the larger cities on the East Coast, it is the leading cause of death (Cotton & Watts, 1997).

Transmission of the **human immunodeficiency virus (HIV),** a retrovirus, occurs primarily through exchange of body fluids (semen, blood, vaginal secretions). Severe depression of the cellular immune system associated with HIV infection characterizes AIDS. Although behaviors that place women at risk have been well documented, all women should be assessed for the possibility of HIV exposure. Until recently HIV infection has commonly been reported at a later disease stage in women; however, this is changing with revised CDC definitions of AIDS. For both men and women, the most commonly reported opportunistic diseases are pneumocystic carinii pneumonia (PCP), candida esophagitis, and wasting syndrome. Other viral infections such as HSV and cytomegalovirus infections seem to be more prevalent in women than men (Wildschut, Weiner & Peters, 1996). PID may be more severe in HIV-infected women and rates of HPV and cervical dysplasia higher. The clinical course of HPV infection in women with HIV infection is accelerated, and recurrence is more frequent.

Once HIV enters the body, seroconversion to HIV positivity usually occurs within 6 to 12 weeks. Although HIV seroconversion may be totally asymptomatic, it usually is accompanied by a viremic, influenza-like response. Symptoms include fever, headache, night sweats, malaise, generalized lymphadenopathy, myalgias, nausea, diarrhea, weight loss, sore throat, and rash.

Laboratory studies may reveal leukopenia, thrombocytopenia, anemia, and an elevated erythrocyte sedimentation rate. HIV has a strong affinity for surface-marker proteins on T-lymphocytes. This affinity leads to significant T-cell destruction. Both clinical and epidemiologic studies have shown that declining CD4 levels are strongly associated with increasing levels for AIDS-related diseases and death in many different groups of HIV-infected persons (Cotton & Watts, 1997).

HIV testing and counseling. Screening, teaching, and counseling regarding HIV risk factors, indications for being tested, and testing are major roles for nurses caring for women today. A number of behaviors that place women at risk for HIV infection have been identified, including intravenous drug use, high-risk sexual partners, multiple sex partners, and a previous history of multiple STDs. HIV infection is usually diagnosed by using HIV-1 antibody tests. Antibody testing is first done with a sensitive screening test such as the enzyme immunoassay (EIA). Reactive screening tests must be confirmed by an additional test, such as the Western blot (WB) or an immunofluorescence assay (IFA). If a positive antibody test is confirmed by a supplemental test, it means that a woman is infected with HIV and is capable of infecting others. HIV antibodies are detectable in at least 95% of patients within 6 months after infection. Although a negative antibody test usually indicates a person is not infected, antibody tests cannot exclude infection that occurred less than 6 months before the test. Because HIV antibody crosses the placenta, its presence in children younger than 18 months of age is not diagnostic of HIV infection (CDC, 1998).

The CDC (1998) guidelines recommend offering HIV testing to all women whose behavior places them at risk for HIV infection. It may be useful to allow women to self-select for HIV testing. Upon entry to the health care system a woman can be handed written information about the risk factors for the AIDS virus and asked to inform the nurse if she believes she is at risk. She should be told that she does not have to say why she may be at risk, only that she thinks she might be.

Counseling before and after HIV testing is standard nursing practice today. It is the nurse's responsibility to assess a woman's understanding of the information such a test would provide and to be sure the woman thoroughly understands the emotional, legal, and medical implications of a positive or negative test before she is ready to take an HIV test. One's life is profoundly altered by a knowledge of HIV seropositivity. A unique stigma is associated with HIV infection that can have a profound impact on the quality of life of those infected. This stigma extends to those who are asymptomatic but seropositive.

Given the strong social stigma attached to HIV infection, nurses must consider the issue of confidentiality and documentation before providing counseling and offering HIV testing to patients.

| LEGAL TIP | HIV Testing

- *If HIV test results are placed in the patient's chart— the appropriate place for all health information— they are available to all who have access to the chart. The woman must be informed of this before testing. Informed consent must be obtained before an HIV test is performed. In some states written consent is mandated.*
- *Counseling associated with HIV testing has two components: pretest and posttest counseling. During pretest counseling, nurses conduct a personalized risk assessment, explain the meaning of positive and negative test results, obtain informed consent for HIV testing, and help women to develop a realistic plan for reducing risk and preventing infection. Posttest counseling includes informing the patient of the test results, reviewing the meaning of the results, and reinforcing prevention messages. All pretest and posttest counseling should be documented.*

There is generally a 1- to 3-week waiting period after testing for HIV, which can be a very anxious time for the woman. It is helpful if the nurse informs her that this time period between blood drawing and test results is routine. Test results, whatever they are, always must be communicated in person and women informed in advance that such is the procedure. Whenever possible the person who provided the pretest counseling should also tell the woman her test results. Some women when informed of negative results may escalate their risk behaviors because they equate negativity with immunity. Others may believe that negative means "bad" and positive means "good." Women's reactions to a negative test should be explored, asking "How do you feel?" HIV-negative result counseling sessions are another opportunity to provide education. Emphasis can be placed on ways in which a woman can remain HIV-free and encouraged to stay negative. She should be reminded that if she has been exposed to HIV in the past 6 months she should be retested, and that if she continues high-risk behaviors she should have on-going testing.

When providing posttest counseling to an HIV-positive woman, privacy with no interruptions is essential. Adequate time for the counseling sessions should also be provided. The nurse should make sure that the woman understands what a positive test means and review the reliability of the test results. Safer sex guidelines need to be reemphasized. Referral for appropriate medical evaluation and follow-up should be made and the need or desire for psychosocial or psychiatric referrals should be assessed. The importance of early medical evaluation so that a baseline assessment can be made and prophylactic medication begun should be stressed. If possible, the nurse should make a referral or appointment for the woman at the posttest counseling session.

As the number of HIV-infected women escalates, prevention, education, and counseling activities must be directed toward women. It is very difficult to keep abreast of the ever-changing picture of AIDS. Important sources of information are the National AIDS Hotline (1-800-342-2437, 1-800-344-7432 [Spanish] or 1-800-243-7889 [deaf] and National AIDS Information Clearing House, P.O. Box 6003, Rockville, MD 20850 [1-800-458-5231]).

Management. During the initial contact with an HIV-infected woman, the nurse should establish what the woman knows about HIV infection. The nurse should ensure that the woman is being cared for by a medical practitioner or at a facility with expertise in caring for persons with HIV infections, including AIDS. Psychologic referral also may be indicated. Resources such as counseling for financial assistance, legal advocacy, suicide prevention, and death and dying may be appropriate. All women who are drug users should be referred to a substance abuse program. A major focus of counseling is prevention of transmission of HIV to partners.

Nurses counseling seropositive women who wish contraceptive information may recommend oral contraceptive and latex condoms; Norplant implants and latex condoms; or tubal sterilization/vasectomy and latex condoms. Spermicides, female condoms, or abstinence can be offered to women whose partners refuse to use condoms.

There is no cure available for HIV infections at this time. Rare and unusual diseases are characteristic of HIV infections. Opportunistic infections and concurrent diseases should be managed vigorously with treatment specific to the infection or disease. Discussion of the medical care of HIV-positive women or women with AIDS is beyond the scope of this chapter. The reader is referred to CDC AIDS hotlines and Internet websites for current information and recommendations (see Appendix D).

Routine gynecologic care for HIV-positive women should include a pelvic examination every 6 months. Careful Pap screening is essential because of the greatly increased incidence of abnormal findings upon examination. In addition, HIV-positive women should be screened for syphilis, gonorrhea, chlamydia, and other vaginal infections.

Coinfection with syphilis is common in HIV-infected women, and unusual serologic responses have been documented among HIV-infected persons who have syphilis (CDC, 1998). Because treatment failures with benzathine penicillin are common, follow-up and evaluation must be done at 3, 6, 9, 12, and 24 months after therapy. Further, HIV-infection increases susceptibility to neurosyphilis, which is hard to differentiate clinically from HIV dementia.

Vaginal Infections

Vaginal discharge and itching of the vulva and vagina are among the most common reasons a woman seeks help from a health care provider. Indeed, more women complain of vaginal discharge than of any other gynecologic symptom. Vaginal discharge resulting from infection must be distinguished from normal secretions. Normal vaginal secretion or leukorrhea is clear to cloudy in appearance and may turn yellow after drying; the discharge is slightly slimy, nonirritating, and has a mild inoffensive odor. Normal vaginal secretions are acidic, with a pH range of 3.8 to 4.2. The amount of leukorrhea present differs with phases of the menstrual cycle with greater amounts occurring at ovulation and just before menses. Leukorrhea is also increased during pregnancy. Normal vaginal secretions contain lactobacilli and epithelial cells. Women who have adequate endogenous or exogenous estrogen will have vaginal secretions.

Vaginitis or abnormal vaginal discharge is related to infection by a microorganism. The most common vaginal infections are bacterial vaginosis, candidiasis, and trichomoniasis. **Vulvovaginitis,** or inflammation of the vulva and vagina, may be caused by vaginal infection; copious amounts of leukorrhea, which can cause maceration of tissues; and chemical irritants, allergens, and foreign bodies, which may produce inflammatory reactions.

Bacterial vaginosis

Bacterial vaginosis (BV), formerly called nonspecific vaginitis, hemophilus vaginitis, or Gardnerella, is the most common type of vaginitis today (Plourd, 1997). These infections are associated with preterm labor and birth. The exact etiology of BV is unknown. It is a syndrome in which normal, H_2O_2-producing lactobacilli are replaced with high concentrations of anaerobic bacteria (Gardnerella and Mobiluncus). With the proliferation of anaerobes, the level of vaginal amines is raised and the normal acidic pH of the vagina is altered. Epithelial cells slough and numerous bacteria attach to their surfaces (clue cells). When the amines are volatilized, the characteristic odor of BV occurs.

Most women with BV complain of a characteristic "fishy odor;" however, not all note it. The odor may be noticed by the woman or her partner after heterosexual intercourse because semen releases the vaginal amines. When present, the BV discharge is usually profuse, thin, and white or gray, or milky in appearance. Some women also may experience mild irritation or pruritus.

Diagnosis. A careful history may help distinguish BV from other vaginal infections if the woman is symptomatic. Reports of fishy odor and increased thin vaginal discharge are most significant, and a report of increased odor after intercourse is also suggestive of BV. Patients with previous occurrence of similar symptoms, diagnosis, and treatment should be queried, because women with BV often have been treated incorrectly because of misdiagnosis.

Microscopic examination of vaginal secretions is always done. Both normal saline and 10% potassium hydroxide (KOH) smears should be made. The presence of clue cells (vaginal epithelial cells coated with bacteria) by wet saline smear is highly diagnostic because the phenomenon is specific to BV. Vaginal secretions should be tested for pH and amine odor. Nitrazine paper is sensitive enough to detect a pH of 4.5 or greater. The fishy odor of BV will be released when KOH is added to vaginal secretions on the lip of the withdrawn speculum.

Management. Treatment of bacterial vaginosis with oral metronidazole (Flagyl) is most effective (CDC, 1998). Side effects of metronidazole are numerous, including sharp, unpleasant metallic taste in the mouth, furry tongue, central nervous system reactions, and urinary tract disturbances. When oral metronidazole is taken, the woman is advised not to drink alcoholic beverages, or she will experience the severe side effects of abdominal distress, nausea, vomiting, and headache. Gastrointestinal symptoms are common whether alcohol is consumed or not. Treatment of sexual partners is not recommended because sexual transmission of BV has not been proven (CDC, 1998).

Candidiasis

Vulvovaginal candidiasis or yeast infection is the second most common type of vaginal infection in the United States. Although vaginal candidiasis infections are common in healthy women, those seen in women with HIV infection are often more severe and persistent. Genital candidiasis lesions may be painful, coalescing ulcerations necessitating continuous, prophylactic therapy.

The most common organism is *Candida albicans;* it is estimated that 80% to 95% of the yeast infections in women are caused by this organism. However, in the past 10 years, the incidence of nonalbicans infections has risen steadily. Women with chronic or recurrent infections often are infected with a higher percentage of nonalbicans species than are women who are experiencing their first infection or who have few recurrences.

Numerous factors have been identified as predisposing a woman to yeast infections, including antibiotic therapy, particularly broad-spectrum antibiotics such as ampicillin, tetracycline, cephalosporins, and metronidazole; diabetes, especially when uncontrolled; pregnancy; obesity; diets high in refined sugars or artificial sweeteners; use of corticosteroids and exogenous hormones; and immunosuppressed states. Clinical observations and research have suggested that tight fitting clothing and underwear or pantyhose made of nonabsorbent materials create an environment in which vaginal fungus can grow.

The most common symptom of yeast infections is vulvular and possibly vaginal pruritus. The itching may be mild or intense, interfere with rest and activities, and occur during or after intercourse. Some women report a feeling of dryness. Others may experience painful urination as the urine flows over the vulva; this usually occurs in women who have excoriations resulting from scratching. Most often the discharge is thick, white, lumpy, and cottage cheeselike. The discharge may be found in patches on the vaginal walls, cervix, and labia. Commonly the vulva is red and swollen as are the labial folds, vagina, and cervix. Although there is not a characteristic odor with yeast infections, sometimes a yeasty or musty smell occurs.

Diagnosis. In addition to a careful history of the woman's symptoms, their onset and course, the history is a valuable screening tool for identifying predisposing risk factors. Physical examination should include a thorough inspection of the vulva and vagina. A speculum examination is always done. Commonly saline and KOH wet smear and vaginal pH are obtained. Vaginal pH is normal with a yeast infection; if the pH is > 4.5 one should suspect trichomoniasis or BV. The characteristic pseudohyphae (bud or branching of a fungus) may be seen on a wet smear done with normal saline; however, they may be confused with other cells and artifacts.

Management. A number of antifungal preparations are available for the treatment of *C. albicans.* Intravaginal agents include miconazole, clotrimazole, butoconazole, and terconazole; fluconazole is an effective oral agent (CDC, 1998). In 1990, many of these medications (e.g., Monistat and Gyne-Lotrimin) were made available over-the-counter. The first time a woman suspects that she may have a yeast infection, she should see a health care provider for confirmation of the diagnosis and treatment recommendation. If she experiences another infection she may wish to purchase an OTC preparation and self-treat; if she elects to do this, she should always be counseled regarding seeking care for numerous recurrent or chronic yeast infections. If vaginal discharge is extremely thick and copious, vaginal debridement with a cotton swab followed by application of vaginal medication may be useful.

Women who have extensive irritation, swelling, and discomfort of the labia and vulva may find sitz baths helpful in decreasing inflammation and increasing comfort. Adding Aveeno powder to the bath may also increase the woman's comfort. Not wearing underpants to bed may help decrease symptoms and prevent recurrences. Completing the full course of treatment prescribed is essential to removing the pathogen and women are instructed to continue medication even during menstruation. They should be counseled not to use tampons during menses because the medication will be absorbed by the tampon. If possible, intercourse is avoided during treatment; if this is not feasible, the woman's partner should use a condom to prevent introduction of more organisms.

Trichomoniasis

Trichomonas vaginalis is almost always an STD. It is also a very common cause of vaginal infection (up to 25% of all vaginitis) and discharge, and thus is discussed in this section.

Trichomoniasis is caused by *Trichomonas vaginalis,* an anaerobic, one-celled protozoan with characteristic flagellae. Although trichomoniasis may be asymptomatic, commonly women experience characteristically yellowish to greenish, frothy, mucopurulent, copious, malodorous discharge. Inflammation of the vulva, vagina, or both may be present and the woman may complain of irritation and pruritus. Dysuria and dyspareunia are often present. Typically, the discharge worsens during and after menstruation. Often the cervix and vaginal walls will demonstrate the characteristic "strawberry spots" or tiny petechiae, and the cervix may bleed on contact. In severe infections, the vaginal walls, cervix, and occasionally the vulva may be acutely inflamed.

Diagnosis. In addition to obtaining a history of current symptoms, a careful sexual history should be obtained. Any history of similar symptoms in the past and treatment used should be noted. The nurse should determine whether the woman's partner(s) were treated and if she has had subsequent relations with new partners.

A speculum examination is always done, even though it may be very uncomfortable for the woman; relaxation techniques and breathing exercises may help the woman with the procedure. Any of the classic signs may or may not be present on physical examination. The typical one-celled flagellate trichomonads are easily distinguished on a normal saline wet prep. Trichomoniasis also may be identified on Pap smears. Because trichomoniasis is an STD, once diagnosis is confirmed appropriate laboratory studies for other STDs should be carried out.

Management. The recommended treatment is metronidazole, 2 gm orally in a single dose (CDC, 1998) Although the male partner is usually asymptomatic, it is recommended that he receive treatment also because he often harbors the trichomonads in the urethra or prostate. It is important that nurses discuss the importance of partner treatment with their patients. If partners are not treated, it is likely that the infection will recur.

Women with trichomoniasis need to understand the sexual transmission of this disease. It is important that the woman know the organism may be present without symptoms being present, perhaps for several months, and that it is not possible to determine when she became infected.

I CARE MANAGEMENT

Women may delay seeking care for STDs because they fear social stigma, they have little accessibility to health care services, are asymptomatic, or unaware that they have an infection.

Assessment and Nursing Diagnoses

A comprehensive assessment focuses on lifestyle issues that are often personal or sensitive. A culturally sensitive, nonjudgmental approach is essential to facilitate accurate data collection. A history that is accurate, comprehensive, and specific is crucial to sound diagnosis. Because many women are embarrassed or anxious, the history should be taken first, with the woman dressed. Information should be collected in a nonjudgmental manner, using open-ended questions and avoiding assumptions of sexual preference. All partners should be referred to as partners and not by gender. A complete history is essential in identifying possible STDs. Specific areas to address are found in Box 6-2. Factors that may influence the development and management of STDs in women include previous history of STD or PID, number of past or current sexual partners, and types of sexual activity. Lifestyle behaviors that place women at risk for STDs should

---

| BOX 6-2 | *Essential Areas of Assessment for a Woman at Risk for or Who Has an STD* |

CURRENT PROBLEM
What symptoms are present?
 Vaginal discharge
 Lesions
 Rash
 Dysuria
 Fever
 Itching, burning
 Dyspareunia
 Malaise

PAST MEDICAL HISTORY
History of STDs
Allergies, especially to medications

MENSTRUAL HISTORY
Last menstrual period (possibility of pregnancy)

PERSONAL AND SOCIAL HISTORY
Sexual History
Sexual preference
Number of partners (past, present)
Types of sexual activity
Frequency of sexual activity

LIFESTYLE BEHAVIORS
Intravenous drug use (or partner)
Smoking
Alcohol use
Inadequate/poor nutrition
High levels of stress, fatigue

---

be specifically queried. Among these are intravenous drug use (IVDU) or partner IVDU, smoking, alcohol use, inadequate or poor nutrition, and high levels of stress or fatigue.

A thorough assessment of symptoms, including a comprehensive physical examination, is essential to diagnosing STDs. Because the speculum usually is not lubricated before insertion into the vagina because cultures of vaginal secretions may have to be obtained, insertion may be more uncomfortable than usual. Women should be informed of this and reassured that every effort will be made to make the speculum examination as comfortable as possible.

Appropriate laboratory studies will be suggested, in part, by the history and physical examination results. These have been discussed in the previous sections. Selected nursing diagnoses for a woman with an STD or vaginal infection are listed in the accompanying box.

Expected Outcomes of Care

Care of the woman focuses on both physical and psychological needs. Avoidance of reinfection and harmful

❙ Nursing Diagnoses_____

Woman with an STD or Vaginal Infection

Anxiety/situational low self-esteem/body image disturbance related to:

- Perceived effects on sexual relationships and family processes
- Possible effects on pregnancy/fetus
- Long-term sequelae of infection

Knowledge deficit related to:

- Transmission/prevention of infection/reinfection
- Safer sex behaviors
- Management of infection

Pain/impaired tissue integrity related to:

- Effects of infection process
- Scratching (excoriation) of pruritic areas
- Hygiene practices

Sexual dysfunction and altered sexuality pattern

Social isolation and impaired social interaction

HOME CARE *Patient Instructions for Self-Care*

STDs

Take your medication as directed.

Use comfort measures for symptom relief as suggested by your health care provider.

Keep your appointment for repeat cultures or checkups after your treatment to make sure your infection is cured.

Inform your sexual partner(s) to be tested and treated, if necessary.

Abstain from sexual intercourse until your treatment is completed or for as long as you are advised by your health care provider.

Use safer sex practices when sexual intercourse is resumed.

Call your health care provider immediately if you notice bumps, sores, rashes, or discharges.

Keep all future appointments with your health care provider, even if things appear normal.

---

sequelae is critical. Measurable expected outcomes are mutually derived with the woman's input. Outcomes for the woman include that she will:

- Be free of infection or, in the case of viral infection, she will have remission or stabilization of the infection.
- Identify and be able to discuss the etiology, management, and expected course of the infection and its prevention.

Plan of Care and Interventions

The nurse must make sure that the woman understands what disease she has, how it is transmitted, and why it must be treated. Patients should be given a brief description of the disease in language that they can understand. This description should include modes of transmission, incubation period, symptoms, infectious period, and potential complications. Effective treatment of STDs necessitates careful, thorough explanation of treatment regimen and follow-up procedures. Thorough, careful instructions about medications must also be provided, both orally and in writing. Side effects, benefits, and risks of the medication should be discussed. Unpleasant side effects or early relief of symptoms may discourage women from completing their medication course. Patients should be strongly urged to take all the medication and not stop even if their symptoms diminish or disappear in a few days. Comfort measures to decrease symptoms such as pain, itching, or nausea should be suggested. Providing written information is a useful strategy because this is a time of high anxiety for many women and they may not be able to hear or remember what they were told. A number of booklets on STDs are already available, or the nurse may wish to develop literature that is specific to her practice setting and patients.

In general, women will be advised to refrain from intercourse until all treatment is finished and a reculture, if appropriate, is done. After the infection is cured, women should be urged to continue using condoms to prevent repeated infections, especially if they have had one episode of PID or continue to have intercourse with new partners. Women may wish to avoid having sex with partners who have many other sexual partners. All women who have contracted an STD should be taught safer sex practices, if this has not been done already. Follow-up appointments should be made as needed. For additional patient information please see the accompanying Home Care box.

Addressing the psychosocial component of STDs is essential. A woman may be afraid or embarrassed to tell her partner or to ask her partner to seek treatment; she may be embarrassed to admit her sexual practices, or she may be concerned about confidentiality. The nurse may need to help the patient deal with the impact of a diagnosis of an STD on a committed relationship for the woman who is then faced with the necessity of dealing with "uncertain monogamy."

In many instances sexual partners should be treated; thus the infected woman is asked to identify and notify all partners who might have been exposed. Often she will find this difficult to do. Empathizing with the patient's feelings and suggesting specific ways of talking with partners will help decrease anxiety and assist in efforts to control infection. For example, the nurse might suggest that the woman say, "I care about you and I'm concerned about you. That's why I'm calling to tell you that I have an STD. My clinician is _____ and she will be happy to talk with you if you would like." Offering literature and role playing situations with the patient also may be of assistance. It is often helpful to remind the woman that although this is an embarrassing situation, most persons would rather know than not know that they have been exposed. Health professionals who take time to counsel their patients on how to talk with their partner(s) can improve compliance and case finding.

Many STDs are reportable; all states require that the five traditional venereal diseases—gonorrhea, syphilis, chancroid, lymphogranuloma venereum, and granuloma inguinale—be reported to public health officials. Many other states require other STDs such as chlamydial infections, genital herpes, and genital warts be reported. In addition, all states require that AIDS cases be reported; 35 states require that HIV infection be reported. The nurse is legally responsible for reporting all cases of those diseases identified as reportable and should make sure she knows what the requirements are in the state in which she practices. The woman must be informed when a case will be reported and told why. Failure to inform the patient that the case will be reported is a serious breach of professional ethics. Confidentiality is a crucial issue for many patients. When an STD is reportable, women need to be told that they may be contacted by a health department epidemiologist. They should be assured that the information reported to and collected by health authorities is not available to anyone without their permission. Every effort, within the limits of one's public health responsibilities, should be made to reassure patients.

Infection control

Infection control measures are essential to protect care providers and to prevent nosocomial infection of patients, regardless of the infectious agent. The risk for occupational transmission varies with the disease. Even when the risk is low, as with HIV, the existence of any risk warrants reasonable precautions. Precautions against airborne disease transmission are practiced in all health care agencies. **Standard Precautions** (precautions to use in care of all persons for infection control) and additional precautions for labor and birth settings are listed in Box 6-3.

Evaluation

Evaluation is a continuous process. To be effective, evaluation is based on patient-centered outcomes identified during the planning stage of nursing care. The nurse can be reasonably assured that care was effective to the extent that these expected outcomes have been met.

▌ PROBLEMS OF THE BREASTS

Fibrocystic Change

Approximately 50% of women experience a breast problem at some point in their adult life. The most common benign breast problem is fibrocystic change. **Fibrocystic change** is not a disease, as previously believed, but a condition found in varying degrees in healthy women's breasts. Fibrocystic change is characterized by lumpiness, with or without tenderness, and usually occurs with changes in the menstrual cycle (Branch, 1998). When fibrocystic breast changes are present in a woman with a family

history of breast cancer, the relative risk of breast cancer is increased (Fiorica, 1994).

There is no known etiologic agent responsible for benign breast disease, although an imbalance of estrogen and progesterone may be responsible. One theory is that estrogen excess and progesterone deficiency in the luteal phase of the menstrual cycle may cause changes in breast tissue.

Although the usual clinical presentation of fibrocystic change is lumpiness in both breasts, single simple cysts may also occur. Symptoms usually develop about a week before menstruation begins and subside about a week after menstruation ends. Symptoms include dull heavy pain and a sense of fullness and tenderness often in the upper outer quadrants of the breasts. On physical examination there may be excessive nodularity that is described as feeling like a "plate of peas." Larger cysts may be described as feeling like water-filled balloons. Women in their 20s report the most severe pain. Women in their 30s have premenstrual pain and tenderness; small multiple nodules are usually present. Women in their 40s usually do not report severe pain, but cysts will be tender; cysts often regress in size.

Steps in the workup of a breast lump may begin with ultrasonography to determine if it is fluid filled or solid. Fluid-filled cysts are aspirated, and the woman is followed on a routine basis for development of other cysts. If the lump is solid, mammography is obtained if the woman is older than 50 years of age. A fine-needle aspiration (FNA) is performed, regardless of the woman's age, to determine the nature of the lump. In some cases, a core biopsy may need to follow FNA to harvest adequate amounts of tissue for pathologic examination (Mishell et al., 1997).

Management depends on the severity of the symptoms. Diet changes and vitamin supplements comprise one management approach. Although still controversial, some advocate eliminating dimethylxanthines (e.g., caffeine and theophylline). Women are encouraged to stop consuming coffee, cola, tea, and chocolate.

Women also report decreased symptoms with such measures as taking vitamin E supplements and decreasing sodium intake or taking mild diuretics shortly before menses. Other pain relief measures include taking analgesics or NSAIDs (e.g., ibuprofen), wearing a supportive bra, and applying heat to the breasts. Oral contraceptives, danazol, bromocriptine, and tamoxifen have also been used with varying degrees of success (Branch, 1998).

Surgical removal of nodules is done only in rare cases. In the presence of multiple nodules, the surgical approach would involve multiple incisions and tissue manipulation and may not prevent the development of more nodules.

Fibroadenoma

The next most common benign condition of the breast that occurs is a **fibroadenoma.** It is the single most common type of tumor seen in the adolescent population, although it can also occur in women in their 30s. The cause of

---

BOX 6-3 *Standard Precautions*

Medical history and examination cannot reliably identify all persons infected with HIV or other blood-borne pathogens. Standard Precautions should therefore be used consistently in the care of all persons. These precautions apply to blood, body fluids, and all secretions and excretions, except sweat, nonintact skin, and mucous membranes. Standard Precautions are recommended to reduce the risk of transmission of microorganisms from known and unknown sources of infection (CDC & HIC-PAC, 1996).

1. Handwashing is recommended promptly and thoroughly between patient contacts. Hands and other skin surfaces should be washed immediately and thoroughly if contaminated with blood or other body fluids. Hands should be washed immediately after gloves are removed.
2. In addition to handwashing, all health care workers should routinely use appropriate barrier precautions to prevent skin and mucous membrane exposure when contact with blood or other body fluids of any person is anticipated. *Latex gloves* should be worn for touching blood and body fluids, mucous membranes, or nonintact skin of all persons; for handling items or surfaces soiled with blood or body fluids; and for performing venipuncture and other vascular access procedures. Gloves should be changed after contact with each patient. *Masks and protective eyewear* or face shields should be worn during procedures that are likely to generate droplets of blood or other body fluids to prevent exposure of mucous membranes of the mouth, nose, and eyes. *Gowns or aprons* should be worn during procedures that are likely to generate splashes of blood or other body fluids.

    Leg coverings, boots, or shoe covers also can be worn to provide protection against splashes and may be recommended for certain procedures such as surgery.
3. All health care workers should take precautions to prevent injuries caused by needles, scalpels, and other sharp instruments or devices during procedures; when cleaning used instruments; during disposal of used needles; and when handling sharp instruments after procedures. *To prevent needlestick injuries,* needles should not be recapped, purposely bent or broken by hand, removed from disposable syringes, or otherwise manipulated by hand. After they are used, disposable syringes and needles, scalpel blades, and other sharp items should be immediately placed in puncture-resistant containers for disposal; the puncture-resistant containers should be located as close as is practical to the use area.

4. Although saliva has not been implicated in HIV transmission, to minimize the need for emergency mouth-to-mouth resuscitation, mouthpieces, resuscitation bags, or other ventilation devices should be available for use in areas in which the need for resuscitation is predictable.
5. Health care workers who have exudative lesions or weeping dermatitis should refrain from all direct patient care and from handling patient care equipment until the condition resolves.

PRECAUTIONS FOR INVASIVE PROCEDURES

An invasive procedure is surgical entry into tissues, cavities, or organs; or repair of major traumatic injuries (1) in an operating or birthing room, emergency department, or out-of-hospital setting, including both physicians' and dentists' offices; and (2) a vaginal or cesarean birth or other invasive obstetric procedure during which bleeding may occur. Standard Precautions, combined with the following precautions, should serve as minimum precautions for all such invasive procedures:

1. All health care workers who participate in invasive procedures must routinely use appropriate barrier precautions to prevent skin and mucous membrane contact with blood and other body fluids of all patients. Gloves and surgical masks must be worn for all invasive procedures. Protective eyewear or face shields should be worn for procedures that commonly result in the generation of droplets, splashing of blood or other body fluids, or the generation of bone chips. Gowns or aprons made of materials that provide an effective barrier should be worn during invasive procedures that are likely to result in the splashing of blood or other body fluids. All health care workers who perform or assist in vaginal or cesarean births should wear gloves and gowns when handling the placenta or the infant until blood and amniotic fluid have been removed from the infant's skin. Gloves should be worn during infant eye prophylaxis, care of the umbilical cord, circumcision site, parenteral procedures, diaper changes, contact with colostrum and postpartum assessments.
2. If a glove is torn or a needle stick or other injury occurs, the glove should be removed and a new glove used as promptly as patient safety permits; the needle or instrument involved in the incident also should be removed from the sterile field.
3. Any needle stick or injury should be reported and appropriate treatment obtained as specified by the health care facility.

---

fibroadenomas is unknown. Fibroadenomas are characterized by discrete, usually solitary lumps less than 3 centimeters in diameter (Branch, 1998). Occasionally, the woman with a fibroadenoma will experience tenderness in the tumor during the menstrual cycle. Fibroadenomas increase in size during pregnancy and decrease in size as the woman ages.

Diagnosis is made by reviewing patient history and physical examination. Mammography, ultrasound, or magnetic resonance imaging (MRI) may be used to determine the cause of the lesion. FNA may be used to determine underlying pathology. Surgical excision may be necessary if the lump is suspicious or if the symptoms are severe. Periodic observation of masses by professional physical examination and/or mammography may be all that is necessary for those masses not needing surgical intervention. Women should be instructed to perform monthly breast self-examinations (see Chapter 5).

Mammary Duct Ectasia

Mammary duct ectasia is an inflammation of the ducts behind the nipple. The cause of mammary duct ectasia is unknown, although chronic inflammation and dilatation of the lactiferous ducts has been suggested. It occurs most often in perimenopausal women. It is characterized by a nipple discharge that is thick, sticky, and colored white, brown, green or purple. Frequently the woman will experience a burning pain, itching, or a palpable mass behind the nipple.

The workup includes a mammogram and aspiration and culture of fluid. Warm compresses applied to the breast may provide relief. Cleaning the nipple with a povidone-iodine solution may be effective. Often the nipple discharge is self-limiting and does not require surgery (Isaacs, 1994). If a mass is present or an abscess occurs, treatment may include a local excision of the affected duct(s), provided the woman has no future plans to breastfeed.

Intraductal Papilloma

Intraductal papilloma is a rare, benign condition that develops within the terminal nipple ducts. The cause is unknown. It usually occurs in women between the ages of 30 and 50. Usually too small to be palpated, the characteristic sign is nipple discharge that is serous, serosanguinous, or bloody. After the possibility of malignancy is eliminated, the affected segments of the ducts and breasts are surgically excised (Mishell et al., 1997).

Cancer of the Breast

The United States has one of the highest rates of carcinoma in the world. One in eight American women will develop breast cancer in her lifetime (American Cancer Society, 1997). There is no clear method for prevention. Prognosis for and survival of the woman are improved with early detection. Therefore the woman must be educated about risk factors, early detection, and screening.

Although the exact cause of breast cancer continues to elude investigators, certain risk factors that increase a woman's risk for developing a malignancy have been identified. These factors are listed in Box 6-4. There has been much discussion about possible links between breast cancer and hormonal therapy. Up to now, however, most studies do not substantiate a significant link between exogenous estrogen therapy and the development of breast cancer.

Even with identification, risk factors help identify only 25% of women who will eventually develop breast cancer. Although the clinical applicability of risk factors has limits, women at increased risk should be screened at more frequent intervals.

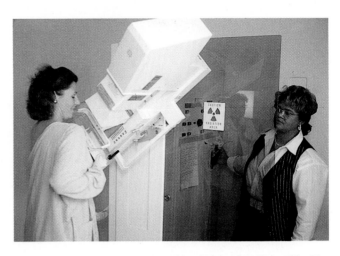

Fig. 6-5 Patient undergoing mammography. (From Edge V & Miller M: *Mosby's clinical nursing series: women's health care*, St Louis, 1994, Mosby.)

BOX 6-4	*Probable Risk Factors for Breast Cancer*

Age over 40
History of breast cancer in one breast
Family history of breast cancer, especially mother or sister
History of ovarian, endometrial, colon, or thyroid cancer
Early menarche
Late menopause
Nulliparity or first pregnancy after age 30
History of fibrocystic breast changes (proliferative lesions with atypical hyperplasia)
Radiation exposure
Excessive alcohol consumption
High-fat diet, obesity

Diagnosis

It is estimated that 90% of all breast lumps are detected by the woman. Of this 90%, only 20% to 25% are malignant. More than half of all lumps are discovered in the upper outer quadrant of the breast. The most common presenting symptom is a lump or thickening of the breast. The lump may feel hard and fixed or soft and spongy. It may have well-defined or irregular borders. It may be fixed to the skin, thereby causing dimpling to occur. A nipple discharge that is bloody or clear also may be present.

Early detection and diagnosis reduce mortality because cancer is found when it is smaller, lesions are more localized, and there tends to be a lower percentage of positive nodes. Regular breast self-examination (BSE) from midadolescence on, a clinical examination by a qualified health care provider, and screening **mammography** (x-ray of the breast) (Fig. 6-5) may aid in the early detection of breast cancers.

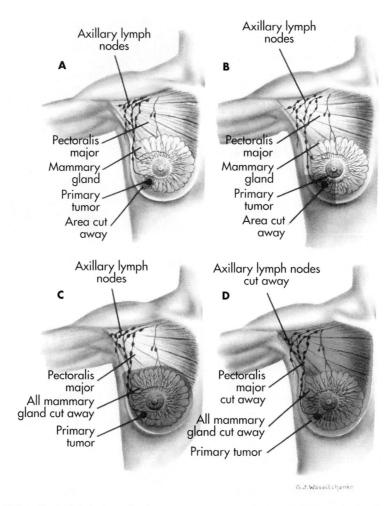

Fig. 6-6 Surgical alternatives for breast cancer. **A,** Lumpectomy (tylectomy). **B,** Quadrectomy (segmental resection). **C,** Total (simple) mastectomy. **D,** Radical mastectomy.

When a suspicious finding on a mammogram is noted or a lump is detected, diagnosis is confirmed by needle aspiration or by a needle localization biopsy. The latter procedure requires the collaborative efforts of both the radiologist and the surgeon. This often requires that the procedure take place in two different environments (radiology and surgery). Therefore patients need specific information regarding procedures, duration, and outcomes.

Laboratory diagnosis of breast cancer and possible cancer metastases includes complete blood count, liver enzyme levels, serum calcium, and alkaline phosphatase level. Elevated liver enzyme levels indicate possible liver metastases and increased serum calcium and alkaline phosphatase levels suggest bone metastases (Shapiro & Clark, 1995).

Nodal involvement and tumor size are the most significant prognostic criteria for long-term survival. One factor that has been helpful in predicting response to therapy and survival is whether the tumor is estrogen-receptor (ER) positive. Women with ER positive tumors tend to respond better to treatment and have higher survival rates.

Management

Controversy continues regarding the best treatment of breast cancer. The women is faced with difficult decisions about the various surgical options (Fig. 6-6). Most health care providers recommend that the malignant mass be removed, as well as the axillary nodes for staging purposes. The treatment can be conservative or more radical. *Breast conserving surgery,* such as a **lumpectomy** (Fig. 6-6, *A*) or quadrectomy (Fig. 6-6, *B*), involves the removal of the tumor and is often followed by radiation therapy. Many women who wish to avoid breast removal because of its psychologic effects may choose this option. A **simple mastectomy** (Fig. 6-6, *C*) is the removal of the breast containing the tumor. A **modified radical mastectomy** is the removal of the breast tissue, skin, fascia of the pectoralis muscle and dissection of the axillary nodes. A **radical mastectomy** is the removal of the breast, underlying pectoralis muscles, and complete axillary node dissection (Fig. 6-6, *D*). These procedures have similar 5-year survival and recurrence rates (Mishell et al., 1997). After surgery, follow-up treatment may include

HOME CARE *Patient Instructions for Self-Care*

Mastectomy

Wash hands well before and after touching incision area or drains.

Empty surgical drains twice a day and as needed, recording the date, time, drain site (if more than one drain is present), and amount of drainage in milliliters in diary you will take to each surgical checkup until your drains are removed. (Before discharge, you may receive a graduated container for emptying drains and measuring drainage.)

Avoid driving, lifting more than 10 pounds, or reaching above your head until given permission by surgeon.

Take medications for pain as soon as pain begins.

Perform arm exercises as directed.

Call physician if inflammation of incision or swelling of the incision or the arm occurs.

Avoid tight clothing, tight jewelry, or other causes of decreased circulation in the affected arm.

Until drains are removed, wear loose-fitting underwear (camisole or half-slip) and clothes, pinning surgical drains inside of clothing. (You will be taught how to do this safely.)

After drains are removed and surgical sites are healing and still tender, wear a mastectomy bra or camisole with a cotton-filled, muslin temporary prosthesis. Temporary prostheses of this type are often available from Reach to Recovery.

Avoid depilatory creams, strong deodorants, and shaving of affected chest area, axilla, and arm.

Sponge bathe until drains are removed.

Return to the surgeon's office for incision check, drain inspection, and possible drain removal as directed.

Contact Reach to Recovery for assistance obtaining external prosthesis and lingerie when dressings, drains, and staples are removed and wound is healing and nontender.

Contact insurance company for information about coverage of prosthesis and wig, if needed. Obtain prescriptions for prosthesis and wig to submit with receipts of purchase for these items to the insurance company. If insurance does not pay for these items, contact hospital or agency social worker or local American Cancer Society for assistance.

Continue with monthly breast self-examination (BSE) of unaffected side and affected surgical site and axilla.

Encourage mother, sisters, and daughters (if applicable) to learn and practice monthly BSE and to have annual professional breast examinations and mammography (if appropriate).

Keep follow-up visits for professional examination, mammography, and testing to detect recurrent breast cancer.

Expect decreased sensation and tingling at incision sites and in the affected arm for weeks to months after surgery.

---

radiation, chemotherapy, or hormonal therapy. The decision to include follow-up therapy is based on the stage of disease, age and menopausal status of the woman, the woman's preference, and her hormonal receptor status. Follow-up treatment is usually used to decrease the risk of recurrence in women who have no evidence of metastasis.

Radiation is usually recommended for women who have stage I or II cancer. Hormone therapy with tamoxifen, an estrogen agonist, is given to women who have ER-positive tumors. Therapy for more advanced tumors is still controversial, but usually includes surgery followed by chemotherapy and/or radiation (Mishell et al., 1997).

Preoperatively women need to be assessed for psychologic preparation and specific teaching needs. A visit from a woman who has had a similar experience may be beneficial preoperatively, as well as postoperatively.

Postoperative nursing care focuses on recovery. Precautions should be taken to avoid taking the blood pressure, giving injections, or taking blood from the arm on the affected side. The woman may have drainage tubes from the incision site that will need to be assessed and drained. Incisional care may include dressing changes. If postoperative arm exercises are appropriate, these may be initiated during the early postoperative period. The woman is usually discharged to home after being given self-care instructions after 24 hours or more, depending on the type of procedure done (see the Home Care box).

Information about reconstruction surgery should be given before surgery, although not all women will be candidates for the procedure or are interested in it. Available options include grafts of muscle and skin from the woman's back, abdomen, or hip, and saline-filled prostheses (Ivey & Gordon, 1994). Silicone gel implants were restricted by the FDA in 1992 to women in safety studies (Logothetis, 1995).

Concerns about appearance after breast surgery may affect the woman's self-concept. Before surgery the woman and her partner need information about what the woman's postoperative appearance will be like. Both the woman and her partner need to be able to discuss feelings and concerns about accepting the changes. Nurses can assist the couple to communicate these feelings and concerns. Information about community resources and support groups such as Reach to Recovery may be beneficial.

Care of the woman with breast cancer is effective if the woman verbalizes satisfaction with the decision-making process about treatment options and if she gets appropriate support from significant others through all stages of treatment and recovery.

KEY POINTS

- Menstrual disorders diminish the quality of life for affected women and their families.
- Premenstrual syndrome is a disorder that begins in the luteal phase of the menstrual cycle and resolves with the onset of menses.
- Premenstrual syndrome is a disorder with both psychologic and physiologic characteristics.
- Endometriosis is characterized by dysmenorrhea, infertility, and less often, alterations in menstrual cycle bleeding and dyspareunia.
- Safer sex practices are key STD prevention strategies.
- HIV is transmitted through body fluids, primarily, blood, semen, and vaginal secretions.
- HPV is the most common viral STD.
- Syphilis has reemerged as a common STD.
- Chlamydia is the most common cause of PID.
- Young sexually active women who do not practice safer sex behaviors and have multiple partners are at greatest risk for STDs and HIV.
- STDs are responsible for substantial mortality and morbidity, personal suffering, and heavy economic burden in the United States.
- STDs and vaginitis are biologic events for which all individuals have a right to expect objective, compassionate, and effective health care.
- The development of breast neoplasms, whether benign or malignant, can have a significant physical and emotional effect on the woman and her family
- The risk of American women developing breast cancer is one in eight.
- An estimated 90% of all breast lumps are detected by women during monthly breast self-examination (BSE).
- Monthly BSE, yearly clinical breast examinations by a health care provider, and routine screening mammograms are recommended for early detection of breast cancer.
- The primary therapy for most women with stages I and II breast cancer is breast conserving surgery followed by radiation therapy.
- Tamoxifen is a common adjunctive therapy for breast cancers that are estrogen-receptor positive.

CRITICAL THINKING EXERCISES

1 *You are asked to teach safer sex practices to a group of girls aged 13 to 16.*
   a *Examine your personal feelings regarding sexual activity in this age group*
   b *Analyze the significance of your reactions in terms of providing this care*
   c *Formulate a teaching plan for this group*
   d *Determine how you evaluate the effects of your care.*

2 *Interview a woman with premenstrual syndrome to determine her response to the disorder.*
   a *What are the woman's perceptions about how others view her disorder?*
   b *Examine how the woman's responses compare with theoretic responses and with your own perceptions.*
   c *Analyze responses to identify positive and negative aspects of premenstrual syndrome*
   d *Investigate counseling or support group options for women with PMS in your community, and prepare a resource list describing the benefits of these resources, costs, if any, and contact information.*

3 *You are assigned to a woman preparing for surgery for breast cancer.*
   a *Identify your own feelings regarding breast cancer or other female reproductive malignancy. How might these feelings affect your ability to provide effective nursing care?*
   b *What type of support system do you believe is needed by women experiencing surgery for breast cancer? What might be the needs of her family?*
   c *Develop a plan of care for this woman and her family.*

4 *You are assigned to the health department STD Clinic.*
   a *What resources are available for counseling women who come to the clinic for testing or treatment?*
   b *Develop information sources that would be helpful in this setting to inform patients about risk factors and safer sex practices.*
   c *Consider how informational sources need to be different for patients of different ages and cultures.*

References

ACOG Committee Opinion: Premenstrual syndrome, *Int J Gynecol Obstet* 50(1):80, 1995.

American Cancer Society: *Cancer facts and figures, 1997,* New York, 1997, American Cancer Society.

Apgar B: Dysmenorrhea and dysfunctional bleeding, *Primary Care* 24(1):161, 1997.

Baker S: Menstruation and related problems and concerns. In Youngkin E & Davis M, editors: *Women's health,* Stamford, Conn, 1998, Appleton & Lange.

Branch L: Breast health. In Youngkin E & Davis M, editors: *Women's health,* Stamford, Conn, 1998, Appleton & Lange.

Carter J & Verhoef M: Efficacy of self-help and alternative treatments of premenstrual syndrome, *Womens Health Issues* 4(3):130, 1994.

Castiglia P: Amenorrhea, *J Pediatr Health Care* 10(5):226, 1996.

Centers for Disease Control and Prevention, DSTD/HIPV (division of STD/HIV Prevention): *Annual Report 1994,* US Department of Health and Human Services, 1995, Atlanta, Centers for Disease Control and Prevention.

Centers for Disease Control and Prevention & Hospital Infection Control Practices Advisory Committee (HIC-PAC): Special communications: guidelines for isolations precautions in hospitals. Part II. Recommendations for isolation precautions in hospitals, *Am J Infection Control* 24(1):24, 1996.

Centers for Disease Control and Prevention: Recommendations of the US Public Health Service Task Force for human immunodeficiency virus counseling and voluntary testing for pregnant women, *MMWR* 44(RR-7):1, 1995.

Centers for Disease Control and Prevention: 1998 guidelines for treatment of sexually transmitted diseases, *MMWR* 47(RR-1):1, 1998.

Chandraiah S: Premenstrual syndrome. In Blackwell R, editor: *Women's medicine,* Cambridge, Mass, 1996, Blackwell Science.

Chuong C, Pearsall-Otey L & Rosenfeld B: A practical guide to relieving PMS, *Contemp Nurse Pract* 1(3):31, 1995.

Cotton D & Watts D: *The medical management of AIDS in women,* New York, 1997, Willey-Liss.

Edge V & Miller M: *Mosby's clinical nursing series: women's health care,* St Louis, 1994, Mosby.

Eng T & Butler W, editors: Institute of Medicine, Committee on Prevention and Control of Sexually Transmitted Diseases: *The hidden epidemic: confronting sexually transmitted diseases.* Washington, DC, 1997, National Academy of Sciences.

Facts and Comparisons: *Loose-leaf drug information service,* St Louis, 1995, Facts and Comparisons.

Fankenauser M: Treatment of dysmenorrhea and premenstrual syndrome, *J Am Pharm Assoc* NS36(8):503, 1996.

Fiorica J: Fibrocystic changes, *Obstet Gynecol Clin North Am* 21(3):461, 1994.

Fogel C: Common symptoms. In Fogel C & Woods N, editors: *Women's health care,* Thousand Oaks, Calif, 1995a Sage.

Fogel C: Sexually transmitted disease. In Fogel C & Woods N, editors: *Women's health care,* Thousand Oaks, Calif, 1995b Sage.

Fogel C: Endocrine causes of amenorrhea, *Primary care practice* 1(5):507, 1997.

Forrest D: Common gynecologic pelvic disorders. In Youngkin E & Davis M, editors: *Women's health,* Stamford, Conn, 1998, Appleton & Lange.

Garner C: Uses of GnRH agonists, *J Obset Gynecal Neonatal Nurs* 23(7):563, 1994.

Garner C: Infertility. In Fogel C & Woods N, editors: *Women's health care,* Thousand Oaks Calif, 1995, Sage.

Golden N & Shenker I: Amenorrhea in anorexia nervosa: neuroendocrine control of hypothalamic dysfunction, *Int J Eating Disorders* 16(1):53, 1994.

Isaacs J: Other nipple discharge, *Clin Obstet Gynecol* 37(4):898, 1994.

Ivey G & Gordon S: Breast reconstruction: new image, new hope, *RN* 57(7):48, 1994.

Kiningham R, Apgar B & Schwenk T: Evaluation of amenorrhea, *Am Fam Physician* 53(4):1185, 1996.

Logothetis M: Women's reports of breast implant problems and silicone-related illness, *J Obstet Gynecol Neonatal Nurs* 24(7):609, 1995.

Lu P & Ory S: Endometriosis: current management, *Mayo Clinic Proc* 70(5):453, 1995.

Mehring P: Dysfunctional uterine bleeding, *Adv Nurse Pract* 5(1):26, 1997.

Mishell D et al.: *Contemporary gynecology,* ed 3, St Louis, 1997, Mosby.

Plourd D: Practical guide to diagnosing and treating vaginitis, *Medscape Womens Health* 2(1):1, 1997.

Rosenfeld R: Treatment of menorrhagia due to dysfunctional uterine bleeding, *Am Fam Physician* 53(1):166, 1996.

Ryan I & Taylor R: Endometriosis and infertility; new concepts, *Obstet Gynecol Sur* 52(6):365, 1997.

Sangi-Haghpeykar H & Poindexter A: Epidemiology of endometriosis among parous women, *Obstet Gynecol* 85(6):983, 1995.

Schaffer S: Vaginitis and sexually transmitted diseases. In Youngkin E & Davis M, editors: *Women's health: a primary care clinical guide,* Stamford, Conn, 1998, Appleton & Lange.

Shapiro T & Clark P: Breast cancer: what the primary care provider needs to know, *Nurs Pract* 20(3):36, 1995.

Speroff L, Glass R & Kase N: *Clinical gynecology, endocrinology, and infertility,* ed 5, Baltimore, 1994, Williams & Wilkins.

Starr W, Lommel L & Shanon M: *Women's primary health care, protocols for practice,* Washington, DC, 1995, American Nurses Publishing.

Wildschut H, Weiner C & Peters T: *When to screen in obstetrics and gynecology,* Philadelphia, 1996, WB Saunders.

Wortley P & Flemming P: AIDS in women in the United States: recent trends, *JAMA* 278(11):911, 1997.

Youngkin E: Sexually transmitted diseases: current and emerging trends, *J Obstet Gynecol Neonatal Nurs* 24(8):743, 1995.

CHAPTER

7

Contraception, Infertility, and Abortion

SHARON E. LOCK

LEARNING OBJECTIVES

- *Define the key terms.*
- *Compare the different methods of contraception.*
- *State the advantages and disadvantages of commonly used methods of contraception.*
- *Explain the common nursing interventions that facilitate contraceptive use.*
- *Recognize the various ethical, legal, cultural, and religious considerations of contraception.*
- *Describe the techniques used for medical and surgical interruption of pregnancy.*
- *Recognize the various ethical and legal considerations of elective abortion.*
- *List common causes of infertility.*
- *Discuss the psychologic impact of infertility.*
- *Identify common diagnoses and treatments for infertility.*
- *Examine the various ethical and legal considerations of infertility.*

KEY TERMS

assisted reproductive therapies (ARTs)
basal body temperature (BBT)
calendar rhythm method
cervical mucus method
contraception
diaphragm
fertility awareness
gamete intrafallopian transfer (GIFT)
impaired fertility
induced abortion
in vitro fertilization–embryo transfer (IVF–ET)
infertility
intrauterine device (IUD)
isoimmunization
periodic abstinence
postcoital test (PCT)
predictor test for ovulation

KEY TERMS—cont'd

semen analysis
spermicide
sterilization
symptothermal method
therapeutic donor insemination (TDI)
toxic shock syndrome (TSS)
vacuum aspiration
zygote intrafallopian transfer (ZIFT)

The reproductive spectrum is the focus of this chapter, covering voluntary control of fertility, interruption of pregnancy, and impaired fertility. The nursing role in the care of women varies, depending on whether management of these fertility-related concerns is associated with assessment of needs, investigation of problems, or implementation of interventions.

▌CONTRACEPTION

Contraception is the voluntary prevention of pregnancy, having both individual and social implications. Today, couples choosing contraception must be informed about prevention of unintended pregnancy, as well as protection against sexually transmitted diseases (STDs). Nurses can be instrumental in the decision-making process.

▌CARE MANAGEMENT

Assessment and Nursing Diagnoses

The woman's knowledge about contraception and her sexual partner's commitment to any particular method are determined. Data are required about the frequency of coitus, number of sexual partners, the level of contraceptive involvement, and her or her partner's objections to any methods. The woman's level of comfort and willingness to touch her genitals and cervical mucus are assessed. Myths are identified, and religious and cultural factors are determined.

The woman's verbal and nonverbal responses to hearing about the various available methods are carefully noted. An individual's reproductive life plan needs to be considered. A history (including menstrual, contraceptive, and obstetric), physical examination (including pelvic examination), and laboratory tests are usually completed.

Informed consent is a vital component in the education of the patient concerning contraception or sterilization. The nurse has the responsibility of documenting information provided and the understanding of that information by the patient. Using the acronym BRAIDED may be useful.

| LEGAL TIP | Informed Consent

B—Benefits: information about advantages and success rates
R—Risks: information about disadvantages and failure rates
A—Alternatives: information on other methods available
I—Inquiries: opportunity to ask questions
D—Decisions: opportunity to decide or change mind
E—Explanations: information about method and how it is used
D—Documentation: information given and patient's understanding

Nursing diagnoses reflect analysis of the assessment findings. Examples of nursing diagnoses that may emerge are listed in the accompanying box.

Nursing Diagnoses

Contraception
Risk for decisional conflict related to:
- Contraceptive alternatives
- Partner's willingness to agree on contraceptive method
Fear related to:
- Contraceptive method side effects
Risk for infection related to:
- Being sexually active
- Use of certain contraceptive methods
- Broken skin or mucous membrane secondary to surgery, IUD insertion, hormonal implant
Risk for altered sexuality patterns related to:
- Fear of pregnancy
Pain related to:
- Postoperative recovery after sterilization
Spiritual distress related to:
- Discrepancy between religious or cultural beliefs and choice of contraception

Expected Outcomes of Care
Planning is a collaborative effort among the woman, her sexual partner (when appropriate), the primary health care provider, and the nurse. The expected outcomes are determined and phrased in patient-centered terms and may include that the woman/couple will do the following:
- Verbalize understanding about contraceptive methods.
- State comfort and satisfaction with the chosen method.
- Use the contraceptive method correctly.
- Achieve pregnancy when planned, if further childbearing is desired.
- Experience no adverse sequelae as a result of the chosen method of contraception.
- Verbalize understanding of all information necessary to give informed consent.

Plan of Care and Interventions
Unbiased patient teaching is fundamental to initiating and maintaining any form of contraception. A care provider relationship based on trust is an important facet in patient compliance. The nurse counters myths with facts, clarifies misinformation, and fills in gaps of knowledge. There are various contraceptive techniques used in North America. The ideal contraceptive should be safe, easily available, economical, acceptable, simple to use, and promptly reversible. Although no method may ever achieve all these objectives, impressive progress has been made.

Contraceptive failure rate refers to the percentage of contraceptive users expected to experience an accidental pregnancy during the first year, even when they use a method consistently and correctly. Contraceptive effectiveness varies from couple to couple (Box 7-1) and depends on both the properties of the method and the characteristics of the user (Hatcher et al., 1998). Failure rates decrease over time either because a user gains experience and uses a method more appropriately or because the less effective users stop using the method.

Safety of a method depends on the patient's medical history, tobacco use, and age. Barrier methods offer some protection from STDs, and oral contraceptives may lower the incidence of ovarian and endometrial cancer, but increase the risk of thromboembolic problems.

Methods of contraception
The following discussion of contraceptive methods provides the nurse with information needed for patient teaching. After implementing the appropriate teaching for

---

BOX 7-1 | *Factors Affecting Method Effectiveness*

Frequency of intercourse
Motivation to prevent pregnancy
Understanding of how to use the method
Compliance with method
Provision of short-term or long-term protection
Likelihood of pregnancy for the individual woman

contraceptive use, the nurse supervises return demonstrations and practice to assess patient understanding. The woman is given written instructions and phone numbers for questions. If the woman has difficulty understanding written instructions, she (and her partner, if available) is offered graphic material and a phone number to call as necessary or an offer to return for further instruction.

Coitus interruptus. *Coitus interruptus* (withdrawal) involves the male partner withdrawing the penis from the woman's vagina before he ejaculates. Although coitus interruptus has been criticized as being an ineffective method of contraception, it is a good choice for couples who do not have another contraceptive available (Hatcher et al., 1998). Effectiveness is similar to barrier methods and depends on the man's ability to withdraw his penis before ejaculation. The failure rate for the typical user of withdrawal is about 19% (Hatcher et al., 1998). Coitus interruptus does not protect against STDs or human immunodeficiency virus (HIV) infection.

Periodic abstinence. Periodic abstinence, or *natural family planning (NFP),* provides contraception by using methods that rely on avoidance of intercourse during fertile periods. It is the only method of contraception acceptable to the Roman Catholic Church. **Fertility awareness** is the combination of charting signs and symptoms of the menstrual cycle with the use of abstinence or other contraceptive methods during fertile periods (Geerling, 1995). Signs and symptoms most commonly used are menstrual bleeding, cervical mucus, and basal body temperature (Hatcher et al., 1998).

Knowledge of the menstrual cycle is basic to the practice of NFP. To review, the human ovum can be fertilized no later than 16 to 24 hours after ovulation. Motile sperm have been recovered from the uterus and the oviducts as long as 60 hours after coitus. However, their ability to fertilize the ovum probably lasts no longer than 24 to 48 hours. Pregnancy is unlikely to occur if a couple abstains from intercourse for 4 days before and for 3 or 4 days after ovulation (fertile period). Unprotected intercourse on the other days of the cycle (safe period) should not result in pregnancy. However, there are two principal problems with this method: the exact time of ovulation cannot be predicted accurately, and couples may find it difficult to exercise restraint for several days before and after ovulation. Women with irregular menstrual periods have the greatest risk of failure with this form of contraception. Therefore NFP methods are not recommended until regular menses has resumed postpartum (Geerling, 1995; Hatcher et al., 1998). The typical failure rate is 20% during the first year of use (Hatcher et al., 1998).

Ovulation usually occurs about 14 days before the onset of menstruation. Therefore variations in the length of menstrual cycles are usually a result of differences in the length of the preovulatory phases. The fertile period can be anticipated by the following:

- Calculating the time at which ovulation is likely to occur based on the lengths of previous menstrual cycles (calendar method)
- Recording the rise in basal body temperature (BBT), a result of the thermogenic effect of progesterone (temperature method)
- Recognizing the changes in cervical mucus at different phases of the menstrual cycle (ovulation or Billings method)
- Using a predictor test for ovulation
- Using a combination of several methods (symptothermal method)

Calendar rhythm method. Practice of the **calendar rhythm method,** (also known as the rhythm method or menstrual cycle charting), is based on the number of days in each cycle counting from the first day of menses (Geerling, 1995). With the calendar method the fertile period is determined after accurately recording the lengths of menstrual cycles for 6 months. The beginning of the fertile period is estimated by subtracting 18 days from the length of the shortest cycle. The end of the fertile period is determined by subtracting 11 days from the length of the longest cycle. If the shortest cycle is 24 days and longest is 30 days, application of the formula is as follows:

Shortest Cycle	Longest Cycle
24	30
−18	−11
6th day	9th day

To avoid conception the couple would abstain during the fertile period—days 6 through 19. If the woman has very regular cycles of 28 days each, the formula indicates the fertile days to be

Shortest Cycle	Longest Cycle
28	28
−18	−11
10th day	17th day

To avoid pregnancy, the couple abstains from day 10 through 17 because ovulation occurs on day 14 ± 2 days. A major drawback of the calendar method is trying to predict future events with past data. The unpredictability of the menstrual cycle is also not taken into consideration.

The method is most useful as an adjunct to the BBT or cervical mucus method.

Basal body temperature method. The **basal body temperature (BBT)** is the lowest body temperature of a healthy person that is taken immediately after waking and before getting out of bed. The BBT usually varies

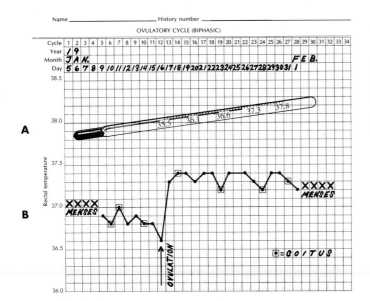

Fig. **7-1 A,** Special thermometer for recording BBT, marked in tenths to enable person to read more easily. **B,** Basal temperature record shows drop and sharp rise at time of ovulation. Biphasic curve indicates ovulatory cycle.

from 36.2° to 36.3° C during menses and for about 5 to 7 days afterward (Fig. 7-1).

If ovulation fails to occur, this pattern of lower body temperature continues throughout the cycle. Infection, fatigue, less than 3 hours sleep per night, awakening late, and anxiety may cause temperature fluctuations, altering the expected pattern. If a new BBT thermometer is purchased, this fact is noted on the chart because the readings may vary slightly. Jet lag, alcohol taken the evening before, or sleeping in a heated waterbed must also be noted on the chart because each affects the BBT.

About the time of ovulation a slight drop in temperature (approximately 0.05° C) may be seen; after ovulation, in concert with the increasing progesterone levels of the early luteal phase of the cycle, the BBT rises slightly (approximately 0.2° to 0.4° C) (Speroff & Darney, 1996). The temperature remains on an elevated plateau until 2 to 4 days before menstruation. Then it drops to the low levels recorded during the previous cycle, unless pregnancy has occurred and the temperature remains elevated.

The drop and subsequent rise in temperature are referred to as the *thermal shift.* When the entire month's temperatures are recorded on a graph, the pattern described is more apparent. It is more difficult to perceive day-to-day variations without the entire picture. Therefore the BBT alone is not a reliable method to predict ovulation (Hatcher et al., 1998; Speroff & Darney, 1996). To determine if a rise in

temperature is indeed the thermal shift, the woman must be aware of other signs approaching ovulation while she continues to assess the BBT (see later discussion of symptothermal method for other indicators of ovulation).

Most counselors advise the couple who wish to prevent conception to avoid unprotected intercourse from the day of the drop in the BBT and for 3 days of elevated temperature (Hatcher et al., 1998) (see the Teaching Guidelines box).

Cervical mucus method. The **cervical mucus method** (also called the Billings method and the Creighton model ovulation method) requires that the woman recognize and interpret the characteristic cyclic changes in the amount and consistency of cervical mucus (see the Teaching Guidelines box on the next page). Each woman has her own unique pattern of mucus changes. The cervical mucus that accompanies ovulation is necessary for viability and motility of sperm. Without adequate cervical mucus, coitus does not result in conception. To ensure an accurate assessment of changes, the cervical mucus should be free from semen, contraceptive gels or foams, and blood or discharge from vaginal infections for at least one full cycle. Other factors that create difficulty in identifying mucus changes include douches and vaginal deodorants, being in the sexually aroused state (which thins the mucus), and taking medications such as antihistamines, which dry up the mucus.

Some women may find this method unacceptable if they are uncomfortable touching their genitals. Whether or not the individual wants to use this method for contraception, it is to the woman's advantage to learn to recognize mucus characteristics at ovulation. Self-evaluation of cervical mucus

TEACHING GUIDELINES
Cervical Mucus Characteristics

SETTING THE STAGE

Show charts of menstrual cycle along with changes in the cervical mucus.

Have woman practice with raw egg white.

Supply her with a BBT log and graph if she doesn't already have one.

Explain that assessment of cervical mucus characteristics is best when mucus is not mixed with semen, contraceptive jellies or foams, or discharge from infections. Douching should not be done before assessment.

CONTENT RELATED TO CERVICAL MUCUS

Explain to woman (couple) how cervical mucus changes throughout the menstrual cycle.

Right before ovulation, the watery, thin, clear mucus becomes more abundant and thick. It feels like a lubricant and can be stretched 5+ cm between the thumb and forefinger; this is called *spinnbarkheit*. This indicates the period of maximum fertility. Sperm deposited in this type of mucus can survive until ovulation occurs.

ASSESSMENT TECHNIQUE

Stress that good hand washing is imperative to begin and end all self-assessment.

Start observation from last day of menstrual flow.

Assess cervical mucus several times a day for several cycles. Mucus can be obtained from vaginal introitus; no need to reach into vagina to cervix.

Record findings on the same record on which BBT is entered.

---

can be highly accurate (Fehring et al., 1994) and can be useful diagnostically for any of the following purposes:

- To alert the couple to the reestablishment of ovulation while breastfeeding and after discontinuation of oral contraception
- To note anovulatory cycles at any time and at the commencement of menopause
- To assist couples in planning a pregnancy

Symptothermal method. The **symptothermal method** combines the BBT and cervical mucus methods with awareness of secondary, cycle phase–related symptoms. The woman gains fertility awareness as she learns the psychologic and physiologic symptoms that mark the phases of her cycle. Secondary symptoms include increased libido, midcycle spotting, mittelschmerz, pelvic fullness or tenderness, and vulvar fullness. The woman is taught to palpate the cervix to assess for changes indicating ovulation; that is, the os dilates slightly, the cervix softens and

rises in the vagina, and cervical mucus is copious and slippery (Trent & Clark, 1997). The woman notes days on which coitus, changes in routine, illness, and so on have occurred (Fig. 7-2). Calendar calculations and cervical mucus changes are used to estimate the onset of the fertile period; changes in cervical mucus or the BBT are used to estimate its end.

Effectiveness of the symptothermal method with abstinence during the fertile period ranges between 73% and 97% (Geerling, 1995).

Predictor test for ovulation. All of the preceding discussion is about assessments that are indicative of but do not prove the occurrence and exact timing of ovulation. The predictor test for ovulation is a major addition to the periodic abstinence methods to help women who want to plan the time of their pregnancies and those who are trying to conceive. The **predictor test for ovulation** detects the sudden surge of luteinizing hormone (LH) that occurs approximately 12 to 24 hours before ovulation. Unlike BBT, the test is not affected by illness, emotional upset, or physical activity. Available for home use, a test kit contains sufficient material for several days' testing of urine during each cycle. A positive response indicative of an LH surge is noted by an easily readable color change. Directions for use of this home test kit vary with the manufacturer.

Barrier methods. Barrier contraceptives are currently receiving great attention and increased use (Speroff & Darney, 1996). This method has the additional distinct advantage of reducing the spread of STDs. Chemical barriers such as nonoxynol-9 have been shown to protect against *Neisseria gonorrhoeae*, *Chlamydia*, and HIV (Hatcher et al., 1998; Heath & Sulik, 1997). Male and female condoms provide a mechanical barrier to STDs (Hatcher et al., 1998).

Spermicides. A vaginal **spermicide** is a physical barrier to sperm penetration that also has a chemical action on sperm. Nonoxynol-9 (N-9) and octoxynol-9 are the most commonly used spermicidal chemicals. Intravaginal spermicides are marketed as aerosol foams, foaming tablets, suppositories, creams, films, and gels (Fig. 7-3). Preloaded, single-dose applicators small enough to be carried in a small purse are available. Typical failure rate in the first year of use is 5% to 50% (Hatcher et al., 1998). Box 7-2 provides patient teaching information about spermicide use.

Condoms. The male *condom* is a thin, stretchable sheath that covers the penis (Fig. 7-4, *B*). In addition to three available sizes, four basic features differ among condoms marketed in the United States. These features are material, shape, lubricants, and spermicides. Ninety-five percent are made of latex rubber. A functional difference in condom shape is the presence or absence of a sperm reservoir tip. To enhance vaginal stimulation, some condoms are contoured and rippled or have ribbed or roughened surfaces. Thinner construction increases heat transmission and sensitivity; a

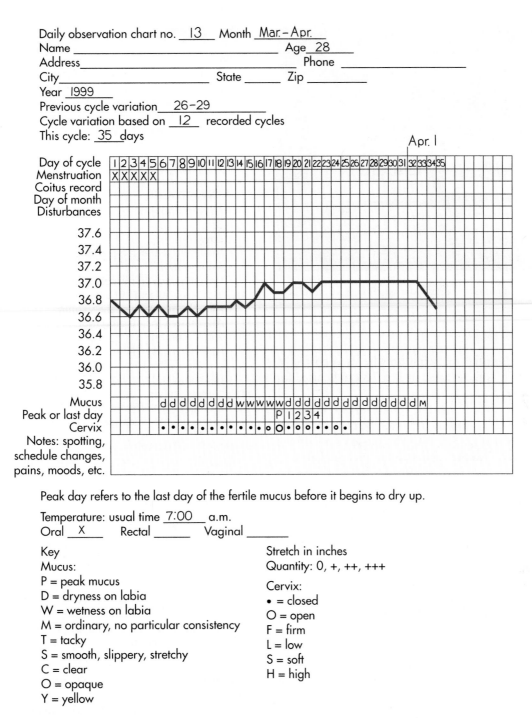

Daily observation chart no. __13__ Month __Mar.–Apr.__
Name _____ Age __28__
Address_____ Phone _____
City_____ State _____ Zip _____
Year __1999__
Previous cycle variation__26–29_____
Cycle variation based on __12__ recorded cycles
This cycle: __35__ days

Fig. 7-2 Example of a completed symptothermal chart.

Peak day refers to the last day of the fertile mucus before it begins to dry up.

Temperature: usual time __7:00__ a.m.
Oral __X__   Rectal _____   Vaginal _____

Key
Mucus:
P = peak mucus
D = dryness on labia
W = wetness on labia
M = ordinary, no particular consistency
T = tacky
S = smooth, slippery, stretchy
C = clear
O = opaque
Y = yellow

Stretch in inches
Quantity: 0, +, ++, +++

Cervix:
• = closed
O = open
F = firm
L = low
S = soft
H = high

variety of colors increases their acceptability and attractiveness (Hatcher et al., 1998). A wet jelly or dry powder lubricates some condoms. Since 1982 spermicide (0.5 g of nonoxynol-9) has been added to the interior or exterior surfaces of some condoms. The addition of nonoxynol-9 to latex condoms not only increases contraceptive effective-

ness, it also increases protection against transmission of STDs, including HIV. Typical failure rate for first year of use is 14% (Hatcher et al., 1998).

For years, health care providers assumed that everyone knew how to use condoms, so proper instruction was not provided. To prevent unintended pregnancy and the spread

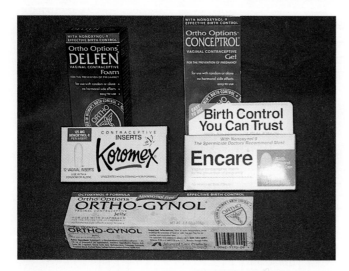

Fig. 7-3 Spermicides. (Courtesy Marjorie Pyle, RNC, Lifecircle, Costa Mesa, Calif.)

of STDs, it is essential that condoms be used correctly. Instructions such as those listed in Box 7-3 can be used for patient teaching.

The vaginal sheath (female condom) is made of polyurethane and has flexible rings at both ends (Speroff & Darney, 1996) (Fig. 7-4, *A*). The closed end of the pouch is inserted into the vagina and is anchored around the cervix: the open ring covers the labia. It can be applied well in advance of intercourse so that spontaneity is unaffected. Before intercourse, a spermicide is added. Since it is a relatively loose sheath, it tends to heighten sensation for the man. Both women and men report that intercourse with the sheath is generally about as satisfying as intercourse without the sheath. Application of this disposable barrier requires no special training. It comes in one size and is available over the counter. Typical failure rate is 21% in the first year of use (Hatcher et al., 1998).

Diaphragm. The vaginal **diaphragm** is a shallow, dome-shaped rubber device with a flexible wire rim that covers the cervix (Fig. 7-4, *C*). There are three main styles of diaphragms, available in a wide range of diameters (50 to 95 mm). Diaphragms differ in the inner construction of the circular rim. The four types of rims are flat spring, coil spring, arcing spring, and wide-seal rim.

The diaphragm should feel comfortable. It should be the largest size the woman can wear without her being aware of its presence. The use of a contraceptive gel or cream with the diaphragm offers both mechanical and chemical barriers to pregnancy.

The diaphragm is a mechanical barrier preventing the meeting of the sperm with the ovum. The diaphragm holds the spermicide in place against the cervix for the 6 hours it

---

BOX 7-2   *Spermicides*

MODE OF ACTION

Spermicides provide a physical and chemical barrier that prevents viable sperm from entering the cervix. The effect is local, within the vagina. The spermicide is placed deeply into the vagina in contact with the cervix before each incidence of coitus.

FAILURE RATE

Typical failure: 5% to 50%

ADVANTAGES

- Easy to apply
- Safe
- Low cost
- Available without a prescription or previous medical examination
- Delicate vaginal mucosa is not harmed unless the woman is allergic to a particular preparation
- Aid in lubrication of the vagina
- Alternative for nursing mothers (does not interfere with lactation)
- Alternative for the premenopausal woman (to prevent masking symptoms of onset of the climacteric)
- Backup when the woman forgets her oral contraceptive
- Increases the effectiveness of condoms and other forms of contraception

STD PROTECTION

Spermicides containing nonoxynol-9 provide some protection against STDs through bacteriostatic action. Need to be used with condoms if protection from STDs is needed.

DISADVANTAGES

- Maximum spermicidal effectiveness lasts usually no longer than 1 hour.
- If intercourse is to be repeated, reapplication of additional spermicide must precede it.
- Some users complain that it is messy and has an unpleasant fizz and taste.
- Allergic response or irritation of vaginal or penile tissue may occur.
- Possible decreased tactile sensation.

NURSING CONSIDERATIONS/PATIENT TEACHING

Can must be shaken to distribute foam spermicide before use.

Tablets and suppositories take from 10 to 30 minutes to dissolve.

Douching must be avoided for at least 6 hours after coitus.

Encourage open communication between sexual partners to discuss intravaginal contraception.

Provide opportunity to see and handle a variety of samples.

Provide anatomic model to practice insertion into the vagina.

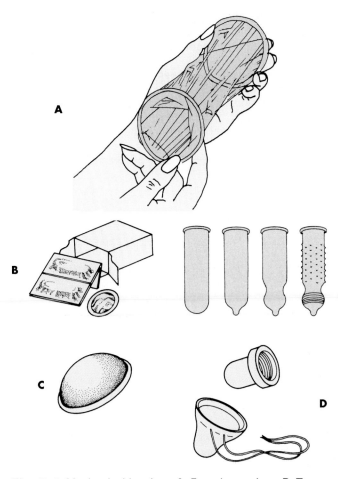

Fig. **7-4** Mechanical barriers. **A,** Female condom. **B,** Types of male condoms. **C,** Diaphragm. **D,** Cervical cap.

takes to destroy the sperm. Typical failure rate of the diaphragm alone is 20% in the first year of use. Effectiveness of the diaphragm can be increased when combined with a spermicide (Hatcher et al., 1998).

Nursing considerations. The woman is informed that she needs an annual gynecologic examination during which the fit of the diaphragm should be assessed. The device may need to be refitted after significant weight loss or weight gain (more than 22 to 33 kg), term birth, or second trimester abortion (Hatcher et al., 1998; Speroff & Darney, 1996). Because there are various types of diaphragms on the market, the nurse uses the package insert for teaching the woman how to use and care for the diaphragm (see Home Care box).

Except for occasional allergic responses to the diaphragm or spermicide, there are no side effects from a well-fitted device. The diaphragm can be inserted as long as 6 hours before intercourse to increase spontaneity, but spermicide must be inserted into the vagina each time intercourse is repeated (Hatcher et al., 1998). The diaphragm must be left in place for at least 6 hours after the last intercourse. The

woman who engages in intercourse infrequently may choose this barrier method. The spermicide does offer additional lubrication if it is needed. A decreased incidence of vaginitis, cervicitis (including cervicitis caused by *Chlamydia trachomatis* and *Neisseria gonorrhoeae),* pelvic inflammatory disease (PID), and cervical intraepithelial neoplasia is noted among women who use contraceptive creams, foams, and gels with the diaphragm.

This method is contraindicated for the woman with relaxation of her pelvic support (uterine prolapse) or a large cystocele.

Disadvantages include the reluctance of some women to insert and remove the diaphragm. A cold diaphragm and a cold gel temporarily reduce vaginal response to sexual stimulation if insertion of the diaphragm occurs immediately before intercourse. Some women or couples object to the "messiness" of the spermicide. These annoyances of diaphragm use, along with failure to insert the device once foreplay has begun, are the most common reasons for failures of this method. Side effects may include irritation of tissues related to contact with spermicides. Urethritis and recurrent cystitis caused by upward pressure of the diaphragm rim against the urethra may be increased by the use of the contraceptive diaphragm (Hatcher et al., 1998).

Toxic shock syndrome (TSS) is a potentially life-threatening system disorder. Although reported in small numbers, TSS can occur in association with the use of the contraceptive diaphragm (Hatcher et al., 1998). The nurse should instruct the woman about ways to reduce her risk for TSS. These measures include prompt removal 6 to 8 hours after intercourse, not using the diaphragm during menses, thorough handwashing before handling and removing the diaphragm, and learning and watching for danger signs of TSS.

> **NURSE ALERT** *The nurse should be alert for signs of TSS in women who use a diaphragm or cervical cap as a contraceptive method. The most common signs include fever of sudden onset greater than 38.4° C, hypotension (systolic less than 90 mm Hg or orthostatic dizziness), and a rash.*

Cervical cap. The *cervical cap* has a 22 mm to 31 mm soft, natural rubber dome with a firm but pliable rim (Fig. 7-4, *D*). It fits snugly around the base of the cervix close to the junction of the cervix and vaginal fornices (Hatcher et al., 1998). The device is available in four sizes. It is recommended that the cap remain in place no less than 8 hours and not more than 48 hours at a time (Secor, 1992). It is left in place 6 to 8 hours after the last act of intercourse. The seal provides a physical barrier to sperm: spermicide inside the cap adds a chemical barrier. The extended period of wear is an added convenience for women who previously used the diaphragm. Instructions for the actual insertion and use of

BOX 7-3   *Male Condoms*

MECHANISM OF ACTION

Sheath is applied over the erect penis before insertion or loss of preejaculatory drops of semen. Used correctly, condoms prevent sperm from entering the cervix. Spermicide-coated condoms cause ejaculated sperm to be immobilized rapidly, thus increasing contraceptive effectiveness.

FAILURE RATE

Typical users, 14%
Correct and consistent users, 3%

ADVANTAGES

Safe
No side effects
Readily available
Premalignant changes in cervix can be prevented or ameliorated in women whose partners use condoms
Method of male nonsurgical contraception

DISADVANTAGES

Must interrupt lovemaking to apply sheath.
Sensation may be altered.
If used improperly, spillage of sperm can result in pregnancy.
Occasionally, condoms may tear during intercourse.

STD PROTECTION

If a condom is used throughout the act of intercourse and there is no unprotected contact with female genitals, a latex rubber condom, which is impermeable to viruses, can act as a protective measure against STDs. The addition of nonoxynol-9 increases protection against transmission of STDs, including HIV.

NURSING CONSIDERATIONS

Teach male to:
- Use a new condom (check expiration date) for each act of sexual intercourse or other acts between partners that involve contact with the penis.

- Place condom after penis is erect and before intimate contact.
- Place condom on head of penis (Fig. A) and unroll it all the way to the base (Fig. B).
- Leave an empty space at the tip (Fig. A); remove any air remaining in the tip by gently pressing air out toward the base of the penis.

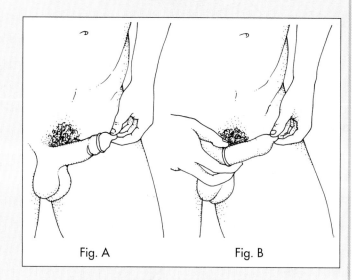

Fig. A   Fig. B

- If a lubricant is desired, use water-based products such as K-Y Jelly. Do not use petroleum-based products because they can cause the condom to break.
- After ejaculation, carefully withdraw the still erect penis from the vagina, holding onto condom rim; remove and discard the condom.
- Store unused condoms in cool, dry place.
- Do not use condoms that are sticky, brittle, or obviously damaged.

---

the cervical cap closely resemble the instructions for the use of the contraceptive diaphragm. Some of the differences are that the cervical cap can be inserted hours before sexual intercourse without a need for additional spermicide later, no additional spermicide is required for repeated acts of intercourse when the cap is used, and the cervical cap requires less spermicide than the diaphragm when initially inserted (Secor, 1992). If the cap is left in place more than 48 hours, it will produce an odor.

Some women are not good candidates for wearing the cervical cap. They include women with abnormal Pap test results, women who cannot be fitted properly with the existing cap sizes, women who find the insertion and removal of the device too difficult, women with a history of TSS, women with vaginal or cervical infections (Hatcher et al.,

1998), and women who experience allergic responses to the cap or spermicide.

Nursing considerations. The angle of the uterus, the vaginal muscle tone, and the shape of the cervix may interfere with the cervical cap's ease of fitting and use. Correct fitting requires time, effort, and skill from both the woman and the clinician (Secor, 1992). The woman must check the cap's position before and after each act of intercourse. Cervical cap use has been associated with abnormal Pap smears (Hatcher et al., 1998). These abnormalities may be manifestations of the human papillomavirus (HPV). Women using the cap should have a Pap test at least every year.

Because of the risk of TSS associated with the use of the cervical cap, another form of birth control is recommended for use during menstrual bleeding and up to at least 6 weeks

HOME CARE *Patient Instructions for Self-Care*

Use and Care of the Diaphragm

POSITIONS FOR INSERTION OF DIAPHRAGM

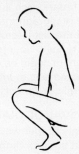

Squatting
Squatting is the most commonly used position, and most women find it satisfactory.

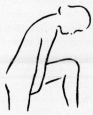

Leg-up Method
Another position is to raise the left foot (if right hand is used for insertion) on a low stool and in a bending position insert the diaphragm.

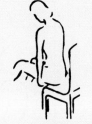

Chair Method
Another practical method for diaphragm insertion is to sit far forward on the edge of a chair.

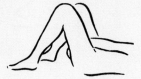

Reclining
You may prefer to insert the diaphragm while in a semi-reclining position in bed.

INSPECTION OF DIAPHRAGM

Your diaphragm must be inspected carefully before each use. The best way to do this is as follows:

Hold the diaphragm up to a light source. Carefully stretch the diaphragm at the area of the rim, on all sides, to make sure there are no holes. Remember, it is possible to puncture the diaphragm with sharp fingernails.

Another way to check for pinholes is to carefully fill the diaphragm with water. If there is any problem, it will be seen immediately.

If your diaphragm is puckered, especially near the rim, this could mean thin spots.

The diaphragm should not be used if you see any of the above; consult your health care provider.

PREPARATION OF DIAPHRAGM

Rinse off cornstarch. Your diaphragm must always be used with a spermicidal lubricant to be effective. Pregnancy cannot be prevented effectively by the diaphragm alone.

Always empty your bladder before inserting the diaphragm. Place about 2 teaspoonfuls of contraceptive jelly or contraceptive cream on the side of the diaphragm that will rest against the cervix (or whichever way you have been instructed). Spread it around to coat the surface and the rim. This aids in insertion and offers a more complete seal. Many women also spread some jelly or cream on the other side of the diaphragm (Fig. A).

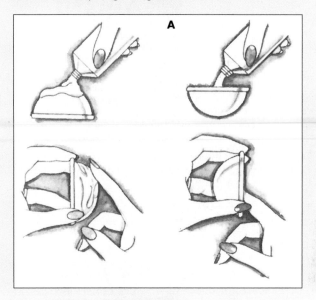

INSERTION OF DIAPHRAGM

The diaphragm can be inserted as long as 6 hours before intercourse. Hold the diaphragm between your thumb and fingers. The dome can either be up or down, as directed by your health care provider. Place your index finger on the outer rim of the compressed diaphragm (Fig. B). Use the fingers of the other hand to spread the labia (lips of the vagina). This will assist in guiding the diaphragm into place.

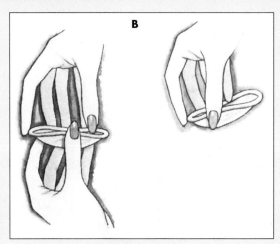

Continued

HOME CARE *Patient Instructions for Self-Care—cont'd*

Use and Care of the Diaphragm —cont'd

Insert the diaphragm into the vagina. Direct it inward and downward as far as it will go to space behind and below the cervix (Fig. C).

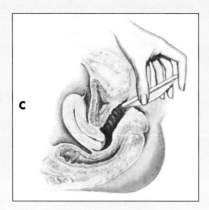

Tuck the front of the rim of the diaphragm behind the pubic bone so that the rubber hugs the front wall of the vagina (Fig. D).

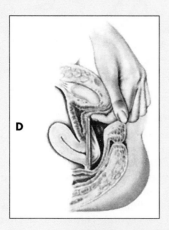

Feel for your cervix through the diaphragm to be certain it is properly placed and securely covered by the rubber dome (Fig. E).

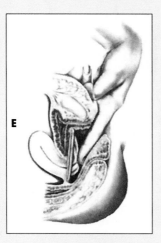

GENERAL INFORMATION

Regardless of the time of the month, you must use your diaphragm each and every time intercourse takes place. Your diaphragm must be left in place for at least 6 hours after the last intercourse. If you remove your diaphragm before the 6-hour period, your chance of becoming pregnant could be greatly increased. If you have repeated acts of intercourse, you need to add more spermicide for each act of intercourse.

REMOVAL OF DIAPHRAGM

The only proper way to remove the diaphragm is to insert your forefinger up and over the top side of the diaphragm and slightly to the side.

Next, turn the palm of your hand downward and backward hooking the forefinger firmly on top of the inside of the upper rim of the diaphragm, breaking the suction.

Pull the diaphragm down and out. This avoids the possibility of tearing the diaphragm with the fingernails. You should not remove the diaphragm by trying to catch the rim from below the dome (Fig. F).

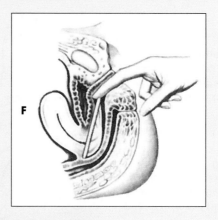

CARE OF DIAPHRAGM

When using a vaginal diaphragm, avoid using products that may contain petroleum, such as certain body lubricants, vaginal lubricants, or vaginitis preparations. These products can weaken the rubber.

A little care means longer wear for your diaphragm. After each use the diaphragm should be washed in warm water and mild soap. Do not use detergent soaps, cold cream soaps, deodorant soaps, and soaps containing petroleum, since they can weaken the rubber.

After washing, the diaphragm should be dried thoroughly. All water and moisture should be removed with a towel. The diaphragm should then be dusted with *cornstarch*. Scented talc, body powder, baby powder, and the like should not be used because they can weaken the rubber.

To clean the introducer (if one is used), wash with mild soap and warm water, rinse, and dry thoroughly.

The diaphragm should be placed back in the plastic case for storage. It should not be stored near a radiator or heat source or exposed to light for an extended period.

postpartum. The cap should be refitted after any gynecologic surgery or birth and after major weight losses or gains. Otherwise, the size should be checked at least once a year (Secor, 1992).

Strong patient motivation is the most important criterion for successful cap use. First-year failure rates range from 5 to 26 pregnancies per 100 women who initiate the use of this method (Hatcher et al., 1998). That failure rate is similar to that of the diaphragm.

The woman must be given the information available for this product as previously presented. The nurse needs to assess the woman's understanding and skill in the use of the cervical cap (see the Home Care box at right).

Hormonal methods. Over 30 different oral contraceptive formulations are available in the United States today. General classes are described in Table 7-1. Because of the wide variety of preparations available, the woman and nurse need to read the package insert for information about specific products prescribed. Formulations include combined estrogen-progestin steroidal medications, progestational agents, and an estrogenic agent. The formulations are administered orally, subdermally, or by implantation.

Combined estrogen-progestin oral contraceptives

Mode of action. The normal menstrual cycle is maintained by a feedback mechanism. Follicle-stimulating hormone (FSH) and luteinizing hormone (LH) are secreted in response to fluctuating levels of ovarian estrogen and progesterone. Regular ingestion of combined oral contraceptive pills (OCPs) suppresses the action of the hypothalamus and anterior pituitary leading to inappropriate secretion of FSH and LH. Therefore follicles do not mature and ovulation is inhibited.

Other contraceptive effects are induced by the combined steroids. Maturation of the endometrium is altered, making it a less favorable site for implantation should ovulation and conception occur. It also has a direct effect on the endometrium, so that from 1 to 4 days after the last steroid tablet is taken, the endometrium sloughs and bleeds as a result of hormone withdrawal. The *withdrawal bleeding* usually is less profuse than that of normal menstruation and may last only 2 to 3 days. Some women have no bleeding at all.

The cervical mucus remains thick as a result of the effect of the progestin. Cervical mucus under the effect of progesterone does not provide as suitable an environment for sperm penetration as does the thin, watery mucus at ovulation (Hatcher et al., 1998).

The possible effect, if any, of altered tubal and uterine motility induced by the steroidal hormones is not clear. Nevertheless, oral hormonal contraceptives, if taken daily for 3 weeks of every 4, provide virtually absolute protection against conception (Cunningham et al., 1997). *Monophasic* pills provide fixed dosages of estrogen and progestin. *Phasic* pills (e.g., biphasic, triphasic, and multiphasic

HOME CARE *Patient Instructions for Self-Care*
Use of the Cervical Cap
Push cap up into vagina until it covers cervix.

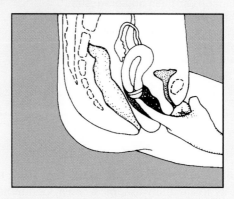

Press rim against cervix to create a seal.

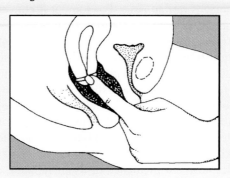

To remove, push rim toward right or left hip to loosen from cervix and then withdraw.

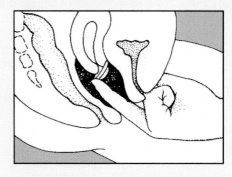

The woman can assume several positions to insert the cervical cap. See the four positions shown for inserting the diaphragm.

oral contraceptives) alter the amount of progestin and sometimes the amount of estrogen within each cycle. These preparations reduce the total dosage of hormones in a single cycle without sacrificing contraceptive efficacy or cycle control (Cunningham et al., 1997).

Advantages. For motivated women it is easy to take an oral contraceptive at about the same time each day. Taking

TABLE 7-1 *Hormonal Contraception*

COMPOSITION	ROUTE OF ADMINISTRATION	DURATION OF EFFECT
Combination estrogen and progestin (synthetic estrogens and progestins in varying doses and formulations)	Oral	24 hours
Progestin only		
Norethindrone, norgestrel	Oral	24 hours
Medroxyprogesterone acetate	Intramuscular injection	3 months
Levonorgestrel	Subdermal implant	Up to 5 years
Progesterone	Intrauterine device	1 year

the pill does not relate directly to the sexual act; this fact increases its acceptability to some women. Commonly there is an improvement in sexual response once the possibility of pregnancy is not an issue. For some it is convenient to know when to expect the next menstrual flow.

Oral contraceptives are considered to be a safe option for older, nonsmoking women until menopause. Perimenopausal women can benefit from regular bleeding cycles, a regular hormonal pattern, and the noncontraceptive health benefits of oral contraceptives (Hatcher et al., 1998).

The noncontraceptive health benefits of oral contraceptives include decreased menstrual blood loss and decreased iron-deficiency anemia, regulation of menorrhagia and irregular cycles, lowered incidence of dysmenorrhea and premenstrual syndrome (PMS). Oral contraceptives also offer protection against endometrial adenocarcinoma and possibly ovarian cancer, reduced incidence of benign breast disease, protection against the development of functional ovarian cysts and some types of pelvic inflammatory disease (PID), and decreased risk of ectopic pregnancy (Contraception Report, 1997; Hatcher et al., 1998; Speroff & Darney, 1996).

Women taking steroidal contraceptives are examined before the medication is prescribed and yearly thereafter. The examination includes medical and family history, weight, blood pressure, general physical and pelvic examination, screening cervical cytologic analysis (Pap smear). Consistent monitoring by the health care provider is valuable in the detection of noncontraception-related disorders as well, so that timely treatment can be initiated.

Use of oral hormonal contraceptives is usually initiated on one of the first 7 days of the menstrual cycle (day 1 of the cycle is the first day of menses). Women can start their use after childbirth or abortion. With a "Sunday start" pack, patients begin taking pills on the first Sunday after the start of their menstrual period (Moore, 1994). If contraceptives are to be started at any time other than during normal menses, or within 3 weeks after birth or abortion, another method of contraception should be used throughout the first week to avoid the risk of pregnancy (Hatcher et al.,

1998). The combined estrogen-progestin pill taken daily 3 weeks out of every 4 is the most effective reversible form of contraception available (Cunningham et al., 1997). Taken exactly as directed, oral contraceptives prevent ovulation, and pregnancy cannot occur; the overall effectiveness rate is almost 100%. Almost all failures (i.e., pregnancy occurs) are caused by omission of one or more pills during the regimen. The typical failure rate due to omission is 5%.

Disadvantages and side effects. Since hormonal contraceptives have come into use, the amount of estrogen and progestational agent contained in each tablet has been reduced considerably (Cunningham et al., 1997). This is important because adverse effects are somewhat dose related.

Women must be screened for conditions that present absolute or relative contraindications to oral contraceptive use. *Absolute contraindications* include a history of thromboembolic disorders, cerebrovascular or coronary artery disease, breast cancer, estrogenic-dependent tumors, pregnancy, impaired liver function, liver tumor, undiagnosed vaginal bleeding, and smokers over 35 years old. Strong relative contraindications include migraine headaches, hypertension, elective surgery, epilepsy, sickle cell disease, diabetes mellitus, and gall bladder disease (Hatcher et al., 1998; Speroff & Darney, 1996).

Certain side effects of OCPs are attributable to estrogen and progestin or both. Side effects of estrogen excess include nausea and vomiting, dizziness, edema, leg cramps, increase in breast size, chloasma (mask of pregnancy), visual changes, hypertension, and vascular headache. Side effects of estrogen deficiency include early spotting (days 1 to 14), hypomenorrhea, nervousness, and atrophic vaginitis leading to painful intercourse (dyspareunia). Side effects of progestin excess include increased appetite, tiredness, depression, breast tenderness, vaginal yeast infection, oily skin and scalp, hirsutism, and postpill amenorrhea. Side effects of progestin deficiency include late spotting and breakthrough bleeding (days 15 to 21), heavy flow with clots, and decreased breast size. One of the most common side effects is bleeding irregularities (Contraception Report, 1997; Hatcher et al., 1998).

In the presence of side effects, especially those that are bothersome, a different product, a different drug content, or another method of contraception may be required. The "right" product for a woman contains the lowest dose of sex steroid hormones that prevents ovulation and that has the fewest and least harmful side effects. There is no way to predict the right dosage for any particular woman; trial and error is the main method for prescribing oral contraceptives, starting with the lowest possible estrogen dose. The changes in glucose tolerance that occur in some women taking oral contraceptives are similar to those changes that occur during pregnancy. The dosage, type, and potency of progestin (not estrogen) produce some deterioration of glucose tolerance in normal women, as well as in those with a history of gestational diabetes (Hatcher et al., 1998; Speroff & Darney, 1996). The effectiveness of oral contraceptives is decreased when the following medications are taken simultaneously (Hatcher et al., 1998).

- Barbiturates (e.g., phenobarbital)
- Anticonvulsants (phenytoin sodium, carbamazepine, primidone)
- Antifungals (e.g., griseofulvin)
- Antibiotics (ampicillin, tetracycline, rifampin)

Also the use of oral contraceptives can decrease the effectiveness of several medications (e.g., oral hypoglycemics and oral anticoagulants) (Hatcher et al., 1998).

Research findings on use of oral contraceptives and risk of breast cancer have been inconsistent (Speroff & Darney, 1996); investigation continues on this important concern. Women who discontinue oral contraception for a planned pregnancy commonly ask whether they should wait before attempting to conceive. Although data are controversial, studies indicate that these infants have no greater chance of being born with any type of birth defect than do infants born to women in the general population, even if conception occurred in the first month after the medication was discontinued (Hatcher et al., 1998; Speroff & Darney, 1996).

After discontinuing oral contraception there is usually a delay before ovulation and menstrual cycles recur, similar to that experienced by a new mother. However, amenorrhea exceeding 6 months after discontinuing use of OCPs should be investigated.

Nursing considerations. There are many different preparations of oral hormonal contraceptives. The nurse reviews the prescribing information in the package insert with the woman. Because of the wide variations, each woman must be clear about the unique dosage regimen for the preparation prescribed for her. Directions for care after missing one or two tablets also vary. Recent findings indicate that if one or two tablets are missed, another form of contraception needs to be used until the required regimen is reestablished (Fig. 7-5). Withdrawal bleeding tends to be short and scanty

signs of POTENTIAL COMPLICATIONS

ORAL CONTRACEPTIVES

Before oral contraceptives are prescribed and periodically throughout hormone therapy the woman is alerted to stop taking the pill and to report any of the following symptoms to the health care provider immediately. The word *aches* helps in retention of this list:

A—Abdominal pain: may indicate a problem with the liver or gallbladder

C—Chest pain or shortness of breath: may indicate possible clot problem within lungs or heart

H—Headaches (sudden or persistent): may be caused by cardiovascular accident or hypertension

E—Eye problems: may indicate vascular accident or hypertension

S—Severe leg pain: may indicate a thromboembolic process

when some combination pills are taken. A woman may see no fresh blood at all. Some women may have only a drop of blood or a brown smudge on their tampon or underwear. This counts as a period. This fact may explain why some women have difficulty remembering the first day of their last period.

No more than 50% to 75% of women who start taking oral contraceptives are still taking them after 1 year (Hatcher et al., 1998). It is therefore important that nurses recommend that all women choosing to use oral contraceptives also be provided with a second method of birth control and that women be instructed and comfortable with this backup method. Most women stop taking oral contraceptives for nonmedical reasons.

The nurse also reviews the signs of potential complications associated with the use of oral contraceptives (see Signs of Potential Complications box).

Oral contraceptives do not protect a woman against STDs. A barrier method such as condoms and spermicide should be used as well if protection is desired (O'Connell, 1996).

Progestin-only contraception. Progestin-only methods impair fertility by inhibiting ovulation, thickening and decreasing the amount of cervical mucus, and thinning the endometrium (Hatcher et al., 1998).

Oral progestins (Minipill). Progestin-only pills are less effective than combined OCPs. Failure rates for typical users is 5% (Hatcher et al., 1998). Effectiveness is increased if minipills are taken correctly. Because minipills contain such a low dose of progestin, the minipill must be taken at the same time each day (Speroff & Darney, 1996). Users often complain of irregular vaginal bleeding.

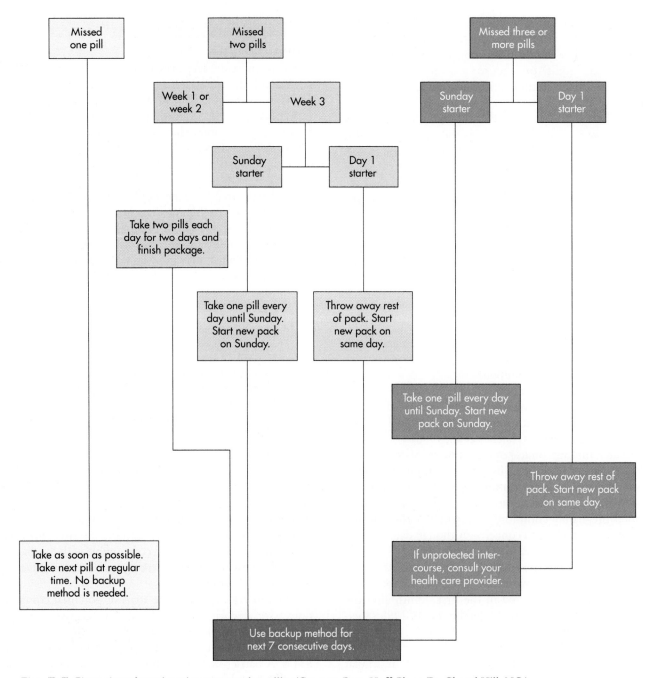

Fig. **7-5** Flow chart for missed contraceptive pills. (Courtesy Patsy Huff, PharmD., Chapel Hill, NC.)

Injectable progestins. The advantages of medroxyprogesterone (DMPA, Depo-Provera) include a contraceptive effectiveness comparable to combined oral contraceptives, longlasting effects, required injections only 4 times a year, and lactation is not likely to be impaired (Cunningham et al., 1997; Hickey & Fraser, 1995). Disadvantages are prolonged amenorrhea or uterine bleeding, increased risk of venous thrombosis and thromboembolism, and no protection against STDs. Some women experience weight gain.

NURSE ALERT *When administering an intramuscular injection of progestin (e.g., Depo-Provera), the site should not be massaged after the injection because this action can hasten the absorption and shorten the period of effectiveness.*

Implantable progestins (Norplant). The Norplant system consists of six flexible, nonbiodegradable Silastic capsules. They contain progestin providing up to 5 years of contraception. Insertion and removal of the capsules are minor

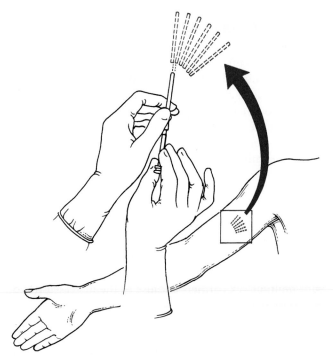

Fig. 7-6 Norplant contraceptive system.

TABLE 7-2 *Dosages for Emergency Contraception*

DRUG	FIRST DOSE (WITHIN 72 HOURS)	SECOND DOSE (12 HOURS LATER)
Ovral	2 white tablets	2 white tablets
Lo/Ovral	4 white tablets	4 white tablets
Nordette	4 light orange tablets	4 light orange tablets
Levlen	4 light orange tablets	4 light orange tablets
Triphasil	4 yellow tablets	4 yellow tablets
Tri-Levlen	4 yellow tablets	4 yellow tablets
Alesse	5 pink tablets	5 pink tablets
Ovrette*	20 yellow tablets†	20 yellow tablets

From Chez R & Chapin J: Emergency contraception: the pill's little-known secret goes public, *Lifelines* 1(5):28, 1997; Lindberg C: Emergency contraception: the nurse's role in providing postcoital options, *J Obstet Gynecol Neonatal Nurs* 26(2):145, 1997.
*Contains only progestin.
†Take within 48 hours.

surgical procedures involving a local anesthetic, a small incision, and no sutures. The capsules are placed subdermally in the inner aspect of the upper arm (Fig. 7-6). The progestin prevents some, but not all, ovulatory cycles and thickens cervical mucus. The effectiveness is greater than 99% over 5 years. Other advantages include long-term continuous contraception not coitus-related and reversibility. Irregular menstrual bleeding is the most common side effect. Other side effects, including headaches, nervousness, nausea, skin changes, and vertigo, are less common. Changes in glucose and insulin values have occurred after 6 months, especially in women who are diabetic (Konje et al., 1992). No STD protection is provided with the Norplant method, so condoms should be used if protection is desired.

Emergency contraception. Emergency contraception is used within 72 hours of unprotected intercourse to prevent pregnancy.

The most common method of emergency contraception is the use of combined oral estrogen and progestin pills. How pregnancy is prevented is not clearly established, although prevention of implantation is the likely mode of action. Recommended medication regimens for emergency contraception are presented in Table 7-2. Contraindications for emergency contraception are the same as for oral contraceptives. Effectiveness of emergency contraception is about 75% (Hatcher et al., 1998).

Oral contraception for emergency contraception can be offered to a woman who has had unprotected sexual intercourse and requests treatment within 72 hours of that event.

To minimize the side effect of nausea that occurs with high doses of estrogen and progestin the woman can be advised to take an over-the-counter antiemetic 1 hour before each dose.

NURSE ALERT *A woman should be told to take pills of only the colors listed for each brand (see Table 7-2) because they are the only ones that contain active hormones.*

If the woman does not begin menstruation within 21 days after taking the pills, she should be evaluated for pregnancy (Chez & Chapin, 1997; Lindberg, 1997).

Intrauterine devices containing copper provide another emergency contraception option. The intrauterine device should be inserted within 7 days of unprotected intercourse (Hatcher et al., 1998). This method is suggested only for women who also wish to have the benefit of long-term contraception.

Contraceptive counseling should be provided to all women requesting emergency contraception, including a discussion of modification of risky sexual behaviors to prevent STDs and unwanted pregnancy.

Mifepristone. Progesterone is essential for maintaining pregnancy. Mifepristone (RU 486) is a progesterone antagonist that prevents implantation of a fertilized egg by blocking the development of the endometrium. It is most effective in early gestation, during the luteal phase, within 10 days of the expected onset of what would be the first missed period after conception. A dose of 600 mg of mifepristone within 24 hours of unprotected intercourse is usually effective in preventing pregnancy (Reifsnider, 1997).

Intrauterine devices. An **intrauterine device (IUD)** is a small, T-shaped device inserted into the uterine cavity. Medicated IUDs are loaded with either copper or progestational

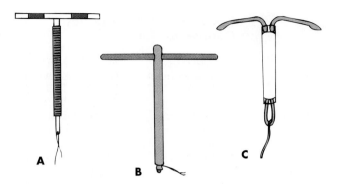

Fig. **7-7** Intrauterine devices. **A,** Copper T-380A. **B,** Progesterone T (Progestasert). **C,** Levonorgestrel-releasing IUD.

agent (Fig. 7-7). These chemically active substances are released continuously for extended periods of time (e.g., copper-bearing devices for 4 to 8 years [at present] and progesterone devices for 1 year) (Hatcher et al., 1998; Speroff & Darney, 1996). IUDs are impregnated with barium sulfate for radiopacity.

Evidence strongly supports a true contraceptive effect in preventing fertilization (Contraception Report, 1992). The copper-bearing IUD damages sperm in transit to the uterine tubes and few sperm reach the ovum, thus preventing fertilization (Speroff & Darney, 1996) (Fig. 7-7, *A*). The progesterone-bearing IUD causes progestin-related effects on cervical mucus and endometrial maturation (Fig. 7-7, *B*). Because the effect is local, there is no disruption of the woman's ovulatory pattern. Copper-bearing IUDs have a lower failure rate than the progesterone-releasing IUDs (Hatcher et al., 1998). The typical failure rate of the IUD ranges from 0.1% to 2.0% (Hatcher et al., 1998).

The IUD offers constant contraception without the need to remember to take pills each day or engage in other manipulation before or between coital acts. If pregnancy can be excluded, an IUD may be placed at any time during the menstrual cycle. An IUD may be inserted immediately after childbirth or abortion (Hatcher et al., 1998; Speroff & Darney, 1996).

The absence of interference with hormonal regulation of menstrual cycles makes the IUD more appropriate than hormonal contraception for heavy smokers, women over 35, women who have hypertension, or those with a history of vascular disease or familial diabetes. Contraceptive effects are reversible. When pregnancy is desired, the IUD may be removed by the health care provider.

The intrauterine progesterone contraception system offers two important noncontraceptive progesterone-related advantages: less blood loss during menstruation and decreased primary dysmenorrhea. The mean blood loss is increased for the copper IUD. This blood loss may be clinically significant in undernourished populations.

The use of an IUD is contraindicated for women with a history of PID, known or suspected pregnancy, undiagnosed genital bleeding, suspected genital malignancy, or a distorted intrauterine cavity. It should not be used by women with multiple sex partners because of the increased risk of exposure to STDs.

Disadvantages of IUD use include risk of PID, especially within 3 months of insertion, and risk of bacterial vaginosis, uterine perforation, and infection at time of insertion. The IUD offers no protection against STDs. The IUD is not recommended for teenagers, but primarily for women who have had at least one child and who are involved in stable monogamous relationships (Hatcher et al., 1998).

Nursing considerations. The woman should be taught to check for the presence of the IUD thread after menstruation and at the time of ovulation, as well as before coitus to rule out expulsion of the device. If pregnancy occurs with the IUD in place, the IUD should be removed immediately, if possible. Retention of the IUD during pregnancy increases the risk of ectopic pregnancy and septic spontaneous abortion (Hatcher et al., 1998). Some women allergic to copper develop a rash, necessitating the removal of the copper-bearing IUD. Signs of potential complications to be taught to the woman are listed in the accompanying box.

Sterilization. **Sterilization** refers to surgical procedures intended to render the person infertile. Most procedures involve the occlusion of the passageways for the ova and sperm (Fig. 7-8). For the female, the uterine tubes are occluded; for the male, the sperm ducts (vas deferens) are occluded. Only surgical removal of the ovaries (oophorectomy) or uterus (hysterectomy) or both will result in absolute sterility for the woman. All other sterilization procedures have a small but definite failure rate; that is, pregnancy may result.

Female sterilization. Female sterilization may be done immediately after childbirth (within 24 to 48 hours), concomitantly with abortion, or as an interval procedure (during any phase of the menstrual cycle). Most sterilization procedures are performed immediately after a pregnancy,

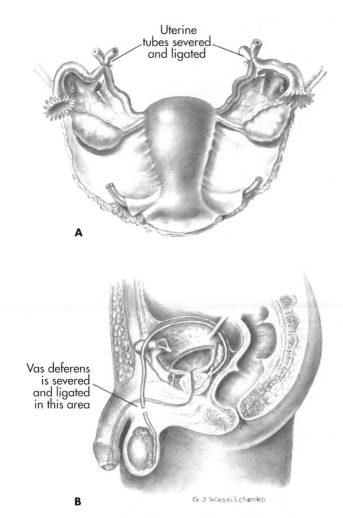

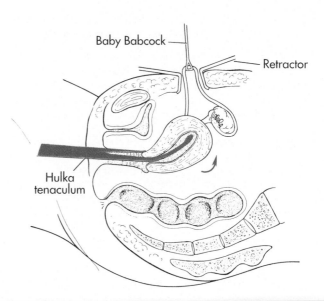

Fig. **7-9** Use of minilaparotomy to gain access to uterine tubes for occlusion procedures. Tenaculum is used to lift uterus upward *(arrow)* toward incision.

Fig. **7-8** Sterilization. **A,** Uterine tubes severed and ligated (tubal ligation). **B,** Sperm duct severed and ligated (vasectomy).

probably because of heightened motivation or increased practicality. Sterilization procedures can be safely done on an outpatient basis.

Tubal occlusion. The operation used commonly is the laparoscopic tubal fulguration (destruction of tissue by means of an electric current [electrocoagulation]). A minilaparotomy may be used for tubal ligation (Fig. 7-9) or for the application of bands or clips (e.g., Hulka-Clemens). Fulguration and ligation are considered to be permanent methods. Use of the bands or clips has the theoretic advantage of possible removal and return of tubal patency. Transcervical approaches to inject occlusive material into the tubes are being investigated (Reifsnider, 1997).

For the minilaparotomy approach the woman is admitted the morning of surgery, having received nothing by mouth (NPO) since midnight. Preoperative sedation is given. The procedure may be carried out with a local anesthetic, but a regional or general anesthetic may also be used.

A small, vertical incision is made in the abdominal wall below the umbilicus. The woman may experience sensations of tugging, but no pain, and the operation is completed within 20 minutes. She may be discharged several hours later if she has recovered from anesthesia. Any abdominal discomfort usually can be controlled with a mild analgesic (e.g., acetaminophen). Within days the scar is almost invisible (see Home Care box). As occurs with any surgery, there is always a possibility of complications of anesthesia, infection, hemorrhage, and trauma to other organs.

Tubal reconstruction. Restoration of tubal continuity (reanastomosis) and function is technically feasible except after laparoscopic tubal fulguration. However, sterilization reversal is costly, difficult (requiring microsurgery), and uncertain (Cunningham et al., 1997). The success rate varies with the extent of tubal destruction and removal. The incidence of successful pregnancy after reanastomosis is only about 15%. The loss of a segment of tube necessary for sperm capacitation and fertilization is the probably the reason for low pregnancy rates and for increased risk of ectopic pregnancy.

Male sterilization. Vasectomy is the easiest and most commonly employed operation for male sterilization. In the United States 500,000 men undergo vasectomy each year (Cunningham et al., 1997). Vasectomy can be carried out with local anesthesia and on an out-of-hospital basis.

In vasectomy small right and left incisions are made into the anterior aspect of the scrotum above and lateral to each testis over the spermatic cord (see Fig. 7-8, *B*). Each vas deferens is identified and doubly ligated with fine, nonabsorbable sutures. Then each vas deferens is severed between

---

HOME CARE *Patient Instructions for Self-Care*

What to Expect after Tubal Ligation
You should expect no change in hormones and their
    influence.
Your menstrual period will be about the same as before
    the sterilization.
You may feel pain at ovulation.
The ovum disintegrates within the abdominal cavity.
It is highly unlikely that you will get pregnant.
You should not experience a change in sexual
    functioning; in fact, you may enjoy sexual relations
    more because you won't be concerned about getting
    pregnant.
Sterilization offers no protection against STDs;
    therefore you may need to use condoms.

---

the ligatures. Occasionally the surgeon cauterizes the cut stumps of the sperm ducts. Many surgeons bury the cut ends into scrotal fascia to lessen the chance of reunion. Then the skin incisions are closed. Usually one nonabsorbable suture is used for closure of each skin incision, and a dressing is applied.

The man is instructed in self-care to promote a safe return to routine activities. To reduce swelling and relieve discomfort, ice packs are applied to the scrotum intermittently for a few hours postoperatively. A scrotal support may be applied to decrease discomfort. Moderate inactivity for about 2 days is advisable because of local scrotal tenderness. The skin suture can be removed 5 to 7 days postoperatively. Sexual intercourse may be resumed as desired.

Sterility is not immediate. Some sperm will remain in the proximal portions of the sperm ducts after vasectomy. One week to several months are required to clear the ducts of sperm (i.e., after approximately 15 ejaculations). Therefore some form of contraception is needed until the sperm count in the ejaculate on two consecutive tests is down to zero (Cunningham et al., 1997).

Vasectomy has no effect on potency (ability to achieve and maintain erection) or volume of ejaculate. Endocrine production of testosterone continues so that secondary sex characteristics are not affected. Sperm production continues. Men occasionally may develop a hematoma, infection, or epididymitis (Hatcher et al., 1998). Less common are painful granulomas from accumulation of sperm. Sperm unable to leave the epididymis are lysed by the immune system. Complications after bilateral vasectomy are uncommon and usually not serious (Giovannucci, 1992). They include bleeding (usually external), suture reaction, and reaction to anesthetic agent. Sterilization failures are rare, occurring in about 2 per 1,000 men.

Tubal reconstruction. Microsurgery to reanastomose the sperm ducts (restoration of tubal continuity) can be accomplished successfully in 81% to 98% of cases (i.e., sperm in the ejaculate); however, the fertility rate is much lower (16% to 79%) (Hatcher et al., 1998). The rate of success decreases as the time since the procedure increases. The vasectomy may result in permanent changes in the testes that leave men unable to father children. The changes are those ordinarily seen only in the elderly (e.g., interstitial fibrosis [scar tissue between the seminiferous tubules]). Some men develop antibodies against their own sperm (autoimmunization). The role of antisperm antibodies in fertility after vasectomy reversal has not been completely determined.

Laws and regulations

All states have strict regulations for informed consent. Many states permit voluntary sterilization of any mature, rational woman without reference to her marital or pregnancy status. Although the partner's consent is not required by law, the woman is encouraged to discuss the situation with the partner, and health care providers may request the partner's consent. Sterilization of minors or mentally incompetent females is restricted by most states. The operation often requires the approval of a board of eugenicists or other court-appointed individuals.

LEGAL TIP Sterilization

- *If federal or state funds are used for sterilization, the person must be at least 21 years old.*
- *Informed consent must include an explanation of the risks, benefits, and alternatives; a statement that describes sterilization as a permanent, irreversible method of birth control; and a statement that mandates a 30-day waiting period between giving consent and the performance of the sterilization. Informed consent must be in the person's native language or an interpreter must be provided.*

Nursing considerations

The nurse plays an important role in assisting people with decision making so that all requirements for informed consent are met. The nurse also provides information about alternatives to sterilization, such as contraception.

The nurse acts as a "sounding board" for people who are exploring the possibility of choosing sterilization and their feelings about and motivation for this choice. The nurse records this information, which may be the basis for referral to a family planning clinic, a psychiatric social worker, or another professional health care provider.

Information must be given about what is entailed in various procedures, how much discomfort or pain can be expected, and what type of care is needed. Many individuals fear sterilization procedures because of the imagined effect on their sexual life. They need reassurance concerning the hormonal and psychologic basis for sexual function and the fact that uterine tube occlusion or vasectomy has no biologic sequelae in terms of sexual adequacy (Hatcher et al., 1998).

Preoperative care includes health assessment, which includes a psychologic assessment, physical examination, and laboratory tests. The nurse assists with the health assessment, answers questions, and confirms the patient's understanding of printed instructions (e.g., nothing by mouth [NPO] after midnight). Ambivalence and extreme fear of the procedure are reported to the health care provider.

Postoperative care depends on the procedure performed, for example, laparoscopy, laparotomy for tubal occlusion, or vasectomy. General care includes recovery after anesthesia, vital signs, fluid and electrolyte balance (intake and output, laboratory values), prevention of or early identification and treatment for infection or hemorrhage, control of discomfort, and assessment of emotional response to the procedure and recovery.

Discharge planning depends on the type of procedure performed. In general, the patient is given written instructions about observing for and reporting symptoms and signs of complications, the type of recovery to be expected, and the date and time for a follow-up appointment.

Evaluation. Evaluation of the effectiveness of care of the woman using a contraceptive method is based on the previously stated outcomes.

Future trends

Contraceptive options are more limited in the United States and Canada than some other industrialized countries. Lack of funding for research, governmental regulations, conflicting values about contraception, and high costs of liability coverage for contraception have been cited as blocks to new and improved methods. However, existing methods of contraception are being improved, and a variety of new ones are being developed.

New formulations of progestin oral contraceptives that have low androgenic and low antiestrogenic effects are in clinical trials as are gonadotropin-releasing hormone methods. A one-size-fits-all diaphragm or shield that is placed in the posterior fornix of the vagina is being tested as is a disposable diaphragm that releases nonoxynol-9. Mifepristone (RU 486) has been tested as a contraceptive by being administered as a single large dose in the follicular phase of the menstrual cycle to inhibit ovulation (Reifsnider, 1997).

New developments in hormonal implants that reduce the number of rods to one or two are being tested, as are biodegradable implants and pellets. Transdermal progestins and vaginal rings that contain estrogen and progestin or progestin only are being investigated. Once-a-month progestin injections and new IUDs containing copper or levonorgestrel are already available outside the United States. Newer versions of the vaginal sponge that contain antiviral spermicides are being tested, as are disposable diaphragms containing spermicide. Chemical forms of male and female sterilization are being studied. Male contraceptives are also being investigated, including hormonal injections (testosterone), gonadotropin-releasing hormone antagonists, calcium channel blockers, and contraceptive vaccines (Hatcher et al. 1998; Reifsnider, 1997).

ABORTION

Induced abortion is the purposeful interruption of pregnancy before 20 weeks' gestation. If the abortion is performed at the woman's request, the term *elective abortion* is used; if performed for reasons of maternal or fetal health or disease, the term *therapeutic abortion* applies. There are many factors that contribute to a woman's decision to have an abortion. Indications include (1) preservation of the life or health of the mother, (2) genetic disorders of the fetus, (3) rape or incest, and (4) the pregnant woman's request. The control of birth, dealing as it does with human sexuality and the question of life and death, is one of the most emotional components of health care and has been the most controversial social issue in the last half of the 20th century (Soriano, 1998). Abortion as a surgical alternative to contraception is regulated in most countries (World Health Organization, 1995). These regulations exist to protect the mother from the complications of abortion.

Most women having abortions are Caucasian, younger than 24 years old, and unmarried (CDC, 1996). Only one fourth of abortions are obtained by married women (Wallach & Zacur, 1995). Sixty percent of women having abortions say they used a contraceptive, but it failed. The U.S. Supreme Court set aside previous antiabortion laws in January 1973, holding that first-trimester abortion is permissible inasmuch as the mortality from interruption of early gestation is now less than the mortality after normal term birth; 90% of abortions are performed at this point in pregnancy (Wallach & Zacur, 1995). Second-trimester abortion was left to the discretion of the individual states (Hatcher et al., 1998). Hospitals maintained by Roman Catholics and some of those maintained by strict fundamentalists forbid abortion (and often sterilization) despite legal challenge.

LEGAL TIP Induced Abortion

It is important for nurses to know the laws regarding abortion in their state of practice before they offer abortion counseling or nursing care to a woman choosing an abortion. Many states enforce a mandatory delay or state-directed counseling before a woman may legally obtain an abortion.

Before the legalization of abortion, many illegal abortions took place, with little documented sequelae other than death from infection or hemorrhage or both. Although studies indicate that biologic sequelae do occur after abortion (e.g., ectopic pregnancy), rates of biologic complications tend to be low, especially if the woman aborts during the first trimester (Speroff & Darney, 1996). Major psychologic sequelae of abortion are rare (Stotland, 1992). Sequelae may be related to circumstances and support systems surrounding the pregnant woman, such as the attitudes reflected by friends, family, and health care workers. Some researchers suggest that emotional distress exhibited by some women after an abortion may be a continuation of symptoms exhibited before the abortion (Grimes, 1995). It must be remembered that the woman facing an abortion is pregnant and may exhibit the emotional responses shared by all pregnant women, including postbirth depression.

Nurses often struggle with the same values and moral convictions as those of the pregnant woman. The conflicts and doubts of the nurse can be readily communicated to women who are already anxious and overly sensitive. Health care professionals need assistance to identify and come to terms with their own feelings. It is not uncommon for confusion to arise as beliefs are challenged by the reality of care. Nurses whose religions or moral beliefs do not support abortion have the right to refuse such an assignment. In reality, reassignment is usually an option so that the abortion patient receives the needed care.

I CARE MANAGEMENT

Assessment and Nursing Diagnoses

A thorough assessment is conducted through history, physical examination, and laboratory tests, including a pregnancy test. The length of pregnancy and the condition of the woman need to be determined to select the appropriate type of abortion procedure. An ultrasound should be performed before a second trimester abortion is done. If the woman is Rh negative and the pregnancy is greater than 8 weeks' gestation, she is a candidate for prophylaxis against Rh isoimmunization. She will receive Rho (D) immune globulin within 72 hours after the abortion if she is D negative and if Coombs' test results are negative (if the woman is unsensitized or isoimmunization has not developed) (Cunningham et al., 1997).

The woman's understanding of alternatives, the types of abortions, and expected recovery is assessed. Misinformation and gaps in knowledge are identified and corrected. The record is reviewed for the signed informed consent, and the woman's understanding is verified. General preoperative, operative, and postoperative assessments are performed.

Analysis of data leads to identification of the appropriate nursing diagnoses for the woman undergoing elective abortion. Potential nursing diagnoses are listed in the box.

I Nursing Diagnoses

Induced Abortion
Decisional conflict related to:
- Perceived conflict related to value system

Fear related to:
- Abortion procedure
- Potential complications
- Implications for future pregnancies
- What others might think

Anticipatory grieving related to:
- Distress at loss or feelings of guilt

Risk for infection related to:
- Effects of the procedure
- Lack of understanding of preoperative and postoperative self-care

Pain related to:
- Effects of the procedure or postoperative events

Expected Outcomes of Care

Planning is a collaborative effort among the woman, her sexual partner (as appropriate), the physician, and the nurse. Expected outcomes are established collaboratively, should be stated in patient-centered terms, and may include that the woman will do the following:

- Verbalize understanding of the information necessary to give informed consent.
- Undergo a successful procedure and uneventful recovery.
- Continue to be satisfied with the decision for induced abortion, the procedure, and her experience with the health care team.

Plan of Care and Interventions

Counseling about abortion includes help for the woman in identifying how she perceives the pregnancy, information about the choices available (i.e., having an abortion or carrying the pregnancy to term and then either keeping the infant or placing the baby for adoption), and information about the types of abortion procedures.

First-trimester abortion

Methods for performing early abortion include vacuum aspiration, medical methods (mifepristone with prostaglandin), and methotrexate with misoprostol.

Vacuum aspiration. Vacuum aspiration (curettage) is the most common procedure in the first trimester, with about 97% of all procedures being performed by suction curettage. Very early abortions (menstrual extraction, endometrial aspiration) can be done with a small flexible plastic cannula without cervical dilatation or anesthesia. The insertion of a small laminaria tent (cone of dried seaweed that swells as it absorbs moisture and dilates the cervix) retained by a vaginal tampon for 4 to 24 hours will usually facilitate the purposeful interruption of a first-trimester pregnancy greater than 8 weeks' gestation by dilating the cervix atraumatically (Wallach & Zacur, 1995). On removal of the moist, expanded laminaria tent the cervix will have dilated two or three times its original diameter. Rarely will further mechanical dilatation of the cervix be required. The insertion of an adequate-sized aspiration cannula (8.5 to 10.5 mm) is almost always possible. Cervical laceration and bleeding are reduced by the use of laminaria. A disadvantage is the delay necessary and the need for an additional visit to the physician's office or clinic. Prostaglandin gel may also be used to soften the cervix (Cunningham et al., 1997).

Aspiration abortion may be performed in the physician's office, the clinic, or the hospital. For the procedure, the vaginal area is cleansed (shaving is not necessary). The suction procedure for performing an early elective abortion (ideal time is 8 to 12 weeks since the last menstrual period) usually requires less than 5 minutes. During the procedure the nurse or physician keeps the woman informed about what to expect next (e.g., menstrual-like cramping and sounds of the suction machine). The nurse assesses the woman's vital signs. The aspirated uterine contents must be carefully inspected to ascertain whether all fetal parts and adequate placental tissue have been evacuated. After the abortion the woman rests on the table until she is ready to stand. Then she remains in the waiting room until she feels she can travel. The woman may remain in the health care facility for 1 to 3 hours for detection of excessive cramping or bleeding; then she is discharged. She may be discharged alone or in the company of a relative or friend, depending on the anesthetic used and policies of the clinic.

Bleeding after the operation is normally about the equivalent of a heavy menstrual period, and cramps are rarely severe. Excessive vaginal bleeding and infection, such as endometritis or salpingitis, are the most common complications of elective abortion. Retained products of conception are the primary cause of vaginal bleeding. Evacuation of the uterus, uterine massage, and administration of oxytocin and/or methylergonovine (Methergine) may be necessary (Hatcher et al., 1998; World Health Organization, 1995). Prophylactic antibiotics have been shown to decrease the risk of infection and should be considered (Grimes, 1995).

Postabortal instructions differ among health care providers (e.g. tampons should not be used for at least 3 days or should be avoided for up to 3 weeks, and resumption of sexual intercourse may be permitted within 1 week or discouraged for 3 weeks). The woman may shower daily. Instruction is given to watch for excessive bleeding (that is, more than one large pad per hour for 4 hours), cramps, or fever and to avoid douches of any type. The woman may expect her menstrual period to resume 4 to 6 weeks from the day of the procedure. The nurse offers information about the birth control method the woman prefers, if this has not been done previously during the counseling interview that usually precedes the decision to have an abortion. The woman must be strongly encouraged to return for her follow-up visit so that complications can be detected and an acceptable contraceptive method prescribed. A pregnancy test may also be performed to determine if the pregnancy has been successfully terminated (Mishell et al., 1997).

Other first-trimester methods

Mifepristone. Mifepristone (RU 486) can be taken up to 5 weeks after conception. The effectiveness of mifepristone is inversely related to gestational age as determined by β-human chorionic gonadotropin levels and the duration of amenorrhea (Donaldson, Briggs & McMaster, 1994). However, it is considered to be an effective and safe method for termination of early pregnancy.

Uterine bleeding begins within 4 days of administration of the first dose. Usually a period of painless heavy bleeding is reported. Termination of pregnancy occurs for most women. When mifepristone is combined with administration of a prostaglandin agent 36 to 48 hours later, the rate of spontaneous abortion increases.

Supporters of this method feel that even with known disadvantages, mifepristone offers a reasonable alternative to surgical abortion, which carries the risks of anesthesia, surgical complications, infertility, and psychologic sequelae (Donaldson, Briggs & McMaster, 1994; Thong & Baird, 1992; World Health Organization Task Force, 1993). Others have taken a strong stand against the use of mifepristone. In the United States it is still not readily available for terminating pregnancy.

Methotrexate. Methotrexate can be given intramuscularly followed by vaginal placement of misoprostol (prostaglandin analog). If abortion does not occur by the next day, misoprostol is repeated (Creinin et al., 1996).

Second-trimester abortion

Second-trimester abortion is associated with an increase of complications and costs (Toppozada, 1995). Dilatation and evacuation, induction of uterine contractions, and major operations are the methods used.

Dilatation and evacuation. Dilatation and evacuation (D & E) can be performed up to 20 weeks' gestation (Hatcher et al., 1994). It is the predominant method of abortion used beyond the first trimester (Wallach & Zacur, 1995). The cervix requires more dilatation because the products of conception are larger. Often laminaria are inserted several hours or several days preceding the procedure. Nursing care includes monitoring vital signs, providing emotional support, administering analgesics, and postoperative monitoring. Disadvantages of D & E may be possible long-term harmful effects on the cervix.

Prostaglandins. The most common technique for medical termination in the second trimester is the administration of prostaglandins (Mishell et al., 1997).

Prostaglandins can be administered in suppository form, as a gel, or by intrauterine injection. Unpleasant side effects (e.g., nausea, vomiting, and diarrhea) usually occur. Repeated doses may be needed for expulsion of the products of conception.

Other second-trimester methods. Other techniques used infrequently are instillation of hypertonic sodium chloride, hypertonic glucose, and urea into the uterine cavity. Uterine contractions usually begin within 12 to 24 hours, and abortion occurs a few hours later. Use of laminaria or oxytocin may facilitate the process. Complications of hypertonic solution injection for second-trimester abortion may occur. Complications include infection, need for dilatation and curettage to remove retained tissue, failure to abort, and excessive bleeding necessitating transfusion.

Hysterotomy and hysterectomy are infrequently used as methods of abortion because of increased morbidity and mortality.

Complications after abortion

The most common complications after abortion include infection, retained products of conception or intrauterine blood clots, continuing pregnancy, cervical or uterine trauma, and excessive bleeding (Hatcher et al., 1998; Wallach & Zacur, 1995). Preoperative antibiotic prophylaxis has been effective in reducing the risk of infection. Women are advised to report fever, pelvic pain, and excessive bleeding. Prophylactic treatment for *Chlamydia trachomatis* and *Neisseria gonorrhoeae* and the use of an oral ergonovine postoperatively may reduce the incidence of infection and retained products of conception.

Nursing considerations

The woman will need help to explore the meaning of the various alternatives and consequences to herself and her significant others. It is often difficult for a woman to express her true feelings (e.g., what abortion means to her now and in the future and what support or regret her friends and peers may demonstrate). A calm, matter-of-fact approach on the part of the nurse can be helpful (e.g., "Yes, I know you are pregnant. I am here to help. Let's talk about alternatives."). Listening to what the woman has to say and encouraging her to speak are essential. Neutral responses such as "Oh," "Uh-huh," and "Umm" and nonverbal encouragement such as nodding, maintaining eye contact, and use of touch are helpful in setting an open, accepting environment. Clarifying, restating, and reflecting statements; open-ended questions; and feedback are communication techniques that can be used to maintain a realistic focus on the situation and bring the woman's problems into the open. Once a decision has been made, the woman must be assured of continued support. Information about what is entailed in various procedures, how much discomfort or pain can be expected, and what type of care is needed must be given. If family or friends cannot be involved, scheduling time for nursing personnel to give the necessary support is an essential component of the care plan.

Evaluation

Evaluation of the effectiveness of care of the woman having an induced abortion is based on the previously stated outcomes.

I IMPAIRED FERTILITY

The inability to conceive and bear a child comes as a surprise to 15% to 20% of otherwise healthy adults (Speroff, Glass & Kase, 1994). Couples requesting assistance with impaired fertility have already decided that they want a child. They seek acceptance and assistance from the health care provider in coping with and possibly resolving this problem.

The traditional definition of **impaired fertility** or **infertility** is the inability to conceive after at least 1 year of unprotected intercourse. Impaired fertility is *primary* if the woman has never been pregnant or the man has never impregnated a woman. It is *secondary* if the woman has been pregnant at least once but has not been able to conceive again or sustain a pregnancy.

An estimated one out of 12 women in the United States experiences some form of infertility (Wilcox & Mosher 1994). Probable causes include the increased incidence of sexually transmitted diseases and endometriosis (tissue occurs in the pelvic cavity or other areas of the body) and the trend to delay pregnancy until later in life when fertility decreases naturally. Cigarette smoking and alcohol use have also been associated with infertility (Speroff, Glass & Kase, 1994; Trantham, 1996). Diagnosis and treatment of impaired fertility require considerable physical, emotional, and financial investment over an extended period.

The attitude, sensitivity, and caring nature of health team members who are involved in the assessment of impaired fertility lay the foundation for the couple's ability to cope with the subsequent therapy and management. All members of the health care team must respect the couple's rights to privacy and the confidentiality of the patient records.

Factors Associated with Infertility

The couple is a biologic unit of reproduction. Many factors, both male and female, contribute to normal fertility. A normally developed reproductive tract in both the male and female partner is essential. Normal functioning of an intact hypothalamic-pituitary-gonadal axis supports gametogenesis—the formation of sperm and ova. The life span of the sperm and ovum is short. Although sperm remain viable in the female's reproductive tract for 48 hours or more, probably only a few retain fertilization potential for more than 24 hours. Ova remain viable for about 24 hours, but the optimum time for fertilization may be no more than 1 to 2 hours (Cunningham et al., 1997). Thus timing of intercourse becomes critical.

The male must produce sperm that are normal, adequate in number, and motile. Accessory glands must provide secretions supportive to the sperm to form semen. The tube system to the urethra must be patent. Ejaculation must deposit semen around the cervix at the appropriate time of the female's menstrual cycle. After being deposited, sperm must undergo capacitation to prepare for fertilization. Then they migrate through the uterus to the ampulla of the uterine tube to fertilize a receptive normal ovum.

In the female, a graafian follicle must mature and release a healthy ovum able to be fertilized. The ovum must be drawn by the fimbria into a healthy, patent uterine tube and fertilized within a few hours. The conceptus must migrate down the tube into a well-developed normal uterus. Implantation of the blastocyst must occur within 7 to 10 days in a hormone-prepared endometrium. The conceptus must develop normally, reach viability, and be born in good condition for extrauterine life.

An alteration in one or more of these structures, functions, or processes results in some degree of impaired fertility. Causes of impaired fertility are sometimes difficult to assign to either the male or female. In general a female factor is responsible for infertility in 40% to 55% of infertile couples. Anovulation accounts for 10% to 15% of the causes, while pelvic factors account for 30% to 40%. The incidence of infertility increases with increasing age of the woman so that the probability of conception is greatly reduced as a result of delayed childbearing until later in life. A male factor (sperm and semen abnormalities) is responsible for infertility in about 30% to 40% of couples. Couple factors (cervical factors associated with abnormal sperm–cervical mucus penetration) are responsible for 10% to 15% of infertility. Unexplained factors account for 10% to 25% of infertility (Mishell et al., 1997). However, unexplained infertility and recurrent (habitual) spontaneous abortion may be the result of aberrations of the immune system (e.g., antisperm antibodies, failure of implantation and growth of a blastocyst) (Gleicher, 1993; Timbers & Feinberg, 1996).

Female infertility

Congenital or developmental factors. Congenital factors rarely cause impaired fertility. If the woman has abnormal external genitals, surgical reconstruction of abnormal tissue and construction of a functional vagina may permit normal intercourse. However, if internal reproductive tract structures are absent, there is no hope for fertility. Vaginal and uterine anomalies and their surgical repair vary from individual to individual. If a functional uterus can be reconstructed, pregnancy may be possible.

Ovarian factors. Anovulation may be primary or secondary. Primary anovulation may be caused by a pituitary or hypothalamic hormone disorder or an adrenal gland disorder such as congenital adrenal hyperplasia. Secondary anovulation may be caused by ovarian disease. In amenorrheic states and instances of anovulatory cycles, hormone studies usually reveal the problem.

Tubal/peritoneal factors. The motility of the tube and its fimbriated end may be reduced or absent as a result of infections, adhesions, scarring, or tumors. Chlamydial infection negatively influences tubal function and impedes fertility (Speroff, Glass & Kase, 1994). In rare instances there may be congenital absence of one tube. It is also possible to find one tube relatively shorter than the other. This condition is often associated with an abnormally developed uterus.

Inflammation within the tube or involving the exterior of the tube or the fimbriated ends represents a major cause of impaired fertility. Tubal adhesions resulting from pelvic infections (e.g., ruptured appendix, STDs) may impair fertility. When infection with purulent discharge eventually heals, scar tissue adhesions form. In the process the tube may be blocked anywhere along its length. It can be closed off at the fimbriated end, or it can be distorted and kinked by adhesions. Adhesions may permit the tiny sperm to pass through the tube but may prevent a fertilized egg from completing the journey into the intrauterine cavity. This results in an ectopic pregnancy that may completely destroy the tube. In other cases, adhesions of the tubes to the ovary or bowel may follow endometriosis.

Uterine factors. Abnormalities of the uterus are more common than might be expected. Minor developmental anomalies of the uterus are fairly common; major anomalies occur rarely. Hysterosalpingography may reveal double uteri or other anomalous congenital variations. Endometrial and myometrial tumors (e.g., polyps or myomas) may also be revealed by x-ray studies of infertile women.

Asherman's syndrome (uterine adhesions or scar tissue) is characterized by hypomenorrhea. The adhesions, which may partially or totally obliterate the uterine cavity, are sequelae to surgical interventions such as too vigorous curettage (scraping) after an abortion (elective or spontaneous). The hysteroscope is useful in the verification of intrauterine anomalies.

Endometritis (inflammation of the endometrium) may result from any of the causes of infection of the cervix or uterine tubes (e.g., *Chlamydia*). Women who have numerous sexual partners are more susceptible to endometrial infection than are women in monogamous relationships.

Vaginal-cervical factors. Vaginal-cervical infections (e.g., *trichomoniasis vaginitis*) increase the acidity of the vaginal fluid and reduce the alkalinity of the cervical mucus. Thus vaginal infection often destroys or drastically reduces the number of viable motile sperm before they enter the cervical canal. The amount of mucus and its physical changes are influenced by the presence of blood, pathogenic bacteria, and irritants such as an IUD or a tumor. Severe emotional stress, antibiotic therapy, and diseases such as diabetes mellitus alter the acidity of mucus.

Some infertile women have sperm antibodies. The production of antibodies by one member of a species against something that is commonly found within that species is termed **isoimmunization.** Sperm may be immobilized within the cervical mucus, or they become incapable of migration into the uterus (see postcoital test). A greater incidence of sperm agglutination occurs in women with otherwise unexplained impaired fertility. However, the true significance and reliability of tests for sperm immobilization or agglutination are uncertain.

Male infertility

Male infertility can be caused by structural and hormonal disorders such as undescended testes, hypospadias, varicoceles (varicose vein of the scrotum), and low testosterone levels. Mumps, especially after adolescence, can result in permanent damage to the testes. Male infertility may also be caused by factors that also affect women, such as nutrition, endocrine disorders, psychologic disorders, and STDs (Greendale et al., 1993; Liel et al., 1993; Schill & Haidl, 1993; Stauber & Brucker, 1993). Exposure to hazards in the workplace such as radiation can also affect sperm production; exposure of the scrotum to high temperatures can both decrease and cause abnormal sperm production.

Substance abuse can be a major factor in male infertility. Alcohol consumption can cause erectile problems (impotence) (Liel et al., 1993). In addition, cigarette smoking has been associated with abnormal sperm, a decreased number of sperm, and chromosome damage. The degree of abnormality is related to the number of cigarettes smoked per day (Liel et al., 1993). Heroin and marijuana use may depress the number and motility of sperm and increase the percentage of abnormally formed sperm. Monoamine oxidase (MAO), an antidepressant, adversely affects spermatogenesis. Amyl nitrate, butyl nitrate, ethyl chloride, and methaqualone (used to prolong orgasm) cause changes in spermatogenesis. Heroin, methadone, selective serotonin reuptake inhibitors (SSRIs), and barbiturates decrease libido. In addition, some antihypertensives may cause impotence (Liel et al., 1993).

CARE MANAGEMENT

Assessment and Nursing Diagnoses

The nurse assists in the assessment by obtaining data relevant to fertility through interview and physical examination. The database needs to include information to identify whether infertility is primary or secondary. Religious, cultural, and ethnic data are noted (see Box 7-4 and the Cultural Considerations box).

Some of the data needed to investigate impaired fertility are of a sensitive, personal nature. Obtaining these data may be viewed as an invasion of privacy. The tests and examinations are occasionally painful and intrusive and can take the romance out of lovemaking. A high level of motivation is needed to endure the investigation.

BOX 7-4   *Religious Considerations of Infertility*

Civil laws and religious proscriptions about sex must always be kept in mind by the health care provider. For example, the Orthodox Jewish husband and wife may face infertility investigation and management problems because of religious laws that govern marital relations. For example, according to Jewish law, the Orthodox couple may not engage in marital relations during menstruation and through the following 7 "preparatory days." The wife then is immersed in a ritual bath (Mikvah) before relations can resume. Fertility problems can arise when the woman has a short cycle (i.e., a cycle of 24 days or fewer; when ovulation would occur on day 10 or earlier).

The Roman Catholic Church regards the embryo as a human being from the first moment of existence and regards technical procedures such as in vitro fertilization, therapeutic donor insemination, and freezing embryos as unacceptable (Fryday, 1995). Both Orthodox Jewish and Roman Catholic women may at times question proposed diagnostic and therapeutic procedures because of religious proscriptions. These women are encouraged to consult their rabbi or priest for a ruling.

Other religious groups may also have ethical concerns about infertility tests and treatments.

CULTURAL CONSIDERATIONS
Fertility/Infertility

Worldwide cultures continue to employ symbols and rites that celebrate fertility. One fertility rite that persists today is the custom of throwing rice at the bride and groom. Other fertility symbols and rites include passing out of congratulatory cigars, candy, or pencils by a new father and baby showers held in anticipation of a child's birth.

In many cultures the responsibility for infertility is usually attributed to the woman. A woman's inability to conceive may be due to her sins, to evil spirits, or to the fact that she is an inadequate person. The virility of a man in some cultures remains in question until he demonstrates his ability to reproduce by having at least one child (Geissler, 1994).

Many couples have already visited various physicians and have read extensively on the subject. Their previous experiences are recorded, and the depth and breadth of their knowledge base are explored.

Because multiple factors involving both partners are common, the investigation of impaired fertility is conducted systematically and simultaneously for both male and female partners. Both partners must be interested in the solution to

BOX 7-5   *Assessment of the Woman*

HISTORY

1. Age
2. Duration of infertility: length of contraceptive and noncontraceptive exposure
3. Obstetric
   a. Number of pregnancies and abortions
   b. Length of time required to initiate each pregnancy
   c. Complications of any pregnancy
   d. Duration of lactation
4. Gynecologic: detailed menstrual history, including age at onset, interruptions in regular menstruation, and any menstrual pain
5. Previous tests and therapy for infertility
6. Medical: general medical history, including chronic and hereditary disease (such as endocrine dysfunction); medications, including vitamins and over-the-counter medications; family history, especially of endocrine disorders; normal sexual development; any galactorrhea when not lactating
7. Surgical: especially abdominal or pelvic surgery
8. Sexual history: frequency of intercourse; number of lifetime sexual partners, previous history of STDs, types of sexual practices; pain or discomfort with intercourse; use of vaginal lubricants
9. Occupational and environmental exposure to chemicals or radiation; physical nature of occupation or hobbies; vacations and work habits
10. Personal: motivation for childbearing; attitude toward partner; reason for seeking advice regarding infertility at this time; support system available; amount of exercise; stress level; use of alcohol, recreational drugs, caffeine, or tobacco; weight changes

PHYSICAL EXAMINATION

1. General: complete physical examination
2. Genital tract: state of hymen (full penetration); clitoris; vaginal infection, including trichomoniasis and candidiasis; cervical tears, polyps, infection, patency of os, accessibility to insemination; uterus, including size and position, mobility; adnexae, tumors, evidence of endometriosis

LABORATORY DATA

1. *Chlamydia* test and gonorrhea culture; additional laboratory studies as indicated (e.g., urine test, complete blood cell count, serologic test for syphilis)
2. For women with irregular menstrual cycles or amenorrhea: serum prolactin level with tomographic x-rays of skull if prolactin level elevated, endometrial biopsy, FSH and LH determination. Other laboratory tests added as desired for a more complete diagnosis of endocrine problems: 17-ketosteroid assay test, 17-hydroxycorticosteroid test, glucose tolerance test
3. Rh factor and antibody titer tests—important in cases of ectopic pregnancy, abortion, and preterm birth problems
4. Sperm antibody agglutination studies: special laboratory procedure involves obtaining a fresh semen specimen from the man and a blood sample from the woman; sperm are incubated in the blood serum of the woman and checked at intervals for agglutination; the result is negative if no agglutinated sperm are found
5. Chromosome studies when indicated

the problem. The medical investigation requires time (3 to 4 months) and considerable financial expense, and it causes emotional distress and strain on the couple's interpersonal relationship. Nurses can be instrumental in providing information about the latest tests and treatment.

Investigation of impaired fertility begins for the woman with a complete history and physical examination (Box 7-5). The history explores the duration of infertility and past obstetric events and contains a detailed sexual history. Medical and surgical conditions are evaluated. Exposure to reproductive hazards in the home (e.g., mutagens such as plastic-vinyl chlorides, teratogens such as alcohol, and emotional stresses) and workplace are explored.

A complete general physical examination is followed by a specific assessment of the reproductive tract. Evidence of endocrine system abnormalities is sought. Inadequate development of secondary sex characteristics (e.g., inappropriate distribution of body fat and hair) may point to problems with the hypothalamic-pituitary-ovarian axis or genetic aberrations (e.g., polycystic ovarian syndrome, Turner's syndrome).

A woman may have an abnormal uterus and tubes as a result of exposure to diethylstilbestrol (DES) in utero. Evidence of past infection of the genitourinary system is sought. Bimanual examination of internal organs may reveal lack of mobility of the uterus or abnormal contours of the uterus and adnexa. Laboratory data are assembled. Data from routine urine and blood tests are obtained along with other diagnostic tests.

Diagnostic tests

Assessment of female infertility. There are several examinations and tests for impaired fertility in the woman. The basic infertility survey involves evaluation of the cervix, uterus, tubes, and peritoneum; detection of ovulation; assessment of immunologic compatibility; and evaluation of psychogenic factors (Morell, 1997; Speroff, Glass & Kase, 1994). The nurse can alleviate some of the anxiety associated with diagnostic testing by explaining to patients the timing and rationale for each test (Table 7-3). Test findings that are favorable to fertility are summarized in Box 7-6.

TABLE 7-3 *Tests for Impaired Fertility*

TEST/EXAMINATION	TIMING (MENSTRUAL CYCLE DAYS)	RATIONALE
Hysterosalpingogram	7 to 10	Late follicular, early proliferative phase; will not disrupt a fertilized ovum; may open uterine tubes before time of ovulation
Postcoital test	1 to 2 days before ovulation	Ovulatory late proliferative phase; look for normal motile sperm in cervical mucus
Sperm immobilization antigen-antibody reaction	Variable, ovulation	Immunologic test to determine sperm and cervical mucus interaction
Assessment of cervical mucus	Variable, ovulation	Cervical mucus should have low viscosity, high spinnbarkeit
Ultrasound diagnosis of follicular collapse	Ovulation	Collapsed follicle is seen after ovulation
Serum assay of plasma progesterone	20 to 25	Midluteal midsecretory phase; check adequacy of corpus luteal production of progesterone
BBT	Chart entire cycle	Elevation occurs in response to progesterone, documents ovulation
Endometrial biopsy	26 to 27	Late luteal, late secretory phase; check endometrial response to progesterone and adequacy of luteal phase
Sperm penetration assay	After 2 days but no more than 1 week of abstinence	Evaluation of ability of sperm to penetrate an egg

BOX 7-6 *Summary of Findings Favorable to Fertility*

1. Follicular development, ovulation, and luteal development are supportive of pregnancy:
   a. BBT (presumptive evidence of ovulatory cycles) is biphasic, with temperature elevation that persists for 12 to 14 days before menstruation
   b. Cervical mucus characteristics change appropriately during phases of menstrual cycle
   c. Laparoscopic visualization of pelvic organs verifies follicular and luteal development
2. The luteal phase is supportive of pregnancy:
   a. Levels of plasma progesterone are adequate
   b. Findings from endometrial biopsy samples are consistent with day of cycle
3. Cervical factors are receptive to sperm during expected time of ovulation:
   a. Cervical os is open
   b. Cervical mucus is clear, watery, abundant, and slippery and demonstrates good spinnbarkeit and arborization (fern pattern)
   c. Cervical examination does not reveal lesions or infections
   d. Postcoital test findings are satisfactory (adequate number of live, motile, normal sperm present in cervical mucus)
   e. No immunity to sperm demonstrated

4. The uterus and uterine tubes are supportive of pregnancy:
   a. Uterine and tubal patency are documented by
      (1) Spillage of dye into peritoneal cavity
      (2) Outlines of uterine and tubal cavities of adequate size and shape, with no abnormalities
   b. Laparoscopic examination verifies normal development of internal genitals and absence of adhesions, infections, endometriosis, and other lesions
5. The male partner's reproductive structures are normal:
   a. No evidence of developmental anomalies of penis, testicular atrophy, or varicocele (varicose veins on the spermatic vein in the groin)
   b. No evidence of infection in prostate, seminal vesicles, and urethra
   c. Testes are more than 4 cm in largest diameter
6. Semen is supportive of pregnancy:
   a. Sperm (number per milliliter) are adequate in ejaculate
   b. Most sperm show normal morphology
   c. Most sperm are motile, forward moving
   d. No autoimmunity exists
   e. Seminal fluid is normal

Detection of ovulation. Documentation of time of ovulation is important in the investigation of impaired fertility. Direct proof of ovulation is pregnancy or the retrieval of an ovum from the uterine tube. However, there are several indirect or presumptive methods for detection of ovulation. These include assessment of BBT and cervical mucus characteristics, as well as endometrial biopsy and pelvic ultrasound. A serum progesterone level may be obtained in the latter half of the menstrual cycle as part of ovulation testing. These clinical tests more or less determine whether progesterone is secreted in significant amounts to accommodate implantation and maintain pregnancy. Occurrence of mittelschmerz and midcycle spotting provides unreliable presumptive evidence of ovulation.

Hormone analysis. Hormone analysis is performed to assess endocrine function of the hypothalamic-pituitary-ovarian axis when menstrual cycles are absent or irregular. Determination of blood levels of prolactin, FSH, LH, and the thyroid hormones may be necessary to diagnose the cause of irregular or absent menstrual cycles.

Timed endometrial biopsy. Endometrial biopsy is scheduled after ovulation, during the luteal phase of the menstrual cycle. Late in the menstrual cycle, 2 to 3 days before expected menses, a small cannula is introduced into the uterus, and a small portion of the endometrium is removed for histologic evaluation. To assess the response of the endometrium to progesterone production, the tissue is dated with respect to expected normal menstrual development. Tissue that is "out of phase" with expected development signifies either abnormal function of the corpus luteum or abnormal response of the endometrium.

Findings favorable to fertility include endometrial tissue that shows no signs of tuberculosis, polyps, or inflammatory conditions and that reflects secretory changes normally seen in the presence of adequate luteal (progesterone) phase.

Hysterosalpingography. Radiographic (x-ray) film allows visualization of the uterine cavity and tubes after the instillation of radiopaque contrast material through the cervix (Fig. 7-10). It is possible to see abnormalities of the uterus such as congenital defects or defects produced by submucous myomas and endometrial polyps. Distortions of the uterine cavity or uterine tubes as a result of current or past pelvic inflammatory disease (PID) are identified. Scar tissue and adhesions from inflammatory processes can immobilize the uterus and tubes, kink the tubes, and surround the ovaries. PID may follow infection from STDs or rupture of an inflamed appendix.

Hysterosalpingography is scheduled 2 to 5 days after menstruation to avoid flushing a potential fertilized ovum out through a uterine tube into the peritoneal cavity. Also at this time there are no open vessels, and all menstrual debris has been discharged. This decreases the risk of embolism or of forcing menstrual debris out through the tubes into the peritoneal cavity. If the woman has PID, she is treated with antimicrobials and the test is rescheduled in 2 to 3 months.

Referred shoulder pain may occur during this procedure. The referred pain is indicative of subphrenic irritation from the contrast media if it is spilled out of the patent uterine tubes. The discomfort can be managed with position change and mild analgesics. Pain usually subsides within 12 to 14 hours. Women with blocked tubes may have cramping up to 48 hours.

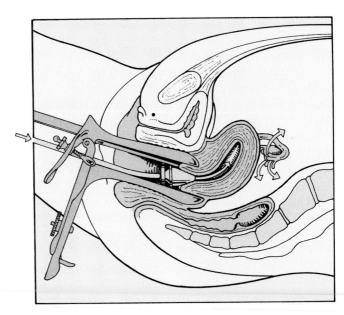

Fig. **7-10** Hysterosalpingography. Note contrast medium flows through intrauterine cannula and out through the uterine tubes.

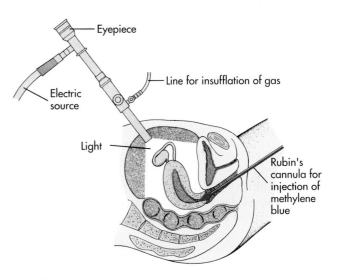

Fig. **7-11** Laparoscopy.

This procedure may be both therapeutic and diagnostic. The passage of contrast medium may clear tubes of mucous plugs, straighten kinked tubes, or break up adhesions within the tubes (caused by salpingitis). The procedure may stimulate cilia in the lining of the tubes to facilitate transport of the ovum. It also may aid healing as a result of the bacteriostatic effect of the iodine within the contrast medium.

Laparoscopy. Laparoscopy is usually scheduled early in the menstrual cycle. During the procedure a small endoscope is inserted through a small incision in the anterior abdominal wall. Cold fiberoptic light sources allow for superior visualization of the internal pelvic structures (Fig. 7-11). The woman is usually admitted shortly before surgery, having taken nothing by mouth (NPO) for 8 hours. She voids before surgery. A general anesthetic is usually given and the woman is placed in the lithotomy position. Her pubic hair is shaved only if this examination is likely to be followed by laparotomy. A needle is inserted and carbon dioxide gas is pumped into the peritoneum to elevate the abdominal wall from the organs, thereby creating an empty space that permits visualization and exploration with the laparoscope. If tubal patency is being assessed, a cannula is used to instill a dye contrast medium through the cervix.

Visualization of the peritoneal cavity in infertile women may reveal endometriosis, pelvic adhesions, tubal occlusion, or polycystic ovaries. Fulguration (destruction of tissue by means of electricity) of small endometrial implants, lysis of adhesions, and taking ovarian biopsies are some of the procedures possible through the use of a laparoscope.

After surgery, deflation of most gas is done by direct expression. Trocar and needle sites are closed with a single subcuticular absorbable suture or skin clip, and an adhesive bandage is applied. Postoperative recovery requires taking vital signs, assessing level of consciousness, preventing aspiration, monitoring intravenous fluids, and reassuring the patient regarding referred shoulder discomfort. Discharge from the hospital usually occurs in 4 to 6 hours. Referred shoulder pain or subcostal discomfort usually lasts only 24 hours and is relieved with a mild analgesic. Severe pain may be relieved when the woman assumes a knee-chest position. The woman must be cautioned against heavy lifting or strenuous activity for 4 to 7 days, at which time she is usually asymptomatic.

Ultrasonography. Abdominal or transvaginal ultrasound is also used to assess pelvic structures (Fig. 7-12). This procedure is used to visualize pelvic tissues for a variety of reasons (e.g., to identify abnormalities, to verify follicular development and maturity, or to confirm intrauterine versus ectopic pregnancy).

Assessment of male infertility

The systematic investigation of infertility in the male patient begins with a thorough history and physical examination (Box 7-7). Assessment of the male patient proceeds in a manner similar to that of the female patient, starting with noninvasive tests. Male reproductive failure may be caused by physiologic, developmental, or endocrine disorders. Infertile men report lower self-esteem, higher anxiety, and more somatic symptoms than fertile men (Amar, 1991). Male fertility declines slowly after the age of 40 years. There is, however, no cessation of sperm production analogous to menopause in women.

Semen analysis. The basic test for male infertility is the **semen analysis.** Examination of semen is an important

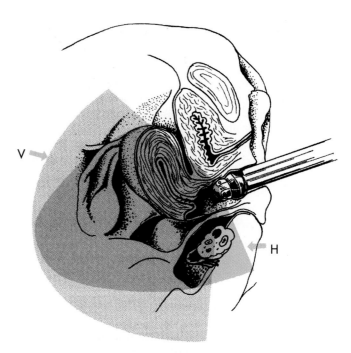

Fig. **7-12** Vaginal ultrasonography. Major scanning planes of transducer. *H*, Horizontal; *V*, vertical.

part of investigation of impaired fertility, since the male is often at least partially responsible (Ross & Niederberger, 1995; Speroff, Glass & Kase, 1994). A complete semen analysis, study of the effects of cervical mucus on sperm forward motility and survival, and evaluation of the sperm's ability to penetrate an ovum provide basic information. Sperm counts vary from day to day and are dependent on emotional and physical status and sexual activity. Therefore a single analysis may be inconclusive. Usually several specimens taken at monthly intervals are evaluated (Trantham, 1996).

Semen is collected by ejaculation into a clean container or a plastic sheathe that does not contain a spermicidal agent (Speroff, Glass & Kase, 1994). The specimen is usually collected by masturbation following 2 to 5 days of abstinence from ejaculation. The semen is taken to the laboratory in a sealed container within 2 hours of ejaculation. Exposure to excessive heat or cold is avoided. Normal values for semen characteristics are given in Box 7-8.

The fertility potential of sperm is difficult to evaluate solely by semen analysis, which gives little insight into sperm survival, cervical penetration, migration to the uterine tubes, or capacity for ovum penetration and fertilization. There is insufficient knowledge regarding if or how male and female antibodies can act to inhibit fertility potential of sperm (autoimmunization) (Speroff, Glass & Kase, 1994).

Seminal deficiency may be attributable to one or more of a variety of factors. The male is assessed for these factors: hypopituitarism, nutritional deficiency, debilitating or chronic disease, trauma, exposure to environmental hazards such as radiation and toxic substances, gonadotropic inadequacy,

BOX 7-7   *Assessment of the Man*

HISTORY

1. Age
2. Fertility in this and other sexual relationships
3. Medical: general medical history, including infections (such as STDs, mononucleosis), mumps, orchitis after adolescence, chronic diseases, recent fever, medications, weight changes, undescended testes after 3 months of age, normal sexual development at puberty
4. Surgical: herniorrhaphy, injuries to genitals, or other surgery in genital area
5. Occupational and environmental exposure to chemicals or radiation, physical nature of occupation and hobbies, vacations and work habits
6. Previous tests and therapy done for study of infertility, duration of infertility in this and previous relationships
7. Sex history in detail: libido, coital history (such as frequency and ability to ejaculate), adequacy of erection, number of lifetime sex partners, attitudes toward masturbation
8. Personal: motivation for childbearing; attitude toward partner; support system available, reason for seeking advice regarding infertility at this time; amount of exercise and stress level; use of alcohol, recreational drugs, caffeine, tobacco, anabolic steroids

PHYSICAL EXAMINATION

1. General: complete physical examination, with special attention given to physical condition and fat and hair distribution
2. Genital tract: penis and urethra; scrotal size; position, size, and consistency of testes; epididymides and vasa deferentia; prostate size and consistency
3. Careful search for varicocele, with man in both supine and upright positions

LABORATORY DATA

1. Routine urine test, gonorrhea and *Chlamydia* tests; serologic test for syphilis
2. Complete semen analysis essential (see Box 7-8)
3. Additional laboratory studies as indicated
   a. Basic endocrine studies indicated in men with oligospermia or aspermia:
      (1) Serum FSH, LH, and testosterone levels
      (2) T_3, T_4, TSH
      (3) Test for sperm antibodies, autoimmunization: autoimmune antibodies (produced by the man against his own sperm) agglutinate or immobilize sperm in fewer than 5% of men who have infertility problems
      (4) 17-hydroxycorticoids and 17-ketosteroids
      (5) Buccal smear and chromosome studies (e.g., Klinefelter's syndrome, XXY sex chromosomes)
   b. Testicular biopsy where correct interpretation is available (may give a more accurate diagnosis and prognosis in cases of azoospermia and severe oligospermia), vasography if indicated and available

---

BOX 7-8   *Semen Analysis*

- Liquefaction usually complete within 10 to 20 minutes
- Semen volume 2 to 5 ml (range 1 to 7 ml)
- Semen pH 7.2 to 7.8
- Sperm density 20 to 200 million cells/ml
- Normal morphology, ≥ 60% normal oval
- Motility (important consideration in sperm evaluation), percentage of forward-moving sperm estimated with respect to abnormally motile and nonmotile sperm ≥ 50%
- Ovum penetration test (may be done if further evaluation necessary)

Note: These values are not absolute, only relative to final evaluation of the couple as a single reproductive unit.

and obstructive lesions of the epididymis and vas deferens (Ross & Niederberger, 1995). Hormone analyses are done for testosterone, gonadotropin, FSH, and LH. The sperm penetration assay may be used to evaluate the ability of sperm to penetrate an egg. Because human oocytes are not readily available, hamster eggs have been used as a substitute to evaluate sperm penetration abilities (no actual fertilization occurs) (Amar, 1991). In addition, testicular biopsy may be warranted.

Assessment of the couple

Postcoital test. The **postcoital test (PCT)** is one method used to test for adequacy of coital technique, cervical mucus, sperm, and degree of sperm penetration through cervical mucus. The test is performed within several hours after ejaculation of semen into the vagina. A specimen of cervical mucus is obtained. Intercourse is synchronized with the expected time of ovulation (as determined from evaluation of BBT, cervical mucus changes, and usual length of menstrual cycle or use of LH detection kit to determine LH surge). It is performed only in the absence of vaginal infection. Couples may experience some difficulty abstaining from intercourse for 2 to 4 days before expected ovulation and then having intercourse with ejaculation on schedule. Sex on demand may strain the couple's interpersonal relationship. A problem may arise if the expected day of ovulation occurs when facilities or the physician is unavailable (such as over a weekend or holiday). If no sperm is found, the coital technique used must be evaluated (e.g., extreme obesity may prevent adequate penile penetration).

Nursing diagnoses are derived from the database. Examples of nursing diagnoses related to impaired fertility are listed in the box.

Nursing Diagnoses

Impaired Fertility

Anxiety related to:
- Unknown outcome of diagnostic workup

Body image or self-esteem disturbance related to:
- Impaired fertility

Risk for ineffective individual/family coping related to:
- Methods used in the investigation of impaired fertility

Decisional conflict related to:
- Therapies for impaired fertility
- Alternatives to therapy: childfree living or adoption

Altered family processes related to:
- Unmet expectations for pregnancy

Anticipatory grieving related to:
- Expected poor prognosis

Pain related to:
- Effects of diagnostic tests (or surgery)

Powerlessness related to:
- Lack of control over prognosis

Altered patterns of sexuality related to:
- Loss of libido secondary to medically imposed restrictions

Risk for social isolation related to:
- Impaired fertility, its investigation and management

Knowledge deficit related to:
- Preconception risk factors
- Factors surrounding ovulation
- Factors surrounding fertility

Expected Outcomes of Care

Planning requires sensitivity to the couple's needs. Equipped with a knowledge of impaired fertility, the nurse can help develop a plan of care for the couple with impaired fertility. The expected outcomes are phrased in patient-centered terms and may include that the couple will do the following:

- Verbalize understanding of the anatomy and physiology of the reproductive system.
- Verbalize understanding of treatment for any abnormalities identified through various tests and examinations (e.g., infections, blocked uterine tubes, sperm allergy, and varicocele) and will be able to make an informed decision about treatment.
- Verbalize understanding of their potential to conceive.
- Resolve guilt feelings and will not need to focus blame.
- Conceive or, failing to conceive, decide on an alternative acceptable to both of them (e.g., childfree living or adoption).
- Demonstrate acceptable methods for handling pressure they may feel from peers and relatives regarding their childless state.

Plan of Care and Interventions
Psychosocial

Within the United States, feelings connected to impaired fertility are numerous and complex. The origin of some of these feelings are myths, superstitions, and misinformation about the causes of infertility. Other feelings arise from the need to undergo many tests and examinations and from being different from others.

Infertility is recognized as a major life stressor that can affect self-esteem, relations with the spouse, family and friends, and careers. Couples often need assistance in separating their concepts of success and failure related to treatment for infertility from personal success and failure. Recognizing the significance of infertility as a loss and resolving these feelings are crucial to putting infertility into perspective, even if treatment is successful (Boxer, 1996).

Nurses can help couples express and discuss their feelings as honestly as possible. Ventilation may help couples unburden themselves of negative feelings. Referral for mental health counseling may be beneficial.

The myriad of psychologic responses to a diagnosis of infertility may tax a couple's giving and receiving of physical and sexual closeness. The prescriptions and proscriptions for achieving conception may add tension to a couple's sexual functioning. Couples may report decreased desire for intercourse, orgasmic dysfunction, or midcycle erectile disorders.

To be able to deal comfortably with a couple's sexuality, nurses must be comfortable with their own sexuality so that they can better help couples understand why the private act of lovemaking needs to be shared with health care professionals. Nurses need up-to-date factual knowledge about human sexual practices and must be (1) able to accept the preferences and activities of others without being judgmental, (2) skilled in interviewing and in therapeutic use of self, sensitive to the nonverbal cues of others, and (3) knowledgeable regarding each couple's sociocultural and religious tenets (Johnson, 1996).

The woman or couple facing infertility exhibits behaviors of the grieving process that are associated with other types of loss. The loss of one's genetic continuity with the generations to come leads to a loss of self-esteem, to a sense of inadequacy as a woman or man, to a loss of control over one's destiny, and to a reduced sense of self (Schoener & Krysa, 1996). Infertile individuals have impaired self-concept and greater dissatisfaction with their marriages (Hirsch & Hirsch, 1995). The investigative process leads to a loss of spontaneity and control over the couple's marital relationship, and sometimes a loss of control over progress toward career and life goals. All people do not have all the reactions described, nor can it be predicted how long any one reaction will last for an individual.

The support systems of the couple with impaired fertility need to be explored. This exploration should include persons available to assist, their relationship to the couple, their ages, their availability, and the cultural or religious support that is available.

If the couple conceives, nurses need to be aware that the concerns and problems of the previously infertile couple may not be over. Many couples are overjoyed with the pregnancy; however, some are not. Some couples rearrange their lives, sense of self, and personal goals within their acceptance of their infertile state. The couple may feel that those who worked with them to identify and treat impaired fertility expect them to be happy with the pregnancy. The couple may be shocked to find that they themselves feel resentment because the pregnancy, once a cherished dream, now necessitates another change in goals, aspirations, and identities. The normal ambivalence toward pregnancy may be perceived as reneging on the original choice to become parents. The couple might choose to abort the pregnancy at this time. Other couples worry about spontaneous abortion. If the couple wishes to continue with the pregnancy, they will need the care other expectant couples need. The couple may need extra preparation for the realities of pregnancy, labor, and parenthood, because they have developed fantasies about childbearing when they thought it was beyond their reach. A history of impaired fertility is considered to be a risk factor for pregnancy. If the couple does not conceive, they are assessed regarding their desire to be referred for help with adoption, therapeutic intrauterine insemination, other reproductive alternatives, or choosing a child-free state. The couple may find a list of agencies, support groups, and other resources in their community helpful (see Appendix D).

Medical. Pharmacologic therapy is often an important but expensive component of patient care for female infertility. Ovulatory stimulants may be warranted to induce ovulation. Clomiphene (Clomid, Serophene), an oral preparation, stimulates the ovarian follicle. It is used to treat anovulation caused by hypothalamic suppression when the hypothalamic-pituitary-ovarian axis is intact. Multifetal pregnancy rates are less than 10%, with most being twin gestations. Bromocriptine (Parlodel), a synthetic ergot alkaloid that inhibits the release of prolactin, is used to treat anovulation caused by elevated levels of prolactin. Thyroid stimulating hormone (Synthroid) is indicated if the woman has hypothyroidism.

Human menopausal gonadotropin (Pergonal) or pure FSH (Metrodin) is used when clomiphene citrate fails to induce ovulation or when pregnancy has not been achieved in 6 to 12 ovulatory cycles. These medications are extremely potent and require daily monitoring with ovarian ultrasonography and monitoring of estradiol levels to prevent hyperstimulation (Hahn, Butkowski & Capper, 1994). The prevalence of multiple pregnancy is greater than 25%. When ovulation is caused either by hypothalamic-pituitary dysfunction or failure, or failure to respond to clomiphene, gonadotropin-releasing hormone (Gn-RH) may be used.

Hormone replacement therapy may be indicated. The woman who has low estrogen levels is a candidate for conjugated estrogens and medroxyprogesterone. A hypoestrogenic condition may result from a high stress level or decreased percentage of body fat as a result of an eating disorder (e.g., anorexia nervosa) or excessive exercise. Hydroxyprogesterone supplementation with vaginal suppositories or intramuscular injection is used to treat luteal phase defects. The nurse may encounter other medications as well. In the presence of adrenal hyperplasia, prednisone, a glucocorticoid, is taken orally. Treatment of endometriosis may include Danazol, progesterones, combined oral contraceptives, or gonadotropin-releasing hormone agonists (Forrest, 1994; Speroff, Glass & Kase, 1994). Infections are treated with appropriate antimicrobial formulations.

Treatment is available for women who have immunologic reactions to sperm. The use of condoms during genital intercourse for 6 to 12 months will reduce female antibody production in most women who have elevated antisperm antibody titers. After the serum reaction subsides, condoms are used at all times except at the expected time of ovulation. Approximately one third of couples with this problem conceive by following this course of action.

Simple changes in lifestyle may be effective in the treatment of subfertile men. Only water-soluble lubricants should be used during intercourse because many commonly used lubricants contain spermicides or have spermicidal properties. High scrotal temperatures may be caused by daily hot tub bathing or saunas in which the testes are kept at temperatures too high for efficient spermatogenesis. It must be remembered that these conditions lead only to lessened fertility and should not be employed as a means of contraception.

Drug therapy may be indicated for male infertility. Problems with the thyroid or adrenal glands are corrected with appropriate medications. Clomiphene may be given for idiopathic subfertility, although its effectiveness in enhancing fertility rates has been poorly documented. Infections are identified and treated promptly with antimicrobials.

Surgical repair of varicocele (enlargement of the veins of the spermatic cord) has been relatively successful in increasing sperm count but not fertility rates. A varicocele on the left side is found in a substantial number of subfertile men.

The primary care provider is responsible for informing patients fully about the prescribed medications. However, the nurse must be ready to answer patients' questions and to confirm their understanding of the drug, its administration, potential side effects, and expected outcomes. Because information varies with each drug, the nurse needs to consult the medication package inserts, pharmacology references, physician, and pharmacist as necessary.

Surgical. A number of surgical procedures can be used for problems causing female infertility. Ovarian tumors must be excised. Whenever possible, functional ovarian tissue is left intact. Scar tissue adhesions caused by chronic infections may cover much or all of the ovary. These adhesions usually necessitate surgery to free and expose the ovary so that ovulation can occur.

Hysterosalpingography is useful for identification of tubal obstruction and also for the release of blockage. During laparoscopy, delicate adhesions may be divided and removed and endometrial implants may be destroyed by electrocoagulation or laser. Laparotomy and even microsurgery may be required to do extensive repair of the damaged tube. Prognosis is dependent on the degree to which tubal patency and function can be restored.

A woman with a relatively small uterus may become pregnant, but the uterus may be incapable of accommodating the enlarging fetus, and a spontaneous abortion may result. In such cases recurrent or habitual (three or more) spontaneous abortions often occur. No medical therapy has been effective for the enlargement of an abnormally small uterus. Observation suggests that women who do become pregnant, but who miscarry, often abort at a later time with each successive pregnancy. Finally, after two or three pregnancy losses, they may give birth to a viable infant. Apparently actual growth of the uterus occurs with each pregnancy. Reconstructive surgery—for example, the unification operation for bicornuate uterus—often improves a woman's ability to conceive and carry the fetus to term.

Surgical removal of tumors or fibroids involving the endometrium or uterus often improves the woman's chance of conceiving and maintaining the pregnancy to viability. Surgical treatment of uterine tumors or maldevelopment that results in successful pregnancy usually requires birth by cesarean surgery near term gestation. The uterus may rupture as a result of weakness of the area of surgical healing.

Radial chemocautery (destruction of tissue with chemicals) or thermocautery (destruction of tissue with heat, usually electrical) of the cervix, cryosurgery (destruction of tissue by application of extreme cold, usually liquid nitrogen), or conization (excision of a cone-shaped piece of tissue from the endocervix) is effective in eliminating chronic inflammation and infection. When the cervix has been deeply cauterized or frozen or when extensive conization has been performed, extreme limitation of mucous production by the cervix may result. Therefore sperm migration may be difficult or impossible because of the absence of a mucous bridge from the vagina to the uterus. Therapeutic intrauterine insemination may be necessary to carry the sperm directly through the internal os of the cervix.

Surgical procedures may also be used for problems causing male infertility. Surgical repair of varicocele has been relatively successful. Ligation of the varicocele does lead to improvement of the sperm quality and commonly to pregnancy.

Microsurgery to reanastomose (restoration of tubal continuity) the sperm ducts can result in pregnancy rates greater than 50% (Speroff, Glass & Kase, 1994). The rate of success decreases as the time since the procedure increases.

Reproductive alternatives. There have been remarkable developments in reproductive medicine. **Assisted reproductive therapies (ARTs)** are creating ethical and legal issues (Box 7-9). The lack of information or misleading information about success rates and the risks and benefits of treatment alternatives prevents couples from making informed decisions. Nurses can provide information so that couples have an accurate understanding of their chances for a successful pregnancy and live birth. Nurses can also provide anticipatory guidance about the moral and ethical dilemmas regarding the use of ARTs. Some of the ARTs for treatment of infertility include in vitro fertilization–embryo transfer (IVF–ET), gamete intrafallopian transfer (GIFT), zygote intrafallopian transfer (ZIFT), ovum transfer (oocyte donation), embryo adoption, embryo hosting, and surrogate parenting. Table 7-4 describes these procedures and the possible indications for the ARTs. Other options include therapeutic donor insemination, adoption, and surrogate mothering.

In vitro fertilization and embryo transfer. **In vitro fertilization and embryo transfer (IVF–ET)** has become a common approach for women with blocked or absent fallopian tubes or with unexplained infertility, and for men with very low sperm counts. As few as 560 to 1,600 sperm are needed for in vitro fertilization. Generally only three or fewer embryos are transferred, to minimize the risk of

---

BOX 7-9	*Ethical Considerations*

ASSISTED REPRODUCTIVE THERAPIES (ARTs)

Issues	Questions
The right to reproduce	Should IVF be available only to married couples?
Ownership of embryo	Should the embryo be frozen for later use? Who has ownership—the woman, the man, or both?
Parenthood and parent-child bonding	Who are the parents—the biologic or adoptive parents?
Rights of research subjects and research initiatives	Is compensation for egg donors acceptable?
Truth telling and confidentiality	Should donors be anonymous?
Intergenerational responsibilities	What are the long-term effects of the medications and treatments on women, children, and families?

TABLE 7-4 *Assisted Reproductive Therapies (ARTs)*

PROCEDURE	DEFINITION	INDICATIONS
In vitro fertilization and embryo transfer (IVF–ET)	A woman's eggs are collected from her ovaries, fertilized in the laboratory with sperm, and transferred to her uterus after normal embryo development has occurred.	Tubal disease or blockage; severe male infertility; endometriosis; unexplained infertility; cervical factor; immunologic infertility
Gamete intrafallopian transfer (GIFT)	Oocytes are retrieved from the ovary, placed in a catheter with washed motile sperm, and immediately transferred into the fimbriated end of the uterine tube. Fertilization occurs in the uterine tube.	Same as for IVF–ET, *except* there must be normal tubal anatomy, patency and absence of previous tubal disease in at least one uterine tube
IVF–ET and GIFT with donor sperm	This process is the same as described above except in cases where the husband's fertility is severely compromised and donor sperm can be used; if donor sperm are used, the wife must have indications for IVF and GIFT.	Severe male infertility; azoospermia; indications for IVF–ET or GIFT
Zygote intrafallopian transfer (ZIFT)	This process is similar to IVF–ET; after in vitro fertilization the ova are placed in one uterine tube during the zygote stage.	Same as for GIFT
Donor oocyte	Eggs are donated by an IVF procedure and the donated eggs are inseminated. The embryos are transferred into the recipient's uterus, which is hormonally prepared with estrogen/progesterone therapy.	Premature ovarian failure; surgical removal of ovaries; congenitally absent ovaries; autosomal or sex-linked disorders; lack of fertilization in repeated IVF attempts because of subtle oocyte abnormalities or defects in oocyte/spermatozoa interaction
Donor embryo (embryo adoption)	A donated embryo is transferred to the uterus of an infertile woman at the appropriate time (normal or induced) of the menstrual cycle.	Infertility not resolved by less aggressive forms of therapy; absence of ovaries; male partner is azoospermic or is severely compromised
Gestational carrier (embryo host); surrogate mother	A couple undertakes an IVF cycle and the embryo(s) is transferred to another woman's uterus (the carrier) who has contracted with the couple to carry the baby to term. The carrier has no genetic investment in the child. Surrogate motherhood is a process by which a woman is inseminated with semen from the infertile woman's partner and then carries the baby until birth.	Congenital absence or surgical removal of uterus; a reproductively impaired uterus, myomas, uterine adhesions, or other congenital abnormalities; a medical condition that might be life-threatening during pregnancy, such as diabetes, immunologic problems, or severe heart, kidney, or liver disease
Therapeutic donor insemination	Donor sperm are used to inseminate the female partner.	Male partner is azoospermic or has a very low sperm count; couple has a genetic defect; male partner has antisperm antibodies

Data from Braverman A & English M: Creating brave new families with advanced reproductive technologies, *NAACOG's Clin Issu Perinat Womens Health Nurs* 3(2):354, 1992; Edge V & Miller M: *Women's health care,* St Louis, 1994, Mosby; Mishell D: *Comprehensive gynecology,* ed 3, St Louis, 1997, Mosby.

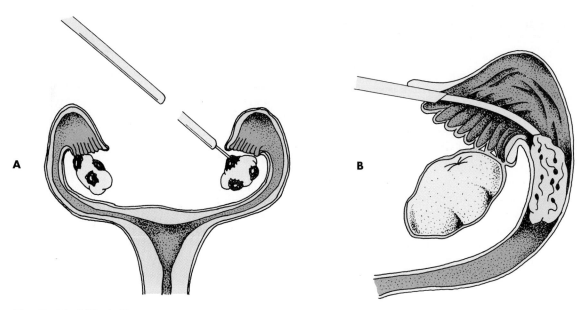

Fig. **7-13** GIFT. **A,** Through laparoscopy, a ripe follicle is located and fluid containing the egg is removed. **B,** The sperm and egg are placed separately in the uterine tube where fertilization occurs. (From Lowdermilk D, Perry S & Bobak I: *Maternity & Women's health care,* ed 6, St Louis, 1997, Mosby.)

multiple pregnancy. When more than three embryos develop in the culture media, the extra embryos can be cryopreserved. If necessary, they can be thawed in a subsequent cycle for later uterine transfer.

Success rates vary widely from center to center. Each couple's physical status and age factor into their individual chances for pregnancy. Rates range from 10% to 40% per cycle and are highly individual. In vitro fertilization costs from $6,000 to $9,000 per treatment.

Gamete intrafallopian transfer. **Gamete intrafallopian tube transfer (GIFT)** is similar to IVF–ET. Ovulation is induced as in IVF–ET, and the oocytes are aspirated from follicles via laparoscopy (Fig. 7-13, *A*). Semen is collected before laparoscopy, and sperm are capacitated by the same technique used for IVF–ET. The ova and sperm are then transferred to one tube (Fig. 7-13, *B*), permitting natural fertilization and cleavage, with subsequent successful pregnancies possible (Rabar, 1991). A 20% to 30% pregnancy rate per cycle has been reported for this technique. GIFT requires women to have at least one normal uterine tube.

Zygote intrafallopian transfer. **Zygote intrafallopian transfer (ZIFT)** is also similar to IVF–ET. In ZIFT, after in vitro fertilization, the ova are placed in the uterine tube during the zygote stage. Success rates for ZIFT are similar to those for GIFT.

Complications. Other than the established risks associated with laparoscopy and general anesthesia, few risks are associated with IVF–ET, GIFT, and ZIFT. The more common transvaginal needle aspiration requires only local or intravenous analgesia. Congenital anomalies occur no more frequently than among naturally conceived embryos.

Ectopic pregnancies do occur more often, however, and these carry a significant maternal risk.

Oocyte donation. Women who have ovarian failure or oophorectomy, who have a genetic defect, or who fail to achieve pregnancy with their own oocytes may be eligible for the use of donor oocytes. Donors who are younger than 35 years and healthy are recruited and paid to undergo ovarian stimulation and oocyte retrieval. The donor eggs are then fertilized in the laboratory with the male partner's sperm. The recipient woman undergoes hormonal stimulation to allow development of the uterine lining. Embryos are then transferred. Pregnancy rates vary from 5% to 20%. The psychosocial issues are similar to those in therapeutic donor insemination. Historically the courts have upheld the gestational mother as the legal mother. It is expected that the egg donor will have no rights or responsibilities in relation to the offspring.

Donor embryos. On occasion, a couple decides that they do not want their frozen embryos, and they release these for "adoption" by other infertile couples. Infertility centers are struggling to develop guidelines and protocols to address the various legal and ethical issues associated with these procedures.

Therapeutic donor insemination. **Therapeutic donor insemination (TDI),** previously referred to as artificial insemination by donor, is used when the male partner has no sperm or a very low sperm count (less than 20 million motile sperm per milliliter), the couple has a genetic defect, or when the male partner has antisperm antibodies. Couples need to be counseled extensively regarding the mutuality of their decision, their ability (particularly of the male partner) to grieve the loss of a biologic child, and long-term issues relating to parenting the child conceived through TDI (Prattke & Gass-Sternas, 1993). Couples also need to be aware of the legal status of TDI in their particular state.

In TDI, donor semen is subjected to laboratory testing to reduce the possibility of life-threatening illnesses for the recipient and her fetus, as well as for factors that could jeopardize the woman's future fertility or compromise the chance of the success of the procedure. Donor semen is tested for serology, serum hepatitis B antigen, *Neisseria gonorrhoeae*, *Chlamydia trachomatis*, cytomegalovirus antibodies, and HIV antibodies (Speroff, Glass & Kase, 1994).

Assuming normal female fertility, intrauterine TDI at or about the time of ovulation has resulted in pregnancy in as many as 70% of cases. If pregnancy has not occurred within six cycles of well-timed insemination, further investigation of the female partner is warranted. The couple must know that there is no guarantee of pregnancy and that the spontaneous abortion rate is approximately the same as in a control population. There is no increase in maternal or perinatal complications; the same frequencies of anomalies (about 5%) and obstetric complications (between 5% and 10%) that accompany natural insemination (through sexual intercourse) apply also to TDI.

Adoption. Couples may choose to build their family by adopting children who are not their own biologically. However, with increased availability of birth control and abortion and increasing numbers of single mothers keeping their babies, the adoption of caucasian infants is extremely limited. Minority infants and infants with special needs, older children, and foreign adoptions are other options.

Most adults assume that they will be able to have children of their own. The discovery that they are unable to do so is often accompanied by feelings of inferiority, doubts about masculinity or femininity, and feelings of guilt or blame in relation to the partner. These feelings and frustrations, combined with the anxiety of waiting for pregnancies, feelings of loss, and the endless medical procedures to investigate infertility create a unique situation for the adoptive couple who is preparing for parenthood (Hahn, 1991).

Hahn (1991) has proposed the following questions to aid couples in their soul searching regarding adoption as an alternative. Can you deal with having little or no information about your child's background? How will you feel if you become pregnant later? Are you willing to accept a child of school age or of different nationality or color? Can you be proud of him or her? Are you willing to tolerate differences? Is it important that your child look like you? Can you encourage talents, skills, and preferences that are very different from your own? How do you feel about knowing the child's birth mother or father? How does your extended family feel about adopted children?

Nurses should have information on adoption available for couples and should use positive language when discussing this option.

Surrogate mothers. Surrogate motherhood can be achieved by two methods. The first is to have the surrogate mother inseminated with semen from the infertile woman's partner and carry the baby until the birth. The baby is then formally adopted by the infertile couple. A less common method is to retrieve an ovum from the infertile woman, fertilize it with her partner's sperm, and place it into the uterus of a surrogate, who becomes a gestational carrier. These newer interventions raise considerable legal and ethical issues that require extensive counseling of couples and the women who choose to become pregnant.

Evaluation

Evaluation of the effectiveness of care of the couple experiencing impaired fertility is based on the previously stated outcomes.

KEY POINTS

- A variety of contraceptive methods are available with various effectiveness rates, advantages, and disadvantages.
- Nurses need to help couples choose the contraceptive method or methods best suited to them.
- Effective contraceptives are available through both prescription and nonprescription sources.
- A variety of techniques are available to enhance the effectiveness of periodic abstinence in motivated couples who prefer this natural method.
- Hormonal contraception includes both precoital and postcoital prevention through various modalities and requires thorough patient education.
- The most widely used emergency contraceptive method is ingestion of high doses of estrogen and progestin oral contraceptive pills taken in 2 doses, 12 hours apart.
- The barrier methods of diaphragm and cervical cap provide safe and effective contraception for women or couples motivated to use them consistently and correctly.
- Proper concurrent use of spermicides and latex condoms provides protection against STDs.
- Tubal ligations and vasectomies are permanent sterilization methods used by increasing numbers of women and men.

Continued

KEY POINTS —cont'd

- Elective abortion performed in the first trimester is safer than an abortion performed in the second trimester.
- The most common complications of elective abortion include infection, retained products of conception, and excessive vaginal bleeding.
- Major psychologic sequelae of elective abortion are rare.
- Infertility is the inability to conceive and carry a child to term gestation at a time the couple has chosen to do so.
- Infertility affects between 15% to 20% of otherwise healthy adults. Infertility increases in women older than 35 years.
- In the United States, 40% to 55% of infertility is related to female causes; 30% to 40% is related to male causes; 10% to 15% is related to couple causes; and 10% to 20% of the causes are unexplained.
- Common etiologic factors of infertility include decreased sperm production, ovulation disorders, tubal occlusion, and endometriosis.
- Reproductive alternatives for family building include IVF–ET, GIFT, ZIFT, oocyte donation, embryo donation, TDI, surrogate motherhood, and adoption.

CRITICAL THINKING EXERCISES

1 *Explore the options in your community for diagnosis, treatment alternatives, and support services for couples experiencing infertility. Discuss your findings in a clinical conference, including the ease or difficulty a couple would have in getting help with their problem.*

2 *You are interviewing a 45-year-old woman in the local health department family planning clinic. She is seeking information about her risks of pregnancy at this time in her life.*

   a *What information will you need from her to respond?*

   b *How might you answer her question based on the answers you may receive in a above?*

   c *Assuming that contraceptive measures are necessary, what methods are appropriate for this woman?*

   d *What further information may you need from this woman to make a contraceptive recommendation?*

CRITICAL THINKING EXERCISES—cont'd

   e *What alterations would you make in a teaching plan for her based on her age and previous experiences with contraception?*

3 *You are working in a health department clinic. A 16-year-old, unmarried woman comes in requesting information about options for an unwanted pregnancy.*

   a *Examine your values about teenage pregnancy. Explore your beliefs about options for an unwanted pregnancy. How might these values and beliefs affect your ability to provide information about options in a nonjudgmental manner?*

   b *What patient information do you need to know before counseling a woman about her options?*

   c *What information is needed by the pregnant woman in making a decision about her unwanted pregnancy?*

   d *What are the laws in your state related to abortion, informed consent, and treatment of minors?*

   e *Select one option for this hypothetical patient and justify your choice.*

References

Amar L: Male infertility. In Garner C, editor: *Principles of infertility nursing,* Boca Raton, Fla, 1991, CRC Press.

Bancroft J: Impact of environment, stress, occupational, and other hazards on sexuality and sexual behavior, *Environ Health Perspect* 101(suppl 2):101, 1993.

Boxer A: Images of infertility, *Nurse Pract Forum* 7(2):60, 1996.

Braverman A & English M: Creating brave new families with advanced reproductive technologies, *NAACOG's Clin Issu Perinat Womens Health Nurs* 3(2):354, 1992.

Centers for Disease Control and Prevention: CDC Surveillance Summaries (Abortion Surveillance–United States, 1991), *MMWR* 45(SS-3):1, 1996.

Chez R & Chapin J: Emergency contraception: the pill's little-known secret goes public, *AWHONN Lifelines* 1(5):28, 1997.

Contraception Report: Contraception choices for women over age 35: focus on benefits and risks, *Contracept Rep* 3(2):4, May 1992.

Contraception Report: Trends in oral contraceptive development and utilization, *Contracept Rep* 7(5):4, 1997.

Creinin M et al.: Methotrexate and misoprostol for early abortion: a multicenter trial. I. Safety and efficacy, *Contraception* 53(6):321, 1996.

Cunningham F et al.: *Williams obstetrics,* ed 20, Stamford, Conn, 1997, Appleton & Lange.

Donaldson K, Briggs J & McMaster D: RU 486: an alternative to surgical abortion, *J Obstet Gynecol Neonatal Nurs* 23(7): 555, 1994.

Edge V & Miller M: *Women's health care,* St Louis, 1994, Mosby.

Fehring R et al.: Use effectiveness of the Creighton model ovulation method of natural family planning, *J Obstet Gynecol Neonatal Nurs* 23(4):303, 1994.

Forrest D: Common gynecologic pelvic disorders. In Youngkin E & Davis M, editors: *Women's health: a primary care clinical guide,* Norwalk, Conn, 1994, Appleton & Lange.

Fryday M: Treating infertility in Roman Catholics, *Nursing Standard* 10(5):31, 1995 .

Geerling J: Natural family planning, *Am Fam Physician* 52(6):1749, 1995.

Geissler E: *Pocket guide to cultural assessment,* St Louis, 1994, Mosby.

Giovannucci E et al.: A long-term study of mortality in men who have undergone vasectomy, *N Eng J Med* 326(21):1392, 1992.

Gleicher N: Immunological infertility & its diagnosis. In Insler V & Lunesfeld B, editors: *Infertility: male and female,* ed 2, Edinburgh, 1993, Churchill Livingston.

Greendale G et al.: The relationship of *Chlamydia trachomatis* infection and male infertility, *Am J Public Health* 83(7):996, 1993.

Grimes D: Sequelae of abortion. In Baird D, Grimes D & Van Look P, editors: *Modern methods of inducing abortion,* London, 1995, Blackwell Science.

Hahn S: Caring for couples considering alternatives in family building. In Garner C, editor: *Principles of infertility nursing,* Boca Raton, Fla, 1991, CRC Press.

Hahn S, Butkowsk C & Capper L: Ovarian hyperstimulation syndrome: protocols for nursing care, *J Obstet Gynecol Neonatal Nurs* 23(3):217, 1994.

Hatcher R et al.: *Contraceptive technology,* ed 17, New York, 1998, Ardent Media, Inc.

Heath C & Sulik S: Contraception and preconception counseling, *Women's Health* 24(10):123, 1997.

Hickey M & Fraser I: The contraceptive use of depot medroxyprogesterone acetate, *Clin Obstet Gynecol* 38(4):849, 1995.

Hirsch A & Hirsch S: The long-term psychosocial effects of infertility, *J Obstet Gynecol Neonatal Nurs* 24(6):517, 1995.

Johnson C: Regaining self-esteem: strategies and interventions for the infertile woman, *J Obstet Gynecol Neonatal Nurs* 25(4):291, 1996.

Konje J et al.: The effect of continuous subdermal levonorgestrel (Norplant) on carbohydrate metabolism, *Am J Obstet Gynecol* 166(1):15, 1992.

Liel Y et al.: Medical conditions leading to infertility. In Insler V & Lunesfeld B, editors: *Infertility: male and female,* ed 2, Edinburgh, 1993, Churchill Livingston.

Lindberg C: Emergency contraception: the nurse's role in providing postcoital options, *J Obstet Gynecol Neonatal Nurs* 26(2):145, 1997.

Lowdermilk D, Perry S & Bobak I: *Maternity and women's health care,* ed 6, St Louis, 1997, Mosby.

Mattison D et al.: Reproductive toxicity: male and female reproductive systems as targets for chemical injury, *Med Clin North Am* 74(2):391, 1990.

Mishell D et al.: *Comprehensive gynecology,* ed 3, St Louis, 1997, Mosby.

Moore R: *Contraception issues and options for young women: contemporary studies in women's health,* Fairlawn, NJ, 1994, MPE Communications.

Morell V: Basic infertility assessment, *Women's Health* 24(1):195, 1997.

O'Connell M: The effect of birth control methods on sexually transmitted disease/HIV risk, *J Obstet Gynecol Neonatal Nurs* 25(6): 476, 1996.

Prattke T & Gass-Sternas K: Appraisal, coping, and emotional health of infertile couples undergoing artificial insemination, *J Obstet Gynecol Neonatal Nurs* 22(6):516, 1993.

Rabar F: Gamete intrafallopian transfer, *AORN J* 53(6):1466, 1991.

Reifsnider E: On the horizon: new options for contraception, *J Obstet Gynecol Neonatal Nurs* 26(1):91, 1997.

Ross L & Niederberger C: Male infertility: diagnosis & treatment, *Compr Ther* 21(6):276, 1995.

Schill W & Haidl G: Medical treatment of male infertility. In Insler V & Lunesfeld B, editors: *Infertility: male and female,* ed 2, Edinburgh, 1993, Churchill Livingston.

Schoener C & Krysa L: The comfort and discomfort of infertility, *J Obstet Gynecol Neonatal Nurs* 25(2):167, 1996.

Secor R: The cervical cap, *NAACOG Clin Issues Perinat Women's Health Nurs* 3(2):236, 1992.

Soriano C: Abortion: new common ground, *USA Weekend* Jan 9-11, 1998.

Speroff L & Darney P: *A clinical guide for contraception,* ed 2, Baltimore, Md, 1996, Williams & Wilkins.

Speroff L, Glass R & Kase N: *Clinical gynecologic endocrinology & infertility,* Baltimore, Md, 1994, Williams & Wilkins.

Stauber M & Brucker C: Psychosomatic aspects of infertility. In Insler V & Lunesfeld B, editors: *Infertility: male and female,* ed 2, Edinburgh, 1993, Churchill Livingston.

Stotland N: The myth of the abortion trauma syndrome, *JAMA* 268(15):1078, 1992.

Thong K & Baird D: Induction of abortion with mifepristone and misoprostol in early pregnancy, *Br J Obstet Gynaecol* 99(12):1004, 1992.

Timbers K & Feinberg R: Recurrent pregnancy loss: a review, *Nurse Pract Forum* 7(2):64, 1996.

Toppozada M: Termination of pregnancy after 14 weeks. In Baird D, Grimes D & Van Look P, editors: *Modern methods of inducing abortion,* London, 1995, Blackwell Science.

Trantham P: The infertile couple, *Am Fam Physician* 54(3):1001, 1996.

Trent A & Clark E: What nurses should know about natural family planning, *J Obstet Gynecol Neonatal Nurs* 26(6):643, 1997.

Wallach E & Zacur H: *Reproductive medicine and surgery,* St Louis, 1995, Mosby.

Wilcox L & Mosher W: Characteristics associated with impaired fecundity in the United States, *Fam Plan Perspect* 26(5):218, 1994.

World Health Organization Task Force: Termination of pregnancy with reduced doses of mifepristone, *Br Med J* 307(6903):532, 1993.

World Health Organization: *Complications of abortion,* Geneva, 1995, World Health Organization.

CHAPTER

8

Conception and Fetal Development

SHANNON E. PERRY

LEARNING OBJECTIVES

- *Define the key terms.*
- *Summarize the process of fertilization.*
- *Explain basic principles of genetics.*
- *Describe the development, structure, and functions of the placenta.*
- *Describe the composition and functions of the amniotic fluid.*
- *Identify three organs or tissues arising from each of the three primary germ layers.*
- *Summarize the significant changes in growth and development of the embryo and fetus.*
- *Identify the potential effects of teratogens during vulnerable periods of embryonic and fetal development.*
- *Describe the Human Genome Project.*
- *Describe the nurse's role in genetic counseling.*
- *Examine ethical dimensions of genetic screening.*

KEY TERMS

amniotic fluid
blastocyst
cephalocaudal development
chorionic villi
chromosome
conception
decidua basalis
dizygotic twins
ductus arteriosus
embryo
fertilization
fetal membranes
fetus
foramen ovale
gamete
gene
genome
hematopoiesis
human chorionic gonadotropin (hCG)
implantation
karyotype

KEY TERMS—cont'd

karyotyping
lecithin/sphingomyelin (L/S) ratio
meconium
meiosis
monozygotic twins
morula
mutation
placenta
quickening
sex chromosome
surfactants
teratogens
umbilical cord
viability
zygote

This chapter presents an overview of the process of fertilization and the development of the normal embryo and fetus. A brief discussion of genetics and genetic counseling is included.

▌ CONCEPTION

Conception, defined as the union of a single egg and sperm, marks the beginning of a pregnancy. Conception occurs not as an isolated event, but as part of a sequential process. This sequential process includes **gamete** (egg and sperm) formation, ovulation (release of the egg), fertilization (union of the gametes), and implantation in the uterus.

Cell Division

Cells are reproduced by two different methods: mitosis and meiosis. In mitosis, body cells replicate to yield two cells with the same genetic makeup as the parent cell. First the cell makes a copy of its deoxyribonucleic acid (DNA); then it divides, and each daughter cell receives one copy of the genetic material. The purpose of mitotic division is for growth and development or cell replacement.

Meiosis produces gametes. Each homologous pair of chromosomes receives one chromosome from the mother and the other from the father; meiosis results in cells containing one of each of the 23 pairs of chromosomes. Because these

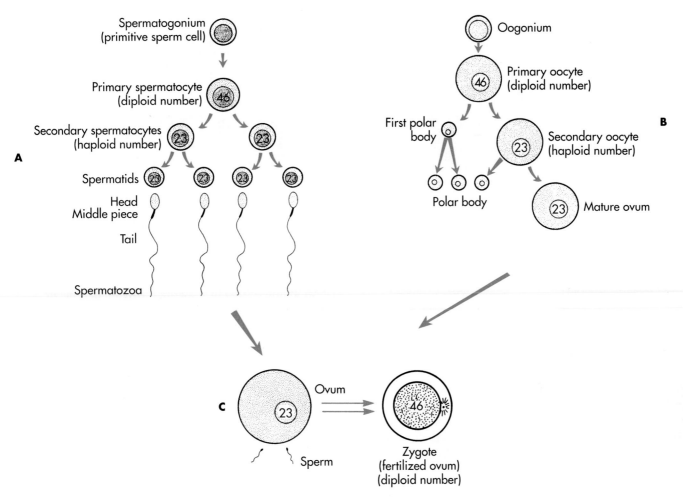

Fig. **8-1 A,** Spermatogenesis. Gametogenesis of the male produces four mature gametes, the sperm. **B,** Oogenesis. Gametogenesis in the female produces one mature ovum and three polar bodies. Note the relative difference in overall size between the ovum and sperm. **C,** Fertilization results in the single-cell zygote and the restoration of the diploid number of chromosomes.

germ cells contain 23 single chromosomes, half of the genetic material of a normal somatic cell, they are called haploid. This halving of the genetic material is accomplished by replicating the DNA once and then dividing twice. In mitosis, the DNA is replicated once and followed by a single cell division. When the female gamete (egg or ovum) and the male gamete (spermatozoan) unite to form the zygote, the diploid number of human chromosomes (46 or 23 pairs) is restored.

The process of DNA replication and cell division in meiosis allows different alleles for genes to be distributed at random by each parent and then rearranged on the paired chromosomes. The chromosomes then separate and proceed to different gametes. Many combinations of genes are possible on each chromosome because parents have genotypes derived from four different grandparents. This random mixing of alleles accounts for the variation of traits seen in the offspring of the same parents (see discussion later in this chapter).

Gametogenesis

When a male reaches puberty, his testes begin the process of spermatogenesis. The cells that undergo meiosis in the male are called spermatocytes. The primary spermatocyte, which undergoes the first meiotic division, contains the diploid number of chromosomes. Remember, however, that the cell has already copied its DNA before division, so four alleles for each gene are actually present. The cell is still considered diploid because the copies are bound together—one allele plus its copy on each chromosome. During the first meiotic division, two haploid secondary spermatocytes are formed. Each secondary spermatocyte contains 22 autosomes and one sex chromosome; one contains the X chromosome (plus its copy), and the other has the Y chromosome (plus its copy). During the second meiotic division, the male produces two gametes with an X chromosome and two gametes with a Y chromosome, all of which will develop into viable sperm (Fig. 8-1, *A*).

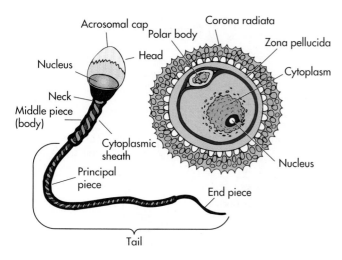

Fig. **8-2** Sperm and ovum.

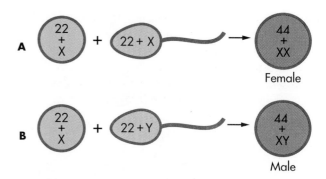

Fig. **8-3** Fertilization. **A,** Ovum fertilized by X-bearing sperm to form female zygote. **B,** Ovum fertilized by Y-bearing sperm to form male zygote. (From Lowdermilk D, Perry S & Bobak I: *Maternity & women's health care,* ed 6, 1997, Mosby.)

Oogenesis, the process of egg (ovum) formation, begins in the female's fetal life. At birth, a woman's ovaries contain all of the cells that may undergo meiosis in her lifetime. The majority of the estimated 2 million primary oocytes (the cells that undergo the first meiotic division) degenerate spontaneously. Only 400 to 500 ova will mature during the approximately 35 years of a woman's reproductive life. The primary oocytes begin the first meiotic division (i.e., they replicate their DNA) during fetal life, but remain suspended at this stage until puberty (Fig. 8-1, *B*). Then usually monthly, one primary oocyte matures and completes the first meiotic division, yielding two unequal cells, the secondary oocyte and a small polar body. Both contain 22 autosomes and one X sex chromosome. At ovulation, the second meiotic division begins, however, the ovum does not complete the second meiotic division unless fertilization occurs. At fertilization, a second polar body and the zygote (the united egg and sperm) are produced (Fig. 8-1, *C*). If fertilization does not occur, the ovum degenerates.

Ovum

Meiosis is the process by which germ cells divide and decrease their chromosomal number by half. In the female this meiotic process produces an ovum (egg) and occurs in the ovarian follicles. Each month one ovum matures with a host of surrounding supportive cells.

At ovulation the ovum is released from the ruptured ovarian follicle. High estrogen levels increase the motility of the uterine tubes so their cilia are able to capture the ovum and propel it through the tube toward the uterine cavity. An ovum cannot move by itself.

Two protective layers surround the ovum (Fig. 8-2). The inner layer is a thick, acellular layer, the zona pellucida. The [ou]ter layer, the corona radiata, is composed of elongated [cell]'s.

Ova are considered fertile for about 24 hours after ovulation. If unfertilized by a sperm, the ovum degenerates and is reabsorbed.

Sperm

Ejaculation during sexual intercourse normally propels almost a teaspoon of semen (containing as many as 200 to 500 million sperm) into the vagina. The sperm swim with the flagellar movement of their tails. Some sperm can reach the site of fertilization within 5 minutes, but the average transit time is 4 to 6 hours. Sperm remain viable within the woman's reproductive system for an average of 2 to 3 days. Most sperm are lost in the vagina, within the cervical mucus, or in the endometrium, or they enter the uterine tube that contains no ovum.

As the sperm travel through the female reproductive tract, enzymes are produced to aid in capacitation of the sperm. Then, small perforations form in the acrosome (a cap on the sperm) and allow enzymes (e.g., hyaluronidase) to escape (see Fig. 8-1). These enzymes are necessary for the sperm to penetrate the protective layers of the ovum before fertilization.

Fertilization

Fertilization takes place in the ampulla (outer third) of the fallopian tube. When a sperm successfully penetrates the membrane surrounding the ovum, both sperm and ovum are enclosed within the membrane, and the membrane becomes impenetrable to other sperm; this process is termed the *zona reaction*. The second meiotic division of the secondary oocyte is then completed, and the ovum nucleus becomes the female pronucleus. The head of the sperm enlarges to become the male pronucleus, and the tail degenerates. The nuclei fuse and the chromosomes combine, restoring the diploid number (46) (Fig. 8-3). Conception, the formation of the **zygote** (the first cell of the new individual), is now complete.

Mitotic cellular replication, called *cleavage,* begins as the zygote travels the length of the uterine tube into the uterus.

This transit time takes 3 to 4 days. Because the fertilized egg divides rapidly without an increase in size, successively smaller cells, *blastomeres,* are formed with each division. A 16-cell **morula,** a solid ball of cells, is produced within 3 days still surrounded by the protective zona pellucida (Fig. 8-4, *A*). Further development occurs as the morula floats freely within the uterus. Fluid passes through the zona pellucida into the intercellular spaces between the blastomeres separating them into two parts; the trophoblast (gives rise to the placenta) and the embryoblast (which gives rise to the embryo). A cavity forms within the cell mass as the spaces come together, forming a structure called the *blastocyst cavity.* When the cavity becomes recognizable, the whole structure of the developing embryo is known as the **blastocyst.** The outer layer of cells surrounding the cavity is the *trophoblast* (the feeding layer).

Implantation

The zona pellucida degenerates, and the trophoblast cells displace endometrial cells at the implantation site and the blastocyst embeds in the endometrium, usually in the anterior or posterior fundal region. Between 6 and 10 days after conception, the trophoblast secretes enzymes that enable it to burrow into the endometrium until the entire blastocyst is covered. This is known as **implantation.** Endometrial blood vessels erode, and some women experience slight implantation bleeding (slight spotting or bleeding during the time of the first missed menstrual period). **Chorionic villi,** finger-like processes or projections, develop out of the trophoblast and extend into the blood-filled spaces of the endometrium. These villi obtain oxygen and nutrients from the maternal bloodstream and dispose of carbon dioxide and waste products into the maternal blood.

After implantation, the endometrium is called the *decidua.* The portion directly under the blastocyst, where the chorionic villi tap into the maternal blood vessels, is the **decidua basalis.** The portion covering the blastocyst is the *decidua capsularis,* and the portion lining the rest of the uterus is the *decidua vera* (Fig. 8-5).

THE EMBRYO AND FETUS

A human pregnancy that reaches term is said to have had a duration of 10 lunar months, 9 calendar months, 40 weeks, or 280 days. Length of pregnancy is computed from the first day of the last menstrual period (LMP) until the day of birth (see discussion of Nägele's rule and adjustment for longer and shorter cycles). However, conception occurs approximately 2 weeks after the first day of the LMP. Thus the postconception age of the fetus is 2 weeks less for a total of 266 days, or 38 weeks. Postconceptional age will be used in the discussion of fetal development.

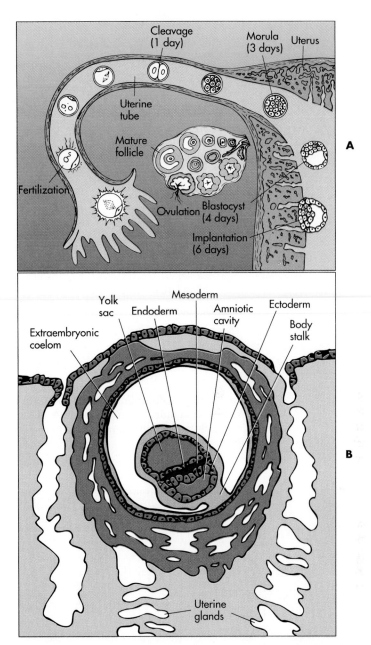

Fig. 8-4 First week of human development. **A,** Follicular development in the ovary, ovulation, fertilization, and transport of the early embryo down the uterine tube and into the uterus where implantation occurs. **B,** Blastocyst embedded in endometrium. Germ layers forming. (*A,* from Carlson B: *Human embryology and developmental biology,* St Louis, 1994, Mosby; *B,* adapted from Langley L et al.: *Dynamic human anatomy and physiology,* ed 5, New York, 1980, McGraw-Hill.)

Intrauterine development is divided into three stages: ovum or preembryonic, embryonic, and fetal (Fig. 8-6). The stage of the ovum lasts from conception until day 14. This period covers cellular replication, blastocyst formation, initial development of the embryonic membranes, and establishment of the primary germ layers.

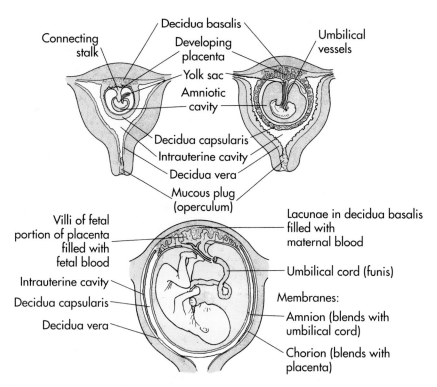

Fig. 8-5 Development of fetal membranes. Note gradual obliteration of intrauterine cavity as decidua capsularis and decidua vera meet. Also note thinning of uterine wall. Chorionic and amniotic membranes are in apposition to each other but may be peeled apart.

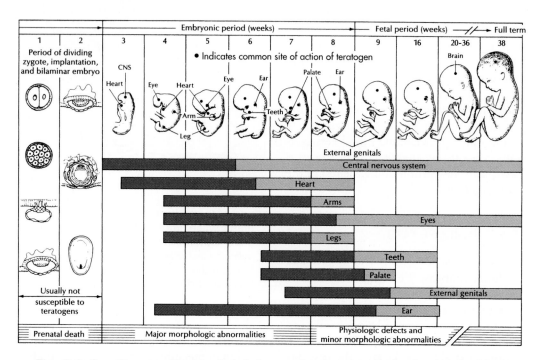

Fig. 8-6 Sensitive, or critical, periods in human development. Dark color denotes highly sensitive periods; light color indicates stages that are less sensitive to teratogens. (From Moore K: *Before we are born: essentials of embryology and birth defects,* ed 3, Philadelphia, 1998, WB Saunders.)

Primary Germ Layers

During the third week after conception the embryonic disk differentiates into three primary germ layers: the ectoderm, mesoderm, and endoderm (or entoderm) (see Fig. 8-4, *B*). All tissues and organs of the embryo develop from these three layers.

The *ectoderm*, the upper layer of the embryonic disk, gives rise to the epidermis, glands (anterior pituitary, cutaneous, and mammary), nails and hair, the nervous system, lens of the eye, tooth enamel, and the floor of the amniotic cavity.

The middle layer, the *mesoderm*, develops into the bones and teeth, muscles (skeletal, smooth, and cardiac), dermis, and connective tissue, cardiovascular system and spleen, and urogenital system.

The lower layer, the *endoderm*, gives rise to the epithelium lining the respiratory tract, digestive tract, and glandular cells of associated organs, including the oropharynx, liver and pancreas, urethra, bladder, and vagina. The endoderm forms the roof of the yolk sac.

Development of the Embryo

The embryonic stage lasts from day 15 until approximately 8 weeks after conception or until the **embryo** measures 3 cm from crown to rump. This embryonic stage is the most critical time in the development of organ systems and the main external features. Developing areas with rapid cell division are the most vulnerable to malformation by environmental **teratogens** (something that causes abnormal development). At the end of the eighth week, all organ systems and external structures are present, and the embryo is unmistakably human (see Fig. 8-6).

Membranes

At the time of implantation, two **fetal membranes,** which will surround the developing embryo, begin to form. The *chorion* develops from the trophoblast and contains the chorionic villi on its surface. The villi burrowing into the decidua basalis increase in size and complexity as the vascular processes develop into the placenta. The chorion becomes the covering of the fetal side of the placenta. It contains the major umbilical blood vessels as they branch out over the surface of the placenta. As the embryo grows, the decidua capsularis becomes stretched. The chorionic villi on this side atrophy and degenerate leaving a smooth chorionic membrane.

The inner cell membrane, the *amnion*, develops from the interior cells of the blastocyst. The cavity that develops between this inner cell mass and the outer layer of cells (trophoblast) is the amniotic cavity (see Fig. 8-4, *B*). As it grows larger, the amnion forms on the side opposite to the developing blastocyst (see Figs. 8-4 and 8-5). The developing embryo draws the amnion around itself, forming a fluid-filled sac. The amnion becomes the covering of the umbilical cord and covers the chorion on the fetal surface of the placenta. As the embryo grows larger, the amnion enlarges to accommodate both the embryo/fetus and its surrounding **amniotic fluid.** The amnion eventually comes in contact with the chorion surrounding the fetus.

Amniotic fluid

Initially, the amniotic cavity derives its fluid by diffusion from the maternal blood. The amount of fluid increases weekly, so that normally 800 and 1,200 ml of transparent amniotic liquid are present at term. The amniotic fluid volume changes constantly. The fetus swallows fluid, and fluid flows into and out of the fetal lungs. The fetus urinates into the fluid, greatly enhancing its volume.

Many functions are served by amniotic fluid for the embryo/fetus. Amniotic fluid helps maintain a constant body temperature. It serves as a source of oral fluid and as a repository for waste. Amniotic fluid cushions the fetus from trauma by blunting and dispersing the forces. It allows freedom of movement for musculoskeletal development. The fluid keeps the embryo from tangling with the membranes, facilitating symmetric growth of the fetus.

The volume of amniotic fluid is an important factor in assessing fetal well-being (Hallak et al., 1993). Having less than 300 ml of amniotic fluid (oligohydramnios) is associated with fetal renal abnormalities. Having greater than 2 L of amniotic fluid (hydramnios) is associated with gastrointestinal and other malformations.

Amniotic fluid contains albumin, urea, uric acid, creatinine, lecithin, sphingomyelin, bilirubin, fructose, fat leukocytes, proteins, epithelial cells, enzymes, and lanugo hair. Study of fetal cells in amniotic fluid through amniocentesis yields much information about the fetus. Genetic studies (**karyotyping**) provide knowledge about the sex and normality of chromosome number and structure. Other studies such as L/S ratio determine the health or maturity of the fetus.

Yolk sac

At the same time as the amniotic cavity and amnion are forming, another blastocyst cavity has formed on the other side of the developing embryonic disk (see Fig. 8-4, *B*). This cavity becomes surrounded by a membrane, forming the yolk sac. The yolk sac aids in transferring maternal nutrients and oxygen, which have diffused through the chorion to the embryo. Blood vessels form to aid transport. Blood cells and plasma are manufactured in the yolk sac during the second and third weeks while uteroplacental circulation is being established and forming primitive blood cells until hematopoietic activity begins. At the end of the third week, the primitive heart begins to beat and circulate the blood through the embryo, connecting stalk, chorion, and yolk sac.

The folding in of the embryo during the fourth to eighth weeks results in part of the yolk sac being incorporated into the embryo's body as the primitive digestive system. Primordial germ cells arise in the yolk sac and move into the embryo. The shrinking remains of the yolk sac degenerate. By the fifth or sixth week, the remnant has separated from the embryo.

Umbilical cord

By day 14 after conception the embryonic disk, amniotic sac, and yolk sac are attached to the chorionic villi by a connecting stalk. During the third week the blood vessels develop to supply the embryo with maternal nutrients and oxygen. During the fifth week, after the embryo has curved inward on itself from both ends bringing the connecting stalk to the ventral side of the embryo, the connecting stalk becomes compressed from both sides by the amnion, forming the narrower **umbilical cord** (see Fig. 8-5). Two arteries carry blood from the embryo to the chorionic villi, and one large vein returns blood to the embryo. One percent of umbilical cords contain only two vessels: one artery and one vein. This occurrence is sometimes associated with congenital malformations.

The cord rapidly increases in length. At term, the cord ranges in length from 30 to 90 cm (average 55 cm) and is approximately 2 cm in diameter. It twists spirally on itself and loops around the embryo/fetus. A true knot is rare, but false knots occur as folds or kinks in the cord and may jeopardize circulation to the fetus. Connective tissue, called *Wharton's jelly*, prevents compression of the blood vessels. This helps to ensure continued nourishment of the embryo/fetus. Compression can occur if the cord lies between the fetal head and the pelvis or is twisted around the fetal body. When the cord is wrapped around the fetal neck, it is called a *nuchal cord*.

As the placenta develops from the chorionic villi, the umbilical cord is usually located centrally. The blood vessels are arrayed out from the center to all parts of the placenta.

Placenta

Structure. During the third week after conception the trophoblast cells of the chorionic villi continue to invade the decidua basalis. As the uterine capillaries are tapped, the endometrial spiral arteries fill with maternal blood. The chorionic villi grow into the spaces with two layers of cells: the outer syncytium and the inner cytotrophoblast. A third layer develops into anchoring septa, dividing the projecting decidua into separate areas called *cotyledons*. In each of the 15 to 20 cotyledons, the chorionic villi branch out and a complex system of fetal blood vessels forms. Each cotyledon is a functional unit. The whole structure is the **placenta** (Fig. 8-7).

The maternal-placental-embryonic circulation is in place by day 17, when the embryonic heart starts beating. By the end of the third week, embryonic blood is circulating ~~between~~ ween the embryo and the chorionic villi. In the inter~~villous~~ us spaces, maternal blood supplies oxygen and nutrients

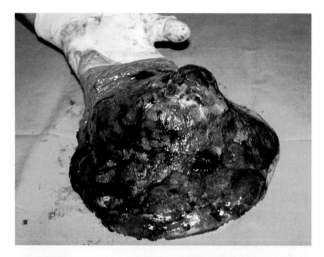

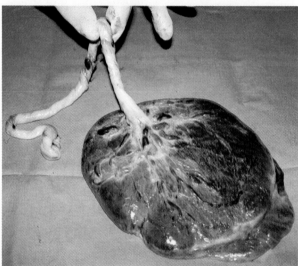

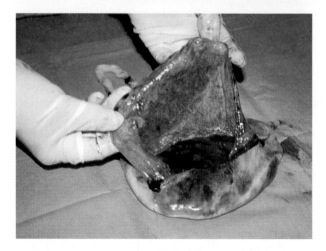

Fig. **8-7** Full-term placentas. **A,** Maternal (or uterine) surface, showing cortyledons and grooves. **B,** Fetal (or amniotic) surface, showing blood vessels running under amnion and converging to form umbilical vessels at attachment of umbilical cord. **C,** Amnion and smooth chorion are arranged to show that they are (1) fused and (2) continuous with margins of placenta. (Courtesy Marjorie Pyle, RNC, Lifecircle, Costa Mesa, Calif.)

to the embryonic capillaries in the villi. Waste products and carbon dioxide diffuse into the maternal blood.

The placenta functions as a means of metabolic exchange. Exchange is minimal at this time because the two cell layers of the villous membrane are too thick. Permeability increases as the cytotrophoblast thins and disappears by the fifth month, leaving only the single layer of syncytium between the maternal blood and the fetal capillaries. The syncytium is the functional layer of the placenta. By the eighth week, genetic testing may be done by obtaining a sample of chorionic villi by aspiration biopsy; however, limb defects have been associated with chorionic villus sampling done before 10 weeks (Hsieh et al., 1995). The structure of the placenta is complete by the twelfth week. The placenta continues to grow wider until 20 weeks when it covers about one half of the uterine surface; it then continues to grow thicker. The branching villi continue to develop within the body of the placenta, increasing the functional surface area.

Functions. One of the early functions of the placenta is as an endocrine gland, which produces the four hormones described below that are necessary to maintain the pregnancy and support the embryo/fetus. These hormones are produced in the syncytium.

The protein hormone, **human chorionic gonadotropin** (hCG), can be detected in the maternal serum by 8 to 10 days after conception, shortly after implantation. This hormone is the basis for pregnancy tests. The hCG preserves the function of the ovarian corpus luteum, ensuring a continued supply of estrogen and progesterone needed to maintain the pregnancy. Spontaneous abortion occurs if the corpus luteum stops functioning before the placenta is producing sufficient estrogen and progesterone. The hCG reaches its maximum level at 50 to 70 days and then begins to decrease.

The other protein hormone produced by the placenta is human placental lactogen (hPL). This substance is similar to a growth hormone and stimulates maternal metabolism to supply needed nutrients for fetal growth. This hormone increases the resistance to insulin, facilitates glucose transport across the placental membrane, and stimulates breast development to prepare for lactation.

The placenta eventually produces more of the steroid hormone progesterone than the corpus luteum does during the first few months of pregnancy. Progesterone maintains the endometrium, decreases the contractility of the uterus, and stimulates development of breast alveoli and maternal metabolism.

By 7 weeks after fertilization, the placenta is producing most of the maternal estrogens, or steroid hormones. The major estrogen secreted by the placenta is estriol, while the ovaries produce mostly estradiol. Measuring estriol levels is a clinical assay for placental functioning. Estrogen stimulates uterine growth and uteroplacental blood flow. It causes a proliferation of the breast glandular tissue and stimulates myometrial contractility. Placental estrogen production increases greatly toward the end of pregnancy. One theory for the initiation of the onset of labor is the decrease in circulating levels of progesterone and the increased levels of estrogen.

The metabolic functions of the placenta may be summarized as respiration, nutrition, excretion, and storage. Oxygen diffuses from the maternal blood across the placental membrane into the fetal blood, and carbon dioxide diffuses in the opposite direction. In this way, the placenta functions as lungs for the fetus.

Carbohydrates, proteins, calcium, and iron are stored in the placenta for ready access to meet fetal needs. Water, inorganic salts, carbohydrates, proteins, fats, and vitamins pass from the maternal blood supply across the placental membrane into the fetal blood, supplying nutrition. Water and most electrolytes with a molecular weight less than 500 readily diffuse through the membrane. Hydrostatic and osmotic pressures aid the flow of water and some solutions. Facilitated and active transport assist in the transfer of glucose, amino acids, calcium, iron, and substances with higher molecular weight. Amino acids and calcium are transported against the concentration gradient between the maternal blood and fetal blood.

The fetal concentration of glucose is lower than the glucose level in the maternal blood because of the rapid metabolism of glucose by the fetus. This fetal requirement demands larger concentrations of glucose than simple diffusion can provide. Therefore, maternal glucose moves into the fetal circulation by active transport.

Pinocytosis is a mechanism used for transferring large molecules, such as albumin and gamma globulins, across the placental membrane. This mechanism conveys the maternal immunoglobulins that provide early passive immunity to the fetus.

Metabolic waste products of the fetus cross the placental membrane from the fetal blood into the maternal blood. The maternal kidneys then excrete them. Many viruses can cross the placental membrane and infect the fetus. Some bacteria and protozoa first infect the placenta and then infect the fetus. Drugs can also cross the placental membrane and may harm the fetus. Caffeine, alcohol, nicotine, carbon monoxide and other toxic substances in cigarette smoke, as well as prescription and recreational drugs (e.g., cocaine, marijuana) readily cross the placenta (Box 8-1).

Although no direct link exists between the fetal blood in the vessels of the chorionic villi and the maternal blood in the intervillous spaces, only one cell layer separates them. Breaks in the placental membrane occasionally occur. Fetal erythrocytes can then leak into the maternal circulation, causing the mother to develop antibodies to the fetal red blood cells. This is often how the Rh-negative mother becomes sensitized to the erythrocytes of her Rh-positive fetus. (See discussions of isoimmunization.)

BOX 8-1	*Developmentally Toxic Exposures in Humans*

Aminopterin	Lead
Androgens	Lithium
Angiotensin-converting	Methimazole
enzyme inhibitors	Methyl mercury
Carbamazepine	Parvovirus B19
Cigarette smoking	Penicillamine
Cocaine	Phenytoin
Coumarin anticoagulants	Radioiodine
Cytomegalovirus	Rubella
Diethylstilbestrol	Syphilis
Ethanol (>/=1 drink/day)	Tetracycline
Etretinate	Thalidomide
Hyperthermia	Toxoplasmosis
Iodides	Trimethadione
Ionizing radiation (>10 rads)	Valproic acid
Isotretinoin	Varicella

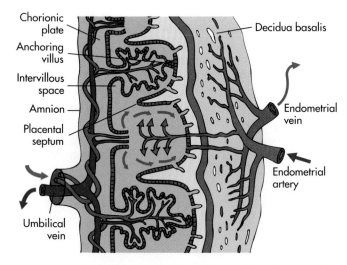

Fig. **8-8** Schematic drawing of the placenta illustrating how the placenta supplies oxygen and nutrition to the embryo and removes its waste products. Deoxygenated blood leaves the fetus in the umbilical arteries and enters the placenta where it is oxygenated. Oxygenated blood leaves the placenta in the umbilical vein, which enters the fetus via the umbilical cord. (From Moore K: *Essentials of human physiology,* Philadelphia, 1988, BC Decker.)

Even though the placenta and fetus are living tissue transplants, they are not destroyed by the host mother (Cunningham et al., 1997). The placental hormones suppress the immunologic response or the tissue evokes no response (Willson & Carrington, 1991).

Placental function depends on the maternal blood pressure supplying circulation. Maternal arterial blood, under pressure in the small uterine spiral arteries, spurts into the intervillous spaces (Fig. 8-8). As long as rich arterial blood continues to be supplied, pressure is exerted on the blood already in the intervillous spaces, pushing it toward drainage by the low-pressure uterine veins. At term gestation, 10% of the maternal cardiac output goes to the uterus.

If there is interference with the circulation to the placenta, the placenta cannot supply the embryo/fetus. Vasoconstriction, such as that caused by hypotension and cocaine use, diminishes uterine blood flow. Decreased maternal blood pressure or cardiac output also diminishes uterine blood flow. When a woman lies on her back with the pressure of the uterus compressing the vena cava (vena caval syndrome), blood return to the right atrium is diminished (see discussion of supine hypertension). Excessive maternal exercise that diverts blood to the muscles away from the uterus also compromises placental circulation. Optimal circulation is achieved when the woman is lying at rest on her side. Decreased uterine circulation may lead to infants who are small for gestational age or intrauterine restriction of the growth of the fetus.

It is believed that *Braxton Hicks contractions* enhance the movement of blood through the intervillous spaces, aiding placental circulation. However, prolonged contractions or too-short intervals between contractions during labor reduce blood flow to the placenta.

Fetal Maturation

The stage of the **fetus,** recognizable as a human being, lasts from 9 weeks until the pregnancy ends. Changes during the fetal period are not as dramatic, since refinement of structure and function are taking place. The fetus is less vulnerable to teratogens except for those affecting central nervous system functioning.

Viability refers to the capability of the fetus to survive outside the uterus. In the past, the earliest age at which fetal survival could be expected was 28 weeks after conception. With modern technology and advancements in maternal and neonatal care, viability is now possible at 20 weeks after conception (22 weeks since LMP; fetal weight of 500 g or more). The limitations on survival outside the uterus are based on central nervous system function and oxygenation capability of the lungs.

Fetal circulatory system

The cardiovascular system is the first organ system to function in the developing human. Blood vessel and blood cell formation begin in the third week to supply the embryo with oxygen and nutrients from the mother. By the end of the third week, the tubular heart begins to beat, and the primitive cardiovascular system links the embryo, connecting stalk, chorion, and yolk sac. During the fourth and fifth weeks, the heart develops into the four-chambered organ. By the end of the embryonic stage, the heart is developmentally complete.

The fetal lungs do not function for respiratory gas exchange, so a special circulatory pathway, the **ductus arteriosus,** exists that bypasses the lungs. Oxygen-rich blood

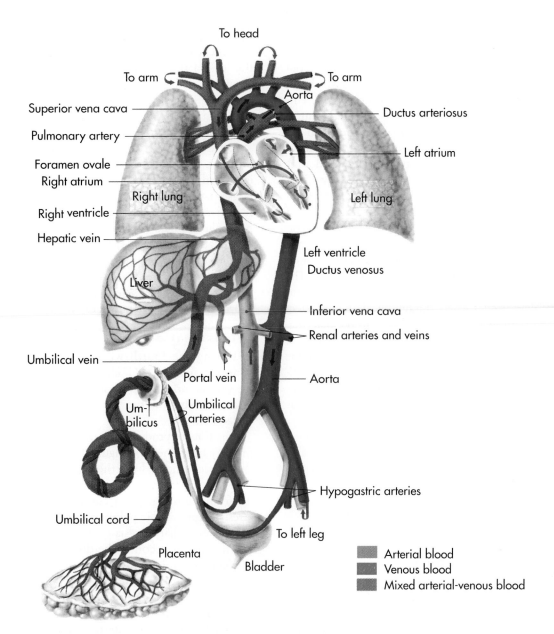

Fig. **8-9** Fetal circulation. *Before birth:* Arterialized blood from the placenta flows into the fetus through the umbilical vein and passes rapidly through the liver into the inferior vena cava; it flows through the foramen ovale into the left atrium, soon to appear in the aorta and arteries of the head. A portion bypasses the liver through the ductus venosus. Venous blood from the lower extremities and head passes predominantly into the right atrium, the right ventricle, and then into the descending pulmonary artery and ductus arteriosus. Thus the foramen ovale and the ductus arteriosus act as bypass channels, allowing a large part of the combined cardiac output to return to the placenta without flowing through the lungs. Approximately 55% of the combined ventricular output flows to the placenta; 35% perfuses body tissues; and the remaining 10% flows through the lungs. *After birth:* The foramen ovale closes, the ductus arteriosus closes and becomes a ligament, the ductus venosus closes and becomes a ligament, and the umbilical vein and arteries close and become ligaments. (Courtesy Ross Laboratories, Columbus, Ohio.)

from the placenta flows rapidly through the umbilical vein into the fetal abdomen (Fig. 8-9). When the umbilical vein reaches the liver, it divides into two branches; one circulates some oxygenated blood through the liver. Most of the blood passes through the ductus venosus into the inferior vena cava. There it mixes with the deoxygenated blood from the fetal legs and abdomen on its way to the right atrium. Most of this blood passes straight through the right atrium and through the **foramen ovale,** an opening into the left atrium. There it mixes with the small amount of blood returning deoxygenated from the fetal lungs through the pulmonary veins.

The blood flows into the left ventricle and is squeezed out into the aorta, where the arteries supplying the heart, head, neck, and arms receive most of the oxygen-rich blood. This pattern of supplying the highest levels of oxygen and nutrients to the head, neck, and arms enhances the **cephalocaudal** (head-to-rump) **development** of the embryo/fetus.

Deoxygenated blood returning from the head and arms enters the right atrium through the superior vena cava. This blood is directed downward into the right ventricle, where it is squeezed into the pulmonary artery. A small amount of blood circulates through the resistant lung tissue, but the majority follows the path with less resistance through the ductus arteriosus into the aorta, distal to the point of exit of the arteries supplying the head and arms with oxygenated blood. The oxygen-poor blood flows through the abdominal aorta into the internal iliac arteries where the umbilical arteries direct most of it back through the umbilical cord to the placenta. There the blood gives up its wastes and carbon dioxide in exchange for nutrients and oxygen. The blood remaining in the iliac arteries flows through the fetal abdomen and legs, ultimately returning through the inferior vena cava to the heart.

The following three special characteristics enable the fetus to obtain sufficient oxygen from the maternal blood:
- Fetal hemoglobin carries 20% to 30% more oxygen than maternal hemoglobin.
- The fetal hemoglobin concentration is about 50% greater than that of the mother.
- The fetal heart rate (FHR) is 120 to 160 beats/minute, making the fetal cardiac output per unit of body weight higher than that of an adult.

Hematopoietic system

Hematopoiesis, the formation of blood, occurs in the yolk sac (see Fig. 8-4, *B*) beginning in the third week. Hematopoietic stem cells seed the fetal liver during the fifth week, and hematopoiesis begins there during the sixth week. This accounts for the relatively large size of the liver between the seventh and ninth weeks. Stem cells seed the fetal bone marrow, spleen and thymus, and lymph nodes between weeks 8 and 11.

The antigenic factors that determine blood type are present in the erythrocytes soon after the sixth week. For this reason, the Rh-negative woman is at risk for isoimmunization in any pregnancy that lasts longer than 6 weeks after fertilization.

Hepatic system

The liver and biliary tract develop from the foregut during the fourth week of gestation. The embryonic liver is prominent and occupies most of the abdominal cavity. Bile, a constituent of meconium, begins to form in the twelfth week.

Glycogen is stored in the fetal liver beginning at week 9 or 10. At term, glycogen stores are twice those of the adult.

Glycogen is the major source of energy for the fetus and neonate who is stressed by in utero hypoxia or by extrauterine loss of the maternal glucose supply, by the work of breathing, or by cold stress.

Iron is stored in the fetal liver. If the maternal intake is sufficient, the fetus can store enough iron to last for up to 5 months after birth.

During fetal life, the liver does not have to conjugate bilirubin for excretion because the unconjugated bilirubin is cleared by the placenta. Therefore the glucuronyl transferase enzyme needed for conjugation that is present in the fetal liver is less than is required after birth. This predisposes the neonate to hyperbilirubinemia.

Coagulation factors II, VII, IX, and X cannot be synthesized in the fetal liver because of the lack of vitamin K synthesis in the sterile fetal gut. This coagulation deficiency persists after birth for several days and is the rationale for the prophylactic administration of vitamin K to the newborn.

Gastrointestinal system

During the fourth week, the embryo changes from almost straight to a "C" shape as both ends fold in toward the ventral surface. A portion of the yolk sac is incorporated into the body from head to tail as the primitive gut (digestive system).

The foregut produces the pharynx, part of the lower respiratory tract, the esophagus, the stomach, the first half of the duodenum, the liver, the pancreas, and the gallbladder. These structures evolve over the fifth and sixth weeks. The malformations that can occur in these areas are esophageal atresia, hypertrophic pyloric stenosis, duodenal stenosis or atresia, and biliary atresia.

The midgut becomes the distal half of the duodenum, the jejunum and ileum, the cecum and appendix, and the proximal half of the colon. The midgut loop projects into the umbilical cord between weeks 5 and 10. A malformation (omphalocele) results if the midgut fails to return to the abdominal cavity, and intestines protrude from the umbilicus. Meckel's diverticulum is the most common malformation of the midgut. It occurs when a remnant of the yolk stalk that has failed to degenerate attaches to the ileum, leaving a blind sac.

The hindgut develops into the distal half of the colon, the rectum and parts of the anal canal, the urinary bladder, and the urethra. Anorectal malformations are the most commonly occurring abnormalities of the digestive system.

The fetus swallows amniotic fluid beginning in the fifth month. Gastric emptying and intestinal peristalsis occur. Fetal nutrition and elimination needs are taken care of by the placenta. As the fetus nears term, fetal waste products accumulate in the intestines as dark green to black, tarry **meconium.** Normally, this substance is passed through the rectum within 48 hours of birth. Sometimes with a breech birth or fetal hypoxia, meconium is passed in utero into the amniotic fluid. The failure to pass meconium after birth can be indicative of atresia somewhere in the digestive tract, an imperforate anus, or a meconium ileus with a firm meconium plug blocking passage. Meconium ileus is seen in infants with cystic fibrosis.

The metabolic rate of the fetus is relatively low, but the infant has great growth and development needs. Beginning in week 9, the fetus synthesizes glycogen for storage in the liver. Between 26 and 30 weeks, the fetus begins to lay down stores of brown fat in preparation for extrauterine cold stress. Thermoregulation in the neonate requires increased metabolism and adequate oxygenation.

The gastrointestinal system is mature by 36 weeks. Digestive enzymes, except pancreatic amylase and lipase, are present in sufficient quantity to facilitate digestion. The neonate cannot digest starches or fats efficiently. Little saliva is produced.

Respiratory system

The respiratory system begins development during embryonic life and continues through fetal life and into childhood until about 8 years of age. The development of the respiratory tract begins during week 4 and continues through week 17 with the formation of the larynx, trachea, bronchi, and lung buds. Between 16 and 24 weeks the bronchi and terminal bronchioles enlarge, and vascular structures and primitive alveoli are formed. Between 24 weeks and term birth, more alveoli form. Specialized alveolar cells, Type I and Type II cells, secrete pulmonary **surfactants** to line the interior of the alveoli. After 32 weeks, sufficient surfactant is present in developed alveoli to provide infants with a good chance of survival. Surfactant production peaks around 35 weeks.

Pulmonary surfactants. The detection of the presence of pulmonary surfactants, surface-active phospholipids, in amniotic fluid has been used to determine the degree of fetal lung maturity, or the ability of the lungs to function after birth. **Lecithin (L)** is the most critical alveolar surfactant required for postnatal lung expansion. It increases in amount after the twenty-fourth week. Another pulmonary phospholipid, **sphingomyelin (S),** remains constant in amount. Thus the measure of lecithin in relation to sphingomyelin, or the **L/S ratio,** is used to determine fetal lung maturity. When the L/S ratio reaches 2:1, the infant's lungs are considered to be mature. This occurs at approximately 35 weeks of gestation (Creasy & Resnik, 1994).

Certain maternal conditions alter the development of the fetal lungs. Those conditions that accelerate lung maturity generally cause decreased maternal placental blood flow. The resulting fetal hypoxia apparently stresses the fetus, increasing blood levels of corticosteroids that accelerate alveolar and surfactant development. Conditions such as maternal hypertension, placental dysfunction, infection, or corticosteroid use accelerate fetal lung maturity. Conditions such as gestational diabetes and chronic glomerulonephritis can retard fetal lung maturity. The use of intrabronchial

synthetic surfactant in the treatment of respiratory distress syndrome in the newborn has greatly improved the chances of survival of preterm infants.

Fetal respiratory movements have been seen on ultrasound as early as the eleventh week. These fetal respiratory movements are believed to aid in development of the chest wall muscles and regulate lung fluid volume. The fetal lungs produce fluid that expands the air spaces in the lungs. The fluid drains into the amniotic fluid or is swallowed by the fetus.

Before birth, secretion of lung fluid decreases. The normal birth process squeezes out approximately one third of the fluid. Infants of cesarean births do not benefit from this squeezing process; thus they may have more respiratory difficulty at birth. The fluid remaining in the lungs at birth is usually reabsorbed into the infant's bloodstream within 2 hours of birth.

Renal system

The permanent kidneys form during the fifth week and begin to function approximately 4 weeks later. Urine formation is present during the third month. Urine is excreted into the amniotic fluid and forms a major part of the amniotic fluid volume. Oligohydramnios, an abnormally small amount of amniotic fluid, is indicative of renal dysfunction. Because the placenta acts as the organ of excretion and maintains fetal water and electrolyte balance, the fetus does not need functioning kidneys while in utero. At birth, however, the kidneys are required immediately for excretory and acid-base regulatory functions.

A fetal renal malformation can be diagnosed in utero. Corrective or palliative fetal surgery may treat the malformation successfully, or plans can be made for treatment immediately after birth (Adzick & Harrison, 1994; Collins, 1995; Howell, 1994).

At term, the fetus has fully developed kidneys. However, the glomerular filtration rate (GFR) is low, and the kidneys lack the ability to concentrate urine. This makes the newborn more susceptible to both overhydration and dehydration and acid-base imbalances.

Most newborns void within 24 hours of birth. With the loss of the swallowed amniotic fluid and the metabolism of nutrients provided by the placenta, voidings for the first days of life are scanty until fluid intake increases.

Neurologic system

The nervous system originates from the ectoderm (the neural plate) during the third week after fertilization. The open neural tube forms during the fourth week. It initially closes at what will be the junction of the brain and spinal cord, leaving both ends open. The embryo folds in on itself lengthwise at this time, forming a head fold in the neural tube at this junction. The cranial end of the neural tube closes, then the caudal end closes. During week 5, different growth rates cause more flexures in the neural tube, delineating three brain areas: the forebrain, midbrain, and hindbrain. Both the forebrain and hindbrain partially divide into two vesicles.

The forebrain develops into the eyes (cranial nerve II) and cerebral hemispheres. The development of all areas of the cerebral cortex continues throughout fetal life and into childhood. The olfactory system (cranial nerve I) and thalamus also develop from the forebrain. Cranial nerves III and IV (oculomotor and trochlear) form from the midbrain. The hindbrain forms the medulla, pons, cerebellum, and the remainder of the cranial nerves. Brain waves can be recorded on an electroencephalogram by week 8.

The spinal cord develops from the long end of the neural tube. Another ectodermal structure, the neural crest, develops into the peripheral nervous system. By the eighth week, nerve fibers traverse throughout the body. By week 11 or 12, the fetus makes respiratory movements, moves all extremities, and changes position in utero. The fetus can suck his or her thumb and swim in the amniotic fluid pool, turn somersaults, and sometimes tie a knot in the umbilical cord. Box 8-2 describes the major types of fetal movements. Sometime between 16 and 20 weeks, when the movements are strong enough to be perceived by the mother as "the baby moving," **quickening** has occurred. The perception of movement occurs earlier in multiparas than in primiparas. The mother also becomes aware of the sleep and wake cycles of the fetus.

Sensory awareness. Purposeful movements of the fetus have been demonstrated in response to a firm touch transmitted through the mother's abdomen. Invasive procedures to be done on a fetus require anesthesia.

Fetuses respond to sound by 24 weeks. Different types of music evoke different movements. The fetus can be soothed by the sound of the mother's voice. Acoustic stimulation can be used to evoke an FHR response (Bar-Hava & Barnhardt, 1994). The fetus becomes accustomed to noises heard repeatedly. Hearing is fully developed at birth.

The fetus is able to distinguish taste. By the fifth month, when the fetus is swallowing amniotic fluid, a sweetener added to the fluid causes the fetus to swallow twice as fast (Poole, 1986). The fetus also reacts to temperature changes. A cold solution placed into the amniotic fluid can cause fetal hiccups.

The fetus reacts to light. Eyes have both rods and cones in the retina by the seventh month. A bright light shone on the mother's abdomen in late pregnancy causes abrupt fetal movements. During sleep time, rapid eye movements (REMs) have been observed similar to those occurring in children and adults while dreaming (Cole, 1997).

At term, the fetal brain is approximately one fourth the size of an adult brain. Neurologic development continues. Stressors on the fetus and neonate, such as chronic poor nutrition or hypoxia, drugs, environmental toxins, trauma, or disease, cause damage to the central nervous system long after the vulnerable embryonic time for malformations in other organ systems. Neurologic insult can result in cerebral palsy, neuromuscular impairment, mental retardation, and learning disabilities.

BOX 8-2	*Major types of fetal movements*

General movements: These slow, gross movements involve the whole body. Their duration is from several seconds to a minute.

Startle movements: These quick (less than 1 second), generalized movements always start in the limbs and may spread to the trunk and neck.

Hiccups: These are repetitive phasic contractions of the diaphragm. A bout may last several minutes.

Fetal breathing movements: These are paradoxic movements in which the thorax moves inward and the abdomen outward with each contraction of the diaphragm.

Isolated arm or leg movements: These movements of extremities occur without movement of the trunk.

Hand-face contact: This occurs any time the moving hand makes contact with the face or mouth.

Retroflexion of the head: This is a slow to jerky backward bending of the head.

Lateral rotation of the head: This involves isolated turning of the head from side to side.

Anteflexion of the head: This is a normally slow, forward bending of the head.

Opening of mouth: This isolated movement may be accompanied by protrusion of the tongue.

Yawn: Mouth is slowly opened and rapidly closed after a few seconds.

Sucking: This burst of rhythmic jaw movements is sometimes followed by swallowing. With this movement, the fetus may be drinking amniotic fluid.

Stretch: This complex movement involves overextension of the spine, retroflexion of the head, and elevation of the arms.

From Carlson B: *Human embryology and developmental biology,* St Louis, 1994, Mosby.

Endocrine system

The thyroid gland develops with structures in the head and neck during the third and fourth weeks. The secretion of thyroxine begins during the eighth week. Maternal thyroxine does not readily cross the placenta; therefore, the fetus who does not produce thyroid hormones will be born with congenital hypothyroidism. If untreated, hypothyroidism can result in severe mental retardation. Screening for hypothyroidism is typically included in the testing when screening for phenylketonuria (PKU) after birth.

The adrenal cortex is formed during the sixth week and produces hormones by the eighth or ninth week. As term approaches, the fetus produces more cortisol. This is believed to aid in initiation of labor by decreasing the maternal progesterone and stimulating production of prostaglandins.

The pancreas forms from the foregut during the fifth through eighth weeks. The islets of Langerhans develop during the twelfth week. Insulin is produced by the twentieth week. In infants of mothers with uncontrolled diabetes, maternal hyperglycemia produces fetal hyperglycemia, stimulating hyperinsulinemia and islet-cell hyperplasia. This results in macrosomia (large-sized fetus). The hyperinsulinemia also blocks lung maturation, placing the neonate at risk for respiratory distress and hypoglycemia when the maternal glucose source is lost at delivery. Control of the maternal glucose level before and during pregnancy minimizes problems for the infant.

Reproductive system

Until the seventh week, no sex differentiation exists in the embryo. Distinguishing characteristics appear approximately the ninth week and are fully differentiated by the twelfth week. When a Y chromosome is present, testes are formed. By the end of the embryonic period, testosterone is being secreted and causes formation of the male genitalia. By week 28, the testes begin descending into the scrotum. After birth, low levels of testosterone continue to be secreted until the pubertal surge.

The female, with two X chromosomes, forms ovaries and female external genitalia. Female and male external genitalia are indistinguishable until after the ninth week. By the sixteenth week, oogenesis has been established. At birth, the ovaries contain the female's lifetime supply of ova. Most female hormone production is delayed until puberty. However, the fetal endometrium responds to maternal hormones, and withdrawal bleeding or vaginal discharge (pseudomenstruation) may occur at birth when these hormones are lost. The high level of maternal estrogen also stimulates mammary engorgement and secretion of fluid ("witch's milk") in newborn infants of both sexes.

Immunologic system

During the third trimester, albumin and globulin are present in the fetus. The only immunoglobulin that crosses the placenta is IgG, providing passive acquired immunity to specific bacterial toxins. The fetus produces IgM immunoglobulins by the end of the first trimester. These are produced in response to blood group antigens, gram-negative enteric organisms, and some viruses. IgA immunoglobulins are not produced by the fetus. However, colostrum, the precursor to breast milk, contains large amounts of IgA and can provide passive immunity to the neonate.

The normal term neonate can fight infection, but not as effectively as an older child. The preterm infant is at much greater risk for infection.

Musculoskeletal system

Bones and muscles develop from the mesoderm by the fourth week of embryonic development. At that time, the cardiac muscle is already beating. The mesoderm next to the neural tube forms the vertebral column and ribs. The parts of the vertebral column grow toward each other to enclose the developing spinal cord. Ossification, or bone formation, begins. If there is a defect in the bony fusion, various forms of spina bifida may occur. A large defect affecting several vertebrae may allow the membranes and spinal cord to pouch out from the back, producing neurologic deficits and skeletal deformity.

The flat bones of the skull develop during the embryonic period, and ossification continues throughout childhood. At birth, connective tissue sutures exist where the bones of the skull meet. The areas where more than two bones meet, called *fontanels,* are especially prominent. The sutures and fontanel allow the bones of the skull to mold, or move during birth, enabling the head to pass through the birth canal.

The bones of the shoulders, arms, hips, and legs appear in the sixth week as a continuous skeleton with no joints. Differentiation occurs, producing separate bones and joints. Ossification will continue through childhood to allow growth. Beginning during the seventh week, muscles contract spontaneously. Arm and leg movements are visible on ultrasound, although the mother does not perceive them until the sixteenth to the twentieth week.

Integumentary system

The epidermis begins as a single layer of cells derived from the ectoderm at 4 weeks. By the seventh week, there are two layers of cells. The cells of the superficial layer are sloughed and become mixed with the sebaceous gland secretions to form the white, cheesy vernix caseosa. This material protects the skin of the fetus. The vernix is thick at 24 weeks but continually decreases until term.

The basal layer of the epidermis is the germinal layer, which replaces the lost cells. Until 17 weeks the skin is very thin and wrinkled, with blood vessels visible underneath. The skin thickens, and all layers are present by term. After 32 weeks, as subcutaneous fat is deposited under the dermis, the skin becomes less wrinkled, translucent, and red in appearance.

By 16 weeks, the epidermal ridges are present on the palms of the hands, the fingers, the bottom of the feet, and the toes. This makes the hand and footprints unique to that infant.

Hairs form from hair bulbs in the epidermis, which project into the dermis. Cells in the hair bulb keratinize to form the hair shaft. As the cells at the base of the hair shaft proliferate, the hair grows to the surface of the epithelium. The very fine hairs, called *lanugo,* appear first at 12 weeks on the eyebrows and upper lip. By 20 weeks, they cover the entire body. At this time, the eyelashes, eyebrows, and scalp hair are beginning to grow. By 28 weeks, the scalp hair is longer than the lanugo, which is thinning and may disappear by term gestation.

Fingernails and toenails develop from thickened epidermis at the tips of the digits beginning during the tenth week. They grow slowly. Fingernails usually reach the fingertips by 32 weeks, and toenails reach toetips by 36 weeks. Table 8-1 summarizes embryonic and fetal development.

TABLE 8-1 *Milestones in Human Development before Birth since Last Menstrual Period (LMP)*

4 WEEKS	8 WEEKS	12 WEEKS
EXTERNAL APPEARANCE		
Body flexed, C shaped; arm and leg buds present; head at right angles to body	Body fairly well formed; nose flat, eyes far apart; digits well formed; head elevating; tail almost disappeared; eyes, ears, nose, and mouth recognizable	Nails appearing; resembles a human; head erect but disproportionately large; skin pink, delicate
CROWN-TO-RUMP MEASUREMENT; WEIGHT		
0.4 to 0.5 cm; 0.4 g	2.5 to 3 cm; 2 g	6 to 9 cm; 9 g
GASTROINTESTINAL SYSTEM		
Stomach at midline and fusiform; conspicuous liver; esophagus short; intestine a short tube	Intestinal villi developing; small intestines coil within umbilical cord; palatal folds present; liver very large	Bile secreted; palatal fusion complete; intestines have withdrawn from cord and assume characteristic positions
MUSCULOSKELETAL SYSTEM		
All somites present	First indication of ossification—occiput, mandible, and humerus; fetus capable of some movement; definitive muscles of trunk, limbs, and head well represented	Some bones well outlined, ossification spreading; upper cervical to lower sacral arches and bodies ossify; smooth muscle layers indicated in hollow viscera
CIRCULATORY SYSTEM		
Heart develops, double chambers visible, begins to beat; aortic arch and major veins completed	Main blood vessels assume final plan; enucleated red cells predominate in blood	Blood forming in marrow
RESPIRATORY SYSTEM		
Primary lung buds appear	Pleural and pericardial cavities forming; branching bronchioles; nostrils closed by epithelial plugs	Lungs acquire definite shape; vocal cords appear
RENAL SYSTEM		
Rudimentary ureteral buds appear	Earliest secretory tubules differentiating; bladder-urethra separates from rectum	Kidney able to secrete urine; bladder expands as a sac
NERVOUS SYSTEM		
Well-marked midbrain flexure; no hind-brain or cervical flexures; neural groove closed	Cerebral cortex begins to acquire typical cells; differentiation of cerebral cortex, meninges, ventricular foramina, cerebrospinal fluid circulation; spinal cord extends entire length of spine	Brain structural configuration almost complete; cord shows cervical and lumbar enlargements; fourth ventricle foramina (pl) developed; sucking present
SENSORY ORGANS		
Eye and ear appearing as optic vessel and otocyst	Primordial choroid plexuses develop; ventricles large relative to cortex; development progressing; eyes converging rapidly; internal ear developing	Earliest taste buds indicated; characteristic organization of eye attained
GENITAL SYSTEM		
Genital ridge appears (fifth week)	Testes and ovaries distinguishable; external genitalia sexless but begin to differentiate	Sex recognizable; internal and external sex organs specific

TABLE 8-1 *Milestones in Human Development before Birth—cont'd*

16 WEEKS	20 WEEKS	24 WEEKS
EXTERNAL APPEARANCE		
Head still dominant; face looks human; eyes, ears, and nose approach typical appearance on gross examination; arm/leg ratio proportionate; scalp hair appears	Vernix caseosa appears; lanugo appears; legs lengthen considerably; sebaceous glands appear	Body lean but well proportioned; skin red and wrinkled; vernix caseosa present; sweat glands forming
CROWN-TO-RUMP MEASUREMENT; WEIGHT		
11.5 to 13.5 cm; 100g	16 to 18.5 cm; 300 g	23 cm; 600g
GASTROINTESTINAL SYSTEM		
Meconium in bowel; some enzyme secretion; anus open	Enamel and dentine depositing; ascending colon recognizable	
MUSCULOSKELETAL SYSTEM		
Most bones distinctly indicated throughout body; joint cavities appear; muscular movements can be detected	Sternum ossifies; fetal movements strong enough for mother to feel	
CIRCULATORY SYSTEM		
Heart muscle well developed; blood formation active in spleen		Blood formation increases in bone marrow and decreases in liver
RESPIRATORY SYSTEM		
Elastic fibers appear in lungs; terminal and respiratory bronchioles appear	Nostrils reopen; primitive respiratory-like movement begins	Alveolar ducts and sacs present; lecithin begins to appear in amniotic fluid (weeks 26 to 27)
RENAL SYSTEM		
Kidney in position; attains typical shape and plan		
NERVOUS SYSTEM		
Cerebral lobes delineated; cerebellum assumes some prominence	Brain grossly formed; cord myelination begins; spinal cord ends at level of first sacral vertebra (S-1)	Cerebral cortex layered typically; neuronal proliferation in cerebral cortex ends
SENSORY ORGANS		
General sense organs differentiated	Nose and ears ossify	Can hear
GENITAL SYSTEM		
Testes in position for descent into scrotum; vagina open		Testes at inguinal ring in descent to scrotum

Continued

| TABLE 8-1 | *Milestones in Human Development before Birth—cont'd* |

28 WEEKS	30 TO 31 WEEKS	36 AND 40 WEEKS
EXTERNAL APPEARANCE		
Lean body, less wrinkled and red; nails appear	Subcutaneous fat beginning to collect; more rounded appearance; skin pink and smooth; has assumed birth position	*36 weeks* Skin pink, body rounded; general lanugo disappearing; body usually plump *40 weeks* Skin smooth and pink; scant vernix caseosa; moderate to profuse hair; lanugo on shoulders and upper body only; nasal and alar cartilage apparent

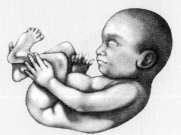

28 WEEKS	30 TO 31 WEEKS	36 AND 40 WEEKS
CROWN-TO-RUMP MEASUREMENT; WEIGHT		
27 cm; 1,110g	31 cm; 1,800 to 2,100 g	*36 weeks* 35 cm; 2,200 to 2,900 g *40 weeks* 40 cm; 3,200+ g
MUSCULOSKELETAL SYSTEM		
Astragalus (talus, ankle bone) ossifies; weak, fleeting movements, minimum tone	Middle fourth phalanxes ossify; permanent teeth primordia seen; can turn head to side	*36 weeks* Distal femoral ossification centers present; sustained, definite movements; fair tone; can turn and elevate head *40 weeks* Active, sustained movement; good tone, may lift head
RESPIRATORY SYSTEM		
Lecithin forming on alveolar surfaces	L/S ratio = 1.2:1	*36 weeks* L/S ratio > 2:1 *40 weeks* Pulmonary branching only two thirds complete
RENAL SYSTEM		
		36 weeks Formation of new nephrons ceases
NERVOUS SYSTEM		
Appearance of cerebral fissures, convolutions rapidly appearing; indefinite sleep-wake cycle; cry weak or absent; weak suck reflex		*36 weeks* End of spinal cord at level of third lumbar vertebra (L-3); definite sleep-wake cycle *40 weeks* Myelination of brain begins; patterned sleep-wake cycle with alert periods; cries when hungry or uncomfortable; strong suck reflex
SENSORY ORGANS		
Eyelids reopen; retinal layers completed, light receptive; pupils capable of reacting to light	Sense of taste present; aware of sounds outside mother's body	
GENITAL SYSTEM		
	Testes descending to scrotum	*40 weeks* Testes in scrotum; labia major well developed

From Wong D & Perry S: *Maternal child nursing care,* St Louis, 1998, Mosby.

Multifetal Pregnancy

Twins

When two mature ova are produced in one ovarian cycle, both have the potential to be fertilized by separate sperm. This results in two zygotes or **dizygotic twins** (Fig. 8-10). There are always two amnions, two chorions, and two placentas that may be fused together. These dizygotic or fraternal twins may be the same sex or different sexes and are genetically no more alike than siblings born at different times. Dizygotic twinning occurs in families, more often among African-American women than Caucasian women, and least often among Asian women. Twinning increases in frequency with maternal age up to 35 years, with parity, and with the use of fertility drugs.

Identical twins (**monozygotic twins**) develop from one fertilized ovum, which then divides (Fig. 8-11). They are the same sex and have the same genotype. If division occurs soon after fertilization, two embryos, two amnions, two chorions, and two placentas that may be fused will develop. Most often, division occurs between 4 and 8 days after fertilization, and there are two embryos, two amnions, one chorion, and one placenta. In this case there are two embryos within a common amnion and a common chorion with one placenta. This often causes problems in circulation

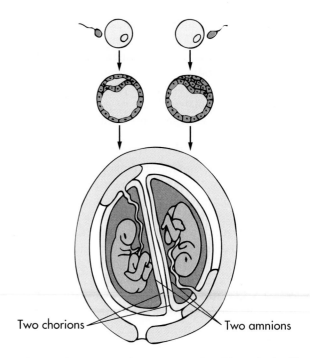

Fig. **8-10** Formation of dizygotic twins. There is fertilization of two ova, two implantations, two placentas, two chorions, and two amnions.

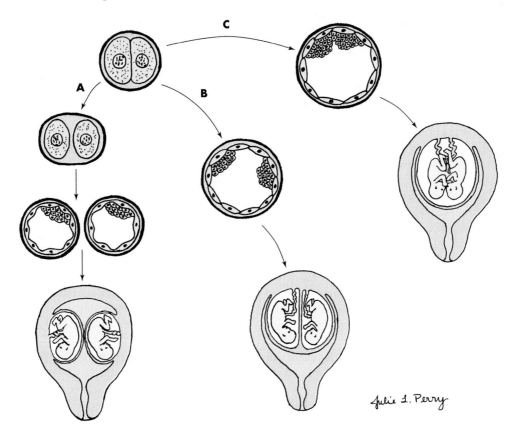

Fig. **8-11** Formation of monozygotic twins. **A,** One fertilization: blastomeres separate, resulting in two implantations, two placentas, and two sets of membranes. **B,** One blastomere with two inner cell masses, one fused placenta, one chorion, and separate amnions. **C,** One blastomere with incomplete separation of cell mass resulting in conjoined twins. (From Wong D & Perry S: *Maternal child nursing care,* St Louis, 1998, Mosby.)

because the umbilical cords may tangle together, and one or both fetuses may die. If division occurs very late, cleavage may not be complete, and conjoined twins could result. Monozygotic twinning occurs in approximately 1 of 250 births (Cunningham et al., 1997). There is no association with race, heredity, maternal age, or parity. Fertility drugs increase the incidence of multiple births.

Other multifetal pregnancies

The occurrence of multifetal pregnancies with three or more fetuses has increased with the use of fertility drugs and in vitro fertilization. Triplets occur once in about 7,600 pregnancies. They can occur from the division of one zygote into two, with one of the two dividing again, producing identical triplets. Triplets can also be produced from two zygotes, one dividing into a set of identical twins and the second zygote a single fraternal sibling, or from three zygotes. Quadruplets, quintuplets, sextuplets, and so on, likewise, have similar possible derivations.

Nongenetic Factors Influencing Development

Not all congenital disorders are inherited. *Congenital* means that the condition was present at birth. Some congenital malformations may be the result of teratogens, defined as environmental substances or exposures that result in functional or structural disability. In contrast to other forms of developmental disabilities, disabilities caused by teratogens are theoretically totally preventable (Hoyme, 1990). Known human teratogens are drugs and chemicals, infections, exposure to radiation (Scialli, 1997), and certain maternal conditions such as diabetes and PKU (see Box 8-1). A teratogen has the greatest effect on the organs and parts of an embryo during its periods of rapid growth and differentiation. This occurs during the embryonic period, specifically from days 15 to 60. During the first 2 weeks of development, teratogens either have no effect or effects so severe that they cause spontaneous abortion. Brain growth and development continue during the fetal period, and teratogens can severely affect mental development throughout gestation (see Fig. 8-5).

Besides the genetic makeup and the influence of teratogens, the adequacy of maternal nutrition also influences development. The embryo and fetus must obtain the nutrients they need from the mother's diet; they cannot tap the maternal reserves. Malnutrition during pregnancy produces low-birth-weight (LBW) newborns who are susceptible to infection. Malnutrition also affects brain development during the latter half of gestation and may result in learning disabilities in the child.

The field of behavioral genetics is engaged in discovering links between genetics and environment in explaining normal and deviant behavior (Sherman et al., 1997). This represents a movement away from the belief that human behavior is almost completely the result of influences of the environment. For example, memory and intelligence, activity level, sociability, and shyness have some degree of genetic influence (Sherman et al., 1997).

I GENETICS AND GENETIC COUNSELING

Importance of Genetics in Maternity Care

Genetic causes of disease have assumed increasing importance as the incidence of communicable diseases has decreased. Rapid expansion in the identification, understanding, and diagnosis of genetic disease has been accompanied by effective medical or surgical therapies in a small number of disorders. For most genetic conditions, therapeutic or preventive measures are nonexistent or disappointingly limited. Consequently, the most useful means of reducing the incidence of these disorders is by preventing their transmission. With the accumulation of knowledge about genetic disorders, the probability of recurrence in any given situation can be predicted with increased accuracy. At present the best means for reducing the number of children born with genetic defects is for health professionals to provide families with genetic information and services.

For all pregnancies, it is standard practice to assess for heritable disorders to identify potential problems (Creasy & Resnik, 1994). The interviewer inquires about the health status of family members, abnormal reproductive outcomes, history of maternal disorders (e.g., diabetes, PKU, cystic fibrosis), drug exposures, and illness. Advanced maternal and paternal ages are noted. Ethnic origin should be recorded, since some disorders appear more often in some groups (Creasy & Resnik, 1994). Examples include Tay-Sachs disease in Jewish individuals of Ashkenazic or Sephardic descent, (β-thalassemia in Italians and Greeks, sickle cell anemia in African-Americans, (α-thalassemia in Southeast Asians and Filipinos, and tyrosinemia in French Canadians from the Lac St. Jean-Chicoutimi region of Quebec.

Genetic Transmission

Human development is a complicated process that depends on the systematic unraveling of instructions found in the genetic material of the egg and sperm. Development from conception to birth of a normal, healthy baby occurs without incident in most cases; occasionally, however, some anomaly in the genetic code of the embryo creates a birth defect or disorder. The science of genetics seeks to explain the underlying causes of congenital disorders (disorders present at birth) and the patterns in which inherited disorders are passed from generation to generation.

Genes and chromosomes

The hereditary material carried in the nucleus of each of the somatic (body) cells determines an individual's physical characteristics. This material, called deoxyribonucleic acid (DNA), forms threadlike strands known as **chromosomes.**

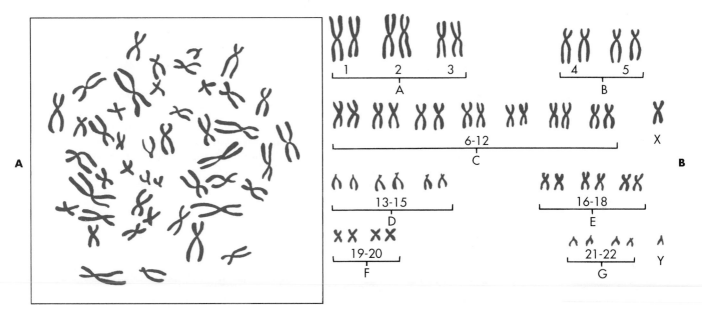

Fig. 8-12 Chromosomes during cell division. **A,** Example of photomicrograph. **B,** Chromosomes arranged in karyotype; female and male sex-determining chromosomes.

Each chromosome is composed of many smaller segments of DNA referred to as **genes.** Genes, or combinations of genes, contain coded information that determines an individual's unique characteristics. The "code" is found in the specific linear order of the molecules that combine to form the strands of DNA.

All normal human somatic cells contain 46 chromosomes arranged as 23 pairs of homologous (matched) chromosomes; one chromosome of each pair is inherited from each parent. There are 22 pairs of autosomes, which control most traits in the body, and one pair of **sex chromosomes,** which primarily control sex determination. The large female chromosome is called the X; the tiny male chromosome is the Y. Generally, the presence of a Y chromosome causes an embryo to develop as a male; in the absence of a Y chromosome, the individual develops as a female. Thus in a normal female the homologous pair of sex chromosomes would be XX, and in a normal male the homologous pair would be XY.

Each person has two genes for every trait, because each gene occupies a specific chromosome location, and because chromosomes are inherited as homologous pairs. In other words, if an autosome has a gene for hair color, its partner will also have a gene for hair color, and they will be in the same location on the chromosome. Although both genes code for hair color, they may not code for the *same* hair color. Different genes coding for different variations of the same trait are called alleles. An individual having two copies of the same allele for a given trait is said to be homozygous for that trait; with two different alleles, the person is heterozygous for the trait.

Some genes are dominant, and their characteristics are expressed even if another allele is present on the other chromosome. Other genes are recessive, and their characteristics will be expressed only if they are carried by both homologous chromosomes. When an egg and a sperm unite, the combination of alleles becomes that individual's entire genetic makeup, or genotype, which includes all the genes that the person carries and that can be passed to offspring. The genotype determines an individual's physical appearance, or phenotype, but this determination is affected by the nature of the dominant or recessive allele.

The pictorial analysis of the number, form, and size of an individual's chromosomes is known as a **karyotype.** A karyotype can be obtained from a blood sample that has been specially treated and stained to make the replicating chromosomes visible under a microscope. The photographed chromosomes are cut out and arranged in a specific numeric order according to their length and shape. Figure 8-12 illustrates the chromosomes in a body cell. Karyotypes can be used to determine what sex the child will be, and whether any gross chromosomal abnormalities are present.

Heritable characteristics are those that can be passed on to offspring. The patterns by which genetic material is transmitted to the next generation are affected by the number of genes involved in the expression of the trait. Many phenotypic characteristics result from two or more genes on different chromosomes acting together (referred to as multifactorial inheritance); others are controlled by a single gene (unifactorial inheritance). Defects at the gene level cannot be determined by conventional laboratory

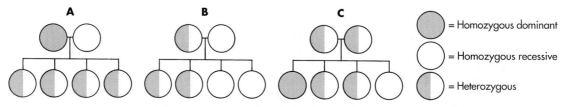

Fig. **8-13** Possible offspring in three types of matings. **A,** Homozygous-dominant parent and homozygous-recessive parent. Children all heterozygous, displaying dominant trait. **B,** Heterozygous parent and homozygous-recessive parent. Children 50% heterozygous displaying dominant trait; 50% homozygous displaying recessive trait. **C,** Both parents heterozygous. Children 25% homozygous displaying dominant trait; 25% homozygous displaying recessive trait; 50% heterozygous displaying dominant trait.

methods such as karyotyping. Instead, genetic counselors predict the probability of the presence of an abnormal gene from the known occurrence of the trait in the individual's family and the known patterns by which the trait is inherited.

Most common congenital malformations result from multifactorial inheritance: a combination of genetic and environmental factors. Examples are cleft lip, cleft palate, congenital heart disease, neural tube defects, and pyloric stenosis. Each malformation may range from mild to severe, depending on the number of genes for the defect present or the amount of environmental influence. Some malformations occur more often in one sex or the other. Multifactorial disorders also tend to occur in families.

Other patterns of inheritance include autosomal dominant and autosomal recessive inheritance. Autosomal dominant inheritance disorders are those in which the abnormal gene for the trait is expressed even when the other member of the pair is normal. The abnormal gene may appear as a result of a **mutation,** a spontaneous and permanent change in the normal gene structure, in which case the disorder occurs for the first time in the family. Usually, an affected individual comes from multiple generations having the disorder. Examples are Marfan's syndrome, achondroplasia, polydactyly, and polycystic kidney disease. Autosomal recessive inheritance disorders are those in which both genes of a pair must be abnormal for the disorder to be expressed. Heterozygous individuals have only one abnormal gene and are unaffected clinically because their normal gene overshadows the abnormal gene. They are known as carriers of the recessive trait. In order for the trait to be expressed, two carriers must each contribute the abnormal gene to the offspring (Fig. 8-13, *C*). There is a 25% chance of the trait occurring in each child. A clinically normal offspring may be a carrier of the gene. Males and females are equally affected. Most inborn errors of metabolism, such as PKU, galactosemia, maple syrup urine disease, Tay Sachs disease, sickle cell anemia, and cystic fibrosis, are autosomal-recessive inherited disorders.

X-linked inheritance

X-linked dominant inheritance disorders occur in both males and heterozygous females. Because the females also have a normal gene, the effects are less severe than in affected males. Affected males transmit the abnormal gene only to their daughters on the X chromosome. Heterozygous females have a 50% chance of transmitting the abnormal gene to each offspring. Vitamin D–resistant rickets and fragile-X syndrome are X-linked dominant disorders. In X-linked recessive inheritance, females may be heterozygous or homozygous for traits carried on the X chromosome because they have two X chromosomes. Males are hemizygous because they have only one X chromosome carrying genes with no alleles on the Y chromosome. Therefore X-linked recessive disorders are most commonly manifested in the male with the abnormal gene on his single X chromosome. Hemophilia, color blindness, and Duchenne's muscular dystrophy are all X-linked recessive disorders.

The Human Genome Project (Box 8-3), funded by the National Institutes of Health, is involved in mapping and sequencing the genetic make-up of humans (Mahowald, 1997). This map will facilitate study of hereditary diseases and will provide the potential for making changes at the gene level to treat or prevent hereditary diseases (Fig. 8-14).

Genetic Counseling

It is expected that by the year 2005, the entire human **genome** (the copy of the genetic material in humans) will be mapped and that all of the 70,000 to 100,000 genes will be identified (Jones, 1996). There are more than 5,000 single-gene disorders that are known (Jones, 1996). This explosion in knowledge has implications for nurses working with mothers and infants, especially those who are involved in genetic counseling.

Purposes of genetic counseling

The purposes of genetic counseling are to (1) advise couples before conception of the probability of conception of

The Human Genome Project

J JENKINS, RN, MSN, AND F COLLINS, MD, PHD

The Human Genome Project is a federally funded, coordinated effort to assemble data on the genetic instructions found within human DNA and within DNA of several model organisms (Collins, 1995; Guyer & Collins, 1995). The ultimate goal of the project is the complete sequencing of all 3 billion base pairs of human DNA. This includes the development of genetic and physical maps that facilitate the identification of human disease genes by positional cloning. This strategy allows the identification of human disease genes without prior information about their biologic function. The focus of genetics specialists has previously been on rare genetic disorders; however, virtually every disease (except trauma) has a genetic component. Medical genetics is now poised to uncover these genetic predispositions, opening the possibility of highly sophisticated diagnostic and therapeutic strategies. Genes that contribute to common polygenic conditions such as diabetes, hypertension, most forms of cancer, and the major mental illnesses will be identified by this approach. These gene discoveries will lead to molecular insights that will revolutionize the treatment of disease, using gene therapy or "designer drug" strategies. For many diseases, however, health care professionals will be able to predict risks but will not be able to intervene with effective treatment for some time (Scanlon & Fibison, 1995). This creates a dilemma for all health care providers. As genetic testing becomes available for risk prediction for diseases such as cancer or Alzheimer's disease, many questions will arise. How reliable is the test? What do these results mean in terms of the actual risk of developing the disease? How useful is this information? What preventive or treatment recommendations will be available based on test results? Laboratories providing genetic testing need to be monitored for quality control of genetic test results: criteria must be established to define when a test should be done only in a research setting. DNA testing, like the administration of a drug, has potential side effects and risks that need to be studied in clinical trials and managed appropriately (Andrews et al., 1994).

Until now, most physicians and nurses have not had the opportunity to incorporate genetics into their practice. An imminent challenge is to prepare providers to be able to include components of genetic risk assessment in all health care delivery, including screening, counseling, education, surveillance, and treatment and to use this information wisely. Because of widespread concerns about misuse of information gained through genetic testing, 5% of the Human Genome Project budget is designated for research into the Ethical, Legal, and Social Implications (ELSI) Program of the project (U.S. Department of Health and Human Services, 1995). Issues of high priority for ELSI have included genetic privacy, the safety and efficacy of genetic testing, informed consent , and the potential for genetic discrimination in health insurance and employment. A recent ruling of the Equal Employment Opportunities Commission (EEOC) renders employment discrimination on the basis of future genetic susceptibility illegal, based on the provisions of the Americans with Disabilities Act. Legislation is urgently needed to address discrimination in health insurance (Hudson et al., 1995).

All health care specialties will be required to distill this evolving body of knowledge and use the genetics information to facilitate consumer decision making. Nurses, with their long tradition of combining clinical skills and attention to the whole person, are in a critical position to lead the way.

---

an infant with a genetic disorder; (2) advise couples after conception and fetal screening of whether or not the fetus has a genetic disorder; and (3) inform the couple of the options that are available to them, including choosing not to become pregnant (Chadwick, 1993).

Genetic counseling services

The most efficient counseling services are associated with the larger universities and major medical centers where support services are available (e.g., biochemistry and cytology laboratories) and consist of a group of specialists under the leadership of a physician trained in medical genetics. Many of these regional centers maintain satellite clinics or services in outlying areas to provide contact with both consumers and health professionals. A number of specialized groups provide clinics and services for people with a specific genetic disorder such as cystic fibrosis, muscular dystrophy, hemophilia, or diabetes. Health professionals should become familiar with people who provide genetic counseling and places in which counseling services are available to patients in their area of practice (Inati, Lazar & Haskin-Leahy, 1994) (Box 8-4).

Management of Genetic Disorders

At this time, there are no cures for genetic disorders, although remedies can be implemented to prevent or reduce the harmful effects of a few disorders. Structural defects can sometimes be modified to produce normal or near-normal function. Research is being conducted to devise methods to influence or change the genes directly by placing substitute DNA in the cells of those with a genetic mutation, thereby preventing or curing the disease process or relieving symptoms (Crombleholme & Bianchi, 1994). Successful treatment of adenosine deaminase deficiency and cystic fibrosis has been reported (Pickler & Munro, 1995). The major thrust in therapy is modification of the internal or external environment to minimize the effects of the disorder.

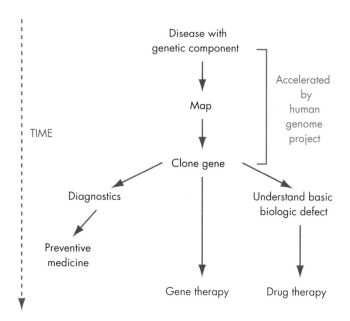

Fig. **8-14** Progress in molecular medicine. The Human Genome Project has accelerated the time required to clone a disease gene. Gene discovery often results in improved diagnostic capabilities. The timeline to develop effective drug or gene therapies is less predictable. (From Collins F: Positional cloning moves from perditional to traditional, *Nature Genetics* 9:347, April 1995.)

BOX 8-4 *Ethical Considerations*

APPLICATION OF GENETIC TECHNOLOGY
Researchers have proposed using fetal neurologic, liver, and pancreatic tissues to treat adults with Parkinson's disease, metabolic disorders, or head and spinal cord injury. The use of fetal tissue in research was banned for several years, but the ban was lifted in 1993. In part, opposition to use of fetal tissue in research was due to the belief of some that women would be encouraged or coerced to become pregnant and abort fetuses to provide material for use in this research. Elective abortion continues to be a controversial issue with compelling arguments both for and against such abortions.

BOX 8-5 *Fetal Malformations Treatable by Open Fetal Surgery*

Posterior urethral valves
CCAM (congenital cystic adenomatoid malformation of the lung)
CDH (congenital diaphragmatic hernia)
Twin-twin transfusion syndrome
Sacrococcygeal teratoma
Complete heart block

From Crombleholme T: Invasive fetal sugery: current status and future directions, *Semin Perinatol* 18(4):385, 1994.

Surgical therapy is employed for congenital heart defects and cosmetic defects such as cleft lip. Advances in fetal surgery are occurring (Box 8-5). Other conditions are treated with product replacement (thyroid for hereditary cretinism), diet modification (low phenylalanine diet for PKU), and corrective devices for missing limbs.

People with some disorders, such as glucose-6-phosphate dehydrogenase (G6PD) deficiency or the porphyrias, can prevent the disease simply by avoiding the specific chemical agent that precipitates the symptoms. Avoiding circumstances that reduce tissue oxygenation can reduce the sickling of red blood cells in sickle cell anemia.

Researchers continue to develop therapies for heritable diseases. Some possible methods of future management include replacement or stabilization by oral or parenteral medications or other methods, altering intracellular DNA, and other projected feats of genetic engineering. Rapid progress is evident in the field of genetic engineering (Dickler & Collier, 1994). Molecular techniques provide infinite possibilities for altering human genes through gene splicing. Thus, it will be possible to use altered genes in ova and sperm for in vitro fertilization.

Estimation of risk

The risks of recurrence of a genetic disorder are determined by the mode of inheritance. The risk of recurrence for disorders caused by a factor that segregates during cell division (genes and chromosomes) can be estimated with a high degree of accuracy by application of the mendelian principles. In a dominant disorder the risk is 50%, or one in two, that a subsequent offspring will be affected; an autosomal-recessive disease carries a one-in-four risk of recurrence; and an X-linked disorder is related to the sex of the child. Translocation chromosomes have a high risk of recurrence.

Disorders in which a subsequent pregnancy would carry no more risk than there would be for pregnancy (estimated at 1 in 30) include those resulting from isolated incidences not likely to be present in another pregnancy. These disorders include maternal infections (e.g., rubella or toxoplasmosis), maternal ingestion of drugs, most chromosomal abnormalities, and a disorder determined to be the result of a fresh mutation.

The risk of recurrence for multifactorial conditions can be estimated empirically. An empiric risk is not based on genetic theory, but rather on experience and observation of the disorder in other families. Recurrence risks are determined by applying the frequency of a similar disorder in other families to the case under consideration.

Interpretation of risk

Counselors explain the risk estimates to patients without making recommendations or decisions and avoid allowing their own biases to interfere. The counselor provides appropriate information about the nature of the disorder, the extent of the risks in the specific case, the probable consequences, and (if appropriate) alternative options available, but the final decision to become pregnant or to continue a pregnancy must be left to the family. An important nursing role is reinforcing the information the families are given, continuing to interpret this information on their level of understanding, and remaining nonjudgmental of the family decision.

The most important concept that must be emphasized to families is that *each pregnancy is an independent event.* For example, in monogenic disorders in which the risk factor is one in four that the child will be affected, the risk remains the same no matter how many affected children are already in the family. Families may maintain the erroneous assumption that the presence of one affected child ensures that the next three will be free of the disorder. However, "chance has no memory." The risk is one in four for each pregnancy. On the other hand, in a family with a child who has a disorder with multifactorial causes, the risk increases with each subsequent child born with the disorder.

Role of Nurse in Genetic Counseling

All nurses, especially those involved in the care of mothers and children, need to (1) have an understanding of genetic theory and the nature of more common genetic disorders to recognize cues that may indicate a genetically related problem, (2) be able to help families obtain counseling services, (3) augment the counseling process (Stringer, Librizzi & Weiner, 1991), and (4) be aware of the legal and ethical issues involved (Penticuff, 1996). Although diagnosis and treatment of genetic disorders require medical skills and determination of risk factors for many disorders requires the expertise of a geneticist, nurses with advanced preparation in genetics and counseling are assuming an increasingly important role in counseling people about genetically transmitted or genetically influenced conditions. Key competencies suggested for genetics nurses are that they must be able to (1) understand and communicate information on the basis of genetic disease, the patterns of inheritance, and testing options; (2) obtain an accurate family history and understand the implications of the medical history; (3) provide an environment for counseling so that patients can explore safely the condition's implications and the family's choices; and (4) be aware of their own capabilities and the need to seek guidance and refer appropriately as necessary (Skirton et al., 1997). See Box 8-6 for information on genetic resources.

Follow-up care

Maintaining contact with the family after genetic counseling, testing, or therapy is one of the most important nursing responsibilities because the success of counseling is measured by the way the family uses the information presented to them. Most counseling services try to schedule at least one postdiagnostic or postcounseling visit to assess how well the family is beginning to incorporate this

---

> **BOX 8-6** **Resources on Genetics**
>
> **THE NATIONAL SOCIETY OF GENETIC COUNSELORS**
> http://members.aol.com/nsgcweb/nsgchome.htm
>
> **THE INTERNATIONAL SOCIETY OF NURSES IN GENETICS (ISONG)**
> *http://nursing.creighton. edu/* (Click on PROFESSIONAL ORGANIZATION and then ISONG.)
>
> **THE NATIONAL CENTER FOR HUMAN GENOME RESEARCH**
> *http://www.nchgr.nih.gov*

---

new information into their lives and value systems. Follow-up visits to the counseling service or visits to the home provide additional opportunities to reexplore all aspects of the situation and to answer any questions that may have occurred to the family since the previous contacts. Clarifying information is an important nursing function.

Referral to appropriate agencies is an essential part of the follow-up management. Many organizations and foundations, such as the Cystic Fibrosis Foundation and the Muscular Dystrophy Association, provide services and equipment for affected children. Early Infant Stimulation Foundation programs are available for children born with Down syndrome. There are also numerous parent groups with which the family can share experiences and derive mutual support from other families with similar problems. Nurses should become familiar with services available in their community that provide assistance and education to families with these special problems. (See Appendix D.)

Emotional support

Probably the most important of all nursing functions is providing emotional support to the family during all aspects of the counseling process. Feelings that are generated under the real or imagined threat posed by a genetic disorder are as varied as the people being counseled. Responses may include a variety of stress reactions, such as apathy, denial, anger, hostility, fear, embarrassment, grief, and loss of self-esteem. Guilt and self-blame are universal reactions. Many look on the disorder as a stigma, especially if the disorder is visible to others. Old wives' tales, superstitions, and long-held misconceptions are all factors that may influence a family's reaction to a genetic disorder.

The attitude of other family members and relatives can have a significant impact on some people, especially in situations where the cause can be identified (such as a dominant or an X-linked disorder). Recessive disorders are less likely to cause blaming, since both partners carry the defective gene. A genetic disorder may cause a family to alter plans for marriage or childbearing even when the probability of recurrence is no more than a random risk.

Factors such as religious beliefs, intellectual level, and prior attitudes toward the disorder affect the way in which families respond to counseling information. Sometimes counselors and other health personnel create barriers through their own attitudes toward a specific disorder. It is often difficult to be nonjudgmental and objective, and nurses may intentionally or unintentionally influence families in making decisions. Families may pressure the nurse to make decisions for them with questions such as, "What would you do if you were me?" Families and individuals need education, guidance, and support throughout the counseling process. They should be given the facts and possible consequences and all of the assistance they need in problem solving, but the final decision regarding a course of action must be their own.

Ethical Dimensions of Genetic Screening

Although genetic screening has the potential for great benefits, there is also a potential for harm. Genetic information may be used to discriminate against individuals in insurance decisions or employment. Conflicts about who will receive scarce genetic service resources may occur and some individuals may experience social stigmatization. Others may experience emotional distress when diagnosed with lethal, untreatable diseases or when the genetic information forces choices that are agonizing (Penticuff, 1996).

There is concern that prenatal screening and diagnosis will challenge our values about the kind of infants that will be born as parents with an affected fetus make the choice to continue or terminate the pregnancy (Penticuff, 1996). Some fear social pressures to make decisions contrary to personal beliefs. Newborn screening presents other dilemmas. The Institute of Medicine Committee on Assessing Genetic Risks "has recommended that newborn screening not be done when early detection will not alter the course of the disease, effective treatment is not available, or there is no effective treatment and testing is being done only to give information to guide their future reproductive plans" (Penticuff, 1996). Detecting carrier status can be used by parents in reproductive planning but it has the potential to result in bias or discrimination. Public demand for genetic testing is expected to increase. Principles of choice and confidentiality must be adhered to by health professionals involved (Penticuff, 1996).

RESEARCH

Pregnancy Interruption for Fetal Anomalies

Recent advances in ultrasound and genetic testing have made it possible to detect fetal anomalies early in gestation. However, in some instances no therapy is available for the problem identified, and couples must make a decision to terminate a planned or unwanted pregnancy. Because many anomalies are not identified until the second trimester, this is when many pregnancy terminations must be performed. A qualitative pilot study was conducted using phenomenologic methods to systematically explore the processes operating within the experience of women undergoing second-trimester pregnancy interruption for fetal anomalies. The study was conducted during a 2-month period with a convenience sampling of three women 4 to 6 weeks after undergoing pregnancy interruptions for fetal anomalies in the second trimester. The researcher described the experience of women undergoing second-trimester pregnancy interruption as "one day you're pregnant, and one day you're not." This summarizes the changes involved in the transition from being pregnant with hopes for the infant and the future to a woman dealing with a loss. The transition was described in two intertwined processes entitled "The Hardest Thing We Ever Did" and "Saying Hello and Goodbye."

CLINICAL APPLICATION OF THE STUDY

When caring for women who must decide whether to interrupt pregnancy for fetal anomalies, nurses should provide as much information as possible, as soon as possible, about the abnormal findings. They should also assist with the decision-making process by encouraging exploration of feelings surrounding religion, pregnancy interruption, and effects of the decision on the family, and assess and identify potential sources of emotional support. Nurses should provide resources specifically associated with second-trimester pregnancy interruption and assist the patient with the making of memories to affirm the existence and importance of the pregnancy.

Source: Bryar S: One day you're pregnant and one day you're not: pregnancy interruption for fetal anomalies, *J Obstet Gynecol Neonatal Nurs* 26(5):599, 1997.

KEY POINTS

- Human gestation is approximately 280 days after the last menstrual period or 266 days after conception.
- Fertilization occurs in the uterine tube within 24 hours of ovulation. The zygote undergoes mitotic divisions, creating a 16-cell morula.
- Implantation begins 6 days after fertilization.
- The organ systems and external features develop during the embryonic period, that is, the third to the eighth week after fertilization.
- Refinement of structure and function occur during the fetal period, and the fetus becomes capable of extrauterine survival.
- There are critical periods in human development during which the embryo-fetus is vulnerable to environmental teratogens.
- The best means for reducing the number of children born with genetic defects is to provide families with genetic information and services.
- Advances in genetics have ethical dimensions.

CRITICAL THINKING EXERCISES

1 *Monica Andrade confides in you that there have been several infants born into her family with serious anomalies. From previous conversations, you know that she is opposed to abortion and would never consider having one. Monica is currently 6 weeks pregnant, and her physician has urged her to have chorionic villus sampling (CVS). Monica asks you for information about CVS and the implications of a finding that her fetus has serious anomalies. Describe your response keeping in mind genetics, the social and moral implications of genetic testing, and Monica's ethical and moral beliefs. What other information do you need? To whom could you refer her? What options does she have?*

2 *Select five household chemicals used in your home. Identify the purpose of the chemicals, and describe the reasons why they are hazardous to the reproductive health of women, men, and a developing embryo-fetus. List alternatives that can be substituted to accomplish the same purpose as the chemicals.*

References

Adzick N & Harrison M: Fetal surgical therapy, *Lancet* 343(8902):897, 1994.

Andrews L et al., editors: *Assessing genetic risks: implications for health and social policy,* Washington, DC, 1994, National Academy Press (Institute of Medicine).

Bar-Hava I & Barnhardt Y: Fetal vibracoustic stimulation, *Female Patient* 19(5):63, 1994.

Carlson B: *Human embryology and developmental biology,* St Louis, 1994, Mosby.

Chadwick R: What counts as success in genetic counselling? *J Med Ethics* 19:43, 1993.

Cole J: What can babies see at birth? *Mother Baby J* 2(4):45, 1997.

Collins F: Positional cloning moves from perditional to traditional, *Nature Genetics* 9:347, April 1995.

Collins J: Fetal surgery: changing the outcome before birth, *J Obstet Gynecol Neonatal Nurs* 23(2):166, 1994.

Creasy R & Resnik J, editors: *Maternal-fetal medicine: principles and practice,* ed 3, Philadelphia, 1994, WB Saunders.

Crombleholme T: Invasive fetal surgery: current status and future directions, *Semin Perinatol* 18(4):385, 1994.

Crombleholme T & Bianchi D: In utero hematopoietic stem cell transplantation and gene therapy, *Semin Perinatol* 18(4):376, 1994.

Cunningham F et al.: *Williams obstetrics,* ed 20, Stamford, Conn, 1997, Appleton & Lange.

Dickler H & Collier E: Gene therapy in the treatment of disease, *J Allergy Clin Immunol* 96:942, 1994.

Fine B: Genetic counseling and women, *Women's Health Issues* 7(4):220, 1997.

Guyer M & Collins F: How is the human genome project doing, and what have we learned so far? *Proc Natl Acad Sci* USA 92(10):841, 1995.

Hallak M et al.: Amniotic fluid index: gestational age-specific values for normal human pregnancy, *J Reprod Med* 38:853, 1993.

Howell L: The unborn surgical patient: a nursing frontier, *Nurs Clin North Am* 29(4):681, 1994.

Hoyme H: Teratogenically induced fetal anomalies, *Clin Perinatol* 17(3):547, 1990.

Hsieh F et al.: Limb defects after chorionic villus sampling, *Obstet Gynecol* 85(1):84, 1995.

Hudson K et al.: Genetic discrimination and health insurance: an urgent need for reform, *Science* 270:391, 1995.

Inati M, Lazar E & Haskin-Leahy L: The role of the genetic counselor in a perinatal unit, *Semin Perinatol* 18:133, 1994.

Jones S: Genetics: changing health care in the 21st century, *J Obstet Gynecol Neonatal Nurs* 25(6):777, 1996.

Langley L et al.: *Dynamic human anatomy and physiology,* ed 5, New York, 1980, McGraw-Hill.

Mahowald M: An overview of the Human Genome Project and its implications for women, *Women's Health Issues* 7(4):206, 1997.

Monsen R: Nursing takes leading role in genetics education, *Am Nurse* 28(8):11, 1996.

Moore K: *Essentials of human physiology,* Philadelphia, 1988, BC Decker.

Moore K: *Before we are born: basic embryology and birth defects,* ed 3, Philadelphia, 1989, WB Saunders.

Penticuff J: Ethical dimensions in genetic screening: a look into the future, *J Obstet Gynecol Neonatal Nurs* 25(6):785, 1996.

Pickler R & Munro C: Gene therapy for inherited disorders, *J Pediatr Nurs* 10(8):40, 1995.

Poole R, editor: *The incredible machine,* Washington, DC, 1986, National Geographic Society.

Scanlon C & Fibison W: *Managing genetic information: implications for nursing practice,* Washington, DC, 1995, American Nurses Association.

Scialli A: Toxicology, *Contemp OB GYN* 42(5):15, 1997.

Sherman S et al.: Behavioral genetics '97: ASHG Statement. Recent developments in human behavioral genetics: past accomplishments and future directions, *Am J Hum Genet* 60(6):1265, 1997.

Skirton H et al.: The role and practice of the genetic nurse: report of the AGNC working party, *J Med Genet* 34(2):141, 1997.

Stringer M, Librizzi R & Weiner S: Establishing a prenatal genetic diagnosis: the nurse's role *MCN Am J Matern Child Nurs* 16(3):152, 1991.

US Department of Health and Human Services: *The human genome project progress report fiscal years 1993-1994,* Washington, DC, 1995, National Institutes of Health.

Willson J & Carrington E: *Obstetrics and gynecology,* ed 9, St Louis, 1991, Mosby.

Wong D & Perry S: *Maternal child nursing care,* St Louis, 1998, Mosby.

CHAPTER

Anatomy and Physiology of Pregnancy

DEITRA LEONARD LOWDERMILK

LEARNING OBJECTIVES

- *Define the key terms.*
- *Describe gravidity and parity using the five- and four-digit systems.*
- *Describe the various types of pregnancy tests.*
- *Explain the expected maternal anatomic and physiologic adaptations to pregnancy.*
- *Differentiate among presumptive, probable, and positive signs of pregnancy.*
- *Identify the maternal hormones produced during pregnancy, their target organs, and their major effects on pregnancy.*
- *Compare the characteristics of the abdomen, vulva, and cervix of the nullipara and multipara.*

KEY TERMS

amenorrhea
ballottement
Braxton Hicks sign
Chadwick's sign
chloasma
colostrum
diastasis recti abdominis
epulis
friability
funic souffle
Goodell's sign
gravida
gravidity
Hegar's sign
human chorionic gonadotropin (hCG)
leukorrhea
lightening
linea nigra
mean arterial pressure (MAP)
Montgomery's tubercles
multigravida
multipara
nulligravida
nullipara
operculum
palmar erythema
parity
physiologic anemia

KEY TERMS—cont'd

postdate birth
preterm
primigravida
primipara
ptyalism
pyrosis
quickening
signs and symptoms of pregnancy
  presumptive
  probable
  positive
striae gravidarum
term
uterine souffle
viability

The goal of maternity care is a healthy pregnancy with a physically safe and emotionally satisfying outcome for mother, infant, and family. Consistent health supervision and surveillance are of utmost importance in achieving this outcome. However, many maternal adaptations are unfamiliar to pregnant women and their families. Helping the pregnant woman recognize the relationship between her physical status and the plan for her care assists her in making decisions and encourages her to participate in her own care.

❙ GRAVIDITY AND PARITY

An understanding of the following terms used to describe pregnancy and the pregnant woman is essential to the study of maternity care:

- **Gravida** A woman who is pregnant.
- **Gravidity** Pregnancy.
- **Multigravida** A woman who has had two or more pregnancies.
- **Multipara** A woman who has completed two or more pregnancies to the stage of fetal viability.
- **Nulligravida** A woman who has never been pregnant.
- **Nullipara** A woman who has not completed a pregnancy with a fetus or fetuses who have reached the stage of fetal viability.

185

TABLE 9-1	*Gravidity and Parity Using Five-Digit (GTPAL) System*				
CONDITION	GRAVIDITY PREGNANCIES	TERM BIRTH	PRETERM BIRTH	ABORTIONS	LIVING CHILDREN
Sarah is pregnant for the first time.	1	0	0	0	0
She carries the pregnancy to term, and the neonate survives.	1	1	0	0	1
She is pregnant again.	2	1	0	0	1
Her second pregnancy ends in abortion.	2	1	0	1	1
During her third pregnancy, she gives birth to preterm twins.	3	1	1	1	3

From Lowdermilk D, Perry S & Bobak I: *Maternity and women's health care*, ed 6, St Louis, 1997, Mosby.

- **Parity**   The number of pregnancies in which the fetus or fetuses have reached viability, not the number of fetuses (e.g., twins) born. Whether the fetus is born alive or is stillborn (fetus who shows no signs of life at birth) after viability is reached does not affect parity.
- **Postterm birth**   Birth of an infant after 42 weeks of gestation.
- **Preterm**   Term used to describe an infant who is born after 20 weeks of gestation but before completion of 37 weeks of gestation.
- **Primigravida**   A woman who is pregnant for the first time.
- **Primipara**   A woman who has completed one pregnancy with a fetus or fetuses who have reached the stage of fetal viability.
- **Term**   Used to describe an infant who is born between the beginning of the thirty-eighth week of gestation and the end of the forty-second week of gestation.
- **Viability**   Capacity to live outside the uterus; approximately 22 to 24 weeks since last menstrual period, or greater than 500 g.

Gravidity and parity information is obtained during history taking interviews and may be recorded in patient records in several ways. One abbreviation commonly used in maternity centers consists of five digits separated by hyphens. The first digit represents the total number of pregnancies, including the present one (*gravidity*); the second digit represents the total number of *full-term* births; the third indicates the number of *preterm* births; the fourth identifies the number of *abortions* (spontaneous or elective termination of pregnancy before viability); and the fifth is the number of children currently *living*. The acronym "GTPAL" may be helpful in remembering this system of notation. For example, if a woman pregnant only once with twins gives birth at the thirty-fifth week and the babies survive, the abbreviation that represents this information is "1-0-1-0-2."

BOX 9-1	*Using TPAL to Define Parity*

T—term birth(s)
P—preterm birth(s)
A—abortions(s)
L—living children

During her next pregnancy the abbreviation is "2-0-1-0-2." Additional examples are given in Table 9-1.

Others prefer a four-digit system. The first digit of the five-digit system, which signifies gravidity, is dropped. The acronym "TPAL" is helpful in remembering what the four digits stand for (Box 9-1).

PREGNANCY TESTS

Early detection of pregnancy allows for early initiation of care. **Human chorionic gonadotropin (hCG)** is the biologic marker on which pregnancy tests are based. Production of hCG begins as early as the day of implantation and can be detected in the blood as early as 6 days after conception or approximately 20 days since the last menstrual period (LMP), and in urine approximately 26 days after conception (Cunningham et al., 1997). The level of hCG rises until it peaks at approximately 60 to 70 days of gestation and then begins to decline. The lowest level is reached between 100 to 130 days of gestation and remains constant until birth (Varney, 1997).

Serum and urine pregnancy tests are performed in clinics, offices, women's health centers, and laboratory settings. Serum tests are more sensitive and can provide earlier and more accurate results than urine tests. Approximately 7 to 10 ml of venous blood is collected for serum testing. Most urine tests require a first-voided morning urine specimen because it contains levels of hCG approximately the same as those in serum. Random urine samples usually have lower levels (Edge & Miller, 1994).

Many different pregnancy tests are available, but they all depend on recognition of hCG or a beta subunit of hCG. The wide variety of tests precludes discussion of each; however, several categories of tests are described here. More complete information can be found in the manufacturer's directions for each test.

Immunoassay tests use the principle of agglutination inhibition and depend on an antigen-antibody reaction between hCG and an antiserum. Usually the antiserum is mixed with urine, and hCG-coated particles (e.g., latex or blood cells) are added. If hCG is present in the urine, agglutination does not occur because the hCG neutralizes the hCG antibody, and the test is considered positive (Cunningham et al., 1997). Latex agglutination inhibition (LAI) tests are easy to do, and results are available in 2 minutes. A positive test is indicated by a clear, milky solution on a slide or in a test tube. LAI tests are accurate from 4 to 10 days after a missed period. Hemagglutination inhibition (HAI) tests are accurate from 4 days after a missed period but require 1 to 2 hours to obtain results (Barkauskas et al., 1994). A positive test is indicated by a ring (blood cells) at the bottom of the test tube.

Radioreceptorassay (RRA) tests are 1-hour serum tests that use radioiodine-labeled hCG and measure the ability of the blood sample to inhibit the bonding of radio-labeled hCG to cell membrane. These tests are usually accurate at the time of missed menses (14 days after conception) (Pagana & Pagana, 1996).

Radioimmunoassay (RIA) pregnancy tests for the beta subunit of hCG use radioactively labeled markers and are usually performed in a laboratory. The test time ranges from 1 to 5 hours. Radioimmunoassays are the most sensitive pregnancy tests available today (Pagana & Pagana, 1996) and can confirm pregnancy 1 week after conception (Varney, 1997).

Enzyme-linked immunosorbent assay (ELISA) testing is the most popular method of testing for pregnancy (Scott et al., 1994). It uses a specific monoclonal antibody (anti-hCG) with enzymes to bond with hCG in urine. The test can detect levels of hCG as low as 25 mIU/ml. As an office or home procedure it requires minimal time and offers results in 5 minutes. A positive test is indicated by a simple color-change reaction.

ELISA technology is the basis for most over-the-counter home pregnancy tests. With these one-step tests, the woman usually applies urine to a strip and reads the results. The test kits come with directions for collection of the specimen, the testing procedure, and reading of the results. Most manufacturers of the kits provide a toll-free telephone number to call if users have concerns and questions about test procedures or results (see Teaching Guidelines box).

Interpreting the results of pregnancy tests requires some judgment. The type of pregnancy test and its degree of sensitivity (ability to detect low levels of a substance) and specificity (ability to detect the absence of a substance) have to be considered in conjunction with the woman's history.

TEACHING GUIDELINES

Home Pregnancy Testing

Follow the manufacturer's instructions carefully. Do not omit steps.

Review the manufacturer's list of food, medications and other substances that can affect the test results.

Use a first-voided morning urine specimen.

If the test done at the time of your missed period is negative, repeat the test in 1 week if you still have not had a period.

If you have questions about the test, contact the manufacturer.

Contact your health care provider for follow-up if the test is positive or if the test is negative and you still have not had a period.

This includes the date of her last normal menstrual period (LNMP), her usual cycle length, and results of previous pregnancy tests. It is important to know if the woman is a substance abuser and what medications she is taking because drugs such as anticonvulsants and tranquilizers can give false results. Improper collection of the specimen, hormone-producing tumors, and laboratory errors also may cause false results (Pagana & Pagana, 1996). Whenever the results are questionable, retesting may be appropriate.

ADAPTATIONS TO PREGNANCY

Maternal physiologic adaptations are attributed to the hormones of pregnancy and to mechanical pressures arising from the enlarging uterus and other tissues. These adaptations protect the woman's normal physiologic functioning, meet the metabolic demands pregnancy imposes on her body, and provide a nurturing environment for fetal development and growth. Although pregnancy is a normal phenomenon, problems can occur. The nurse needs a foundation in normal maternal physiology to accomplish the following:

- Identify potential or actual deviation from normal adaptation to initiate care.
- Help the woman understand the anatomic and physiologic changes during pregnancy.
- Allay the woman's (and family's) anxiety, possibly resulting from a lack of knowledge.
- Teach the woman (and family) signs and symptoms that should be reported to the health care provider.

Signs of Pregnancy

Some of the physiologic adaptations are recognized as signs and symptoms of pregnancy. Three categories of **signs and symptoms of pregnancy** that are commonly used are **presumptive**, those changes felt by the woman (e.g., amenorrhea, fatigue, nausea and vomiting, breast changes); **probable,**

TABLE 9-2 *Signs of Pregnancy*

TIME OF OCCURRENCE (GESTATIONAL AGE)	SIGN	OTHER POSSIBLE CAUSE
PRESUMPTIVE SIGNS		
3-4 weeks	Breast changes	Premenstrual changes, oral contraceptives
4 weeks	Amenorrhea	Stress, vigorous exercise, early menopause, endocrine problems, malnutrition
4-14 weeks	Nausea, vomiting	Gastrointestinal virus, food poisoning
6-12 weeks	Urinary frequency	Infection, pelvic tumors
12 weeks	Fatigue	Stress, illness
16-20 weeks	Quickening	Gas, peristalsis
PROBABLE SIGNS		
5 weeks	Goodell's sign	Pelvic congestion
6-8 weeks	Chadwick's sign	Pelvic congestion
6-12 weeks	Hegar's sign	Pelvic congestion
4-12 weeks	Positive pregnancy test (serum)	Hydatidiform mole, choriocarcinoma
6-12 weeks	Positive result to pregnancy test (urine)	False-positive results may be caused by pelvic infection, tumors
16 weeks	Braxton Hicks contractions	Myomas, other tumors
16-28 weeks	Ballottement	Tumors, cervical polyps
POSITIVE SIGNS		
5-6 weeks	Visualization of fetus by real-time ultrasound examination	No other causes
16 weeks	Visualization of fetus by x-ray study	
6 weeks	Fetal heart tones detected by ultrasound examination	
8-17 weeks	Fetal heart tones detected by Doppler ultrasound stethoscope	
17-19 weeks	Fetal heart tones detected by fetal stethoscope	
19-22 weeks	Fetal movements palpated	
Late pregnancy	Fetal movements visible	

From Lowdermilk D, Perry S & Bobak I: *Maternity and women's health care,* ed 6, St Louis, 1997, Mosby.

those changes observed by an examiner (e.g., Hegar's sign, ballottement, pregnancy tests); and **positive,** those signs that are attributed only to the presence of the fetus (e.g., hearing fetal heart tones, visualization of the fetus, and palpating fetal movements). Table 9-2 summarizes these signs of pregnancy in relation to when they might occur and other causes for their occurrence.

REPRODUCTIVE SYSTEM AND BREASTS

Uterus

Changes in size, shape, and position

The phenomenal uterine growth in the first trimester is stimulated by high levels of estrogen and progesterone. Early uterine enlargement results from increased vascularity and dilatation of blood vessels, hyperplasia (production of new muscle fibers and fibroelastic tissue) and hypertrophy (enlargement of preexisting muscle fibers and fibroelastic

tissue), and development of the decidua. By 7 weeks' gestation the uterus is the size of a large hen's egg; by 10 weeks, the size of an orange (twice its nonpregnant size); by 12 weeks, the size of a grapefruit. After the third month uterine enlargement is primarily the result of mechanical pressure of the growing fetus (Varney, 1997). In the nonpregnant woman, the uterine cavity holds approximately 10 ml of fluid; during pregnancy, its capacity increases to 5 L or more (Cunningham et al., 1997). Table 9-3 compares uterine measurements for the nonpregnant and pregnant uterus at 40 weeks' gestation.

As the uterus enlarges, it also changes in shape and position. At conception the uterus is shaped like an upside-down pear. During the second trimester, as the muscular walls strengthen and become more elastic, the uterus becomes spherical or globular. Later, as the fetus lengthens, the uterus becomes larger and more ovoid and rises out of the pelvis into the abdominal cavity.

The pregnancy may "show" after the fourteenth week, although this depends to some degree on the woman's

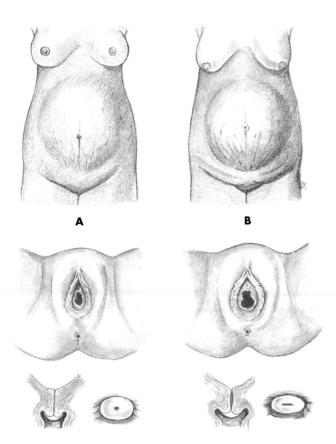

Fig. **9-1** Comparison of abdomen, vulva, and cervix in **A**, nullipara, and **B**, multipara at the same stage of pregnancy.

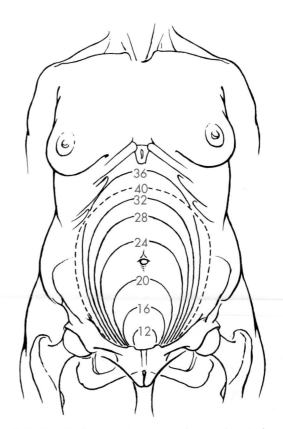

Fig. **9-2** Height of fundus by weeks of normal gestation with a single fetus. *Dashed line* indicates heights after lightening. (From Barkauskas V et al.: *Health and physical assessment*, St Louis, 1994, Mosby.)

TABLE 9-3	Comparison of Measurements for Nonpregnant and Pregnant Uterus at 40 Weeks*	
MEASUREMENT	**NONPREGNANT**	**PREGNANT (40 WEEKS)**
Length	6.5 cm	32 cm
Width	4 cm	24 cm
Depth	2.5 cm	22 cm
Weight	60-70 g	1,100-1,200 g
Volume	≥10 ml	5,000 ml

Data from Lowdermilk D, Perry S & Bobak I: *Maternity and women's health care*, ed 6, St Louis, 1997, Mosby.
*Note that references vary as to the exact values, but all references agree on the magnitude of the growth of the uterus during pregnancy.

height and weight. Abdominal enlargement may be less apparent in the nullipara with good abdominal muscle tone (Fig. 9-1). Posture also influences the type and degree of abdominal enlargement that occurs. In normal pregnancies the uterus enlarges at a predictable rate. Uterine enlargement is determined by measuring fundal height. This measurement is commonly used to estimate the duration of

pregnancy. However, variation in the position of the fundus or the fetus, variations in the amount of amniotic fluid present, the presence of more than one fetus, maternal obesity, and variation in examiner techniques can reduce the accuracy of this estimation of the duration of pregnancy.

As the uterus grows and fills the pelvic cavity, it is elevated out of the pelvic area and may be palpated above the symphysis pubis some time between the twelfth and fourteenth weeks of pregnancy (Fig. 9-2). The uterus rises gradually to the level of the umbilicus at 22 to 24 weeks and nearly reaches the xiphoid process at term. Between weeks 38 and 40, fundal height drops as the fetus begins to descend and engage in the pelvis (**lightening**) (see dashed lines in Fig. 9-2). Generally, lightening occurs in the nullipara approximately 2 weeks before the onset of labor and at the start of labor in the multipara.

Generally the uterus rotates to the right as it elevates, probably because of the presence of the rectosigmoid colon on the left side. However, the extensive hypertrophy (enlargement) of the round ligaments keeps the uterus in the midline. Eventually the growing uterus touches the anterior abdominal wall and displaces the intestines to either side of the abdomen (Fig. 9-3). Whenever a pregnant woman is standing, most of her uterus rests against

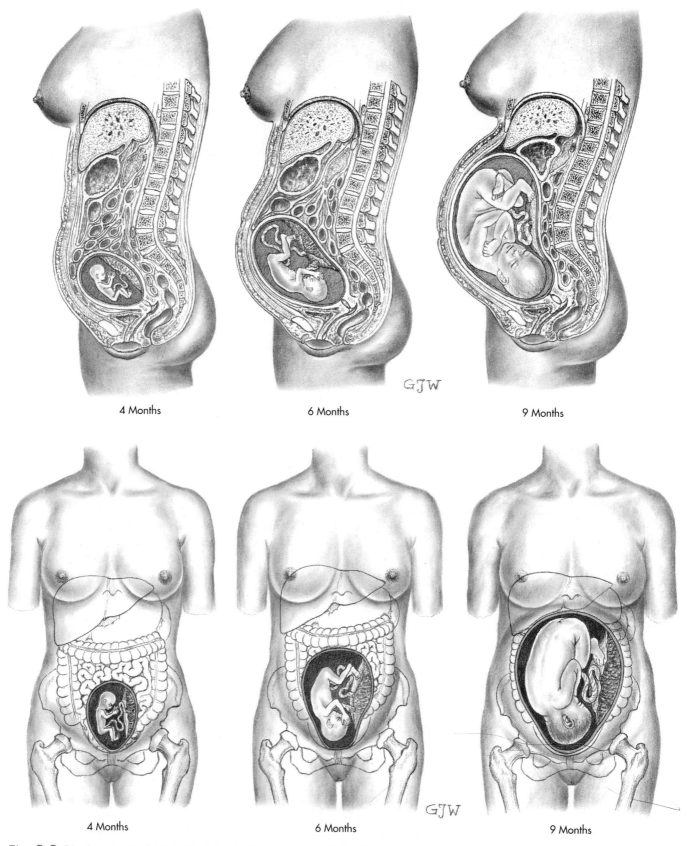

4 Months   6 Months   9 Months

GJW

4 Months   6 Months   9 Months

GJW

Fig. **9-3** Displacement of internal abdominal structures and diaphragm by the enlarging uterus at 4, 6, and 9 months of gestation. (From Lowdermilk D, Perry S & Bobak I: *Maternity and women's health care,* ed 6, St Louis, 1997, Mosby.)

blood flow through the intervillous spaces of the placenta and thereby promote oxygen delivery to the fetus. Although Braxton Hicks contractions are not painful, some women do complain that they are annoying. After the twenty-eighth week, these contractions become much more definite, but they usually cease with walking or exercise. Braxton Hicks contractions can be mistaken for true labor; however, they do not increase in intensity or frequency or cause cervical dilatation.

Uteroplacental blood flow

Placental perfusion depends on the maternal blood flow to the uterus. Blood flow increases rapidly as the uterus increases in size. Although uterine blood flow increases twentyfold, the feto-placental unit grows more rapidly. Consequently, more oxygen is extracted from the uterine blood during the latter part of pregnancy (Cunningham et al., 1997). In a normal term pregnancy, one sixth of the total maternal blood volume is within the uterine vascular system. The rate of blood flow through the uterus averages 500 ml/min, and oxygen consumption of the gravid uterus averages 25 ml/min. A low maternal arterial pressure, contractions of the uterus, and maternal supine position are three factors known to decrease blood flow. Estrogen stimulation may increase uterine blood flow. Doppler ultrasound can be used to measure uterine blood flow velocity, especially in pregnancies at risk because of conditions associated with decreased placental perfusion such as hypertension, intrauterine growth restriction, diabetes mellitus, and multiple gestation (Scott et al., 1994).

Using an ultrasound device or a fetal stethoscope, the health care provider may hear the **uterine souffle,** or bruit, a rushing or blowing sound of maternal blood flowing through uterine arteries to the placenta that is synchronous with the maternal pulse. The **funic souffle,** which is synchronous with the fetal pulse rate and caused by fetal blood coursing through the umbilical cord, may also be heard, as well as the actual fetal heart tones.

Cervical changes

A softening of the cervical tip may be observed at approximately the beginning of the sixth week in a normal, unscarred cervix. This probable sign of pregnancy, **Goodell's sign,** is brought about by increased vascularity, slight hypertrophy, and hyperplasia (increase in number of cells) of the muscle and its collagen-rich connective tissue, which becomes loose, edematous, highly elastic, and increased in volume. The glands near the external os proliferate beneath the stratified squamous epithelium, giving the cervix the velvety appearance characteristic of pregnancy (Fig. 9-5). **Friability** is increased; that is, the cervix bleeds easily when scraped or touched. Increased friability is the cause of the few drops of blood seen after coitus with deep penetration or after vaginal examination. These few

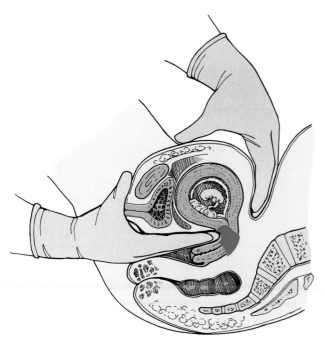

Fig. 9-4 Hegar's sign. Bimanual examination for assessing compressibility, softening of isthmus (lower uterine segment) while the cervix is still firm.

the anterior abdominal wall and this contributes to altering her center of gravity.

During the early weeks of pregnancy an increase in uterine blood flow and lymph causes pelvic congestion and edema. As a result the uterus, cervix, and isthmus soften perceptibly and progressively, and the cervix takes on a bluish color (**Chadwick's sign,** a probable sign of pregnancy) (Scott et al., 1994).

At approximately 6 weeks' gestation, softening and compressibility of the lower uterine segment (the uterine isthmus) occurs (**Hegar's sign**). This results in exaggerated uterine anteflexion during the first 3 months of pregnancy (Fig. 9-4). In this position the uterine fundus presses on the urinary bladder, causing the woman to experience urinary frequency.

Early uterine enlargement may not be symmetrical, depending on the site of implantation. For example, if cornual implantation occurred, a soft irregular bulge (Piskacek's sign) may be detected during a pelvic examination (Varney, 1997).

Changes in contractility

Soon after the fourth month of pregnancy, uterine contractions can be felt through the abdominal wall. These contractions are referred to as the **Braxton Hicks sign,** a probable sign of pregnancy. Braxton Hicks contractions are irregular, painless contractions that occur intermittently throughout pregnancy. These contractions facilitate uterine drops are usually within normal limits. Pregnancy can also cause the squamocolumnar junction, the site for obtaining cells for cervical cancer screening, to be located away from the cervix. Because of all these changes, evaluation of abnormal Papanicolaou tests during pregnancy can be complicated (Kost et al., 1993).

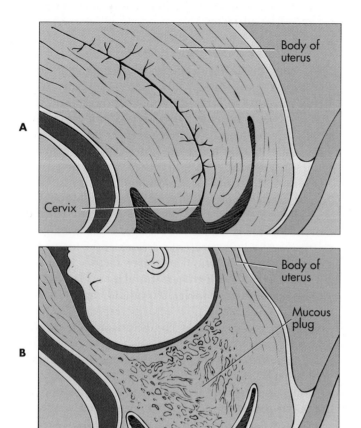

A, Body of uterus

Cervix

B, Body of uterus

Mucous plug

Cervix

Fig. **9-5 A,** Cervix in nonpregnant woman. **B,** Cervix during pregnancy. (From Lowdermilk D, Perry S & Bobak I: *Maternity and women's health care,* ed 6, St Louis, 1997, Mosby.)

The cervix of the nullipara is rounded. Lacerations of the cervix almost always occur during the birth process. With or without lacerations, however, after childbirth the cervix becomes more oval in the horizontal plane, and the external os appears as a transverse slit (see Fig. 9-1).

Changes related to the presence of the fetus

Passive movement of the unengaged fetus is called **ballottement** and can be identified generally between the sixteenth and eighteenth week. Ballottement is a technique of palpating a floating structure by bouncing it gently and feeling it rebound. In the technique used to palpate the fetus, the examiner places a finger in the vagina and taps gently upward causing the fetus to rise. The fetus then sinks, and a gentle tap is felt on the finger (Fig. 9-6). Internal ballottement of a fetus within a uterus is a probable objective sign of pregnancy.

The first recognition of fetal movements, or "feeling life," by the multiparous woman may occur as early as the fourteenth to sixteenth week. The nulliparous woman may not notice these sensations until the eighteenth week or later. **Quickening,** a presumptive sign of pregnancy, is commonly described as a flutter and is difficult to distinguish from peristalsis. Gradually, fetal movements increase in intensity and frequency. The week when quickening occurs provides a tentative clue in dating the duration of gestation.

Vagina and Vulva

Pregnancy hormones prepare the vagina for stretching during labor and birth by causing the vaginal mucosa to thicken, connective tissue to loosen, smooth muscle to hypertrophy, and the vaginal vault to lengthen. Increased vascularity results in a violet-bluish color of the vaginal mucosa and cervix. The deepened color, termed Chadwick's sign, may be evident as early as the sixth week, but is easily noted at the eighth week of pregnancy.

Leukorrhea is a white or slightly gray mucoid discharge with a faint musty odor. This copious mucoid fluid occurs

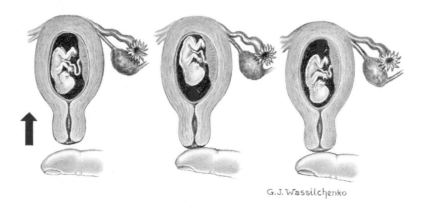

G.J. Wassilchenko

Fig. **9-6** Internal ballottement (18 weeks).

in response to cervical stimulation by estrogen and progesterone. The fluid is whitish because of the presence of many exfoliated vaginal epithelial cells caused by hyperplasia of normal pregnancy. This vaginal discharge is never pruritic or blood stained. Because of the progesterone effect, ferning usually does not occur in the dried cervical mucous smear as it would in a smear of amniotic fluid. Instead, a beaded or cellular crystallizing pattern formed in the dried mucus is seen (Cunningham et al., 1997). The mucus fills the endocervical canal, resulting in the formation of the mucous plug (**operculum**) (see Fig. 9-5). The operculum acts as a barrier against bacterial invasion during pregnancy.

During pregnancy, the pH of vaginal secretions rises from approximately 4 to approximately 6.5. The rise in pH is a result of increased production of lactic acid in the vaginal epithelium, which is probably caused by increased estrogen levels. The pregnant woman is more vulnerable to vaginal infections, especially yeast infections (Mishell et al., 1997).

The increased vascularity of the vagina and other pelvic viscera results in a marked increase in sensitivity. The increased sensitivity may lead to a high degree of sexual interest and arousal, especially during the second trimester of pregnancy. The increased congestion plus the relaxed walls of the blood vessels and the heavy uterus may result in edema and varicosities of the vulva. The edema and varicosities usually resolve during the postpartum period.

External structures of the perineum are enlarged during pregnancy because of an increase in vasculature, hypertrophy of the perineal body, and deposition of fat (Fig. 9-7). The labia majora of the nullipara approximate and obscure the vaginal introitus; those of the parous woman separate and gape after childbirth and perineal or vaginal injury.

Figure 9-1 compares the perineum of the nullipara and the multipara in relation to the pregnant abdomen, vulva, and cervix.

Breasts

Fullness, heightened sensitivity, tingling, and heaviness of the breasts begin in the early weeks of gestation in response to increased levels of estrogen and progesterone. These changes are considered presumptive signs of pregnancy because other factors can cause them to occur. Breast sensitivity varies from mild tingling to sharp pain. Nipples and areolae become more pigmented, secondary pinkish areolae develop, extending beyond the primary areolae, and nipples become more erectile. Hypertrophy of the sebaceous (oil) glands embedded in the primary areolae, called **Montgomery's tubercles** (see Fig. 5-6), may be seen around the nipples. These sebaceous glands may have a protective role in that they keep the nipples lubricated for breastfeeding. Suppleness of the nipples is jeopardized if the protective oils are washed off with soap.

The richer blood supply causes the vessels beneath the skin to dilate. Once barely noticeable, the blood vessels become visible, often appearing in an intertwining blue network beneath the surface of the skin. Venous congestion in the breasts is more obvious in primigravidas. Striae gravidarum (stretch marks) may appear at the outer aspects of the breasts.

During the second and third trimesters, growth of the mammary glands accounts for the progressive breast enlargement. The high levels of luteal and placental hormones in pregnancy promote proliferation of the lactiferous ducts and lobule-alveolar tissue, so that palpation of the breasts reveals a generalized, coarse nodularity. Glandular tissue

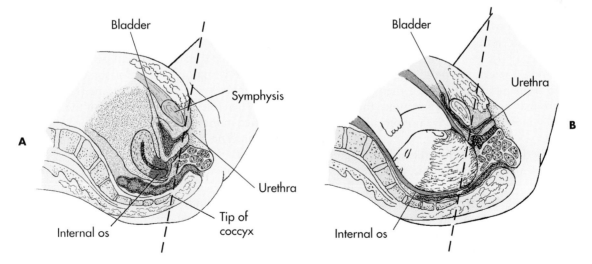

Fig. 9-7 **A,** Pelvic floor in nonpregnant woman. **B,** Pelvic floor at end of pregnancy. Note marked hypertrophy and hyperplasia below dotted line joining tip of coccyx and inferior margin of symphysis. Note elongation of bladder and urethra as a result of compression. Fat deposits are increased.

displaces connective tissue, and as a result the tissue becomes softer and looser.

Although development of the mammary glands is functionally complete by midpregnancy, lactation is inhibited until a drop in estrogen level occurs after the birth. A thin, clear, viscous secretory material (precolostrum) can be found in the acini cells by the third month of gestation. **Colostrum,** the creamy, white-to-yellowish to orange premilk fluid, may be expressed from the nipples as early as 16 weeks of gestation (Lawrence, 1994). See Chapter 21 for discussion of lactation.

GENERAL BODY SYSTEMS

Cardiovascular System

Maternal adjustments to pregnancy involve extensive changes in the cardiovascular system, both anatomic and physiologic. Cardiovascular adaptations protect the woman's normal physiologic functioning, meet the metabolic demands pregnancy imposes on her body, and provide for fetal developmental and growth needs.

Slight cardiac hypertrophy (enlargement) is probably secondary to the increased blood volume and cardiac output that occurs. The heart returns to its normal size after childbirth. As the diaphragm is displaced upward by the enlarging uterus, the heart is elevated upward and rotated forward to the left (Fig. 9-8). The apical impulse, a point of maximum intensity (PMI), is shifted upward and laterally approximately 1 to 1.5 cm. The degree of shift depends on the duration of pregnancy and the size and position of the uterus. The changes in heart size and position and increases in blood volume and cardiac output contribute to auscultatory changes common in pregnancy. There is more audible splitting of S1 and S2, and S3 may be readily heard after 20 weeks of gestation. Additionally, systolic and diastolic murmurs may be heard over the pulmonic area. These are transient and disappear shortly after the woman gives birth (Cunningham et al., 1997).

Between 14 and 20 weeks, the pulse increases approximately 10 to 15 beats per minute, which then persists to term. Palpitations may occur. In twin gestations, the maternal heart rate may increase 40% above nonpregnant levels (Fuschino, 1992).

The cardiac rhythm may be disturbed. The pregnant woman may experience sinus arrhythmia, premature atrial contractions, and premature ventricular systole. In the healthy woman with no underlying heart disease, no therapy is needed; however, women with preexisting heart disease will need close medical and obstetric supervision during pregnancy (see Chapter 23).

Blood pressure

Arterial blood pressure (brachial artery) is affected by age, activity level, and presence of health problems. Additional factors must be considered during pregnancy. These

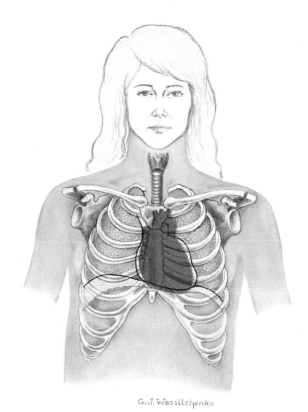

G. J. Wassilchenko

Fig. 9-8 Changes in position of heart, lungs, and thoracic cage in pregnancy. *Broken line,* Nonpregnant; *solid line,* change that occurs in pregnancy.

factors include maternal anxiety, maternal position, and size and type of blood pressure apparatus.

Maternal anxiety can elevate readings. If an elevated reading is found, the woman is given time to rest, and the reading is repeated.

Maternal position affects readings. Brachial blood pressure is highest when the woman is sitting, lowest when she is lying in the lateral recumbent position, and intermediate when she is supine, except for some women who experience supine hypotensive syndrome (see following discussion). Therefore at each prenatal visit the reading should be obtained in the same arm and with the woman in the same position. The position and arm used should be recorded along with the reading.

The proper size cuff is absolutely necessary for accurate readings. The cuff should be 20% wider than the diameter of the arm around which it is wrapped, or approximately 12 to 14 cm for average-sized individuals and 18 to 20 cm for obese persons. Too small a cuff yields a false high reading; too large a cuff yields a false low reading. Caution should also be used when comparing auscultatory and oscillatory blood pressure readings because discrepancies can occur (Green & Froman, 1996).

In the first trimester, blood pressure usually remains the same as the prepregnancy level. During the second trimester,

BOX 9-2	*Calculation of MAP*

Blood pressure: 106/70

$$\text{Formula: } \frac{(\text{systolic}) + 2\,(\text{diastolic})}{3} =$$

$$\frac{(106) + 2(70)}{3} =$$

$$\frac{106 + 140}{3} =$$

$$246/3 = 82 \text{ mm Hg}$$

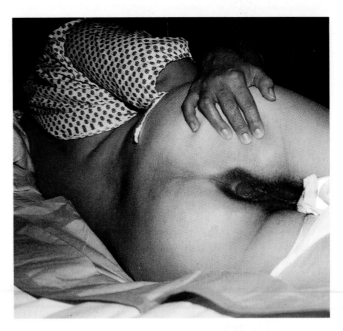

Fig. **9-9** Varicosities of rectal area (hemorrhoids). (Courtesy Marjorie Pyle, RNC, Lifecircle, Costa Mesa, Calif.)

there is a decrease in both systolic and diastolic pressure of 5 to 10 mm Hg. This decrease is probably the result of peripheral vasodilation caused by hormonal changes that occur during pregnancy. During the third trimester, maternal blood pressure should return to the first trimester levels.

Calculating the **mean arterial pressure (MAP)** (mean of the blood pressure in the arterial circulation) can increase the diagnostic value of the findings. Normal MAP readings in the nonpregnant woman are 86.4 mm Hg plus or minus 7.5 mm Hg. MAP readings for a pregnant woman are slightly higher (Scott et al., 1994). One way to calculate a MAP is illustrated in Box 9-2.

Some degree of compression of the vena cava occurs in all women who lie on their backs during the second half of pregnancy (see Fig. 15-4). Some women experience a fall in their systolic blood pressure of more than 30 mm Hg. After 4 to 5 minutes a reflex bradycardia is noted, cardiac output is reduced by half, and the woman feels faint. This condition is referred to as *supine hypotensive syndrome* (Cunningham et al., 1997).

Compression of the iliac veins and inferior vena cava by the uterus causes increased venous pressure and reduced blood flow in the legs (except when the woman is in the lateral position). These alterations contribute to the dependent edema, varicose veins in the legs and vulva, and hemorrhoids that develop in the latter part of term pregnancy (Fig. 9-9).

Blood volume and composition

The degree of blood volume expansion varies considerably. Blood volume increases by approximately 1,500 ml or 40% to 50% above nonpregnancy levels (Cunningham et al., 1997). This increase consists of 1,000 ml plasma plus 450 ml red blood cells (RBCs). The blood volume starts to increase during the tenth to twelfth week, peaks at the thirty-second to thirty-fourth week, then decreases slightly at the fortieth week. The increase in volume of a multiple gestation is greater than that for a pregnancy with a single fetus (Fuschino, 1992). Increased volume is a protective mechanism. It is essential for meeting the blood needs of the hypertrophied vascular system of the enlarged uterus, adequately hydrating fetal and maternal tissues when the woman assumes an erect or supine position, and providing a fluid reserve to compensate for blood loss during birth and the puerperium. Peripheral vasodilation maintains a normal blood pressure despite the increased blood volume in pregnancy.

During pregnancy there is an accelerated production of RBCs (normal 4.2 to 5.4 million/mm3). The percentage of increase depends on the amount of iron available. The RBC mass increases by 30% to 33% by term if an iron supplement is taken. The average increase is 18% in women if no supplement is taken (Bennett & Brown, 1993).

Because the plasma increase exceeds the increase in RBC production, there is a decrease in normal hemoglobin values (12 to 16 g/dl blood) and hematocrit values (37% to 47%). This state of hemodilution is referred to as **physiologic anemia.** The decrease is more noticeable during the second trimester, when rapid expansion of blood volume takes place faster than RBC production. If the hemoglobin value drops to 10 g/dl or less or if the hematocrit drops to 35% or less, the woman is considered anemic.

The total white cell count increases during the second trimester and peaks during the third trimester. This increase is primarily in the granulocytes; the lymphocyte count stays approximately the same throughout pregnancy. See Appendix A for laboratory values during pregnancy.

Cardiac output

Cardiac output increases from 30% to 50% over the nonpregnant rate by the thirty-second week of pregnancy; it declines to approximately a 20% increase at 40 weeks. This

BOX 9-3	*Cardiovascular Changes in Pregnancy*
Heart rate	Increases 10-15 bpm
Blood pressure	Remains at prepregnancy levels in first trimester
	Slight decrease in second trimester
	Returns to prepregnancy levels in third trimester
Blood volume	Increased by 1,500 ml or 40% to 50% above prepregnancy level
Red blood cell mass	Increased 18% to 33%
Hemoglobin	Decreased
Hematocrit	Decreased
White blood cell count	Increases in second and third trimester
Cardiac output	Increases 30% to 50%

elevated cardiac output is largely a result of increased stroke volume and in response to increased tissue demands for oxygen (nonpregnant value is 5 to 5.5 L/min; pregnant value is 6 to 7 L/min) (Scott et al., 1994). Cardiac output in late pregnancy is appreciably higher when the woman is in the lateral recumbent position than when she is supine. In the supine position, the large, heavy uterus often impedes venous return to the heart and affects blood pressure. Cardiac output increases with any exertion, such as labor and birth. Box 9-3 summarizes cardiovascular changes in pregnancy.

Circulation and coagulation times

The circulation time decreases slightly by week 32. It returns to near normal at term. There is a greater tendency for blood to coagulate (clot) during pregnancy because of increases in various clotting factors (Factors VII, VIII, IX, X, and fibrinogen). This, combined with the fact that fibrinolytic activity (the splitting up or the dissolving of a clot) is depressed during pregnancy and the postpartum period, provides a protective function to decrease the chance of bleeding but also makes the woman more vulnerable to thrombosis, especially after cesarean birth.

Respiratory System

Structural and ventilatory adaptations occur during pregnancy to provide for maternal and fetal needs. Maternal oxygen requirements increase in response to the acceleration in the metabolic rate and the need to add to the tissue mass in the uterus and breasts. In addition, the fetus requires oxygen and a way to eliminate carbon dioxide.

Elevated levels of estrogen cause the ligaments of the rib cage to relax, permitting increased chest expansion (see Fig. 9-8). The transverse diameter of the thoracic cage increases by approximately 2 cm, and the circumference increases to 6 cm (Cunningham et al., 1997). The costal angle increases

and the lower rib cage appears to flare out. The chest may not return to its prepregnant state after birth (Seidel et al., 1998).

The diaphragm is displaced by as much as 4 cm during pregnancy. As pregnancy advances, thoracic (costal) breathing replaces abdominal breathing, and it becomes less possible for the diaphragm to descend with inspiration. Thoracic breathing is primarily accomplished by the diaphragm rather than by the costal muscles (Blackburn & Loper, 1992).

The upper respiratory tract becomes more vascular in response to elevated levels of estrogen. As the capillaries become engorged, edema and hyperemia develop within the nose, pharynx, larynx, trachea, and bronchi. This congestion within the tissues of the respiratory tract gives rise to several conditions commonly seen during pregnancy. These conditions include nasal and sinus stuffiness, epistaxis (nosebleed), changes in the voice, and a marked inflammatory response that can develop into a mild upper respiratory infection.

Increased vascularity of the upper respiratory tract also can cause the tympanic membranes and eustachian tubes to swell, giving rise to symptoms of impaired hearing, earaches, or a sense of fullness in the ears.

Pulmonary function

The pregnant woman breathes deeper or increases her tidal volume, which is the volume of gas moved into or out of the respiratory tract with each breath. Her respiratory rate is only slightly increased (approximately two breaths per minute). The increase in respiratory tidal volume associated with the normal respiratory rate causes the respiratory minute volume to increase by approximately 40% (Blackburn & Loper, 1992). The expiratory reserve volume and residual volume decrease progressively during pregnancy. The inspiratory capacity increases slightly while the vital capacity remains unchanged. The total lung capacity decreases slightly. These changes are related to the elevation of the diaphragm and chest wall changes (Fuschino, 1992) (see Box 9-4 for respiratory changes in pregnancy).

During pregnancy, changes in the respiratory center result in a lowered threshold for carbon dioxide. The actions of progesterone and estrogen are presumed responsible for the increased sensitivity of the respiratory center to carbon dioxide. In addition, pregnant women become more aware of the need to breathe; some may even complain of dyspnea at rest.

Although pulmonary function is not impaired by pregnancy, diseases of the respiratory tract may be more serious during this time (Cunningham et al., 1997). One important factor responsible for this may be the increased oxygen requirement.

Basal metabolism rate

The basal metabolism rate (BMR) usually rises by the fourth month of gestation. It is increased by 15% to 20%

BOX 9-4 | **Respiratory Changes in Pregnancy**

Respiratory rate	Unchanged or slightly increased
Tidal volume	Increased 30% to 40%
Vital capacity	Unchanged
Inspiratory capacity	Increased
Expiratory volume	Decreased
Total lung capacity	Unchanged to slightly decreased
Oxygen consumption	Increased 15% to 20%

BOX 9-5 | *Acid-Base Values in Arterial Blood of Pregnant Women*

Pco_2	27 to 32 mm Hg (decreased)
Sodium bicarbonate	18 to 21 mEq/L (decreased)
Blood pH	Slight increase (more alkaline)

by term (Worthington-Roberts & Williams, 1993). The BMR returns to nonpregnant levels by 5 to 6 days postpartum. The elevation in BMR during pregnancy reflects increased oxygen demands of the uterine-placental-fetal unit, as well as oxygen consumption from increased maternal cardiac work. Peripheral vasodilation and acceleration of sweat-gland activity help dissipate the excess heat resulting from the increased BMR during pregnancy. Pregnant women may experience heat intolerance, which is annoying to some women. Lassitude and fatigability after only slight exertion are experienced by many women in early pregnancy. These feelings, along with a greater need for sleep, may persist and may be caused in part by the increased metabolic activity.

Acid-base balance

By approximately the tenth week of pregnancy, there is a decrease of approximately 5 mm Hg in the partial pressure of carbon dioxide (Pco_2). Progesterone may be responsible for increasing the sensitivity of the respiratory center receptors, so that tidal volume is increased and Pco_2 falls, the base excess (HCO_3, or bicarbonate) falls, and pH increases slightly. These alterations in acid-base balance indicate that pregnancy is a state of respiratory alkalosis compensated by mild metabolic acidosis (Fuschino, 1992). These changes also facilitate the transport of CO_2 from the fetus, as well as facilitate O_2 release from the mother to the fetus. Box 9-5 lists acid-base values during pregnancy.

Renal System

The kidneys are responsible for maintaining electrolyte and acid-base balance, regulating extracellular fluid volume, excreting waste products, and conserving essential nutrients.

Anatomic changes

Changes in renal structure during pregnancy result from hormonal activity (estrogen and progesterone), pressure from an enlarging uterus, and an increase in blood volume. As early as the tenth week of pregnancy, the renal pelvis and the ureters dilate. Dilatation of the ureters is more pronounced above the pelvic brim, in part because they are compressed between the uterus and the pelvic brim. In most women the ureters below the pelvic brim are of normal size. The smooth-muscle walls of the ureters undergo hyperplasia and hypertrophy and muscle tone relaxation. The ureters elongate, become tortuous, and form single or double curves. In the latter part of pregnancy, the renal pelvis and ureter are dilated more on the right side than on the left because the heavy uterus is displaced to the right by the sigmoid colon.

Because of these changes, a larger volume of urine is held in the pelves and ureters, and urine flow rate is slowed. The resulting urinary stasis or stagnation has the following consequences:

- There is a lag between the time urine is formed and when it reaches the bladder. Therefore clearance test results may reflect substances contained in glomerular filtrate several hours before.
- Stagnated urine is an excellent medium for the growth of microorganisms. In addition, the urine of pregnant women contains more nutrients, including glucose, thereby increasing the pH (making the urine more alkaline). This makes pregnant women more susceptible to urinary tract infection.

Bladder irritability, nocturia, and urinary frequency and urgency (without dysuria) commonly are reported in early pregnancy. Near term, bladder symptoms may return, especially after lightening occurs.

Urinary frequency results initially from increased bladder sensitivity and later from compression of the bladder (see Fig. 9-7). In the second trimester the bladder is pulled up out of the true pelvis into the abdomen. The urethra lengthens to 7.5 cm as the bladder is displaced upward. The pelvic congestion that occurs in pregnancy is reflected in hyperemia of the bladder and urethra. This increased vascularity causes the bladder mucosa to be traumatized and bleed easily. Bladder tone may decrease, which increases the bladder capacity to 1,500 ml. At the same time the bladder is compressed by the enlarging uterus, resulting in the urge to void even if the bladder contains only a small amount of urine.

Functional changes

In normal pregnancy, renal function is altered considerably. Glomerular filtration rate (GFR) and renal plasma flow (RPF) increase early in pregnancy (Cunningham et al., 1997). These changes are caused by pregnancy hormones, an increase in blood volume, the woman's posture, physical activity, and nutritional intake. The woman's kidneys must manage the increased metabolic and circulatory demands of the maternal body and also excretion of fetal waste products.

Renal function is most efficient when the woman lies in the lateral recumbent position and least efficient when the woman assumes a supine position. A side-lying position increases renal perfusion, which increases urinary output and decreases edema. When the pregnant woman is lying supine, the heavy uterus compresses the vena cava and the aorta, and cardiac output decreases. As a result, blood flow to the brain and heart is continued at the expense of other organs, including the kidneys and uterus.

Fluid and electrolyte balance

Selective renal tubular reabsorption maintains sodium and water balance regardless of changes in dietary intake and losses through sweat, vomitus, or diarrhea. From 500 to 900 mEq of sodium are normally retained during pregnancy to meet fetal needs. To prevent excessive sodium depletion, the maternal kidneys undergo a significant adaptation by increasing tubular reabsorption. Because of the need for increased maternal intravascular and extracellular fluid volume, additional sodium is needed to expand fluid volume and to maintain an isotonic state. As efficient as the renal system is, it can be overstressed by excessive dietary sodium intake or restriction or by use of diuretics. Severe hypovolemia and reduced placental perfusion are two consequences of using diuretics during pregnancy.

The capacity of the kidneys to excrete water during the early weeks of pregnancy is more efficient than later in pregnancy. As a result, some women feel thirsty in early pregnancy because of the greater amount of water loss. The pooling of fluid in the legs in the latter part of pregnancy decreases renal blood flow and GFR. This pooling of blood in the lower legs is sometimes referred to as *physiologic edema* or dependent edema and requires no treatment. The normal diuretic response to the water load is triggered when the woman lies down, preferably on her side, and the pooled fluid reenters general circulation.

Normally the kidney reabsorbs almost all of the glucose and other nutrients from the plasma filtrate. In pregnant women, however, tubular reabsorption of glucose is impaired so that glycosuria occurs at varying times and to varying degrees. Normal values range from 0 to 20 mg/dl, meaning that during any one day the urine is sometimes positive and sometimes negative. In nonpregnant women, blood glucose levels must be at 160 to 180 mg/dl before glucose is "spilled" into the urine (not reabsorbed). During pregnancy, glycosuria occurs when maternal glucose levels are lower than 160 mg/dl. Why glucose, as well as other nutrients such as amino acids, is wasted during pregnancy is not understood, nor has the exact mechanism been discovered. Although glycosuria may be found in normal pregnancies (1+ levels on dipstick may be seen with increased anxiety states), the possibility of diabetes mellitus and gestational diabetes must be kept in mind.

BOX 9-6	*Renal Changes in Pregnancy*
Bladder capacity	Increased to 1,500 ml
Glomerular filtration rate (GFR)	Increased 30% to 50%
Renal plasma flow (RPF)	Increased 30%

RENAL LABORATORY VALUES

Serum

Blood Urea Nitrogen	Decreased (normal: 8-20 mg/dl)
Creatinine	Decreased (normal: 0.6-1.2 mg/dl)
Uric acid	Decreased first and second trimesters (normal: 4.5-5.8 mg/dl) Returns to prepregnancy levels in third trimester

Urine

Glucose	Present in urine of 20% of pregnant women (normal: 0-20 mg/dl)

Proteinuria usually does not occur in normal pregnancy except during labor or after birth (Cunningham et al., 1997). However, the increased amount of amino acids that needs to be filtered may exceed the capacity of the renal tubules to absorb it, so that small amounts of protein are then lost in the urine. Values of trace to 1+ (plus) protein (dipstick assessment) or less than 300 mg per 24 hours are acceptable during pregnancy (Blackburn & Loper, 1992). The amount of protein excreted is not an indication of the severity of renal disease, nor does an increase in protein excretion in a pregnant woman with known renal disease necessarily indicate a progression in her disease. However, a pregnant woman with hypertension and proteinuria must be carefully evaluated, since she may be at greater risk for an adverse pregnancy outcome (see Box 9-6 for renal changes during pregnancy).

Integumentary System

Alterations in hormonal balance and mechanical stretching are responsible for several changes in the integumentary system during pregnancy. General changes include increases in skin thickness and subdermal fat, hyperpigmentation, hair and nail growth, accelerated sweat and sebaceous gland activity, and increased circulation and vasomotor activity. Cutaneous elastic tissues are more fragile, resulting in striae gravidarum, or stretch marks. Cutaneous allergic responses are enhanced as well.

Hyperpigmentation is stimulated by the anterior pituitary hormone melanotropin, which is increased during pregnancy. Darkening of the nipples, areolae, axillae, and vulva occurs at approximately the sixteenth week of gestation.

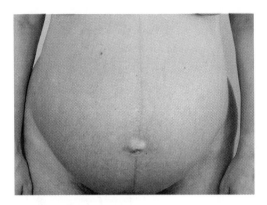

Fig. 9-10 Linea nigra. (From Seidel H et al.: *Mosby's guide to physical examination,* ed 4, St Louis, 1998, Mosby.)

CULTURAL CONSIDERATIONS

Skin Assessment during Pregnancy

Integumentary system changes vary greatly among women of different racial backgrounds. For example, vascular spiders and palmar erythema are seen more often in Caucasian women than in African-American women. Areolar pigmentation varies by race. African-American women have the darkest areolae, Caucasian women have the lightest, and Asian and Native American women have intermediate pigmentation. When performing physical assessments, the color of the woman's skin should be noted along with any changes that may be attributed to pregnancy.

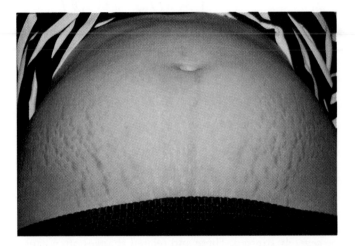

Fig. 9-11 Striae gravidarum, or "stretch marks." (Courtesy Michael S. Clement, MD, Mesa, Ariz.)

Facial melasma, also called **chloasma** or mask of pregnancy, is a blotchy, brownish hyperpigmentation of the skin over the cheeks, nose, and the forehead, especially in dark-complexioned pregnant women. Chloasma appears in 50% to 70% of pregnant women, beginning after the sixteenth week and increasing gradually until term. The sun intensifies this pigmentation in susceptible women. Chloasma caused by normal pregnancy usually fades after birth.

The **linea nigra** (Fig. 9-10) is a pigmented line extending from the symphysis pubis to the top of the fundus in the midline; this line is known as the *linea alba* before hormone-induced pigmentation. In primigravidas the extension of the linea nigra, beginning in the third month, keeps pace with the rising height of the fundus; in multigravidas the entire line often appears earlier than the third month. Not all pregnant women develop linea nigra.

Striae gravidarum, or stretch marks (seen over lower abdomen in Fig. 9-11), which appear in 50% to 90% of pregnant women during the second half of pregnancy, may be caused by action of adrenocorticosteroids. Striae reflect separation within the underlying connective (collagen) tissue of the skin. These slightly depressed streaks tend to occur over areas of maximum stretch (i.e., abdomen, thighs, and breasts). The stretching sometimes causes a sensation that resembles itching. The tendency to develop striae may be familial. After birth they usually fade, although they never disappear completely. Color of striae varies depending on the pregnant woman's skin color. The striae appear pinkish on a woman with light skin, and are lighter than surrounding skin in dark-skinned women. In the multipara, in addition to the striae of the present pregnancy, glistening silvery lines (in light-skinned women) or purplish lines (in dark-skinned women) are commonly seen. These represent the scars of striae from previous pregnancies.

Angiomas are commonly referred to as vascular spiders. They are tiny, star-shaped or branched, slightly raised and pulsating end-arterioles usually found on the neck, thorax, face, and arms. They occur as a result of elevated levels of circulating estrogen. The spiders are bluish in color and do not blanch with pressure. Vascular spiders appear during the second to the fifth month of pregnancy in 65% of Caucasian women and 10% of African-American women. The spiders usually disappear after birth.

Pinkish-red, diffuse mottling or well-defined blotches are seen over the palmar surfaces of the hands in approximately 60% of Caucasian women and 35% of African-American women during pregnancy (Cunningham et al., 1997). These color changes called **palmar erythema** are related primarily to increased estrogen levels. (See Cultural Considerations box for skin assessment during pregnancy.)

Gum hypertrophy may occur. An **epulis** (gingival granuloma gravidarum) is a red, raised nodule on the gums that bleeds easily. This lesion may develop around the third month and usually continues to enlarge as pregnancy progresses. It is usually managed by avoiding trauma to the gums (e.g., using a soft toothbrush). An epulis usually regresses spontaneously after birth.

Nail growth may be accelerated. Some women may notice thinning and softening of the nails. Oily skin and

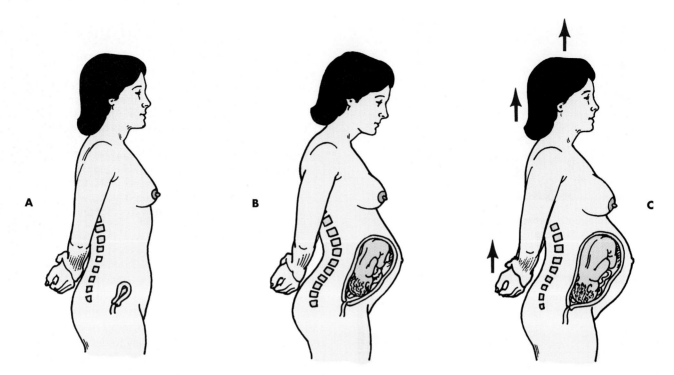

Fig. **9-12** Postural changes during pregnancy. **A,** Nonpregnant. **B,** Incorrect posture during pregnancy. **C,** Correct posture during pregnancy.

acne vulgaris may occur during pregnancy. For some women the skin clears and looks radiant. Hirsutism, the excessive growth of hair or growth of hair in unusual places, is commonly reported. An increase in fine hair growth may occur but tends to disappear after pregnancy. However, growth of coarse or bristly hair does not usually disappear after pregnancy.

Increased blood supply to the skin leads to increased perspiration. Women feel hotter during pregnancy, possibly related to a progesterone-induced increase in body temperature and the increased basal metabolic rate (BMR).

Musculoskeletal System

The gradually changing body and increasing weight of the pregnant woman cause noticeable alterations in her posture (Fig. 9-12) and way of walking. The great abdominal distention that gives the pelvis a forward tilt, decreased abdominal muscle tone, and increased weight bearing require a realignment of the spinal curvatures late in pregnancy. The woman's center of gravity shifts forward. An increase in the normal lumbosacral curve (lordosis) develops, and a compensatory curvature in the cervicodorsal region (exaggerated anterior flexion of the head) develops to help her maintain her balance. Aching, numbness, and weakness of the upper extremities may result. Large breasts and a stoop-shouldered stance will further accentuate the lumbar and dorsal curves. Walking is more difficult, and the waddling

gait of the pregnant woman, called "the proud walk of pregnancy" by Shakespeare, is well known. The ligamentous and muscular structures of the middle and lower spine may be severely stressed. These and related changes often cause musculoskeletal discomfort.

The young, well-muscled woman may tolerate these changes without complaint. However, older women or those with a back disorder or a faulty sense of balance may have a considerable amount of back pain during and just after pregnancy.

Slight relaxation and increased mobility of the pelvic joints are normal during pregnancy. They are secondary to the exaggerated elasticity and softening of connective and collagen tissue caused by increased circulating steroid sex hormones, especially estrogen. Relaxin, an ovarian hormone, assists in this relaxation and softening. These adaptations permit enlargement of pelvic dimensions to facilitate labor and birth. The degree of relaxation varies, but considerable separation of the symphysis pubis and the instability of the sacroiliac joints may cause pain and difficulty in walking. Obesity and multifetal pregnancy tend to increase the pelvic instability. Peripheral joint laxity also increases as pregnancy progresses, but the cause is not known (Schauberger et al., 1996).

The muscles of the abdominal wall stretch and ultimately lose some tone. During the third trimester the rectus abdominis muscles may separate (Fig. 9-13), allowing abdominal

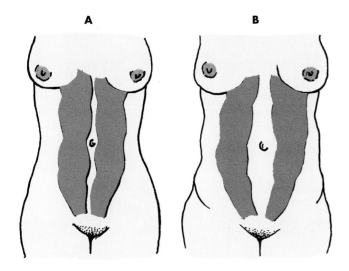

Fig. 9-13 Possible change in rectus abdominis muscles during pregnancy. **A,** Normal position in nonpregnant woman. **B,** Diastasis recti abdominis in pregnant woman.

contents to protrude at the midline. The umbilicus flattens or protrudes. After birth, the muscles gradually regain tone. However, separation of the muscles (**diastasis recti abdominis**) may persist.

Neurologic System

Little is known regarding specific alterations in function of the neurologic system during pregnancy, aside from hypothalamic-pituitary neurohormonal changes. Specific physiologic alterations resulting from pregnancy may cause the following neurologic or neuromuscular symptoms:

- *Compression* of pelvic nerves or vascular stasis caused by enlargement of the uterus may result in sensory changes in the legs.
- *Dorsolumbar lordosis* may cause pain because of traction on nerves or compression of nerve roots.
- *Edema* involving the peripheral nerves may result in carpal tunnel syndrome during the last trimester. The edema compresses the median nerve beneath the carpal ligament of the wrist. The syndrome is characterized by paresthesia (abnormal sensation such as burning or tingling) and pain in the hand, radiating to the elbow. The dominant hand is usually affected most, although as many as 80% of women experience symptoms in both hands. Symptoms usually regress after pregnancy. In some cases, surgical treatment may be necessary (Cunningham et al., 1997).
- *Acroesthesia* (numbness and tingling of the hands) is caused by the stoop-shouldered stance (see Fig. 9-12, *B*) assumed by some women during pregnancy. The condition is associated with traction on segments of the brachial plexus.

- *Tension headache* is common when anxiety or uncertainty complicates pregnancy. However, vision problems, sinusitis, or migraine may also be responsible for headaches.
- *"Lightheadedness," faintness,* and even *syncope* (fainting) are common during early pregnancy. Vasomotor instability, postural hypotension, or hypoglycemia may be responsible.
- *Hypocalcemia* may cause neuromuscular problems such as muscle cramps or tetany.

Gastrointestinal System

A variety of gastrointestinal system changes occur during pregnancy. The appetite fluctuates, intestinal secretion is reduced, liver function is altered, and absorption of nutrients is enhanced. The colon is displaced laterally upward and posteriorly. Peristaltic activity (motility) decreases. As a result bowel sounds are diminished, and constipation, nausea, and vomiting are common. Blood flow to the pelvis increases as does venous pressure, contributing to hemorrhoid formation in later pregnancy.

Appetite

During pregnancy, the pregnant woman's appetite and food intake fluctuate. Early in pregnancy, some women experience "morning sickness" in response to increasing levels of hCG and altered carbohydrate metabolism. *Morning sickness* refers to nausea with or without vomiting; it can occur any time of the day. It appears at approximately 4 to 6 weeks gestation and usually subsides by the end of the third month (first trimester) of pregnancy. Severity varies from mild distaste for certain foods to more severe vomiting. The condition may be triggered by the sight or odor of various foods. Fatigue may also be responsible for severe nausea, but further research is needed to determine the role of this factor (O'Brien & Zhou, 1995). By the end of the second trimester, appetite increases in response to increasing metabolic needs. Rarely does morning sickness have harmful effects on the embryo/fetus or the woman. Whenever the vomiting is severe or persists beyond the first trimester, or when it is accompanied by fever, pain, or weight loss, further evaluation is necessary and medical intervention is likely.

Women may also experience changes in their sense of taste, leading to cravings and changes in dietary intake. Some women have pica (nonfood cravings such as ice, clay, and laundry starch). Usually these cravings, if consumed in moderation, are not harmful to the pregnancy if the woman has adequate nutrition otherwise (Cunningham et al., 1997).

Mouth

Epulis is a condition in which the gums become hyperemic, spongy, and swollen during pregnancy. They tend to bleed easily because the rising levels of estrogen cause selective increased vascularity and connective tissue proliferation (a nonspecific gingivitis). Some pregnant women complain of **ptyalism** (excessive salivation), which may be caused by the decrease in unconscious swallowing by the woman when nauseated or from stimulation of salivary glands by eating starch (Cunningham et al., 1997). Epulis and bleeding gums are discussed in the section on the integumentary system.

Esophagus, stomach, and intestines

Herniation of the upper portion of the stomach (hiatal hernia) occurs after the seventh or eighth month of pregnancy in approximately 15% to 20% of pregnant women. This condition results from upward displacement of the stomach, which causes the hiatus of the diaphragm to widen. It occurs more often in multiparas and older or obese women.

Increased estrogen production causes decreased secretion of hydrochloric acid. Therefore peptic ulcer formation or flare-up of existing peptic ulcers is uncommon during pregnancy.

Increased progesterone production causes decreased tone and motility of smooth muscles so that there is esophageal regurgitation, slower emptying time of the stomach, and reverse peristalsis. As a result the woman may experience "acid indigestion" or heartburn **(pyrosis).**

Iron is absorbed more readily in the small intestine in response to increased needs during pregnancy. Even when the woman is deficient in iron, it will continue to be absorbed in sufficient amounts for the fetus to have a normal hemoglobin level.

Increased progesterone (causing loss of muscle tone and decreased peristalsis) results in an increase in water absorption from the colon and may cause constipation. Constipation can also result from hypoperistalsis (sluggishness of the bowel), food choices, lack of fluids, iron supplementation, decreased activity level, abdominal distention by the pregnant uterus, and displacement and compression of the intestines. If the pregnant woman has hemorrhoids (see Fig. 9-9) and is constipated, the hemorrhoids may evert or may bleed during straining at stool. A mild ileus (sluggishness and lack of movement of the intestines) that follows birth, as well as postbirth fluid loss and perineal discomfort, contribute to continuing constipation.

Gallbladder and liver

The gallbladder is quite often distended because of its decreased muscle tone during pregnancy. Increased emptying time and thickening of bile caused by prolonged retention are typical changes. These features, together with slight hypercholesterolemia from increased progesterone levels, may account for the development of gallstones during pregnancy.

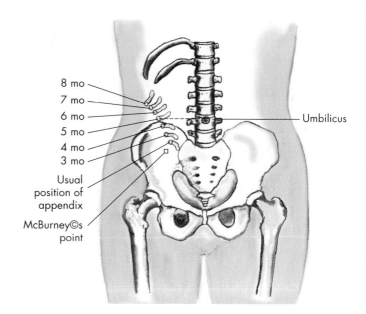

Fig. **9-14** Change in position of appendix in pregnancy. Note McBurney's point.

Hepatic function is difficult to appraise during pregnancy. However, only minor changes in liver function develop. Occasionally, intrahepatic cholestasis (retention and accumulation of bile in the liver, caused by factors within the liver) occurs late in pregnancy in response to placental steroids and may result in pruritus gravidarum (severe itching) with or without jaundice. These distressing symptoms subside soon after birth.

Abdominal discomfort

Intraabdominal alterations that can cause discomfort include pelvic heaviness or pressure, round ligament tension, flatulence, distention and bowel cramping, and uterine contractions. In addition to displacement of intestines, pressure from the expanding uterus causes an increase in venous pressure in the pelvic organs. Although most abdominal discomfort is a consequence of normal maternal alterations, the health care provider must be constantly alert to the possibility of disorders such as bowel obstruction or an inflammatory process.

Appendicitis may be difficult to diagnose in pregnancy because the appendix is displaced upward and laterally, high and to the right, away from McBurney's point (Fig. 9-14).

Endocrine System
Pituitary and placental hormones

During pregnancy, the elevated levels of estrogen and progesterone (produced first by the corpus luteum in the ovary until approximately 14 weeks and then by the placenta) suppress secretion of follicle-stimulating hormone

(FSH) and luteinizing hormone (LH) by the anterior pituitary. The maturation of a follicle and ovulation do not occur. Although the majority of women experience **amenorrhea** (absence of menses), at least 20% have some slight, painless spotting during early gestation. Implantation bleeding and bleeding following intercourse related to cervical friability can occur. Most of the women experiencing slight gestational bleeding continue to full term and have normal infants. However, all instances of bleeding should be reported and evaluated.

After implantation, the fertilized ovum and the chorionic villi produce hCG, which maintains the corpus luteum's production of estrogen and progesterone until the placenta takes over their production (Scott et al., 1994).

Progesterone is essential for maintaining pregnancy by relaxing smooth muscles, resulting in decreased uterine contractility and prevention of spontaneous abortion. Progesterone and estrogen cause fat to deposit in subcutaneous tissues over the maternal abdomen, back, and upper thighs. This fat serves as an energy reserve for both pregnancy and lactation. Estrogen also promotes the enlargement of the genitals, uterus, and breasts and increases vascularity, causing vasodilation. Estrogen causes relaxation of pelvic ligaments and joints. It also alters metabolism of nutrients by interfering with folic acid metabolism, increasing the level of total body proteins, and promoting retention of sodium and water by kidney tubules. Estrogen may decrease secretion of hydrochloric acid and pepsin, which may be responsible for digestive upsets such as nausea.

Serum prolactin produced by the anterior pituitary begins to rise early in the first trimester and increases progressively to term. It is responsible for initial lactation; however, the high levels of estrogen and progesterone inhibit lactation by blocking the binding of prolactin to breast tissue, until after birth (Guyton & Hall, 1997).

Oxytocin is produced by the posterior pituitary in increasing amounts as the fetus matures. This hormone can stimulate uterine contractions during pregnancy, but high levels of progesterone prevent contractions until near term. Oxytocin also stimulates the let-down or milk-ejection reflex after birth in response to the infant sucking at the mother's breast.

Human placental lactogen (hPL) or human chorionic somatomammotropin produced by the placenta acts as a growth hormone and contributes to breast development. It decreases the maternal metabolism of glucose and increases the amount of fatty acids for metabolic needs (Guyton & Hall, 1997).

Thyroid gland

During pregnancy gland activity and hormone production increases. The increased activity is reflected in a moderate enlargement of the thyroid gland caused by hyperplasia of the glandular tissue and increased vascularity (Cunningham et al., 1997). Thyroxine-binding globulin (TBG) increases as a result of increased estrogen levels. This increase begins at approximately 20 weeks of gestation. The level of total (free and bound) thyroxine (T_4) increases between 6 and 9 weeks' gestation and plateaus at 18 weeks. Free thyroxine (T_4) and free triiodothyronine (T_3) returns to nonpregnant levels after the first trimester. Despite these changes in hormone production, the pregnant woman usually does not develop hyperthyroidism (Cunningham et al., 1997).

Parathyroid gland

Parathyroid hormone controls calcium and magnesium metabolism. Pregnancy induces a slight hyperparathyroidism, a reflection of increased fetal requirements for calcium and vitamin D. The peak level of parathyroid hormone occurs between 15 and 35 weeks' gestation when the needs for growth of the fetal skeleton are greatest. Levels return to normal after birth.

Pancreas

The fetus requires significant amounts of glucose for its growth and development. To meet its need for fuel, the fetus not only depletes the store of maternal glucose but also decreases the mother's ability to synthesize glucose by siphoning off her amino acids. Maternal blood glucose levels fall. Maternal insulin does not cross the placenta to the fetus. As a result, in early pregnancy, the pancreas decreases its production of insulin.

As pregnancy continues, the placenta grows and produces progressively larger amounts of hormones (i.e., hPL, estrogen, and progesterone). Cortisol production by the adrenals also increases. Estrogen, progesterone, hPL, and cortisol collectively decrease the mother's ability to use insulin. Cortisol stimulates increased production of insulin but also increases the mother's peripheral resistance to insulin (i.e., the tissues cannot use the insulin). Decreasing the mother's ability to use her own insulin is a protective mechanism that ensures an ample supply of glucose for the needs of the fetoplacental unit. The result is an added demand for insulin by the mother that continues to increase at a steady rate until term. The normal beta cells of the islets of Langerhans in the pancreas can meet this demand for insulin.

Adrenal glands

The adrenal glands change little during pregnancy. Secretion of aldosterone is increased, resulting in reabsorption of excess sodium from the renal tubules. Cortisol levels are also increased.

These profound endocrine changes are essential for pregnancy maintenance, normal fetal growth, and postpartum recovery.

RESEARCH

Psychosocial Adjustment of Mature Gravidas during Pregnancy

Although most pregnancies occur in women younger than 35 years of age, there is an increasing number of women 35 years of age and older giving birth for the first time. Many of these women are in their later reproductive years and have delayed childbearing. Historically, older gravidas were considered at greater risk for maternal and fetal complications. In addition to some greater medical risks associated with age, older gravidas also face psychosocial challenges. A static group comparison design was used to determine if gravidas age 35 years or older have greater conflict in adapting to pregnancy than do younger gravidas. A convenience sample of 116 women in their third trimester of pregnancy were given two questionnaires to complete. The first questionnaire measured demographic and obstetric information, and the second questionnaire, the Prenatal Self-Evaluation Questionnaire II, measured conflict in the seven developmental tasks of pregnancy. Participants were asked to complete the questionnaires during their prenatal care office visit and prenatal education classes. The conflicts an older gravida may have about her maternal role are not diminished or accentuated by age or previous experience with pregnancy and birth. Older gravidas had significantly less fear of helplessness and loss of control in labor than did younger gravidas.

CLINICAL APPLICATION OF THE STUDY

Nurses caring for older gravidas should assess concerns throughout pregnancy. Older gravidas need labor preparation although they maintain control and cope with labor. An older gravida may have fewer peers who are pregnant with whom she can share similar experiences.

Source: Stark M: Psychosocial adjustment during pregnancy: the experience of mature gravidas, *J Obstet Gynecol Neonatal Nurs* 26(2):207, 1997.

KEY POINTS

- The biochemical, physiologic, and anatomic adaptations that occur during pregnancy are profound and revert back to the nonpregnant state following birth and lactation.
- Maternal adaptations are attributed to the hormones of pregnancy and to mechanical pressures exerted by the enlarging uterus and other tissues.
- The ability to recognize the beta subunit of hCG through the use of monoclonal antibody technology has revolutionized endocrine tests for pregnancy.

KEY POINTS—cont'd

- Presumptive, probable, and positive signs of pregnancy aid in the diagnosis of pregnancy; only positive signs (identification of a fetal heart beat, verification of fetal movements, and visualization of the fetus) can establish the diagnosis of pregnancy.
- Adaptations to pregnancy protect the woman's normal physiologic functioning, meet the metabolic demands pregnancy imposes, and provide for fetal development and growth needs.
- The rise in pH of the pregnant woman's vaginal secretions makes her more vulnerable to vaginal infections.
- Increased vascularity and sensitivity of the vagina and other pelvic viscera may lead to a high degree of sexual interest and arousal.
- Some adaptations to pregnancy result in discomforts such as fatigue, urinary frequency, nausea, and breast sensitivity.
- As pregnancy progresses, balance and coordination are affected by changes in the woman's joints and her center of gravity.

CRITICAL THINKING EXERCISES

1 *Interview three pregnant women (and partners, if present) at 12 weeks, 24 weeks and 36 weeks of gestation:*
   a *How does each pregnant woman feel about changes in her body?*
   b *Has her partner expressed any feelings/opinions about these changes? If so, how have these feelings/opinions affected the woman?*
   c *Which changes do they find pleasant?*
   d *Which changes do they find uncomfortable or troublesome?*
   e *What is their level of understanding of these changes?*
   f *Use your findings to develop a teaching plan for each woman. Provide rationale for your choices of topics to include.*
2 *Go to a local pharmacy and get information on at least three different home pregnancy test kits. (The pharmacist may be able to provide product information.) Compare the directions for use, how to interpret test results, and the costs. In a group conference, discuss the pros and cons of using the different types of kits. Develop a plan to counsel a teenager who thinks she is pregnant and wants information about home pregnancy tests.*

CRITICAL THINKING EXERCISES—cont'd

3 *During your experience in a prenatal clinic or physician/midwife office, ask the pregnant women that you meet if they used a home pregnancy test to confirm pregnancy. Compare women who did home testing with those who had pregnancy tests done by their health care provider in terms of when the woman's first prenatal visit occurred. Discuss your findings with those of the other students in your clinical group.*

References

Barkauskas V et al.: *Health and physical assessment,* St Louis, 1994, Mosby.

Bennett V & Brown L: *Myles textbook for midwives,* ed 12, Edinburgh, 1993, Churchill Livingstone.

Blackburn S & Loper D: *Maternal, fetal, and neonatal physiology: a clinical perspective,* Philadelphia, 1992, WB Saunders.

Cunningham F et al.: *Williams obstetrics,* ed 20, Stamford, Conn, 1997, Appleton & Lange.

Edge V & Miller M: *Women's health care, Mosby's clinical nursing series,* St Louis, 1994, Mosby.

Fuschino W: Physiologic changes of pregnancy: impact on critical care, *Crit Care Nurs Clin North Am* 4(4):691, 1992.

Green L & Froman R: Blood pressure measurement during pregnancy: auscultating versus oscillatory methods, *J Obstet Gynecol Neonatal Nurs* 25(2):155, 1996.

Guyton A & Hall J: *Human physiology and mechanism of disease,* ed 6, Philadelphia, 1997, WB Saunders.

Kost E et al.: The "less than optimal" cytology: important in obstetric patients and a routine gynecologic population, *Obstet Gynecol* 81:127, 1993.

Lawrence R: *Breastfeeding: a guide for the medical profession,* ed 4, St Louis, 1994, Mosby.

Lowdermilk D, Perry S & Bobak I: *Maternity and women's health care,* ed 6, St Louis, 1997, Mosby.

Mishell D et al.: *Comprehensive gynecology,* ed 3, St Louis, 1997, Mosby.

O'Brien B & Zhou Q: Variables related to nausea and vomiting during pregnancy, *Birth* 22(2):93, 1995.

Pagana K & Pagana T: *Mosby's diagnostic and laboratory test reference,* ed 3, St Louis, 1996, Mosby.

Schauberger C et al.: Obstetrics: peripheral joint laxity increases in pregnancy but does not correlate with serum relaxin levels, *Am J Obstet Gynecol* 174(2):667, 1996.

Scott J et al.: *Danforth's obstetrics and gynecology,* ed 7, Philadelphia, 1994, JB Lippincott.

Seidel H et al.: *Mosby's guide to physical examination,* ed 4, St Louis, 1998, Mosby.

Varney H: *Varney's midwifery,* ed 3, Sudbury, Mass, 1997, Jones and Bartlett.

Worthington-Roberts B & Williams S: *Nutrition in pregnancy and lactation,* ed 5, St Louis, 1993, Mosby.

CHAPTER

Nursing Care During Pregnancy

REBECCA BURDETTE SAUNDERS

LEARNING OBJECTIVES

- *Define the key terms.*
- *Describe the process of confirming pregnancy and estimating the date of birth.*
- *Summarize the physical, psychosocial, and behavioral changes that usually occur as the mother and other family members adapt to pregnancy.*
- *Outline the patterns of health care provided to assess maternal and fetal health status at the initial and follow-up visits during pregnancy.*
- *Describe the nursing assessments, diagnoses, interventions, and methods of evaluation that are typical when providing care for the pregnant woman.*
- *Discuss education needed by pregnant women to understand physical discomforts related to pregnancy and to recognize signs and symptoms of potential complications.*
- *Explain the impact of culture, age, parity, and number of fetuses on the response of the family to the pregnancy and on the prenatal care provided.*
- *Discuss the purpose of childbirth education and strategies used to provide appropriate information.*
- *Compare the options expectant families have in choice of care providers, birth plans, and birth settings.*
- *Summarize the care of a woman who is battered during pregnancy.*

KEY TERMS

alternative birth centers (ABCs)
ambivalence
attachment
battering
birth plan
Bradley method
breast shells
couvade
conscious relaxation
cultural prescriptions
cultural proscriptions
Dick-Read method
effleurage
emotional lability
epulis
estimated date of birth (EDB)
freestanding birth centers
fundal height
gingivitis
home birth
Kegel exercises
Lamaze method
morning sickness
multifetal pregnancy
Nägele's rule
pelvic tilt (rock)
pinch test
quickening
round ligament pain
supine hypotension
trimesters

The prenatal period is a time of physical and psychologic preparation for birth and parenthood. Becoming a parent is considered one of the maturational crises of adult life, and as such it is a time of intense learning for both parents and those close to them. The prenatal period provides a unique opportunity for nurses and other members of the health care team to influence family health. During this period, essentially healthy women seek regular care and guidance. The nurse's

health promotion interventions can affect the well-being of the woman, her unborn child, and the rest of her family for many years to come.

Regular prenatal visits, ideally beginning soon after the first missed menstrual period, offer opportunities to ensure the health of the expectant mother and her infant. Prenatal health care permits diagnosis and treatment of maternal disorders that may have preexisted or may develop during the pregnancy. Care is designed to monitor the growth and development of the fetus and to identify abnormalities that may interfere with the course of normal labor. The woman and her family can seek support for stress and learn parenting skills.

Pregnancy spans 9 calendar months, 10 lunar months, or approximately 40 weeks. Pregnancy is divided into three 3-month periods called **trimesters.** The first trimester lasts from weeks 1 through 13; the second, weeks 14 through 26; the third, weeks 27 through term gestation (38 to 40 weeks). The focus of this chapter is on meeting the health needs of the expectant family over the prenatal period.

DIAGNOSIS OF PREGNANCY

Women may suspect pregnancy when they miss a menstrual period. Many women come to the first prenatal visit after a positive home pregnancy test. However, the clinical diagnosis of pregnancy before the second missed period may be difficult in some women. Physical variability, lack of relaxation, obesity, or tumors, for example, may confound even the experienced obstetrician or midwife. Accuracy is important, however, because emotional, social, medical, or legal consequences of an inaccurate diagnosis, either positive or negative, can be extremely serious. A correct date for the last (normal) menstrual period (LMP), the date of intercourse, and a basal body temperature (BBT) record may be of great value in the accurate diagnosis of pregnancy.

Signs and Symptoms

Great variability is possible in the subjective and objective symptoms of pregnancy. Therefore the diagnosis of pregnancy may be uncertain for a time. Many of the indicators of pregnancy are clinically useful in the diagnosis of pregnancy, and they are classified as presumptive, probable, or positive.

Presumptive indicators of pregnancy include subjective symptoms and objective signs. Subjective symptoms may include amenorrhea, nausea and vomiting **(morning sickness),** breast fullness and sensitivity, urinary frequency, lassitude or fatigue, weight gain, and mood swings. Quickening may be noted between weeks 16 and 20. Objective signs include a variety of physical changes including elevation of BBT, skin changes such as striae gravidarum and deeper pigmentation of the face and abdomen (chloasma, linea nigra), breast changes, abdominal enlargement, and changes in the uterus and vagina.

The *presumptive indicators of pregnancy* can be caused by conditions other than gestation. Therefore these signs alone are not reliable for diagnosis. For example, amenorrhea may be caused by an endocrine disorder; lassitude and fatigue may signify anemia or infection; fibroids may cause enlargement of the uterus; and nausea or vomiting may be caused by a gastrointestinal upset or allergy.

Probable indicators of pregnancy are observed by an examiner. When combined with presumptive signs and symptoms, they strongly suggest pregnancy. Objective signs include uterine enlargement, Braxton Hicks contractions, uterine souffle, ballottement, and positive pregnancy test results. The positive indicators of pregnancy are the presence of a fetal heartbeat distinct from that of the mother, fetal movement felt by someone other than the mother, and visualization of the fetus with a technique such as ultrasound (Scott et al., 1994). See also Table 8-2.

Estimating Date of Birth

Following the diagnosis of pregnancy the woman's first question usually concerns when she will give birth. This date has traditionally been termed the estimated date of confinement (EDC). To promote a more positive perception of both pregnancy and birth, however, the term **estimated date of birth (EDB)** is usually used. Because the precise date of conception generally is unknown, several formulas or rules of thumb have been suggested for calculating the EDB. None of these guides are infallible, but **Nägele's rule** is reasonably accurate and is the method usually used.

Nägele's rule is as follows: add 7 days to the first day of the LMP, subtract 3 months, and add 1 year. For example, if the first day of the LMP was July 10, 1998, the EDB is April 17, 1999. In simple terms, add 7 days to the LMP and count forward 9 months. Nägele's rule assumes that the woman has a 28-day cycle and that the pregnancy occurred on the fourteenth day. An adjustment is in order if the cycle is longer or shorter than 28 days. With the use of Nägele's rule, only about 4% to 10% of pregnant women give birth spontaneously on the EDB. Most women give birth during the period extending from 7 days before to 7 days after the EDB.

ADAPTATION TO PREGNANCY

Pregnancy affects all family members, and each family member must adapt to the pregnancy and interpret its meaning in light of his or her own needs. This process of family adaptation to pregnancy takes place within a cultural environment that is influenced by societal trends. Dramatic changes have occurred in Western society in recent years, and the nurse must be prepared to support single-parent families, reconstituted families, and dual-career families, as well as traditional families in the childbirth experience.

Much of the research on family dynamics in pregnancy and childbirth preparation in the United States and Canada has been done with white, middle-class families, and findings may not apply to families who do not fit the traditional American model. The terms spouse, husband, and wife, for example, are used consistently in family literature. The nurse may have to adapt these terms to apply to corresponding roles in many expectant families.

Maternal Adaptation

Women of all ages use the months of pregnancy to adapt to the maternal role, a complex process of social and cognitive learning. Early in pregnancy nothing seems to be happening, and much time is spent sleeping. With the perception of fetal movement in the second trimester, the woman turns her attention inward to her pregnancy and to relationships with her mother and other women who have been or who are pregnant.

Pregnancy is a maturational crisis that can be stressful but rewarding as the woman prepares for a new level of caring and responsibility. Her self-concept changes in readiness for parenthood as she prepares for her new role. Gradually, she moves from being self-contained and independent to being committed to a lifelong concern for another human being. This growth requires mastery of certain developmental tasks: accepting the pregnancy, identifying with the role of mother, reordering the relationships between herself and her mother and between herself and her partner, establishing a relationship with the unborn child, and preparing for the birth experience (Wayland & Tate, 1993; Zachariah, 1994). The partner's emotional support is an important factor in the successful accomplishment of these developmental tasks.

Accepting the pregnancy

The first step in adapting to the maternal role is accepting the idea of pregnancy and assimilating the pregnant state into the woman's way of life (Mercer, 1995). The degree of acceptance is reflected in the woman's readiness for pregnancy and her emotional responses.

Many women are dismayed initially at finding themselves pregnant. However, eventual acceptance of pregnancy parallels the growing acceptance of the reality of a child. Nonacceptance of the pregnancy should not be equated with rejection of the child. A woman may dislike being pregnant but feel love for the child to be born.

Women who are happy and pleased about their pregnancy often view it as biologic fulfillment and part of their life plan. They have high self-esteem and tend to be confident about outcomes for themselves, their babies, and other family members.

Although a general state of well-being predominates, many women are surprised to experience **emotional lability,** the rapid and unpredictable changes in mood. These swings in emotions and increased sensitivity to others are disconcerting to the expectant mother and those around her. Increased irritability, explosions of tears and anger, and feelings of great joy and cheerfulness alternate, apparently with little or no provocation.

Profound hormonal changes that are part of the maternal response to pregnancy may be responsible for mood changes, much as they are before menstruation or during menopause. Other reasons such as sexual concerns or fear of pain during the birth have also been postulated to explain this seemingly erratic behavior.

Pregnant women are affected emotionally by changes that occur in the physical contours and functions of their bodies. During the first trimester body shape changes little, but by the second trimester obvious bulging of the abdomen, thickening of the waist, and enlargement of the breasts proclaim the state of pregnancy. The woman develops a feeling of an overall increase in the size of her body and of occupying more space.

The woman's attitude about her body is thought to be influenced by her values and personality traits. This attitude often changes as pregnancy progresses. A positive body attitude usually is expressed during the first trimester. As the pregnancy advances, however, the feelings become more negative. For most women the feeling of liking or not liking their bodies in the pregnant state is temporary and does not cause permanent changes in their self-perceptions.

Most women experience ambivalent feelings during pregnancy. **Ambivalence,** having conflicting feelings simultaneously, is considered a normal response for people preparing for a new role. During pregnancy, women may, for example, feel great pleasure that they are fulfilling a lifelong dream, but they also may feel great regret that life as they now know it is ending.

Even women who are pleased to be pregnant may experience feelings of hostility toward the pregnancy or unborn child from time to time. Such things as a partner's chance remark about the attractiveness of a slim, nonpregnant woman or news of a colleague's promotion if her decision to have a child means relinquishing a job can give rise to ambivalent feelings. Body sensations, feelings of dependence, or the realization of the responsibilities of child care also can trigger such feelings.

Intense feelings of ambivalence that persist through the third trimester may indicate an unresolved conflict with the motherhood role (Mercer, 1995). After the birth of a healthy child, however, memories of these ambivalent feelings usually are dismissed. If the child is born with a defect, however, a woman may look back at the times when she did not want the child and feel intensely guilty. She may believe that her ambivalence caused the birth defect. She will then need assurance that her feelings were not responsible for the problem.

Identifying with mother role

The process of identifying with the mother role begins early in each woman's life at the time she is being mothered as a child. Her social group's perception of what constitutes the feminine role can subsequently influence her toward choosing between motherhood or a career, being married or single, or being independent rather than interdependent. Practice roles, such as playing with dolls, baby-sitting, and taking care of siblings, may increase her understanding of what being a mother entails.

Many women have always wanted a baby, liked children, and looked forward to motherhood. Their high motivation to become a parent promotes acceptance of pregnancy and eventual prenatal and parental adaptation. Other women apparently have not considered in any detail what motherhood means to them. During pregnancy conflicts such as not wanting the pregnancy and child-related or career-related decisions need to be resolved.

Reordering personal relationships

Close relationships held by the pregnant woman undergo change during pregnancy as she prepares emotionally for the new role of mother. As family members learn their new roles, periods of tension and conflict may occur. An understanding of the typical patterns of adjustment can help the nurse to reassure the pregnant woman and explore issues related to social support. Promoting effective communication patterns between the expectant mother and her own mother and between the expectant mother and her partner are common nursing interventions provided during the prenatal visits.

The woman's relationship with her mother is significant in adaptation to pregnancy and motherhood. Important components in the pregnant woman's relationship with her mother are the mother's availability (past and present), her reactions to the daughter's pregnancy, respect for her daughter's autonomy, and the willingness to reminisce (Mercer, 1995).

The mother's reaction to the daughter's pregnancy signifies her acceptance of the grandchild and of her daughter. If the mother is supportive, the daughter has an opportunity to discuss pregnancy and labor and her feelings of joy or ambivalence with a knowledgeable and accepting woman. Rubin (1975) noted that if the pregnant woman's mother is not pleased with the pregnancy, the daughter begins to have doubts about her self-worth and the eventual acceptance of her child by others.

Mothers who respect their daughters' autonomy prompt feelings of self-confidence in their daughters. Parents who have helped their adult children become independent are seen as being willing to help rather than interfering or dominating (Fig. 10-1).

Reminiscing about the pregnant woman's early childhood and sharing the grandmother-to-be's account of her childbirth experience help the daughter anticipate and prepare for labor and birth. Hearing about themselves as young children makes pregnant women feel loved and wanted. They draw closer to their parents and begin to feel that, despite the errors they might make in their own mothering experiences, they will continue to be loved by their children.

Although the woman's relationship with her mother is significant in considering her adaptation in pregnancy, the most important person to the pregnant woman is usually the father of her child. A woman who is nurtured by her partner during pregnancy has fewer emotional and physical symptoms, fewer labor and childbirth complications, and an

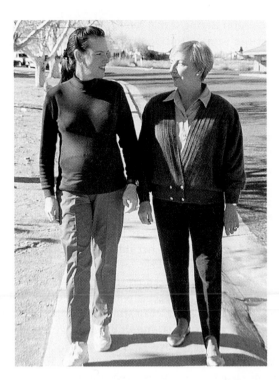

Fig. **10-1** A pregnant woman and her mother enjoying their walk together. (Courtesy Michael S. Clement, MD, Mesa, Ariz.)

easier postpartum adjustment. Women express two major needs within this relationship during pregnancy: feeling loved and valued and having the child accepted by the partner (Richardson, 1983).

The marital or committed relationship is not static but evolves over time. The addition of a child changes forever the nature of the bond between partners. Couples grow closer during pregnancy, and pregnancy has a maturing effect on the partners' relationship as they assume new roles and discover new aspects of one another. Partners who trust and support each other are able to share mutual-dependency needs (Mercer, 1995).

Sexual expression during pregnancy is highly individual. The sexual relationship is affected by physical, emotional, and interactional factors, including myths about sex during pregnancy, sexual dysfunction, and physical changes in the woman.

Myths about body functions and fantasies about the influence of the fetus as a third party in lovemaking are commonly expressed. An individual may also inaccurately attribute anomalies, mental retardation, and other injuries to the mother and fetus to sexual relations during pregnancy. Some couples fear that the woman's genitals will be drastically changed by the birth process. Couples may not express their concerns to the health care provider because of embarrassment or because they do not want to appear foolish.

Discomfort during sexual activity may be caused by pressure on the woman's abdomen and deep penetration or thrusting. Postcoital cramping and backache may occur (see Sexual Counseling, p. 241).

As pregnancy progresses, changes in body shape, body image, and levels of discomfort influence both partners' desire for sexual expression. During the first trimester the woman's sexual desire may decrease, especially if she experiences breast tenderness, nausea, fatigue, or sleepiness. As she progresses into the second trimester, however, her sense of well-being combined with the increased pelvic congestion that occurs at this time may increase her desire for sexual release. In the third trimester, somatic complaints and physical bulkiness may increase her physical discomfort and diminish her interest in sex (Rynerson & Lowdermilk, 1993).

Partners need to feel free to discuss their sexual responses during pregnancy. Their sensitivity to each other and willingness to share concerns can strengthen their sexual relationship. Partners who do not understand the rapid physiologic and emotional changes of pregnancy can become confused by the other's behavior. By talking to each other about the changes they are experiencing, couples can define problems and then offer the needed support. Nurses can facilitate communication between partners by talking to expectant couples about possible changes in feelings and behaviors they may experience as pregnancy progresses (Rynerson & Lowdermilk, 1993).

Establishing relationship with the fetus

Emotional **attachment** to the child begins during the prenatal period as women use fantasizing and daydreaming to prepare themselves for motherhood (Rubin, 1975). They think of themselves as mothers and imagine maternal qualities they would like to possess. Expectant parents desire to be warm, loving, and close to their child. They try to anticipate changes in their lives that the child will bring and wonder how they will react to noise, disorder, less freedom, and caregiving activities. The mother-child relationship progresses through pregnancy as a developmental process. Three phases in the developmental pattern become apparent.

In Phase 1 the woman accepts the biologic fact of pregnancy. She needs to be able to state, "I am pregnant" and incorporate the idea of a child into her body and self-image.

Early in pregnancy the mother's thoughts center around herself and the immediate reality of the pregnancy itself. The child is viewed as part of herself, and most women think of their fetus as unreal during the early period of pregnancy (Lumley, 1980, 1982).

In Phase 2 the woman accepts the growing fetus as distinct from herself and as a person to nurture. She can now say, "I am going to have a baby." By the fifth month, there usually is a growing awareness of the child as a separate being. This differentiation of the child from the woman's

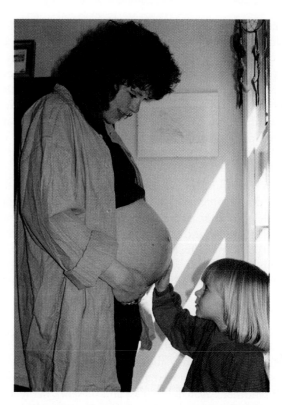

Fig. **10-2** Sibling feeling movement of fetus. (Courtesy Kim Molloy, San Jose, Calif.)

self permits the beginning of the mother-child relationship that involves not only caring but also responsibility. Women whose pregnancies are planned are pleased with their pregnancy and develop attachment to the child earlier than other women (Koniak-Griffin, 1988).

With acceptance of the reality of the child (hearing the heartbeat and feeling the child move) and an overall feeling of well-being, the woman enters a quiet period and becomes more introspective. A fantasy child becomes precious to the woman. As the woman seems to withdraw and to concentrate her interest on the unborn child, her partner sometimes feels left out. If there are children in the family, they may become more demanding in their efforts to redirect the mother's attention to themselves.

During Phase 3 of the attachment process, the woman prepares realistically for the birth and parenting of the child. She expresses the thought "I am going to be a mother" and defines the nature and characteristics of the child. She may, for example, speculate about the child's sex and personality traits based on patterns of fetal activity.

Although the mother alone experiences the child within, both parents and siblings believe the unborn child responds in a very individualized, personal manner. Family members may interact a great deal with the unborn child by talking to the fetus and stroking the mother's abdomen, especially when the fetus shifts position (Fig. 10-2). More research is necessary to help nurses understand the factors that promote early attachment and the benefits of those feelings.

Preparing for childbirth

Many women actively prepare for birth. They read books, view films, attend parenting classes, and talk to other women. They seek the best caregiver possible for advice, monitoring, and caring (Patterson, Freese & Goldenberg, 1990). The multipara has her own history of labor and birth, which influences her approach to preparation for this childbirth experience.

Anxiety can arise from concern about a safe passage for herself and her child during the birth process (Mercer, 1995; Rubin, 1975). This concern may not be expressed overtly, but cues are given as the nurse listens to plans women make for care of the new baby and other children in case "anything should happen." These feelings persist despite statistical evidence about the safe outcome of pregnancy for mothers and their infants. Many women fear the pain of childbirth or mutilation because they do not understand anatomy and the birth process. Education by the nurse can alleviate many of these fears. Women also express concern over what behaviors are appropriate during the birth process and how the persons who will be caring for them will accept them and their actions. The best preparation for labor is "a healthy sense of the realistic— an awareness of work, pain, and risk balanced by a sense of excitement and expectation of the final reward" (Lederman, 1984).

Toward the end of the third trimester breathing is difficult and movements of the fetus become vigorous enough to disturb the mother's sleep. Backaches, frequency and urgency of urination, constipation, and varicose veins can become troublesome. The bulkiness and awkwardness of her body interfere with the woman's ability to care for other children, perform routine work-related duties, and assume a comfortable position for sleep and rest. By this time most women become impatient for labor to begin, whether the birth is anticipated with joy, dread, or a mixture of both. A strong desire to see the end of pregnancy, to be over and done with it, makes women at this stage ready to move on to childbirth.

Paternal Adaptation

The father's beliefs and feelings about the ideal mother and father and his cultural expectation of appropriate behavior during pregnancy affect his response to his partner's need for him. One man may engage in nurturing behavior. Another may feel lonely and alienated as the woman becomes physically and emotionally engrossed in the unborn child. He may seek comfort and understanding outside the home or become interested in a new hobby or involved with his work. Some men view pregnancy as proof of their masculinity and their dominant role. To others, pregnancy has no meaning in terms of responsibility to either mother or child. However, for most men pregnancy can be a time of preparation for the parental role with intense learning.

Accepting the pregnancy

The ways fathers adjust to the parental role is the subject of increasing research (Holditch-Davis et al., 1994; Jordan, 1990; Palkovitz, 1992). In older societies the man enacted the ritual **couvade;** that is, he behaved in specific ways and respected taboos associated with pregnancy and giving birth. In this way the man's new status was recognized and endorsed. His behavior acknowledged his psychosocial and biologic relationship to the mother and child. In Western societies the participation of fathers in childbirth has risen dramatically over the past 20 years, and the father in the role of labor coach is common.

A man's readiness for fatherhood may be reflected in the way he views the couple's relative financial security and the stability of their relationship and in the way he deals with the realization that the upcoming birth marks the end of the childless period. Many men express concern for the family's economic security. Today most young married women are employed outside the home but have a phase of unemployment for childbearing and child care. The length of unemployment is determined by the couple's economic status, the policies of the woman's employer, and the couple's value system. Some men compensate for anticipated needs by keeping their current jobs even though they had planned a change, by working overtime, or by taking on extra work. Some men acquire new or additional insurance at this time.

The man's emotional responses to becoming a father, his concerns, and informational needs change during the course of pregnancy. Phases of the developmental pattern become apparent. May (1982b) described three phases characterizing the three developmental tasks experienced by the expectant father: the announcement phase, the moratorium phase, and the focusing phase.

The early period, the announcement phase, may last from a few hours to a few weeks. The developmental task is to accept the biologic fact of pregnancy. Men react to the confirmation of pregnancy with joy or dismay, depending on whether the pregnancy is desired or unplanned or unwanted.

If pregnancy is unplanned or unwanted, some men find the alterations in life plans and lifestyles difficult to accept. Some men engage in extramarital affairs for the first time during their partner's pregnancy. Others batter their partners (McFarlane et al., 1992).

The second phase, the moratorium phase, is the period when he adjusts to the reality of pregnancy. The developmental task is to accept the pregnancy. Men appear to put conscious thought of the pregnancy aside for a time. They become more introspective and engage in many discussions about their philosophy of life, religion, childbearing, and child-rearing practices and their relationships with family members and friends. Depending on the man's readiness for the pregnancy, this phase may be relatively short or persist until the last trimester.

The third phase, called the focusing phase, begins in the last trimester and is characterized by the father's active involvement in both the pregnancy and his relationship with his child. The developmental task is to negotiate with his partner the role he is to play in labor and to prepare for parenthood. In this phase the man concentrates on his experience of the pregnancy and begins to think of himself as a father.

Men are involved in pregnancy in a variety of ways. May (1980, 1982a) described three styles of involvement in the pregnancy exhibited by men during their wives' first pregnancy: the observer style, the expressive style, and the instrumental style.

The observer style is exhibited by those fathers who are happy about the pregnancy and supportive of their wives. However, because of cultural values or shyness, they avoid involvement in activities such as parent education classes, decisions about breastfeeding, or the choice of professional care. Other fathers who are ambivalent about pregnancy and the role of father need time to adjust to the idea of pregnancy and fatherhood. Some men cope by becoming involved in careers and resisting their wives' attempts to involve them in preparations for the coming child.

Men who show the expressive style display a strong emotional response to pregnancy and a desire to be a full partner in the project (Fig. 10-3). These men are aware of their partner's needs for support. They experience the same emotional lability and ambivalence as that experienced by

pregnant women. Some fathers report having physical discomforts such as nausea and fatigue usually experienced by pregnant women (Klein, 1991). The psychosomatic symptoms of expectant fathers have long been recognized as a phenomenon of expectant fatherhood.

The instrumental style is adopted by men who see tasks they can perform in their role as manager of the pregnancy. They ask questions; are interested in the role of labor coach; and plan for photographs during pregnancy, birth, and the neonatal period. They feel responsible for the outcome of pregnancy and are protective and supportive of their wives.

The three styles of involvement provide examples of the different ways men can experience pregnancy. Each man needs to feel free to define his role in pregnancy, just as the woman does. Because of cultural conditioning, personality, or a different supportive style, however, not all men are able or willing to attend childbirth classes or act as labor coaches. More research is needed to determine whether similar styles of involvement occur in the partners of multiparous women, in men from various cultural groups, and in same-sex partners, and what the effects on the relationship are when the partners' expectations do not coincide.

Identifying with father role

Each father brings to pregnancy attitudes that affect the way in which he adjusts to the pregnancy and parental role. His memories of the fathering he received from his own father, the experiences he has had with child care, and the perceptions of the male and father roles within his social group will guide his selection of the tasks and responsibilities he will assume. Some men are highly motivated to nurture and love a child. They may be excited and pleased about the anticipated role of father. Others may be more detached or even hostile to the idea of fatherhood.

Reordering personal relationships

The partner's main role in pregnancy is to nurture and respond to the pregnant woman's feelings of vulnerability. The partner must also deal with the reality of the pregnancy (Jordan, 1990). The partner's support indicates involvement in the pregnancy and preparation for attachment to the child.

Some aspects of a partner's behavior indicate rivalry. Direct rivalry with the fetus may be evident, especially during sexual activity. Men may protest that fetal movements prevent sexual gratification or that they are being watched by the fetus during sexual activity.

The woman's increased introspection may cause her partner to feel uneasy as she becomes preoccupied with thoughts of the child and of her motherhood, with her growing dependence on her physician or midwife, and with her reevaluation of the couple's relationship.

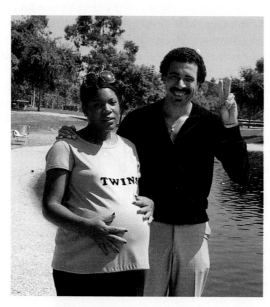

Fig. **10-3** Mother and father walk together. Women respond positively to their partner's interest and concern. (Courtesy Marjorie Pyle, RNC, Lifecircle, Costa Mesa, Calif.)

Deciding on the infant's feeding method is of concern when the partners' preferences differ or one partner has intense opinions about a method. The recognized benefits and disadvantages of one method over another appear to be irrelevant. Some partners insist that the woman breastfeed; others are adamantly opposed to breastfeeding. If one partner refuses to voice an opinion, the other may experience uneasiness or uncertainty.

Establishing relationship with the fetus

The father-child attachment can be as strong as the mother-child relationship, and fathers can be as competent as mothers in nurturing their infants. The father-child attachment also begins during pregnancy. A father may rub or kiss the maternal abdomen, try to listen to the fetus, or play with the fetus as he notes fetal movement.

Men prepare for fatherhood in many of the same ways as women do for motherhood—by reading, fantasizing, and daydreaming about the baby. They may adjust work commitments or plan vacations so that they can spend time with their new family.

Daydreaming about their role as father is common in the last weeks before the birth; men rarely describe their daydreams unless they are reassured that such daydreams are normal.

Nurses can help fathers identify concerns and prepare for the reality of a baby by asking questions such as the following:

- What do you expect the baby to look and act like?
- What do you think being a father will be like?
- Have you thought about the baby's crying? Changing diapers? Burping the baby? Being awakened at night? Sharing your partner with the baby?

The father may not wish to answer such questions when they are asked but may need time to think them through or discuss them with his partner.

If an expectant father can only imagine an older child and has difficulty visualizing or talking about an infant, this situation needs to be explored. The nurse can tell the father about the unborn child's ability to respond to light, sound, and touch and encourage him to feel and talk to the fetus. Plans for seeing, holding, and examining the newborn can be made.

As the birth day approaches, fathers have more questions about fetal and newborn behaviors. Some fathers are shocked or amazed at how small the clothes and furniture for the baby are.

Some fathers become involved by picking the child's name and anticipating the child's sex, if it is not already known. Some couples select the name of the child as early as the first month of pregnancy. Family tradition, religious customs, and the continuation of the parent's name or names of relatives or friends are important in the selection process.

At the time of birth, most parents are able to accept the sex of the child, but occasionally show or voice disappoint-ment. The parents may experience a grief reaction and sense of loss at birth as they release their fantasized image of the child and begin to accept the real child. These negative responses toward a normal, healthy baby may be difficult for nurses to understand. However, most such responses are temporary. Providing an accepting environment for parental reactions will facilitate the parent's ability to move beyond disappointment to acceptance.

Preparing for childbirth

The days and weeks immediately before the expected day of birth are characterized by anticipation and anxiety. Boredom and restlessness are common as the couple focuses on the birth process.

During the last 2 months of pregnancy, many expectant fathers experience a surge of creative energy at home and on the job. They may become dissatisfied with their present living space. If possible, they tend to act on the need to alter the environment. This activity may be overt evidence of his sharing in the childbearing experience but doing so by channeling the anxiety or other feelings experienced during the final weeks before birth into other productive activities. This behavior earns recognition and compliments from friends, relatives, and the partner.

The father's anxieties may also be expressed by his refusal to think about the birth, planning other activities during his partner's labor, or sleeping and resting to the exclusion of all else. The expectant mother may become concerned about possibly being deserted physically or emotionally at a time when she is feeling most vulnerable.

The father's major concerns are getting the mother to a medical facility in time for the birth and not appearing ignorant. Many fathers want to be able to recognize labor and determine when it is appropriate to leave for the hospital or call the physician or midwife. They may fantasize different situations and plan what they will do in response to them, or they may rehearse taking various routes to the hospital, timing each route at different times of the day.

Many fathers have questions about the labor suite's furniture, nursing staff, and location, as well as the availability of the physician and anesthesiologist. Others want to know what is expected of them when their partners are in labor. The father may also have fears concerning safe passage of his partner and the mutilation and death of his partner and child. While he harbors these fears, he cannot help his mate deal with her own unspoken or overt apprehension.

With the exception of childbirth preparation classes, a father has few opportunities to learn ways to be an involved and active partner in this rite of passage into parenthood. The tensions and apprehensions of the unprepared, unsupportive father are readily transmitted to the mother and may increase her fears. His own self-doubts and fear of inadequacy may be realized if he is not supported. Self-confidence comes from achieving realistic goals and earning the approval of others.

The same fears, questions, and concerns may affect birth partners who are not the biologic fathers. Birth partners need to be kept informed, supported, and included in all activities in which the mother desires their participation.

Sibling Adaptation

Sharing the spotlight with a new brother or sister may be the first major crisis for a child. The older child often experiences a sense of loss or feels jealous at being "replaced" by the new sibling. Some of the factors that influence the child's response are age, the parents' attitudes, the role of the father, the length of separation from the mother, the hospital's visitation policy, and the way the child has been prepared for the change (Mackey & Miller, 1992).

The mother with other children must devote time and effort to reorganizing her relationships with existing children. She needs to prepare siblings for the birth of the child (Fig. 10-4 and Box 10-1) and begin the process of role tran-

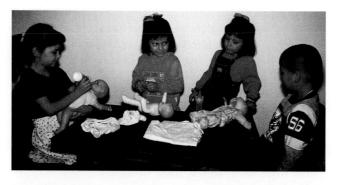

Fig. 10-4 Sibling class of preschoolers learning infant care using dolls. (Courtesy Michael S. Clement, MD, Mesa, Ariz.)

sition in the family by including the children in the pregnancy and being sympathetic to older children's protests against losing their places in the family hierarchy. No child willingly gives up a familiar position.

Siblings' responses to pregnancy vary with their age and dependency needs. The 1-year-old infant seems largely unaware of the process, but the 2-year-old child notices the change in his or her mother's appearance and may comment that "Mommy's fat." The 2-year-old child's need for sameness in the environment makes the child aware of any change. Toddlers may exhibit more "clinging" behavior and revert to dependent behaviors in toilet training or eating.

By the third or fourth year of age children like to be told the story of their own beginning and accept its being compared to the present pregnancy. They like to listen to heartbeats and feel the baby moving in utero (see Fig. 10-2). Sometimes they worry about how the baby is being fed and what it wears.

School-age children take a more clinical interest in their mother's pregnancy. They may want to know in more detail, "How did the baby get in there?" and "How will it get out?" Children in this age group notice pregnant women in stores, churches, and schools and sometimes seem shy if they need to approach a pregnant woman directly. On the whole they look forward to the new baby, see themselves as "mothers" or "fathers," and enjoy buying baby supplies and readying a place for the baby. Because they still think in concrete terms and base judgments on the here and now, they respond positively to their mother's current good health.

Early and middle adolescents preoccupied with the establishment of their own sexual identity may have difficulty

---

BOX 10-1　*Tips for Sibling Preparation*

PRENATAL

1. Take your child on a prenatal visit. Let the child listen to the fetal heart beat and feel the baby move.
2. Involve the child in preparations for the baby, such as helping decorate the baby's room.
3. Move the child to a bed (if still sleeping in a crib) at least 2 months before the baby is due.
4. Read books, show videos, and/or take child to sibling preparation classes, including a hospital tour.
5. Answer your child's questions about the coming birth, what babies are like, and any other questions.
6. Take your child to the homes of friends who have babies so that the child has realistic expectations of what babies are like.

DURING THE HOSPITAL STAY

1. Have someone bring the child to the hospital to visit you and the baby (unless you plan to have the child attend the birth).
2. Don't force interactions between the child and the baby. Often the child will be more interested in seeing you and being reassured of your love.

3. Help the child explore the infant by showing how and where to touch the baby.
4. Give the child a gift (from you or you, the father, and baby).

GOING HOME

1. Leave the child at home with a relative or baby-sitter.
2. Have someone else carry the baby from the car so that you can hug the child first.

ADJUSTMENT AFTER THE BABY IS HOME

1. Arrange for a special time with the child alone with each parent.
2. Don't exclude the child during infant feeding times. The child can sit with you and the baby and feed a doll or drink juice or milk with you or sit quietly with a game.
3. Prepare small gifts for the child so that when the baby gets gifts, the sibling won't feel left out. The child can also help open the baby gifts.
4. Praise the child for acting age appropriately (so that being a baby does not seem better than being older).

accepting the overwhelming evidence of the sexual activity of their parents. They reason that if they are too young for such activity, certainly their parents are too old. They seem to take on a critical parental role and may ask, "What will people think?" or "How can you let yourself get so fat?" Many pregnant women with teenage children will confess that the attitudes of their teenagers are the most difficult aspect in their current pregnancy.

Late adolescents do not appear to be unduly disturbed. They realize that they soon will be gone from home. Parents usually report they are comforting and act more as other adults than as children.

Grandparent Adaptation

Every pregnancy affects all family relationships. For expectant grandparents, a first pregnancy in a child is undeniable evidence that they are growing older. Many think of a grandparent as old, white-haired, and becoming feeble of mind and body; however, some people face grandparenthood while still in their 30s or 40s. A mother-to-be announcing her pregnancy to her mother may be greeted by a negative response that indicates that she is not ready to be a grandmother. Daughter and mother both may be startled and hurt by the response.

Some expectant grandparents not only are nonsupportive but also use subtle means to decrease the self-esteem of the young parents-to-be. Mothers may talk about their terrible pregnancies; fathers may discuss the endless cost of rearing children; and mothers-in-law may complain that their sons are neglecting them because their concern is now directed toward the pregnant daughters-in-law.

However, most grandparents are delighted at the prospect of a new baby in the family. It reawakens the feelings of their own youth, the excitement of giving birth, and their delight in the behavior of the parents-to-be when they were infants. They set up a memory store of the child's first smiles, first words, and first steps, which they can use later for "claiming" the newborn as a member of the family. Their and the parents' satisfaction comes with the realization that the continuity between past and present is guaranteed.

In addition, the grandparent is the historian who transmits the family history, a resource person who shares knowledge based on experience; a role model; and a support person. The grandparent's presence and support can strengthen family systems by widening the circle of support and nurturance (Fig. 10-5). Other sources of information cannot replace the unique contribution that grandparents make. The parent in turn acts as a negotiator in establishing the grandparent-grandchild relationship.

Many women report that their pregnancies bridged the final gap between them and their own mothers. The estrangement that began in adolescence disappears as the now-pregnant daughter experiences joys, concerns, and anxieties similar to those her mother felt before her.

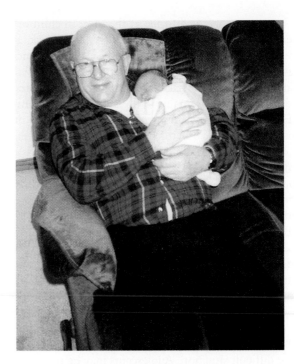

Fig. 10-5 Grandfather relaxing with grandson. (Courtesy Kathryn Schweer, Waterloo, Iowa.)

Expectant grandparenthood also can represent a maturational crisis for the parent of an expectant parent. To be truly family oriented, maternity care must include the grandparent in the implementation of the nursing process with childbearing families. A class for grandparents is one method of incorporating the grandparents into the family system and encouraging communication between the generations.

Grandparents' anxieties and concerns and their relationships with expectant parents and grandchildren should be discussed during courses for expectant parents. The expectant parents may use this opportunity to begin to resolve conflicts and perceived differences with their parents, a task that can also enhance their ability to relate to their own children.

Battering during Pregnancy

Pregnancy often is the beginning or escalation of violence (Chescheir, 1992). Besides physical abuse being harmful to the mother, the risk of fetal injury is very high. Studies have demonstrated that **battering** during pregnancy also results in a higher rate of low-birth-weight newborns and maternal complications of low weight gain, infections, and anemia. In addition, the woman may smoke or use alcohol or other drugs as means of coping (McFarlane, Parker & Soeken, 1996).

If the pregnant woman remains with her partner, she is at additional risk for repeated physical and psychologic trauma. The potential for child abuse is great, especially if the batterer's anger is directed at the unborn child or if he is jealous of the fetus (Campbell, Oliver & Bullock, 1993). After birth the mother may be so physically and emotionally drained that she may have difficulty bonding with her infant. She may be at risk of becoming an abusive mother whether or not she remains in the abusive relationship.

During pregnancy, the target body parts change during abusive episodes. Women report physical blows directed to the head, breasts, abdomen, and genitalia. Sexual assault is common (McFarlane, 1993). The battered pregnant woman should be treated as a high-risk obstetric patient because she is prone to anxiety, depression, alcohol and drug use, and inadequate and late prenatal care (Campbell et al., 1992).

Bullock (1993) reports pregnant women experience difficulties that may assist the nurse in identifying battering during pregnancy. These difficulties include consumption of an inadequate diet, lack of sleep, inadequate consumption of milk and milk products, and minimal forms of self-relaxation; in essence the battered pregnant woman may not take proper care of herself.

Battering and pregnancy in teenagers constitute a particularly difficult situation. Adolescents may be more trapped in the abusive relationship because of their inexperience. Many professionals and the adolescents themselves ignore the violence because it may not be believable, because relationships are transient, and because the jealous and controlling behavior is interpreted as love and devotion. Routine screening for abuse and sexual assault is recommended for pregnant adolescents (Parker, 1993). Because pregnancy in young adolescent girls is commonly the result of sexual abuse, the nurse should assess the desire to maintain the pregnancy. (See Chapter 4 for assessment for battering.)

I CARE MANAGEMENT

The professionals who provide health care for the pregnant woman and her family include nurses, physicians, midwives, nutritionists, and social workers. Collaboration among these individuals is necessary to provide holistic care. The case management model, which makes use of care maps and critical pathways, is one system that promotes comprehensive care with limited overlap in services. To emphasize the nursing role, care management here is organized around the central elements of the nursing process: assessment, nursing diagnoses, expected outcomes, plan of care and interventions, and evaluation.

Assessment and Nursing Diagnoses

Once the presence of pregnancy has been confirmed and the woman's desire to continue the pregnancy has been validated, prenatal care is begun. The assessment process begins at the initial prenatal visit and is continued throughout the pregnancy. Assessment techniques include the interview, physical examination, and laboratory tests. Because the initial visit and follow-up visits are distinctly different in content and process, they are described separately below.

Initial visit

The pregnant woman and family members who may be present should be told that the first prenatal visit is more lengthy and in-depth than future visits. The initial evaluation includes a comprehensive health history emphasizing the current pregnancy, previous pregnancies, the family, a psychosocial profile, a physical assessment, diagnostic testing, and an overall risk assessment. A prenatal history form (Fig. 10-6) is the best way to document information obtained. To be useful in communicating with other care providers, entries on the form should be made with attention to neatness and clarity. Some early teaching is provided at this time.

Interview. The therapeutic relationship between the nurse and the woman is established during the initial assessment interview. It is a time for planned, purposeful communication that focuses on specific content. The data collected are of two types: the woman's subjective appraisal of her health status and the nurse's objective observations. During the interview the nurse observes the woman's affect, posture, body language, skin color, and other physical and emotional signs.

Often the pregnant woman is accompanied by one or more family members. The nurse needs to build a relationship with these people as part of the social context of the patient. In addition, family members help recall and validate information related to the woman's health. With her permission, those accompanying the woman can be included in the initial prenatal interview, and the observations and information about the woman's family form part of the database (Fig. 10-7). For example, if the woman is accompanied by small children, the nurse can ask about her plans for child care during the time of labor and birth. Special needs are noted at this time (i.e., wheelchair access, assistance in getting on and off the examining table, cognitive deficits).

Reason for seeking care. Although pregnant women are scheduled for "routine" prenatal visits, they often come to the health care provider seeking information or reassurance about a particular concern. When the patient is asked a broad, open-ended question such as, "How have you been feeling?" she may reveal problems that could otherwise be overlooked. The woman's chief concerns should be recorded in her own words to alert other personnel to the priority of needs as identified by her. At the initial visit, the desire for information about what is normal in the course of pregnancy is typical.

Current pregnancy. The presumptive signs of pregnancy may be of great concern to the woman. A review of symptoms she is experiencing, and how she is coping with them, helps establish a database to develop a plan of care.

Obstetric/gynecologic history. Data are gathered on the woman's age at menarche, menstrual history, and contraceptive history; the nature of any infertility or gynecologic conditions (e.g., fibroids); her history of any sexually transmitted diseases (STDs); her sexual history; and the history of all her pregnancies, including the present pregnancy, and their outcomes. The date of the last Papanicolaou test and

FAIRFAX HOSPITAL

PRENATAL RECORD

Name		Religion	Date

Address		Telephone

Occupation	Business Address		Business Telephone

Husband's Name	Business Address		Business Telephone

Husband's Occupation		Referred by

Age	Gravida	Para	Term	Premature	Abortions	Living

LMP	PMP	Quickening	EDB

Significant History

Significant Findings

Date													
Wt. ( )													
BP													
Edema													
Ht. of Fundus													
Position													
FH	+	+	+	+	+	+	+	+	+	+	+	+	+
Urine	Sug/Pro												
Gestation													
Movement													
Initials													
RTC													

Blood Group	Rh	STS	Hgb. HCT.	Pap	HBsAg

Rubella	Glucola	Alpha Feto Protein	GC	HIV

PPD	Chest X-Ray	Vitamin Supplement	Breast Bottle	Anesthesia Preference	Pediatrician

PROBLEM LIST

☐ Family Planning Information

Form 922
R91

Fig. **10-6** Sample prenatal history form.

Continued

FAIRFAX HOSPITAL

PRENATAL RECORD Continuation

Name _____

PRESENT PREGNANCY

Nausea		Vomiting		Other Symptoms of Pregnancy		
Bleeding		Cramping		Pain		Edema
Pregnancy Test	Date					

PREVIOUS PREGNANCIES

No.	Date Delivered	Feeding	Sex	Wt.	Wks. Preg.	Condition Birth	Condition Now	Duration of Labor	Type of Delivery	Remarks
1										
2										
3										
4										
5										
6										

HISTORY

Menstruation Onset	Frequency	Duration	Flow	Pain
Usual Childhood Illnesses	Rheumatic Fever		Heart Disease	Pulmonary Disease
Convulsions	Venereal Disease		Allergies	Blood Transfusion
Injuries	Operations		Urinary Disease	
Alcohol	Smoking		Drugs	Medication

FAMILY HISTORY

Mother	Father	Siblings	Other
Diabetes		Twins	

PHYSICAL EXAMINATION

General	Ht.	BP	Eyes	Fundi
Ears	Mouth	Teeth	Throat	Thyroid
Chest	Breasts	Nipples	Heart	Lungs
Abdomen	Extremities			

Ext. Genitalia		Perineum	
Vagina		Cervix	
Uterus			
Adnexa			
BI c.m.	DC c.m.	Arch	
Sacrum		Spines	
Post. Sagittal	SS Ligaments	Coccyx	

_____ , MD
SIGNATURE   Form 923
                 R87

Fig. **10-6—Cont'd** Sample prenatal history form.

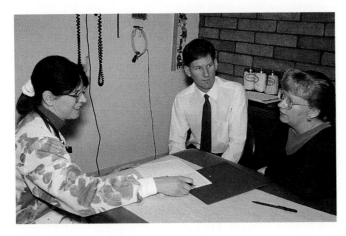

Fig. **10-7** Prenatal interview. (Courtesy Michael S. Clement, MD, Mesa, Ariz.)

the result are noted. The date of her LMP is obtained to establish the EDB. (See the Guidelines box.)

Medical history. The medical history includes those medical or surgical conditions that may affect the pregnancy or that may be affected by the pregnancy. For example, a pregnant woman who has diabetes or epilepsy requires special care. Because most women are anxious during the initial interview, the nurse's reference to cues, such as a Medic-Alert bracelet, prompts the woman to explain allergies, chronic diseases, or medications being taken (e.g., cortisone, insulin, or anticonvulsants).

The nature of previous surgical procedures should also be described. If a woman has undergone uterine surgery or extensive repair of the pelvic floor, a cesarean birth may be necessary; appendectomy rules out appendicitis as a cause of right lower quadrant pain; spinal surgery may contraindicate the use of spinal or epidural anesthesia. Any injury involving the pelvis is noted.

Often women who have chronic or handicapping conditions forget to mention them during the initial assessment because they have become so adapted to them. Special shoes or a limp may indicate the existence of a pelvic structural defect, which is an important consideration in pregnant women. The nurse who observes these special characteristics and inquires about them sensitively can obtain individualized data that will provide the basis for a comprehensive nursing care plan. Observations are vital components of the interview process because they prompt the nurse and woman to focus on the specific needs of the woman and her family.

Nutritional history. The woman's nutritional history is an important component of the prenatal history because her nutritional status has a direct effect on the growth and development of the fetus. A dietary assessment can reveal special diet practices, food allergies, eating behaviors, and other factors related to her nutritional status. Pregnant women are usually motivated to learn about good nutrition and respond well to the feedback regarding good nutrition generated by this assessment.

GUIDELINES/GUÍAS

Have you had a pregnancy test?
¿Se ha hecho la prueba de embarazo?

When was your last menstrual cycle?
¿Cuándo fue su última regla?

Have you been pregnant before?
¿Estuvo embarazada antes?

How many times?
¿Cuántas veces?

How many children do you have?
¿Cuántos hijos tiene usted?

Have you ever had a spontaneous abortion?
¿Ha tenido un aborto natural?

Have you ever had a therapeutic abortion?
¿Ha tenido un aborto provocado?

Have you ever had a stillborn?
¿Ha tenido un niño que nació muerto?

Have you ever had cesarean?
¿Ha tenido una cesárea?

Have you had any problems with past pregnancies?
¿Ha tenido algún problema en sus embarazos previos?

Do you take drugs? Prescription medicine?
¿Usa drogas? ¿Medicina recetada?

If so, which type of medicine do you use and for what?
¿Cuál medicina usa y para qué?

Do you drink alcohol? Do you smoke?
¿Toma licor o bebidas alcohólicas? ¿Fuma?

Drug use. A woman's past and present use of legal (over-the-counter [OTC], prescription, caffeine, alcohol, nicotine) and illegal (marijuana, cocaine, heroin) drugs needs to be assessed because many substances cross the placenta and may therefore harm the developing fetus. Periodic urine toxicology screening tests are often recommended during the pregnancies of women who have a history of illegal drug use.

Family history. The family history provides information about the woman's immediate family, including parents, siblings, and children. These data help identify familial or genetic disorders or conditions that could affect the present health status of the woman or her fetus.

Social and experiential history. Situational factors such as the family's ethnic and cultural background and socioeconomic status are determined during the social and experiential history-taking. The following information may be obtained over several encounters. The woman's perception of this pregnancy is explored by asking her such questions as the following: Is this pregnancy wanted or not, planned or not? Is the woman pleased, displeased, accepting, or nonaccepting? What problems may arise because of the pregnancy: financial, career, and living accommodations? The family support system is determined by asking her such questions as the following: What primary support is available to her? Are changes needed to promote adequate support? What are the existing relationships among the mother, father/partner, siblings, and in-laws? What preparations are being made for her care and that of dependent family members during labor and for the care of the infant after birth? Is community support needed, for example, financial or educational? What are the woman's ideas about childbearing, her expectations of the infant's behavior, and her outlook on life and the female role? Other such questions that need to be asked include: What does the woman think it will be like to have a baby in the home? How is her life going to change by having a baby? What plans does having a baby interrupt? During interviews throughout the pregnancy the nurse should remain alert to the appearance of potential parenting problems, such as depression, lack of family support, and inadequate living conditions. The nurse needs to assess what the woman's attitude toward health care is, particularly during childbearing; what she expects of the health care provider; and her view of the relationship between the woman and nurse.

Coping mechanisms and patterns of interacting are also identified. Early in the pregnancy the nurse should determine the woman's knowledge of pregnancy; maternal changes; fetal growth; self-care; and care of the newborn, including feeding. Asking about attitudes toward unmedicated or medicated childbirth and about her knowledge of the availability of parenting skills classes is important. Before planning for nursing care the nurse needs information about the woman's decision-making abilities and living habits (e.g., exercise, sleep, diet, diversional interests, personal hygiene, clothing). Common stressors during childbearing that have been identified include the baby's welfare, labor and birth process, behaviors of the newborn, woman's relationship with the baby's father, changes in body image, and physical symptoms (Affonso & Mayberry, 1990).

Attitudes concerning the range of acceptable sexual behavior during pregnancy should also be explored by asking questions such as the following: What has your family (partner, friends) told you about sex during pregnancy? The woman's sexual self-concept is given more emphasis by asking questions such as the following: How do you feel about the changes in your appearance? How does your partner feel about your body now? Do maternity clothes make pregnant women attractive?

All women should be assessed for a history or risk of physical abuse, particularly because the likelihood of abuse can increase during pregnancy. Although visual cues from the woman's appearance or behavior may suggest the possibility, if questioning is limited to those women who fit the supposed profile of the battered woman, many women will be missed (McFarlane et al., 1992; Norton et al., 1995; Stewart & Cecutti, 1993).

Review of systems. During this portion of the interview, the woman is asked to identify and describe preexisting or concurrent problems with any of the body systems, and her mental status is assessed. The woman is questioned about physical symptoms she has experienced, such as shortness of breath or pain. Pregnancy affects and is affected by all body systems; therefore information on the present status of the body systems is important in planning care. For each sign or symptom described, the following additional data should be obtained: body location, quality, quantity, chronology, setting, aggravating or alleviating factors, and associated manifestations (onset, character, course) (Seidel et al., 1998).

Physical examination. The initial physical examination provides the baseline for assessing subsequent changes. The examiner should determine the patient's needs for basic information regarding the structure of the genital organs and provide this information, along with a demonstration of the equipment that may be used and an explanation of the procedure itself. The interaction requires an unhurried, sensitive, and gentle approach with a matter-of-fact attitude.

The physical examination begins with assessment of vital signs including blood pressure, height, and weight. The bladder should be empty before pelvic examination.

Each examiner develops a routine for proceeding with the physical examination; most choose the head-to-toe progression. Heart and breath sounds are evaluated, and extremities are examined. Distribution, amount, and quality of body hair is of particular importance because the findings reflect nutritional status, endocrine function, and general emphasis on hygiene. The thyroid gland is assessed carefully. The height of the fundus is noted if the first examination is done after the first trimester of pregnancy. The typical basic examination is usually completed without much discomfort for the healthy woman. During the examination, the examiner needs to remain alert to the woman's clues that give direction to the remainder of the assessment and that indicate imminent untoward response such as supine hypotension. See Chapter 5 for a detailed description of the physical examination.

Whenever a pelvic examination is performed, the tone of the pelvic musculature and the need for the woman's knowledge of Kegel exercises (p. 229) are assessed. Particular attention is paid to the size of the uterus because this is an indication of the timing of gestation. The nurse present during the examination can coach the woman in breathing and relaxation techniques at this time, as needed.

Laboratory tests. The laboratory data yielded by the analysis of the specimens obtained during the examination provide important information concerning the symptoms of pregnancy and the woman's health status. Such information is used for making nursing and medical diagnoses.

Specimens are collected at the initial visit so that the cause of any abnormal findings can be treated (Table 10-1). Tine or purified protein derivative tuberculin (PPD) tests are administered to assess for exposure to tuberculosis. The woman is tested for hepatitis B surface antigen (HBsAG) and hepatitis B surface antibody (HbsAB), if she has not received hepatitis B vaccine. During the pelvic examination, cervical and vaginal smears are obtained for cytologic studies and for diagnosis of infection (e.g., *Chlamydia*, gonorrhea). Blood is drawn for a variety of tests: RPR/VDRL test for syphilis; complete

TABLE 10-1 *Laboratory Tests in Prenatal Period*

LABORATORY TEST	PURPOSE
Hemoglobin/hematocrit/WBC, differential	Detects anemia/detects infection
Hemoglobin electrophoresis	Identifies women with hemoglobinopathies (e.g., sickle cell anemia, thalassemia)
Blood type, Rh, and irregular antibody	Identifies those fetuses at risk for developing erythroblastosis fetalis or hyperbilirubinemia in neonatal period
Rubella titer	Determines immunity to rubella
Tuberculin skin testing; chest film after 20 weeks' gestation in women with reactive tuberculin tests	Screens for exposure to tuberculosis
Urinalysis, including microscopic examination of urinary sediment; pH, specific gravity, color, glucose, albumin, protein, RBC, WBC, casts, acetone; hCG	Identifies women with unsuspected diabetes mellitus, renal disease, hypertensive disease of pregnancy; infection; pregnancy
Urine culture	Identifies women with asymptomatic bacteriuria
Renal function tests: BUN, creatinine, electrolytes, creatinine clearance, total protein excretion	Evaluates level of possible renal compromise in women with a history of diabetes, hypertension, or renal disease
Pap test	Screens for cervical intraepithelial neoplasia, herpes simplex type 2, and HPV
Vaginal or rectal smear for *Neisseria gonorrhoeae*, *Chlamydia*, HPV, GBS	Screens high-risk population for asymptomatic infection. GBS done at 35-37 weeks
RPR/VDRL/FTA-ABS	Identifies women with untreated syphilis
HIV* antibody, hepatitis B surface antigen, toxoplasmosis	Screens for infection
1-hour glucose tolerance	Screens for gestational diabetes; done at initial visit for women with risk factors; done at 28 weeks for all pregnant women
3-hour glucose tolerance	Screens for diabetes in women with elevated glucose level after 1-hour test; must have two elevated readings for diagnosis
Cardiac evaluation: ECG, chest x-ray film, and echocardiogram	Evaluates cardiac function in women with a history of hypertension or cardiac disease

BUN, Blood urea nitrogen; *ECG,* electrocardiogram; *FTA-ABS,* fluorescent treponemal antibody absorption test; *GBS,* group B streptococcus; *hCG,* human chorionic gonadotropin; *HIV,* human immunodeficiency virus; *HPV,* human papillomavirus; *RPR,* rapid plasma reagin.
*With patient permission.

blood cell count (CBC) with hematocrit, hemoglobin, and differential values; tests for blood type and Rh factor; antibody screen (Kell, Duffy, rubella, toxoplasmosis, and anti-Rh); test for sickle cell anemia; and measurement of the folacin level, when indicated. Urine is tested for glucose (diabetes), protein (pregnancy-induced hypertension), and nitrites and leukocytes (urinary tract infection); culture and sensitivity tests are ordered as necessary. Testing for antibody to the human immunodeficiency virus (HIV) is strongly recommended for all pregnant women (Box 10-2).

The finding of risk factors during pregnancy may indicate the need to repeat some tests at other times. For example, exposure to tuberculosis or an STD would necessitate repeat testing.

Follow-up Visits

Monthly visits are scheduled routinely during the first and second trimesters, although additional appointments may be made as the need arises. During the third trimester, however, the relative quietness of the first and second trimesters gives way to an active period in which the practical realities

BOX 10-2 *Ethical Considerations for HIV Screening*

Pregnant women are ethically obligated to seek reasonable care during pregnancy and to avoid causing harm to the fetus. Maternity nurses should be advocates for the fetus, but not at the expense of the pregnant woman.

Mandatory HIV screening involves ethical issues related to privacy invasion, discrimination, social stigma, and reproductive risks to the pregnant woman. Incidence of perinatal transmission from an HIV-positive mother to her fetus ranges from 25% to 35%. Methods of preventing maternal-fetal transmission are not available. However, Zidovudine decreases perinatal transmission (Connor et al., 1994). Until there is a change in technology that alters the diagnosis or treatment of the fetus, testing of the pregnant woman should be voluntary, although some professional groups now advocate mandatory testing. Health care providers have an obligation to make sure the pregnant woman is well informed about HIV symptoms and testing.

of expectant parenthood are considered. Starting with week 28, maternity visits are scheduled every 2 weeks until week 36, and then every week until birth. The pattern of interviewing the woman first and then assessing physical changes and performing laboratory tests is maintained.

Interview

Follow-up visits are less intensive than the initial prenatal visit. At each of these follow-up visits, the woman is asked to summarize relevant events that have occurred since the previous visit. She is asked about her general emotional and physiologic well-being, complaints or problems, or questions she may have. Personal and family needs are also identified and explored.

Because the woman's emotional state affects her general well-being and that of her family, her and her family's emotional well-being is assessed at each visit. Emotional changes are common during pregnancy, and therefore it is reasonable for the nurse to ask whether the woman has experienced any mood swings, reactions to changes in her body image, bad dreams, or worries. Positive feelings (her own and those of her family) are also noted. The reactions of family members to the pregnancy and the woman's emotional changes are recorded.

How the woman is progressing through the developmental tasks of pregnancy is also assessed. By the beginning of the second trimester, most women have accepted the biologic fact of pregnancy. Usually by the fifth month, pregnant women are experiencing a growing awareness of the child as a separate being, distinct from themselves; women can say, "I am going to have a baby." With quickening, she turns her attention inward (becomes introspective) to her pregnancy and toward her relationships with others (e.g., her mother and partner).

During the third trimester, current family situations and their effect on the mother are assessed, for example, siblings' and grandparents' responses to the pregnancy and the coming child. In addition, the following questions are addressed:

- What anticipatory planning is in progress concerning new parenting responsibilities, sibling rivalry, recuperation from pregnancy and birth, and fertility management?
- What successes or frustrations with diet, rest and relaxation, sexuality, and emotional support is the mother experiencing?
- What is the mother's understanding of her family's needs in relation to the pregnancy and the unborn child?
- How well prepared are the parents for coping with an emergency? That is, does the mother know the warning signs, understand what they represent, and the way and to whom to report them?
- Does the mother know the signs of preterm and term labor?

- What is the mother's understanding of the labor process and expectations of herself and others during labor; does she know what to bring to the hospital or birthing center?
- If she is having a home birth, have all the necessary supplies been obtained?
- What plans have the mother and her family made for labor?
- What anxieties are the mother or her family experiencing regarding labor or the unborn child?
- What does the mother wish to know about the control of discomfort during labor?
- Is the mother (and her partner or support person) planning to attend any parent education classes?
- Does the mother have questions about fetal development and methods to assess fetal well-being?

A review of the woman's physical systems is appropriate at each meeting, and any suspicious signs or symptoms are assessed in depth. Discomforts reflecting adaptations to pregnancy are identified. Special inquiries are made about possible infections (e.g., genitourinary tract, respiratory tract). The woman's knowledge of self-care measures is assessed, as well as the success of these and prescribed therapy.

Physical examination

Reevaluation is a constant aspect of a pregnant woman's care. Each woman reacts differently to pregnancy. As a result, careful monitoring of the pregnancy and her reactions to care is vital. The database is updated at each time of contact with the pregnant woman. Physiologic changes are documented as the pregnancy progresses because this makes it possible for any deviations from normal progress to be identified.

At each visit, pulse and respirations are measured; blood pressure (same arm with woman sitting) is taken; her weight is determined and whether the weight gain (or loss) is compatible with the overall plan for weight gain is evaluated; urine may be checked by dipstick; and the presence and degree of edema are noted. Abdominal inspection and palpation and measurement of fundal height are aspects of the examination at each visit; these are discussed in more detail in the following section. While assessing the pregnant woman's abdomen with the woman in the lithotomy position during the second and third trimesters, the nurse must watch for the occurrence of **supine hypotension** (see the Emergency box). When a woman is lying in this position, the weight of abdominal contents may compress the vena cava and aorta, causing a drop in blood pressure.

The findings revealed during the interview and physical examination reflect the status of maternal adaptations. When any of the findings are suspicious, an in-depth examination is performed.

Careful interpretation of blood pressure is important in the risk factor analysis of all pregnant women. Blood pressure is evaluated on the basis of absolute values and the length of gestation and is interpreted in the light of modifying factors.

An absolute systolic blood pressure of 140 mm Hg or more and diastolic blood pressure of 90 mm Hg or more indicate the existence of hypertension. A rise in the systolic blood pressure of 30 mm Hg more than the baseline pressure or in the diastolic blood pressure of 15 mm Hg more than the baseline pressure is also a significant finding, regardless of whether the absolute values are less than 140/90 mm Hg. For example, if a woman's blood pressure normally is 105/60

mm Hg, a change to 120/75 mm Hg indicates a heightened risk for hypertension. The blood pressure decreases slightly in midpregnancy, then returns to baseline by term (Duvekot & Peeters, 1994). An increase in the systolic blood pressure is a better indicator of the risk for pregnancy-induced hypertension (PIH) than is an increase in the diastolic pressure (Sibai et al., 1995a).

In assessing blood pressure the nurse needs to always keep in mind that an increase in blood pressure could indicate the onset of either PIH or the HELLP syndrome (*h*emolysis, *e*levated *l*iver enzymes, and *l*ow *p*latelet count). Either of these could result in devastating consequences for the woman or her fetus (Sibai et al., 1995b). See Chapter 24 for a further discussion of these two disorders.

The mother is monitored continuously for signs and symptoms of potential complications. Persistent and excessive vomiting and ketonuria may indicate the development of hyperemesis gravidarum. Uterine cramping and vaginal bleeding are signs of threatened abortion. Chills and fever are symptoms of infection. The cause of hypertension must be investigated. Discharge from the vagina may be amniotic fluid or associated with infection (see the Signs of Potential Complications box).

EMERGENCY

Supine Hypotension

SIGNS/SYMPTOMS

Pallor
Dizziness, faintness, breathlessness
Tachycardia
Nausea
Clammy (damp, cool) skin; sweating

INTERVENTIONS

Position woman on her side until her signs/symptoms subside and vital signs stabilize within normal limits (WNL).

signs of POTENTIAL COMPLICATIONS

FIRST TRIMESTER

Signs/Symptoms	Possible Causes
Severe vomiting	Hyperemesis gravidarum
Chills, fever	Infection
Burning on urination	Infection
Diarrhea	Infection
Abdominal cramping; vaginal bleeding	Spontaneous abortion, ectopic pregnancy

SECOND AND THIRD TRIMESTERS

Signs/Symptoms	Possible Causes
Persistent, severe vomiting	Hyperemesis gravidarum
Amniotic fluid discharge from vagina	Premature rupture of membranes (PROM)
Vaginal bleeding, severe abdominal pain	Spontaneous abortion, placenta previa, placental separation
Chills, fever, burning on urination, diarrhea	Infection
Severe backache or flank pain	Kidney infection or stones; preterm labor
Change in fetal movements: absence of fetal movements after quickening, any unusual change in pattern or amount	Fetal jeopardy or intrauterine fetal death
Uterine contractions; pressure; cramping	Preterm labor
Visual disturbances: blurring, double vision, or spots	Hypertensive conditions, pregnancy-induced hypertension (PIH)
Swelling of face or fingers and over sacrum	Hypertensive conditions, PIH
Headaches: severe, frequent, or continuous	Hypertensive conditions, PIH
Muscular irritability or convulsions	Hypertensive conditions, PIH
Epigastric pain (perceived as severe stomachache)	Hypertensive conditions, PIH
Glycosuria, positive glucose tolerance test reaction	Gestational diabetes mellitus
Sudden weight gain 2 + kg/wk	PIH

GUIDELINES/GUÍAS

Get up on the scale.
Súbase a la báscula/la pesa.

I need a urine sample.
Necesito una muestra de orina.

Go to the bathroom.
Vaya al baño.

I need to take your blood pressure.
Necesito tomarle la presión arterial.

I am going to listen to the baby's heartbeat.
Voy a escuchar el latido del corazón del bebé.

The doctor is going to examine you.
El doctor le va a hacer un examen.

Don't be afraid.
No tenga miedo.

Lie down, please.
Acuéstese, por favor.

Open your legs, please.
Separe las piernas, por favor.

Relax.
Relájese/cálmese.

Go to the laboratory for a blood test.
Vaya al laboratorio para un análisis de sangre.

Go to this office for your ultrasound.
Vaya a esta oficina para que le hagan el sonagrama.

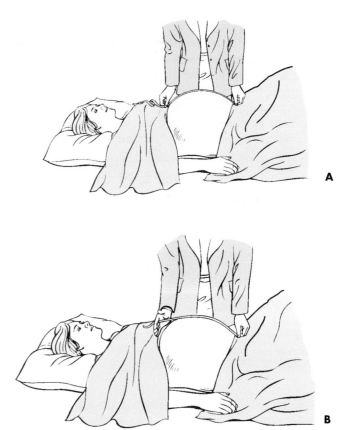

Fig. **10-8** Measurement of fundal height from symphysis that **A,** includes the upper curve of the fundus, and **B,** does not include the upper curve of the fundus. Note position of hands and measuring tape.

Fetal assessment

Toward the end of the first trimester, before the uterus is an abdominal organ, the fetal heart tones (FHTs) can be heard with an ultrasound fetoscope or an ultrasound stethoscope. To hear the FHTs the instrument is placed in the midline just anterior to the symphysis pubis and firm pressure applied. The woman and her family should be offered the opportunity to listen to the FHTs. The health status of the fetus is assessed at each visit for the remainder of the pregnancy. (See the Guidelines box.)

Fundal height. During the second trimester the uterus becomes an abdominal organ. Measurement of the height of the uterus above the symphysis pubis is used as one indicator of fetal growth progress. The measurement also provides a gross estimate of the duration of pregnancy. In addition, it may aid in the identification of high-risk factors. A stable or decreased fundal height may indicate the presence of intrauterine growth restriction; an excessive increase could indicate the presence of multifetal gestation or hydramnios.

A paper tape measure or a pelvimeter may be used to measure **fundal height.** To increase the reliability of the measurement, the same person could examine the pregnant woman at each of her prenatal visits, but often this is not possible because different clinicians may see the woman at prenatal visits. All clinicians who examine a particular pregnant woman should be consistent in their measurement technique. Ideally a protocol should be established for the health

care setting in which the measurement technique is explicitly set forth and the woman's position on the examining table, the measuring device, and method of measurement used are specified. Conditions under which the measurements are taken can also be described in the woman's records, including whether the bladder was empty and whether the uterus was relaxed or contracted at the time of measurement.

Various positions for measuring fundal height have been described. The woman can be supine, have her head elevated, have her knees flexed, or have both her head elevated and knees flexed. Measurements obtained with the woman in the various positions differ, making it even more important to standardize the fundal height measurement technique (Engstrom et al., 1993).

Placement of the tape measure can also vary. The tape can be placed in the middle of the woman's abdomen and the measurement made from the upper border of the symphysis pubis to the upper border of the fundus with the tape measure held in contact with the skin for the entire length of the uterus (Fig. 10-8, *A*). In another measurement technique, the upper curve of the fundus is not included in the measurement. Instead, one end of the tape measure is held at the upper border of the symphysis pubis with one hand and the other hand is placed at the upper border of

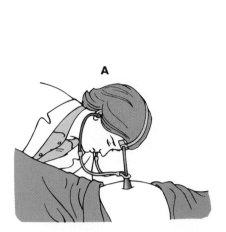
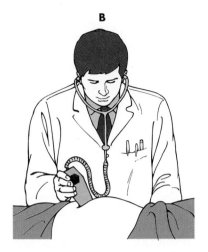
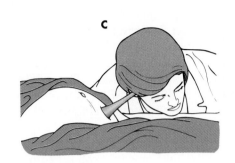

Fig. **10-9** Detecting fetal heartbeat. **A,** Fetoscope (18 to 20 weeks). **B,** Doppler ultrasound stethoscope (12 weeks). **C,** Pinard's stethoscope. NOTE: Hands should not touch stethoscope while nurse is listening.

the fundus. The tape is placed between the middle and index fingers of the other hand and the point where these fingers intercept the tape measure is taken as the measurement (Fig. 10-8, *B*) (Engstrom & Sittler, 1993).

During the second and third trimesters (weeks 18 to 30), the height of the fundus in centimeters is approximately the same as the number of weeks of gestation, if the woman's bladder is empty at the time of measurement (Cunningham et al., 1997).

Gestational age. In an uncomplicated pregnancy, fetal gestational age is estimated after the duration of pregnancy and the expected date of birth (EDB) are determined. Fetal gestational age is determined from the menstrual history, contraceptive history, pregnancy test result, and the following findings obtained during the clinical evaluation:

- First uterine size estimate: date, size
- Fetal heart (FH) first heard: date, Doppler stethoscope, fetoscope
- Date of quickening
- Current fundal height, estimated fetal weight (EFW)
- Current week of gestation by history of LMP and/or ultrasound
- Ultrasound: date, week of gestation, biparietal diameter (BPD)
- Reliability of dates

Quickening ("feeling of life") refers to the mother's first perception of fetal movement. It usually occurs between the sixteenth and twentieth weeks of gestation.

In some centers, ultrasonography is performed routinely in all pregnant women, and this allows a more exact estimation of gestational age. It may also be used to establish the duration of pregnancy if the woman cannot give a precise date for her last menstrual period (LMP) or if the size of the uterus does not conform to the stated date of the LMP. The routine use of sonography in low-risk pregnancies has not been documented to be associated with improved fetal outcome, however (Garmel & D'Alton, 1994).

Health status. The assessment of fetal health status includes consideration of fetal movement, the fetal heart rate (FHR) and rhythm, and abnormal maternal or fetal symptoms.

The mother is instructed to note the extent and timing of fetal movements and to report immediately if the pattern changes or if movement ceases. Regular movement has been found to be a reliable determinant of fetal health (Wilailak et al., 1992). The FHR is checked on routine visits once it has been heard (Fig. 10-9). Early in the second trimester the heartbeat may be heard with the Doppler stethoscope (Fig. 10-9, *B*). To detect the heartbeat before the fetus can be palpated by Leopold's maneuvers (see Fig. 15-5), the scope is moved around the abdomen until the heartbeat is heard. Each nurse develops a set pattern for searching the abdomen for the heartbeat; for example, she may start first in the midline about 2 to 3 cm above the symphysis, then move to the left lower quadrant, and so on. The heartbeat is counted and the quality and rhythm noted. Later in the second trimester the FHR can be determined with the fetoscope or Pinard's stethoscope (Fig. 10-9, *A* and *C*). A normal rate and rhythm are other good indicators of fetal health. Once the heartbeat is noted, its absence is cause for immediate investigation.

Fetal health status is intensively investigated if any maternal or fetal complications arise (e.g., maternal hypertension, intrauterine growth restriction [IUGR], premature rupture of membranes [PROM], irregular or absent FHR, or absence of fetal movements after quickening). Careful, precise, and concise recording of patient responses and laboratory results contributes to the continuous supervision vital to ensuring the well-being of the mother and fetus.

Laboratory tests

The number of routine laboratory tests done during pregnancy is limited. A clean-catch urine specimen is obtained to test for glucose, protein, and nitrites and leukocytes at each follow-up visit. Urine specimens for culture and sensitivity, as well as blood samples, are obtained only if signs and symptoms warrant. A hematocrit determination is done at each visit in some offices. A blood specimen is obtained at 16 weeks to determine the alpha-fetoprotein level.

The multiple-marker, or triple-screen, test is used to detect Down syndrome. Done between 16 and 18 weeks' gestation, it measures the maternal serum level of alpha-fetoprotein (MSAFP), human chorionic gonadotropin (hCG), and unconjugated estriol. Adjusted values are combined to yield the risk for Down syndrome (Heyl, Miller & Canick, 1990). Low levels may be associated with Down syndrome and other chromosomal abnormalities (Cunningham et al., 1997).

The following blood tests are repeated as necessary: RPR/VDRL test for syphilis; complete blood cell count with hematocrit, hemoglobin, and differential values; antibody screen (Kell, Duffy, rubella, toxoplasmosis, anti-Rh, HIV; sickle cell; and level of folacin when indicated). If not done earlier in pregnancy, a glucose screen is performed in women over 25 years of age. A glucose challenge is usually done between 24 and 28 weeks' gestation. Cervical and vaginal smears are repeated as necessary to examine for *Chlamydia* organisms, gonorrhea, and herpes simplex virus types 1 and 2. Group B streptococcus (GBS) testing is done between 35 and 37 weeks' gestation; cultures collected earlier will not accurately predict GBS status at time of birth.

Other tests

Other diagnostic tests are available to assess the health status of both the pregnant woman and the fetus. Ultrasonography, for example, may be performed to determine the status of the pregnancy and to confirm gestational age of the fetus. Amniocentesis, a procedure used to obtain amniotic fluid for analysis, may be needed to evaluate the fetus for genetic disorders or gestational maturity. These and other tests that are used to determine health risks for the mother and infant are described in Chapter 22.

After obtaining information through the assessment process, the data are analyzed to identify deviations from the norm and unique needs of the pregnant woman and her family. Although comprehensive health care requires collaboration among professionals from several disciplines, nurses are in an excellent position to formulate diagnoses that can be used to guide independent interventions. The diagnoses in the accompanying box are examples of the nursing diagnoses that may be appropriate in the prenatal period.

❙ Nursing Diagnoses

The Prenatal Period

Anxiety related to:
- Increased knowledge and understanding in the care of mothers and infants.
- Physical discomforts of pregnancy

- Ambivalent and labile emotions
- Changes in family dynamics
- Fetal well-being
- Ability to manage anticipated labor

Altered family processes related to:
- Changing roles and responsibilities
- Inadequate understanding of physical and emotional changes in pregnancy
- Increased concern about labor

Altered nutrition: less than body requirements related to:
- Morning sickness

Body image disturbance related to:
- Anatomic and physiologic changes of pregnancy

Altered health maintenance related to knowledge deficit regarding self-care measures for:
- Posture and body mechanics
- Rest and relaxation
- Personal hygiene
- Activity and exercise
- Safety

Impaired individual coping related to knowledge deficit regarding:
- Recognizing onset of complications
- Distinguishing between true and false labor
- Emergency arrangements

Sleep pattern disturbance related to:
- Discomforts of late pregnancy
- Anxiety about approaching labor

Expected Outcomes of Care

The plan of nursing care for women and their families during pregnancy is given direction by the diagnoses that have been formulated during prenatal visits. Individualized plans that are developed mutually with the pregnant woman are more likely to result in desirable outcomes than those developed by the nurse for the woman. Below are examples of outcomes that may be expected. The pregnant woman will:
- Indicate decreased anxiety about the health of her fetus and herself.
- Describe improved family dynamics.
- Show appropriate weight gain patterns.
- Report increasing acceptance of changes in body image.
- Demonstrate knowledge for self-care.
- Ask for clarification of information about pregnancy and birth.
- Report signs and symptoms of complications.
- Describe appropriate measures taken to relieve physical discomforts.
- Develop a realistic birth plan.
- Indicate satisfaction with health care providers and processes.

Plan of Care and Interventions

The nurse-patient relationship is critical in setting the tone for further interaction. The techniques of listening with an attentive expression, touching, and using eye contact have their place, as does recognizing the woman's feelings and her right to express these feelings. The interaction may occur in various formal or informal settings. The clinic, home visits, or telephone conversations all provide opportunities for contact and can be used effectively for this purpose. Sometimes women repeatedly seek information about a particular problem. At other times, there may be another underlying problem the woman is hesitant to broach. The nurse needs to be astute in identifying such unvoiced needs and can help the woman by asking for a patient-generated solution and a subsequent report of its effectiveness.

In supporting a patient the nurse must remember that both the nurse and the woman are contributing to the relationship. The nurse has to accept the woman's responses as a factor in trying to be of help. An example of one nurse-patient relationship is as follows:

> Mrs. _____ had been very forthright in saying that this pregnancy was unplanned but had countered this observation with comments such as, "All things happen for the best," and "Children bring their own love." Over time, as our relationship developed to one of mutual trust, she complained increasingly of her fear of pain, of hating to wear maternity clothes, and of having to give up helping the family. Finally I ventured to say, "Sometimes when a pregnancy is unplanned, women resent it and are angry about it." Her relief was evident. She said, "Oh, you don't know how angry I've been." As a result, the whole tenor of support being offered changed, and the plan was adjusted to meet her real needs.

The nurse also needs to accept that the woman must be a willing partner in a purely voluntary relationship. As such, the relationship can be refused or terminated at any time by the pregnant woman or her family.

Supportive care involves developing, augmenting, or changing the mechanisms used by women and their families in coping with stress. The nurse tries to promote active participation by the people in the solution of their own problems. The nurse can help a woman gather pertinent information, explore alternative actions, decide on a course of action, and assume responsibility for the outcomes. These outcomes may be any or all of the following: living with a problem as it is, easing the effects of a problem so that it can be accepted more readily, or eliminating the problem by effecting change.

At other times a successful outcome can be documented readily. For example, a woman who early in her pregnancy had predicted a severe depressive state in the postbirth period was elated when such a state did not materialize. She remarked to the nurse who had provided support during the pregnancy and birth, "You're the best nerve medicine I've ever had!"

Care paths

Today there is emphasis on better coordination of prenatal care services for childbearing families. Because a large number of health care professionals are involved in care of the expectant mother, unintentional gaps or overlaps in care may occur. Care paths are used to improve the consistency of care provided. Although the Care Path on p. 228 focuses only on prenatal education, it is one example of the type of form that might be developed to guide health care providers in carrying out the appropriate assessments and interventions in a timely way. Use of care paths may contribute to improved satisfaction of families with the prenatal care that is provided, and members of the health care team may function more efficiently and effectively.

Education about maternal and fetal changes

Expectant parents are typically curious about the growth and development of the fetus and the consequent changes that occur in the mother's body. Mothers in particular are sometimes more tolerant of the discomforts related to the continuing pregnancy if they understand the underlying causes. Literature that describes the fetal and maternal changes is often available and can be used in explaining changes as they occur. Table 8-1 summarizes fetal development.

Education for self-care

Health maintenance is an important aspect of prenatal care. Patient participation in the care ensures prompt reporting of untoward responses to pregnancy. Patient assumption of responsibility of health maintenance is assisted by the nurse's understanding of maternal adaptations to the growth of the unborn child and a readiness to learn. Nurses in their role of teacher provide patients with the information necessary for compliance with health care measures.

The expectant mother needs information about many subjects. The nurse who is observant, listens, and knows typical concerns of expectant parents can anticipate questions that will be asked and prompt mothers and fathers to discuss what is on their minds. Many times, printed literature can be given to supplement the individualized teaching the nurse provides, and women often avidly read books and pamphlets related to their own experience. When nurses read the literature before they distribute it, they have an opportunity to point out areas that may not correspond with local health care practices. Patients who receive conflicting advice or instruction are likely to grow increasingly frustrated with members of the health care team and the care provided. Several topics that may cause concerns in pregnant women are discussed in the following sections.

Nutrition. Proper nutrition is an important factor in the maintenance of maternal health during pregnancy and the provision of adequate nutrients for embryonic and fetal development. Assessing a woman's nutritional status and

CARE PATH *Prenatal Care Pathways*

ST. MARY'S HEALTH CENTER
St Louis, Missouri

PRENATAL EDUCATION CLINICAL PATHWAY

INITIAL VISIT AND ORIENTATION: _____   SOCIAL SERVICE: _____   DIETICIAN: _____

I. EARLY PREGNANCY (WEEKS 1-20) *(initial and date after education given)*

Fetal Growth and Development _____   Testing: Labs _____   Ultrasound _____

Maternal Changes _____

Lifestyle: Exercise/Stress/Nutrition _____   Possible Complications:
Drugs, OTC, Tobacco, Alcohol _____   a. Threatened AB _____
STDs _____   b. Diabetes _____
c. _____ _____

Psycho/Social Adjustments: Introduction to Breastfeeding _____
Acceptance _____   and Childbirth Preparation
FOB Involved/Accepts _____
Baby for adoption _____   Dietary Follow-Up _____

II. MID-PREGNANCY (WEEKS 21-27) *(initial and date after education given)*

Fetal Growth and Development _____   Breast or Bottle Feeding _____

Maternal Changes _____   Birth Plan Initiated _____

Daily Fetal Movement _____   Childbirth Preparation _____

Possible Complications: _____
a. Preterm Labor Prevention _____
b. PIH Symptoms _____
c. _____ _____   Dietary Follow Up _____

III. LATE PREGNANCY (WEEKS 28-40) *(initial and date after education given)*

Fetal Growth and Development _____   Childbirth Preparation:
S/S of Labor; Labor Process _____
Fetal Evaluation: Pain Management: natural childbirth, _____
Meds, Epidural
Daily Movement _____ NSTs _____   cesarean; VBAC _____
Kick Counts _____ BPPs _____   Birth Plan Complete _____
Review Hospital Policies _____

Maternal Changes _____   Parenting Preparation:
Pediatrician _____   Childcare _____
Possible Complications: Siblings _____   Immunizations _____
a. Preterm Labor Prevention _____   Car Seat/Safety _____
b. PIH Symptoms _____
c. _____ _____

Breastfeeding Preparation: Post-Partum:
Nipple Assessment _____   P.P. Care/Check-Up _____
Emotional Changes _____
Dietary Follow-Up _____   B.C. Options _____
Safe Sex/STDs _____

Signature: _____   _____

providing information on nutrition are part of the nurse's responsibilities in rendering prenatal care. In some settings, a registered dietitian conducts classes for pregnant women on the topics of nutritional status and nutrition during pregnancy or interviews them to assess their knowledge of these topics. Nurses can refer women to a registered dietitian if a need is revealed during the nursing assessment. (For detailed information concerning maternal and fetal nutritional needs and related nursing care, see Chapter 11).

Personal hygiene. During pregnancy, the sebaceous (sweat) glands are highly active because of hormonal influences, and women often perspire freely. They may be reassured that the increase is normal and that their previous patterns of perspiration will return after the postpartum period. Washing the body regularly is basic to good personal hygiene. Baths and warm showers can be therapeutic because they relax tense, tired muscles, help counter insomnia, and make the pregnant woman feel fresh. Tub bathing is permitted even in late pregnancy because little water enters the vagina unless under pressure. However, late in pregnancy, when the woman's center of gravity lowers, she is at risk for falling. Tub bathing is contraindicated after rupture of the membranes.

Prevention of urinary tract infections. Because of dramatic changes that occur in the renal system during pregnancy (see Chapter 9), urinary tract infections are common, but they may be asymptomatic. Women should know, however, to inform their health care provider if blood or pain occurs on urination. These infections pose a risk to the mother and fetus, and thus the prevention and early treatment of these infections are essential.

The nurse can assess the woman's understanding and use of good handwashing techniques before and after urinating and whether she knows to wipe from front to back. Soft, absorbent toilet tissue, preferably white and unscented, should be used, because harsh, scented, or printed toilet paper may cause irritation. Bubble bath or other bath oils should be avoided because these may be irritating to the urethra. Women should wear underpants and panty hose with a cotton crotch and avoid wearing tight-fitting slacks or jeans for long periods, because anything that allows a build-up of heat and moisture in the genital area may foster the growth of bacteria.

Some women do not consume enough fluid and food. After discovering her food preferences, the nurse should advise the woman to drink 2 to 3 L (8 to 12 glasses) of liquid a day to maintain an adequate fluid intake that ensures frequent urination. Pregnant women should not limit fluids in an effort to reduce the frequency of urination. Women need to know that if urine looks dark (concentrated), they need to increase their fluid intake. Cranberry juice may be suggested because it is more acidic than other fluids and makes the urinary tract less hospitable to bacteria by lowering the pH. The consumption of yogurt and acidophilus milk may also help prevent urinary tract and vaginal infections.

The nurse should review healthy urination practices with the woman. Women should be told not to ignore the urge to urinate because holding urine lengthens the time bacteria are in the bladder and thus allows them to multiply. Women should plan ahead when they are faced with situations that may require them to delay urination (e.g., a long car ride). They always should urinate before going to bed at night. Bacteria also can be introduced during intercourse. Therefore, women are advised to urinate before and after intercourse, then drink a large glass of water to promote additional urination.

Kegel exercises. **Kegel exercises** (exercises for the pelvic floor) strengthen the muscles around the reproductive organs and improve muscle tone. Many women are not aware of the muscles of the pelvic floor (see Fig. 5-2) until it is pointed out that these are the muscles used during urination and sexual intercourse and therefore can be consciously controlled. Inasmuch as the muscles of the pelvic floor encircle the outlet through which the baby must pass, it is important that they be exercised, because an exercised muscle can then stretch and contract readily at the time of birth.

Kegel exercises should also be done immediately after giving birth to help the pelvic floor muscles return to normal functioning. They can then strengthen these muscles and improve muscle tone. If practiced on a regular basis, the exercises can help prevent a prolapsed uterus and stress incontinence from occurring later in life.

Several ways of performing Kegel exercises have been described. The method that is suggested by nurse researchers involved in a research utilization project for continence in women is described in the Teaching Guidelines box, p. 58. The nurse can be reasonably assured that the teaching has been effective if the woman reports an increased ability to control urine flow and greater muscular control during sexual intercourse.

Preparation for breastfeeding the newborn. Pregnant women are usually eager to discuss their plans for feeding the newborn. Breast milk is the food of choice, in part because breastfeeding is associated with a decreased incidence of perinatal morbidity and mortality. The American Academy of Pediatrics recommends breastfeeding for at least a year. However, a deep-seated aversion to breastfeeding on the part of the mother or partner, the mother's need for certain medications, and certain medical complications, such as active tuberculosis, newly diagnosed breast cancer, and hepatitis C, are contraindications to breastfeeding (Lawrence, 1994). Although hepatitis B antigen has not been shown to be transmitted via breast milk, as an added precaution it is recommended that infants born to hepatitis B antigen–positive women receive the hepatitis B vaccine and hepatitis B immune globulin (HBIG) immediately after birth. HIV-infected women in countries where infant mortality exceeds 50% as the result of diarrhea and other infectious diseases (excluding AIDS) are advised to breastfeed. In developed countries, women who are HIV positive are discouraged from nursing because the risk of HIV transmission outweighs the risk of the infant dying from another cause (Lawrence, 1994).

The woman and her partner are encouraged to decide which method of feeding is suitable for them; however, the benefits of breastfeeding should be emphasized. Once the couple has been given information about the advantages and disadvantages of bottle feeding and breastfeeding, they can make an informed choice. Health care providers support their decisions and provide any needed assistance.

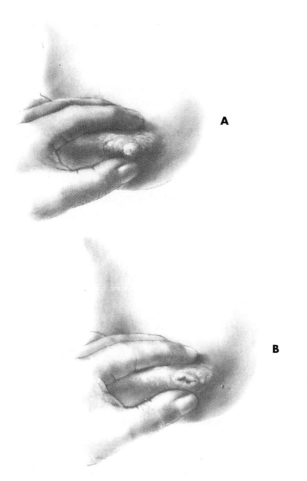

Fig. **10-10** **A,** Normal nipple everts with gentle pressure. **B,** Inverted nipple inverts with gentle pressure. (Modified from Lawrence R: *Breastfeeding: a guide for the medical profession,* ed 4, St Louis, 1994, Mosby.)

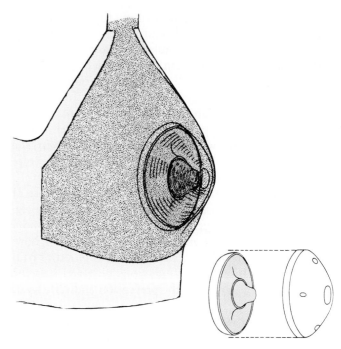

Fig. **10-11** Breast shell in place inside bra to evert nipple. (Modified from Lawrence R: *Breastfeeding: a guide for the medical profession,* ed 4, St Louis, 1994, Mosby.)

The **pinch test** is done to determine whether the nipple is everted or inverted (Fig. 10-10). The nurse shows the woman the way to perform the pinch test. It involves having the woman place her thumb and forefinger on her areola and gently press inward. This will cause her nipple to stand erect or invert. Most nipples will stand erect.

Exercises to break the adhesions that cause the nipple to invert do not work and may in fact precipitate uterine contractions (Lawrence, 1994). The use of **breast shells** by women with flat or inverted nipples is recommended (Fig. 10-11). Breast shells work by exerting a continuous, gentle pressure around the areola that pushes the nipple through a central opening in the inner shield. Breast shells should be worn for 1 to 2 hours daily during the last trimester of pregnancy. They should be worn for gradually increased lengths of time (Lawrence, 1994). Breast stimulation is contraindicated in women at risk for preterm labor. Therefore, the decision to recommend the use of breast shells to women with flat or inverted nipples must

be made judiciously. Continuous support and guidance must be given to the woman as part of the nursing care plan.

The woman is taught to cleanse the nipples with warm water to keep the ducts from being blocked with dried colostrum. Soap, ointments, alcohol, and tinctures should not be applied because they remove protective oils that keep the nipples supple. The use of these substances may cause the nipples to crack during early lactation (Lawrence, 1994).

The woman who plans to breastfeed should purchase a nursing bra that will accommodate her increased breast size during the last few months of pregnancy and during lactation. If her breasts are very heavy, or if the woman feels uncomfortable with the weight unsupported, the bra can be worn day and night.

Dental care. Dental care during pregnancy is especially important because nausea during pregnancy may lead to poor oral hygiene, allowing dental caries to develop. No physiologic alteration during gestation can cause dental caries, however. Because calcium and phosphorus in the teeth are fixed in enamel, the old adage "for every child a tooth" is not true.

There is no scientific evidence that filling teeth or even dental extraction involving the administration of local or nitrous oxide-oxygen anesthesia precipitates abortion or premature labor. Antibacterial therapy should be considered for sepsis, however, especially in pregnant women who have had rheumatic heart disease or nephritis. Emergency dental surgery is not contraindicated during pregnancy. However, the risks and benefits of dental surgery need to be explained to the mother (Papp et al., 1990).

HOME CARE *Patient Instructions for Self-Care*

Exercise Tips for Pregnant Women

Consult your health care provider when you know or suspect you are pregnant. Discuss your medical and obstetric history, your current exercise regimen, and the exercises you would like to continue throughout pregnancy.

Seek help in determining an exercise routine that is well within your limit of tolerance, especially if you have not been exercising regularly.

Consider decreasing weight-bearing exercises (jogging, running) and concentrating on non–weight-bearing activities such as swimming, cycling, or stretching. If you are a runner, starting in your seventh month, you may wish to walk instead.

Avoid risky activities such as surfing, mountain climbing, skydiving, and racquetball because such activities that require precise balance and coordination may be dangerous. Avoid activities that require holding your breath and bearing down (Valsalva's maneuver). Jerky, bouncy motions also should be avoided.

Exercise regularly at least three times a week, as long as you are healthy, to improve muscle tone and increase or maintain your stamina. If you do exercises sporadically, this may put undue strain on your muscles. Limit activity to shorter intervals. Exercise for 10 to 15 minutes, rest for 2 to 3 minutes, then exercise for another 10 to 15 minutes.

Decrease your exercise level as your pregnancy progresses. The normal alterations of advancing pregnancy, such as decreased cardiac reserve and increased respiratory effort, may produce physiologic stress if you exercise strenuously for a long time.

Take your pulse every 10 to 15 minutes while you are exercising. If it is more than 140 beats/min, slow down until it returns to a maximum of 90 beats/min. You should be able to converse easily while exercising. If you cannot, you need to slow down.

Avoid becoming overheated for extended periods of time. It is best not to exercise for more than 35 minutes, especially in hot, humid weather. As your body temperature rises, the heat is transmitted to your fetus. Prolonged or repeated elevation of fetal temperature may result in birth defects, especially

during the first 3 months. Your temperature should not exceed 38° C.

Avoid the use of hot tubs and saunas.

Warm-up and stretching exercises prepare your joints for more strenuous exercise and lessen the likelihood of strain or injury to your joints. After the fourth month of gestation you should not perform exercises flat on your back.

A cool-down period of mild activity involving your legs after an exercise period will help bring your respiration, heart, and metabolic rates back to normal and prevent the pooling of blood in the exercised muscles.

Rest for 10 minutes after exercising, lying on your side. As the uterus grows, it puts pressure on a major vein in your abdomen, which carries blood to your heart. Lying on your side removes the pressure and promotes return circulation from your extremities and muscles to your heart, thereby increasing blood flow to your placenta and fetus. You should rise gradually from the floor to prevent dizziness or fainting (orthostatic hypotension).

Drink two or three 8-ounce glasses of water after you exercise to replace the body fluids lost through perspiration. While exercising, drink water whenever you feel the need.

Increase your caloric intake to replace the calories burned during exercise and provide the extra energy needs of pregnancy. (Pregnancy alone requires an additional 300 kcal/day.) Choose such high-protein foods as fish, milk, cheese, eggs, or meat.

Take your time. This is not the time to be competitive or train for activities requiring long endurance.

Wear a supportive bra. Your increased breast weight may cause changes in posture and put pressure on the ulnar nerve.

Wear supportive shoes. As your uterus grows, your center of gravity shifts and you compensate for this by arching your back. These natural changes may make you feel off balance and more likely to fall.

Stop exercising immediately if you experience shortness of breath, dizziness, numbness, tingling, pain of any kind, more than four uterine contractions per hour, decreased fetal activity, or vaginal bleeding, and consult your health care provider.

Modified from Artal R & Subak-Sharpe G: *Pregnancy & exercise,* New York, 1992, Delacorte Press; Fishbein E & Phillips M: How safe is exercise during pregnancy? *J Obstet Gynecol Neonatal Nurs* 19(1):45, 1990; ACOG: Exercise during pregnancy and the postpartum period, *Technical Bulletin* 189, Feb, 1994; Pivarnik J: Maternal exercise in pregnancy, *Sports Med* 18:215, 1994.

Physical activity. Physical activity promotes a feeling of well-being in the pregnant woman. It improves circulation, promotes relaxation and rest, and counteracts boredom, as it does in the nonpregnant woman. Detailed exercise tips for pregnancy are presented in the Home Care box above. Exercises that help relieve the low back pain that often arises during the second trimester because of the increased weight of the fetus are demonstrated in Fig. 10-12.

Posture and body mechanics. Many maternal adaptations predispose the woman to suffering backache and

incurring possible injury. The pregnant woman's center of gravity changes, pelvic joints soften and relax, and stress is placed on abdominal musculature as pregnancy progresses. Poor posture and body mechanics contribute to the discomfort and potential for injury. To minimize these problems, women can acquire a kinesthetic sense for good body posture (Fig. 10-13). The activities described in the Home Care box on p. 233 can also promote greater physical comfort.

Rest and relaxation. The pregnant woman is encouraged to plan regular rest periods, particularly as pregnancy

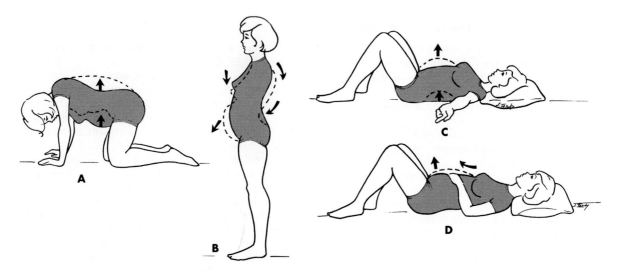

Fig. **10-12** Exercises. **A to C,** Pelvic rocking relieves low backache (excellent for relief of menstrual cramps as well). **D,** Abdominal breathing aids relaxation and lifts abdominal wall off uterus.

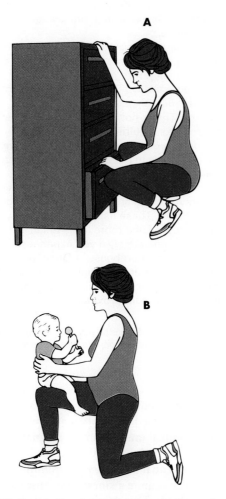

Fig. **10-13** Correct body mechanics. **A,** Squatting. **B,** Lifting.

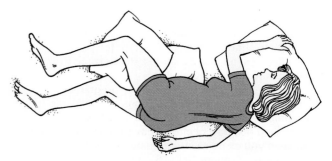

Fig. **10-14** Side-lying position for rest and relaxation. Some women prefer to support upper part of leg with pillows.

advances. The side-lying position is recommended because it promotes uterine perfusion and fetoplacental oxygenation by eliminating pressure on the ascending vena cava and descending aorta, which can lead to supine hypotension (Fig. 10-14). The mother should also be shown the way to rise slowly from a side-lying position to prevent placing strain on the back and to minimize the orthostatic hypotension caused by changes in position common in the latter part of pregnancy. To stretch and rest back muscles at home or work, the nurse can show the woman the way to do the following exercises:

Stand behind a chair. Support and balance self using the back of the chair (Fig. 10-15). Squat for 30 seconds; stand for 15 seconds. Repeat six times, several times per day, as needed.

While sitting in a chair, lower head to knees for 30 seconds. Raise head up. Repeat six times, several times per day, as needed.

HOME CARE *Patient Instructions for Self-Care*

Posture and Body Mechanics

To prevent or relieve backache

Do pelvic tilt:
- **Pelvic tilt (rock)** on hands and knees (see Fig.10-12, *A*) and while sitting in straight-back chair.
- Pelvic tilt (rock) in standing position against a wall, or lying on floor (see Fig. 10-12, *B* and *C*).
- Perform abdominal muscle contractions during pelvic tilt while standing, lying, or sitting to help strengthen rectus abdominis muscle (see Fig. 10-12, *D*).
- Use good body mechanics.
- Use leg muscles to reach objects on or near floor. Bend at the knees, not the back. Knees are bent to lower body to squatting position. Feet are kept 12 to 18 inches apart to provide a solid base to maintain balance (see Fig. 10-13, *A*).
- Lift with the legs. To lift heavy object (young child), one foot is placed slightly in front of the other and kept flat as woman lowers herself onto one knee. She lifts the weight holding it close to her body and never higher than the chest. To stand up or sit down, one leg is placed slightly behind the other as she raises or lowers herself (see Fig. 10-13, *B*).

To restrict the lumbar curve

For prolonged standing (e.g., ironing, out-of-home employment), place one foot on low footstool or box; change positions often.

Move car seat forward so that knees are bent and higher than hips. If needed, use a small pillow to support low back area.

Sit in chairs low enough to allow both feet to be placed on floor and preferably with knees higher than hips.

To prevent round ligament pain and strain on abdominal muscles

Implement suggestions given in Table 10-2.

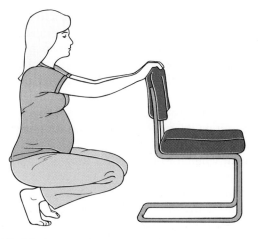

Fig. **10-15** Squatting for muscle relaxation and strengthening and for keeping leg and hip joints flexible.

Conscious relaxation is the process of releasing tension from the mind and body through conscious effort and practice. The ability to relax consciously and intentionally can be beneficial for the following reasons:
- It can relieve the normal discomforts related to pregnancy.
- It can reduce stress and therefore diminish pain perception during the childbearing cycle.
- It can heighten self-awareness and trust in one's own ability to control one's responses and functions.
- It can help the woman cope with stress in everyday life situations, whether she is pregnant or not.

The techniques for conscious relaxation are numerous and varied. The guidelines given in Box 10-3 can be used by anyone.

Employment. Employment of pregnant women has been shown to have no adverse effects on pregnancy outcomes (Henriksen et al., 1994; Messersmith-Heroman, Heroman & Moore, 1994; Seneviratne & Fernando, 1994). Job discrimination that is based strictly on pregnancy is illegal. However, some job environments pose potential risk to the fetus (e.g., dry cleaning plants, chemistry laboratories, parking garages).

Activities that depend on a good sense of balance should be discouraged, however, especially during the latter half of pregnancy. Commonly, excessive fatigue is the deciding factor in the termination of employment. Women in sedentary jobs need to walk around at intervals to counter the usual sluggish circulation in the legs that can cause varices and thrombophlebitis to develop. They should neither sit nor stand in one position for long periods and they should avoid crossing their legs at the knees because these foster such conditions. Standing for long periods of time also increases the risk of preterm labor. The pregnant woman's chair should provide adequate back support. Use of a footstool can prevent pressure on veins, relieve strain on varicosities, and minimize swelling of feet.

Clothing. Comfortable, loose clothing is best. Washable fabrics (e.g., absorbent cottons) are often preferred.

BOX 10-3   *Conscious Relaxation Tips*

Preparation: Loosen clothing, assume a comfortable sitting or side-lying position with all parts of body well supported with pillows.

Beginning: Allow self to feel warm and comfortable. Inhale and exhale slowly, and imagine peaceful relaxation coming over each part of the body, starting with the neck and working down to the toes. Often people who learn conscious relaxation speak of feeling relaxed even if some discomfort is present.

Maintenance: Use imagery (fantasy or daydream) to maintain the state of relaxation. Using *active imagery*, imagine yourself moving or doing some activity and experiencing its sensations. Using *passive imagery*, imagine yourself watching a scene, such as a lovely sunset.

Awakening: Return to the wakeful state gradually. Slowly begin to take in stimuli from the surrounding environment.

Further retention and development of the skill: Practice regularly for some periods each day, for example, at the same hour for 10 to 15 minutes each day, to feel refreshed, revitalized, and invigorated.

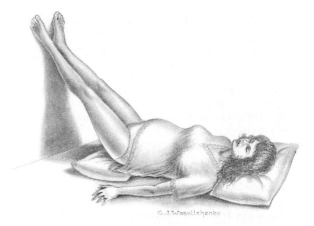

Fig. **10-16** Position for resting legs and for reducing edema and varicosities. Encourage woman with vulvar varicosities to include pillow under her hips.

Maternity clothes may be purchased new or found at thrift shops or garage sales in good condition because they rarely wear out. Tight bras and belts, stretch pants, garters, tight-top knee socks, panty girdles, and other constrictive clothing should be avoided because tight clothing over the perineum encourages vaginitis and miliaria (heat rash), and impaired circulation in the legs can cause varicosities.

Maternity bras are constructed to accommodate the increased breast weight, chest circumference, and the size of breast tail tissue (under the arm). These bras also have drop-flaps over the nipples to facilitate breastfeeding. A good bra can help prevent neckache and backache.

Elastic hose have been shown to give considerable comfort and to promote greater venous emptying in women with large varicose veins (Nilsson, Austrell & Norgren, 1992; Priollet et al., 1994). Ideally, support stockings should be put on before the woman gets out of bed in the morning. Fig. 10-16 demonstrates a position for resting the legs and reducing swelling and varicosities.

Comfortable shoes that provide firm support and promote good posture and balance are also advisable. Very high heels and platform shoes are not recommended because of the woman's changed center of gravity, which can cause her to lose her balance. In addition, in the third trimester the woman's pelvis tilts forward and her lumbar curve increases. The resulting leg aches and cramps are only aggravated by nonsupportive shoes.

Travel. Travel is not contraindicated in low-risk pregnant women, but those with high-risk pregnancies are advised to avoid long-distance travel after fetal viability has been reached so as to avert the economic and psychologic consequences of giving birth to a preterm infant far from home (Easa et al., 1994). Travel to areas where medical care is poor, water is untreated, or malaria is prevalent should be avoided if possible (Bia, 1992). Another thing to be borne in mind by women contemplating foreign travel is that many health insurance carriers do not cover a birth in a foreign setting or even hospitalization for preterm labor (Barry & Bia, 1989).

Pregnant women who travel for long distances should schedule periods of activity and rest. While sitting the woman can practice deep breathing, foot circling, and alternately contracting and relaxing different muscle groups. She should avoid becoming fatigued. Although travel in itself is not a cause of adverse outcomes such as spontaneous abortion or preterm labor, certain precautions are recommended while traveling in a car. A woman who does not wear automobile restraints risks injury to herself and her fetus (Hammond et al., 1990). Maternal death as a result of injury is the most common cause of fetal death. The next most common cause is placental separation. This occurs because body contours change in reaction to the force of a collision. The uterus as a muscular organ can adapt its shape to that of the body, but the placenta is not resilient, so that at the impact of collision placental separation can occur. A combination lap belt and shoulder harness is the most effective automobile restraint (Fig. 10-17), and both should be used. The lap belt should be worn low across the pelvic bones and as snug as is comfortable. The shoulder harness should be worn above the

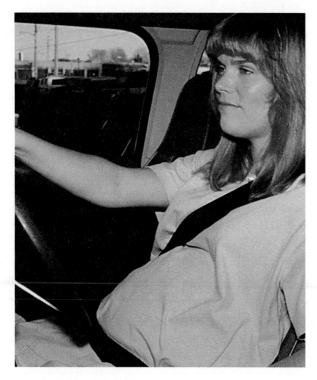

Fig. **10-17** Proper use of seat belt and head rest. (Courtesy Michael S. Clement, MD, Mesa, Ariz.)

gravid uterus and below the neck to prevent chafing. The pregnant woman should sit upright. The headrest should be used to prevent a whiplash injury.

For pregnant women traveling in high-altitude regions, lowered oxygen levels may cause fetal hypoxia, especially if the pregnant woman is anemic (Barry & Bia, 1989). However, the current information on this is limited, and there are as of yet, no set recommendations regarding the exposure of pregnant women to high altitudes (Nicholas, 1993).

Airline travel in large commercial jets usually poses little risk to the pregnant woman, but policies vary from airline to airline, so the pregnant woman is advised to inquire about restrictions or recommendations from her carrier (Skjenna et al., 1991). Magnetometers (metal detectors) used at airport security checkpoints are not harmful to the fetus. The 8% humidity at which the cabins of commercial airlines are maintained may result in some water loss; hydration (with water) should therefore be maintained under these conditions (Barry & Bia, 1989). Sitting in the cramped seat of an airliner for prolonged periods may increase the risk of superficial and deep thrombophlebitis. A pregnant woman is encouraged to take a 15-minute walk around the aircraft during each hour of travel to minimize this risk. A seat in the nonsmoking section of flights on which smoking is permitted is advised to prevent her car-

boxyhemoglobin levels from becoming elevated (see the Teaching Guidelines box).

Medications. Although much has been learned in recent years about fetal drug toxicity (see Box 8-1), the possible teratogenicity of many medications, prescription and OTC, is still unknown. This is especially true for new medications and combinations of drugs. Moreover, certain subclinical errors or deficiencies in intermediate metabolism in the fetus may cause an otherwise harmless drug to be converted into a hazardous one. The greatest danger of drug-caused developmental defects in the fetus extends from the time of fertilization through the first trimester, a time when the woman may not realize she is pregnant. Self-treatment must be discouraged. The use of all drugs, including OTC medications and vitamins, should be limited and a careful record kept of all therapeutic agents used (ACOG, 1994a).

Immunizations. There has been some concern over the safety of various immunization techniques during pregnancy (Cunningham et al., 1997). Immunization with live or attenuated live viruses is contraindicated during pregnancy because of its potential teratogenicity. Live-virus vaccines include those for measles (rubeola and rubella), chickenpox, and mumps, as well as the Sabin's (oral) poliomyelitis vaccine. Vaccines consisting of killed viruses may be used. Those that may be administered during pregnancy include tetanus, diphtheria, recombinant hepatitis B, and rabies vaccines.

Alcohol, cigarette smoke, and other substances. A safe level of alcohol consumption during pregnancy has not yet been established. Although the consumption of occasional alcoholic beverages may not be harmful to the mother or her developing embryo or fetus, complete abstinence is strongly advised (ACOG, 1994a). Maternal alcoholism is associated with high rates of spontaneous abortion and fetal alcohol syndrome; the risk for spontaneous abortion in the first trimester is dose related (three or more drinks per day) (Cook, Petersen & Moore, 1990).

Cigarette smoking or continued exposure to a smoke-filled environment (even if the mother does not smoke) is associated with fetal growth restriction and an increase in perinatal and infant morbidity and mortality. Exposure to nicotine has been shown to have a negative effect on the growth of the fetus (Bardy et al., 1993). Smoking is also associated with an increased frequency of preterm labor, premature rupture of membranes (PROM), abruptio placentae, placenta previa, and fetal death resulting possibly from decreased placental perfusion. Laboratory studies have revealed that smoking causes fetal hypoxia (ACOG, 1993; Cook, Petersen & Moore, 1990; Wilcox, 1993). All pregnant women who smoke should be strongly encouraged to quit or at least cut down. Pregnant women need to be told about the negative effects of even secondhand smoke on the fetus (ACOG, 1993; Economides & Braithwaite, 1994; Sanyal, Li & Belanger, 1994). Research has shown that early intervention may be effective in helping the woman cut down or quit smoking (Kendrick et al., 1994).

Most studies of human pregnancy have revealed no association between caffeine consumption and birth defects or low birth weight (Cunningham et al., 1997; Mills et al., 1993). Because other effects are unknown, however, pregnant women are advised to limit their caffeine intake.

Any drug or environmental agent that enters the pregnant woman's bloodstream has the potential to cross the placenta and harm the fetus (Brody et al., 1994). Marijuana, heroin, and cocaine are common examples of such substances (see Chapter 23).

Normal discomforts. Women pregnant for the first time are confronted with symptoms that would be considered abnormal in the nonpregnant state. Much of the prenatal care requested by such women is prompted by the need for explanations of the causes of the discomforts and for advice on ways to relieve the discomforts. The discomforts of the first trimester are fairly specific. Information about the physiology and prevention of and self-care

for discomforts experienced during the three trimesters is given in Table 10-2. Nurses can do much to allay a first-time mother's anxiety about such symptoms by telling her about them in advance, using terminology that the woman (or couple) can understand. Women who understand the physical discomforts of pregnancy are less apt to become overly anxious about their health. In addition, understanding the rationale for treatment promotes their participation in their care.

Recognizing potential complications. One of the most important responsibilities of persons involved in the care of the pregnant woman is to alert her to signs and symptoms that indicate a potential complication of pregnancy. The woman needs to know how to report such warning signs (see Signs of Potential Complications box, p. 223). When one is stressed by a disturbing symptom, it is difficult to remember specifics. Therefore the pregnant woman and her family are reassured if they receive a printed form listing the signs and symptoms that warrant an investigation and the phone numbers to call in an emergency.

The nurse needs to answer questions honestly as they arise during pregnancy. It is often difficult for the pregnant woman to know when to report signs and symptoms. The mother is encouraged to refer to the printed list of potential complications and to listen to her body. If she senses that something is wrong, she should call her care provider. Several signs and symptoms need to be discussed more extensively. These include vaginal bleeding, alteration in fetal movements, symptoms of pregnancy induced hypertension (PIH), rupture of membranes, and preterm labor.

If *vaginal bleeding* occurs in the third trimester, it is important to differentiate brownish spotting occurring 48 hours after vaginal examination or after intercourse from the "show" of pinkish mucus. The woman is to come to the hospital's emergency area immediately for diagnosis and treatment if bleeding is other than one of the preceding types.

Should the pregnant woman notice cessation, noticeable diminution, or acceleration in the amount of *fetal movement,* she is to notify her health care provider.

Appearance of *edema* of the hands and around the eyes, severe *headaches, visual changes,* or feelings of *jitteriness* require immediate evaluation for PIH.

A gush or trickle of clear *watery discharge* that appears to come from the vagina may indicate rupture of membranes. The diagnosis requires a visit to the clinic or hospital for evaluation.

Recognizing preterm labor. Teaching each mother-to-be to recognize preterm labor is necessary. Preterm labor is that which occurs after the twentieth week but before the thirty-seventh week of pregnancy. It is a condition in which uterine contractions cause the cervix to open earlier than normal, and it can result in preterm birth. Although certain

Text continued on p. 241

TABLE 10-2 *Discomforts Related to Pregnancy*

First Trimester

DISCOMFORT	PHYSIOLOGY	EDUCATION FOR SELF-CARE
Breast changes, new sensation: pain, tingling, tenderness	Hypertrophy of mammary glandular tissue and increased vascularization, pigmentation, and size and prominence of nipples and areolae caused by hormonal stimulation	Wear supportive maternity bras with pads to absorb discharge, may be worn at night; wash with warm water and keep dry; breast tenderness may interfere with sexual expression/foreplay but is temporary
Urgency and frequency of urination	Vascular engorgement and altered bladder function caused by hormones; bladder capacity reduced by enlarging uterus and fetal presenting part	Empty bladder regularly; perform Kegel exercises; limit fluid intake before bedtime; wear perineal pad; report pain or burning sensation to primary health care provider
Languor and malaise; fatigue (early pregnancy, usually)	Unexplained; may be caused by increasing levels of estrogen, progesterone, and hCG or by elevated BBT; psychologic response to pregnancy and its required physical/psychologic adaptations	Rest as needed; eat well-balanced diet to prevent anemia
Nausea and vomiting, morning sickness—occurs in 50% to 75% of pregnant women; starts between first and second missed periods and lasts until about fourth missed period; may occur any time during day; fathers also may have symptoms	Cause unknown; may result from hormonal changes, possibly hCG; may be partly emotional, reflecting pride in, ambivalence about, or rejection of pregnant state	Avoid empty or overloaded stomach; maintain good posture—give stomach ample room; stop smoking; eat dry carbohydrate on awakening; remain in bed until feeling subsides, or alternate dry carbohydrate 1 hour with fluids such as hot herbal decaffeinated tea, milk, or clear coffee the next hour until feeling subsides; eat five to six small meals per day; avoid fried, odorous, spicy, greasy, or gas-forming foods; consult primary health care provider if intractable vomiting occurs
Ptyalism (excessive salivation) may occur starting 2 to 3 weeks after first missed period	Possibly caused by elevated estrogen levels; may be related to reluctance to swallow because of nausea	Use astringent mouth wash; chew gum
Gingivitis and **epulis** (hyperemia, hypertrophy, bleeding, tenderness); condition will disappear spontaneously 1 to 2 months after birth	Increased vascularity and proliferation of connective tissue from estrogen stimulation	Eat well-balanced diet with adequate protein and fresh fruits and vegetables; brush teeth gently and observe good dental hygiene; avoid infection; see dentist
Nasal stuffiness; epistaxis (nosebleed)	Hyperemia of mucous membranes related to high estrogen levels	Use humidifier; avoid trauma; normal saline nose drops or spray may be used
Leukorrhea: often noted throughout pregnancy	Hormonally stimulated cervix becomes hypertrophic and hyperactive, producing abundant amount of mucus	Not preventable; do not douche; wear perineal pads; perform hygienic practices such as wiping front to back; report to primary health care provider if accompanied by pruritus, foul odor, or change in character or color
Psychosocial dynamics, mood swings, mixed feelings	Hormonal and metabolic adaptations; feelings about female role, sexuality, timing of pregnancy, and resultant changes in life and lifestyle	Participate in pregnancy support group; communicate concerns to partner, family, and others; request referral for supportive services if needed (financial assistance)

Continued

TABLE 10-2 *Discomforts Related to Pregnancy—cont'd*

Second Trimester

DISCOMFORT	PHYSIOLOGY	EDUCATION FOR SELF-CARE
Pigmentation deepens, acne, oily skin	Melanocyte-stimulating hormone (from anterior pituitary)	Not preventable; usually resolves during puerperium
Spider nevi (angiomas) appear over neck, thorax, face, and arms during second or third trimesters	Focal networks of dilated arterioles (end-arteries) from increased concentration of estrogens	Not preventable; they fade slowly during late puerperium; rarely disappear completely
Palmar erythema occurs in 50% of pregnant women; may accompany spider nevi	Diffuse reddish mottling over palms and suffused skin over thenar eminencies and fingertips may be caused by genetic predisposition or hyperestrogenism	Not preventable; condition will fade within 1 week after giving birth
Pruritus (noninflammatory)	Unknown cause; various types as follows: nonpapular; closely aggregated pruritic papules	Keep fingernails short and clean; contact primary health care provider for diagnosis of cause
	Increased excretory function of skin and stretching of skin possible factors	Not preventable; symptomatic: Keri baths; mild sedation
		Distraction; tepid baths with sodium bicarbonate or oatmeal added to water; lotions and oils; change of soaps or reduction in use of soap; loose clothing
Palpitations	Unknown; should not be accompanied by persistent cardiac irregularity	Not preventable; contact primary health care provider if accompanied by symptoms of cardiac decompensation
Supine hypotension (vena cava syndrome) and bradycardia	Induced by pressure of gravid uterus on ascending vena cava when woman is supine; reduces uterine-placental and renal perfusion	Side-lying position or semisitting posture, with knees slightly flexed (see supine hypotension, p. 222)
Faintness and, rarely, syncope (orthostatic hypotension) may persist throughout pregnancy	Vasomotor lability or postural hypotension from hormones; in late pregnancy may be caused by venous stasis in lower extremities	Moderate exercise, deep breathing, vigorous leg movement; avoid sudden changes in position* and warm crowded areas; move slowly and deliberately; keep environment cool; avoid hypoglycemia by eating 5 to 6 small meals per day; wear elastic hose; sit as necessary; if symptoms are serious, contact primary health care provider
Food cravings	Cause unknown; craving determined by culture or geographic area	Not preventable; satisfy craving unless it interferes with well-balanced diet; report unusual cravings to primary health care provider
Heartburn (pyrosis or acid indigestion): burning sensation, occasionally with burping and regurgitation of a little sour-tasting fluid	Progesterone slows GI tract motility and digestion, reverses peristalsis, relaxes cardiac sphincter, and delays emptying time of stomach; stomach displaced upward and compressed by enlarging uterus	Limit or avoid gas-producing or fatty foods and large meals; maintain good posture; sip milk for temporary relief; hot herbal tea, chewing gum; primary health care provider may prescribe antacid between meals; contact primary health care provider for persistent symptoms
Constipation	GI tract motility slowed because of progesterone, resulting in increased resorption of water and drying of stool; intestines compressed by enlarging uterus; predisposition to constipation because of oral iron supplementation	Drink six glasses of water per day; include roughage in diet; moderate exercise; maintain regular schedule for bowel movements; use relaxation techniques and deep breathing; do not take stool softener, laxatives, mineral oil, other drugs, or enemas without first consulting primary health care provider

*Caution woman to rise slowly and sit on edge of bed or to assume hands-and-knee posture before rising, and to get up slowly after sitting or squatting.

TABLE 10-2 *Discomforts Related to Pregnancy—cont'd*		
Second Trimester—cont'd		
DISCOMFORT	**PHYSIOLOGY**	**EDUCATION FOR SELF-CARE**
Flatulence with bloating and belching	Reduced GI motility because of hormones, allowing time for bacterial action that produces gas; swallowing air	Chew foods slowly and thoroughly; avoid gas-producing foods, fatty foods, large meals; exercise; maintain regular bowel habits
Varicose veins (varicosities): may be associated with aching legs and tenderness; may be present in legs and vulva; hemorrhoids are varicosities in perianal area	Hereditary predisposition; relaxation of smooth muscle walls of veins because of hormones causing tortuousdilated veins in legs and pelvic vasocongestion; condition aggravated by enlarging uterus, gravity, and bearing down for bowel movements; thrombi from leg varices rare but may be produced by hemorrhoids	Avoid obesity, lengthy standing or sitting, constrictive clothing, and constipation and bearing down with bowel movements; moderate exercises; rest with legs and hips elevated (see Fig. 10-16); wear support stocking; thrombosed hemorrhoid may be evacuated; relieve swelling and pain with warm sitz baths, local application of astringent compresses
Leukorrhea: often noted throughout pregnancy	Hormonally stimulated cervix becomes hypertrophic and hyperactive,producing abundant amount of mucus	Not preventable; do not douche; maintain good hygiene; wear perineal pads; report to primary health care provider if accompanied by pruritus, foul odor, or change in character or color
Headaches (through week 26)	Emotional tension (more common than vascular migraine headache); eye strain (refractory errors); vascular engorgement and congestion of sinuses resulting from hormone stimulation	Conscious relaxation; contact primary health care provider for constant "splitting" headache, to assess for pregnancy-induced hypertension (PIH)
Carpal tunnel syndrome (involves thumb, second, and third fingers, lateral side of little finger)	Compression of median nerve resulting from changes surrounding tissues; pain, numbness, tingling, burning; loss of skilled movements (typing); dropping of objects	Not preventable; elevate affected arms; splinting of affected hand may help; regressive after pregnancy; surgery is curative
Periodic numbness, tingling of fingers (acrodysesthesia) occurs in 5% of pregnant women	Brachial plexus traction syndrome resulting from drooping of shoulders during pregnancy (occurs especially at night and early morning)	Maintain good posture; wear supportive maternity bra; condition will disappear if lifting and carrying baby does not aggravate it
Round ligament pain (tenderness)	Stretching of ligament caused by enlarging uterus	Not preventable; rest, maintain good body mechanics to avoid overstretching ligament; relieve cramping by squatting or bringing knees to chest, sometimes heat helps
Joint pain, backache, and pelvic pressure; hypermobility of joints	Relaxation of symphyseal and sacroiliac joints because of hormones, resulting in unstable pelvis; exaggerated lumbar and cervicothoracic curves caused by change in center of gravity resulting from enlarging abdomen	Maintain good posture and body mechanics; avoid fatigue; wear low-heeled shoes; abdominal supports may be useful; conscious relaxation; sleep on firm mattress; apply local heat or ice; get back rubs; do pelvic rock exercise; rest; condition will disappear 6 to 8 weeks after birth

Continued

TABLE 10-2　*Discomforts Related to Pregnancy—cont'd*

Third Trimester

DISCOMFORT	PHYSIOLOGY	EDUCATION FOR SELF-CARE
Shortness of breath and dyspnea occur in 60% of pregnant women	Expansion of diaphragm limited by enlarging uterus; diaphragm is elevated about 4 cm; some relief after lightening	Good posture; sleep with extra pillows; avoid overloading stomach; stop smoking; contact health care provider if symptoms worsen to rule out anemia, emphysema, and asthma
Insomnia (later weeks of pregnancy)	Fetal movements, muscle cramping, urinary frequency, shortness of breath, or other discomforts	Reassurance; conscious relaxation; back massage or **effleurage** (Fig. 10-18); support of body parts with pillows; warm milk or warm shower before retiring
Psychosocial responses: mood swings, mixed feelings, increased anxiety	Hormonal and metabolic adaptations; feelings about impending labor, birth, and parenthood	Reassurance and support from significant other and nurse; improved communication with partner, family, and others
Gingivitis and epulis (hyperemia, hypertrophy, bleeding, tenderness): condition will disappear spontaneously 1 to 2 months after birth	Increased vascularity and proliferation of connective tissue from estrogen stimulation	Well-balanced diet with adequate protein and fresh fruits and vegetables; gentle brushing and good dental hygiene; avoid infection; see dentist for teeth cleaning
Urinary frequency and urgency return	Vascular engorgement and altered bladder function caused by hormones; bladder capacity reduced by enlarging uterus and fetal presenting part	Empty bladder regularly, Kegel exercises; limit fluid intake before bedtime; reassurance; wear perineal pad; contact health care provider for pain or burning sensation
Perineal discomfort and pressure	Pressure from enlarging uterus, especially when standing or walking; multifetal gestation	Rest, conscious relaxation, and good posture; contact health care provider for assessment and treatment if pain is present
Braxton Hicks contractions	Intensification of uterine contractions in preparation for work of labor	Reassurance; rest; change of position; practice breathing techniques when contractions are bothersome; effleurage
Leg cramps (gastrocnemius spasm), especially when reclining	Compression of nerves supplying lower extremities because of enlarging uterus; reduced level of diffusible serum calcium or elevation of serum phosphorus; aggravating factors: fatigue, poor peripheral circulation, pointing toes when stretching legs or when walking, drinking more than 1 L (1 qt) of milk per day	Check for Homans' sign; if negative, use massage and heat over affected muscle; dorsiflex foot until spasm relaxes (Fig. 10-19); stand on cold surface; oral supplementation with calcium carbonate or calcium lactate tablets; aluminum hydroxide gel, 30 ml, with each meal removes phosphorus by absorbing it
Ankle edema (nonpitting) to lower extremities	Edema aggravated by prolonged standing, sitting, poor posture, lack of exercise, constrictive clothing (e.g., garters), or by hot weather	Ample fluid intake for natural diuretic effect; put on support stockings before arising; rest periodically with legs and hips elevated (see Fig. 10-16), exercise moderately; contact health care provider if generalized edema develops; *diuretics are contraindicated*

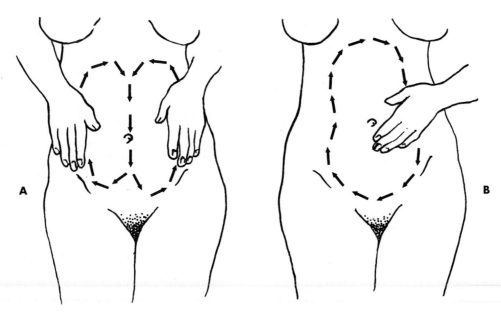

Fig. **10-18** Pattern for effleurage, a light, rhythmic stroking useful for inducing relaxation. **A,** Self-effleurage. **B,** Effleurage by another.

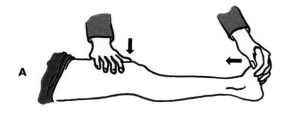

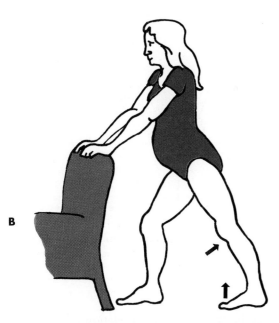

Fig. **10-19** Relief of muscle spasm (leg cramps). **A,** Another person dorsiflexes foot with knee extended. **B,** Woman stands and leans forward, thereby dorsiflexing foot of affected leg.

factors, such as multifetal pregnancy, may increase a woman's chances of going into preterm labor, the specific cause (or causes) is not known. If the woman knows the warning signs and symptoms of preterm labor and seeks care early enough, should they occur, it may be possible to prevent a preterm birth. Warning signs and symptoms of preterm labor are given in the Home Care box. Figure 10-20 shows where in the body the symptoms of preterm labor may be located.

Sexual counseling

The sexual counseling of expectant couples includes countering misinformation, providing reassurance of normality, and suggesting alternative behaviors. The uniqueness of each couple is considered within a biopsychosocial framework (see the Home Care box).

Counseling couples concerning sexual adjustments that must be made during pregnancy demands self-assessment on the part of the nurse, as well as a knowledge of the physical, social, and emotional responses to sex during pregnancy (Rynerson & Lowdermilk, 1993). Not all maternity nurses are comfortable dealing with the sexual concerns of their patients. Therefore those nurses who are aware of their personal strengths and limitations in dealing with sexual content are better prepared to make referrals if necessary.

Many women merely need permission to be sexually active during pregnancy. Many other women, however, need to be given information about the physiologic changes that occur during pregnancy and have the myths associated with sex during pregnancy dispelled. Such tasks are within the purview of the nurse and should be an integral component of the health care rendered.

HOME CARE *Patient Instructions for Self-Care*

How to Recognize Preterm Labor

Because the onset of preterm labor is subtle and often hard to recognize, it is important to know how to feel your abdomen for uterine contractions. You can feel for contractions in the following way. While lying down, place your fingertips on the top of your uterus. A contraction is the periodic tightening or hardening of your uterus. If your uterus is contracting, you will actually feel your abdomen get tight or hard and then feel it relax or soften when the contraction is over.

If you think you are having any of the other signs and symptoms of preterm labor, empty your bladder, drink three to four glasses of water for hydration, lie down tilted toward your side, and place a pillow at your back for support.

Check for contractions for 1 hour. To tell how often contractions are occurring, check the minutes that elapse from the beginning of one contraction to the beginning of the next.

It is *normal* to have some uterine contractions throughout the day. They usually occur when a woman changes positions. These usually irregular and mild contractions are called Braxton Hicks contractions. They help with uterine tone and uteroplacental perfusion.

It is *not normal* to have frequent uterine contractions (every 10 minutes or more often for 1 hour).

Contractions of labor are regular, frequent, and hard. They also may be felt as a tightening of the abdomen or a backache. This type of contraction causes the cervix to efface and dilate.

Call your doctor, nurse-midwife, clinic, or labor and birth unit, or go to the hospital if any of the following signs occur:
- You have uterine contractions every 10 minutes or more often for 1 hour *or*
- You have any of the other signs and symptoms for 1 hour *or*
- You have any bloody spotting or leaking of fluid from your vagina

It is often difficult to identify preterm labor. Accurate diagnosis requires assessment by the health care provider, usually in the hospital or clinic.

Post these instructions where they can be seen by everyone in the family.

HOME CARE *Patient Instructions for Self-Care*

Sexuality in Pregnancy

- Be aware that maternal physiologic changes, such as breast enlargement, nausea, fatigue, abdominal changes, perineal enlargement, leukorrhea, pelvic vasocongestion, and orgasmic responses, may affect sexuality and sexual expression.
- Discuss responses to pregnancy with your partner.
- Keep in mind that cultural prescriptions (dos) and proscriptions (don'ts) may affect your responses.
- Although your libido may be depressed during the first trimester, it increases during the second and third trimesters.
- Discuss and explore with your partner:
  - Alternative behaviors (e.g., mutual masturbation, foot massage, cuddling)
  - Alternative positions (e.g., female superior, side-lying) for sexual intercourse
- Intercourse is safe as long as it is not uncomfortable. There is no correlation between intercourse and spontaneous abortion, but observe the following precautions:
  - Abstain from intercourse if you experience uterine cramping or vaginal bleeding; report event to your caregiver as soon as possible.
  - Abstain from intercourse (or any activity that results in orgasm) if you have a history of cervical incompetence, until it is corrected.
- Continue to use "safer sex" behaviors. Women at risk for acquiring or transmitting sexually transmitted diseases are encouraged to use condoms during sexual intercourse throughout pregnancy.

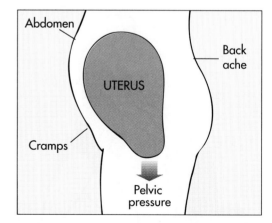

Fig. **10-20** Symptoms of preterm labor. (From Lowdermilk D, Perry S & Bobak I: *Maternity and women's health care*, ed 6, St Louis, 1997, Mosby.)

Some couples need to be referred for sex therapy or family therapy. Couples with long-standing problems with sexual dysfunction that are intensified by pregnancy are candidates for sex therapy. Whenever a sexual problem is a symptom of a more serious relationship problem, the couple would benefit from family therapy.

Using the history. The couple's sexual history provides a basis for counseling, but history-taking is also an ongoing process. The couple's receptivity to changes in attitudes, body image, partner relationships, and physical status are relevant topics throughout pregnancy. Whenever changes occur, unexpected problems may arise that require intervention. The history reveals the patient's knowledge of female anatomy and physiology and her attitudes about sex during pregnancy, as well as her perceptions of the pregnancy, the health status of the couple, and the quality of their relationship. An understanding of the couple's subjective experience provides the direction and focus for sexual counseling.

Countering misinformation. Many myths and much of the misinformation related to sex and pregnancy are masked by seemingly unrelated issues. For example, a question about the baby's ability to hear and see in utero may be prompted by questions about the baby being an observer of lovemaking. The counselor must be extremely sensitive to the questions behind such questions when counseling in this highly charged emotional area.

Suggesting alternative behaviors. At this time research has not demonstrated conclusively that coitus and orgasm are contraindicated at any time during pregnancy for the obstetrically and medically healthy woman (Cunningham et al., 1997; Scott et al., 1994). However, a history of more than one spontaneous abortion or a threatened abortion in the first trimester; impending spontaneous abortion in the second trimester; and PROM, bleeding, or abdominal pain during the third trimester warrant precaution when it comes to coitus and orgasm (Rynerson & Lowdermilk, 1993).

Solitary and mutual masturbation and oral-genital intercourse may be used by couples as alternatives to penile-vaginal intercourse. Partners who enjoy cunnilingus may feel "turned off" by the normal increase in the amount and odor of vaginal discharge during pregnancy. Couples who practice cunnilingus should be cautioned against the blowing of air into the vagina, particularly during the last few weeks of pregnancy when the cervix may be slightly open. An air embolism can occur if air is forced between the uterine wall and the fetal membranes and enters the maternal vascular system through the placenta.

Showing the woman or couple pictures of possible variations of coital position is often helpful (Fig. 10-21). The female-superior, side-by-side, and rear-entry positions are possible alternative positions to the traditional male-superior position. The woman astride (superior position) allows her to control the angle and depth of penile penetration, as well as to protect her breasts and abdomen. The side-by-side position is the preferred one, especially during the third trimester, because it requires less energy and places less pressure on the pregnant abdomen.

Multiparous women sometimes experience severe breast tenderness in the first trimester. A coital position that avoids direct pressure on the woman's breasts and decreased breast fondling during love play can be recommended to such couples. The woman should also be reassured that this condition is normal and temporary.

Some women complain of lower abdominal cramping and backache after orgasm during the first and third trimesters. A back rub can often relieve some of the

Fig. **10-21** Positions for sexual intercourse during pregnancy. **A,** Female superior; **B,** side by side; **C,** rear entry. (From Lowdermilk D, Perry S & Bobak I: *Maternity and women's health care,* ed 6, St Louis, 1997, Mosby.)

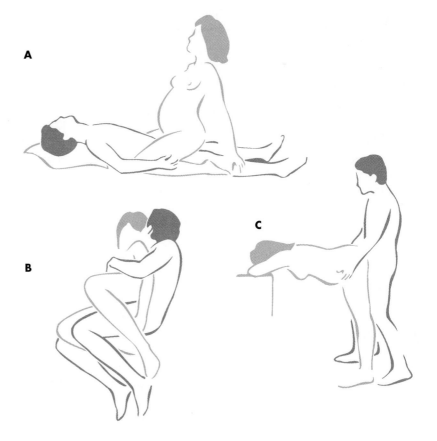

discomfort and provide a pleasant experience. A tonic uterine contraction, often lasting up to a minute, replaces the rhythmic contractions of orgasm during the third trimester. Changes in the fetal heart rate without fetal distress have also been reported.

The objective of "safer sex" is to provide prophylaxis against the acquisition and transmission of STDs (e.g., herpes simplex virus [HSV], HIV). Because these diseases may be transmitted to the woman and her fetus, the use of condoms is recommended throughout pregnancy if the woman is at risk for acquiring an STD.

Well-informed nurses who are comfortable with their own sexuality and the sexual counseling needs of expectant couples can offer counseling in this valuable but often neglected area. They can establish an open environment in which couples can feel free to introduce their concerns about sexual adjustment and seek support and guidance. This is important for lesbian women and their partners, as well as for women partnered by men.

Psychosocial support

Esteem, affection, trust, concern, consideration of cultural and religious responses, and listening are all components of the emotional support given the pregnant woman and her family. The woman's satisfaction with her relationships and support, her feeling of competence, and her sense of being in control are important issues to be addressed in the third trimester. A discussion of the unborn child's responses to stimuli, such as sound, light, maternal posture, and tension, as well as the child's patterns of sleeping and waking can be helpful. Also discussed are emotional tensions that can arise related to the childbirth experience, such as those stemming from fear of pain, loss of control, and possible birth of child before reaching hospital; anxieties about the recognized responsibilities and tasks of parenthood; parental concerns about the safety of the mother and unborn child; parental concerns about siblings and their acceptance of the new baby; parental concerns about social and economic responsibilities; and parental concerns arising from conflicts in cultural, religious, or personal value systems. (Sequin et al., 1995; Starn, 1991a, 1991b).

The father's or partner's commitment to the pregnancy, the couple's relationship, and their concerns about sexuality and sexual expression can emerge as issues for many expectant parents. Validation, feedback, and social comparison characterize the support given.

Providing the mother- and father-to-be an opportunity to discuss their concerns, providing a listening ear, and validating the normality of their responses can meet their needs to varying degrees. Nurses must also recognize that men feel more vulnerable during their partner's pregnancy. Female partners may also have these feelings. Anticipatory guidance and health promotion strategies can help partners cope with their concerns. Nursing intervention may either directly help them deal with such concerns in the event that such intimate feelings are confided or do so indirectly through the education of the mothers. Health care providers can stimulate and encourage open dialogue between the couple.

Evaluation

Evaluation of the effectiveness of care of the woman during pregnancy is based on the previously stated outcomes.

I VARIATIONS IN PRENATAL CARE

The course of prenatal care described thus far may seem to suggest that the experiences of childbearing women are similar and that nursing interventions are uniformly consistent across all populations. Although typical patterns of response to pregnancy are easily recognized and many aspects of prenatal care indeed are consistent, pregnant women enter the health care system with individual concerns and needs. The ability of the nurse to assess unique needs and to tailor interventions to the individual are hallmarks of expertise in providing care. Variations that influence prenatal care include culture, age, and number of fetuses.

Cultural Influences

Prenatal care as we know it is a phenomenon of Western medicine. In the Western biomedical model of care, women are encouraged to seek prenatal care as early as possible in their pregnancy by visiting a physician, nurse-midwife, or office or clinic. Such visits are usually routine and, as already mentioned, follow a systematic sequence, with the initial visit followed by monthly, then semimonthly, then weekly visits. Monitoring weight and blood pressure; testing blood and urine; teaching specific information about diet, rest, and activity; and preparing for childbirth are common components of prenatal care. This model is not only unfamiliar but seems strange to many groups (Green, 1990; Kulig, 1990).

Many cultural variations in prenatal care exist (Meikle et al., 1995). Even if the prenatal care described is familiar to a woman, some practices may conflict with the beliefs and practices of a subculture group to which she belongs. Because of these and other factors, such as lack of money, lack of transportation, and poor communication on the part of health care providers, women from many such groups do not participate in the prenatal care system (Lazarus & Philipson, 1990; Leatherman, Blackburn & Davidhizar, 1990; Scupholme, Robertson & Kamons, 1991). Such behavior may be misinterpreted by nurses as uncaring, lazy, or ignorant.

A concern for modesty is also a deterrent to many women's seeking prenatal care. For some women, exposing body parts, especially to a man, is considered a major violation of their modesty. For many women, invasive procedures, such as a vaginal examination, may be so threatening that they cannot be discussed, even with their own husbands. Thus many women prefer a female to a male health care provider (Geissler, 1994; Hutchinson & Baqi-Aziz, 1994). Too often, health care providers assume women lose this modesty during pregnancy and labor, but actually most women value and appreciate efforts to maintain their modesty.

For numerous cultural groups a physician is deemed appropriate only in times of illness, and because pregnancy is considered a normal process and the woman is in a state of health, the services of a physician are considered inappropriate. Even if problems with pregnancy do develop from the standpoint of Western medicine, they may not be perceived as problems but considered normal by members of these cultural groups.

Although pregnancy is considered normal by many, certain practices are expected of women of all cultures to ensure a good outcome. **Cultural prescriptions** tell women what to do, and **cultural proscriptions** establish taboos. The purposes of these practices are to prevent maternal illness resulting from a pregnancy-induced imbalanced state and to protect the vulnerable fetus. Prescriptions and proscriptions regulate the woman's emotional response, clothing, activity and rest, sexual activity, and dietary practices.

To provide culturally sensitive care, the nurse must be knowledgeable about practices and customs, although it is not possible to know all there is to know about every culture and subculture, as well as the many lifestyles that exist. The nurse can question patients about cultural beliefs and childbearing, and the nurse can support and nurture those beliefs that promote physical or emotional adaptation. However, if potentially harmful beliefs are identified, the nurse should carefully explore such beliefs with the patient and use them in the reeducation and modification process.

Emotional response

Virtually all cultures emphasize the importance of maintaining a socially harmonious and agreeable environment for a pregnant woman. An absence of stress is important in ensuring a successful outcome for the mother and baby. Harmony with other people must be fostered, and visits from extended family members may be required to demonstrate pleasant and noncontroversial relationships. If discord exists in a relationship, it is usually dealt with in culturally prescribed ways.

Besides proscriptions regarding food, other proscriptions involve imitative magic. Many Mexicans believe pregnant women should not witness an eclipse of the moon because it may cause a cleft palate in the infant. They also believe that exposure to an earthquake may precipitate preterm birth, miscarriage, or even a breech presentation. In some cultures a pregnant woman must not ridicule someone with an affliction for fear her child might be born with the same handicap. A mother should not hate a person

lest her child resemble that person, and dental work should not be done because it may cause a baby to have a "harelip." A widely held folk belief in many cultures is that the pregnant woman should refrain from raising her arms above her head and tying knots so that the umbilical cord does not wrap around the baby's neck or knot. Other cultures believe placing a knife under the bed of a laboring woman will "cut" her pain.

Clothing

Although most cultural groups do not prescribe specific clothing to be worn during pregnancy, modesty is an expectation of many. Some Mexican women of the Southwest wear a cord beneath the breast and knotted over the umbilicus. This cord, called a *muneco*, is thought to prevent morning sickness and ensure a safe birth. Amulets, medals, and beads may also be worn to ward off evil spirits (Spector, 1996).

Physical activity and rest

Norms that regulate the physical activity of mothers during pregnancy vary tremendously. Many groups, including Native Americans and some Asian groups (Lee, 1989), encourage women to be active, to walk, and to engage in normal although not strenuous activities to ensure that the baby is healthy and not too large. On the other hand, other groups such as the Filipino culture believe that any activity is dangerous, and others willingly take over the work of the pregnant woman. Some Filipinos believe that this inactivity protects the mother and child. The mother is encouraged simply to produce the succeeding generation. If health care providers do not know of this belief, they could misinterpret this behavior as laziness or noncompliance with the desired prenatal health care regimen. Again, it is important for the nurse to find out the way each pregnant woman views activity and rest.

Sexual activity

In most cultures, sexual activity is not prohibited until the end of pregnancy. Mexican-Americans view sexual activity as necessary to keep the birth canal lubricated (Geissler, 1994). On the other hand, some Vietnamese may have definite proscriptions against sexual intercourse, requiring abstinence throughout the pregnancy because it is thought that sexual intercourse may harm the mother and fetus (Geissler, 1994).

Diet

Nutritional information given by Western health care providers may also be a source of conflict for many cultural groups, but such a conflict commonly is not known by the health care providers unless they understand the dietary beliefs and practices of the particular people for whom they are caring. For example, Muslims must eat meat slaughtered in accordance with Muslim law. If this is not possible, they will accept Kosher or vegetarian foods (Hutchinson & Baqi-Aziz, 1994). Many cultures permit pregnant women to eat only warm foods (Geissler, 1994).

Age Differences

The age of the childbearing couple may have a significant influence on their physical and psychosocial adaptation to pregnancy. Normal developmental processes that occur in both very young and older mothers are interrupted by pregnancy and require a different type of adaptation to pregnancy than that of the woman of typical childbearing age. Although the individuality of each pregnant woman is recognized, special needs of expectant mothers 15 years of age or younger or those 35 years or older are summarized below.

Adolescent mothers

Over one million teenage girls in the United States become pregnant annually (AGI, 1994). About 9% of sexually active 14 year olds, 18% of 15 to 17 year olds, and 22% of 18 to 19 year olds become pregnant every year (AGI, 1994). Most of the teenage births are the result of unintended pregnancies. Only 14% were intended (Moore, Snyder & Glei, 1995).

The United States has the highest teenage birth rate in the industrialized world (Moore, Snyder & Glei, 1995). In contrast, although other industrialized nations have similar levels of sexually experienced adolescents, the numbers of teenage births and abortions are less than those in the United States. Thus it would appear that teenagers in other industrialized countries are using effective contraception more consistently than teenagers in the United States (AGI, 1994).

The motivation to avoid pregnancy is probably related to the adolescent's perception of the benefits of postponing parenthood, and this perception is in turn influenced by her present situation and her belief in future life options. Adolescents from a lower socioeconomic status (SES) have fewer choices. Therefore, instead of striving for high educational attainment and a professional career, they may have to choose other ways of accomplishing the transition to adulthood. Sexual intercourse and having a baby may seem to be more viable alternatives than attending college.

The risk for problems during pregnancy and childbirth is greatest in the pregnant adolescent girl younger than 15 years. The incidence of low-birth-weight infants and spontaneous abortion, as well as infant mortality, are two to three times higher for girls in this age group than they are for women older than 25 years (Leland et al., 1995; National Center for Health Statistics, 1990).

The very young adolescent is at particular risk during pregnancy because she tends to enter prenatal care later than do older adolescents and women. Such late entry into prenatal care may be the result of late recognition of pregnancy, denial of pregnancy, or confusion about available services (Kinsman & Slap, 1992). Such a delay in care may leave an inadequate time before the birth to attend to cor-

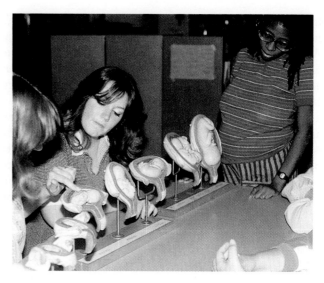

Fig. **10-22** Pregnant adolescents reviewing fetal development. (Courtesy Marjorie Pyle, RNC, Lifecircle, Costa Mesa, Calif.)

rectable problems. The very young pregnant adolescent is at higher risk for each of the confounding variables associated with poor pregnancy outcomes and for those conditions associated with a first pregnancy (e.g., pregnancy-induced hypertension). When prenatal care is initiated early and consistently, and confounding variables (e.g., socioeconomic factors) are controlled, very young pregnant adolescents are at no greater risk (nor are their infants) for an adverse outcome than older pregnant women. The role of the nurse in reducing the risks and consequences of adolescent pregnancy is thus twofold: first, to encourage early and continued prenatal care, and second, to refer the adolescent, if necessary, for appropriate social support services, which can help reverse the effects of a negative socioeconomic environment (Fig. 10-22).

Older mothers

Two groups of older parents have emerged in the population of women having a child late in their childbearing years. One group consists of women who have many children or who have a child during the menopausal period. The other group consists of relative newcomers to maternity care. These are women who have deliberately delayed childbearing until their late 30s or early 40s (Duchon & Muise, 1993).

Multiparous mothers. Multiparous women may be those who have never used contraceptives because of personal choice or lack of knowledge concerning contraceptives, or they may be women who have used contraceptives successfully during the childbearing years but, as menopause approaches, they may cease menstruating regularly or stop using contraceptives and consequently become pregnant. The older multiparous woman may feel that pregnancy separates her from her peer group and that her age is a hindrance to close associations with young mothers. Other parents welcome the unexpected infant as evidence of continuing maternal and paternal roles.

Primiparous mothers. The number of first-time pregnancies in women between the ages of 35 and 40 years has increased by 37% over the past 10 years. It is not uncommon now to see women in their late 30s or even in their early 40s pregnant for the first time. Reasons for delaying pregnancy include advanced education, career priorities, better contraceptive measures, and infertility.

These women choose parenthood as opposed to a child-free lifestyle. They often are successfully established in a career and a lifestyle with a partner that includes time for self-attention, the establishment of a home with accumulated possessions, and freedom to travel. When asked the reason they choose pregnancy later in life, many reply, "because time is running out."

The dilemma of choice includes the recognition that being a parent will have positive and negative consequences (Chervenak & Kardon, 1991). Couples need to discuss the consequences of childbearing and child rearing before committing themselves to this lifelong venture. Partners in this group seem to share the preparation for parenthood, planning for a family-centered birth, and desire to be loving and competent parents. However, the reality of child care may prove difficult for such parents.

As with mothers of all ages, the mother over 35 who is accustomed to the stimulation of the contact with other adults may find the isolation with her infant difficult to accept. Anger and resentment toward the father (or infant) can result, even with "preparation" for these aspects of parenting.

First-time mothers older than 35 years select the "right time" for pregnancy; this right time is influenced by their awareness of the increasing possibility of infertility or of genetic defects in the infants of older women. Such women seek information about pregnancy from books and friends. They actively try to prevent fetal disorders and are careful in searching for the best possible maternity care. They identify sources of stress in their lives. They have concerns about having enough energy and stamina to meet the demands of parenting and their new roles and relationships.

If they become pregnant after treatment for infertility, they may suddenly have negative or ambivalent feelings about the pregnancy. They may experience a multifetal pregnancy that may create emotional and physical problems. Adjusting to parenting two or more infants requires adaptability and additional resources.

During pregnancy, parents explore the possibilities and responsibilities of changing identities and new roles. They must prepare a safe and nurturing environment during pregnancy and after birth. They must integrate the child into an established family system and negotiate new roles (parent roles, sibling roles, grandparent roles) for family members.

Multifetal pregnancy

A **multifetal pregnancy** places the mother and fetuses at risk. The maternal blood volume is increased, resulting in an increased strain on the maternal cardiovascular system. Anemia often develops because of a greater demand for iron by the fetuses. Marked uterine distention and increased pressure on the adjacent viscera and pelvic vasculature and diastasis of the two recti abdomini muscles (in the midline) may occur. Placenta previa develops more commonly in multifetal pregnancies because of the large size or placement of the placentas (Cunningham et al., 1997; Scott et al., 1994). Premature separation of the placenta may occur before the second and any subsequent fetuses are born.

Twin pregnancies often end in prematurity. Spontaneous rupture of membranes before term is common (Buckley & Kulb, 1990). Congenital malformations are twice as common in monozygotic twins as in singletons, though there is no increase in the incidence of congenital anomalies in dizygotic twins. In addition, two-vessel cords—that is, cords with a single umbilical artery—occur more often in twins than in singletons, but this abnormality is most common in monozygotic twins. However, the most serious problem for the fetus is the local shunting of blood between placentas (twin-to-twin transfusion), causing the recipient twin to be larger and the donor twin to be small, pallid, dehydrated, malnourished, and hypovolemic. However, congenital heart failure may develop in the larger twin during the first 24 hours after birth.

The clinical diagnosis of multifetal pregnancy is accurate in about 90% of cases. The likelihood of a multifetal pregnancy is increased if any one or a combination of the following factors is revealed during a careful assessment (Buckley & Kulb, 1990):

- History of dizygous twins in the female lineage
- Use of fertility drugs
- More rapid uterine growth for time in pregnancy
- Hydramnios
- The palpation of an excessive number of small or large parts
- Asynchronous fetal heartbeats or more than one fetal electrocardiographic tracing
- Ultrasonographic evidence of more than one fetus

The diagnosis of a twin pregnancy can come as a shock to many expectant parents, and they may need additional support and education to help them cope with the changes they face. The mother will need nutrition counseling so that she gains more weight than that needed for a singleton birth, counseling that maternal adaptations will probably be more uncomfortable, and information about the possibility of a preterm birth.

The prenatal care given women with multifetal pregnancies includes changes in the pattern of care and modifications in other aspects such as the amount of weight gained and the diet observed. The prenatal visits of these mothers are scheduled at least every 2 weeks in the second trimester and weekly thereafter. No specific recommendation for weight gain for women with multifetal pregnancies has been made. In twin gestations, reports of gains of 20 kg have been associated with positive outcomes. Iron and vitamin supplementation is desirable. Attempts are made to prevent preeclampsia and eclampsia, which occur more commonly during multifetal pregnancies, and vaginitis; if they cannot be prevented, they are treated.

The considerable uterine distention involved can cause the backache commonly experienced by pregnant women to be even worse. Elastic stockings or maternity tights may be worn to control leg varicosities. If there are risk factors for preterm birth (e.g., premature dilatation of the cervix), abstinence from orgasm and nipple stimulation during the last trimester is recommended to help avert preterm labor. Frequent ultrasound examinations and heart rate monitoring will occur. Some practitioners recommend bed rest beginning at 20 weeks in women carrying twins to prevent preterm labor. Other practitioners question the value of prolonged bed rest. If bed rest is recommended, the mother needs to assume a lateral position to promote increased placental perfusion. If birth is delayed until after the thirty-sixth week, the risk of morbidity and mortality for the neonates decreases.

Multiple newborns will likely place a strain on finances, space, workload, and the mother's and family's coping capability. Lifestyle changes may be necessary. Parents will need assistance in making realistic plans for the care of the babies, for example, whether to breastfeed and whether to raise them as "alike" or as separate persons. Parents should be referred to national organizations such as Parents of Twins, Mothers of Multiples, and the La Leche League for further support (see Appendix D).

CHILDBIRTH EDUCATION

Content taught in the American educational system does little to prepare individuals for becoming parents. Informal preparation, especially through participation in care of younger siblings or relatives, is increasingly uncommon. Many individuals facing parenthood therefore have little information about what to expect and have few skills necessary to deal effectively with pregnancy and parenthood. Childbirth education classes are one way to fill this void.

Because of their knowledge, communication skills, acceptability to couples, and position in the health care system, nurses provide much of the education available for couples about reproduction, both informally and through courses focusing on aspects of the transition to parenthood. All professional nurses are prepared by their education and practice to participate in such teaching, particularly the immediate, situation-based teaching needed in clinic and hospital settings. Advanced preparation for childbirth education is also available and is especially useful for the nurse teaching in group situations or in cases in which a more

sophisticated psychologic approach is used and involves exploration of feelings and adjustment of expectations.

In a comprehensive preparation-for-parenthood educational program, expectant parents and their families are recognized as having different interests and needing different information as the pregnancy progresses. Consequently such programs are designed to meet the informational needs of parents during the three major stages of pregnancy and after birth—first-trimester classes, second-trimester classes, third-trimester classes, and postpartum ("fourth-trimester") classes.

First-trimester ("early bird") classes provide fundamental information and focus on the following topics: (1) early fetal development; (2) physiologic and emotional changes that occur early in pregnancy; (3) human sexuality; (4) birth settings and types of health care providers; (5) rest, exercise, and measures for relieving common discomforts; (6) the nutritional needs of the mother and fetus; and (7) the development of a birth plan. Environmental and workplace hazards have become important concerns in recent years, so even though pregnancy is considered a normal process, exercises, warning signs, drugs, and self-medication are topics of interest and concern.

Second-trimester classes emphasize the woman's participation in self-care and provide information about preparation for breastfeeding and formula feeding; basic hygiene; common complaints and simple, safe remedies; continued fetal development; infant health; and parenting. Support systems that are available during pregnancy and after birth are discussed throughout the series of classes. Such support systems can help parents function independently and effectively. During all the classes, participants are encouraged to openly express their feelings and concerns about any aspect of pregnancy, birth, and parenting.

During the third trimester, childbirth education focuses on preparation for the experiences of labor and birth. A study of 800 women in England found that receipt of information and a feeling of control were important components of women's satisfaction with the birth and their subsequent emotional well-being (Hetherington, 1990). Physiologic effects of length of labor and anesthesia/analgesia on mother and infant vary; formal preparation may assist in reducing the use of analgesia and anesthesia. Obstetric, postnatal, and neonatal complications may be reduced by combining a multidisciplinary team and comprehensive health services with childbirth education. Classes tailored to the needs of varied groups may be essential for effective outcomes.

Some women or couples want primarily to learn what to expect from medications. Others have a strong desire to use their own resources rather than pharmacotherapeutics to manage labor discomfort. Couples need information about the advantages and disadvantages of pain medication and other techniques for coping with labor. Although neither partner should feel guilty *if* pain medication is required during a particular labor experience, an emphasis on nonpharmacologic pain management strategies helps couples manage the labor and birth with dignity and increased comfort. Currently, most instructors teach a flexible approach, which helps couples learn and master many techniques that can be used during labor. Women are encouraged to incorporate their natural responses into coping with the pain of labor and birth. Couples are taught gate-control techniques such as massage, pressure on the palms or soles of the feet, hot compresses to the perineum, perineal massage, applications of heat or cold, breathing patterns, and focusing of attention on visual or other stimuli as ways to increase coping and decrease the distress from labor pain. (See Chapter 13 for further discussion of methods of managing pain.)

Program Types

An English physician, Grantly Dick-Read, published two books in which he theorized that pain in childbirth is socially conditioned and caused by a fear-tension-pain syndrome. His first book, *Natural Childbirth*, was published in 1933. Dick-Read's second book, *Childbirth without Fear*, was published in the United States in 1944. The work of Dick-Read became the foundation for organized programs of preparation for childbirth and teacher training throughout the United States, Canada, Great Britain, and South Africa. In 1960, the nurses prepared through such programs established the International Childbirth Education Association (ICEA). The **Dick-Read method,** referred to as *childbirth without fear,* basically recommended three techniques: deep breathing during abdominal thoracic respirations, shallow breathing, and breath holding for the second stage of labor. As knowledge about the effects of breath holding for pushing has grown, contemporary teachers of the Dick-Read method have altered this recommendation. Relaxation is an important part of the Dick-Read method (Dick-Read, 1987). Women are taught to consciously and progressively relax different muscle groups through the entire body until a high degree of skill at relaxation is achieved. Consequently, a woman is able to relax completely between contractions and keep all muscles except the uterus relaxed during contractions.

During the 1960s the **Lamaze method,** also known as the psychoprophylactic method (PPM), gained popularity in the United States. PPM offered new perspectives on preparation for childbirth by emphasizing mind control. Marjorie Karmel introduced PPM to the United States in her book, *Thank You, Dr. Lamaze,* which was published in the United States in 1959. PPM combines controlled muscular relaxation and breathing techniques. Active relaxation is an integral part of the Lamaze method (Lamaze, 1970). The woman is taught to contract specific muscle groups (neuromuscular control) while relaxing the remainder of her body. She thus learns to relax the uninvolved muscles in her body while her uterus contracts. Instead of tensing during

uterine contractions, women respond with conditioned relaxation and breathing patterns. In 1960 the American Society for Psychoprophylaxis in Obstetrics (ASPO) was formed in New York as a national organization to promote use of the Lamaze method and prepare teachers of the method. It continues to be an active organization, training large numbers of childbirth educators.

A Denver obstetrician, Robert Bradley, published *Husband-Coached Childbirth* in 1965. In the book he advocates what he calls true "natural" childbirth, without any form of anesthesia or analgesia and with a husband-coach and breathing techniques for labor. The American Academy of Husband-Coached Childbirth (AAHCC) was founded to make the **Bradley method** available and prepare teachers. This method of partner-coached childbirth uses breath control, abdominal breathing, and general body relaxation. Working in harmony with the body is emphasized (Bradley, 1981). Bradley's technique emphasizes environmental variables such as darkness, solitude, and quiet to make childbirth a more natural experience. Women using the Bradley method often appear to be sleeping during labor because they are in such a deep state of mental relaxation.

These methods incorporate intellectual and physical components. However, the Dick-Read and Bradley methods emphasize the naturalness of childbirth, whereas Lamaze emphasizes active mental and physical conditioning. Each program educates women to exchange fear of the unknown for confidence and understanding. Adequate prenatal education includes information on maternal adaptation, nutrition, sexuality, basic hygiene, and labor and birth. Support for the woman in labor is provided by her husband or another support person chosen by the expectant mother. Specially trained labor attendants, termed *monitrices,* sometimes provide support for the laboring woman using the Lamaze method.

In the holistic approach to childbirth education the emphasis is on the way the mind, body, and spirit are related and affect one another. Some specially trained professionals incorporate a variety of techniques and psychotherapeutic methodologies designed to promote self-awareness and identify attitudes, traumas, and anxieties that may interfere in the process of labor (Peterson, 1991; Wilberg, 1992). Dealing with these issues during pregnancy may promote more satisfying labor and assist people in becoming more effective, happier parents.

A variety of approaches to childbirth education have evolved as educators attempt to meet learning needs. In addition to classes designed specifically for pregnant adolescents and their partners and/or parents, classes have begun for other groups with special learning needs such as first-time mothers over 35, single women, adoptive parents, and parents of twins. Refresher classes for parents with children review coping techniques for labor and birth and help couples prepare for sibling reactions and adjustments to a new baby. Cesarean birth classes are offered for couples who may be at risk for an operative birth. Because many women successfully give birth vaginally after a previous cesarean birth, some classes focus on vaginal birth after cesarean (VBAC).

Because environmental influences and maternal behavior greatly affect newborn health, preconception and early pregnancy classes have been developed. These typically provide information about behaviors such as nutrition and exercise that promote improved pregnancy outcomes and the risks of environmental hazards, smoking, alcohol, and drugs.

Because of the multicultural composition of the population, great diversity exists in attitudes, expectations, and behaviors judged appropriate during pregnancy and early parenthood. No one approach can meet all needs. For example, classes for new immigrants are particularly effective when taught in class members' primary language. For classes to be meaningful, childbirth educators must understand the value systems in other cultures and their influence on issues such as nutrition, early prenatal care, maternal weight gain, and infant feeding practices. Parent educators must establish rapport, be understood, and build on cultural practices, reinforcing the positive and promoting change only if a practice (e.g., pica) is directly harmful (USDA & USDHHS, 1990; Waxler-Morrison, Anderson & Richardson, 1990).

Most childbirth education classes are attended by the pregnant woman and her partner, although a friend, teenage daughter, or parent may be the selected support person. When family-centered care is practiced, other family members may be present for the birth. Classes may be offered for grandparents and siblings to prepare them for their attendance at birth and/or the arrival of the baby. Classes focus on preparing families intellectually, emotionally, and physically for childbirth and promote wellness and improved lifestyle behaviors during the childbearing years (ASPO/Lamaze, 1990). Most childbirth preparation classes include content on pain management and relaxation.

Childbirth educators have a unique opportunity to influence positively the course of labor and birth. The ability of the educator to communicate effectively and to engage class members in the learning process determines to a large extent how much time and effort the couple is willing to invest in serious preparation. Creative teaching strategies are needed, and with the wealth of media now available, childbirth educators should have no difficulty designing classes that meet a wide variety in learning styles and educational needs of class participants. Educators that focus on immediate concerns of the couple are more likely to pique their interest and get them involved in class activities.

Informal Teaching

Not all expectant mothers and support people attend formal classes in preparation for childbirth. For those who do attend, extensive preparation is possible. However, many

do not take advantage of classes for a variety of reasons: employment; inaccessibility because of time; cultural, ethnic, or religious orientation; cost; lack of knowledge regarding choices in prenatal education classes; or lack of readiness. For these women, clinicians need to provide information that includes the following:

- Process of labor: admission, examination, care in labor
- Plans to get to hospital (when to go and where); care of other children
- Methods to control pain (e.g., analgesia and anesthesia, breathing and relaxing techniques)
- Supplies to have in a suitcase already packed for the trip to the hospital or birthing center: personal items for grooming, items for labor as desired (e.g., warm socks, focal point), supportive bra, slippers
- Responsibilities of the partner, family member, or friend who will be supporting the woman during labor and birth
- Emergency arrangements (e.g., precipitous birth)

Even if the woman or couple have attended parent education classes, the nurse should review the following topics to further ensure their preparation for childbirth:

- Symptoms of impending labor
- Breathing and relaxation techniques
- Involvement of partner
- Plans to get to hospital
- Plans during labor, terminology involved, and what care to expect
- Preparation for baby
- Preparation of grandparents and siblings

If a hospital birth is planned, often the woman must pre-register at the hospital of choice. Most hospitals now provide pamphlets containing information such as where to report when labor begins and the policies pertaining to visitors and visiting hours. Many facilities also conduct tours.

OPTIONS FOR CHILDBEARING FAMILIES

Today, childbearing couples are faced with an array of options including what type of professional will provide health care services, the development of a birth plan, and choice of birth settings. More than ever, nurses have a unique opportunity to provide information and assist couples in making informed choices.

Care Provider

Often the first decision the woman makes is who will be her primary health care provider for the pregnancy and birth. This decision is doubly important because it usually affects where the birth will take place. The nurse can provide information about the different types of health care providers and the kind of care to expect from each type. Physicians (obstetricians and family practice physicians) attend about 95% of births in the United States and Canada

(National Center for Health Statistics, 1993). They see low- and high-risk patients. Care often includes pharmacologic and medical management of problems and the use of technologic procedures. Family practice physicians may need backup by obstetricians if a specialist is needed for a problem such as a cesarean birth. Most physicians manage births in a hospital setting.

Nurse-midwives are registered nurses with additional education and training in the care of obstetric patients. They provide care for about 4% of the births in the United States and Canada (National Center for Health Statistics, 1993). Certified nurse-midwives may practice with physicians or independently with an arrangement for physician backup. They usually see low-risk obstetric patients. Care is often noninterventional, and the woman and family are usually encouraged to be active participants in the care. Nurse-midwives must refer patients to physicians for complications. Most births are managed in hospital settings or alternative birth centers; a small percentage may be managed in a home setting.

Independent midwives (also called lay midwives) are nonprofessional caregivers. Their training varies greatly, from formal training to self-teaching. They manage about 1% of births in the United States and Canada (National Center for Health Statistics, 1993). Patients who develop problems need to be seen by a physician. Almost all births managed by lay midwives occur in the home setting.

Birth Plan

The **birth plan** is a natural evolution of the contemporary wellness-oriented lifestyle. It is a tool by which parents can explore their childbirth options and choose those that are most important to them. Many parents already indicate some of their preferences by the type of health care provider and birth setting (hospital, free-standing birth center, or home) they have chosen. Some pregnant women enlist the services of a health care provider only after an interview and a tour of the birth facility. Others do not give conscious thought to the conduct of their pregnancies, the labor and birth process, recovery, and early parenthood. These women may need help with decision making. After the confirmation of pregnancy, couples tend to focus on the reality of their situation and their emotional responses. However, it is acceptable for the nurse to initiate a discussion of a birth plan during the first and second prenatal visits. Some maternity clinics provide printed material describing available options and giving answers to commonly asked questions. In addition, tours of the birth setting are offered by almost all facilities that provide perinatal services.

Patients' expectations must be reasonable and in keeping with the resources available in the community. The nurse can provide couples with pertinent information so that they can make informed decisions, alerting them to various options and the advantages and consequences of each.

The nurse needs to assess patients' readiness to learn and avoid overloading them with information. Some health care providers provide birth plan lists. A discussion of the printed list can serve as a means of getting couples to start thinking about, discussing, and identifying what is personally important to them. However, it is important to remember that some options may only be appropriate for low-risk women. The options of women with a high-risk pregnancy or those in whom complications develop during labor may be severely limited.

The birth plan can serve as a means of open communication between the pregnant woman and her partner and between the couple and health care providers. An early introduction to the idea of a birth plan allows the couple time to think about events or situations that could make their childbearing experience more meaningful and those they would prefer to avoid. The nurse-patient discussion of the birth plan needs to take place in an accepting atmosphere in which the patients can see themselves as unique and yet normal.

Topics for discussion and decision making may include any or all of the following:

- Partner's participation: Attend prenatal visits? Childbirth/parent education classes? Present during labor? During birth? During cesarean birth?
- Birth setting: Hospital delivery room or birthing room (if available)? A birthing center? Home?
- Labor management: Would you like to walk around during labor? Use a rocking chair? Use a shower? Use a jacuzzi, if available? Consider an electronic fetal monitor? Be interested in having music or dimmed lighting? Have older children or other people present? Is telemetry monitoring available? Consider stimulation of labor? Consider medication—what kind?
- Birth: Have you considered the various positions for birth—side lying? On hands and knees, kneeling, or squatting? Use a birthing bed? Or delivery table? Will you be photographing, videotaping, or recording any of the labor or birth? Who would you like to be present—partner, older siblings, other family members, or friends? What do you know about the use of forceps? episiotomies? Will your partner want to cut the umbilical cord?
- Immediately after birth: Do you want to hold the baby right away? To breastfeed immediately?
- Newborn care: What about circumcision for your baby (if male)? Will the baby be breastfed or bottle fed?
- Postpartum care: What kind of care do you anticipate—LDRP, mother-baby coupling, "request" coupling (newborn cared for in nursery while mother rests)? How long does your insurance company allow you to stay? Would you like to attend self-care classes or prefer to get such information from videotapes? On which subjects?

If older siblings are to be included in the labor and birth process, this needs to be reviewed and cleared with the physician or nurse-midwife, as well as with the staff at the birth setting. This should be done long before the EDB so that the stress this type of negotiation could cause during labor can be avoided. Some facilities require that a sibling present at a birth attend preparation classes. The woman needs to specify who will be responsible for the sibling during labor and birth because this is a requirement at many facilities.

Birth Setting

With careful thought, the concept of family-centered maternity care can be implemented in any setting. The three primary options of birth settings today are the hospital, an alternative birth center, and home. Women consider several factors in choosing a setting for childbirth, including the preference of their health care provider, characteristics of the birthing unit, and preference of their third-party payer (Mackey, 1990).

Hospital

Approximately 98% of all births in the United States take place in a hospital setting (National Center for Health Statistics, 1993). However, the types of labor and birth services vary greatly, from the traditional labor and delivery rooms with separate postpartum and newborn units to in-hospital birthing centers where all or almost all care takes place in a single unit.

Labor, delivery, recovery (LDR) and labor, delivery, recovery, postpartum (LDRP) rooms offer families a comfortable, private space for childbirth (see Fig. 15-15). Few admission or risk criteria exist for the use of these rooms. Some hospitals incorporate labor support by highly trained nurses, monitrices, or doulas (Greek, meaning "woman's servant"). Women labor, give birth, and spend the first bonding time with their families in the LDR room. If they are not in an LDRP room, transfer to a postpartum room is usually the only room change they have to make. The woman and her family may choose this environment because it is more homelike, but also because assistance is immediately available in case of emergencies.

Alternative birth center

Alternative birth centers (ABCs) may be physically separate from or part of the traditional obstetrics department. Delivery and operating rooms and medical or neonatal intensive care facilities should be easily accessible for use if serious problems arise. Hospital ABCs and freestanding birth centers are intended to offer families an alternative to home birth, providing a compromise between hospital and home. These birth-setting choices have been shown to be safe alternatives to birth in a traditional delivery setting (Alden & Harris, 1995). In addition, they can be designed to ensure quality control and be cost effective, two significant issues in the delivery of health care today.

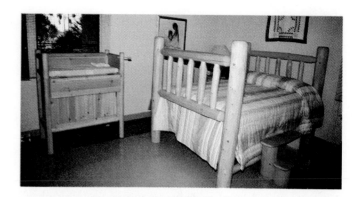

A

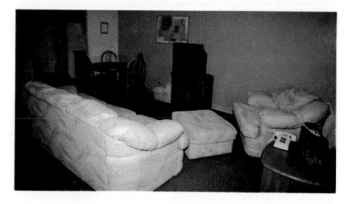

B

Fig. **10-23** Alternative birth center. **A,** Note double bed and crib in homelike surroundings. **B,** Lounge and kitchen. (Courtesy Michael S. Clement, MD, Mesa, Ariz.)

ABCs typically have homelike accommodations, including a double bed for the couple and a crib for the newborn (Fig. 10-23). Emergency equipment and medications are discreetly stored within cupboards, out of view but easily accessible. Private bathroom facilities are incorporated into each birth unit in the center. An early labor lounge or a living room and small kitchen may be available. Careful screening of each applicant ensures that only low-risk and prepared women or couples participate in ABC births.

The family is admitted to the ABC where labor and birth will occur. Family members may remain there until discharge if the time interval and requirements for room use permit. If the family has to remain in the ABC for more than 24 hours after the birth, the demand for use of the ABC by other families may require transfer of the first family to a postpartum room in the hospital setting.

Although most ABCs and LDR/LDRP rooms are located in hospitals, a growing number of **freestanding birth centers** have been developed. Most freestanding birth centers are staffed by physicians who have privileges at the local hospital and certified nurse-midwives who are equipped to attend low-risk women.

Services provided by the freestanding birth centers include those necessary for safe management during the childbearing cycle. In addition, attendance at childbirth and parenting classes is required of all patients. Prenatal supervision of the woman, whose nutritional and health status must be good and who must be experiencing a low-risk pregnancy, begins in the first trimester. Patients must understand that situations may require transfer to a hospital and must agree to abide by those guidelines.

Birth centers may have resources such as a lending library for parents, reference files on related topics, recycled maternity clothes and baby clothes and equipment, and supplies and reference materials for childbirth educators. The centers may also have referral files for community resources that offer services relating to childbirth and early parenting, including support groups (such as single parents, postbirth support groups, and parents of twins), genetic counseling, women's issues, and consumer action. These centers are often close to a major hospital so that quick transfer to that institution is possible if necessary. Ambulance service and emergency procedures must be readily available. Fees vary with the services provided but typically are less than or equal to those charged by local hospitals. Some centers base fees on the ability of the family to pay (reduced-fee sliding scale). Several third-party payers, Medicaid, and CHAMPUS recognize and reimburse these clinics. Patients should check with insurers to see what services are covered.

Home birth

Home birth has always been popular in countries such as Sweden and the Netherlands. In developing countries, hospitals or adequate lying-in facilities are often unavailable to most pregnant women and home birth is a necessity.

National groups supporting home birth are the Home Oriented Maternity Experience (HOME) and the National Association of Parents for Safe Alternatives in Childbirth (NAPSAC). These groups work to foster more humane childbearing practices at all levels, integrating the alternatives for childbirth to meet the needs of the total population. The literature on childbirth demonstrates that medically directed home birth services with skilled nurse-midwives and medical backup have statistically excellent outcomes (Jones, 1991).

The first advantage of home birth is that the family is in control of the experience. Another is that the birth may be more physiologically natural in familiar surroundings. The mother may be more relaxed than she would be in the hospital environment. The family can assist in and be a part of the happy event, and mother-father (partner)-infant (and sibling-infant) contact is immediate and sustained. In addition, home birth may be less expensive than a hospital confinement. Serious infection may be less likely, assuming strict aseptic principles are followed, since people generally are relatively immune to their own home bacteria (Jones, 1991).

Although some physicians, nurse-midwives, and nurses support home births that use good medical and emergency backup systems, many regard this practice as exposing the mother and fetus to unnecessary danger. Thus home births are not widely accepted by the medical community, making it difficult for a family to find a qualified health care provider to give prenatal care and attend the birth. Also, backup emergency care by a physician in a hospital may be difficult to arrange in advance. If an emergency delivery is necessary, no effective way to do this rapidly exists in the home setting.

Most health care providers agree that if home birth is the woman's choice, certain criteria must be met for a safe home birth experience. The woman must be comfortable with her decision to have her baby at home. She should be in good health. Home birth is not indicated for women with a high-risk pregnancy, such as when the woman has diabetes, heart disease, or preeclampsia. A drive to the hospital (if needed) should take no more than 10 to 15 minutes. Finally, the woman should be attended by a well-trained physician or midwife with adequate medical supplies and resuscitation equipment, including oxygen (Jones, 1991).

Facilities and supplies can approximate those available in hospitals if the family works closely with the physician, nurse, or midwife to complete preparations well in advance of the birth. Childbirth education classes should include instructions on assisting with the birth of the infant without the midwife, physician, or other attendant present and should be attended by both expectant parents. Classes for siblings and grandparents are recommended if they will be present at birth. These activities add to the competence and pleasure of the parents and other family members.

Detailed descriptions for preparation are needed and may be obtained from the physician's office, the midwife, or local health agencies. Some agencies may provide some equipment and supplies. If a home birth is planned, obtaining and storing the necessary articles in advance is usually possible. In contrast, if birth in the home or elsewhere is an emergency or determined by unforeseen circumstances, considerable improvisation may be necessary.

A visit to the home by the physician or midwife who will be present during the birth is recommended well before the expected date of birth. At that time the process of birth can be discussed so that everyone is aware of the characteristics of normal labor and birth, the newborn stage, deviations from normal, and the plan of care for each stage.

Home birth is a selected alternative to hospital birth for some women and couples and a necessity for others. A physically and emotionally safe outcome can be anticipated for most women and couples and their infants, especially if they are prepared and have adequate health care support.

RESEARCH

Physical Abuse, Smoking, and Substance Use during Pregnancy

Smoking, physical abuse, and substance use during pregnancy are recognized as public health problems that have damaging effects on maternal and infant health. The purpose of this study was to establish the singular and combined occurrence of physical abuse, smoking, and substance use during pregnancy and their effect on birth weight. The sample consisted of an ethnically stratified cohort of 1,203 African-American, Hispanic, and Caucasian pregnant women from public prenatal clinics. Data were collected using the Abuse Assessment Screen, which consists of five questions to determine the frequency, severity, perpetrator, and body sites of injury. In private examination rooms without the male partner present, each pregnant woman was invited to participate in the study. Women were reimbursed for their participation. The assessment screen was administered three times to each woman during her pregnancy. All women were entered into the study at their first prenatal visit and followed until delivery. After delivery, the medical records of the mothers were evaluated for recorded use of tobacco, alcohol, and illicit drugs. Researchers found the incidence of physical abuse was 16%; smoking, 29.5%; and alcohol/illicit drug use, 11.9%. Significant relationships existed between physical abuse and smoking for African-American and Caucasian women. Physical abuse, smoking, and alcohol/illicit drug use were significantly related to birth weight.

CLINICAL APPLICATION OF STUDY

Nurses should be aware that physical abuse during pregnancy is common and can be readily detected with the appropriate screening tool. As part of their baseline assessment, nurses should screen for physical abuse and use of tobacco, alcohol, and illicit drugs. Nurses can use clinical protocols that integrate assessment and intervention for women presenting with problems.

Source: McFarlane J, Parker B & Soeken K: Physical abuse, smoking, and substance abuse during pregnancy: prevalence, interrelationships, and effects on birth weight, *J Obstet Gynecol Neonatal Nurs* 25(4):313, 1996.

KEY POINTS

- The prenatal period is a preparatory one both physically, in terms of fetal growth and parental adaptations, and psychologically, in terms of anticipation of parenthood.
- Discomforts and changes of pregnancy can cause anxiety to the woman and her family and require sensitive attention and a plan for teaching self-care measures.
- Education about healthy ways of using the body (e.g., exercise, body mechanics) is essential given maternal anatomic and physiologic responses to pregnancy.

KEY POINTS—cont'd

- Important components of the initial prenatal visit include detailed and carefully recorded findings from the interview, a comprehensive physical examination, and selected laboratory tests.
- Even in normal pregnancy the nurse must remain alert to hazards such as supine hypotension, warning signs and symptoms, and signs of potential parenting problems.
- Blood pressure is evaluated on the basis of absolute values and length of gestation and interpreted in the light of modifying factors.
- The quiet period of the second trimester gives way to an active period more oriented to the reality of impending childbirth and parenting responsibilities; attention to prebirth preparation is a necessary component of prenatal care.
- Each pregnant woman needs to know how to recognize and report preterm labor.
- Childbirth education is a process designed to help parents make the transition from the role of expectant parents to the role and responsibilities of parents of a new baby.
- Perpetuation of violence against women is influenced by the historical and societal norm of valuing women.
- Nurses must explore their values and beliefs concerning violence against women in order to identify and intervene effectively.

CRITICAL THINKING EXERCISES

1 *You are presenting a childbirth preparation class. The members of the class appear to be from various cultural and ethnic groups. The topic for today's discussion is the discomforts of pregnancy. What information do you need to prepare for the class? What questions can you ask the couples to ensure that the content of the class is culturally relevant?*

2 *Brenda Baer is a primigravida who comes with her husband for the first prenatal visit during her second month of pregnancy. You know that assessing family relationships is important in providing comprehensive nursing care. What observations are important? What questions might you ask? What anticipatory guidance might you provide?*

CRITICAL THINKING EXERCISES—cont'd

3 You are providing clinic care for a 15-year-old adolescent, Juanita, in her seventh month of pregnancy who has come for her first prenatal visit. Juanita is living at home with her mother and 17-year-old sister, who has a 2-year-old girl. Her mother works in the food services department of the local hospital and has told Juanita that she may live at home with her baby but that she will have to be responsible for the infant's care. Juanita describes the father of the baby as a 22-year-old who works at a fast-food restaurant, but she complains that during the past month, he has lost interest in their relationship. What are the physical risks associated with adolescent pregnancy? What are the likely psychosocial needs of Juanita? What long-term outcomes may be expected as you consider Juanita's future? How can an interdisciplinary approach to care benefit the patient? What community resources should be investigated? What legal issues are involved?

References

Affonso D & Mayberry L: Common stressors reported by a group of childbearing American women, *Health Care Women Int* 11(3):331, 1990.

Alan Guttmacher Institute (AGI): *Sex and America's teenagers*, New York, 1994, Alan Guttmacher Institute.

Alden K & Harris B: Choices in child bearing. In Fogel C & Woods N, editors: *Women's health care*, Thousand Oaks, Calif, 1995, Sage.

American College of Obstetricians and Gynecologists: Smoking and reproductive health, *Technical Bulletin* 180, Washington, DC, 1993, ACOG.

American College of Obstetricians and Gynecologists: *Precis V: an update in obstetrics and gynecology*, Washington, DC, 1994a, ACOG.

American College of Obstetricians and Gynecologists: Exercise during pregnancy and the postpartum period, *Technical Bulletin* 189, Washington, DC, 1994b, ACOG.

American Society for Psychoprophylaxis in Obstetrics/Lamaze: *Candidate guide: childbirth educator certification program*, Arlington, Va, 1990, The Society ASPO/Lamaze.

Bardy A et al.: Objectively measured tobacco exposure during pregnancy: neonatal effects and relation to maternal smoking, *Br J Obstet Gynaecol* 100(8):721, 1993.

Barry M & Bia F: Pregnancy and travel, *JAMA* 261(5):728, 1989.

Bia F: Medical considerations for the pregnant traveler, *Infect Dis Clin North Am* 6(2):371, 1992.

Bradley R: *Husband-coached childbirth*, ed 3, New York, 1981, Harper & Collins.

Brody T et al.: *Human pharmacology: molecular to clinical*, St Louis, 1994, Mosby.

Buckley K & Kulb N: *High-risk maternity nursing manual*, Baltimore, 1990, Williams & Wilkins.

Bullock L: Nursing interventions for abused women on obstetrical units, *AWHONN Clin Issues Perinat Women's Health Nurs* 4(3):371, 1993.

Campbell J et al.: Correlates of battering during pregnancy, *Res Nurs Health* 15(3):219, 1992.

Campbell J, Oliver C & Bullock L: Why battering during pregnancy? *AWHONN Clin Issues Perinat Women's Health Nurs* 4(3):343, 1993.

Chervenak J & Kardon N: Advancing maternal age: the actual risks, *Female Patient* 16:17, 1991.

Chescheir N: Domestic violence, *Curr Pract* 14(2):2, 1992.

Connor E et al.: Reduction of maternal-infant transmission of human immunodeficiency virus type 1 with zidovudine treatment, *N Engl J Med* 331(18):1173, 1994.

Cook P, Petersen R & Moore D: *Alcohol, tobacco, and other drugs may harm the unborn*, US Department of Health and Human Services, DHHS Pub. No. (ADM)90-1711, Rockville, Md, 1990, Office for Substance Abuse Prevention.

Cunningham F et al.: *Williams obstetrics*, ed 20, Stamford, Conn, 1997, Appleton & Lange.

Dick-Read G: *Childbirth without fear*, ed 5, New York, 1987, Harper & Collins.

Duchon M & Muise K: Pregnancy after age 35, *Physician Assistant* 17(7):27, 1993.

Duvekot J & Peeters L: Maternal cardiovascular hemodynamic adaptation to pregnancy, *Obstet Gynecol Surv* 49(suppl 12):S1, 1994.

Easa D et al.: Unexpected preterm delivery in tourists: implications for long-distance travel during pregnancy, *J Perinatol* 14(4):264, 1994.

Economides D & Braithwaite J: Smoking, pregnancy and the fetus, *J Royal Society Health* 114(4):198, 1994.

Engstrom J et al.: Fundal height measurement, *J Nurse Midwifery* 38(1):23, 1993.

Engstrom J & Sittler C: Fundal height measurement. Part I–Technique for measuring fundal height, *J Nurse Midwifery* 38(1):5, 1993.

Fishbein E & Phillips M: How safe is exercise during pregnancy? *J Obstet Gynecol Neonatal Nurs* 19(1):45, 1990.

Garmel S & D'Alton M: Diagnostic ultrasound in pregnancy: an overview, *Semin Perinatol* 18(3):117, 1994.

Geissler E: *Pocket guide to cultural assessment*, St Louis, 1994, Mosby.

Green N: Stressful events related to childbearing in African-American women: a pilot study, *J Nurse Midwifery* 35(4):231, 1990.

Hammond T et al.: The use of automobile safety restraint systems during pregnancy, *J Obstet Gynecol Neonatal Nurs* 19(4):339, 1990.

Henriksen T et al.: Employment during pregnancy in relation to risk factors and pregnancy outcome, *Br J Obstet Gynaecol* 101(10):858, 1994.

Hetherington S: A controlled study of the effect of prepared childbirth classes on obstetric outcome, *Birth* 17(2):89, 1990.

Heyl P, Miller W & Canick J: Maternal serum screening for aneuploid pregnancy, alphafetoprotein, hCG, and unconjugated estriol, *Obstet Gynecol* 76(6):1025, 1990.

Holditch-Davis D et al.: Beyond couvade: pregnancy symptoms in couples with a history of infertility, *Health Care Women Int* 15(6):537, 1994.

Hutchinson M & Baqi-Aziz M: Nursing care of the childbearing Muslim family, *J Obstet Gynecol Neonatal Nurs* 23(9):767, 1994.

Jones C: *Alternative birth: the complete guide*, Los Angeles, 1991, Jeremy P Tarcher.

Jordan P: Laboring for relevance: expectant and new fatherhood, *Nurs Res* 39(1):11, 1990.

Kendrick J et al.: Integrating smoking cessation into routine public prenatal care: the smoking cessation in pregnancy project, *Am J Public Health* 82(2):217, 1994.

Kinsman S & Slap G: Barriers to adolescent prenatal care, *J Adolesc Health* 13(2):146, 1992.

Klein H: Couvade syndrome: male counterpart to pregnancy, *Int J Psychiatry Med* 21(1):57, 1991.

Koniak-Griffin D: The relationship between social support, self-esteem, and maternal-fetal attachment in adolescents, *Res Nurs Health* 11(4):269, 1988.

Kulig J: Childbearing beliefs among Cambodian refugee women, *West J Nurs Res* 12(1):108, 1990.

Lamaze F: *Painless childbirth: the Lamaze method*, Chicago, 1970, Regnery Books.

Lawrence R: *Breastfeeding: a guide for the medical profession*, St Louis, 1994, Mosby.

Lazarus E & Philipson E: A longitudinal study comparing the prenatal care of Puerto Rican and white women, *Birth* 17(1):6, 1990.

Leatherman, J, Blackburn D & Davidhizar R: How postpartum women explain their lack of obtaining adequate prenatal care, *J Adv Nurs* 15(3):256, 1990.

Lederman R: *Psychological adaptation in pregnancy: assessment of seven dimensions of maternal development*, Englewood Cliffs, NJ, 1984, Prentice-Hall.

Lee R: Understanding Southeast-Asian mothers-to-be, *Childbirth Educ* 8:32, 1989.

Leland N et al.: Variations in pregnancy outcomes by race among 10-14 year old mothers in the United States, *Public Health Rep* 110(1):53, 1995.

Lumley J: The image of the fetus in the first trimester, *Birth Fam J* 17:5, 1980.

Lumley J: Attitudes to the fetus among primigravidas, *Aust Pediatr J* 18(2):106, 1982.

Mackey M: Women's choices of childbirth setting, *Health Care Women Int* 11(2):175, 1990.

Mackey M & Miller H: Women's views of postpartum sibling visitation, *Matern Child Nurs J* 20(1):40, 1992.

May K: A typology of detachment and involvement styles adopted during pregnancy by first-time expectant fathers, *West J Nurs Res* 2(2):445, 1980.

May K: Father participation in birth: fact and fiction, *J Calif Perinat Assoc* 2:41, 1982a.

May K: Three phases of father involvement in pregnancy, *Nurs Res* 31(6):337, 1982b.

McFarlane J: Abuse during pregnancy: the horror and the hope, *AWHONN Clin Issues Perinat Women's Health Nurs* 4(3):350, 1993.

McFarlane J et al.: Assessing for abuse during pregnancy: severity and frequency of injuries and associated entry into prenatal care, *JAMA* 267(23):3176, 1992.

McFarlane J, Parker J & Soeken K: Physical abuse, smoking, and substance use during pregnancy: prevalence, interrelationships, and effects on birth weight, *J Obstet Gynecol Neonatal Nurs* 25(4):313, 1996.

Meikle S et al.: Women's reasons for not seeking prenatal care: racial and ethnic factors, *Birth* 22(2):81, 1995.

Mercer R: *Becoming a mother,* Springer, 1995, New York.

Messersmith-Heroman K, Heroman W & Moore T: Pregnancy outcome in military and civilian women, *Mil Med* 159(8):577, 1994.

Mills J et al.: Moderate caffeine use and the risk of spontaneous abortion and intrauterine growth retardation, *JAMA* 269(5):5593, 1993.

Moore K, Snyder N & Glei D: *Facts at a glance,* Flint, Mich, 1995, Charles Stewart Mott Foundation.

National Center for Health Statistics: *Advance report of the monthly vital statistics,* Washington, DC, 1990, US Dept of Health and Human Services, Public Health Service.

National Center for Health Statistics: Advance report of final natality statistics, 1991, *Monthly Vital Statistics Report* 42(suppl):1 1993.

Nicholas R: High altitude sojourn in pregnancy and childhood, *Ther Umsch* 50(4):246, 1993.

Nilsson L, Austrell C & Norgren L: Venous function during late pregnancy: the effect of elastic compression hosiery, *Vasa* 21(2):203, 1992.

Norton L et al.: Battering in pregnancy: an assessment of two screening methods, *Obstet Gynecol* 85(3):321, 1995.

Palkovitz R: Changes in father-infant bonding beliefs across couples' first transition to parenthood, *Matern Child Nurs J* 20(3,4):141, 1992.

Papp E et al.: Longitudinal study of the dental status of pregnant women under prenatal care, *Fogorv Sz* 83(7):199, 1990.

Parker B: Abuse of adolescents: what can we learn from pregnant teenagers? *AWHONN Clin Issues Perinat Women's Health Nurs* 4(3):363, 1993.

Patterson E, Freese M & Goldenberg R: Seeking safe passage: utilizing health care during pregnancy, *Image J Nurs Sch* 22(1):27, 1990.

Peterson G: *An easier childbirth: a mother's workbook for health and emotional well-being during pregnancy and delivery,* Los Angeles, 1991, Jeremy P Tarcher.

Priollet P et al.: Study and treatment of varicose veins: truths and countertruths, *Ann Cardiol Angeiol Paris* 43(5):275, 1994.

Richardson P: Women's perceptions of change in relationships shared with children during pregnancy, *Matern Child Nurs J* 12(2):75, 1983.

Rubin R: Maternal tasks in pregnancy, *Matern Child Nurs J* 4(3):143, 1975.

Rynerson B & Lowdermilk D: Sexual intimacy in pregnancy. In Knuppel R & Drukker J, editors: *High-risk pregnancy: a team approach,* ed 2, Philadelphia, 1993, Saunders.

Sanyal M, Li Y & Belanger K: Metabolism of polynuclear aromatic hydrocarbon in human term placenta influenced by cigarette smoke exposure, *Reprod Toxicol* 8(5):411, 1994.

Scott J et al.: *Danforth's obstetrics and gynecology,* ed 7, Philadelphia, 1994, Lippincott.

Scupholme A, Robertson E & Kamons A: Barriers to prenatal care in multiethnic, urban sample, *J Nurse Midwifery* 36(2):111, 1991.

Seguin L et al.: Chronic stressors, social support, and depression during pregnancy, *Obstet Gynecol* 85(4):583, 1995.

Seidel H et al.: *Mosby's guide to physical examination,* ed 4, St Louis, 1998, Mosby.

Seneviratne S & Fernando O: Influence of work on pregnancy outcome, *Int J Gynaecol Obstet* 45(1):35, 1994.

Sibai B et al.: Risk factors for preeclampsia in healthy nulliparous women: a prospective multicenter study, the National Institute of Child Health and Human Development Network of Maternal-Fetal Medicine Units, *Am J Obstet Gynecol* 172(2 Pt 1):642, 1995a.

Sibai B et al.: Pregnancies complicated by HELLP syndrome (hemolysis, elevated liver enzymes and low platelets): subsequent pregnancy outcome and long-term prognosis, *Am J Obstet Gynecol* 172(1 Pt 1):125, 1995b.

Skjenna O et al.: Helping patients travel by air, *Can Med Assoc J* 144(3):287, 1991.

Spector R: *Cultural diversity in health and illness,* ed 4, Stamford, Conn, 1996, Appleton & Lange.

Starn J: Childbirth classroom: labor after birth, *Childbirth Instr* 1:27, 1991a.

Starn J: Cultural childbearing: beliefs and practices, *Int J Childbirth Edu* 6(3):38, 1991b.

Stewart D & Cecutti A: Physical abuse in pregnancy, *Can Med Assoc J* 149(9):1257, 1993.

USDA and USDHHS: *Cross-cultural counseling: a guide for nutrition and health counselors,* Washington, DC, 1990, US Government Printing Office.

Wayland J & Tate S: Maternal-fetal attachment and perceived relationships with important others in adolescents, *Birth* 20(4):198, 1993.

Waxler-Morrison N, Anderson J & Richardson E, editors: *Cross-cultural nursing*, Vancouver, Canada, 1990, University of British Columbia Press.

Wilailak S et al.: Assessment of fetal well-being: fetal movement and count versus non stress test, *Int J Gynaecol Obstet* 38(1)23, 1992.

Wilberg G: *Preparing for birth and parenthood: an awareness training and teaching manual for childbirth professionals*, Boston, 1992, Butterworth-Heinemann.

Wilcox A: Birth weight and perinatal mortality: the effects of maternal smoking, *Am J Epidemiol* 137(10):1098, 1993.

Zachariah R: Maternal-fetal attachment: influence of mother-daughter and husband-wife relationships, *Res Nurs Health* 17(1):37, 1994.

CHAPTER

11

Maternal and Fetal Nutrition

MARY COURTNEY MOORE

LEARNING OBJECTIVES

- *Define the key terms.*
- *Explain recommended maternal weight gain during pregnancy (total amount gained and rate of gain) based on prepregnancy weight for height.*
- *State recommended dietary allowance for energy sources, protein, and key vitamins and minerals during pregnancy and lactation.*
- *Give examples of the food sources that provide the nutrients required for optimal maternal nutrition during pregnancy and lactation.*
- *Examine the role of nutritional supplements during pregnancy.*
- *List five nutritional risk factors during pregnancy.*
- *Compare the dietary needs of adolescent and mature pregnant women.*
- *Give examples of cultural food patterns and possible dietary problems for two ethnic groups or for two alternative eating patterns.*
- *Assess nutritional status during pregnancy.*
- *Apply the nursing process to maternal and fetal nutrition.*

KEY TERMS

anemia
anthropometric measurements
body mass index (BMI)
diet history
energy (kcal)
food cravings
intrauterine growth restriction (IUGR)
lactose intolerance
low birth weight (LBW)
physiologic anemia
pica
pyrosis
Recommended Dietary Allowances (RDA)
small for gestational age (SGA)
vegetarian diet
WIC (Women, Infants, and Children Program)

Nutrition is one of the many factors that influence the outcome of pregnancy (Fig. 11-1). Poverty, a deprived environment, limited education, unhealthy or bizarre food habits, and chronic illnesses have adverse effects on the nutritional health of pregnant women. Currently 19 industrialized nations report infant mortality rates lower than that of the United States (Wegman, 1996), and at least 20% of infant deaths are related to **low birth weight (LBW),** which is defined as a birth weight of 2,500 g or less, to preterm births, or to both. Many factors contribute to the occurrence of LBW or preterm birth, but good maternal nutrition before and during pregnancy is believed to be one of the most important preventive measures. As a result, it is essential that the importance of good nutrition be emphasized to all women of childbearing potential. Therefore the nurse must have a thorough understanding of nutrient needs during pregnancy, and nutrition assessment, intervention, and evaluation must be an integral part of the nursing care given to pregnant women.

NUTRIENT NEEDS DURING PREGNANCY

Pregnant women need more of some nutrients than do nonpregnant women. These nutrient needs are determined, at least in part, by the stage of gestation in that the amount of fetal growth varies during the different stages of pregnancy. During the first trimester the synthesis of fetal tissues places relatively few demands on maternal nutrition. Therefore during the first trimester when the embryo/fetus is very small, the needs are only slightly greater than those before pregnancy. In contrast, the last trimester is a period of noticeable fetal growth when most of the deposition of the fetal stores of energy sources and minerals occurs. Therefore as fetal growth progresses during the second and third trimesters, the pregnant woman's need for some nutrients increases greatly. Factors that contribute to the increase in nutrient needs include the following:

- The uterine-placental-fetal unit—Placentas of well-nourished mothers are able to provide adequate nutrients to the fetus. Placentas of poorly nourished

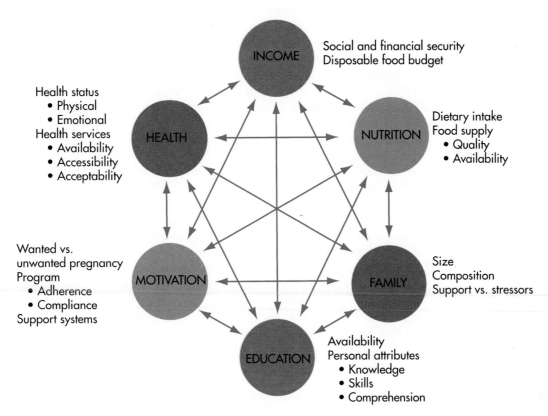

Fig. **11-1** Web of influences that can affect outcome of pregnancy. Much more than luck goes into having a healthy baby. (From Wardlaw G & Insel P: *Perspectives in nutrition,* St Louis, 1993, Mosby.)

mothers often contain fewer and smaller cells. The ability of such poorly developed placentas to synthesize substances needed by the fetus, facilitate the flow of needed nutrients, and inhibit the passage of potentially harmful substances is reduced. Understandably, the infant of a poorly nourished mother may be poorly nourished and **small for gestational age (SGA).** Fig. 11-2 shows a possible mechanism by which maternal malnutrition may lead to **intrauterine growth restriction (IUGR),** or impaired fetal growth.

- Maternal blood volume and constituents–During pregnancy the total blood volume increases by about 33% more than the normal volume. The plasma volume increases by 50% in women in their first pregnancies and more than this in multiparas. Red blood cell (RBC) production is stimulated during pregnancy, but although the number of RBCs increases gradually, the expansion of the plasma volume proceeds rapidly.
- Maternal mammary changes–A noticeable increase in the lactiferous ducts and lobule-alveolar tissue takes place.

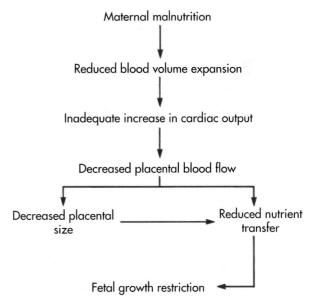

Fig. **11-2** Possible mechanism for fetal and placental growth restriction seen with maternal malnutrition in animal models and human subjects. (From Rosso P: Placental growth, development and function in relation to maternal nutrition, *Fed Proc* 39(2):250, 1980.)

- Metabolic needs—Basal metabolic rates, when expressed as kilocalories (kcal) per minute, are approximately 20% higher in pregnant women than in nonpregnant women. This increase includes the energy cost for tissue synthesis.

The National Research Council has made recommendations for the increased intake of specific nutrients during pregnancy in the form of **Recommended Dietary Allowances (RDAs)**. The RDAs for pregnancy and lactation are given in Table 11-1. The RDAs were developed for use with groups of people, and they should therefore not be confused with requirements. However, they do provide a guideline on which to base individualized nutrition counseling. A margin of safety has been built into these allowances to cover a wide range of individual needs. The reference woman for the typical RDA is 25 to 50 years old, weighs 58 kg, is 164 cm tall, lives in a temperate climate, and is a normally active, healthy woman. Variations from this state would need to be considered when individualizing counseling. The woman's age, activity level, current weight, number of fetuses, and alterations in health are examples of such variations.

Energy Needs

Energy (kcal) needs are met by carbohydrate, fat, and protein in the diet. No specific recommendations exist for the amount of carbohydrate and fat in the diet of the pregnant woman. However, the intake of these nutrients should be adequate to support the recommended weight gain. Although protein can be used to supply energy, its primary role is to provide amino acids for the synthesis of new tissues (see discussion later in chapter). The RDA (in kilocalories) during the second and third trimesters of pregnancy is 300 kcal greater than the prepregnancy needs. Longitudinal assessment of weight gain during pregnancy is the best way to determine whether the kilocalorie intake is adequate; very underweight or active women may require more than the additional 300 kcal to sustain the desired rate of weight gain.

Weight gain

The optimal weight gain during pregnancy is not known precisely. It is known, however, that the amount of weight gained by the mother during pregnancy has an important bearing on the course and outcome of the pregnancy. Although an adequate weight gain does not necessarily indicate that the diet is nutritionally adequate, it reduces the risk of delivering an SGA or preterm infant.

The desirable weight gain during pregnancy varies among women. The primary factor to consider in making a weight gain recommendation is the appropriateness of the prepregnancy weight for the woman's height, that is, whether the woman's weight was normal before pregnancy,

or whether she was underweight or overweight. Maternal and fetal risks in pregnancy are increased when the mother is significantly underweight or overweight before pregnancy and when weight gain during pregnancy is either too low or too high. Severely underweight women are more likely to experience preterm labor and to give birth to LBW infants. Moreover, for infants of normal-weight and underweight women, birth weight is directly related to maternal weight gain during pregnancy, and inadequate gain increases the risk of delivering an infant with IUGR (Cogswell & Yip, 1995). Greater-than-expected weight gain during pregnancy may occur for many reasons, including multiple gestation, edema, pregnancy-induced hypertension (PIH), and overeating. When obesity is present (either preexisting obesity or obesity that develops during pregnancy), there is an increased likelihood of macrosomia and fetopelvic disproportion, operative delivery, birth trauma, and infant mortality. Obese women are more likely than normal-weight women to have hypertension and diabetes, and their risk of giving birth to a child with a major congenital defect is double that of normal-weight women (Prentice & Goldberg, 1996). The cost of pregnancy in an obese woman has been estimated to be triple that of a normal-weight woman (Prentice & Goldberg, 1996).

A commonly used method of evaluating the appropriateness of weight for height is the **body mass index (BMI),** which is calculated by the following formula:

$$BMI = Weight/height^2$$

where the weight is in kilograms and height is in meters. Thus, for a woman who weighed 51 kg before pregnancy and is 1.57 m tall:

$$BMI = 51/(1.57),^2 \text{ or } 20.7$$

The BMI can be classified into the following categories: less than 19.8, underweight or low; 19.8 to 26.0, normal; 26.0 to 29.0, overweight or high; and greater than 29.0, obese (Institute of Medicine, 1992). Figure 11-3 provides an easy way of estimating and categorizing the BMI.

Women with a low BMI should gain approximately 12.5 to 18 kg during pregnancy (Fig. 11- 4). Women with a normal BMI should gain 11.5 to 16 kg, and those with a high BMI should gain 7 to 11.5 kg. Obese women should gain at least 7 kg. Adolescents and African-American women should be encouraged to aim for the upper portion of their recommended weight gain range because their infants tend to be smaller than those of adult Caucasian women (Institute of Medicine, 1992). Adolescents who are less than 2 to 3 years postmenarche are believed to be at greatest nutritional risk, because it is postulated that the fetus and still-growing mother are then competing for nutrients. Evidence of nutritional competition exists even during the pregnancies of older adolescents (up to 19 years of age), however, which emphasizes the need for especially

Text continues on p. 264.

TABLE 11-1 Nutritional Recommendations during Pregnancy and Lactation

NUTRIENT	RDA FOR NONPREGNANT FEMALE (25-50 YR)	RDA DURING PREGNANCY	RDA FOR LACTATION* (FIRST 6 MO/ SECOND 6 MO)	REASONS FOR INCREASED NEED	FOOD SOURCES
Calories	Variable	Same as nonpregnant (first trimester); nonpregnant +300 (second and third trimesters)	Nonpregnant +500; nonpregnant +500	Increased energy needs for fetal growth and milk production	Carbohydrate, fat, protein
Protein (g)	50	60	65/62	Synthesis of the products of conception: fetus, amniotic fluid, placenta; growth of maternal tissue: uterus, breasts, red blood cells, plasma proteins, secretion of milk protein during lactation	Meats, eggs, milk, cheese, legumes (dry beans and peas, peanuts), nuts, grains
MINERALS					
Calcium (mg)	800	1,200	1,200/1,200	Fetal skeleton and tooth bud formation; maintenance of maternal bone and tooth mineralization; prevent mobilization of calcium from bones to maintain calcium in milk	Milk, cheese, yogurt, sardines or other fish eaten with bones left in, deep green leafy vegetables except spinach or Swiss chard† tofu, baked beans
Phosphorus (mg)	15	1,200	1,200/1,200	Fetal skeleton and tooth bud formation	Milk, cheese, yogurt, meats, whole grains, nuts, legumes
Iron (mg)	15	30	15/15	Increased maternal hemoglobin formation, fetal liver iron storage	Liver, meats, whole or enriched breads and cereals, deep green leafy vegetables, legumes, dried fruits

RDA, Recommended dietary allowance.
*Milk production generally declines during the second 6 months of lactation as the infant's diet increasingly begins to include other foods, thus maternal needs for many nutrients decrease.
†Spinach and chard contain calcium but also contain oxalic acid, which inhibits calcium absorption.

Continued

| TABLE 11-1 | *Nutritional Recommendations during Pregnancy and Lactation—cont'd* |

NUTRIENT	RDA FOR NONPREGNANT FEMALE (25-50 YR)	RDA DURING PREGNANCY	RDA FOR LACTATION* (FIRST 6 MO/ SECOND 6 MO)	REASONS FOR INCREASED NEED	FOOD SOURCES
Zinc (mg)	12	15	19/16	Component of numerous enzyme systems; possibly important in preventing congenital malformations	Liver, shellfish, meats, whole grains, milk
Iodine (μg)	150	175	200/200	Increased maternal metabolic rate	Iodized salt, seafood, milk and milk products, commercial yeast breads, rolls, and donuts
Magnesium (μg)	280	320	355/340	Involved in energy and protein metabolism, tissue growth, muscle action	Nuts, legumes, cocoa, meats, whole grains
Selenium (μg)	55	65	75/75	Antioxidant (protects cell membranes), tooth component	Organ meats, seafood, whole grains, legumes, molasses
FAT-SOLUBLE VITAMINS					
A (RE)[†]	800	800	1,300/1,200	Essential for cell development, thus growth; tooth bud formation (development of enamel-forming cells in gum tissue); bone growth	Deep green leafy vegetables, dark yellow vegetables and fruits, chili peppers, liver, fortified margarine and butter
D (μg)[‡]	5	10	10/10	Involved in absorption of calcium and phosphorus, improves mineralization	Fortified milk, fortified margarine, egg yolk, butter, liver, seafood
E (mg)	8	10	12/11	Antioxidant (protects cell membranes from damage), especially important for preventing hemolysis of red blood cells	Vegetable oils, green leafy vegetables, whole grains, liver, nuts and seeds, cheese, fish

*Milk production generally declines during the second 6 months of lactation as the infant's diet increasingly begins to include other foods, thus maternal needs for many nutrients decrease.
[†]RE, Retinol equivalents. Replaces international units (IU). 1 RE = 5 IU.
[‡]As cholecalciferol. 10 μg cholecalciferol = 400 IU of vitamin D.

TABLE 11-1 *Nutritional Recommendations during Pregnancy and Lactation—cont'd*

NUTRIENT	RDA FOR NONPREGNANT FEMALE (25-50 YR)	RDA DURING PREGNANCY	RDA FOR LACTATION* (FIRST 6 MO/ SECOND 6 MO)	REASONS FOR INCREASED NEED	FOOD SOURCES
Water-soluble vitamins					
C (mg)	60	70	95/90	Tissue formation and integrity, formation of connective tissue, enhancement of iron absorption	Citrus fruits, strawberries, melons, broccoli, tomatoes, peppers, raw deep green leafy vegetables
Folic acid (µg)	180	400	280/260	Prevent neural tube defects; increased red blood cell formation; prevention of macrocytic or megaloblastic anemia	Green leafy vegetables, oranges, broccoli, asparagus, artichokes, liver
Thiamin (mg)	1.1	1.5	1.6/1.6	Involved in energy metabolism	Pork, beef, liver, whole or enriched grains, legumes
Riboflavin (mg)	1.3	1.6	1.8/1.7	Involved in energy and protein metabolism	Milk, liver, enriched grains, deep green and yellow vegetables
Pyridoxine (B$_6$) (mg)	1.6	2.2	2.1/2.1	Involved in protein metabolism	Meat, liver, deep green vegetables, whole grains
B$_{12}$ (µg)	2.0	2.2	2.6/2.6	Production of nucleic acids and proteins, especially important in formation of red blood cells and prevention of megaloblastic or macrocytic anemia	Milk, egg, meat, liver, cheese
Niacin (mg)	15	17	20/20	Involved in energy metabolism	Meat, fish, poultry, liver, whole or enriched grains, peanuts

*Milk production generally declines during the second 6 months of lactation as the infant's diet increasingly begins to include other foods; thus maternal needs for many nutrients decrease.

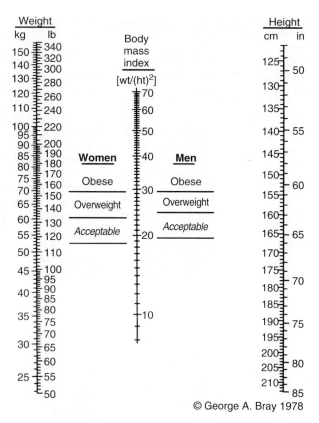

© George A. Bray 1978

Fig. **11-3** Nomogram for body mass index (BMI). To determine BMI, use a straightedge to connect the individual's height and weight. (From Moore M: *Pocket guide to nutritional care,* St Louis, 1997, Mosby.)

careful nutrition teaching and follow-up during all adolescent pregnancies. The weight gain goals of women shorter than 157 cm should be near the lower end of their recommended ranges to reduce the risk of mechanical complications during birth.

No recommendations have been made regarding optimal weight gain based on BMI for multifetal gestations. In twin gestations, gains of approximately 16 to 20 kg have been reported to be associated with the best outcomes (Newman & Ellings, 1995).

Pattern of weight gain

The weight gain should take place throughout pregnancy. The risk of delivering an SGA infant is reported to be greater when the weight gain early in pregnancy has been poor. The likelihood of preterm birth has been observed to be greater when the gains during the last half of pregnancy have been inadequate. These risks were found to exist even when the total gain for the pregnancy was in the recommended range.

The optimal rate of weight gain depends on the stage of pregnancy. During the first and second trimesters, growth takes place primarily in maternal tissues; during the third trimester, growth occurs primarily in fetal tissues. During the first trimester there is an average total weight gain of only 1 to 2.5 kg. Thereafter the recommended weight gain increases to approximately 0.4 kg per week for a woman of normal weight. The recommended weekly weight gain for overweight women during the second and third trimesters is 0.3 kg, and it is 0.5 kg for underweight women. The recommended caloric intake corresponds to this pattern of gain (see Table 11-1). There is no increment for the first trimester; an additional 300 kcal per day over the prepregnant intake is recommended during the second and third trimesters. The amount of food providing 300 kcal is not great. It can be provided by one additional serving from each of the following groups: milk, yogurt, or cheese (all skim milk products); fruits; vegetables; and bread, cereal, rice, or pasta.

A chart has been developed for monitoring weight gain in normal-weight, underweight, and overweight women (see Fig. 11-4). The weight gain measured at each prenatal visit is plotted on this chart to monitor the woman's progress in achieving the weight gain goal. Each pregnant woman should understand the desirable pattern and amount of weight gain. The woman may be more successful with the weight gain recommendations when she participates in establishing her own weight goal within the range recommended for her BMI.

The reasons for an inadequate weight gain (less than 1 kg per month for normal-weight women or less than 0.5 kg per month for obese women during the last two trimesters) or excessive weight gain (more than 3 kg per month) should be thoroughly evaluated. Possible reasons for deviations from the expected rate of weight gain, besides inadequate or excessive dietary intake, include measurement or recording errors, differences in the weight of clothing, the time of day, and the accumulation of fluids. An exceptionally high gain is likely to result from the accumulation of fluids, and a gain of more than 3 kg in a month, especially after the twentieth week of gestation, often heralds the development of PIH.

Hazards of restricting adequate weight gain

An obsession with thinness and dieting pervades the North American culture. Slender, figure-conscious women may find it difficult to make the transition from guarding against weight gain before pregnancy to valuing weight gain during pregnancy. In counseling these women the nurse can emphasize the positive effects of good nutrition, as well as the adverse effects of maternal malnutrition (manifested by poor weight gain) on infant growth and development. This counseling includes information on the components of weight gain during pregnancy (Fig. 11-5) and the amount of this weight that will be lost after the birth. Early in a woman's

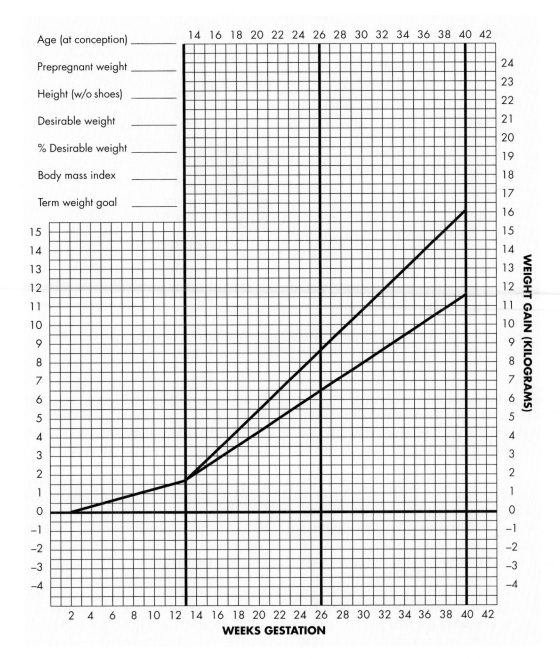

Fig. 11-4 Prenatal weight gain grid for normal weight women. *Note:* Young adolescents, African-American women, and smokers should strive for gains at upper end of recommended ranges; short women (<157 cm) should strive for gains at lower end of range. (From California Department of Health Services, MCH/WIC: *Nutrition during pregnancy and the postpartum period,* June, 1990, California Department of Health Services.)

pregnancy, explaining ways to lose weight in the postpartum period helps relieve her concerns. (Because lactation can help to gradually reduce maternal energy stores, this also provides an opportunity to promote breastfeeding.)

Pregnancy is not a time to diet. Even obese (BMI of 26 to 29) or morbidly obese (BMI of >29) pregnant women need to gain at least enough weight to equal the weight of the products of conception (fetus, placenta, and amniotic fluid). If they limit their caloric intake to prevent weight gain, they may also excessively limit their intake of important nutrients. Moreover, dietary restriction results in the catabolism of fat stores, which in turn augments the production of ketones. The long-term effects of mild ketonemia during pregnancy are not known, but ketonuria has been found

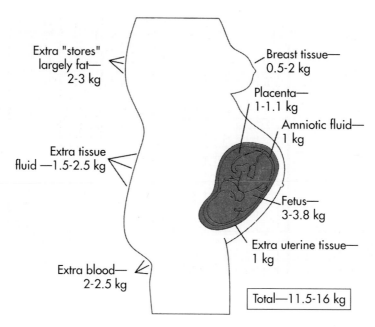

Extra "stores" largely fat— 2-3 kg

Extra tissue fluid —1.5-2.5 kg

Extra blood— 2-2.5 kg

Breast tissue— 0.5-2 kg

Placenta— 1-1.1 kg

Amniotic fluid— 1 kg

Fetus— 3-3.8 kg

Extra uterine tissue— 1 kg

Total—11.5-16 kg

Fig. **11-5** Components of maternal weight gain at 40 weeks' gestation. (Modified from Worthington-Roberts B & Williams S: *Nutrition in pregnancy and lactation,* ed 5, St Louis, 1993, Mosby.)

to be correlated with the occurrence of preterm labor. It should be stressed to obese women, and all pregnant women for that matter, that the quality of the weight gain is important, with emphasis placed on the consumption of nutrient-dense foods and the avoidance of empty-calorie foods. Ideally, obese and morbidly obese women would lose weight before conception.

Weight gain is important, but pregnancy is not an excuse for uncontrolled dietary indulgence. The old saying that the pregnant woman is "eating for two" should not be interpreted to mean that the pregnant woman needs to greatly increase her food intake. Instead she should place an emphasis on the quality of her food intake as she considers her needs and those of her fetus. Excessive weight gained during pregnancy may be difficult to lose after pregnancy, thus contributing to chronic overweight or obesity, an etiologic factor in a host of chronic diseases, including hypertension, diabetes mellitus, and arteriosclerotic heart disease. The woman who gains 18 kg or more is especially at risk.

Protein

Protein, with its essential constituent nitrogen, is the nutritional element basic to growth. An adequate protein intake is essential to meet increasing demands in pregnancy. These demands arise from the rapid growth of the fetus; enlargement of the uterus and its supporting structures, mammary glands, and placenta; increase in the maternal circulating blood volume and the subsequent demand for increased amounts of plasma protein to maintain colloidal osmotic pressure; and formation of amniotic fluid.

Milk, meat, eggs, and cheese are complete protein foods with a high biologic value. Legumes (dried beans and peas), whole grains, and nuts are also valuable sources of protein. In addition, these protein-rich foods are a source of other nutrients such as calcium, iron, and B vitamins; plant sources of protein often provide needed dietary fiber. The recommended daily food plan (Table 11-2 and Fig. 11-6) is a guide to the amounts of these foods that would supply the quantities of protein needed. The RDAs provide for only a modest increase in protein intake over the prepregnant levels in adult women. Protein intake in many people in the United States exceeds the RDA, so many women may not need to increase their protein intake at all during pregnancy. Three servings of milk, yogurt, or cheese (four for adolescents) and 5 to 6 ounces (140 to 168 g) (two servings) of meat, poultry, or fish would supply the RDA of protein for the pregnant woman. Additional protein would be provided by vegetables and breads, cereals, rice, or pasta. Pregnant adolescents, women from impoverished backgrounds, and women adhering to unusual diets, such as a macrobiotic (highly restricted vegetarian) diet, are those whose protein intake is most likely to be inadequate. The use of high-protein supplements is not recommended, because they have been associated with an increased incidence of preterm births.

Fluid

Water plays an important role during pregnancy. Essential during the exchange of nutrients and waste products across cell membranes, water is the main substance of cells, blood,

TABLE 11-2 *Daily Food Guide for Pregnancy and Lactation*

FOOD GROUP	SERVING SIZE	SUGGESTED NUMBER OF SERVINGS		
		NONPREGNANT, NONLACTATING WOMAN	PREGNANT WOMAN	LACTATING WOMAN
GRAIN PRODUCTS Include whole-grain and enriched breads, cereals, pasta, and rice.	1 slice bread; 1/2 bun, bagel, or English muffin; 1-oz ready-to-eat cereal; 1/2 c cooked grains	6-11	6-11	6-11
VEGETABLES Eat dark green leafy and deep yellow often. Eat dried beans and peas often; count 1/2 c cooked dried beans or peas as a serving of vegetables or 1 oz from meat group.	1 c raw leafy greens; 1/2 c of others	3-5	3-5	3-5
FRUITS Include citrus fruits, strawberries, or melons frequently.	1 medium apple, orange, banana, peach, etc; 1/2 c small or diced fruit; 3/4 c juice	2-4	2-4	2-4
MILK AND MILK PRODUCTS	1 c milk or yogurt; 1 1/2 oz cheese	2-3	3 or more	4 or more
MEAT, POULTRY, FISH, DRY BEANS, NUTS, AND EGGS Eat peanut butter or nuts rarely to avoid excessive fat intake. Limit egg intake to reduce cholesterol intake; trim fat from meat, and remove skin from poultry.	1/2 c cooked dried beans, 1 egg, or 1 1/2 T peanut butter is equivalent to 1 oz of meat	Up to 6 oz total	Up to 6 oz total	Up to 6 oz total

From Lowdermilk D, Perry S & Bobak I: *Maternity & women's health care,* ed 6, St Louis, 1997, Mosby.
c, Cup; *T,* tablespoon.

lymph, amniotic fluid, and other vital body fluids. It also aids in maintaining body temperature. A good fluid intake promotes good bowel function, which is sometimes a problem during pregnancy. The recommended daily intake is about 6 to 8 glasses (1,500 to 2,000 ml) of fluid. Water, milk, and fruit juices are good sources. There is evidence that dehydration may increase the risk of cramping/contractions and preterm labor.

Women who consume more than 300 mg of caffeine daily (equivalent to about 500 to 750 ml of coffee) are at increased risk of spontaneous abortion and of delivering infants with IUGR. Caffeine's ill effects have been proposed to result from vasoconstriction of the blood vessels supplying the uterus or interference with cell division in the developing fetus (Hinds et al., 1996). Consequently, caffeine-containing products, including caffeinated coffee, tea, soft drinks, and cocoa beverages, should be avoided or consumed only in limited quantities.

Aspartame (Nutrasweet, Equal) and acesulfame K (Sweet One), two artificial sweeteners commonly used in low- or no-calorie beverages, have not been found to have adverse effects on the normal mother and fetus, but aspartame use should be avoided by the mother homozygous for phenylketonuria (PKU) (Position of the ADA, 1993).

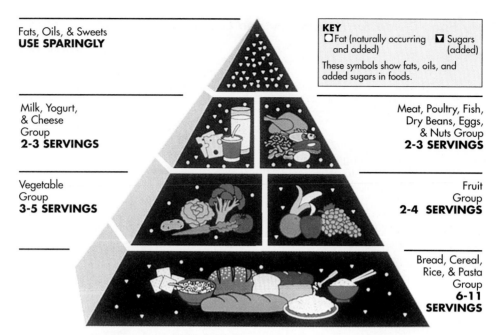

Fats, Oils, & Sweets
USE SPARINGLY

KEY
☐ Fat (naturally occurring   ☑ Sugars
and added)   (added)
These symbols show fats, oils, and
added sugars in foods.

Milk, Yogurt,
& Cheese
Group
2-3 SERVINGS

Meat, Poultry, Fish,
Dry Beans, Eggs,
& Nuts Group
2-3 SERVINGS

Vegetable
Group
3-5 SERVINGS

Fruit
Group
2-4 SERVINGS

Bread, Cereal,
Rice, & Pasta
Group
**6-11
SERVINGS**

Fig. **11-6** Food guide pyramid, a guide to daily food choices. (Courtesy US Department of Agriculture, Washington, DC.)

Minerals and Vitamins

In general the nutrient needs of pregnant women, with perhaps the exception of the iron needs, can be met through dietary sources. Counseling about the need for a varied diet rich in vitamins and minerals should be a part of the early prenatal care of every pregnant woman and should be reinforced throughout pregnancy. However, supplements of certain nutrients (listed in the following discussion) are recommended whenever the woman's diet is very poor or whenever significant nutritional risk factors are present. Nutritional risk factors in pregnancy are listed in Box 11-1.

Iron

Iron is needed both to allow for transfer of adequate iron to the fetus and to permit expansion of the maternal RBC mass. Beginning in the latter part of the first trimester the blood volume of the mother increases steadily, peaking at about 1,500 ml more than in the nonpregnant state. In twin gestations, the increase is at least 500 ml greater than in pregnancies with single fetuses (Newman & Ellings, 1995). Plasma volume increases more than RBC mass, with the difference between plasma and RBCs being greatest during the second trimester. The relative excess of plasma causes a modest decrease in the hemoglobin concentration and hematocrit, known as **physiologic anemia** of pregnancy. This is a normal adaptation during pregnancy.

However, poor iron nutriture, which can result in iron deficiency anemia, is relatively common among women in

BOX 11-1	*Indicators of Nutritional Risk in Pregnancy*

Adolescence
Frequent pregnancies: 3 within 2 years
Poor fetal outcome in a previous pregnancy
Poverty
Poor diet habits with resistance to change
Use of tobacco, alcohol, or drugs
Weight at conception under or over normal weight
Problems with weight gain
  Any weight loss
  Weight gain of less than 1 kg/mo after the first trimester
  Weight gain of more than 1 kg/wk after the first trimester
Multifetal pregnancy
Low hemoglobin and/or hematocrit values

the childbearing years. It affects nearly one fifth of the pregnant women in industrialized countries. The maternal mortality rate is increased among anemic women, who are poorly prepared to tolerate hemorrhage at the time of birth. In addition, anemic women may have a greater likelihood of cardiac failure during labor, postpartum infections, and/or poor wound healing (Allen, 1997). The fetus is also affected by maternal anemia. The risk of preterm birth is about threefold greater in anemic women, and fetal iron stores may also be reduced by maternal anemia (Allen, 1997). Anemia is more common among adolescents and African-American women than among adult Caucasian women.

The Institute of Medicine (1992) recommends that all pregnant women receive a supplement of 30 mg of ferrous iron daily, starting by 12 weeks of gestation. (Iron supplements may be poorly tolerated during the nausea prevalent in the first trimester.) However, if iron-deficiency anemia, manifested by a low hematocrit value or low serum hemoglobin and ferritin levels, is present, increased dosages (60 to 120 mg daily) are required. It must also be borne in mind that certain foods taken with an iron supplement can promote or inhibit the absorption of iron from the supplement. See the Home Care box on p. 278 regarding iron supplementation. Even when a woman is taking an iron supplement, however, she should also include good food sources of iron in her daily diet (see Table 11-1). Milk and milk products contain little iron and interfere with its absorption; therefore, they should not be taken with the supplement.

Calcium

Fetal calcification is the reason for most of the increased calcium needs during pregnancy. Milk is the richest source of calcium; 1,200 mg—precisely the RDA for pregnant women—is contained in 1 L. Cottage cheese and ice cream contain less calcium than milk, yogurt, and cheese do. However, one problem that can interfere with milk consumption is **lactose intolerance,** which is the inability to digest milk sugar (lactose) because of the lack of the enzyme lactase in the small intestine. It is relatively common in adults, particularly African-Americans, Asians, Native Americans, and Eskimos. Milk consumption may cause abdominal cramping, bloating, and diarrhea in such people. Yogurt, sweet acidophilus milk, buttermilk, cheese, chocolate milk, and cocoa may be tolerated even when fresh fluid milk is not. Commercial products that contain lactase (e.g., Lactaid) are available in pharmacies and many supermarkets. The lactase in these products hydrolyzes, or digests, the lactose in the milk, making it possible for lactose-intolerant people to drink milk. Supermarkets often carry milk that has been pretreated with lactase.

In some cultures it is uncommon for adults to drink milk. For example, Puerto Ricans and other Hispanic people may use it only as an additive in coffee. Pregnant women from these cultures may need to consume nondairy sources of calcium. Vegetarian diets may also be deficient in calcium (Box 11-2). If calcium intake appears low and the woman does not change her diet habits despite counseling, a supplement containing 600 mg of elemental calcium may be needed daily. Calcium supplements may also be recommended when a pregnant woman experiences leg cramps that are caused by an imbalance in the calcium-phosphorus ratio.

Sodium

During pregnancy the need for sodium increases slightly, primarily because the body water is expanding

---

BOX 11-2 **Calcium Sources for Women Who Do Not Drink Milk**

Each of the following provides approximately the same amount of calcium as 1 cup of milk:

FISH
3 oz can of sardines
4 1/2 oz can of salmon
  (if bones are eaten)

BEANS AND LEGUMES
3 cups of cooked dried beans
2 1/2 cups of refried beans
2 cups of baked beans with molasses
1 cup of tofu (calcium added in processing)

GREENS
1 cup of collards
1 1/2 cups of kale or turnip greens

BAKED PRODUCTS
3 pieces of cornbread
3 English muffins
4 slices of French toast
2 (7-inch diameter) waffles

FRUITS
11 dried figs
1 1/8 cups of orange juice with calcium added

SAUCES
3 oz of pesto sauce
5 oz of cheese sauce

(e.g., the expanding blood volume). Sodium is essential for maintaining body water balance. In the past, dietary sodium was routinely restricted in an effort to control the peripheral edema that commonly occurs during pregnancy. However, it is now recognized that moderate peripheral edema is normal in pregnancy, occurring as a response to the fluid-retaining effects of elevated levels of estrogen. An excessive emphasis on sodium restriction may also make it difficult for pregnant women to achieve an adequate diet. Grain, milk, and meat products, which are good sources of the nutrients needed during pregnancy, are significant sources of sodium. In addition, sodium restriction may stress the adrenal glands and kidneys as they attempt to retain adequate sodium. In general, sodium restriction is necessary only if the woman has a medical condition such as renal or liver failure or hypertension.

Excessive intake of sodium is discouraged during pregnancy, just as it is in nonpregnant women, because it may contribute to abnormal fluid retention and edema. Table salt (sodium chloride) is the richest source of sodium. Most canned foods contain added salt, unless the label states otherwise. Large amounts of sodium are also found in many processed foods, including meats (e.g., smoked or cured meats, cold cuts, and corned beef), baked goods, mixes for casseroles or grain products, soups, and condiments. Products low in nutritive value and excessively high in sodium include pretzels, potato and other chips, pickles, catsup, prepared mustard, steak and Worcestershire sauces, some soft drinks, and bouillon. A specific RDA for sodium does not exist, but an intake of 2 to 3 g per day seems reasonable. This can usually be achieved by salting food lightly during cooking, adding no additional salt at the table, and also by avoiding low-nutrient/high-sodium foods.

Zinc

Zinc is a constituent of numerous enzymes involved in major metabolic pathways. Zinc deficiency is associated with malformations of the central nervous system in infants. When large amounts of iron and folic acid are consumed, the absorption of zinc is inhibited and the serum zinc levels are reduced as a result. Because iron and folic acid supplements are commonly prescribed during pregnancy, pregnant women should therefore be encouraged to consume good sources of zinc daily (see Table 11-1). Women with anemia who receive high-dose iron supplements also need supplements of zinc and copper (Institute of Medicine, 1992).

Fluoride

The role of fluoride in the prenatal development of teeth is not well understood. A long-term, prospective study is currently underway at the Eastman Dental Center in Rochester, in which the effectiveness of prenatal fluoride supplementation on the incidence of tooth decay in 5-year-old children is being evaluated (Worthington-Roberts & Williams, 1993). The effect of prenatal fluoride supplementation on the development of caries-resistant teeth in the infant is unknown.

Fat-soluble vitamins

Fat-soluble vitamins—A, D, E, and K—are stored in the body tissues; in the event of chronic overdoses, these vitamins can reach toxic levels. Because of the high potential for toxicity, pregnant women are therefore advised to take fat-soluble vitamin supplements only as prescribed. Vitamins A and D deserve special mention, however.

Adequate intake of vitamin A is needed so that sufficient amounts of the vitamin can be stored in the fetus. However, dietary sources can readily supply sufficient amounts. Congenital malformations have occurred in infants of mothers who took excessive amounts of vitamin A during pregnancy, and thus supplements are not recommended for pregnant women (Institute of Medicine, 1992). Vitamin A analogs (e.g., isotretinoin [Accutane]), which are prescribed for the treatment of cystic acne, are a special concern. Isotretinoin use during early pregnancy has been associated with an increased incidence of heart malformations, facial abnormalities, cleft palate, hydrocephalus, and deafness and blindness in the infant, as well as an increased risk of spontaneous abortion. Topical agents such as tretinoin (Retin-A) do not appear to enter the circulation in any substantial amounts, but their safety in pregnancy has not been confirmed.

Vitamin D plays an important role in the absorption and metabolism of calcium. The main food sources of this vitamin are enriched or fortified foods such as milk and ready-to-eat cereals. Vitamin D is also produced in the skin by the action of ultraviolet light (in sunlight). A severe deficiency may lead to neonatal hypocalcemia and tetany, as well as to hypoplasia of the tooth enamel. The daily consumption of a quart of milk provides the RDA of vitamin D and calcium for most pregnant women. For this reason, women who do not usually drink milk should be encouraged to do so. It is advisable for women with lactose intolerance and those who refuse to include milk in their diet to take a daily supplement providing 10 μg (400 IU) of vitamin D, particularly during the winter months and in northern latitudes where sunlight exposure is limited (Institute of Medicine, 1992). The risk of deficiency is also increased in dark-skinned women and those who habitually wear clothing that covers most of their skin.

Water-soluble vitamins

Body stores of water-soluble vitamins are much smaller than those of fat-soluble vitamins, and the water-soluble vitamins, in contrast to the fat-soluble ones, are readily excreted in the urine. Therefore good sources of these vitamins must be consumed frequently, and toxicity with overdose is less likely than it is in people taking fat-soluble vitamins.

Because of the augmented maternal erythropoiesis of pregnancy, pregnant women need substantially more folic acid (folacin or folate); this is also necessary to meet the needs of the rapidly growing cells in fetal and placental tissues. In 1992 the U.S. Public Health Service recommended that all women of childbearing potential consume 0.4 mg (400 μg) of folic acid daily. It is estimated that the incidence of neural tube defects (NTDs) could be halved if all women had an adequate folic acid intake during the periconceptual period (Butterworth & Bendich, 1996). In the United States, all enriched grain products (which include most white breads, flour, and pasta) must contain folic acid at a level of 1.4 mg per kg flour. This level of fortification supplies approximately 0.1 mg folic acid daily in the average American diet (U.S. DHHS, FDA, 1996). All women of childbearing potential need careful counseling about including good sources of folic acid in their diet: green leafy vegetables, whole and enriched grains, folic acid–fortified ready-to-eat cereals, and meats (see Table 11-2). However, even women with good eating habits may find it difficult to consume enough dietary folic acid, and therefore a supplement is advisable for women who are or might become pregnant.

Pyridoxine, or vitamin B_6, is involved in protein metabolism. Although levels of a pyridoxine-containing enzyme have been reported to be low in women with PIH, there is no evidence that supplementation prevents or eradicates the condition. No supplement is recommended routinely, but women with poor diets and those at nutritional risk (see Box 11-1) may need a supplement providing 2 mg/day (Institute of Medicine, 1992).

Vitamin C, or ascorbic acid, plays an important role in tissue formation and enhances the absorption of iron. The vitamin C needs of most women are readily met by a diet that includes at least one daily serving of citrus fruit or juice or another good source of the vitamin (see Table 11-2), but women who smoke need more. A supplement of 50 mg/day is recommended for women determined to be at nutritional risk (Institute of Medicine, 1992). However, if the mother should take excessive doses of this vitamin during pregnancy, vitamin C deficiency may develop after birth in the infant.

Nutrient supplements

The consensus of the 1990 Institute of Medicine committee is that food can and should be the normal vehicle to meet the additional needs imposed by pregnancy, except for iron. Recall that a supplemental dose of 30 mg per day is recommended. However, some women chronically consume diets that are deficient in necessary nutrients and, for whatever reason, may be unable to change this intake. For these women a supplement should be considered. It is important that the pregnant woman understand that the use of a vitamin/mineral supplement does not lessen the need to consume a nutritious, well-balanced diet.

Pica and food cravings. Pica, which is the practice of consuming nonfood substances (e.g., clay or laundry starch) or excessive amounts of foodstuffs low in nutritional value (e.g., cornstarch or ice), often is influenced by the woman's cultural background. In the United States it appears to be most common among African-American women, women from rural areas, and women with a family history of pica. The regular and heavy consumption of low-nutrient products may cause more nutritious foods to be displaced from the diet, and the items consumed may also interfere with the absorption of nutrients, especially minerals. The existence of pica, as well as details of the type and amounts of products ingested, is likely to be discovered only by the sensitive interviewer who has developed a relationship of trust with the woman. A patient teaching plan can be formulated after careful assessment of the potential for harm caused by the practice. It has been proposed that pica and **food cravings** (i.e., the urge to have ice cream, pickles, or pizza, for example) during pregnancy are caused by an innate drive to consume nutrients missing from the diet. However, research has not supported this hypothesis.

Adolescent pregnancy. Many adolescent females have diets that fall below the recommended intakes of key nutrients, including energy, calcium, and iron. In one survey, 37% of African-American teens and 42% of Caucasian adolescents were underweight, when classified according to their BMI (Sargent et al., 1994).

Pregnant adolescents and their infants are at increased risk of complications during pregnancy and parturition. Growth of the pelvis is delayed in comparison to growth in stature, and this helps to explain why cephalopelvic disproportion and other mechanical problems associated with labor are common among young adolescents. Competition between the growing adolescent and the fetus for nutrients may also contribute to some of the poor outcomes apparent in teen pregnancies. Growth during pregnancy is difficult to assess because "shrinkage" in height has been observed in very young pregnant women (Scholl & Hediger, 1993). Postural changes may contribute to this apparent shrinkage; whatever the reason, it complicates the assessment of maternal nutritional status. When growth of adolescent females was carefully assessed (using lower leg length, a measurement that was unlikely to undergo shrinkage) during pregnancy, it was determined that the females who were still growing had infants that were significantly smaller than those of mature women (Scholl & Hediger, 1993). Growth was found to occur in both primigravidas and multigravidas. Because it is difficult in a nonresearch setting to determine which adolescents are still growing and which ones have completed their growth, pregnant adolescents are encouraged to choose a weight gain goal at the upper end of the range for their BMI (Institute of Medicine, 1992). The goal is to reduce the prevalence of LBW among infants of teen mothers.

Efforts to improve the nutritional health of pregnant adolescents focus on improving the nutrition knowledge, meal planning, and food preparation/selection skills of young females; promoting access to prenatal care; developing nutrition interventions and educational programs that are effective with adolescents; and striving to understand the factors that create barriers to change in the adolescent population (Story, 1997).

Pregnancy-induced hypertension. The cause of PIH, or preeclampsia, is not known. There has been speculation that the poor intake of several nutrients, including calcium, magnesium, vitamin B_6, and protein, might foster its development, but there is no definite evidence that nutritional deficiencies are causes or that nutritional supplements can help prevent it. At present, a diet adequate in the recommended nutrients (see Table 11-2) appears to be the best means of reducing the risk of PIH.

Exercise during pregnancy. Moderate exercise during pregnancy yields numerous benefits, including improving muscle tone, potentially shortening the course of labor, and promoting a sense of well-being. By observing careful guidelines (ACOG, 1994), most women can safely exercise throughout pregnancy. However, two nutritional concepts are especially important for women who choose to exercise during pregnancy. First, a liberal amount of fluid should be consumed before, during, and after exercise because dehydration can trigger premature labor. Second, the calorie intake should be sufficient to meet the increased needs of pregnancy and the demands of exercise.

NUTRIENT NEEDS DURING LACTATION

Nutritional needs during lactation are similar in many ways to those during pregnancy (see Table 11-2). Needs for energy (calories), protein, calcium, phosphorus, magnesium, iodine, zinc, vitamin D, the B vitamins (thiamine, riboflavin, niacin, pyridoxine, and vitamin B_{12}), and vitamin C remain elevated over nonpregnant needs. The RDA for some of these (e.g., magnesium, vitamin C, zinc, and protein) is slightly to moderately higher than during pregnancy (see Table 11-1). This allowance covers the amount of the nutrient released in the milk, as well as needs of the mother for tissue maintenance. In the case of iron and folic acid, the RDA during lactation is lower than during pregnancy. Both of these nutrients are essential for RBC formation, and thus for maintaining the increase in the blood volume that occurs during pregnancy. With the decrease in maternal blood volume to nonpregnant levels after delivery, maternal iron and folic acid needs also fall. Many lactating women experience a delay in the return of menses, and this also conserves blood cells and reduces iron and folic acid needs. It is especially important that the calcium intake be adequate; if it is not and the woman does not respond to diet counseling, a supplement of 600 mg of calcium per day may be needed (Institute of Medicine, 1992).

The suggested RDA is an increase of 500 kcal more than the woman's nonpregnant intake. The Institute of Medicine (1992) recommends that lactating women consume at least 1,800 kcal per day, because it becomes difficult to obtain adequate nutrients for the maintenance of lactation at levels below that. Because of the deposition of energy stores, the woman who has gained the optimal amount of weight during pregnancy is heavier after birth than at the beginning of pregnancy. As a result of the caloric demands of lactation, however, the lactating mother usually experiences a gradual but steady weight loss. Most women rapidly lose several pounds during the first month postpartum, whether they breastfeed or not. After the first month, the average loss during lactation is 0.5 to 1.0 kg a month, and a woman who is overweight may be able to lose up to 2 kg without decreasing her milk supply (Institute of Medicine, 1992).

Fluid intake must also be adequate to maintain milk production, but the mother's level of thirst is the best guide to the right amount. There is no need to consume more fluids than that needed to satisfy thirst.

Smoking and alcohol and excessive caffeine intake should be avoided during lactation. Smoking may not only impair milk production, but also it exposes the infant to the risk of passive smoking. It is speculated that the infant's psychomotor development may be affected by maternal alcohol use, and alcoholic beverages (two drinks per day) may impair the milk ejection reflex. Coffee intake may lead to a reduced iron concentration in milk and consequently contribute to the development of anemia in the infant. The caffeine concentration in milk is only approximately 1% of the mother's plasma level, but caffeine seems to accumulate in the infant. Some breastfed infants of mothers who drank large amounts of coffee or caffeine-containing soft drinks have been reported to be unusually active and wakeful (Lawrence, 1994).

CARE MANAGEMENT

During pregnancy, nutrition plays a key role in achieving an optimal outcome for the mother and her unborn baby. The motivation to learn about nutrition is usually greater during pregnancy because parents strive to "do what's right for the baby." Optimal nutrition cannot eliminate all the problems that may arise during pregnancy, but it does establish a good foundation for supporting the needs of the mother and her unborn baby.

Assessment and Nursing Diagnoses

Assessment is based on a **diet history** (a description of the woman's usual food and beverage intake and factors affecting her nutritional status, such as medications being taken and the adequacy of income to allow her to purchase the necessary foods) obtained from an interview and review of the woman's health records, physical examination, and laboratory results. Ideally a nutritional assessment is performed before conception so that any recommended changes in diet, lifestyle, and weight can be undertaken before the woman becomes pregnant.

Diet history

Obstetric and gynecologic effects on nutrition. Nutritional reserves may be depleted in the multiparous woman or the one who has had frequent pregnancies (especially 3 pregnancies within 2 years). A history of preterm birth or birth of an LBW or SGA infant may indicate inadequate dietary intake. PIH may also be a factor in poor maternal nutrition. Birth of a large-for-gestational age (LGA) infant may indicate the existence of maternal diabetes mellitus. Previous contraceptive methods may also affect reproductive health. Increased menstrual blood loss often occurs during the first 3 to 6 months after placement of an intrauterine contraceptive device. Consequently the user may have low iron stores or even iron deficiency anemia. Oral contraceptive agents, on the other hand, are associated with decreased menstrual losses and increased iron stores; however, oral contraceptives may interfere with folic acid metabolism.

Medical history. Chronic maternal illnesses such as diabetes mellitus, renal disease, liver disease, cystic fibrosis or other malabsorptive disorders, seizure disorders and the use of anticonvulsant agents, hypertension, and PKU may affect a woman's nutritional status and dietary needs. In women with illnesses that have resulted in nutritional deficits or that require dietary treatment (e.g., diabetes mellitus or PKU), it is extremely important for nutritional care to be started and for the condition to be optimally controlled before conception. The registered dietitian can provide in-depth counseling for the woman who requires a therapeutic diet during pregnancy and lactation.

Usual maternal diet. The woman's usual food and beverage intake, the adequacy of her income and other resources to meet her nutritional needs, any dietary modifications, food allergies and intolerances, and all medications and nutrition supplements being taken, as well as pica and cultural dietary requirements, should be ascertained. In addition, the presence and severity of nutrition-related discomforts of pregnancy, such as morning sickness, constipation, and pyrosis (heartburn), should be determined. These discomforts are discussed in more detail in the section on implementation. The nurse should be alert to any evidence of eating disorders such as anorexia nervosa, bulimia, and frequent and rigorous dieting before or during pregnancy.

The impact of food allergies and intolerances on nutritional status ranges from very important to almost nil. Lactose intolerance is of special concern in pregnant and lactating women because no other food group equals milk and milk products in terms of calcium content. If a woman suffers from lactose intolerance, the interviewer should explore her intake of other calcium sources (see Box 11-2).

The assessment must include an evaluation of the woman's financial status and her knowledge of sound dietary practices. The quality of the diet increases with increasing socioeconomic status and educational level. Poor women may not have access to adequate refrigeration and cooking facilities and may find it difficult to obtain adequate nutritious food. The pregnancy rates are high among homeless women, and many such women cannot or do not take advantage of services such as food stamps.

Box 11-3 provides a simple tool for obtaining diet history information. When potential problems are identified, they should be followed up with a careful interview.

Physical examination

Anthropometric (body) **measurements** provide short- and long-term information on a woman's nutritional status and are thus essential to the assessment. At a minimum, the woman's height and weight must be determined at the time of her first prenatal visit, and her weight should be measured at every subsequent visit (see earlier discussion of BMI).

A careful physical examination can reveal objective signs of malnutrition (Table 11-3). It is important to note, however, that some of these signs are nonspecific and the physiologic changes of pregnancy may complicate the interpretation of physical findings. For example, lower extremity edema often occurs when caloric and protein deficiency are present, but it may also be a normal finding in the third trimester. The interpretation of physical findings is made easier by a thorough health history and by laboratory testing, if indicated.

Laboratory testing

The only nutrition-related laboratory test necessary for most pregnant women is a hematocrit or hemoglobin measurement to screen for the presence of **anemia**. Because of the physiologic anemia of pregnancy, the reference values for hemoglobin and hematocrit must be adjusted during pregnancy. The lower limit of the normal range for hemoglobin during pregnancy is 11 g/dl in the first and third trimesters and 10.5 g/dl in the second trimester (compared with 12 g/dl in the nonpregnant state). The lower limit of the normal range for hematocrit is 33% during the first and third trimesters and 32% in the second trimester (compared with 36% in the nonpregnant state). Cutoff values for anemia are higher in women who smoke or live at high altitudes, because the decreased oxygen-carrying capacity of their RBCs causes them to produce more RBCs than other women (Institute of Medicine, 1992).

A woman's history or physical findings may indicate the need for additional testing, such as a complete blood cell count with a differential to identify megaloblastic or macrocytic anemia and the measurement of levels of specific vitamins or minerals believed to be lacking in the diet.

The assessment gives a basis for making appropriate nursing diagnoses (see the accompanying Nursing Diagnoses box).

▌ Nursing Diagnoses

Maternal Nutrition
Nutrition, altered: less than body requirements related to:
- Inadequate information about nutritional needs and weight gain during pregnancy
- Misperceptions regarding normal body changes during pregnancy and inappropriate fear of becoming fat
- Inadequate income or skills in meal planning and preparation

Nutrition, altered: more than body requirements related to:
- Excessive intake of energy (calories) or decrease in activity during pregnancy
- Use of unnecessary dietary supplements, especially supplements of fat soluble vitamins, protein (if diet is adequate in protein), and therapeutic amounts of iron (in the absence of iron-deficiency anemia)

Constipation related to:
- Decrease in GI motility because of elevated progesterone levels
- Compression of intestines by enlarging uterus
- Oral iron supplementation

Knowledge deficit related to:
- Inadequate information regarding nutritional needs during pregnancy

BOX 11-3   *Nutrition Questionnaire*

What you eat and some of the lifestyle choices you make can affect your nutrition and health now and in the future. Your nutrition can also have an important effect on your baby's health. Please answer these questions by circling the answers that apply to you.

EATING BEHAVIOR

1. Are you frequently bothered by any of the following? (circle all that apply):

    Nausea   Vomiting   Heartburn   Constipation

2. Do you skip meals at least 3 times a week?   No   Yes
3. Do you try to limit the amount or kind of food you eat to control your weight?   No   Yes
4. Are you on a special diet now?   No   Yes
5. Do you avoid any foods for health or religious reasons?   No   Yes

FOOD RESOURCES

1. Do you have a working stove?   No   Yes

    Do you have a working refrigerator?   No   Yes
2. Do you sometimes run out of food before you are able to buy more?   No   Yes
3. Can you afford to eat the way you should?   No   Yes
4. Are you receiving any food assistance now? (circle all that apply):   No   Yes

    Food stamps   School breakfast   School lunch

    WIC   Donated food/commodities

    Food from a food pantry, soup kitchen, or food bank
5. Do you feel you need help in obtaining food?   No   Yes

FOOD AND DRINK

1. Which of these did you drink yesterday?

    (circle all that apply):

Soft drinks	Coffee	Tea	Fruit drink
Orange juice	Grapefruit juice	Other juices	Milk
Kool-Aid	Beer	Wine	Alcoholic drinks
Water	Other beverages (list) _____		

2. Which of these foods did you eat yesterday?

    (circle all that apply):

Cheese	Pizza	Macaroni and cheese
Yogurt	Cereal with milk	

    Other foods made with cheese (such as tacos, enchiladas, lasagna, cheeseburgers)

Corn	Potatoes	Sweet potatoes	Green salad
Carrots	Collard greens	Spinach	Turnip greens
Broccoli	Green beans	Green peas	Other vegetables
Apples	Bananas	Berries	Grapefruit
Melon	Oranges	Peaches	Other fruit
Meat	Fish	Chicken	Eggs
Peanut butter	Nuts	Seeds	Dried beans
Cold cuts	Hot dog	Bacon	Sausage
Cake	Cookies	Doughnut	Pastry
Chips	French fries		

    Other deep-fried foods, such as fried chicken or egg rolls

Bread	Rolls	Rice	Cereal
Noodles	Spaghetti	Tortillas	

    Were any of these whole grain?   No   Yes
3. Is the way you ate yesterday the way you usually eat?   No   Yes

LIFESTYLE

1. Do you exercise for at least 30 minutes on a regular basis (3 times a week or more)?   No   Yes
2. Do you ever smoke cigarettes or use smokeless tobacco?   No   Yes
3. Do you ever drink beer, wine, liquor, or any other alcoholic beverages?   No   Yes
4. Which of these do you take?

    (circle all that apply):

    Prescribed drugs or medications

    Any over-the-counter products (such as aspirin, Tylenol, antacids, or vitamins)

    Street drugs (such as marijuana, speed, downers, crack, or heroin)

Modified from Food and Nutrition Board, Institute of Medicine: *Nutrition during pregnancy and lactation: an implementation guide,* Washington, DC, 1992, National Academic Press.

TABLE 11-3 *Physical Assessment of Nutritional Status*

SIGNS OF GOOD NUTRITION	SIGNS OF POOR NUTRITION
GENERAL APPEARANCE	
Alert, responsive, energetic, good endurance	Listless, apathetic, cachectic, easily fatigued, looks tired
MUSCLES	
Well developed, firm, good tone, some fat under skin	Flaccid, poor tone, undeveloped, tender, "wasted" appearance
NERVOUS CONTROL	
Good attention span, not irritable or restless, normal reflexes, psychologic stability	Inattentive, irritable, confused, burning and tingling of hands and feet, loss of position and vibratory sense, weakness and tenderness of muscles, decrease or loss of ankle and knee reflexes
GASTROINTESTINAL FUNCTION	
Good appetite and digestion, normal regular elimination, no palpable organs or masses	Anorexia, indigestion, constipation or diarrhea, liver or spleen enlargement
CARDIOVASCULAR FUNCTION	
Normal heart rate and rhythm, no murmurs, normal blood pressure for age	Rapid heart rate, enlarged heart, abnormal rhythm, elevated blood pressure
HAIR	
Shiny, lustrous, firm, not easily plucked, healthy scalp	Stringy, dull brittle, dry, thin and sparse, depigmented, can be easily plucked
SKIN (GENERAL)	
Smooth, slightly moist, good color	Rough, dry, scaly, pale, pigmented, irritated, easily bruised, petechiae
FACE AND NECK	
Skin color uniform, smooth, pink, healthy appearance; no enlargement of thyroid gland; lips not chapped or swollen	Scaly, swollen, skin dark over cheeks and under eyes, lumpiness or flakiness of skin around nose and mouth; thyroid enlarged; lips swollen, angular lesions or fissures at corners of mouth
ORAL CAVITY	
Reddish pink mucous membranes and gums; no swelling or bleeding of gums; tongue healthy pink or deep reddish in appearance, not swollen or smooth, surface papillae present; teeth bright and clean, no cavities, no pain, no discoloration	Gums spongy, bleed easily, inflamed or receding; tongue swollen, scarlet and raw, magenta color, beefy, hyperemic and hypertrophic papillae, atrophic papillae; teeth with unfilled caries, absent teeth, worn surfaces, mottled
EYES	
Bright, clear, shiny, no sores at corners of eyelids, membranes moist and healthy pink color, no prominent blood vessels or mound of tissue (Bitot's spots) on sclera, no fatigue circles beneath	Eye membranes pale, redness of membrane, dryness, signs of infection, Bitot's spots, redness and fissuring of eyelid corners, dryness of eye membrane, dull appearance of cornea, soft cornea, blue sclerae
EXTREMITIES	
No tenderness, weakness, or swelling; nails firm and pink	Edema, tender calves, tingling, weakness; nails spoon-shaped, brittle
SKELETON	
No malformations	Bowlegs, knock-knees, chest deformity at diaphragm, beaded ribs, prominent scapulas

Expected Outcomes of Care

An individualized nursing plan of care based on the nursing diagnoses should be developed in collaboration with the woman. For many women with uncomplicated pregnancies, the nurse can serve as the primary source of nutrition education during pregnancy. The registered dietitian, who has specialized training in diet evaluation and planning, nutritional needs during illness, and ethnic and cultural food patterns, as well as in translating nutrient needs into food patterns, frequently serves as a consultant. Pregnant women with serious nutritional problems, those with intervening illnesses such as diabetes (either preexisting or gestational), and any others requiring in-depth dietary counseling should be referred to the dietitian. The nurse, dietitian, physician, and nurse-midwife collaborate in helping the woman achieve nutrition-related expected outcomes. Some common nutrition-related outcomes require the woman to take the following actions:

- Achieve an appropriate weight gain during pregnancy—an appropriate goal for weight gain takes into account such factors as the woman's prepregnancy weight, whether she is overweight/obese or underweight, and whether the pregnancy is single or multifetal
- Consume adequate nutrients from the diet and supplements to meet estimated needs
- Cope successfully with the nutrition-related discomforts associated with pregnancy, such as pyrosis (heartburn), morning sickness, and constipation
- Avoid or reduce potentially harmful practices such as smoking, alcohol consumption, and caffeine intake
- Return to prepregnancy weight (or an appropriate weight for height) within 6 months of giving birth

Plan of Care and Interventions

Nutritional care and teaching generally involve (1) acquainting the woman with the nutritional needs during pregnancy and the characteristics of an adequate diet, if necessary; (2) helping her to individualize her diet so that she achieves an adequate intake while conforming to her personal, cultural, financial, and health circumstances; (3) acquainting her with strategies for coping with the nutrition-related discomforts of pregnancy; (4) helping her use nutrition supplements appropriately; and (5) consulting with and making referrals to other professionals or services as indicated. Two programs that provide nutrition services are the food stamp program and the Special Supplemental Program for **Women, Infants, and Children (WIC),** which provides vouchers for selected foods to pregnant and lactating women, as well as infants and children at nutritional risk. WIC foods include eggs, cheese, milk, juice, and fortified cereals; these are chosen because they provide iron, protein, vitamin C, and other vitamins.

Adequate dietary intake

Diet teaching can take place in a one-on-one interview or in a group setting. In either case, teaching should emphasize the importance of choosing a varied diet composed of readily available foods (rather than specialized diet supplements). Good nutrition practices (and the avoidance of poor practices such as smoking and alcohol or drug use) are essential content for prenatal classes designed for women in early pregnancy.

The food pyramid (see Fig. 11-6) can be used as a guide to making daily food choices during pregnancy and lactation, just as it is during other stages of the life cycle. The pyramid places the bread, cereal, rice, and pasta group at its base. This position was chosen to indicate that this group should serve as the basis for a healthy diet; six to eleven servings are recommended each day. Vegetables (three to five servings) and fruits (two to four servings) are just above the grains group. The milk, yogurt, and cheese group (two to three servings for nonpregnant adults, increasing to three to four servings for pregnant and lactating women) and the meat, poultry, fish, dried beans, eggs, and nuts group (two to three servings) form a narrow band near the top of the pyramid. At the apex are fats, oils , and sweets (not considered a food group), which are to be used sparingly. The importance of consuming adequate amounts from the milk, yogurt, and cheese group needs to be emphasized, especially for adolescents and women under 25 who are still actively adding calcium to their skeletons; adolescents need at least 1 L of milk or the equivalent daily.

Pregnancy. The pregnant woman must understand what an adequate weight gain during pregnancy means, recognize the reasons for its importance, and be able to evaluate her own gain in terms of the desirable pattern. Many women, particularly those who have worked hard to control their weight before pregnancy, may find it difficult to understand the reason the weight gain goal is so high when a newborn is so small. The nurse can explain that the maternal weight gain consists of increments in the weight of many tissues, not just the growing fetus (see Fig. 11-5).

Dietary overindulgence, on the other hand, which may result in excessive fat stores that persist after giving birth, should be discouraged. Nevertheless, it is best not to focus unduly on weight gain, which can result in feelings of stress and guilt in the woman who does not observe the preferred pattern of gain. Teaching regarding weight gain during pregnancy is summarized in Box 11-4.

Postpartum. The need for a varied diet consisting of a representation of foods from all the food groups continues throughout lactation. As mentioned previously, the lactating woman should be advised to consume at least 1,800 kcal daily, and she should receive counseling if her diet appears to be inadequate in any nutrients. Special attention should be given to her calcium, zinc, vitamin B_6, and folic acid intake, because the RDAs for these remain higher than

Weight Gain during Pregnancy

- Progressive weight gain during pregnancy is essential to ensure normal fetal growth and development and the deposition of maternal stores that promote successful lactation.
- Recommended weight gain during pregnancy is determined largely by prepregnancy weight for height.
    Normal-weight women, 11.5-16 kg; underweight women, 12.5-18 kg; overweight women, 7-11.5 kg.
- Weight gain should be achieved through a balanced diet of regular foods chosen from all the different food groups (see Table 11-2).
- The pattern of weight gain is important: approximately 0.4 kg per week during the second and third trimesters for normal-weight women; 0.5 kg per week for underweight women; and 0.3 kg per week for overweight women.

those for nonpregnant women (see Table 11-1), and it may be difficult for her to consume enough without careful diet planning.

The woman who does not breastfeed will lose weight gradually if she consumes a balanced diet that provides slightly less than her daily energy expenditure. Lactating and nonlactating women should know that fat is the most concentrated source of calories in the diet (9 kcal/g vs. 4 kcal/g in carbohydrates and proteins), and fat calories are more efficiently converted into fat stores than calories from carbohydrates or proteins. Therefore the first step in weight reduction (or preventing excessive weight gain) is to evaluate the sources of fat in the diet and explore with the patient ways of reducing them. Even foods such as vegetables that are originally low in fat can become high in fat when fried or sautéed, served with excessive amounts of salad dressing, consumed with high-fat dips or sauces, or seasoned with butter or bacon drippings. A reasonable weight loss goal for nonlactating women is 0.5 to 1 kg per week; a loss of 1 kg per month is recommended for most lactating women.

Daily food guide and menu planning. The daily food plan (see Table 11-2 and Fig. 11-6) can be used as a guide for educating the woman about nutritional needs during pregnancy and lactation. This food plan is general enough to be used by women from a wide variety of cultures, including women following a vegetarian diet. One of the more helpful teaching strategies is to help the patient plan daily menus that follow the food plan and are affordable, are realistic in terms of preparation time, and are compatible with personal preferences and cultural practices. Information regarding cultural food patterns is provided later in this chapter.

Therapeutic diets. During pregnancy and lactation, the food plan for women on special therapeutic diets may

have to be modified. The registered dietitian can instruct these women about their diets and assist them in meal planning. However, the nurse should understand the basic principles of the diet and be able to reinforce the diet teaching.

The nurse should be especially aware of the dietary modifications necessary for women with diabetes mellitus (gestational or preexisting) because this disease is relatively common and because fetal deformity and death occur more often in pregnancies complicated by hyperglycemia or hypoglycemia. Therefore every effort should be made to maintain blood glucose levels in the normal range throughout pregnancy. The food plan of the woman with diabetes usually includes four to six meals and snacks daily, with the daily carbohydrate intake distributed fairly evenly among the meals and snacks. The complex carbohydrates—fibers and starches—should be well represented in the diet of the diabetic woman. To maintain strict control of the blood glucose level, the pregnant diabetic woman usually must monitor her own level daily. Urine glucose and ketone measurements are not sensitive enough to detect hyperglycemia accurately and provide no information about hypoglycemia. The nurse must therefore teach the woman the way to monitor her own blood glucose level, unless she has already been doing this before pregnancy.

Iron supplementation. As mentioned earlier, the nutritional supplement most commonly needed during pregnancy is iron. However, a variety of dietary factors can affect the completeness of absorption of an iron supplement. Bran, milk, egg yolks, coffee, tea, or oxalate-containing vegetables such as spinach and Swiss chard consumed at the same time as iron will inhibit iron absorption. Conversely, iron absorption is promoted by a diet rich in vitamin C (e.g., citrus fruits or melons) or "heme iron" (found in red meats, fish, and poultry). Iron supplements are best absorbed on an empty stomach, thus they can be taken between meals with beverages other than milk, tea, or coffee. However, some women have gastrointestinal discomfort when they take the supplement on an empty stomach; therefore a good time for them to take the supplement is just before bedtime. Constipation is common with iron supplementation. Iron supplements should be kept away from any children in the household because their ingestion could result in acute iron poisoning and even death. The accompanying Home Care box summarizes important points regarding iron supplementation.

Coping with nutrition-related discomforts of pregnancy

The most common nutrition-related discomforts of pregnancy are nausea and vomiting or "morning sickness," constipation, and pyrosis.

HOME CARE *Patient Instructions for Self-Care*

Iron Supplementation

- It is difficult to consume enough iron in the diet to meet iron needs and prevent anemia during pregnancy.
- Vitamin C (in citrus fruits, tomatoes, melons, and strawberries) and heme iron (in meats) increase the absorption of iron supplement. Therefore include these in the diet often.
- Bran, tea, coffee, milk, oxalates (in spinach and Swiss chard), and egg yolk decrease iron absorption. Avoid consuming them at the same time as the supplement.
- Iron is best absorbed if it is taken when the stomach is empty; that is, take it between meals with a beverage other than tea, coffee, or milk.
- Iron can be taken at bedtime if abdominal discomfort occurs when it is taken between meals.
- If an iron dose is missed, take it as soon as it is remembered if that is within 13 hours of the scheduled dose. Do *not* double up on the dose.
- Keep the supplement in a child-proof container and out of the reach of any children in the household.
- The iron may cause stools to be black or dark green.
- Constipation is common with iron supplementation. A diet high in fiber with adequate fluid intake is recommended.

BOX 11-5	*Food Plan for a Woman with Nausea and Vomiting during Early Pregnancy*

BREAKFAST	**AFTERNOON**
Toasted oat bran bagel, plain	Vegetable juice Rice cake
MIDMORNING	**DINNER**
Blueberry muffin Skim milk	Baked chicken with skin removed Spinach salad Butternut squash casserole Skim milk
LUNCH	
Tuna or pasta salad Carrot sticks Melon balls Water	**AFTER DINNER** Wheat bran cereal Strawberries Skim milk

From Lowdermilk D, Perry S & Bobak I: *Maternity & women's health care,* ed 6, St Louis, 1997, Mosby.

Nausea and vomiting. Nausea and vomiting are most common during the first trimester. Most of the time the nausea and vomiting cause only mild to moderate problems nutritionally, although they may be a source of substantial discomfort. The pregnant woman may find the following suggestions helpful in alleviating the problems:

- Eat dry, starchy foods such as dry toast, melba toast, or crackers on awakening in the morning and at other times when nausea occurs.
- Avoid consuming excessive amounts of fluids early in the day or when nauseated (but compensate by drinking fluids at other times).
- Eat small amounts frequently (every 2 to 3 hours) and avoid large meals that distend the stomach.
- Avoid skipping meals and thus becoming extremely hungry, which may worsen nausea. Have a snack such as cereal with milk, a small sandwich, or yogurt before bedtime.
- Avoid sudden movements. Get out of bed slowly.
- Decrease intake of fried and other fatty foods. Good choices are starches such as pastas, rice, and breads and low-fat protein foods (skinless broiled or baked poultry, cooked dried beans or peas, lean meats, and broiled or canned fish).

- Fresh air may help relieve nausea. Keep the environment well ventilated (e.g., open a window), go for a walk outside, or decrease cooking odors by using an exhaust fan.
- During episodes of nausea eat foods served at cool temperatures and foods that give off little aroma.
- Avoid brushing teeth immediately after eating.
- Some women find that salty and tart foods (e.g., potato chips and lemonade) are tolerated during periods of nausea.

A sample daily food plan that follows these guidelines while providing an adequate diet for the pregnant woman is shown in Box 11-5.

Hyperemesis gravidarum, or severe and persistent vomiting causing weight loss, dehydration, and electrolyte abnormalities, occurs in up to approximately 1% of pregnant women. Intravenous fluid and electrolyte replacement is usually necessary for those women who lose 5% of their body weight. Often this is followed by improved tolerance to the oral intake of food; therapy then consists of the frequent consumption of small amounts of low-fat foods. Enteral tube feeding by means of small-bore nasogastric tubes has been successful in some women. Because the pulmonary aspiration of the feeding is a potential complication if vomiting occurs, antiemetic medications are sometimes administered in conjunction with the tube feedings. Tube feedings may be used to supplement oral intake, with the volume of the tube feeding gradually being decreased as oral intake improves. In some instances total parenteral nutrition (balanced intravenous feedings of amino acids, carbohydrates, lipids, vitamins, and minerals) has been used to nourish women with hyperemesis gravidarum when their nutritional status has been severely impaired.

Constipation. Improved bowel function generally results from increasing the intake of fiber (e.g., wheat bran and whole wheat products, popcorn, and raw or lightly steamed vegetables) in the diet, because fiber helps to retain water within the stool, creating a bulky stool that stimulates intestinal peristalsis. The RDA for adults for fiber is 25 g to 35 g. An increase of approximately 15% would be optimal. An adequate fluid intake (at least 50 ml/kg/day) helps to hydrate the fiber and increase the bulk of the stool. Making a habit of regular exercise that uses large muscle groups (walking, swimming, cycling) also helps to stimulate bowel motility.

Pyrosis. Pyrosis, or heartburn, is usually caused by the reflux of gastric contents into the esophagus. This condition can be minimized by the consumption of small, frequent meals, rather than two or three larger meals daily. Because fluids further distend the stomach, they should not be consumed with foods. The woman needs to be sure to drink adequate amounts between meals, however. Avoiding spicy foods may help alleviate the problem. Lying down immediately after eating and wearing clothing that is tight across the abdomen can contribute to the problem of reflux.

Cultural influences

Consideration of a woman's cultural food preferences enhances communication, providing a greater opportunity for compliance with the agreed upon pattern of intake. Women in most cultures are encouraged to eat a diet typical for them. The nurse needs to be aware of what constitutes a typical diet for each cultural or ethnic group. However, within one cultural group several variations may occur. Thus careful exploration of individual preferences is needed. Although ethnic and cultural food beliefs may seem, at first glance, to conflict with the dietary instruction provided by physicians, nurses, and dietitians, it is often possible for the empathic health care provider to identify cultural beliefs that are congruent with the modern understanding of pregnancy and fetal development. Many cultural food practices have some merit or the culture would not have survived. Food cravings during pregnancy are considered normal by many cultures, but the kinds of cravings often are culturally specific. In most cultures women crave acceptable foods, such as chicken, fish, and greens among African-Americans. Cultural influences on food intake usually lessen if the woman and her family become more integrated into the dominant culture. Nutritional beliefs and the practices of selected cultural groups are summarized in Table 11-4.

Vegetarian diets

Vegetarian diets represent another cultural effect on nutritional status. Foods basic to almost all **vegetarian diets** are vegetables, fruits, legumes, nuts, seeds, and grains. However, there are many variations in vegetarian diets. Semi-vegetarians, who are not truly vegetarians, include fish, poultry, eggs, and dairy products in their diets but do not eat beef or pork. Such a diet can be completely adequate for pregnant women. Besides plant products, lactoovovegetarians also eat dairy products. Iron and zinc intake may not be adequate in these women, but such diets can be otherwise nutritionally sound. Strict vegetarians, or vegans, consume only plant products. Because vitamin B_{12} is found only in foods of animal origin, this diet is therefore deficient in vitamin B_{12}. As a result, strict vegetarians should take a supplement or consume vitamin B_{12} fortified foods (e.g., soy milk) regularly. Vitamin B_{12} deficiency can result in megaloblastic anemia, glossitis, and neurologic deficits in the mother. Infants born to affected mothers are likely to have megolablastic anemia and exhibit neurodevelopmental delays. Iron, calcium, zinc, and vitamin B_6 intake may also be low in women on this diet, and some strict vegetarians have excessively low caloric intakes. The protein intake should be assessed especially carefully because plant proteins tend to be "incomplete," in that they lack one or more amino acids required for growth and the maintenance of body tissues. However, the daily consumption of a variety of different plant proteins—grains, dried beans and peas, nuts, and seeds—helps to provide all of the essential amino acids.

Evaluation

It is essential to set concrete, measurable outcomes; evaluate the woman's progress toward these outcomes regularly; and revise the plan of care if the outcomes are not achieved. In evaluating the adequacy of nutritional intake during pregnancy, the patient's weight gain can be compared with standardized grids showing recommended patterns (see Fig. 11-4). These grids are based on mean data and do not always take into account factors such as ethnic or racial variations. To evaluate the adequacy of the woman's diet, her diet can be compared with the plan in Table 11-2. Again, it is essential that individual factors affecting nutritional needs and dietary intake be considered. Physical examination and laboratory testing (see section on assessment) can be used as a means of confirming that a woman's nutritional status is adequate. If an inadequate weight gain is found or nutritional deficits appear, it is essential that the nurse reassess the woman and her understanding of her nutritional needs, reinforce teaching as needed, make referrals as indicated, and continue to reevaluate her nutritional status regularly (see Plan of Care on p. 283).

TABLE 11-4   *Characteristic Food Patterns of Selected Cultures*

MILK GROUP	PROTEIN GROUP	FRUITS AND VEGETABLES	BREADS AND CERALS	POSSIBLE DIETARY PROBLEMS
NATIVE AMERICAN (MANY TRIBAL VARIATIONS; MANY "AMERICANIZED")				
Fresh milk	Pork, beef, lamb, rabbit	Green peas, beans	Refined bread	Obesity, diabetes,
Evaporated milk for cooking	Fowl, fish, eggs	Beets, turnips	Whole wheat	alcoholism,
Ice cream	Legumes	Leafy green and other vegetables	Cornmeal	nutritional
Cream pie	Sunflower seeds	Grapes, bananas, peaches, other fresh fruits	Rice	deficiencies expressed in dental
	Nuts: walnut, acorn, pine, peanut butter	Roots	Dry cereals	problems and iron-deficiency anemia
	Game meat		"Fry" bread	Inadequate amounts of all nutrients
			Tortillas	Excessive use of sugar
MIDDLE EASTERN* (ARMENIAN, GREEK, SYRIAN, TURKISH)				
Yogurt	Lamb	Peppers, tomatoes, cabbage, grape leaves, cucumbers, squash	Cracked wheat and dark bread	Fry many meats and vegetables
Little butter	Nuts	Dried apricots, raisins, dates		Lack of fresh fruits
	Dried peas, beans, lentils			Insufficient foods from milk group
	Sesame seeds			High consumption of sweetenings, lamb fat, and olive oil
AFRICAN-AMERICAN				
Milk†	Pork: all cuts, plus organs, chitterlings	Leafy vegetables	Cornmeal and hominy grits	Extensive use of frying, smothering
Ice cream	Beef, lamb	Green and yellow vegetables	Rice	in gravy, or simmering
Cheese: longhorn, American	Chicken, giblets	Potato: white, sweet	Biscuits, pancakes, white breads	Fats: salt pork, bacon drippings, lard, and gravies
	Eggs	Stewed fruit	Puddings: bread, rice	High consumption of sweets
	Nuts	Bananas and other fresh fruit		Insufficient citrus
	Legumes			Vegetables often boiled for long periods with pork fat and much salt
	Fish, game			Limited amounts from milk group†
CHINESE (CANTONESE MOST PREVALENT)				
Milk: water buffalo	Pork sausage‡	Many vegetables	Rice/rice flour products	Tendency of some immigrants to use
	Eggs and pigeon eggs	Radish leaves	Cereals, noodles	large amounts of grease in cooking
	Fish	Bean, bamboo sprouts	Wheat, corn, millet seed	Limited use of milk and milk products
	Lamb, beef, goat			Often low in protein, calories, or both
	Fowl: chicken, duck			Soy sauce (high sodium)
	Nuts			
	Legumes			
	Soybean curd (tofu)			

MSG, Monosodium L-glutamate.
*Religious holidays may involve fasting, which is believed to increase the likelihood of preterm labor. Fasting requirement may be waived during pregnancy.
†Lactose intolerance relatively common in adults.
‡Lower in fat content than Western sausage.

TABLE 11-4 *Characteristic Food Patterns of Selected Cultures—cont'd*

MILK GROUP	PROTEIN GROUP	FRUITS AND VEGETABLES	BREADS AND CEREALS	POSSIBLE DIETARY PROBLEMS
FILIPINO (SPANISH-CHINESE INFLUENCE)				
Flavored milk Milk in coffee Cheese: gouda, cheddar	Pork, beef, goat, rabbit Chicken Fish Eggs, nuts, legumes	Many vegetables and fruits	Rice, cooked cereals Noodles: rice, wheat	Limited use of milk and milk products Tendency to prewash rice Tendency to have only small portions of protein foods
ITALIAN				
Cheese Some ice cream	Meat Eggs Dried beans	Leafy vegetables Potatoes Eggplant, tomatoes, peppers Fruits	Pasta White breads, some whole wheat Farina Cereals	Prefer expensive imported cheeses; reluctant to substitute less expensive domestic varieties Tendency to overcook vegetables Limited use of whole grains High consumption of sweets Extensive use of olive oil Insufficient servings from milk group
JAPANESE (ISEI, MORE JAPANESE INFLUENCE; NISEI, MORE WESTERNIZED)				
Increasing amounts being used by younger generations	Pork, beef, chicken Fish Eggs Legumes: soya, red, lima beans Tofu Nuts	Many vegetables and fruits Seaweed	Rice, rice cakes Wheat noodles Refined bread, noodles	Excessive sodium: pickles, salty crisp seaweed, MSG, and soy sauce Insufficient servings from milk group May use prewashed rice
HISPANIC, MEXICAN-AMERICAN				
Milk Cheese Flan, ice cream	Beef, pork, lamb, chicken, tripe, hot sausage, beef intestines Fish Eggs Nuts Dry beans: pinto, chickpeas (often eaten more than once daily)	Spinach, wild greens, tomatoes, chilies, corn, cactus leaves, cabbage, avocado, potatoes, Pumpkin, zapote, peaches, guava, papaya, citrus	Rice, cornmeal Sweet bread, pastries Tortilla: corn, flour Vermicelli (fideo)	Limited meats primarily due to cost Limited use of milk and milk products Large amounts of lard Abundant use of sugar Tendency to boil vegetables for long periods

Continued

TABLE 11-4 *Characteristic Food Patterns of Selected Cultures—cont'd*

MILK GROUP	PROTEIN GROUP	FRUITS AND VEGETABLES	BREADS AND CERALS	POSSIBLE DIETARY PROBLEMS
POLISH				

Milk
Sour cream
Cheese
Butter
	Pork (preferred)
	Chicken
		Vegetables—limited
		  fresh
		Cabbage
		Roots—potatoes
		Fruits—limited fresh
			Dark rye	Sodium in ham,
				  sausage, pickles
				High consumption of
				  sweets
				Tendency to
				  overcook vegetables
				Limited fruits, raw
				  vegetables

PUERTO RICAN				

Limited use of milk
  products
Coffee with milk
  (café con leche)
	Pork
	Poultry
	Eggs (Fridays)
	Dried codfish
	Beans (*habichuelas*)
		Avocado, okra
		Eggplant
		Sweet yams
		Starchy vegetables
		  and fruits *(viandas)*
			Rice
			Cornmeal
				Small amounts of
				  pork and poultry
				Extensive use of fat,
				  lard, salt pork, and
				  olive oil
				Lack of milk products

SCANDINAVIAN (DANISH, FINNISH, NORWEGIAN, SWEDISH)				

Cream
Butter
Cheeses
	Wild game
	Reindeer
	Fish (fresh or dried)
	Eggs
		Berries
		Dried fruit
		Vegetables: cole
		  slaw, roots
			Whole wheat, rye,
			  barley, sweets
			  (cookies and sweet
			  breads)
				Insufficient fresh
				  fruits and vegetables
				High consumption of
				  sweets, pickled
				  salted meats, and
				  fish

SOUTHEAST ASIAN (VIETNAMESE, CAMBODIAN)				

Generally not taken
Coffee with
  condensed cow's
  milk
Plain yogurt
Ice cream (rare)
Soybean milk
	Fish (daily): fresh,
	  dried, salted
	Poultry/eggs: duck,
	  chicken
	Pork
	Beef (seldom)
	Dry beans
	Tofu
		Seasonal variety:
		  fresh or preserved
		Green, leafy
		  vegetables
		Yams
		Corn
			Rice: grains, flour,
			  noodles
			French bread
			"Cellophane" (bean
			  starch) noodles
				Fresh milk products
				  generally not
				  consumed
				Poultry/eggs may be
				  limited
				Meat considered
				  "unclean" is
				  avoided
				Preference for a diet
				  high in salt and
				  pepper, as well as
				  rice and pork
				High intake of MSG
				  and soy sauce

JEWISH: ORTHODOX*				

Milk[†]
Cheese[†]
	Meat (bloodless;
	  Kosher prepared):
	  beef, lamb, goat,
	  deer, poultry (all
	  types), no pork
	Fish with fins and
	  scales only
	No crustaceans
		Wide variety	Wide variety	High intake of
				  sodium in meat
				  products

*Religious holidays may involve fasting, which is believed to increase the likelihood of preterm labor. Fasting requirement may be waived during pregnancy.
[†]Milk and milk products not eaten with meat, milk may be taken before the meal or 6 hours after; different sets of dishes and silverware are used to serve milk and meat products.

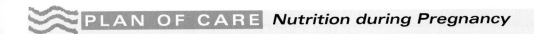

PLAN OF CARE *Nutrition during Pregnancy*

> **NURSING DIAGNOSIS** Knowledge deficit related to nutritional requirements during pregnancy.

Expected Outcomes *The patient will delineate nutritional requirements and exhibit evidence of incorporating requirements into diet.*

Nursing Interventions/*Rationales*

Review basic nutritional requirements for a healthy diet using recommended dietary guidelines and the food guide pyramid *to provide knowledge baseline for discussion.*

Discuss increased nutrient needs (calories, protein, minerals, vitamins) that occur as a result of being pregnant *to increase knowledge needed for altered dietary requirements.*

Discuss the relationship between weight gain and fetal growth *to reinforce interdependence of fetus and mother.*

Calculate the appropriate total weight gain range during pregnancy using the woman's body mass index as a guide and discuss recommended rates of weight gain during the various trimesters of pregnancy *to provide concrete measures of dietary success.*

Review food preferences, cultural eating patterns or beliefs, and prepregnancy eating patterns *to enhance integration of new dietary needs.*

Discuss how to fit nutritional needs into usual dietary patterns and how to alter any identified nutritional deficits or excesses *to increase chances of success with dietary alterations.*

Discuss food aversions or cravings that may occur during pregnancy and strategies to deal with these if they are detrimental to fetus (e.g., pica) *to ensure well-being of fetus.*

Have woman keep a food diary delineating eating habits, dietary alterations, aversions, and cravings *to track eating habits and potential problem areas.*

> **NURSING DIAGNOSIS** Altered nutrition: more than body requirements related to excessive intake and/or inadequate activity levels.

Expected Outcomes *The patient's weekly weight gain will be reduced to the appropriate rate using her body mass index (BMI) and recommended weight gain ranges as guidelines.*

Nursing Interventions/*Rationales*

Review recent diet history (including food cravings) using a food diary, 24-hour recall, or food frequency approach *to ascertain food excesses contributing to excess weight gain.*

Review normal activity and exercise routines *to determine level of energy expenditure;* discuss eating patterns and reasons that lead to increased food intake (e.g., cultural beliefs or myths, increased stress, boredom) *to identify habits that contribute to excess weight gain.*

Review optimal weight gain guidelines and their rationale *to ensure that woman is knowledgeable about healthful weight gain rates.*

Set target weight gains for the remaining weeks of the pregnancy *to establish set goals.*

Discuss with the woman what changes can be made in diet, activity, and lifestyle *to enhance chances of meeting weight gain goals and dietary needs.* (Weight reduction diets should be avoided, since they may deprive mother and fetus of needed nutrients and lead to ketonemia.)

> **NURSING DIAGNOSIS** Altered nutrition: less than body requirements related to inadequate intake of needed nutrients.

Expected Outcomes *The patient's weekly weight gain will be increased to the appropriate rate using her BMI and recommended weight gain ranges as guidelines.*

Nursing Interventions/*Rationales*

Review recent diet history (including food aversions) using a food diary, 24-hour recall, or food frequency approach *to ascertain dietary inadequacies contributing to lack of sufficient weight gain.*

Review normal activity and exercise routines *to determine level of energy expenditure;* discuss eating patterns and reasons that lead to decreased food intake (e.g., morning sickness, pica, fear of becoming fat, stress, boredom) *to identify habits that contribute to inadequate weight gain.*

Review optimal weight gain guidelines and their rationale *to ensure that woman is knowledgeable about healthful weight gain rates.*

Set target weight gains for the remaining weeks of the pregnancy *to establish set goals.*

Review increased nutrient needs (calories, protein, minerals, vitamins) that occur as a result of being pregnant *to ensure woman is knowledgeable about altered dietary requirements.*

Review relationship between weight gain and fetal growth *to reinforce that adequate weight gain is needed to promote fetal well-being.*

Discuss with woman what changes can be made in diet, activity, and lifestyle *to enhance chances of meeting set weight gain goals and nutrient needs of mother and fetus.*

If woman has fear of being fat, if symptoms of an eating disorder are evident, or if problems in adjusting to a changing body image surface, refer woman to the appropriate mental health professional for evaluation, *since intensive treatment and follow-up may be required to ensure fetal health.*

From Wong D & Perry S : *Maternal child nursing care*, St Louis, 1998, Mosby.

RESEARCH

Pica Practices of Pregnant Women

Pica is defined as an unusual craving during pregnancy when women want to ingest typically inedible items such as dirt, clay, grass, and laundry starch. It was hypothesized that an association between pica practices and maternal hemoglobin levels exists. This retrospective cohort study was conducted to determine the prevalence of pica during pregnancy, maternal hemoglobin levels at delivery, and the association of pica with two adverse pregnancy outcomes: low birth weight and preterm birth. The study had 281 women 16 to 30 years of age who had infants younger than 1 year of age and who participated in the Special Supplemental Nutrition Program for Women, Infants and Children (WIC). These women were interviewed at four different clinics. Medical records from 31 hospitals were abstracted. The maternal hemoglobin levels at delivery, mean birth weight, and mean gestational age were compared with women who reported pica and women who did not. There were no differences in mean birth weight or mean gestational age of infants born to women from the pica group and the non-pica group. Pica practices are associated with significantly lower maternal hemoglobin levels at delivery but are not associated with pregnancy outcomes.

CLINICAL APPLICATION OF THE STUDY

The findings from this study can be valuable in counseling women who are anemic. Women who report pica can be informed of the health risks associated with it. Nurses should assess women who have pica cravings during their pregnancy for low hemoglobin levels.

Source: Rainville A: Pica practices of pregnant women are associated with lower maternal hemoglobin level at delivery, *J Am Diet Assoc* 98(3):293, 1998.

KEY POINTS

- A woman's nutritional status before, during, and after pregnancy contributes, to a significant degree, to her well-being and that of her developing fetus.
- Many physiologic changes occurring during pregnancy influence the need for additional nutrients and the efficiency with which the body utilizes them.
- Both the total maternal weight gain and the pattern of weight gain are important determinants of the outcome of pregnancy.
- The appropriateness of the mother's prepregnancy weight for height (BMI) is a major determinant of her recommended weight gain during pregnancy.

KEY POINTS—cont'd

- Nutritional risk factors include adolescent pregnancy; bizarre or faddist food habits; abuse of nicotine, alcohol, or drugs; a low weight for height; and frequent pregnancies.
- Iron supplementation is recommended routinely during pregnancy because it is nearly impossible to obtain adequate intakes from dietary sources alone. Other supplements may be recommended when nutritional risk factors are present.
- The nurse and patient are influenced by cultural and personal values and beliefs during nutrition counseling.
- Pregnancy complications that may be nutrition related include anemia, PIH, gestational diabetes, and intrauterine growth restriction.
- Dietary adaptation can be effective interventions for some of the common discomforts of pregnancy, including nausea and vomiting, constipation, and heartburn.

CRITICAL THINKING EXERCISES

1 *At a prenatal clinic, assess the weight gain patterns of three different women. What advice is indicated based on the patterns seen?*

2 *Interview a pregnant woman at a prenatal clinic. Obtain a diet history using the nutrition questionnaire. With the woman's input, develop an appropriate meal pattern utilizing the food guide pyramid.*

3 *Visit a prenatal clinic in the community. Obtain information about the cultural and ethnic backgrounds of the clients there. Select one ethnic group/culture. Plan a class on nutrition during pregnancy or lactation to be presented at the clinic. In your planning, you should demonstrate both an awareness of specific nutritional needs during pregnancy and lactation and a sensitivity toward food practices and beliefs of the ethnic group/culture you selected.*

4 *Develop an appropriate 1-day menu for a pregnant woman who chooses to use no dairy products or one who is a vegetarian.*

References

Allen L: Pregnancy and iron deficiency: unresolved issues, *Nutr Rev* 5(4):91, 1997

American College of Obstetrics and Gynecology (ACOG): Exercise during pregnancy and the postpartum period, *Technical Bulletin #189*, Washington DC, 1994, ACOG.

Butterworth C Jr & Bendich A: Folic acid and the prevention of birth defects, *Ann Rev Nutr* 16:73, 1996.

Cogswell M & Yip R: The influence of fetal and maternal factors on the distribution of birthweight, *Semin Perinatol* 19(3):222, 1995.

The food guide pyramid, Hyattsville, Md, 1992, US Department of Agriculture.

Hinds T et al.: The effect of caffeine on pregnancy outcome variables, *Nutr Rev* 54(7):203, 1996.

Institute of Medicine: *Nutrition during pregnancy and lactation: an implementation guide,* Washington, DC, 1992, National Academy Press.

Lawrence R: *Breastfeeding: a guide for the medical profession,* ed 4, St Louis, 1994, Mosby.

National Academy of Sciences–Institute of Medicine: *Nutrition during pregnancy,* Washington, DC, 1990, National Academy Press.

Newman R & Ellings J. Antepartum management of the multiple gestation: the case for specialized care, *Semin Perinatol* 19(5):7, 1995.

Position of the American Dietetic Association: Use of nutritive and nonnutritive sweeteners, *J Am Dietet Assoc* 93(10):816, 1993.

Prentice A & Goldberg G: Maternal obesity increases congenital malformations, *Nutr Rev* 54(5):146, 1996.

Rosso P: Placental growth, development and function in relation to maternal nutrition, *Fed Proc* 39(2):250, 1980.

Sargent R et al.: Black and white adolescent females' pre-pregnancy nutrition status, *Adolescence* 29:845, 1994.

Scholl T & Hediger M: A review of the epidemiology of nutrition and adolescent pregnancy: maternal growth during pregnancy and its effect on the fetus, *J Am Coll Nutr* 12(2):101, 1993.

Story M: Promoting healthy eating and ensuring adequate weight gain in pregnant adolescents: issues and strategies, *Ann NY Acad Sci* 817:321, May 28, 1997.

US Department of Health and Human Services, Food and Drug Administration: Food standards: amendment of the standards of identity for enriched grain products to require addition of folic acid, *Federal Register* 61:8781, 1996.

Wardlaw G & Insel P: *Perspectives in nutrition,* ed 2, St Louis, 1993, Mosby.

Wegman M: Infant mortality: some international comparisons, Pediatrics 98(6 Pt 1):1020, 1996.

Worthington-Roberts B & Williams S: *Nutrition in pregnancy and lactation,* ed 5, St Louis, 1993, Mosby.

CHAPTER

Factors and Processes of Labor and Birth

DEITRA LEONARD LOWDERMILK

LEARNING OBJECTIVES

- *Define the key terms.*
- *Explain the five factors that affect the labor process.*
- *Describe the anatomic structure of the bony pelvis.*
- *Recognize the normal measurements of the diameters of the pelvic inlet, cavity, and outlet.*
- *Review the anatomy and the normal measurements of the fetal skull.*
- *Explain the significance of molding of the fetal head during labor.*
- *Describe the cardinal movements of the mechanism of labor.*
- *Assess the maternal anatomic and physiologic adaptations to labor.*
- *Describe fetal adaptations to labor.*

KEY TERMS

asynclitism
attitude
biparietal diameter
bloody show
breech
cephalic
dilatation
effacement
engagement
Ferguson reflex
fontanels
gynecoid pelvis
labor
lie
lightening
mechanism of labor
molding
position
presentation
presenting part
station
suboccipitobregmatic diameter
Valsalva maneuver
vertex

uring late pregnancy, the woman and fetus prepare for the labor process. The fetus has grown and developed in preparation for extrauterine life. The woman has undergone various physiologic adaptations during pregnancy that prepare her for birth and motherhood. Labor and birth represent the end of pregnancy and the beginning of extrauterine life for the newborn.

This chapter discusses the factors affecting labor, the process involved, the normal progression of events, and the adaptations made by both the woman and fetus. This information will provide the theory base necessary for care of the laboring woman and her family.

FACTORS AFFECTING LABOR

Five factors affect the process of labor and birth. These are easily remembered as the five P's: passenger (fetus and placenta), passageway (birth canal), powers (contractions), position of the mother, and psychologic response. The first four factors are presented here as the basis of understanding the physiologic process of labor. The fifth factor is discussed in Chapter 15.

Passenger

The way the passenger, or fetus, moves through the birth canal is determined by several interacting factors: the size of the fetal head, fetal presentation, fetal lie, fetal attitude, and fetal position.

Because the placenta must also pass through the birth canal, it can be considered a passenger along with the fetus. However, the placenta rarely impedes the process of labor in normal vaginal birth.

Size of the fetal head

Because of its size and relative rigidity, the fetal head has a major effect on the birth process. The fetal skull is composed of two parietal bones, two temporal bones, the frontal bone, and the occipital bone (Fig. 12-1, *A*). These bones are united by membranous sutures: the sagittal, lambdoidal, coronal, and frontal (Fig. 12-1, *B*). Membrane-filled spaces

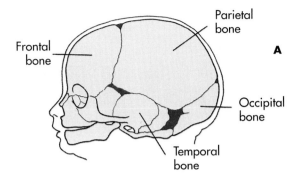

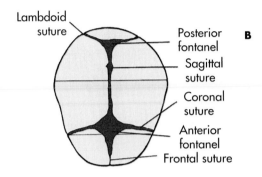

Fig. **12-1** Fetal head at term. **A,** Bones. **B,** Sutures and fontanels.

called **fontanels** are located where the sutures intersect. During labor, after rupture of membranes, palpation of fontanels and sutures during vaginal examination reveals fetal presentation, position, and attitude.

The two most important fontanels are the anterior and posterior ones (see Fig. 12-1, *B*). The larger of these, the anterior fontanel, is diamond shaped, about 3 by 2 cm in size, and lies at the junction of the sagittal, coronal, and frontal sutures. It closes by 18 months after birth. The posterior fontanel lies at the junction of the sutures of the two parietal bones and the one occipital bone, is triangular in shape, and is about 1 by 2 cm in size. It closes 6 to 8 weeks after birth.

Sutures and fontanels make the skull flexible to accommodate the infant brain, which continues to grow for some time after birth. Because the bones are not firmly united, however, slight overlapping of the bones, or **molding** of the shape of the head, occurs during labor. This capacity of the bones to slide over one another also permits adaptation to the various diameters of the maternal pelvis. Molding can be extensive, but the heads of most newborns assume their normal shape within 3 days of birth.

Although the size of the fetal shoulders may affect passage, their position can be altered relatively easily during labor, so that one shoulder may occupy a lower level than the other. This creates a shoulder diameter that is smaller than the skull, facilitating passage through the birth canal.

The circumference of the fetal hips is usually small enough not to create problems.

Fetal presentation

Presentation refers to the part of the fetus that enters the pelvic inlet first and leads through the birth canal during labor at term. The three main presentations are **cephalic** (head first), occurring in 96% of births (Fig. 12-2); **breech** (buttocks first), occurring in 3% of births (Fig. 12-3, *A-C*); and shoulder, seen in 1% of births (Fig. 12-3, *D*). **Presenting part** refers to that part of the fetal body first felt by the examining finger during a vaginal examination. In a cephalic presentation, the presenting part is usually the occiput; in a breech presentation, it is the sacrum; in the shoulder presentation, it is the scapula. When the presenting part is the occiput, the presentation is noted as **vertex** (see Fig. 12-2). Factors that determine the presenting part include fetal lie, fetal attitude, and extension or flexion of the fetal head.

Fetal lie

Lie is the relationship of the long axis (spine) of the fetus to the long axis (spine) of the mother. There are two primary lies: *longitudinal,* or vertical, in which the long axis of the fetus is parallel with the long axis of the mother (see Fig. 12-2); and *transverse,* or horizontal, in which the long axis of the fetus is at a right angle to that of the mother (Fig. 12-3, *D*). Longitudinal lies are either cephalic or breech presentations, depending on the fetal structure that first enters the mother's pelvis. An oblique lie is less common and usually converts to a longitudinal or transverse lie during labor (Cunningham et al., 1997). Vaginal birth cannot occur when the fetus stays in a transverse lie.

Fetal attitude

Attitude is the relationship of the fetal body parts to each other. The fetus assumes characteristic posture (attitude) in utero partly because of the mode of fetal growth and partly because of the way the fetus conforms to the shape of the uterine cavity. Normally, the back of the fetus is markedly flexed so that the head is flexed on the chest, the thighs are flexed on the abdomen, and the legs are flexed at the knees. The arms are crossed over the thorax, and the umbilical cord lies between the arms and the legs. This attitude is called *general flexion* (see Fig. 12-2).

Deviations from the normal attitude may cause difficulties in childbirth. For example, in a cephalic presentation, the fetal head may be extended or flexed in a manner that presents a head diameter that exceeds the limits of the maternal pelvis, leading to prolonged labor, forceps- or vacuum-assisted birth, or cesarean birth.

There are certain critical diameters of the fetal head that are usually measured. The **biparietal diameter,** which is about 9.25 cm at term, is the largest transverse diameter and

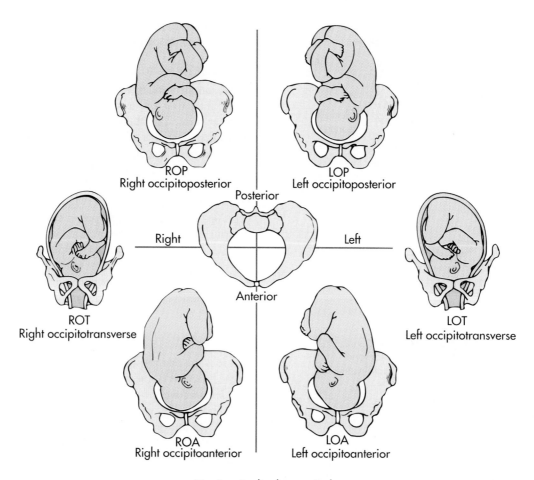

ROP
Right occipitoposterior

LOP
Left occipitoposterior

Posterior

Right — Left

Anterior

ROT
Right occipitotransverse

LOT
Left occipitotransverse

ROA
Right occipitoanterior

LOA
Left occipitoanterior

Lie: Longitudinal or vertical
Presentation: Vertex
Reference point: Occiput
Attitude: Complete flexion

Fig. 12-2 Examples of fetal vertex (occiput) presentations in relation to front, back, or side of maternal pelvis.

an important indicator of fetal head size (Fig. 12-4, *B*). In a well-flexed cephalic presentation, the biparietal diameter is the widest part of the head entering the pelvic inlet. There are several anteroposterior diameters, but the smallest and most critical one is the **suboccipitobregmatic diameter** (about 9.5 cm at term). When the head is in complete flexion, this diameter allows the fetal head to pass through the true pelvis easily (Figs. 12-4, *A*, and 12-5, *A*). As the head is more extended, the anteroposterior diameter widens and the head may not be able to enter the true pelvis (Fig. 12-5, *B* and *C*).

Fetal position

The presentation or presenting part is that portion of the fetus that overlies the pelvic inlet. **Position** is the relationship of the presenting part (occiput, sacrum, mentum [chin], or sinciput [deflexed vertex]), to the four quadrants of the mother's pelvis (see Fig. 12-2). Position is denoted by a three letter abbreviation. The first letter of the abbreviation denotes the location of the presenting part in the right (*R*) or left (*L*) side of the mother's pelvis. The middle letter stands for the specific presenting part of the fetus (*O* for occiput, *S* for sacrum, *M* for mentum [chin], and *Sc* for scapula [shoulder]). The third letter stand for the location of the presenting part in relation to the anterior (*A*), posterior (*P*), or transverse (*T*) portion of the maternal pelvis. For example, ROA means that the occiput is the presenting part and is located in the right anterior quadrant of the maternal pelvis (see Fig. 12-2). LSP means that the sacrum is the presenting part and is located in the left posterior quadrant of the maternal pelvis (see Fig. 12-3, *C*).

Station is the relationship of the presenting part of the fetus to an imaginary line drawn between the maternal ischial spines. The placement of the presenting part is

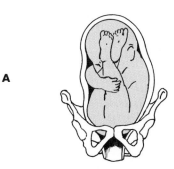

A

Frank breech

Lie: Longitudinal or vertical
Presentation: Breech (incomplete)
Presenting part: Sacrum
Attitude: Flexion, except for legs at knees

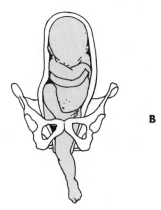

B

Single footling breech

Lie: Longitudinal or vertical
Presentation: Breech (incomplete)
Presenting part: Sacrum
Attitude: Flexion, except for one leg extended
at hip and knee

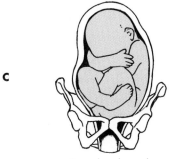

C

Complete breech

Lie: Longitudinal or vertical
Presentation: Breech (sacrum and feet presenting)
Presenting part: Sacrum (with feet)
Attitude: General flexion

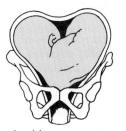

D

Shoulder presentation

Lie: Transverse or horizontal
Presentation: Shoulder
Presenting part: Scapula
Attitude: Flexion

Fig. **12-3** Fetal presentations. **A** to **C,** Breech (sacral) presentation. **D,** Shoulder presentation.

measured in centimeters above or below the spines. For example, when the lowermost portion of the presenting part is 1 cm above the spines, it is noted as being minus (-) 1. At the level of the spines, the station is referred to as 0 (zero). When the presenting part is 1 cm below the spines, the station is said to be plus (+) 1 (Fig. 12-6). Birth is imminent when the presenting part is at +4 to +5 cm. The station of the presenting part should be determined when labor begins so that the rate of descent of the fetus during labor can be accurately determined.

Engagement is the term used to indicate that the presenting part (usually the biparietal diameter) has passed through the maternal pelvic brim or inlet into the true pelvis and usually corresponds to Station 0. Engagement often occurs in the weeks just before labor begins in primigravi-

das and may occur before labor or during labor in multigravidas. Engagement can be determined by abdominal or vaginal examination.

Passageway

The passageway, or birth canal, is composed of the mother's rigid bony pelvis and the soft tissues of the cervix, pelvic floor, vagina, and introitus (the external opening to the vagina). Although the soft tissues, particularly the muscular layers of the pelvic floor, contribute to vaginal birth of the fetus, the maternal pelvis plays a far greater role in the labor process because the fetus must successfully accommodate itself to this relatively rigid passageway. Therefore the size and shape of the pelvis must be determined before childbirth begins.

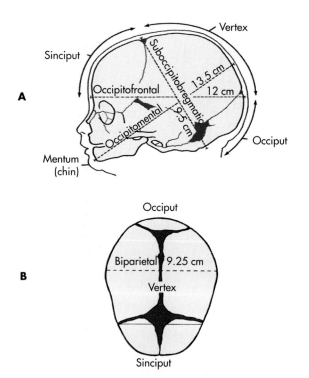

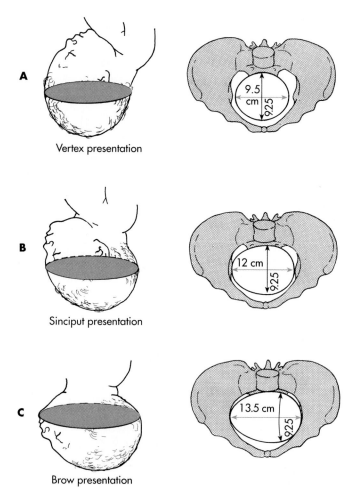

Fig. **12-4** Diameters of the fetal head at term. **A,** Cephalic presentations: occiput, vertex, and sinciput, and cephalic diameters: suboccipitobregmatic, occipitofrontal, and occipitomental. **B,** Biparietal diameter.

Fig. **12-5** Head entering pelvis. Biparietal diameter is indicated with shading (9.25 cm). **A,** Suboccipitobregmatic diameter: complete flexion of head on chest so that smallest diameter enters. **B,** Occipitofrontal diameter: moderate extension (military attitude) so that large diameter enters. **C,** Occipitomental diameter: marked extension (deflection) so that largest diameter, which is too large to permit head to enter pelvis, is presenting.

Bony pelvis

The anatomy of the bony pelvis is described in Chapter 5. The following discussion focuses on the importance of pelvic configurations as they relate to the labor process. (It may be helpful to refer back to Fig. 5-4).

The bony pelvis is formed by the fusion of the ilium, ischium, pubis, and sacral bones. The four pelvic joints are the symphysis pubis, the right and left sacroiliac joints, and the sacrococcygeal joint (Fig. 12-7). The bony pelvis is separated by the brim, or inlet, into two parts: the false pelvis and the true pelvis. The false pelvis is that part above the brim and plays no part in childbearing. The true pelvis, that part involved in birth, is divided into three planes: the inlet, or brim; the midpelvis, or cavity; and the outlet.

The pelvic inlet, which is the upper border of the true pelvis, is formed anteriorly by the upper margins of the pubic bone, laterally by the iliopectineal lines along the innominate bones, and posteriorly by the anterior, upper margin of the sacrum and the sacral promontory.

The pelvic cavity, or midpelvis, is a curved passage having a short anterior wall and a much longer concave posterior wall. It is bounded by the posterior aspect of the symphysis pubis, the ischium, a portion of the ilium, the sacrum, and the coccyx.

The pelvic outlet is the lower border of the true pelvis. Viewed from below, it is ovoid, somewhat diamond-

shaped, bounded by the pubic arch anteriorly, the ischial tuberosities laterally, and the tip of the coccyx posteriorly. In the latter part of pregnancy the coccyx is movable (unless it has been broken in a fall during skiing or skating, for example, and has fused to the sacrum during healing).

The pelvic canal varies in size and shape at various levels. The diameters at the plane of the pelvic inlet, midpelvis, and outlet, plus the axis of the birth canal (Fig. 12-8), determine whether vaginal birth is possible and the manner by which the fetus may pass down the birth canal.

The subpubic angle, which determines the type of pubic arch, together with the length of the pubic rami and the intertuberous diameter, is of great importance. Because the fetus must first pass beneath the pubic arch, a narrow sub-

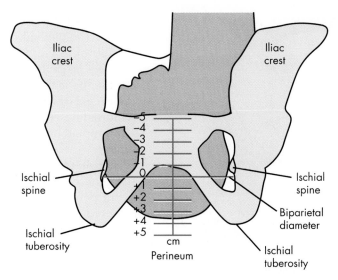

Fig. **12-6** Stations of presenting part, or degree of descent. Biparietal diameter of the fetal head is just below the level of the ischial spines, between station 0 and station +1.

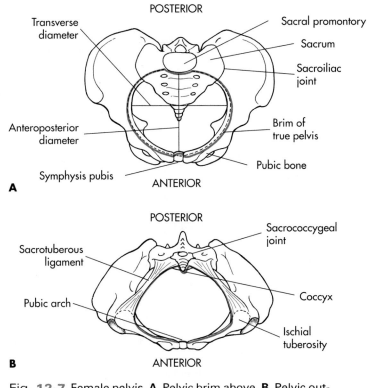

Fig. **12-7** Female pelvis. **A,** Pelvic brim above. **B,** Pelvic outlet from below.

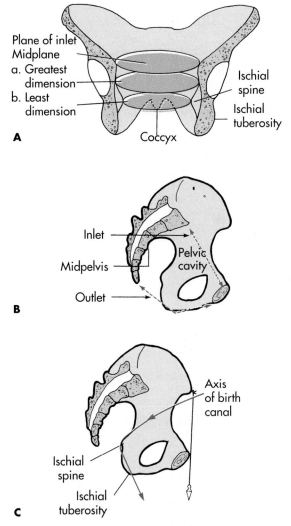

Fig. **12-8** Pelvic cavity. **A,** Inlet and midplane. Outlet not shown. **B,** Cavity of true pelvis. **C,** Note curve of sacrum and axis of birth canal.

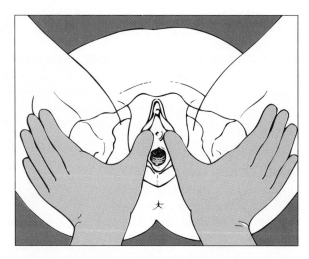

Fig. **12-9** Estimation of angle of subpubic arch. Using both thumbs, examiner externally traces descending rami down to tuberosities. (From Barkauskas V et al.: *Health and physical assessment,* St Louis, 1994, Mosby.)

pubic angle will be less accommodating than a rounded wide arch. The method of measurement of the subpubic arch is shown in Fig. 12-9. A summary of obstetric measurements is given in Table 12-1.

The four basic types of pelvis are classified as follows:
1. Gynecoid (the classic female type)
2. Android (resembling the male pelvis)
3. Anthropoid (resembling the pelvis of anthropoid apes)
4. Platypelloid (the flat pelvis)

The **gynecoid pelvis** is the most common, with major gynecoid pelvic features present in 50% of all women. Anthropoid and android features are less common and platypelloid pelvic features are the least common. Mixed types of pelves are more common than pure types (Cunningham et al., 1997). Examples of pelvic variations and their effects on mode of birth are given in Table 12-2.

Assessment of the bony pelvis can be performed during the first prenatal evaluation and need not be repeated if the

TABLE 12-1 *Obstetric Measurements*		
PLANE	**DIAMETER**	**MEASUREMENTS**

Inlet (superior strait)
  Conjugates
    Diagonal
    Obstetric: measurement that
      determines whether presenting part
      can engage or enter superior strait
    True (vera) (anteroposterior)
	12.5 to 13 cm
	1.5 to 2 cm less than diagonal
	(radiographic)
	
	≥11 cm (12.5) (radiographic)
		Length of diagonal conjugate (*solid colored line*), obstetric conjugate (*broken colored line*) and true conjugate (*black line*)

Midplane
  Transverse diameter
    (interspinous diameter)
  The midplane of the pelvis normally
    is its largest plane and the one of
    greatest diameter.
	10.5 cm	Measurement of interspinous diameter.*

Outlet
  Transverse diameter (intertuberous
    diameter)
  The outlet presents the smallest plane
    of the pelvic canal.
	≥8 cm	Use of Thom's pelvimeter to measure intertuberous diameter.*

*From Barkauskas V et al.: *Health and physical assessment,* St Louis, 1994, Mosby.

pelvis is of adequate size and suitable shape. In the third trimester of pregnancy, the examination of the bony pelvis may be more thorough and the results more accurate because there is relaxation and increased mobility of the pelvic joints and ligaments caused by hormonal influences. Widening of the joint of the symphysis pubis and the resulting instability may cause pain in any or all of the pelvic joints.

Because the examiner does not have direct access to the bony structures and because the bones are covered with varying amounts of soft tissue, estimates of size and shape are approximate. Precise bony pelvis measurements can be determined by use of computed tomography, ultrasound, or x-ray films. However, x-ray examination is rarely done during pregnancy because the x-rays may damage the developing fetus.

Soft tissues

The soft tissues of the passageway include the distensible lower uterine segment, cervix, pelvic floor muscles, vagina, and introitus (external opening to the vagina). Before labor begins, the uterus is composed of the uterine body (corpus) and cervix (neck). After labor has begun, uterine contractions cause the uterine body to have a thick and muscular upper segment and a thin-walled passive muscular lower segment. A physiologic retraction ring separates the two segments (Fig. 12-10). The lower uterine segment gradually distends to accommodate the intrauterine contents as the wall of the upper segment thickens and its accommodating capacity is reduced. The contractions of the uterine body thus exert downward pressure on the fetus, pushing it against the cervix.

The cervix effaces (thins) and dilates (opens) sufficiently to allow the first fetal portion to descend into the vagina. As the fetus descends, the cervix is actually drawn upward and over this first portion.

The pelvic floor is a muscular layer that separates the pelvic cavity above from the perineal space below. This structure helps the fetus rotate anteriorly as it passes through the birth canal. As noted earlier, the soft tissues of the vagina develop throughout pregnancy until at term the vagina can dilate to accommodate the fetus and permit passage of the fetus to the external world.

Powers

Involuntary and voluntary powers combine to expel the fetus and the placenta from the uterus. Involuntary uterine contractions, called the *primary powers,* signal the beginning of labor. Once the cervix has dilated, voluntary bearing-down efforts by the woman, called the *secondary powers,* augment the force of the involuntary contractions.

Primary powers

The involuntary contractions originate at certain pacemaker points in the thickened muscle layers of the upper uterine segment. From the pacemaker points, contractions move downward over the uterus in waves, separated by short rest periods. Terms used to describe these involuntary contractions include frequency (the time from the beginning of one contraction to the beginning of the next); duration (length of contraction); and intensity (strength of contraction).

The primary powers are responsible for the effacement and dilatation of the cervix and descent of the fetus. **Effacement** of the cervix means the shortening and thinning of the cervix during the first stage of labor. The cervix, normally 2 to 3 cm in length and about 1 cm thick, is

---

TABLE 12-2 *Comparison of Pelvic Types*

	GYNECOID (50% OF WOMEN)	ANDROID (23% OF WOMEN)	ANTHROPOID (24% OF WOMEN)	PLATYPELLOID (3% OF WOMEN)
Brim	Slightly ovoid or transversely rounded	Heart shaped, angulated	Oval, wider anteroposteriorly	Flattened anteroposteriorly, wide transversely
	◯ Round	♡ Heart	⬭ Oval	⬭ Flat
Depth	Moderate	Deep	Deep	Shallow
Side walls	Straight	Convergent	Straight	Straight
Ischial spines	Blunt, somewhat widely separated	Prominent, narrow interspinous diameter	Prominent, often with narrow interspinous diameter	Blunted, widely separated
Sacrum	Deep, curved	Slightly curved, terminal portion often beaked	Slightly curved	Slightly curved
Subpubic arch	Wide	Narrow	Narrow	Wide
Usual mode of birth	Vaginal Spontaneous Occipitoanterior position	Cesarean Vaginal Difficult with forceps	Vaginal Forceps Spontaneous Occipitoposterior or occipitoanterior position	Vaginal Spontaneous

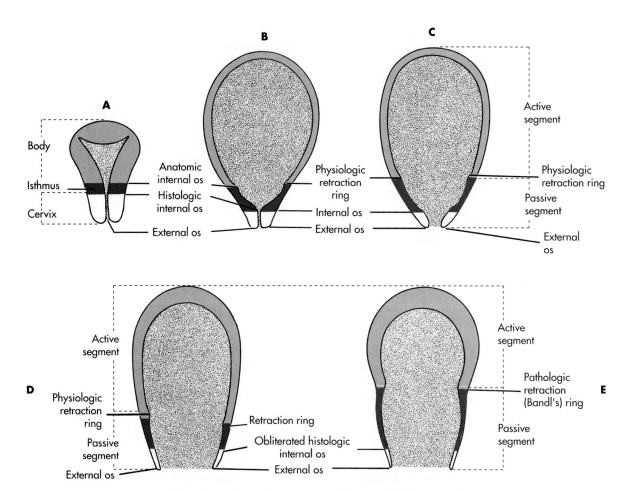

Fig. **12-10** Progressive development of segments and rings of uterus at term. Note differences in **A,** nonpregnant uterus, **B,** uterus at term and uterus in normal labor in early first stage, **C,** and in second stage. **D,** Passive segment is derived from lower uterine segment (isthmus) and cervix, and physiologic retraction ring is derived from anatomic internal os. **E,** Uterus in abnormal labor in second-stage dystocia. Pathologic retraction (Bandl's) ring that forms under abnormal conditions develops from physiologic ring. (Modified from Willson J & Carrington E: *Obstetrics and gynecology,* ed 9, St Louis 1991, Mosby.)

obliterated or "taken up" by a shortening of the uterine muscle bundles during the thinning of the lower uterine segment that occurs in advancing labor. Only a thin edge of the cervix can be palpated when effacement is complete. Effacement generally is advanced in first-time term pregnancy before more than slight dilatation occurs. In subsequent pregnancies, effacement and dilatation of the cervix tend to progress together. Degree of effacement is expressed in percentages from 0% to 100% (e.g., a cervix is 50% effaced) (Fig. 12-11, *A-C*).

Dilatation of the cervix is the enlargement or widening of the cervical opening and the cervical canal that occurs once labor has begun. The diameter of the cervix increases from less than 1 cm to full dilatation (approximately 10 cm) to allow birth of a term fetus. When the cervix is fully dilated (and completely retracted), it can no longer be palpated (Fig. 12-11, *D*). Full cervical dilatation marks the end of the first stage of labor.

Dilatation of the cervix occurs by the drawing upward of the musculofibrous components of the cervix that is caused by strong uterine contractions. Pressure exerted by the amniotic fluid while the membranes are intact or the force applied by the presenting part also can promote cervical dilatation. Scarring of the cervix as a result of prior infection or surgery may slow cervical dilatation.

In the first and second stages of labor increased intrauterine pressure caused by contractions exerts pressure on the descending fetus and the cervix. This results in the mechanical stretching of the cervix, the **Ferguson reflex,** which stimulates uterine contractions and ultimately, expulsion of the fetus.

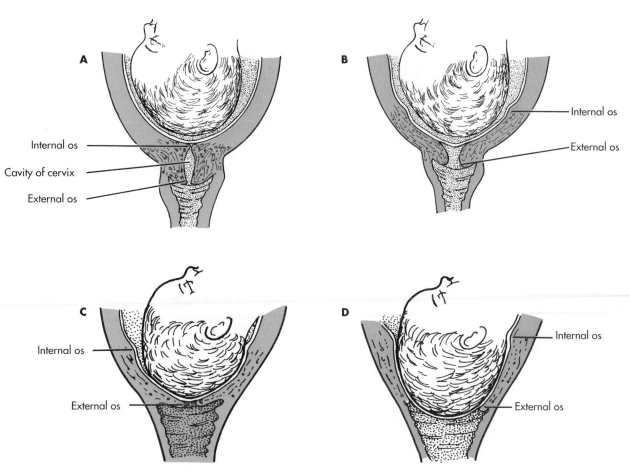

Fig. **12-11** Cervical effacement and dilatation. Note how cervix is drawn up around presenting part (internal os). Membranes are intact, and head is not well applied to cervix. **A,** Before labor. **B,** Early effacement. **C,** Complete effacement (100%). Head is well applied to cervix. **D,** Complete dilatation (10 cm). There is some overlapping of cranial bones, and membranes are still intact.

Uterine contractions are usually independent from external forces. For example, laboring women who are paraplegic will have normal but painless uterine contractions (Cunningham et al., 1997). However, uterine contractions may decrease in frequency and intensity if narcotic analgesic medication or epidural analgesia is given early in labor.

Secondary powers

As soon as the presenting part reaches the pelvic floor the contractions change in character and become expulsive. The laboring woman who has not received nerve block anesthesia experiences an involuntary urge to push. She uses secondary powers (bearing-down efforts) to aid in expulsion of the fetus as she contracts her diaphragm and abdominal muscles and pushes. These bearing down efforts result in increased intraabdominal pressure that compresses the uterus on all sides and adds to the power of the expulsive forces.

The secondary powers have no effect on cervical dilatation, but they are of considerable importance in the expulsion of the infant from the uterus and vagina after the cervix is fully dilated. Studies have shown that pushing in the second stage is more effective and the woman is less fatigued when she begins to push only after she has the urge to do so rather than beginning to push without an urge to do so when she is fully dilated (Roberts & Woolley, 1996).

The way a woman pushes in second stage is a much debated topic. Studies have been done that investigated the effects of spontaneous bearing-down efforts, directed pushing, Valsalva (closed glottis and prolonged bearing-down) pushing, open glottis pushing, 'mini' pushing, and forced methods of pushing (Paine & Tinker, 1992; Thomson, 1995; Woolley & Roberts, 1995). Although no significant differences have been found in the duration of second-stage labor, adverse consequences have been reported with certain pushing techniques. Fetal hypoxia and subsequent acidosis have

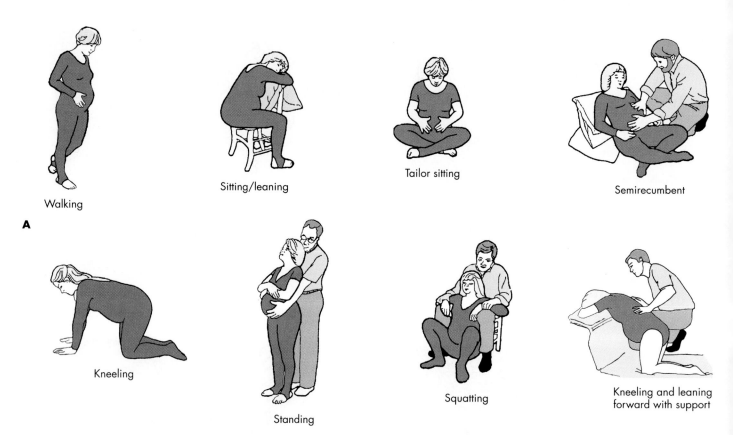

A

Walking

Sitting/leaning

Tailor sitting

Semirecumbent

Kneeling

Standing

Squatting

Kneeling and leaning forward with support

Fig. 12-12 Positions for labor and birth. **A,** Positions for labor.

Continued

been associated with prolonged breath holding and forceful pushing efforts. Perineal tears have been associated with directed pushing. Continued study is needed to determine the effectiveness and appropriateness of teaching strategies used by nurses to teach pushing techniques, the suitability and effectiveness of various pushing techniques related to nonreassuring fetal heart problems, and the standards for length of pushing in terms of maternal and fetal outcomes (Petersen & Besuner, 1997).

Position of the Laboring Woman

Position affects the woman's anatomic and physiologic adaptations to labor. Frequent changes in position relieve fatigue, increase comfort, and improve circulation (Melzack, Belanger & Lacroix, 1991). Therefore, a laboring woman should be encouraged to find positions that are most comfortable to her (see Fig. 12-12).

An upright position (walking, sitting, kneeling, or squatting) offers a number of advantages (Fig. 12-12, *A*). Gravity can promote the descent of the fetus. Uterine contractions are generally stronger and more efficient in effacing and dilating the cervix, resulting in shorter labor (Golay, Vedam & Sorger, 1993; Shermer & Raines, 1997).

An upright position is also beneficial to the mother's cardiac output, which normally increases during labor as uterine contractions return blood to the vascular bed. The increased cardiac output improves blood flow to the uteroplacental unit and the maternal kidneys. Cardiac output is compromised if the descending aorta and ascending vena cava are compressed during labor. Compression of these major vessels may result in supine hypotension and fetal heart rate deceleration. With the woman in an upright position pressure on the maternal vessels is reduced and compression is prevented. If the woman wishes to lie down, a lateral position is suggested (Cunningham et al., 1997).

The "all fours" position (hands and knees) may be used to relieve backache if the fetus is in an occipitoposterior position and may assist in anterior rotation of the fetus (Bennett & Brown, 1993; Simkin, 1995).

Positioning for second-stage labor (Fig. 12-12, *B*) may be determined by the woman's preference, but is constrained by the condition of the woman or fetus, the environment, and the health care provider's confidence in assisting in a birth in a specific position (Bennett & Brown, 1993). A women who pushes in a semirecumbent position needs adequate body support to push effectively because her weight will be on her sacrum, moving the coccyx forward and causing a reduction in the pelvic outlet.

In a sitting or squatting position, abdominal muscles work in greater synchrony with uterine contractions during

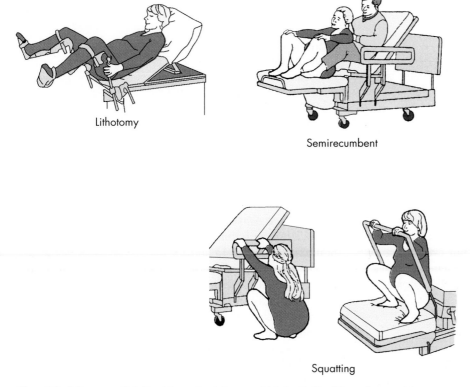

Lithotomy

Semirecumbent

Lateral recumbent

B

Squatting

Fig. **12-12, cont'd** Positions for labor and birth. **B,** Positions for pushing.

bearing-down efforts. Kneeling or squatting moves the uterus forward and straightens the long axis of the birth canal and can facilitate the second stage of labor by increasing the pelvic outlet (Bennett & Brown, 1993).

The lateral position can be used by the woman to help rotate a fetus in a posterior position. It can also be used when there is a need for less force to be used during bearing down such as when there is a need to control the speed of a precipitous birth (Roberts & Woolley, 1996).

There is no evidence that any of these positions suggested for second-stage labor increase the need for use of operative techniques (e.g., forceps- or vacuum-assisted birth, cesarean birth, episiotomy) or cause perineal trauma. There is also no evidence that use of any of these positions adversely affects the newborn (Bennett & Brown, 1993; Biancuzzo, 1993; Golay, Vedam & Sorger, 1993).

PROCESS OF LABOR

Labor is the process of moving the fetus, placenta, and membranes out of the uterus and through the birth canal. Various changes take place in the woman's reproductive system in the days and weeks just before labor begins. Labor itself can be discussed in terms of the mechanisms involved in the process and the stages that the woman moves through.

Signs Preceding Labor

In first-time pregnancies the uterus sinks downward and forward about 2 weeks before term, when the fetus's presenting part (usually the fetal head) descends into the true pelvis. This settling is called **lightening** or "dropping" and usually happens gradually (Fig. 12-13). After lightening, women feel less congested and breathe more easily. However, there is usually more bladder pressure as a result of this shift and consequently a return of urinary frequency. In a multiparous pregnancy, lightening may not take place until after uterine contractions are established and true labor is in progress.

The woman may complain of persistent low backache and sacroiliac distress as a result of relaxation of the pelvic joints. She may identify strong, frequent, but irregular uterine (Braxton Hicks) contractions.

The vaginal mucus becomes more profuse in response to the extreme congestion of the vaginal mucous membranes. Brownish or blood-tinged cervical mucus may be passed (**bloody show**). The cervix becomes soft (ripens) and partially effaced and may begin to dilate. The membranes may rupture spontaneously.

Other phenomena are common in the days preceding labor: (1) loss of 0.5 to 1.5 kg in weight, caused by water loss resulting from electrolyte shifts that in turn are produced by changes in estrogen and progesterone levels, and (2) a surge

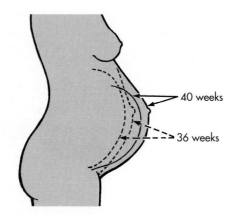

Fig. **12-13** Lightening.

of energy. Women speak of having a burst of energy that they often use to clean the house and put everything in order. Less commonly, some women experience diarrhea, nausea, vomiting, and indigestion (Varney, 1997). Box 12-1 lists signs that may precede labor.

Onset of Labor

The onset of true labor cannot be ascribed to a single cause. Many factors, including changes in the maternal uterus, cervix, and pituitary gland, are involved. Hormones produced by the normal fetal hypothalamus, pituitary, and adrenal cortex probably contribute to the onset of labor. Progressive uterine distention, increasing intrauterine pressure, and aging of the placenta seem to be associated with increasing myometrial irritability. This is a result of increased concentrations of estrogen and prostaglandins, as well as decreasing progesterone levels. The mutually coordinated effects of these factors result in the occurrence of strong, regular, rhythmic uterine contractions. Normally, the outcome of these factors working together is the birth of the fetus and the expulsion of the placenta. However, it is still not completely understood how certain alterations trigger others and how proper checks and balances are maintained.

Oncofetal fibronectin is a newly studied protein found in plasma and cervicovaginal secretions of pregnant women as labor approaches or when there are certain complications of pregnancy such as postterm pregnancy, preterm labor, and pregnancy-induced hypertension. Although the exact significance of oncofetal fibronectin levels is not clear, it may become a clinical marker for true labor and have predictive value for identifying certain complications of pregnancy (Dunn & Feinberg, 1996).

Stages of Labor

Labor is considered "normal" when the woman is at or near term, no complications exist, a single fetus presents by vertex, and labor is completed within 24 hours. The course of normal labor, which is remarkably constant, consists of (1) regular progression of uterine contractions, (2) effacement and progressive dilatation of the cervix, and (3) progress in descent of the presenting part. Four stages of labor are recognized. These stages are discussed in greater detail, along with nursing care for the laboring woman and family, in Chapters 15 and 17.

The first stage of labor is considered to last from the onset of regular uterine contractions to full dilatation of the cervix. Commonly the onset of labor is difficult to establish because the woman may be admitted to the labor unit just before birth and the beginning of labor may be only an estimate. The first stage is much longer than the second and third combined. Great variability is the rule, however, depending on the factors discussed previously in this chapter. Full dilatation may occur in less than 1 hour in some multiparous pregnancies. In first-time pregnancy, complete dilatation of the cervix can take up to 20 hours. There are no absolute values for the normal length of the first stage of labor (ACOG, 1995). Variations may reflect differences in the patient population or in clinical practice.

The first stage of labor has been divided into three phases: a latent phase, an active phase, and a transition phase. During the latent phase there is more progress in effacement of the cervix and little increase in descent. During the active phase and the transition phase there is more rapid dilatation of the cervix and an increased rate of descent of the presenting part.

The second stage of labor lasts from the time the cervix is fully dilated to the birth of the fetus. The second stage takes an average of 20 minutes for a multiparous woman and 50 minutes for a nulliparous woman. Labor of up to 2 hours has been considered within the normal range for the second stage, but there can be significant variations. For example, a woman who has received epidural analgesia may take up to 3 hours (Johnson & Rosenfeld, 1995). As long as there is progress, and the fetal status is reassuring, the length of the second stage is usually not related to adverse perinatal outcomes (ACOG, 1995).

Three phases of the second stage have been identified and described by Simkin and associates (1991). These phases are latent—a period when the woman is not feeling the urge

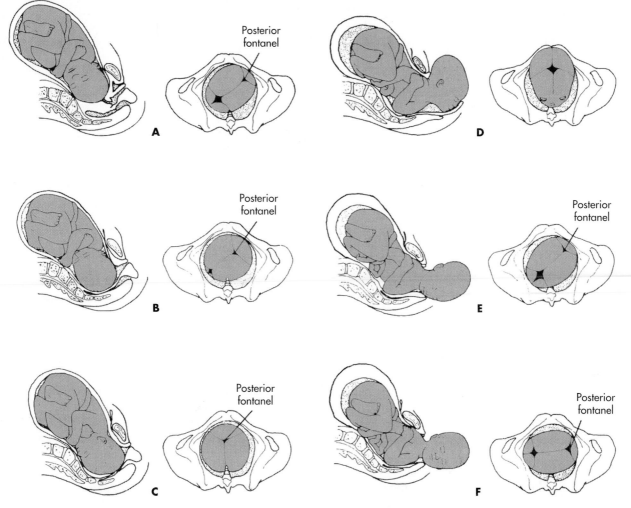

Fig. **12-14** Cardinal movements of the mechanism of labor. Left occipitoanterior (LOA) presentation. **A,** Engagement and descent. **B,** Flexion. **C,** Internal rotation to occipitoanterior position (OA). **D,** Extension. **E,** External rotation beginning (restitution). **F,** External rotation.

to push, is resting, or is only exerting small bearing-down efforts with contractions; active—a period when the woman is making strong bearing-down efforts and the fetal station is advancing; and transition—the time when the fetal head is crowning and the woman may be experiencing more pain and exerting either decreased or increased bearing-down efforts.

The third stage of labor lasts from the birth of the fetus until the placenta is delivered. The placenta normally separates with the third or fourth strong uterine contraction after the infant has been born. After it has separated, the placenta can be delivered with the next uterine contraction. The duration of the third stage may be as short as 3 to 5 minutes, although up to 1 hour is considered within normal limits (Bennett & Brown, 1993). The risk of hemorrhage increases as the length of the third stage increases (Cunningham et al., 1997).

The fourth stage of labor arbitrarily lasts about 2 hours after delivery of the placenta. It is the period of immediate recovery, when homeostasis is reestablished. It serves as an important period of observation for complications, such as abnormal bleeding.

Mechanism of Labor

As already discussed, the female pelvis has varied contours and diameters at different levels, and the presenting part of the passenger is large in proportion to the passage. Therefore, for vaginal birth to occur, the fetus must adapt to the birth canal during the descent. The turns and other adjustments necessary in the human birth process are termed the **mechanism of labor** (Fig. 12-14). The seven cardinal movements of the mechanism of labor that occur in a vertex presentation are engagement, descent, flexion, internal rotation, extension, external rotation (restitution), and finally

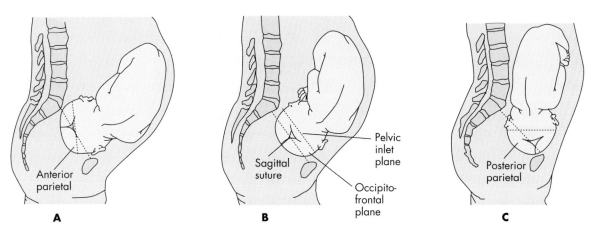

Fig. **12-15** Synclitism and asynclitism. **A,** Anterior asynclitism. **B,** Normal synclitism. **C,** Posterior asynclitism.

birth by expulsion. Although these movements are discussed separately, in actuality a combination of movements occurs simultaneously. For example, engagement involves both descent and flexion.

Engagement

When the biparietal diameter of the head passes the pelvic inlet, the head is said to be engaged in the pelvic inlet (Fig. 12-14, *A*). In most nulliparous pregnancies this occurs before the onset of active labor because the firmer abdominal muscles direct the presenting part into the pelvis. In multiparous pregnancies, in which the abdominal musculature is more relaxed, the head often remains freely movable above the pelvic brim until labor is established.

Asynclitism. The head usually engages in the pelvis in a synclitic position, one that is parallel to the anteroposterior plane of the pelvis. Frequently **asynclitism** occurs (the head is deflected) anteriorly or posteriorly in the pelvis, which can facilitate descent because the head is being positioned to accommodate to the pelvic cavity (Fig. 12-15). However extreme asynclitism can cause cephalopelvic disproportion, even in a normal size pelvis, because the head is positioned so that it cannot descend.

Descent

Descent refers to the progress of the presenting part through the pelvis. Descent depends on at least four forces: (1) pressure exerted by the amniotic fluid, (2) direct pressure exerted by the contracting fundus on the fetus, (3) force of the contraction of the maternal diaphragm and abdominal muscles in the second stage of labor, and (4) extension and straightening of the fetal body. The effects of these forces are modified by the size and shape of the maternal pelvic planes and the size of the fetal head and its capacity to mold.

The degree of descent is measured by the station of the presenting part (see Fig. 12-9). As already mentioned, little descent occurs during the latent phase of the first stage of labor. Descent accelerates in the active phase when the cervix has dilated to 5 to 7 cm. It is especially apparent when the membranes have ruptured.

In a first-time pregnancy descent is usually slow but steady; in subsequent pregnancies descent may be rapid. Progress in descent of the presenting part is determined by abdominal palpation (Leopold's maneuvers) and vaginal examination until the presenting part can be seen at the introitus.

Flexion

As soon as the descending head meets resistance from the cervix, pelvic wall, or pelvic floor, it normally flexes, so that the chin is brought into closer contact with the fetal chest (Fig. 12-14, *B*). Flexion permits the smaller suboccipitobregmatic diameter (9.5 cm) rather than the larger diameters to present to the outlet.

Internal rotation

The maternal pelvic inlet is widest in the transverse diameter. Therefore the fetal head passes the inlet into the true pelvis in the occipitotransverse position. The pelvic outlet is widest in the anteroposterior diameter, however. Therefore, for the fetus to exit, the head must rotate. Internal rotation begins at the level of the ischial spines but is not completed until the presenting part reaches the lower pelvis. As the occiput rotates anteriorly, the face rotates posteriorly. With each contraction the fetal head is guided by the bony pelvis and the muscles of the pelvic floor. Eventually the occiput will be in the midline beneath the pubic arch. The head is almost always rotated by the time it reaches the pelvic floor (Fig. 12-14, *C*). Both the levator ani muscles and the bony pelvis are important for achieving anterior rotation. A previous childbirth injury or regional anesthesia may compromise the function of the levator sling.

Extension

When the fetal head reaches the perineum, it is deflected anteriorly for birth. The occiput passes under the lower border of the symphysis pubis first, then the head emerges by extension: first the occiput, then the face, and finally the chin (Fig. 12-14, *D*).

Restitution and external rotation

After the head is born, it rotates briefly to the position it occupied when it was engaged in the inlet. This movement is referred to as *restitution* (Fig. 12-14, *E*). The 45-degree turn realigns the infant's head with her or his back and shoulders. The head can then be seen to rotate further. This external rotation occurs as the shoulders engage and descend in maneuvers similar to those of the head (Fig. 12-14, *F*). As noted earlier, the anterior shoulder descends first. When it reaches the outlet, it rotates to the midline and is delivered from under the pubic arch. The posterior shoulder is guided over the perineum until it is free of the vaginal introitus.

Expulsion

After birth of the shoulders, the head and shoulders are lifted up toward the mother's pubic bone and the trunk of the baby is born by flexing it laterally in the direction of the symphysis pubis. When the baby has completely emerged, birth is complete, and the second stage of labor ends.

PHYSIOLOGIC ADAPTATION TO LABOR

In addition to the maternal and fetal anatomic adaptations that occur during birth, physiologic adaptations must also occur. Accurate assessment of the mother and fetus requires a knowledge of expected adaptations.

Fetal Adaptation

Several important physiologic adaptations occur in the fetus. These changes occur in fetal heart rate, fetal circulation, respiratory movements, and other behaviors.

Fetal heart rate

Fetal heart rate (FHR) monitoring provides reliable and predictive information about the condition of the fetus related to oxygenation. Stresses to the uterofetoplacental unit result in characteristic FHR patterns. It is important that the nurse have a basic understanding of the factors involved in fetal oxygenation and of the fetal responses that reflect adequate fetal oxygenation. (See Chapter 14 for further discussion.)

The average FHR at term is 140 beats per minute (beats/min). The normal range is 110 to 160 beats/min. Earlier in gestation the FHR is higher, with an average of approximately 160 beats/min at 20 weeks' gestation. The rate decreases progressively as the maturing fetus reaches term. However, temporary accelerations and slight early decelerations of the FHR can be expected in response to spontaneous fetal movement, vaginal examination, fundal pressure, uterine contractions, abdominal palpation, and fetal head compression. Other fetal heart deceleration patterns are not expected and need interventions.

Fetal circulation

Fetal circulation can be affected by many factors. These include maternal position, uterine contractions, blood pressure, and umbilical cord blood flow. Uterine contractions during labor tend to decrease circulation through the spiral arterioles and subsequent perfusion through the intervillous space. Most healthy fetuses are well able to compensate for this stress and the exposure to increased pressure while moving passively through the birth canal during labor. Usually umbilical cord blood flow is undisturbed by uterine contractions or fetal position (Lowe & Reiss, 1996).

Fetal respiration

Certain changes stimulate chemoreceptors in the aorta and carotid bodies to prepare the fetus for initiating respirations immediately after birth (Lowe & Reiss, 1996). These changes include the following:
- Fetal respiratory movements decrease during labor
- Fetal oxygen pressure falls (Po_2)
- Arterial carbon dioxide pressure (Pco_2)
- Arterial pH falls
- Bicarbonate level falls
- Fetal lung fluid clears during labor and vaginal birth

Maternal Adaptation

A thorough understanding of maternal adaptations to pregnancy assists the nurse to anticipate and meet the woman's needs during labor. Further changes occur as the woman progresses through the stages of labor. Various body systems adapt to the process of labor, causing both objective signs and subjective symptoms.

Cardiovascular changes

The nurse can expect some changes in the woman's cardiovascular system during labor. During each contraction, 400 ml of blood is emptied from the uterus into the maternal vascular system. This increases cardiac output by about 10% to 15% in the first stage and by about 30% to 50% in the second stage.

Changes in the woman's blood pressure also occur. Blood flow, which is reduced in the uterine artery by contractions, is redirected to peripheral vessels. As a result, peripheral resistance increases, blood pressure rises, and the pulse rate increases. During the first stage of labor, uterine contractions cause systolic readings to rise by about 10 mm Hg. Therefore assessing blood pressure between contractions provides more accurate readings (Varney, 1997). During the second stage, contractions may cause systolic pressures to increase by 30 mm Hg and diastolic readings to increase by 25 mm Hg, with both systolic and diastolic pressures remaining somewhat elevated even between contractions. Therefore the woman already at risk for hypertension is at increased risk for complications such as cerebral hemorrhage.

Supine hypotension occurs when the ascending vena cava and descending aorta are compressed. The laboring woman is at greater risk for supine hypotension if the uterus is particularly large because of multifetal pregnancy, hydramnios, obesity, or if she is dehydrated or hypovolemic. In addition, anxiety and pain, as well as some medications, can cause hypotension.

The woman should be discouraged from using the **Valsalva maneuver** (holding one's breath and tightening abdominal muscles) for pushing during the second stage. This activity increases intrathoracic pressure, reduces venous return, and increases venous pressure. The cardiac output and blood pressure increase, and the pulse slows temporarily. During the Valsalva maneuver, fetal hypoxia may occur. The process is reversed when the woman takes a breath.

The white blood cell (WBC) count can increase to 25,000/mm^3, although it usually averages an increase to 14,000 to 16,000/mm^3 (Cunningham et al., 1997). Although the mechanism leading to this increase in WBCs is unknown, it may be secondary to physical or emotional stress or to tissue trauma. Labor is strenuous, and physical exercise alone can increase the WBC count.

Some peripheral vascular changes occur, perhaps in response to cervical dilatation or to compression of maternal vessels by the fetus passing through the birth canal. Flushed cheeks, hot or cold feet, and eversion of hemorrhoids may result (Box 12-2).

Respiratory changes

Respiratory system adaptations also are seen. Increased physical activity with greater oxygen consumption is reflected in an increase in the respiratory rate. Hyperventilation may cause respiratory alkalosis (an increase in pH), hypoxia, and hypocapnia (decrease in carbon dioxide). In the unmedicated woman in the second stage, oxygen consumption almost doubles. Anxiety also increases oxygen consumption.

Renal changes

Several renal system changes occur. In the second trimester, the urinary bladder becomes an abdominal organ. When filling, it is palpable above the symphysis pubis.

BOX 12-2	*Maternal Physiologic Changes during Labor*

Cardiac output increases 10% to 15% in first stage; 30% to 50% in second stage
Heart rate slightly increases in first and second stage
Systolic blood pressure increases during uterine contractions in first stage; systolic and diastolic pressures increase during uterine contractions in second stage
White blood cell count increases
Respiratory rate increases
Temperature may be slightly elevated
Proteinuria 1+ may occur
Gastric motility and absorption of solid food is decreased; nausea, vomiting may occur during transition to second stage labor
Blood glucose level decreases

During labor, spontaneous voiding may be difficult for various reasons: tissue edema caused by pressure from the presenting part, discomfort, sedation, and embarrassment. Proteinuria of 1 plus (+) is a normal finding because it can occur in response to the breakdown of muscle tissue from the physical work of labor.

Integumentary changes

The integumentary system changes are evident, especially in the great distensibility (stretching) in the area of the vaginal introitus. The degree of distensibility varies with the individual. Despite this ability to stretch, minute tears in the skin around the vaginal introitus do occur.

Musculoskeletal changes

The musculoskeletal system is stressed during labor. Diaphoresis, fatigue, proteinuria (1+), and perhaps an increased temperature accompany the marked increase in muscle activity. Backache and joint ache (unrelated to fetal position) occur as a result of increased joint laxity at term. The labor process itself and the woman's pointing her toes can cause leg cramps.

Neurologic changes

The neurologic system reflects the stress and discomfort of labor. Sensorial changes occur as the woman moves through phases of the first stage of labor and as she moves from one stage to the next. Initially she may be euphoric. Euphoria gives way to increased seriousness, then to amnesia between contractions during the second stage, and finally to elation or fatigue after giving birth. Endogenous endorphins (a morphinelike chemical produced naturally by the body) raise the pain threshold and produce sedation. In addition, physiologic anesthesia of perineal tissues, caused by pressure of the presenting part, decreases perception of pain.

Gastrointestinal changes

Labor affects the woman's gastrointestinal system. Dry lips and mouth may result from mouth breathing, dehydration, and emotional response to labor. During labor, gastrointestinal motility and absorption of solid foods are decreased, and stomach emptying time is slowed. Nausea and vomiting of undigested food eaten after onset of labor are common. Nausea and belching also occur as a reflex response to full cervical dilatation. The woman may state that diarrhea accompanied the onset of labor, or the nurse may palpate the presence of hard or impacted stool in the rectum.

Endocrine changes

The endocrine system is active during labor. The onset of labor may be triggered by decreasing levels of progesterone and increasing levels of estrogen, prostaglandins, and oxytocin. Metabolism increases, and blood glucose levels may decrease with the work of labor.

RESEARCH

Variability in Breathing Patterns during Latent Labor

Instruction in the use of breathing strategies during childbirth is part of all childbirth education programs. During early latent labor (<4 cm dilatation), women are encouraged to follow a slow and deep pattern of breathing and to accentuate this pattern with the onset of contractions. Research has supported the efficacy of slow-paced respiration in reducing pain and/or distress during contractions. No studies, however, have examined how women breathe during latent labor and whether different patterns of breathing are associated with different outcomes.

The breathing patterns of a small sample of women during latent labor were examined. Breathing and psychologic data were collected from 21 primiparous women recruited through prenatal classes and physician offices. Women were questioned about their thoughts during and between contractions, and their responses were tape recorded. Breathing measures were obtained after the verbal interview by a respiratory inductive plethysmograph system to obtain continuous, noninvasive measures of breathing patterns during latent labor. Considerable variation among women in individual respiratory rate and tidal volume both between and during contractions was reported. The most significant finding was the extreme variability observed in women's breathing.

CLINICAL APPLICATION OF THE STUDY

When nurses are caring for a woman in labor, it is not always easy to implement breathing techniques learned in childbirth classes. Nurses may find it best to determine the breathing pattern of the patient and tailor instructions to fit the style of breathing that each woman finds comfortable.

Source: Hesson K, Hill T & Bakal D: Variability in breathing patterns during latent labor, *J Nurse Midwifery* 42(1):99, 1997.

KEY POINTS

- Labor and birth are affected by the 5 P's—the passenger, passageway, powers, position of the woman, and psychologic responses.
- Because of its size and relative rigidity, the fetal head is a major factor in determining the course of birth.
- The diameters at the plane of the pelvic inlet, midpelvis, and outlet, plus the axis of the birth canal, determine whether vaginal birth is possible and the manner in which the fetus passes down the birth canal.
- Involuntary uterine contractions act to expel the fetus and placenta during the first stage of labor; these are augmented by voluntary bearing-down efforts during the second stage.
- The first stage of labor is from the time dilatation begins to the time when the cervix is fully dilated. The second stage of labor lasts from the time of full dilatation to the birth of the infant. The third stage of labor lasts from the infant's birth to the expulsion of the placenta. The fourth stage is the first 2 hours after birth.
- The cardinal movements of the mechanism of labor are engagement, descent, flexion, internal rotation, extension, restitution and external rotation, and expulsion of the infant.
- Although the events precipitating the onset of labor are unknown, many factors, including changes in the maternal uterus, cervix, and pituitary gland, are thought to be involved.
- An understanding of maternal adaptations to pregnancy is fundamental to ensuring that the pregnant woman's needs are anticipated and met.
- A healthy fetus with an adequate uterofetoplacental circulation will be able to compensate for the stress of uterine contractions.

CRITICAL THINKING EXERCISES

1 *You have been asked by the staff at the local Red Cross office to prepare a childbirth class for a group of first-time pregnant women on the process of labor.*

   a *Identify essential content to be covered and describe how you would collect data about the group's knowledge and educational levels.*

   b *Plan a 30-minute class, including appropriate audiovisuals. Discuss the plan with your faculty.*

CRITICAL THINKING EXERCISES—cont'd

    c *Give the class and ask the group to evaluate it. Discuss this feedback with your faculty and identify modifications for future sessions.*

2 *Visit a prenatal clinic where most of the patients are non-English speaking.*

    a *Investigate (through an interpreter or other means) the knowledge level of women who are at least 36 weeks pregnant regarding signs of labor.*

    b *Formulate a teaching plan that will provide the women with correct information and implement it.*

    c *Evaluate whether or not your teaching was effective.*

References

American College of Obstetricians and Gynecologists: Dystocia, and the augmentation of labor, *Technical Bulletin No. 218,* Washington, DC, 1995, ACOG.

Barkauskas V et al.: *Health and physical assessment,* St Louis, 1994, Mosby.

Bennett V & Brown L: *Myles textbook for midwives,* 12 ed, Edinburgh, 1993, Churchill-Livingstone.

Biancuzzo M: Six myths of maternal posture during labor, *MCN Am J Matern Child Nurs* 18(5):264, 1993.

Cunningham F et al.: *Williams obstetrics,* ed 20, Stamford, Conn, 1997, Appleton & Lange.

Dunn P & Feinberg R: Oncofetal fibronectin: new insight into the physiology of implantation and labor, *J Obstet Gynecol Neonatal Nurs* 25(9):753, 1996.

Golay J, Vedam S & Sorger L: The squatting position for the second stage of labor: effects on labor and on maternal and fetal well-being, *Birth* 20(2):73, 1993.

Johnson S & Rosenfeld J: The effect of epidural anesthesia on the length of labor, *J Fam Pract* 40(4):244, 1995.

Lowe N & Reiss R: Parturition and fetal adaptation, *J Obstet Gynecol Neonatal Nurs* 25(1):339, 1996.

Melzack R, Belanger E & Lacroix R: Labor pain: effect of maternal position on front and back pain, *J Pain Symptom Manage* 6(8):476, 1991.

Paine L & Tinker D: The effect of maternal bearing-down efforts on the actual umbilical cord pH and length of second stage labor, *J Nurse Midwifery* 37(1):61, 1992.

Petersen L & Besuner P: Pushing techniques during labor: issues and controversies, *J Obstet Gynecol Neonatal Nurs* 26(6): 719, 1997.

Roberts J & Woolley D: A second look at the second stage of labor, *J Obstet Gynecol Neonatal Nurs* 25(5):415, 1996.

Shermer R & Raines D: Positioning during the second stage of labor: moving back to the basics, *J Obstet Gynecol Neonatal Nurs* 26(6):727, 1997.

Simkin P: Reducing pain and enhancing progress in labor: a guide to nonpharmacologic methods for maternity care givers, *Birth* 22(3):161, 1995.

Simkin P, Whalley J & Keppler A: *Pregnancy , childbirth and the newborn,* ed 2, Seattle, 1991, Childbirth Education Association of Seattle and Meadowbrook Press Inc.

Thomson A: Maternal behaviors during spontaneous and directed pushing in the second stage of labour, *J Adv Nurs* 22(6):1027, 1995.

Varney H: *Varney's midwifery,* ed 3, Sudbury, Mass, 1997, Jones and Bartlett.

Woolley D & Roberts J: Second stage pushing: a comparison of Valsalva-style pushing with 'mini' pushing, *J Perinat Educ* 4(4):37, 1995.

CHAPTER

13

Management of Discomfort

JEAN A. BACHMAN

LEARNING OBJECTIVES

- Define the key terms.
- Compare the various childbirth preparation methods.
- Describe the breathing and relaxation techniques used for each stage of labor.
- Identify nonpharmacologic strategies to enhance relaxation and decrease discomfort during labor.
- Discuss the types of analgesia and anesthesia used during labor.
- Compare the types of pharmacologic control used to relieve discomfort in the different stages of labor and for different methods of birth.
- Discuss the use of naloxone (Narcan) and naltrexone (Trexan).
- Relate each step of the nursing process to the pharmacologic management of labor discomfort.
- Describe the nursing responsibilities appropriate for a woman receiving analgesia or anesthesia during labor and birth.

KEY TERMS

agonist-antagonist compounds
allergic reaction
analgesia
anesthesia
ataractics
Bradley method
counterpressure
Dick-Read method
effleurage
endorphins
epidural block
epidural blood patch
gate-control theory
hyperventilation
Lamaze (psychoprophylaxis) method
local infiltration anesthesia
narcotic analgesic
narcotic antagonist
neonatal narcosis
paracervical block
pudendal block
referred pain
somatic pain
spinal block
systemic analgesia
visceral pain

Pregnant women commonly worry about the pain they will experience during labor and childbirth and how they will react to and deal with that pain. A wide variety of childbirth preparation methods can provide ways to help the woman cope with the discomfort of labor. However, the interventions selected depend on the situation and the preference of both the woman and her health care provider.

The discomforts experienced during labor are discussed in this chapter, as are the nonpharmacologic and pharmacologic interventions to relieve the discomforts that can be used during the different stages of labor. This information provides the basis for understanding the nurse's role in management of maternal discomfort during labor.

DISCOMFORT DURING LABOR

Neurologic Origins

The discomfort experienced during labor has two origins (Lowe, 1996). During the *first stage of labor* uterine contractions cause cervical dilatation and effacement and uterine ischemia (decreased blood flow and therefore local oxygen deficit) resulting from contraction of the arteries to the myometrium. Pain impulses during the first stage of labor are transmitted through the spinal nerve segment of T11-12 and accessory lower thoracic and upper lumbar sympathetic nerves. These nerves originate in the uterine body and cervix.

The discomfort from cervical changes and uterine ischemia is **visceral pain.** It is located over the lower portion of the abdomen and radiates to the lumbar area of the back and down the thighs. Usually the woman experiences discomfort only during contractions and is free from pain between contractions.

During the *second stage of labor,* the stage of expulsion of the baby, the woman experiences perineal or **somatic pain.** The perineal discomfort results from stretching of perineal tissues to allow passage of the fetus and traction on the peritoneum and uterocervical supports during contractions. Discomfort also can be produced by expulsion forces or from pressure by the presenting part on the bladder, bowel, or other sensitive pelvic structures. Pain impulses during the second stage of labor are carried through S1-4 and spinal nerve segments and the parasympathetic system from perineal tissues.

Pain experienced during the *third stage of labor,* as well as so-called afterpains, is uterine, similar to that experienced early in the first stage of labor. Areas of discomfort during labor are illustrated in Fig. 13-1.

Pain may be *local,* with cramping and a tearing or bursting sensation resulting from distention and laceration of the cervix, vagina, or perineal tissues. The discomfort is commonly perceived as an intense burning sensation that is felt as the tissue stretches. Pain also may be **referred pain,** in which the discomfort is felt in the back, flanks, and thighs.

Perception of Pain

Although the pain threshold is remarkably similar in all persons regardless of gender, social, ethnic, or cultural differences, these differences play a definite role in the individual's *perception of pain.* The effects of factors such as culture, counterstimuli, and distraction in coping with pain are not fully understood. The meaning of pain and the verbal and nonverbal expressions given to pain are apparently learned from interactions within the primary social group. Cultural influences may impose unrealistic expectations. For instance, Asian women believe it shameful to scream or show pain, and they avoid verbal expression (Weber, 1996).

Expression of Pain

Pain results in both psychic responses and reflex physical actions. The quality of physical pain has been described as prickling, burning, aching, throbbing, sharp, nauseating, or cramping. The pain in childbirth gives rise to symptoms that are identifiable. The activity of the sympathetic nervous system may increase in response to pain, resulting in changes in blood pressure, pulse, respiration, and skin color. Pallor and diaphoresis may be seen (Potter & Perry, 1995). Bouts of nausea and vomiting also are commonplace.

Certain *affective expressions* of suffering are often seen. Such changes include increasing anxiety with lessened perceptual field, writhing, crying, groaning, gesturing (hand clenching and wringing), and excessive muscular excitability

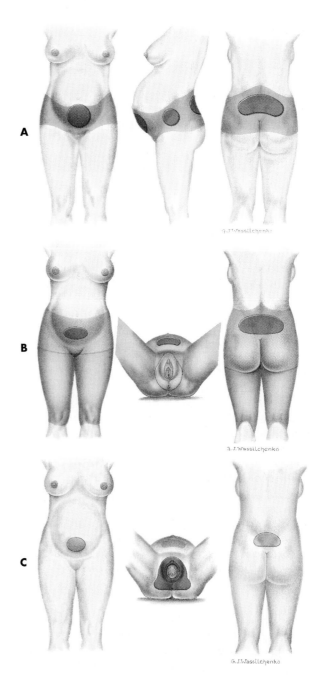

Fig. 13-1 Discomfort during labor. **A,** Distribution of labor pain during first stage. **B,** Distribution of labor pain during transition and early phase of second stage. **C,** Distribution of pain during late second stage and actual birth. (*Gray areas* indicate mild discomfort; *light-colored areas* indicate moderate discomfort; *dark-colored areas* indicate intense discomfort.)

throughout the body. Cultural expression of pain may vary. For example, Native American women may endure pain quietly, whereas Hispanic women may endure pain stoically, as it is expected and esteemed, but consider it acceptable to cry out (Villarruel, 1995).

FACTORS INFLUENCING PAIN RESPONSE

A woman's pain during childbirth is unique to each woman and is influenced by a variety of factors. These factors include culture, anxiety and fear, previous birth experience, childbirth preparation, and support.

America is increasingly becoming a multicultural society, which is reflected in the obstetric population. As nurses care for women and families from a variety of cultural backgrounds in labor and birth, they must have knowledge and understanding of how culture mediates pain (Weber, 1996). An understanding of the beliefs, values, and practices of various cultures helps the nurse provide appropriate culturally sensitive care (see the accompanying Cultural Considerations box). The nurse must take care not to have cultural blindness, an inability to see other courses of action, which may lead to cultural clashes, that result in less-than-optimal-care and less-than-satisfied women who are of a different culture than the nurse (Weber, 1996).

Anxiety and fear are commonly associated with increased pain during labor. Mild anxiety is considered normal for a woman during labor and birth. However, excessive anxiety and fear cause more catecholamine secretion, which increases the stimuli to the brain from the pelvis because of decreased blood flow and increased muscle tension, which in turn magnifies pain (Lowe, 1996). Thus, as fear and anxiety heighten, muscle tension increases, the effectiveness of the uterine contractions decreases, the experience of discomfort increases, and a cycle of increased fear and anxiety begins.

Previous birth experiences may also influence the woman's response to pain. For women who have had a difficult and painful previous birth experience, anxiety and fear from this past experience may lead to increased pain. Conversely, a woman who has experienced a labor and birth where pain coping skills were successful may have increased anxiety because those previous coping skills no longer work because of a more difficult labor and birth.

Women with a history of substance abuse experience as much pain during labor as other women. Although it is usually unnecessary to withhold pain medications, close monitoring for complications associated with each substance is part of the nursing assessment.

At times, particularly intense pain stimuli can be ignored. This is possible because certain nerve cell groupings within the spinal cord, brain stem, and cerebral cortex may have the ability to modulate the pain impulse through a blocking mechanism. This **gate-control theory** helps explain the way pain relief techniques taught in childbirth preparation classes and hypnosis work to relieve the pain in labor. According to this theory, pain sensations travel along sensory nerve pathways to the brain, but only a limited number of sensations or messages can travel through these nerve pathways at one time. By using distraction techniques such as massage

CULTURAL CONSIDERATIONS

Some Cultural Beliefs about Pain

The following are only examples of how women of different cultural backgrounds may react to pain. Because they are generalizations, the nurse needs to assess each woman experiencing pain related to childbirth.

Chinese women may not exhibit reactions to pain. They consider it impolite to accept something when it is first offered; therefore pain interventions may need to be offered more than once. Acupuncture may be used for pain relief.

Iranian women may be vocal in response to labor pain. Japanese women may be stoic in response to labor pain.

Haitian women may demonstrate a high tolerance for pain.

Southeast Asian women may endure severe pain before requesting relief.

Mexican women may be stoic until late in labor when they may then become vocal and request pain relief.

or stroking, music, and imagery, the capacity of the nerve pathways to transmit pain is reduced or completely blocked. These distracters are thought to work by closing down a hypothetic gate in the spinal cord, thus preventing pain signals from reaching the brain. The perception of pain is thereby diminished.

In addition, when the laboring woman engages in neuromuscular and motor activities, the resulting activity within the spinal cord itself further modifies the transmission of pain. Cognitive activities involving concentration on breathing and relaxation require selective and directed cortical activity, which activates and closes the gating mechanism as well. This gate-control theory therefore underscores the need for a supportive birth setting that allows the laboring woman to relax and use the various higher mental activities.

Finally, the critical issue for the nurse is how nursing support can make a difference in the pain experience of the woman during labor and birth. What the nurse must realize is that the pain occurring during childbirth and the management of this pain belongs to the woman experiencing the pain, and the nurse must engage in a cooperative effort to provide whatever external tools the woman requires to manage her pain experience (Lowe, 1996). These tools include both nonpharmacologic and pharmacologic interventions.

NONPHARAMACOLOGIC MANAGEMENT OF DISCOMFORT

It is important to alleviate pain, but commonly it is not the amount of pain the woman experiences, but *whether she meets her goals for herself in coping with the pain* that influences her perception of the birth experience as "good" or "bad." The observant nurse looks for cues to identify the woman's desired level of control in the management of pain and its relief.

The woman who chooses to deal with childbirth pain using nonpharmacologic or a combination of nonpharmacologic and pharmacologic methods needs care and support from nurses and other care providers who are skilled in pain management. Nonpharamcologic methods for relief of discomfort are taught in many different types of prenatal preparation classes. Regardless of whether a woman or couple has attended these classes or read various books and magazines on the subject, the nurse can teach the woman techniques to relieve discomfort while labor is in progress.

Childbirth Preparation Methods

Today most health care providers recommend or offer childbirth preparation classes to expectant parents. Major methods taught in the United States are the **Dick-Read method,** or natural childbirth; the Lamaze, or psychoprophylactic method (PPM); and the Bradley method, or husband-coached childbirth (see Chapter 10).

How childbirth education influences a woman's response to pain is not completely understood. Some data indicate that women who attend childbirth classes report less pain throughout labor and birth than do women who are unprepared, whereas other investigations have not supported this finding (Lowe, 1996). However, combined results of a number of studies suggest that not only is confidence greater after childbirth preparation but that this confidence is related to decreased pain perception and decreased analgesia during labor (Lowe, 1996).

Dick-Read method

To replace fear of the unknown with understanding and confidence, Dick-Read's (1987) program includes information on labor and birth, as well as nutrition, hygiene, and exercise. Classes include practice in three techniques: physical exercise to prepare the body for labor, conscious relaxation, and breathing patterns.

Conscious relaxation involves progressive relaxation of muscle groups in the entire body. With practice, many women are able to relax on command, both during and between contractions. Some women actually sleep between contractions.

Breathing patterns include deep abdominal respirations for most of labor, shallow breathing toward the end of the first stage, and, until recently, breath holding for pushing with contractions in the second stage of labor.

Teachers of the Dick-Read method also contend that the weight of the abdominal musculature on the contracting uterus increases pain. The woman is taught to force her abdominal muscles to rise as the uterus rises forward during a contraction, thus lifting the abdominal muscles off the contracting uterus.

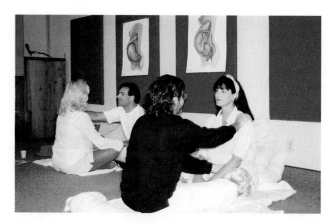

Fig. **13-2** Expectant parents learning relaxation techniques. (Courtesy Marjorie Pyle, RNC, Lifecircle, Costa Mesa, Calif.)

The Dick-Read method has been adapted to include labor support by the father or a support person chosen by the mother.

Lamaze method

The **Lamaze (psychoprophylaxis) method** grew out of Pavlov's work on classical conditioning. According to Lamaze, pain is a conditioned response. Therefore women can also be conditioned not to experience pain in labor; the Lamaze method does this by conditioning women to respond to mock uterine contractions with controlled muscular relaxation and breathing patterns instead of crying out and losing control (Lamaze, 1972). Coping strategies also include concentrating on a focal point, such as a favorite picture or pattern, to keep nerve pathways occupied so they cannot respond to painful stimuli.

The woman is taught to relax uninvolved muscle groups while she contracts a specific muscle group (Fig. 13-2). She applies this during labor by relaxing uninvolved muscles while her uterus contracts. The perception of maintaining control has also been found to be closely associated with ultimate satisfaction with the birth experience (Mackey, 1990).

Lamaze teachers believe that chest breathing lifts the diaphragm off the contracting uterus, thus giving it more room to expand. The chest breathing patterns are varied according to the intensity of the contractions and the progress of labor. Teachers also seek to eliminate fear by increasing the woman's understanding of body functions and the neurophysiology of pain. Support in labor is provided by the woman's partner or other support person or by a specially trained labor attendant termed a *monitrice.*

Bradley method

The **Bradley method,** also called husband-coached childbirth, was devised based on observations of animal behavior during birth and emphasizes working in harmony with the body, using breath control, abdominal breathing, and general body relaxation (Bradley, 1981). The husband or partner takes an active role in assisting the woman to relax and use correct breathing techniques. This method also stresses environmental factors such as darkness, solitude, and quiet to make childbirth a more natural experience.

Comparison of childbirth methods

Most proponents of prepared childbirth agree that the major causes of pain in labor are fear and tension. All childbirth methods attempt to reduce these two factors and eliminate pain by increasing the woman's knowledge of what to expect in labor and birth, enhancing her self-confidence and sense of control, preparing a support person, and educating her in physical conditioning and relaxation breathing.

There are a few fine differences in approach. For example, in the Bradley method, women are discouraged from using medication and encouraged to focus inwardly and to take direction from their own body. In the Lamaze method, the judicious use of pain medication is considered an appropriate adjunct to relaxation techniques, and external focusing and distraction are stressed. In reality, few instructors adhere strictly to one particular method but rather incorporate a variety of strategies aimed at increasing the woman's ability to cope with labor and minimize her need for medication.

Relaxing and Breathing Techniques

Focusing, imagery, and feedback relaxation

Some women bring a favorite object, such as a photograph, to the labor room to focus their attention on during contractions. Others choose some fixed object in the labor room for this purpose. In either event, as the contraction begins, they focus on this object to reduce their perception of pain. With imagery, the woman is encouraged to focus on a pleasant scene, or picture a place she feels relaxed or an activity she enjoys (Cassidy, 1993). These techniques coupled with feedback relaxation, help the woman work with her contractions rather than against them. The support person monitors this process, telling the woman when to begin the breathing techniques (Fig. 13-3). In a common feedback mechanism, the woman and her support person verbalize the word "relax" at the onset of each contraction and throughout it as needed. The nurse can assist the woman by providing a quiet environment and offering cues as needed.

Music. Music can also enhance relaxation during labor. Women should be encouraged to bring their musical preferences and tape or compact disc players to the hospital or birthing center. Using a headset or earphones may increase the music's effectiveness because the sounds around her will not be a distraction.

Breathing techniques

Different approaches to childbirth preparation stress varying techniques for using breathing as a tool to help the woman maintain control through contractions. In the first stage, such breathing techniques can promote relaxation of

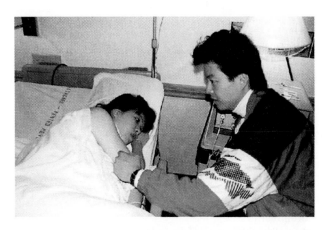

Fig. **13-3** Laboring woman using focusing and breathing techniques during contraction with coaching from her partner. (Courtesy Marjorie Pyle, RNC, Lifecircle, Costa Mesa, Calif.)

abdominal muscles and thereby enlarge the abdominal cavity. This lessens the friction and discomfort between the uterus and the abdominal wall during contractions. Because the muscles of the genital area also become more relaxed, they do not interfere with descent of the fetus. In the second stage, breathing is used to increase abdominal pressure and thereby assist in expelling the fetus. It can also be used to prevent precipitate expulsion of the fetal head.

For those couples who have prepared for labor by practicing such relaxing and breathing techniques, occasional reminders may be all that is necessary to help them along. For those who have had no preparation, instruction in simple breathing and relaxation can be given early in labor and often is surprisingly successful. Motivation is high, and the readiness to learn is enhanced by the reality of labor.

There are various breathing techniques during contractions. The nurse needs to ascertain what, if any, techniques the laboring couple knows before providing them with instruction. Simple patterns are easily learned. All patterns begin with the routine cleansing breath and end with a deep breath exhaled to "blow the contraction away." Generally, slow abdominal breathing, approximately half the woman's normal breathing rate, is initiated when the woman can no longer walk or talk through contractions (Box 13-1). As contractions increase in frequency and intensity, the woman may need to change to chest breathing, which is more shallow and approximately twice her normal rate of breathing.

The most difficult time to maintain control during contractions comes when the cervix dilates to 8 to 10 cm. This period is also called the transition period. Even for the woman who has prepared for labor, concentration on breathing techniques is difficult to maintain. The type used at this stage may be the 4:1 pattern: breath, breath, breath, breath, blow (as though blowing out a candle). This ratio may be increased to 6:1 or 8:1. However, an undesirable side effect of this type of breathing may be **hyperventilation.** The woman and her support person must be aware of the

---

BOX 13-1 *Breathing Techniques*

CLEANSING BREATH
Relaxed breath in through nose and out mouth. Used at the beginning and end of each contraction.

SLOW-PACED BREATHING (approximately 6-8 breaths per minute)
Not less than half normal breathing rate (No. breaths/min divided by 2)
IN-2-3-4/OUT-2-3-4/IN-2-3-4/OUT-2-3-4 . . .

MODIFIED-PACED BREATHING (approximately 32-40 breaths per minute)
Not more than twice normal breathing rate (No. breaths/min × 2)
IN-OUT/IN-OUT/IN-OUT/IN-OUT/ . . .
For more flexibility and variety, the woman may combine the slow and modified breathing by using the slow breathing for beginnings and ends of contractions and modified breathing for more intense peaks. This technique conserves energy and lessens fatigue.

PATTERNED-PACED BREATHING (same rate as modified)
Enhances concentration
a. 3:1 Patterned breathing
   IN-OUT/IN-OUT/IN-OUT/IN-BLOW (repeat through contraction)

b. 4:1 Patterned breathing
   IN-OUT/IN-OUT/IN-OUT/IN-OUT/IN-BLOW (repeat through contraction)
You may do any pattern desired, although ratios of 5:1 or higher tend to be very tiring. Some people like to do patterned breathing to a tune (Yankee Doodle, Old McDonald), to a repeated phrase (I think I can, I think I can), or in a pyramid pattern such as 1:1, 2:1, 3:1, 4:1, 5:1——5:1, 4:1, 3:1, 2:1, 1:1
c. *Coach call:* May be used when woman needs more distraction and concentration (e.g., during transition). The woman's coach signals the breathing ratio with his/her fingers or by verbal cues, changing the ratio after each "IN-BLOW."
Example:

IN-OUT/IN-OUT/IN-BLOW

IN-OUT/IN-OUT/IN-OUT/IN-OUT/IN-BLOW

IN-OUT/IN-BLOW

From Shapiro et al.: *The Lamaze ready reference guide for labor and birth,* ed 2, Washington, DC, 1997, Chapter ASPO/Lamaze.

---

accompanying symptoms of the resultant *respiratory alkalosis:* lightheadedness, dizziness, tingling of fingers, or circumoral numbness. Such alkalosis may be eliminated by having the woman breathe into a paper bag held tightly around the mouth and nose. This causes her to rebreathe carbon dioxide and thus replace the bicarbonate ion. She can breathe into her cupped hands if no bag is available.

Effleurage and counterpressure

Effleurage and counterpressure are two methods that have brought relief to many women during the first stage of labor. The gate-control theory may supply the reason for the effectiveness of these measures. **Effleurage** (see Fig. 10-18), which is a light stroking of the abdomen in rhythm with breathing during contractions, is used to distract the woman from contraction pain. Often the pressure of monitor belts makes it difficult to perform effleurage on the abdomen; thus a thigh or the chest may be used. **Counterpressure** is steady pressure in the sacral area with the fist or heel of the hand, which may help the woman cope with the sensations of internal pressure and pain in the lower back. Although not scientifically evaluated, pressure may also be applied bilaterally to the hips or knees to reduce low back pain (Simkin, 1995).

Water therapy

Although not universally accepted or implemented, bathing, showering, or jet hydrotherapy (whirlpool baths) using warm water are other nonpharmacologic measures that can be used to promote comfort and relaxation during labor (Fig. 13-4). Many birthing units have installed baths with air jets. With or without air jets, however, the buoyancy of the warm water provides support for tense muscles.

There are several immediate benefits of water therapy. The relief from discomfort and general body relaxation it produces reduce the woman's anxiety, which in turn decreases adrenaline production. This triggers an increase in levels of oxytocin (to stimulate labor) and endorphins (to reduce pain perception). In addition, with jet hydrotherapy, the bubbles and gentle lapping of the water stimulate the nipples, which triggers more oxytocin production. This has not been observed to cause hyperstimulation of the uterus. The cervix has often been observed to dilate 2 to 3 cm in 30 minutes of whirlpool therapy. In addition, it promotes diuresis and a decrease in blood pressure (Simkin, 1995). Whirlpool baths in labor have also been found to have positive effects on analgesia requirements, instrumentation rates, condition of the perineum, and personal satisfaction with labor (Rush et al., 1996).

If the woman is experiencing "back labor" secondary to an occiput posterior or transverse position, she is encouraged to assume the hands and knees or the side-lying position in the tub. Because this position decreases pain and increases relaxation and the production of oxytocin, the fetus may spontaneously rotate to the occiput anterior position.

In some settings, jet hydrotherapy may need to be approved by the woman's primary health care provider. The

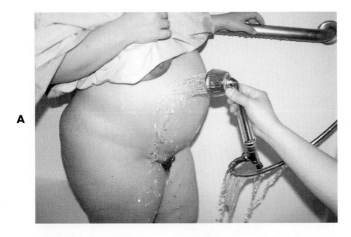

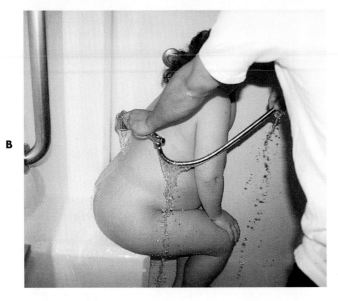

Fig. **13-4** Water therapy during labor. **A,** Use of shower during labor. **B,** Woman experiencing back labor relaxes while husband provides warm water on her back. (Courtesy Marjorie Pyle, RNC, Lifecircle, Costa Mesa, Calif.)

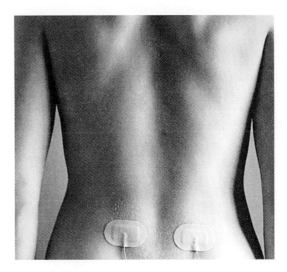

Fig. **13-5** Placement of TENS electrodes on back for relief of labor pain. (Courtesy 3M HealthCare, Minneapolis, Minn.)

woman's vital signs must be within normal limits and she should be in the active phase of the first stage of labor. If she is in the latent phase, her contractions may slow down. Fetal well-being must be established. Fetal heart rate (FHR) monitoring is done by Doppler device or fetoscope. Placement of internal electrodes is contraindicated for jet hydrotherapy. The woman's membranes may be intact or ruptured. If ruptured, the fluid must be clear or only lightly stained with meconium (Simkin, 1995).

There is no limit to the time women can stay in the bath, and often women are encouraged to stay in it as long as desired. However, studies have shown that most women use jet hydrotherapy for 30 to 60 minutes (Shorn, McAllister & Blanco, 1993).

During the bath, if the woman's temperature and FHR increase, the water is cooled down or the woman is asked to

step out of the bath to cool down. The bath water is kept between 36.7° and 37.8° C (Simkin, 1995). The mother's temperature may remain slightly elevated for a short time after the bath. Fluids and ice chips and a cool face cloth are offered during the bath.

The tub must be meticulously cleaned after use. Cleansing solutions vary with institution; however, household bleach (Clorox) is commonly used.

Transcutaneous electrical nerve stimulation

Transcutaneous electrical nerve stimulation (TENS) involves the placement of two pairs of electrodes on either side of the thoracic and sacral spine (Fig. 13-5). Continuous mild electrical currents are applied from a battery-operated device. During a contraction the woman increases the stimulation by turning control knobs on the device. Women describe the resulting sensation as a tingling or buzzing and pain relief as good or very good. The technique poses no risk to the mother or fetus, and is credited with reducing or eliminating the need for analgesia and with increasing the woman's perception of control over the experience. It may be effective because of the placebo effect; that is, confidence in TENS may stimulate the release of endogenous opiates (*endorphins*) in the woman's body and thus alleviate the discomfort (Scott et al., 1994).

The nurse's involvement in the method consists of explaining the device and its use, carefully placing and securing the electrodes, and closely evaluating its effectiveness.

Other Nonpharmacologic Methods

There are various other nonpharmacologic methods for control of discomfort in labor (Box 13-2). Many of these are taught in childbirth preparation classes. Most need

Nonpharmacologic Strategies to Encourage Relaxation and to Relieve Pain

CUTANEOUS STIMULATION STRATEGIES
Counterpressure
Effleurage
Therapeutic touch
Walking
Rocking
Changing positions
Application of heat or cold
TENS
Acupressure
Showers, baths

SENSORY STIMULATION STRATEGIES
Aromatherapy
Breathing techniques
Music
Imagery
Use of focal points

COGNITIVE STRATEGIES
Childbirth education
Hypnosis

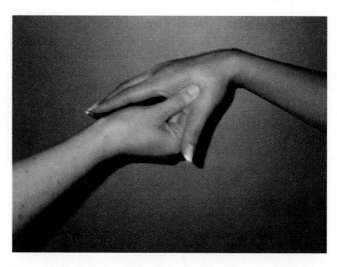

Fig. 13-6 Ho-Ku acupressure point (back of hand where thumb and index finger come together) used to enhance uterine contractions without increasing pain. (From Dickason E, Silverman B & Kaplan J: *Maternal-infant nursing care,* ed 3, St Louis, 1998, Mosby.)

practice for the best results, although the nurse may use some of them successfully without the woman having prior knowledge of the method.

Acupressure

Acupressure techniques can be used in pregnancy, labor, and postpartum to relieve pain and other discomforts. Pressure, heat, or cold is applied to acupuncture points called *tsubos.* These points have an increased density of neuroreceptors and increased electrical conductivity. The effectiveness of acupressure has been attributed to the gate-control theory and an increase in endorphin levels (Jiménez, 1992).

Acupressure should not be applied over the abdomen during pregnancy or before 38 weeks' gestation on the small toenail, anterior or medial aspects of the lower legs, or the tissue between the thumb and forefinger because this action might cause preterm labor (Jiménez, 1992). Acupressure is best applied over bare skin without using lubricants. Pressure is usually applied with the pads of the thumbs and fingers (Fig. 13-6). Synchronized breathing by the giver and the woman is suggested for greater effectiveness. Acupressure points include shoulders, low back, hips, ankles, small toenail, soles of the foot, and sacral points.

Application of heat and cold

Warmed blankets, warm compresses, a warm bath or shower, or use of a moist heating pad can reduce pain during labor. Heat acts to relieve muscle ischemia and increase blood flow to the area of discomfort. Heat application is effective for back pain caused by a posterior presentation or general backache from fatigue (Simkin, 1995).

Cold application such as cool cloths or ice packs may be effective to increase comfort when the woman feels warm or may be applied to areas of pain. Cooling works in relieving pain by lowering the muscle temperature and relieving muscle spasms (Simkin, 1995).

Heat and cold may be used alternately for a greater effect. Neither heat nor cold should be applied over ischemic or anesthetized areas because tissues can be damaged.

Therapeutic touch

Therapeutic touch uses the concept of energy fields within the body called *prana.* Prana are thought to be deficient in people who are in pain. Therapeutic touch uses laying on of the hands of a specially trained person to redirect energy fields associated with pain (Mackey, 1995). Little is known about the use or effectiveness of therapeutic touch for relieving labor pain.

Hypnosis

Hypnosis is not commonly used for pain management in the United States, but it is associated with shorter labors and less analgesic use (Jenkins & Pritchard, 1993). Hypnosis techniques used for labor and birth place an emphasis on relaxation. The woman may be given direct suggestions about pain relief or indirect suggestions that she is experiencing diminished sensations. The woman receives posthypnotic suggestions, such as "you will be able to push the baby out easily," to increase her confidence.

| BOX 13-3 | *Pharmacologic Control of Discomfort by Stage of Labor and Method of Birth* |

FIRST STAGE

Systemic analgesia
  Narcotic analgesic compounds
  Mixed narcotic agonist-antagonist compounds,
    analgesic potentiators
Nerve block analgesia/anesthesia
  Lumbar epidural analgesia

SECOND STAGE

Nerve block analgesia/anesthesia
  Local infiltration anesthesia
  Pudendal block
  Subarachnoid (spinal) anesthesia
  Epidural block
  Epidural and spinal narcotics
Inhalation analgesia/anesthesia
  Nitrous oxide-oxygen
  General anesthesia

VAGINAL BIRTH

Local infiltration
Pudendal block
Lumbar epidural block
  Analgesia
  Anesthesia
Subarachnoid block
  Analgesia
  Anesthesia

CESAREAN BIRTH

Subarachnoid block
  Spinal block
  Saddle block (low spinal)
Lumbar epidural block
  Anesthesia
Inhalation
  General anesthesia

Biofeedback

Biofeedback is another relaxation technique that can be used for labor. Biofeedback is based on the theory that if a person can recognize physical signals, then certain internal physiologic events can be changed (whatever signs the woman has that is associated with her pain). A woman must be educated to become aware of her body and its responses and how to relax for biofeedback to be effective (Alexander & Steeful, 1995).

Aromatherapy

Aromatherapy uses essential oils distilled from plants, flowers, herbs, and trees to promote health and well-being and treat illnesses. The use of herbal teas and vapors is reported to have good effects in pregnancy and labor for some women (Burnes & Blamey, 1994). Lavender, clary sage, and bergamot promote relaxation and can be used by adding a few drops to a warm bath, to warm water used for soaking compresses that can be applied to the body, to an aromatherapy lamp to vaporize a room, or to oil for a back massage (Tisserand, 1990).

PHARMACOLOGIC MANAGEMENT OF DISCOMFORT

Sedatives

Sedatives such as barbiturates relieve anxiety and induce sleep only in prodromal or early latent labor and in the absence of pain. If the woman is experiencing pain, sedatives given without an analgesic may only increase apprehension and cause the mother to become hyperactive and disoriented. Undesirable side effects include respiratory and vasomotor depression affecting both the mother and newborn. Because of these drawbacks, barbiturates are seldom used (Scott et al., 1994).

Analgesia and Anesthesia

The use of analgesia and anesthesia was not generally accepted as part of obstetric management until Queen Victoria used chloroform during the birth of her son in 1853. Since then much study has gone into the development of pharmacologic control of discomfort during the birth period. The goal of researchers is to develop methods that provide adequate pain relief to women without adding to maternal or fetal risk or affecting the progress of labor.

Nursing management of obstetric analgesia and anesthesia combines the nurse's expertise in maternity care with a knowledge and understanding of anatomy and physiology, and of medications and their desired and undesired side effects and methods of administration.

Anesthesia encompasses analgesia, amnesia, relaxation, and reflex activity. It is the abolition of pain perception by interrupting the nerve impulses going to the brain. Loss of sensation may be partial or complete, sometimes with the loss of consciousness.

The term **analgesia** is best reserved to describe the alleviation of the sensation of pain or the raising of the threshold for pain perception without loss of consciousness.

The type of analgesic or anesthetic is determined in part by the stage of labor the woman is in and by the method of birth planned (Box 13-3).

Systemic analgesia

Systemic analgesia remains the major method of analgesia for relieving the pain of labor when personnel trained

TABLE 13-1 *Opioids Used for Labor Analgesia*

DRUG	USUAL DOSE (IV/IM)	ONSET (IV/IM)	DURATION	COMMENTS
Meperidine	25 mg IV/ 50 mg IM	5-10 min IV/ 40-45 min IM	2-3 hr	Active metabolite in normeperidine, neonatal effects most likely if birth occurs between 1 and 4 hr after administration
Morphine	2-5 mg IV/ 10 mg IM	5 min IV/ 20-40 min IM	3-4 hr	Infrequent use during labor, greater respiratory depression in neonate than with meperidine
Fentanyl	25-50 µg IV/ 100 µg IM	2-3 min IV/ 10 min IM	30-60 min	Short-acting, potent respiratory depressant, used as continuous infusion and/or PCA, cumulative effect with large doses over time
Nalbuphine	10-20 mg IV/IM	2-3 min IV/ 15 min IM/SC	3-6 hr	Agonist/antagonist, less nausea and vomiting than with meperidine
Butorphanol	1-2 mg IV/IM	5-10 min IV/IM	3-4 hr	Agonist/antagonist, maternal sedation similar to meperidine plus phenothiazine
Pentazocine	20-40 mg	2-3 min IV/ 15-20 min IM/SC	2-3 hr	Agonist/antagonist, psychomimetic effects possible with usual doses but more frequent after large doses, infrequent use

From Wakefield M: Systemic analgesia: opioids, ketamine, and inhalation agents. In Chestnut D: *Obstetric anesthesia: principles and practice,* St Louis, 1994, Mosby.
IV, Intravenous; *IM,* intramuscular; *PCA,* patient-controlled analgesia; *SC,* subcutaneous.

in administering regional analgesia are not available (Scott et al., 1994). Systemic analgesics cross the blood-brain barrier to provide central analgesic effects. However, they also cross the placental barrier. The effects on the fetus depend on the maternal dosage, the pharmacokinetics of the specific drug, and the route and timing of administration. Intravenous (IV) administration is often preferred over intramuscular (IM) administration because the onset of the drug effect is faster and more reliable. Classes of analgesic drugs used to relieve pain of childbirth include narcotics, narcotic agonist-antagonist compounds, and tranquilizers such as analgesic-potentiating drugs (ataractics) (Table 13-1).

Narcotic analgesic compounds. Narcotic analgesics such as meperidine (Demerol) and fentanyl (Sublimaze) are especially effective for relieving severe, persistent, or recurrent pain. They have no amnesic effect.

Meperidine is the most commonly used narcotic for women in labor (Scott et al., 1994). It overcomes inhibitory factors in labor and may even relax the cervix. After IV injection, the onset is rapid (30 seconds); the maximum effect is reached in 5 to 10 minutes and lasts about 3 hours. The peak effect after IM injection is reached in 40 to 50 minutes. In a randomized controlled study, women who received meperidine IV reported significantly lower levels of pain than those reported by women who received it IM (Isenor & Penny-MacGillivary, 1993). Ideally birth should occur less than 1 hour or more than 4 hours after IM injection so the neonatal CNS depression resulting from meperidine is minimized. Because tachycardia is a possible side effect, meperidine is used cautiously for women with cardiac disease.

Fentanyl is a potent, short-acting narcotic analgesic. The onset of the drug effect after IV injection occurs within 2 minutes and lasts about 30 to 60 minutes. Onset of the drug

effect after IM injection occurs in 7 to 15 minutes; the peak effect is reached in 20 to 30 minutes and lasts for 1 to 2 hours. Additive central nervous system (CNS) and respiratory depression occurs if fentanyl is given with alcohol, antihistamines, antidepressants, or other sedative/hypnotics.

Mixed narcotic agonist-antagonist compounds. An agonist is an agent that activates something; an antagonist is an agent that blocks or prevents something from happening. Mixed narcotic **agonist-antagonist compounds** such as butorphanol (Stadol) and nalbuphine (Nubain), in the doses used during labor, provide analgesia without causing respiratory depression in the mother or neonate. They are administered either IM or IV. Butorphanol (1 to 3 mg IM; 0.5 to 2 mg IV) and nalbuphine (10 to 20 mg IV or IM) may be given during the first stage of labor.

Analgesic potentiators (ataractics). Phenothiazines, so-called tranquilizers, have the property of augmenting most of the desirable but few of the undesirable effects of analgesics or general anesthetics. These **ataractics** do not relieve pain but decrease anxiety and apprehension, as well as potentiate narcotic effects. This potentiation effect causes the two involved drugs to work together more effectively, such that the narcotic dosage can be reduced. The analgesic potentiators include promethazine (Phenergan), propiomazine (Largon), hydroxyzine (Vistaril), and promazine (Sparine).

In addition to potentiating the effects of the analgesic, the ataractic (tranquilizer) also acts as an antinauseant and antiemetic. The combination of agents can be administered safely until the end of the first stage of labor. The following are the usual doses of the various agents: promethazine 25 to 50 mg IM or 15 to 25 mg IV; promazine 50 mg IM or 5 to 10 mg IV; hydroxyzine 25 to 50 mg IM. Because hydroxyzine is given only by IM injection, onset of effect is slower and less predictable. Fetal or neonatal problems rarely develop when the women are given these dosages.

Narcotic antagonists. Narcotics such as meperidine and fentanyl may cause excessive CNS depression in the mother or newborn. **Narcotic antagonists** such as naloxone (Narcan) and naltrexone (Trexan) promptly reverse the narcotic effects. In addition, the antagonist also counters the effect of stress-induced levels of endorphins. **Endorphins** are endogenous opioids secreted by the pituitary gland that act on the central and peripheral nervous systems to reduce pain. Beta-endorphin is the most potent of the endorphins. The physiologic role of endorphins is not completely understood. It is thought that endorphins increase during pregnancy and birth in humans and serve to augment the laboring woman's tolerance of acute pain.

A narcotic antagonist is especially valuable if labor is more rapid than expected, and birth is anticipated when the narcotic is at its peak effect. The antagonist may be given through the woman's IV line, or it can be administered IM. Narcotic antagonists can counteract the maternal and neonatal narcotic effects. The mother needs to be told, however, that the pain will return with administration of an antagonist.

> **NURSE ALERT** *Narcotic antagonists must be administered cautiously to a substance-dependent woman because the drugs may precipitate withdrawal symptoms (see the box on Signs of Potential Complications).*

A narcotic antagonist can be given to the newborn to treat **neonatal narcosis,** which is a state of CNS depression in the newborn produced by a narcotic. Affected infants may exhibit respiratory depression, hypotonia, lethargy, and a delay in temperature regulation. Alterations of neurologic and behavioral responses may be evident for 72 hours after birth. Meperidine may be present in the neonate's urine for up to 3 weeks. Some depression of attention and social responsiveness may be evident for up to 6 weeks.

Nerve block analgesia and anesthesia

A variety of compounds is used in obstetrics to produce regional analgesia (some pain relief and motor block) and anesthesia (pain relief and motor block). Most of these drugs are related chemically to cocaine and end with the suffix *-caine*. This is a way of identifying a local anesthetic.

The principal pharmacologic effect of local anesthetics is the temporary interruption of the conduction of nerve impulses, notably pain. Examples of common agents given in 0.25% to 1% solutions are lidocaine (Xylocaine), bupivacaine (Marcaine), chloroprocaine (Nesacaine), tetracaine (Pontocaine), and mepivacaine (Carbocaine).

Rarely, people are sensitive (allergic) to one or more local anesthetics. Such sensitivity may be determined by administering minute amounts of the drug to test for an allergic reaction. Such a reaction may include respiratory depression, hypotension, and other serious adverse effects. Atropine, antihistamines, oxygen, and supportive measures should reverse these effects.

Local infiltration anesthesia. Local infiltration anesthesia of perineal tissue is commonly used when an episiotomy is to be done and when time or the fetal head position does not permit a pudendal block to be administered (Scott et al., 1994). Rapid anesthesia is produced by injecting an average of 10 to 20 ml of local anesthetic with 1% lidocaine or 2% chloroprocaine into the skin and then subcutaneously into the region to be anesthetized. Epinephrine often is added to the solution to intensify the anesthesia in a limited region and to prevent excessive bleeding and systemic effects by constricting local blood vessels (Clark, Queener & Karb, 1996). Repeated injection prolongs the anesthesia as long as needed.

Pudendal block. Pudendal block is useful for the second stage of labor, episiotomy, and birth. Although it does not relieve pain from uterine contractions, it does relieve pain in the lower vagina and vulva and the perineum (Fig. 13-7, *A*).

A pudendal nerve block needs to be administered 10 to 20 minutes before perineal anesthesia is needed. The pudendal nerve traverses the sacrosciatic notch just medial to the tip of the ischial spine on each side. Injection of an anesthetic solution at or near these points will anesthetize the pudendal nerves peripherally (Fig. 13-8). The transvaginal approach is generally used because it is less painful for the woman, is more successful in blocking pain, and tends to be associated with fewer fetal complications (Chestnut, 1994). Pudendal block does not alter maternal hemodynamic or respiratory functions, vital signs, or FHR. However, it can cause the bearing-down reflex to be lessened or lost completely.

If all branches of the pudendal nerve are anesthetized, the resulting analgesia is sufficient for spontaneous vaginal birth or outlet (low) forceps-assisted birth. A pudendal block does not provide analgesia for uterine exploration or manual removal of the placenta (Scott et al., 1994).

Spinal block. In **spinal block,** local anesthetic is injected through the third, fourth, or fifth lumbar interspace into the subarachnoid space (Fig. 13-9), where the

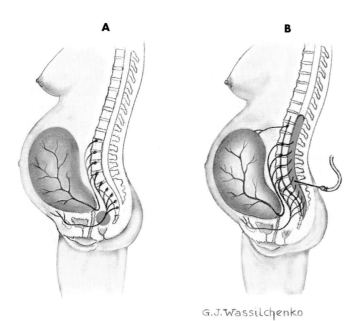

G.J.Wassilchenko

Fig. 13-7 Pain pathways and sites of pharmacologic nerve blocks. **A,** Pudendal block: suitable during second and third stages of labor and for repair of episiotomy or lacerations. **B,** Epidural block: suitable for all stages of labor and for repair of episiotomy and lacerations.

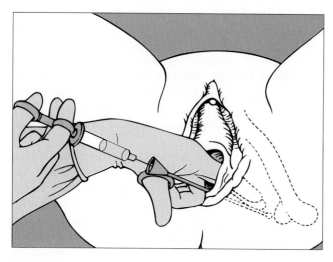

Fig. 13-8 Pudendal block. Use of needle guide (Iowa trumpet) and Luer-Lok syringe to inject medication.

medication mixes with cerebrospinal fluid (CSF). This technique is commonly used for cesarean births. A low spinal block may be used for vaginal birth, but it is not suitable for labor. The spinal block given for cesarean birth provides anesthesia from the nipple (T6) to the feet. If used for a vaginal birth, the anesthesia level is from the hips (T10) to the feet (see Fig. 13-9, *C*).

For a spinal block, the woman is positioned in a sitting or lateral position similar to that for an epidural placement so that the intervertebral space is widened. The nurse sup-

---

EMERGENCY

Maternal Hypotension with Decreased Placental Perfusion

SIGNS/SYMPTOMS

Maternal hypotension (20% drop from preblock level or less than 100 mm Hg systolic)
Fetal bradycardia
Decreased beat-to-beat FHR variability

INTERVENTIONS

Turn woman to lateral position or place pillow or wedge under right hip (see Fig. 15-4) to deflect uterus.
Maintain IV infusion at rate specified, or increase prn per hospital protocol.
Administer oxygen by face mask at 10 to 12 L/min.
Elevate the woman's legs.
Notify the physician/midwife/anesthesiologist/nurse anesthetist.
Administer IV vasopressor (e.g., ephedrine) per protocol
Remain with woman: continue to monitor maternal BP and FHR every 5 minutes until stable or per primary health care provider's order.

---

ports the woman because she must remain still during the placement of the spinal needle. The insertion is made between contractions. After the insertion, the woman may be positioned upright to get the level of anesthesia for a vaginal birth or positioned supine if the level desired is for a cesarean birth. The anesthetic effect usually begins in 1 to 2 minutes after the anesthetic is injected and lasts 1 to 3 hours, depending on the type of agent used (Chestnut, 1994).

Marked hypotension, decreased cardiac output and placental perfusion, and respiratory inadequacy can occur during spinal anesthesia. If signs of serious maternal hypotension or fetal distress develop, emergency care must be given (see the accompanying Emergency box).

Because the woman is not able to sense her contractions, she must be instructed when to bear down if having a vaginal birth. If the birth occurs in a delivery room (rather than a labor-delivery-recovery room), the mother will need assistance in being transferred to a recovery bed after delivery of the placenta.

Advantages of spinal anesthesia include ease of administration, absence of fetal hypoxia with maintenance of maternal normotension, and the woman is conscious.

Disadvantages of spinal anesthesia include drug reactions (e.g., allergy), hypotension, and respiratory paralysis. In addition, when spinal anesthesia is given, the need for operative birth (episiotomy, forceps extraction, or vacuum-assisted birth) tends to be greater because the voluntary expulsive efforts are eliminated. After birth, the woman may experience bladder and uterine atony, as well as postspinal headache.

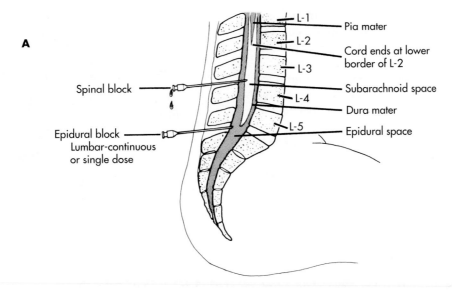

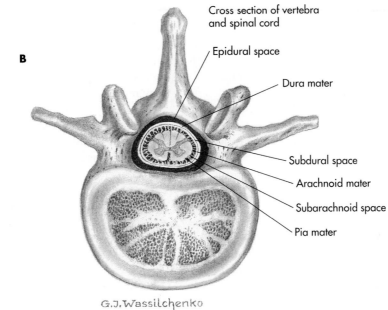

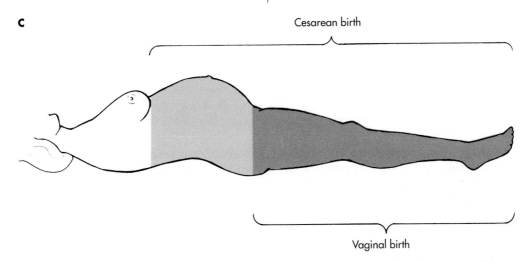

Fig. **13-9 A,** Membranes and spaces of spinal cord and levels of sacral, lumbar, and thoracic nerves. **B,** Cross-section of vertebra and spinal cord. **C,** Level of anesthesia necessary for cesarean and vaginal births. (C is courtesy Ross Laboratories, Columbus, Oh.)

Leakage of CSF from the site of puncture of the meninges (membranous coverings of the spinal cord) is thought to be the major causative factor in postlumbar puncture (postspinal) headache. Presumably, postural changes cause the diminished volume of CSF to exert traction on pain-sensitive CNS structures. The resulting headache, auditory, and visual problems may persist for days or weeks.

The likelihood of headache after lumbar puncture can be reduced if the anesthesiologist uses a small-gauge spinal needle and avoids multiple punctures of the meninges. Positioning the woman flat in bed (with only a small, flat pillow for her head) for at least 8 hours after spinal anesthesia has also been recommended to prevent postspinal headache, but there is no definitive evidence showing this measure is effective. Positioning the woman on her abdomen is thought to decrease the loss of CSF through the puncture site. Hyperhydration has been claimed to be of value in preventing and treating headache, but there is no compelling evidence to support its use (Cunningham et al., 1997). Initial treatment for postlumbar puncture headache usually includes analgesics, bed rest, caffeine, and increased fluid intake (i.e., 150 ml/hr IV) (ACOG, 1996).

An autologous **epidural blood patch** (a patch repairing a tear or a hole in the dura mater around the spinal cord) is often beneficial, and such treatment may be considered if the headache does not resolve spontaneously (Scott et al., 1994). To form a patch, a few milliliters of the woman's blood without anticoagulant is injected epidurally at the site of the spinal tap (Fig. 13-10), which then forms a clot that covers the hole and prevents further fluid loss.

Epidural block. The pain of uterine contractions and birth (vaginal and abdominal) can be relieved by injecting a suitable local anesthetic into the epidural (peridural) space between the fourth and fifth lumbar vertebrae (see Figs. 13-7, *B*, and 13-9, *A*).

Complete lumbar **epidural block** for relieving the discomfort of labor and vaginal birth requires a block from T10 to S5. For cesarean birth, a block from at least T8 to S1 is essential. The diffusion of epidural anesthesia depends on the location of the catheter tip, the dosage and volume of the anesthetic agent used, and the woman's position (e.g., horizontal or head up) (Cunningham et al., 1997).

For the induction of lumbar epidural anesthesia, the woman is positioned as for a spinal injection (i.e., sitting) or in a modified Sims position (Fig. 13-11). For this modified lateral Sims position, the woman is placed on her side, with her shoulders parallel, legs slightly flexed, and back arched.

After the epidural has been started, the woman is positioned preferably on her side so that the uterus does not compress the ascending vena cava and descending aorta, which can impair venous return and decrease placental perfusion. Oxygen should be available to treat hypotension should it occur despite maintenance of IV fluid and

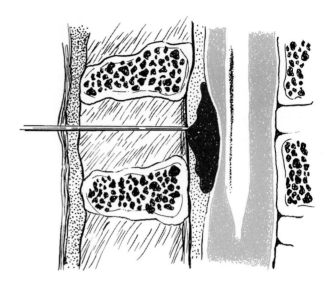

Fig. **13-10** Blood patch therapy for spinal headache.

displacement of the uterus to the side. Ephedrine (a vasopressor used to increase maternal blood pressure) and increased IV fluid infusion rate may be needed (see the Emergency box on p. 316). The FHR and progress in labor must be monitored carefully because the laboring woman may not be aware of changes in the strength of uterine contractions or the descent of the presenting part.

A single injection, intermittent bolus, or continuous infusion (via pump) through an indwelling catheter usually results in excellent analgesia-anesthesia. The *advantages* of an epidural block are numerous: the mother remains alert and cooperative, good relaxation is achieved, airway reflexes remain intact, only partial motor paralysis develops, gastric emptying is not delayed, and blood loss is not excessive. Fetal distress is rare but may occur in the event of rapid absorption or noticeable maternal hypotension. The dose, volume, and type of anesthetic can be modified to allow the mother to push, to produce perineal anesthesia, and to permit forceps or even cesarean birth if required (Cunningham et al., 1997).

The *disadvantages* of an epidural block for the woman include the need for an intravenous line, occasional dizziness, weakness of the legs, difficulty emptying the bladder, and shivering (Youngstrom et al., 1996). Because a considerable amount of the drug must be used, adverse reactions or the rapid absorption of the anesthetic agent may result in maternal hypotension, convulsions, or paresthesia. Epidural analgesia may cause changes in the labor process. Data from retrospective studies and clinical trials suggest there is a relationship between epidural analgesia and longer labor and increased incidence of operative birth (Hawkins et al., 1995; Thorp & Breedlove, 1996). Occasionally, accidental high-spinal anesthesia (and later, postepidural headache) may follow inadvertent perforation of the dural membrane during the administration of lumbar epidural anesthesia.

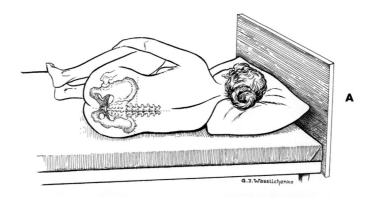

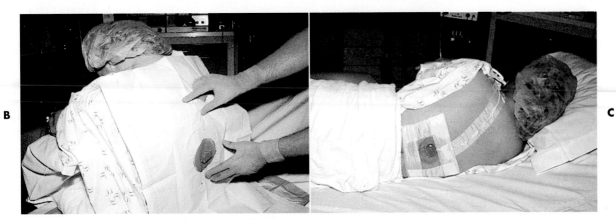

Fig. **13-11** Positioning for spinal and epidural blocks. **A,** Lateral position. **B,** Upright position. **C,** Catheter for epidural taped to woman's back with port segment located near shoulder. (**B** and **C** courtesy Michael S. Clement, MD, Mesa, Ariz.)

For some women the selected anesthetic is ineffective, and a second form of anesthesia is required to establish effective pain relief. For women who progress rapidly in labor, pain relief may not be obtained before birth occurs.

Epidural analgesia and intrathecal narcotics. There is a high concentration of narcotic receptors along the pain pathway in the spinal cord, in the brainstem, and in the thalamus. Because these receptors are highly sensitive to narcotics, a small quantity of narcotic produces marked analgesia lasting for several hours. The medication is injected through a catheter placed in the epidural or subarachnoid space, which communicates with these narcotic receptors. Pain transmission is blocked without compromising motor ability, thus the so-called "walking epidural," which restores the woman's confidence in her ability to master labor no longer dominated by pain (Youngstrom et al., 1996).

The use of epidural or intrathecal narcotics during labor has several advantages. These agents do not cause maternal hypotension or affect vital signs. The woman feels contractions but not pain. Her ability to bear down during the second stage of labor is preserved because the pushing reflex is not lost and motor power remains intact.

Fentanyl, sufentanil, or preservative-free morphine may be used. Fentanyl and sufentanil produce short-acting anal-gesia (1 1/2 to 3 1/2 hours), and morphine may provide pain relief for 4 to 7 hours. Morphine may be combined with fentanyl or sufentanil. The short-acting narcotics are often used with multiparous women, and the morphine may be used with nulliparous women or women with a history of long labors (Manning, 1996). For most women, intrathecal narcotics do not provide adequate analgesia for second-stage labor pain, episiotomy, or birth (Cunningham et al., 1997). Pudendal blocks or local anesthetics may be necessary.

A more common indication for the administration of epidural or intrathecal narcotics is the relief of postoperative pain. For example, women who give birth by cesarean receive fentanyl (Innovar) or morphine through the catheter. The catheter may then be removed, and the women are usually pain free for 24 hours. Occasionally the catheter is left in place in case another dose is needed.

Women who receive epidurally administered morphine after the cesarean birth are up soon after surgery with surprising ease and are able to care for their babies. The early ambulation and freedom from pain also facilitate bladder emptying. To those women who have had a previous cesarean birth and have experienced the usual postoperative pain, the effects of this approach seem miraculous. However, the mother may not understand why she may experience pain after the narcotic wears off.

Side effects of epidural or intrathecal narcotics include nausea, vomiting, pruritus (itching), urinary retention, and delayed respiratory depression. These side effects are more common when morphine is administered. Antiemetics, antipruritics, and narcotic antagonists are used to relieve symptoms. For example, naloxone or naltrexone, nalbuphine hydrochloride (Nubain), promethazine, or metoclopramide (Reglan) may be administered. Hospital protocols should provide specific instructions for the treatment of these side effects. Use of epidural narcotics is not without risks. Respiratory depression is a serious concern; the woman's respiratory rate should be assessed and documented every hour for 24 hours, or per the timing designated by hospital protocol. Naloxone hydrochloride should be readily available if the respiratory rate decreases to 10 breaths per minute or if oxygen saturation drops below 89%. Administration of oxygen by face mask may also be initiated, and an anesthesiologist should be notified.

Contraindications to subarachnoid and epidural blocks. Patient conditions that are contraindications to epidural analgesia include (ACOG, 1996):

- *Antepartum hemorrhage.* Acute hypovolemia leads to increased sympathetic tone to maintain the blood pressure. Any anesthetic technique that blocks the sympathetic fibers can produce significant hypotension that can endanger the mother and baby.
- *Anticoagulant therapy or bleeding disorder.* If a woman is receiving anticoagulant therapy or has a bleeding disorder, injury to a blood vessel may cause the formation of a hematoma that may compress the cauda equina or the spinal cord and lead to serious CNS sequelae.
- *Infection at the injection site.* Infection can be spread through the peridural or subarachnoid spaces if the needle traverses an infected area.
- *Allergy to anesthetic drug.*

Drug effects on neonate. Debate persists concerning the effects of epidural anesthesia on the neonate's neurobehavioral responses. Results from studies of associations between neurobehavioral outcome and epidural anesthesia are far from consistent. For example, studies comparing neonatal neurobehavioral scores of infants born to mothers with and mothers without epidural analgesia either have shown little or no difference in the scores (Hamza, 1994; Scherer & Holzgreve, 1995) or have shown that the neonates of mothers who received epidural anesthesia did not score as well on neurobehavioral tests (Sepkoski et al., 1992).

Paracervical (uterosacral) block. Paracervical blocks can be used to relieve pain from the lower uterine segment and cervix to the upper third of the vagina. They are rarely used for labor because of the potential fetal complications

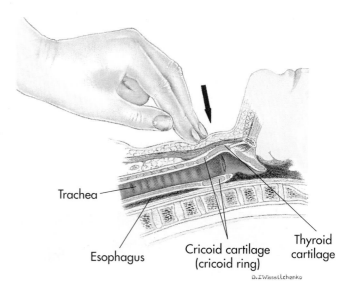

Fig. **13-12** Technique for applying pressure on cricoid cartilage to occlude esophagus to prevent pulmonary aspiration of gastric contents during induction of general anesthesia.

related to rapid absorption of the drug. They may be used for anesthesia during abortion or other gynecologic procedures.

General anesthesia. General anesthesia rarely is used for uncomplicated vaginal birth and is infrequently used for cesarean birth. It may be necessary if there is a contraindication to nerve block analgesia or anesthesia or if the woman is not already receiving regional analgesia or anesthesia when there is an emergency maternal or fetal situation.

If general anesthesia is being considered, the nurse gives the woman nothing by mouth and sees that an IV infusion is established. If time allows, the nurse premedicates the woman with a nonparticulate oral antacid such as sodium citrate (30 ml) to neutralize acid contents of the stomach. If there is sufficient time, some anesthesiologists/physicians also order the administration of a histamine blocker such as cimetidine to decrease the production of gastric acid and metoclopramide to increase gastric emptying (Scott et al., 1994). Before the anesthesia is given, a wedge should be placed under the woman's right hip to displace the uterus to the left. As already noted, such uterine displacement prevents aortal compression, which interferes with placental perfusion. Sometimes the nurse is asked to assist with applying *cricoid pressure* (Fig. 13-12) before intubation.

Priorities for recovery room care are to maintain an open airway, maintain cardiopulmonary functions, and prevent postpartum hemorrhage. Routine postpartum care is organized around facilitating parent-child attachment as soon as possible and answering the mother's questions. Whenever appropriate, the nurse assesses the mother's readiness to see the baby, as well as her response to the anesthesia and to the event that necessitated general anesthesia (e.g., having a cesarean birth when vaginal birth was anticipated).

Inhalation analgesia and anesthesia. Nitrous oxide is the only inhalation agent used for obstetrics in the United States. It is rarely used for labor in the United States but may be used in other countries for this purpose.

Nitrous oxide is commonly used for cesarean births when inhalation anesthesia is needed. It is usually combined with oxygen in a 50/50 mixture. Thiopental, a short-acting barbiturate, combined with succinylcholine, a muscle relaxer, is given IV before tracheal intubation.

Other inhalation agents include halothane, enflurane or isoflurane, and methoxyflurane. These agents relax the uterus quickly and facilitate intrauterine manipulation, version, and extraction. However, these agents cross the placenta readily and can produce narcosis in the fetus. They are rarely used today in the United States.

I CARE MANAGEMENT

The choice of pain relief depends on a combination of factors, including the woman's special needs and wishes, the availability of the desired method, the health care provider's knowledge and expertise in nonpharmacologic and pharmacologic methods of pain relief, and the phase and stage of labor. The nurse is responsible for maintaining continuous maternal and fetal assessment, establishing mutual goals with the woman (and her family), formulating nursing diagnoses, planning and implementing nursing care, and evaluating the effects of care. It is essential for the nurse to carefully document all aspects of care management.

Assessment and Nursing Diagnoses

The assessment of the woman, her fetus, and her labor is a joint effort on the part of the nurse and the primary health care providers who consult with the woman regarding their findings and recommendations. The needs of each woman are different, and many factors must be considered in assessment to determine whether nonpharmacologic, a combination of nonpharmacologic and pharmacologic, or pharmacologic methods of pain management are used (see Cultural Considerations box on p. 307). A self-assessment tool, such as an analog scale, allows the woman to indicate on a line how severe she perceives her pain experience to be. Self-assessment is recommended to ensure pain management is based on the subjective nature of the woman's pain rather than on just the nurse's judgment (Olden et al., 1995).

History

The woman's prenatal record is read and relevant information identified. This includes the woman's parity, estimated date of birth, and complications and medications during pregnancy. If the woman has a history of allergies, this is noted and a warning is carefully displayed in a prominent place. A history of smoking and neurologic and spinal disorders is noted.

Interview

Interview data consist of the time of the woman's last meal; the type of food consumed; the nature of any existing respiratory condition (cold, allergy); and unusual reactions to medications (e.g., allergy), cleansing agents, latex, or tape. The woman is asked whether she attended preparation classes for childbirth and the extent of her preparation, and preferences for management of discomfort are noted. Her knowledge of options for the management of discomfort is also assessed. Information on the woman's perception of discomfort and her expressed need for medication are added to the database. Relevant events that have occurred since the woman's last contact with the primary health care provider are also reviewed (e.g., infections, diarrhea, change in fetal behavior). If verbal and physical signs indicate the existence of substance abuse, the nurse should ask the woman to identify the type of drug used, the last time the drug was used, and the method of administration.

Physical examination

The character and status of the labor and fetal response are assessed during physical examination. The nurse evaluates the woman's hydration status by assessing intake and output measurements, moisture of the mucous membranes, and skin turgor. Bladder distention is noted. Any evidence of skin infection near sites of possible needle insertion is recorded and reported. Signs of apprehension such as fist clenching and restlessness are also noted.

If the woman is in labor, the status of maternal vital signs and FHR; uterine contractions, cervical effacement, and dilatation; station; and the anticipated time until birth are all considered. The length of labor and degree of fatigue are important considerations. If pharmacologic methods are to be used, the type of analgesia and anesthesia chosen varies depending on the phase and stage of labor (see Box 13-3).

Laboratory tests

The results of laboratory tests are reviewed to determine whether the woman is suffering from anemia (hemoglobin and hematocrit), coagulopathy or bleeding disorder (prothrombin time and platelet count), or infection (white blood cell count and differential).

Signs of Potential Problems

Any medication can cause an **allergic reaction** that may be minor or as severe as anaphylaxis. Severe reactions may occur suddenly and lead to shock. The most dramatic form of anaphylaxis is sudden severe bronchospasm, vasospasm, severe hypotension, and death. Signs of anaphylaxis are largely caused by contraction of smooth muscles, and this may be heralded by irritability, extreme weakness, and nausea and vomiting, leading to dyspnea, cyanosis, convulsions, and cardiac arrest. The acute allergic reaction—anaphylaxis—must be diagnosed and treated immediately by the health care team to prevent consequences. Treatment usually consists of 1:1000 epinephrine injected SC or IM, followed by parenteral administration of antihistamines. Supportive care is given to alleviate the symptoms, and the type of care is determined by the rapid assessment of cardiovascular and respiratory response of the woman to primary interventions; CPR may be necessary. The nurse must also be alert to fetal well-being; any FHR decelerations should be noted and reported to the primary health care provider.

Minor reactions consist of a rash, rhinitis, fever, asthma, and pruritus. Management of the less acute allergic response does not constitute an emergency. As a part of the assessment for allergic reactions, the nurse monitors the woman's vital signs, respiratory status, cardiovascular status, platelet count, and white blood cell count. The woman is observed for side effects of drug therapy, especially drowsiness (Clark et al., 1996).

Nursing diagnoses vary from woman to woman. Some nursing diagnoses of relevance in the management of discomfort during the birth period are listed in the accompanying box.

I Nursing Diagnoses_____

Pain Management during Labor and Birth

Risk for altered tissue perfusion related to:
* Effects of analgesia or anesthesia
* Maternal position

Hypothermia related to:
* Effects of analgesia or anesthesia

Pain related to:
* Processes of labor and birth

Situational low self-esteem related to:
* Negative perception of the woman's (or her family's) behavior

Anxiety or fear related to knowledge deficit of:
* Procedure for nerve block analgesia
* Expected sensation during nerve block analgesia
* Mother's role during nerve block analgesia
* Options for analgesia and anesthesia

Risk for maternal injury related to:
* Effects of analgesia and anesthesia on sensation and motor control

Risk for injury to fetus related to:
* Maternal hypotension
* Maternal position (aortocaval compression)

Expected Outcomes of Care

The expected outcomes of nursing care in the management of the discomfort of labor and birth include the following:
* The woman, her partner, and family will verbalize understanding of their needs and rights with regard to the use of nonpharmacologic methods, analgesia, and anesthesia.
* The woman will experience adequate pain relief without increasing maternal risk (e.g., through the use of pharmacologic methods and appropriate medication, including the appropriate dose, timing, and route of administration).
* Fetal well-being will be maintained, and the newborn will adjust to extrauterine life.

Plan of Care and Interventions

A plan of care is developed for each woman that should address her particular clinical and nursing problems. The nurse collaborates with the primary health care provider and laboring woman in selecting those aspects of care relevant to the individual woman and her family.

Nonpharmacologic interventions

The nurse supports and assists the woman as she uses nonpharmacologic interventions for pain relief and relaxation. During labor, the nurse should ask the woman how she feels in order to evaluate the effectiveness of the specific pain management. Appropriate interventions can then be planned or continued for effective care, such as trying other nonpharmacologic methods or combining nonpharmacologic methods with medications.

The woman's *perception* of her behavior during labor is of utmost importance. If she planned a nonmedicated birth but then needs and accepts medication, her self-esteem may falter. The nurse gives verbal and nonverbal reassurance of the acceptability of her behavior as necessary and reinforces after birth if possible. Explanations about the fetal response to maternal discomfort, the effects of maternal fatigue, and the medication itself are supportive measures. The woman may also be experiencing anxiety and stress related to the anticipated or actual pain. Stress can cause increased maternal catecholamine production. Raised levels of catecholamines have been linked to dysfunctional labor and fetal and neonatal distress and illness. Nurses must be able to implement strategies aimed at reducing this stress (Green, 1993).

Pharmacologic interventions

Informed consent. The primary health care provider and anesthesia care provider are responsible for informing women of the alternative methods of pharmacologic pain relief available in the hospital setting. The description of various anesthetic techniques and what they entail is essential to informed consent, even if the woman has received information about analgesia and anesthesia earlier in her pregnancy. This interview should take place just before or early in labor so the woman has time to consider alternatives. Nurses play a part in the informed consent by clarifying and describing the procedures or by acting as a woman's advocate and asking the primary health care provider for further explanations. The procedure and its advantages and disadvantages must be thoroughly explained.

LEGAL TIP **Informed Consent for Anesthesia**

THE WOMAN RECEIVES (IN AN UNDERSTANDABLE MANNER):
- *Explanation of anesthesia and analgesia alternatives available*
- *Description of the anesthetic and procedure for administration*
- *Description of the benefits, discomforts, risks, and consequences to the mother and the fetus of the anesthetic selected*
- *Explanation of how complications can be treated*
- *Information that the anesthetic is not always effective*
- *Indication that the woman may withdraw consent at any time*
- *Opportunity to answer any questions*
- *Opportunity to explain in the mother's own words components of the consent*

CONSENT FORM:
- *Written in woman's primary language*
- *Woman's signature*
- *Date of consent*
- *Signature of anesthesia care provider, certifying that the woman has received and appears to understand the explanation*

Timing of administration

It is often the nurse who notifies the primary health care provider that the woman is in need of pharmacologic measures to relieve her discomfort. Therefore the primary health care provider often writes orders for the administration of pain medication needed based on the nurse's clinical judgment. The pharmacologic measures used to manage discomfort of labor are summarized in Box 13-3 by stage of labor and method of birth.

Preparation for procedures

The nurse reviews the methods of pain relief available to the woman or validates her choices and also clarifies the information as necessary. The procedure and what will be asked of her (e.g., to maintain flexed position during insertion of epidural needle) need to be explained to the woman. The woman can also benefit from knowing the way the medication is to be given, how much discomfort she is likely to experience during administration of the medication, what sensations she can expect, the way the skin is prepared, how long it will take to administer the medication, and how long

it will take for the medication to take effect. The nurse also explains the reason for emptying the bladder before analgesic or anesthetic is given and for keeping the bladder empty. If an indwelling epidural catheter is to be threaded, the woman should be told that she may experience a momentary twinge down her leg, hip, or back and that this feeling is not a sign of injury. A long needle is used for pudendal blocks (see Fig. 13-8). The sight of this needle may be frightening so the woman can be reassured that only the tip of the needle will be inserted.

Administration of medication

Accurate monitoring of the progress of labor forms the basis for nursing judgment of the need for pharmacologic control of discomfort. Knowledge of the medications that are used during childbirth including route, dosage, effects, side effects, and nursing implications is also essential.

Intravenous route. The preferred route of administration of medications such as meperidine or fentanyl is through IV tubing, administered into the port nearest the woman while the infusion of IV solution is stopped. The medication is given slowly in small doses at the *beginning* of three to five consecutive contractions. Because uterine blood vessels are constricted during contractions, the medication stays within the maternal vascular system for several seconds before the uterine blood vessels reopen. The IV infusion is then restarted slowly to prevent a bolus of medication from forming. Using this method of injection, the amount of drug crossing the placenta to the fetus is minimized. With decreased placental transfer the mother's degree of pain relief is maximized. Use of the IV route is associated with the following advantages:
- Onset of pain relief is more immediate.
- Pain relief is obtained with small doses of the drug.
- The duration of effect is more predictable.

Intramuscular route. IM injections of analgesics, although still used, are not the preferred route for administering such agents in the laboring woman. Identified disadvantages of the IM route include the following:
- Onset of pain relief is delayed.
- Higher doses of medication are required.
- Medication is released from the muscle tissue at an unpredictable rate and is available for transfer across the placenta to the fetus.

IM injections are given in the upper portion of the arm (deltoid site) if regional anesthesia is planned later in the labor. This is the preferred site because the autonomic blockage from the regional (e.g., epidural) anesthesia causes blood flow to the gluteal region to be increased and absorption of the drug to be accelerated. The maternal plasma level of the drug necessary to bring pain relief usually is reached 45 minutes after IM injection, followed by a decline in plasma levels. The maternal drug levels (after IM injections) are unequal because of uneven distribution (maternal uptake) and metabolism. The advantage of using the IM route is quick administration.

Nerve blocks. An IV line is established before the induction of nerve blocks such as epidural, spinal, and general anesthesia. Anesthesia protocols usually include the administration of a bolus of IV fluid before epidural and spinal anesthesia for blood volume expansion to prevent maternal hypotension. Lactated Ringer's or Plasma-Lyte A and normal saline solutions are the preferred solutions. Infusion solutions without dextrose are preferred, especially when the solution needs to be infused rapidly (e.g., in the presence of severe dehydration or to maintain blood pressure) because solutions containing dextrose raise the maternal blood glucose levels rapidly. The fetus responds to high blood glucose levels by increasing insulin production, and this can lead to fetal or neonatal hypoglycemia. In addition, dextrose changes the osmotic pressure so that fluid is excreted from the kidneys more rapidly.

The woman needs assistance in assuming and maintaining the correct position for epidural and spinal anesthesia (see Fig. 13-11).

Safety and general care. After administration of a nerve block, the woman is protected from injury by raising the side rails and placing a call bell within easy reach when the nurse is not in attendance. Oxygen and suction should be readily available at the bedside. The nurse must make sure there is no prolonged pressure on an anesthetized part (e.g., lying on one side with weight on one leg; tight bedclothes on feet). If stirrups are to be used, the nurse should place pads on them, adjust both stirrups to the same level and angle, place both of the woman's legs into them simultaneously without putting pressure on the popliteal angle, and apply restraints without restricting circulation.

The nurse monitors and records the woman's response to nonpharmacologic pain relief methods and/or to medication. Response to medication includes the level of pain relief, level of apprehension, return of sensations and perception of pain, and allergic or untoward reactions that occur (e.g., hypotension, respiratory depression, and hypothermia). The nurse continues to monitor maternal vital signs, blood pressure, the strength and the frequency of uterine contractions, changes in the cervix and station of the presenting part, the presence of the bearing-down reflex, bladder filling, and state of hydration. Determining the fetal response after induction of analgesia or anesthesia is of vital importance. The woman is asked if she (or the family) has any questions. The nurse also assesses the woman's and her family's understanding of the need for ensuring her safety (e.g., keeping side rails up, calling for assistance as needed).

The time that elapses between the administration of a narcotic and the baby's birth are noted. Documentation is completed if the newborn was given any medications to reverse narcotic effects. Postpartum, the woman who has had spinal, epidural, or general anesthesia is assessed for return of sensory and motor sensations in addition to the usual postpartum assessments (see Plan of Care).

Special concerns

Two additional concerns about use of analgesia and anesthesia—the use of anesthesia in obese women and postpartum hypothermia—are discussed in the following sections.

Anesthesia in the obese woman. Obesity is defined as an excess of body fat causing weight to be greater than 20% over ideal weight; obesity affects 6% to 10% of pregnant women. Weight more than twice the ideal body weight is considered morbid obesity. A study of anesthesia-related maternal mortality in Michigan between 1972 and 1984 revealed that obesity was a risk factor in 80% of the maternal deaths (Endler et al., 1988). A retrospective study of morbidly obese women covering the years 1978 to 1989 revealed that 62% underwent cesarean birth and 48% underwent emergency cesarean birth (Hood & Dewan, 1993).

As discussed in detail in Chapter 9, the maternal physiologic changes are the product of hormonal influences and mechanical effects. In obese women, the weight of the fat tissue together with the added metabolic demands this involves also affect maternal physiology (Endler, 1990). Both pregnancy and obesity cause blood volume and cardiac output to increase, and in the latter case, they expand in proportion to the amount of fat tissue. During labor and vaginal birth, and in the immediate postpartum period, blood values and cardiac output in obese women reach levels 80% greater than prelabor values. The enlarged uterus and abdominal fat mass also further increase the possibility of aortocaval compression.

The respiratory system is also stressed in obese pregnant women (Endler, 1990), and the pulmonary function of the obese laboring woman is in a precarious state. Therefore the woman's oxygenation must be carefully monitored during birth and the immediate postpartum period. Monitoring by pulse oximeter has been suggested.

The gastric emptying time is delayed, tone in the cardiac sphincter is decreased, and gastric contents are hyperacidic in all pregnant women. However, the obese woman is more likely to have a hiatal hernia and a marked increase in intragastric pressure and volume. Therefore these women are at great risk for regurgitation and aspiration (Endler, 1990).

Management of the obese woman during labor should focus on efforts to minimize oxygen consumption and maximize pulmonary function. Epidural analgesia administered during the first stage of labor can bring about decreased demand on the metabolic and respiratory systems and improved oxygenation. This is because pain causes the catecholamine levels to rise, which in turn causes

PLAN OF CARE *Nonpharmacologic Management of Discomfort*

NURSING DIAGNOSIS Pain related to physiologic response to labor

Expected Outcomes *Woman will express decrease in intensity of discomfort and experience satisfaction with her labor and birth performance.*

Nursing Interventions/*Rationales*

Assess whether woman and significant other have attended childbirth classes, her knowledge of labor process, and her current level of anxiety *to plan supportive strategies.*

Encourage support person to remain with woman in labor *to provide support and increase probability of response to comfort measures.*

Teach and/or review nonpharmacologic techniques available to decrease anxiety and pain during labor (i.e., focusing and feedback, breathing techniques, effleurage and sacral pressure) *to enhance chances of success in using techniques.*

Explore other techniques that the woman or significant other may have learned in childbirth classes (i.e., hypnosis, yoga, acupressure, biofeedback, therapeutic touch, aromatherapy, imaging, vocalizations) *to provide largest repertoire of coping strategies.*

Explore use of jet hydrotherapy if ordered by physician and if woman meets use criteria (i.e., vital signs within normal limits [WNL], cervix 4 to 5 cm dilated, active phase of first stage labor) *to aid relaxation and stimulate production of natural oxytocin.*

Explore use of transcutaneous nerve stimulation per physician order *to provide an increased perception of control over pain and an increase in release of endogenous opiates.*

Assist woman to change positions and to use pillows *to reduce stiffness, aid circulation, and promote comfort.*

Assess bladder for distention and encourage voiding often *to avoid bladder distention and subsequent discomfort.*

Encourage rest between contractions *to minimize fatigue.*

Keep woman and significant other informed about progress *to allay anxiety.*

Guide couple through the labor stages and phases, helping them use and modify comfort techniques that are appropriate to each phase *to ensure greatest effectiveness of techniques employed.*

From Wong D & Perry S: *Maternal child nursing care,* St Louis, 1998, Mosby.

---

cardiac output to increase. Effective epidural analgesia retards this rise in catecholamine levels.

Intravenous narcotics may be used during the first stage of labor. However, the dose and the effects must be monitored carefully because obese women are extremely sensitive to the respiratory depressant effects of narcotics (Endler, 1990). An epidural block during the second stage of labor provides complete pain relief and also supports cardiovascular function.

An epidural block is preferred to general anesthesia in obese women who must give birth by cesarean. Problems associated with general anesthesia in obese women include potential difficulties during intubation, a hypertensive effect of laryngoscopy and intubation, and aspiration and pulmonary complications. A spinal block may be used if there is insufficient time to induce an epidural block. Uterine displacement to prevent aortocaval compression is difficult to achieve in the obese woman in the supine position needed for cesarean birth. If the woman is extremely obese, a wedge may not be able to elevate the right hip enough to prevent compression. In this case, it may be necessary to physically lift the abdominal fat pad off the abdomen until the peritoneal cavity has been entered (Endler, 1990).

Postpartum hypothermia after analgesia and anesthesia. Hypothermia is defined as core body temperature of less than 35° C. During labor and immediately postpartum, women who have received pain medications are predisposed to hypothermia because of the combination of vasodilation that normally occurs during pregnancy and the effects of the administration of the analgesia and anesthesia.

Opiates/narcotics, barbiturates, tranquilizers, and antiemetics are thought to affect thermoregulation by increasing vasodilation and radiant loss; general anesthesia agents are thought to do so by depressing thermoregulation; and epidural and spinal anesthesia are thought to do so by inducing peripheral dilatation (Dunn et al., 1993). During labor, vaginal or cesarean birth, or immediately after birth women may experience shivering, hypotension, and respiratory distress. The hypothermia may result in cardiovascular, pulmonary, circulatory, hematologic, neurologic, or renal complications (Dunn et al., 1993). The nurse can minimize these complications by making sure that the birthing areas are warm, wet drapes and towels are removed, women are covered with warm blankets after birth, and hypothermia is recognized early. Explaining these effects to the woman and her support people will help allay concerns.

Evaluation

Evaluation of the effectiveness of care of the woman needing management of discomfort during labor and birth is based on the previously stated outcomes.

KEY POINTS

- The expected outcome of preparation for childbirth and parenting is "education for choice."
- Nonpharmacologic pain and stress management strategies are valuable for managing labor discomfort alone or in combination with pharmacologic methods.
- The gate-control theory of pain is the basis for many of the nonpharmacologic methods of pain relief.
- The type of analgesic or anesthetic to be used is determined in part by the stage of labor and the method of birth.
- Narcotic effects can be potentiated with ataractics.
- Naloxone and naltrexone are narcotic antagonists that can reverse narcotic effects, especially respiratory depression.
- Pharmacologic control of discomfort during labor requires collaboration among the health care providers and laboring woman.
- The nurse must understand various qualities of the medications, their expected effect, potential side effects, and methods of administration.
- An IV line and maternal hydration are essential during regional nerve blocks.
- Maternal analgesia and anesthesia potentially affect neonatal neurobehavioral response.
- The use of narcotic agonist-antagonist compounds in women with narcotic dependency may cause symptoms of narcotic withdrawal.
- General anesthesia is rarely used for vaginal birth, but it may be used for cesarean birth or whenever rapid anesthesia is needed in an emergency childbirth situation.

CRITICAL THINKING EXERCISES

1 *You are assigned to care for a Mexican woman in active labor who has her fists tightly clenched and is grimacing. She does not speak English. She is not making any kind of request for anything for the pain. You are convinced that discomfort should be avoided if possible.*

  a *Examine the assumptions the nurse may have about how women of different cultures exhibit reactions to pain.*

  b *Examine assumptions that both the nurse and Mexican woman may have about pain relief.*

CRITICAL THINKING EXERCISES—cont'd

  c *Propose arguments for and against use of pharmacologic agents for control of discomfort.*

  d *Formulate a plan of care for pain relief in this situation and justify your choice of interventions.*

2 *Talk to a woman of a culture different from yours who has experienced childbirth. Ask her to describe her reactions to pain, how she sought relief of the pain, the atmosphere of the childbirth setting, and the attitudes of the health care providers.*

  a *Analyze the way the atmosphere of the setting and the attitudes of the health care providers might have influenced the perceptions of pain in the woman.*

  b *Examine the childbirth setting where you are now assigned.*

   1) *What is the atmosphere of the setting, and what are the attitudes of the health care providers regarding the expression of pain by women of various cultures?*

   2) *Analyze the effect when the nurse's culture differs from that of the woman for whom she is caring.*

References

Alexander C & Steeful L: Biofeedback: Listen to the body, *RN* 58(8);51, 1995.

American College of Obstetrics and Gynecology: Obstetric analgesia and anesthesia. *Technical Bulletin, No 225,* Washington DC, 1996, ACOG.

Bradley R: *Husband-coached childbirth,* ed 3, New York, 1981, Harper & Collins.

Burnes E & Blamey C: Using aromatherapy in childbirth, *Nurs Times* 90(9):54: 1994.

Cassidy J: A picture perfect birth: guided imagery interrupts the pain/anxiety cycle, *RN* 56(6):45, 1993.

Chestnut D: Alternative regional anesthetic techniques: paracervical block, lumbar sympathetic block, pudendal block and perineal infiltration. In Chestnut D: *Obstetric anesthesia: principals and practice,* St Louis, 1994, Mosby.

Clark J, Queener S & Karb V: *Pharmacological basis of nursing practice,* ed 5, St Louis, 1996, Mosby.

Cunningham F et al.: *Williams obstetrics,* ed 20, Stamford, Conn, 1997, Appleton & Lange.

Dickason E, Silverman B & Kaplan J: *Maternal-infant nursing care,* ed 3, St Louis, 1998, Mosby.

Dick-Read G: *Childbirth without fear,* ed 5, New York, 1987, Harper & Collins.

Dunn P et al.: Maternal hypothermia: implications for obstetric nurses, *J Obstet Gynecol Neonatal Nurs* 23(3):238, 1993.

Endler G: The risk of anesthesia in obese parturients, *J Perinat* 10(2):175, 1990.

Endler G et al.: Anesthesia-related maternal mortality in Michigan, 1972-1984, *Am J Obstet Gynecol* 159(1):187, 1988.

Green J: Expectations and experiences of pain in labor: findings from a large prospective study, *Birth* 20(2):65, 1993.

Hamza J: Effect of epidural anesthesia on the fetus and the neonate, *Cah Anesthesiol* 42(2):265, 1994.

Hawkins J et al.: A reevaluation of the association between instrument delivery and epidural anesthesia, *Regional Anesthesia* 20(1):50, 1995.

Hood D & Dewan D: Anesthetic and obstetric outcome in morbidly obese parturients, *Anesthesiology* 79(6):1210, 1993.

Isenor L & Penny-MacGillivary T: Intravenous meperidine infusion for obstetric analgesia, *J Obstet Gynecol Neonatal Nurs* 22(4):349, 1993.

Jenkins M & Pritchard M: Hypnosis: practical applications and theoretical considerations, *Br J Obstet Gynecol* 100(3):221, 1993.

Jiménez S: Teaching acupressure for pregnancy and birth, *J Perinat Educ* 11(1):58, 1992.

Lamaze F: *Painless childbirth*, New York, 1972, Pocket Books.

Lowe N: The pain and discomfort of labor and birth, *J Obstet Gynecol Neonatal Nurs* 25(1):82, 1996.

Mackey M: Women's preparation for the childbirth experience, *Matern Child Nurs J* 19(2):143, 1990.

Mackey R: Discovering the healing power of therapeutic touch, *Am J Nurs* 95(4):26, 1995.

Manning J: Intrathecal narcotics: new approach for labor analgesia, *J Obstet Gynecol Neonatal Nurs* 25(3):221, 1996.

Olden A et al.: Patients' versus nurses' assessments of pain and sedation after cesarean section, *J Obstet Gynecol Neonatal Nurs* 24(2):137, 1995.

Potter P & Perry A: *Basic nursing: theory and practice*, ed 3, St Louis, 1995, Mosby.

Rush J et al.: The effects of whirlpool baths in labor: a randomized, controlled trial, *Birth*, 23(3):136, 1996.

Scherer R & Holzgreve W: Influence of epidural analgesia on fetal and neonatal well-being, *Eur J Obstet Gynecol Reprod Biol* 59(suppl):S17, 1995.

Schorn M, McAllister J & Blanco J: Water immersion and the effect on labor, *J Nurse Midwifery* 38(6):336, 1993.

Scott J et al.: *Danforth's obstetrics and gynecology*, ed 7, Philadelphia, 1994, JB Lippincott Co.

Sepkoski C et al.: The effects of maternal epidural anesthesia on neonatal behavior during the first month, *Dev Med Child Neurol* 34(12):1072, 1992.

Shapiro H et al.: *The Lamaze ready reference guide for labor*, ed 2, Washington DC, 1997, Chapter ASPO/Lamaze.

Simkin P: Reducing pain and enhancing progress in labor: a guide to nonpharmacologic methods of maternity caregivers, *Birth* 22(3):161, 1995.

Thorp J & Breedlove G: Epidural analgesia in labor: an evaluation of risks and benefits. *Birth* 23(2):63, 1996.

Tisserand M: *Aromatherapy for women*, London, 1990, Thorsons.

Valnet J: *The practice of aromatherapy*, Rochester, Vt, 1990, Healing Arts Press.

Villarruel A: Mexican-American cultural meanings, expressions, self-care and dependent-care actions associated with experiences of pain, *Res Nurs Health* 18(5):427, 1995.

Wakefield M: Systemic analgesia: opioids, ketamine, and inhalation agents. In Chestnut, D: *Obstetric anesthesia: principles and practice*, St Louis, 1994, Mosby.

Weber S: Cultural aspects of pain in childbearing women, *J Obstet Gynecol Neonatal Nurs* 25(1):67, 1996.

Wong D & Perry S: *Maternal child nursing care*, St Louis, 1998, Mosby.

Youngstrom P et al.: Epidurals redefined in analgesia and anesthesia: a distinction with a difference, *J Obstet Gynecol Neonatal Nurs* 25(4):350, 1996.

CHAPTER

14

Fetal Monitoring

SUSAN M. TUCKER

LEARNING OBJECTIVES

- Define the key terms.
- Explain baseline fetal heart rate and variability and periodic and episodic changes.
- Compare fetal heart rate monitoring by intermittent auscultation and external and internal electronic methods.
- Differentiate between reassuring and nonreassuring fetal heart rate patterns, and identify appropriate nursing interventions.
- Describe the care of the woman with electronic fetal heart rate monitoring.

KEY TERMS

accelerations
amnioinfusion
baseline fetal heart rate (FHR)
bradycardia
decelerations
electronic fetal monitoring (EFM)
episodic changes in FHR
hypoxemia
hypoxia
intermittent auscultation
intrauterine pressure catheter (IUPC)
nonreassuring FHR patterns
periodic changes in FHR
prolonged decelerations
reassuring FHR patterns
spiral electrode
tachycardia
tocolysis
tocotransducer
ultrasound transducer
uteroplacental insufficiency
variability

*S*ince the 1970s, when fetal monitoring first made its debut, considerable expertise has been gained in the assessment of fetal hemodynamic and oxygen status. Evaluation of the baseline fetal heart rate (FHR) remains a complex task,

however, because of the number of factors that must be considered and the variations in the "normal" fetal response to labor. Ways of describing FHR patterns have been based on terminology coined by equipment manufacturers, researchers, and authors and have varied by region in the country, institution, and health care provider.

The lack of agreement on definitions and interpretations of FHR patterns has limited the study of efficacy and validity of electronic fetal monitoring (EFM). In 1995 a research-planning workshop was held to develop research guidelines for EFM interpretation. Experts in the field, including those in medicine, nursing, epidemiology, basic science, and the general public, participated. The first document to be published by the group was a proposed nomenclature system for EFM interpretation. This document presented standardized definitions for fetal heart rate monitoring (National Institute of Child Health and Human Development Research Planning Workshop, 1997). These definitions will be tested for reliability and accuracy and will be refined based on results of the tests.

Even though testing of the definitions has not yet been completed, some effect on clinical practice is likely. For that reason, this chapter includes the new definitions and discussion of the current systems of interpretation of EFM. Practitioners who continue to use the established terminology during this period of transition should continue to use guidelines developed by the Association of Women's Health, Obstetric, and Neonatal Nurses (AWHONN, 1993) and the American College of Obstetricians and Gynecologists (1995). Practitioners who wish to use the new terminology will need to communicate with other health care providers about the use of the new terminology instead of established definitions (Harvey, 1997). They will also need to make changes in their practice as the definitions are refined through testing. All perinatal health care providers need to keep abreast of the new developments in EFM technology and knowledge to ensure the best possible outcomes for mothers and newborns.

▌BASIS FOR MONITORING

The Fetal Response

Because labor represents a period of physiologic stress for the fetus, frequent monitoring of fetal health is part of the nursing care during labor. The fetal oxygen supply must be maintained during labor to prevent fetal compromise and promote newborn health after birth. The fetal oxygen supply can be reduced in a number of ways:

1. Reduction of blood flow through the maternal vessels as a result of maternal hypertension or hypotension (systolic blood pressure of 100 mm Hg in brachial artery is necessary for placental perfusion).
2. Reduction of the oxygen content of the maternal blood as a result of hemorrhagic hypovolemia or severe anemia.
3. Alterations in fetal circulation, occurring with compression of the cord, placental separation, or head compression (head compression causes increased intracranial pressure and vagal nerve stimulation with slowing of the heart rate).
4. Reduction in blood flow to the intervillous space in the placenta secondary to uterine hypertonus (generally caused by excessive exogenous oxytocin) or as a result of placental vasculature deterioration associated with maternal disorders such as hypertension and diabetes.

Fetal well-being during labor can be measured by the *response of the FHR to uterine contractions*. In general, a **reassuring FHR pattern** is characterized by the following:

- A baseline FHR in the normal range of 110 to 160 beats per minute with no periodic changes and a moderate baseline variability
- Early decelerations
- Accelerations with fetal movement

Characteristically, a normal uterine activity pattern in labor includes contractions that occur every 2 to 5 minutes with the following characteristics: duration is less than 90 seconds, intensity is less than 100 mm Hg pressure, time between the end of one and the start of another is 30 seconds or more, and average intrauterine pressure between contractions is 15 mm Hg or less.

Fetal Compromise

The goals of intrapartum FHR monitoring are to identify and differentiate the reassuring patterns from the nonreassuring patterns, which are indicative of fetal compromise.

Nonreassuring patterns are those associated with fetal **hypoxemia,** which is a deficiency of oxygen in the arterial blood and if uncorrected can deteriorate to severe fetal **hypoxia,** which is an inadequate supply of oxygen at the cellular level. Nonreassuring FHR patterns include the following:

- Progressive increase or decrease in baseline rate
- Tachycardia of 160 beats per minute or more
- Progressive decrease in baseline variability
- Severe variable decelerations (FHR less than 70 beats per minute lasting longer than 30 to 60 seconds, with rising baseline, decreasing variability, or slow return to baseline)

- Late decelerations of any magnitude, especially those that are repetitive and uncorrectable, with decreasing variability or rising baseline FHR
- Absence of FHR variability
- Prolonged deceleration (greater than 60 to 90 seconds)
- Severe bradycardia (less than 70 beats per minute.

The nurse's role is to continually assess whether the FHR pattern is reassuring, which reflects adequate fetal oxygenation. When the pattern is nonreassuring the nurse must discriminate between those patterns that are indicative of mild fetal hypoxemia and other nonreassuring patterns that indicate severe fetal hypoxia. The nursing interventions to be taken when encountering nonreassuring patterns are described in detail in this chapter.

MONITORING TECHNIQUES

Intermittent Auscultation

Intermittent auscultation of the fetal heart rate can be performed with a Leff scope, DeLee-Hillis fetoscope, or ultrasound device. If a Leff scope is used, the domed side should be opened to the connective tubing to the ear pieces. The domed side is then applied to the maternal abdomen. The fetoscope is applied over the listener's head because bone conduction amplifies the fetal heart sounds for counting. The ultrasound device transmits ultrahigh frequency sound waves reflecting movement of the fetal heart and converts these sounds into an electronic signal that can be counted (Fig. 14-1).

The procedure for performing auscultation is as follows:

1. Perform Leopold's maneuvers by palpating the maternal abdomen to identify fetal presentation and position.
2. Place the listening device over the area of maximum intensity and clarity of the fetal heart sounds to obtain the clearest and loudest sound, which is easiest to count.

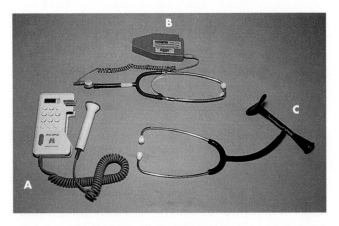

Fig. 14-1 **A**, Ultrasound fetoscope. **B**, Ultrasound stethoscope. **C**, DeLee-Hillis fetoscope. (Courtesy Michael S. Clement, MD, Mesa, Ariz.)

3. Palpate the abdomen for the absence of uterine activity to be able to count the FHR between contractions.
4. Count the maternal radial pulse at the same time as listening to the FHR to differentiate it from the fetal rate.
5. Count the FHR for 30 to 60 seconds between contractions to identify the baseline rate. This rate can only be assessed during the absence of uterine activity.
6. Auscultate the FHR during a contraction and for 30 seconds after the end of the contraction to identify any increases or decreases in FHR in response to the contraction.

The method and frequency of fetal surveillance during labor will vary depending on maternal-fetal risk factors and the preference of the facility. In the absence of risk factors, the standard practice is to auscultate the FHR as follows:

- First stage
  Latent phase: every 60 minutes
  Active phase: every 30 minutes
- Second stage
  Every 15 minutes

If risk factors are present, the FHR is auscultated as follows:

- First stage
  Latent phase: every 30 minutes
  Active phase: every 15 minutes
- Second stage
  Every 5 minutes

> **NURSE ALERT** *When the FHR is auscultated and documented, it is inappropriate to use the descriptive terms associated with electronic fetal monitoring because the majority of the terms are visual descriptions of the patterns produced on the monitor tracing. However, terms that are numerically defined, such as bradycardia and tachycardia, can be used.*

The ideal method of fetal assessment during labor continues to be debated. Results from multiple research studies indicate that both intermittent auscultation of the FHR at the frequencies just given and electronic FHR monitoring are associated with similar fetal outcomes (Thacker, Stroup & Peterson, 1995). However, the advantage of intermittent auscultation is that it is a high-touch, low-technologic method of assessing fetal status during labor that places fewer restrictions on maternal activity. Because childbirth is a natural process, most women and fetuses fare well with minimal intervention and periodic assessment.

Every effort should be made to use the method of fetal assessment the woman desires. However, auscultation of the FHR in accordance with the frequency guidelines just given may be difficult in today's busy labor and birth units. When used as the primary method of fetal assessment, auscultation requires a one-to-one nurse-to-fetus staffing ratio (for example, a woman with twins would require two primary nurses). If acuity and census change so that auscultation standards are no longer met, the nurse must inform the physician or nurse-midwife that continuous EFM will be used until staffing can be arranged to meet the standards.

The woman can become anxious if the examiner cannot readily count the fetal heartbeats. It often takes time for the inexperienced listener to locate the heartbeat and find the area of maximum intensity. If it takes considerable time to locate the fetal heartbeats, the examiner can reassure the mother by offering her an opportunity to also listen to them once they have been heard. If the examiner cannot locate the fetal heartbeat, assistance should be requested. In some cases, ultrasound can be used to help locate the fetal heartbeat. Seeing the FHR on the ultrasound screen will be reassuring to the mother if there was initial difficulty in locating the best area for auscultation.

Electronic Fetal Monitoring

There are two modes of **electronic fetal monitoring** (EFM). The external mode employs the use of external transducers placed on the woman's abdomen to assess heart rate and uterine activity. The internal mode uses a **spiral electrode** applied to the fetal presenting part to assess the fetal ECG and the **intrauterine pressure catheter (IUPC)** to assess uterine activity and pressure. A brief description contrasting the external and internal modes of EFM is provided in Table 14-1.

External monitoring

Separate transducers are used to monitor the FHR and uterine contractions (Fig. 14-2, *A*). The **ultrasound transducer** acts through the reflection of high-frequency sound waves from a moving interface, in this case the fetal heart and valves. Therefore short-term variability and beat-to-beat changes in the FHR cannot be assessed by this method. It is also difficult to reproduce a continuous and precise record of the FHR because of artifacts introduced by fetal and maternal movement. The FHR tracing is printed on a standard formatted FHR monitor paper. The standard paper speed is 3 cm/min. Once the nurse locates the area of maximum intensity of FHR, conductive gel is applied to the surface of the ultrasound transducer, and the transducer is positioned over this area.

The **tocotransducer** (tocodynamometer) measures uterine activity transabdominally. The device is placed over the fundus above the umbilicus. Uterine contractions or fetal movement depress a pressure-sensitive surface on the side next to the abdomen. The tocotransducer can measure and record the frequency, regularity, and duration of uterine contractions but not their intensity. This method is especially valuable during the first stage of labor in women with intact membranes, or it can be used for antepartum testing.

TABLE 14-1 *External and Internal Modes of Monitoring*

EXTERNAL MODE	INTERNAL MODE
FHR	
Ultrasound transducer: High-frequency sound waves reflect mechanical action of the fetal heart. Used during the antepartum and intrapartum period. Noninvasive. Does not require rupture of membranes or cervical dilatation.	*Spiral electrode:* This electrode converts the fetal ECG as obtained from the presenting part of the FHR via a cardiotachometer. This method can only be used when membranes are ruptured and cervix sufficiently dilated during the intrapartum period. Electrode penetrates into fetal presenting part by 1.5 mm and must be attached securely to ensure a good signal.
UTERINE ACTIVITY	
Tocotransducer: This instrument monitors frequency and duration of contractions by means of pressure sensing device applied to the maternal abdomen. Used during both the antepartum and intrapartum periods.	*Intrauterine pressure catheter (IUPC):* This instrument monitors the frequency, duration, and intensity of contractions. There are two types of IUPCs. One is a fluid-filled system, and the other is a solid catheter. Both measure intrauterine pressure at the catheter tip and convert the pressure into millimeters of mercury on the uterine activity panel of the strip chart. Both can be used only when membranes are ruptured and the cervix sufficiently dilated during the intrapartum period.

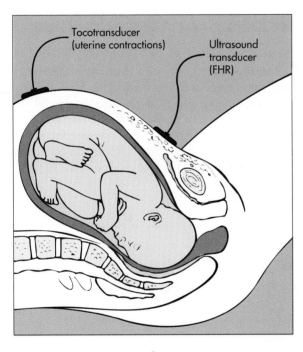

A

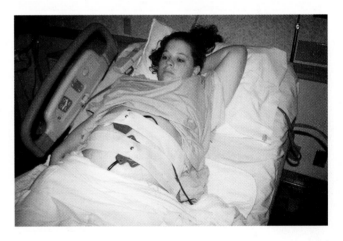

B

Fig. 14-2 **A,** External noninvasive fetal monitoring using tocotransducer and ultrasound transducer. **B,** Ultrasound transducer is placed below umbilicus, over the area where fetal heart rate is best heard, and tocotransducer is placed on uterine fundus. (Courtesy Marjorie Pyle, RNC, Lifecircle, Costa Mesa, Calif.)

The equipment is easily applied by the nurse, but it must be repositioned as the woman or fetus changes position (see Fig. 14-2, *B*). The woman is asked to assume a semisitting position or lateral position. The equipment is removed periodically to wash the applicator sites and to give back rubs.

This type of monitoring confines the woman to bed. Portable telemetry monitors allow observation of the FHR and uterine contraction patterns by means of centrally located electronic display stations. These portable units permit the woman to walk around during electronic monitoring.

Internal monitoring

The technique of continuous internal monitoring provides an accurate appraisal of fetal well-being during labor (Fig. 14-3). For this type of monitoring, the membranes must be ruptured, the cervix sufficiently dilated, and the presenting part low enough for placement of the electrode. A small spiral electrode attached to the presenting part yields a continuous FHR on the fetal monitor strip. Internal monitoring of the FHR may be implemented without internal monitoring of uterine activity.

To monitor uterine activity, a solid or fluid-filled intrauterine pressure catheter (IUPC) is introduced into the uterine cavity. A solid catheter has a pressure-sensitive tip that measures changes in intrauterine pressure. A catheter filled with sterile water can also be used. As the uterus contracts, it compresses the catheter, placing pressure on the monitor strain gauge or pressure transducer. The pressures sensed by both types of catheters are then converted into a pressure reading in millimeters of mercury. The normal range during a contraction is 50 to 75 mm Hg. The display of FHR and uterine activity on the chart paper differs for the two modes of electronic monitoring (Fig. 14-4). Note that each small square represents 10 seconds; each larger box of 6 squares equals 1 minute when the monitor is set to run at 3 cm/min.

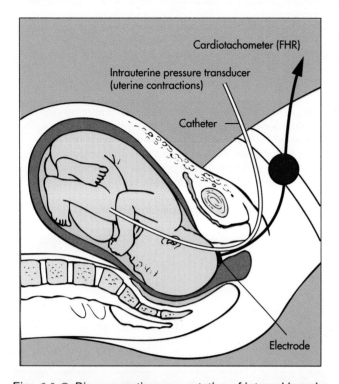

Fig. **14-3** Diagrammatic representation of internal invasive fetal monitoring with intrauterine pressure catheter and spiral electrode in place (membranes ruptured and cervix dilated).

FETAL HEART RATE PATTERNS

Baseline Fetal Heart Rate

The intrinsic rhythmicity of the fetal heart and the fetal autonomic nervous system control the FHR. An increase in sympathetic response results in acceleration of the FHR. An augmentation in parasympathetic response produces a slowing of the FHR. Usually, a balanced increase of sympathetic and parasympathetic response occurs during contractions, with no observable change in the FHR.

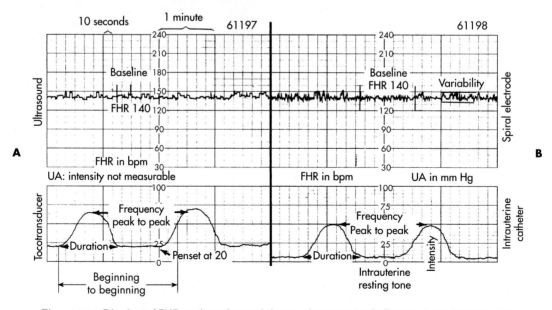

Fig. **14-4** Display of FHR and uterine activity on chart paper. **A,** External mode with ultrasound and tocotransducer as signal source. **B,** Internal mode with spiral electrode and intrauterine catheter as signal source. (From Tucker S: *Pocket guide to fetal monitoring and assessment,* ed 3, St Louis, 1996, Mosby.)

TABLE 14-2 *Tachycardia and Bradycardia*

TACHYCARDIA	BRADYCARDIA
DEFINITION	
FHR above 160 beats per minute lasting longer than 10 min	FHR below 110 beats per minute lasting longer than 10 min
CAUSE	
Early fetal hypoxemia	Late fetal hypoxia/hypoxemia
Maternal fever	Beta-adrenergic blocking drugs (propranolol; anesthetics
Parasympatholytic drugs (atropine, hydroxyzine)	for epidural, spinal, caudal, and pudendal blocks)
Beta-sympathomimetic drugs (ritodrine, isoxsuprine)	Maternal hypotension
Intraamniotic infection	Prolonged umbilical cord compression
Maternal hyperthyroidism	Fetal congenital heart block
Fetal anemia	Maternal hypothermia
Fetal heart failure	Prolonged maternal hypoglycemia
Fetal cardiac dysrhythmias	
Street drugs (cocaine, methamphetamines)	
CLINICAL SIGNIFICANCE	
Persistent tachycardia in absence of periodic changes does not appear serious in terms of neonatal outcome (especially true if tachycardia is associated with maternal fever); tachycardia is a nonreassuring sign when associated with late decelerations, severe variable decelerations, or absence of variability.	Bradycardia with moderate variability and absence of periodic changes is not a sign of fetal compromise if FHR remains above 80 beats per minute; bradycardia caused by hypoxia is a nonreassuring sign when associated with loss of variability and late decelerations.
NURSING INTERVENTION	
Dependent on cause; reduce maternal fever with antipyretics as ordered and cooling measures; oxygen at 8 to 10 L/min per face mask may be of some value; carry out health care provider's orders based on alleviating cause.	Dependent on cause; intervention not warranted in fetus with heart block diagnosed by ECG; oxygen at 8 to 10 L/min per face mask may be of some value; carry out health care provider's orders based on alleviating cause. Scalp stimulation may be performed to determine whether or not the fetus has the ability to compensate physiologically for stress (FHR will accelerate).

Baseline fetal heart rate is the average rate during a 10 minute segment that excludes periodic or episodic changes, periods of marked variability, and segments of the baseline that differ by more than 25 beats per minute (National Institute, 1997). The normal range at term is 110 to 160 beats per minute.

Tachycardia is a baseline FHR above 160 beats per minute. It can be considered an early sign of fetal hypoxia and can result from maternal or fetal infection, such as prolonged rupture of membranes with amnionitis; maternal hyperthyroidism or fetal anemia; or in response to drugs such as atropine, hydroxyzine (Vistaril), terbutaline, or street drugs such as cocaine or methamphetamines.

Bradycardia is a baseline FHR below 110 beats per minute. (Bradycardia should be distinguished from prolonged deceleration patterns, which are periodic changes described later in this chapter.) It can be considered a later sign of fetal hypoxia and is known to occur before fetal demise. Bradycardia can result from placental transfer of drugs such as anesthetics, prolonged compression of the umbilical cord, maternal hypothermia, and maternal

hypotension. Maternal supine hypotensive syndrome, caused by uterine pressure (the weight of the gravid uterus) on the vena cava, decreases the return of blood flow to the maternal heart, which then reduces maternal cardiac output and blood pressure. These responses in the mother subsequently result in a decrease in the FHR and fetal bradycardia. Table 14-2 contrasts tachycardia with bradycardia.

Variability of the FHR can be described as irregular fluctuations in the baseline FHR of 2 cycles per minute or greater (National Institute, 1997). Variability has been described as short term (beat to beat) or long term (rhythmic waves or cycles from baseline). The current definition for research does not distinguish between short-term and long-term variability because in actual practice, they are viewed together (National Institute, 1997). This definition does identify four ranges of variability as seen in Fig. 14-5. These are based on visualization of the amplitude in the peak-to-trough in beats per minute and include the following:
- Absent or undetected variability
- Minimal variability (greater than undetected but not more than 5 beats per minute)

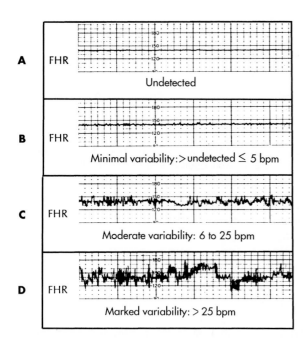

Fig. 14-5 Fetal heart rate variability. **A,** Undetected. **B,** Minimal. **C,** Moderate. **D,** Marked. (Modified from Tucker S: *Pocket guide to fetal monitoring and assessment,* ed 3, St Louis, 1996, Mosby.)

- Moderate variability (6 to 25 beats per minute)
- Marked variability (greater than 25 beats per minute)

A sinusoidal pattern, a regular smooth wavelike pattern, is not included in the current research definition of FHR variability.

Absence of or undetected variability is considered non-reassuring. Decreased variability can result from fetal hypoxemia and acidosis, as well as from certain drugs that depress the central nervous system (CNS), including analgesics, narcotics (meperidine [Demerol]), barbiturates (secobarbital [Seconal] and pentobarbital [Nembutal]), tranquilizers (diazepam [Valium]), ataractics (promethazine [Phenergan]), and general anesthetics. In addition, a temporary decrease in variability can occur when the fetus is in a sleep state. These sleep states do not usually last longer than 30 minutes. Table 14-3 contrasts key differences between increased and decreased variability.

Periodic and Episodic Changes in Fetal Heart Rate

Changes from baseline patterns in FHR are categorized as periodic or episodic. **Periodic changes** are those that occur with uterine contractions. **Episodic** (non-periodic) **changes** are those that are not associated with uterine contractions. These patterns include accelerations and decelerations (National Institute, 1997).

Accelerations

Acceleration of the FHR is defined as a visually apparent abrupt increase in FHR above the baseline rate. The increase is equal to or greater than 15 beats per minute and lasts 15 seconds or more, with the return to baseline less than 2 minutes from the beginning of the acceleration. In preterm gestations, the definition of an acceleration is a peak greater than or equal to 10 beats per minute above baseline for at least 10 seconds. Acceleration of the FHR for more than 10 minutes is considered a baseline change.

Accelerations can be periodic or episodic. Accelerations that are periodic are caused by dominance of the sympathetic nervous response and are usually encountered with breech presentations (Fig. 14-6, *A*). Pressure of the contraction applied to the fetal buttocks results in accelerations, whereas pressure applied to the head results in decelerations. Accelerations may occur, however, during the second stage of labor in cephalic presentations. Accelerations (Fig. 14-6, *B*) of the FHR that are episodic occur during fetal movement and are indications of fetal well-being.

Decelerations

Decelerations, caused by dominance of parasympathetic response, may be benign or nonreassuring. The three types of decelerations encountered during labor are early, late, and variable. FHR decelerations are described by their relation to the onset and the end of a contraction and by their shape.

Early deceleration of the FHR is a visually apparent gradual increase in and return to baseline FHR in response to compression of the fetal head. It is a normal and usually benign finding (Fig. 14-7, *A*) (National Institute, 1997). The deceleration is characterized by a uniform shape and an early onset corresponding to the rise in intrauterine pressure as the uterus contracts. When present, early deceleration usually occurs during the first stage of labor when the cervix is dilated 4 to 7 cm. Early deceleration is sometimes seen during the second stage when the patient is pushing. Early decelerations as a response to fetal head compression can occur during vaginal examinations, as a result of fundal pressure, during placement of the internal mode for fetal monitoring, and during uterine contractions.

Because early decelerations are considered a benign pattern, interventions are not necessary. The value of identifying early decelerations is to be able to distinguish them from late or variable decelerations, which can be nonreassuring and for which interventions are appropriate. Table 14-4 contrasts accelerations of FHR with early decelerations.

Uteroplacental insufficiency causes late decelerations. *Late deceleration* of the FHR is a visually apparent gradual decrease in and return to baseline FHR associated with uterine contractions (National Institute, 1997). The deceleration begins after the contraction has started, and the lowest point of the deceleration occurs after the peak of the contraction. Usually the deceleration does not return to baseline until after the contraction is over (Fig. 14-7).

TABLE 14-3 *Increased and Decreased Variability*

INCREASED VARIABILITY	DECREASED VARIABILITY
CAUSE	
Early mild hypoxia	Hypoxia/acidosis
Fetal stimulation by the following:	CNS depressants
Uterine palpation	Analgesics/narcotics
Uterine contractions	Meperidine (Demerol)
Fetal activity	Alphaprodine (Nisentil)
Maternal activity	Morphine
Street drugs (e.g., cocaine and methamphetamines)	Pentazocine (Talwin)
	Barbiturates
	Secobarbital (Seconal)
	Pentobarbital (Nembutal)
	Amobarbital (Amytal)
	Tranquilizers
	Diazepam (Valium)
	Ataractics
	Promethazine (Phenergan)
	Propiomazine (Largon)
	Hydroxyzine (Vistaril)
	Promazine (Sparine)
	Parasympatholytics
	Atropine
	General anesthetics
	Prematurity
	Fetal sleep cycles
	Congenital abnormalities
	Fetal cardiac arrhythmias
CLINICAL SIGNIFICANCE	
Significance of marked variability not known; increased variability from a previous average variability is earliest FHR sign of mild hypoxemia	Benign when associated with periodic fetal sleep states, which last 20 to 30 min; if caused by drugs, variability usually increases as drugs are excreted
	Decreased variability considered nonreassuring if caused by hypoxia/asphyxia; occurring with late decelerations, decreased variability is associated with fetal acidosis and low Apgar scores
NURSING INTERVENTION	
Observe FHR tracing carefully for any nonreassuring patterns including decreasing variability and late decelerations; if using external mode of monitoring, consider using internal mode (spiral electrode) for a more accurate tracing	Dependent on cause; intervention not warranted if associated with fetal sleep states or temporarily associated with CNS depressants; consider performing external stimulation or scalp stimulation during a vaginal exam to elicit an acceleration of FHR or return to average variability; consider application of internal mode (spiral electrode); assist health care provider with fetal blood sampling for pH if ordered; prepare for birth if so indicated by the primary health care provider

Late deceleration patterns, when persistent or recurrent, usually indicate fetal hypoxia because of deficient placental perfusion. Persistent and repetitive late decelerations are associated with fetal hypoxia and acidosis. They should be considered an ominous sign when they are uncorrectable, especially if they are associated with decreased variability and tachycardia. Late decelerations caused by maternal supine hypotensive syndrome are usually correctable when the woman turns to her side to displace the weight of the gravid uterus off the vena cava. This allows a better return of maternal blood flow to the heart, which increases cardiac output and blood pressure.

Late decelerations caused by uteroplacental insufficiency can result from uterine hyperstimulation with oxytocin, pregnancy-induced hypertension (PIH), postmature syndrome, amnionitis, small-for-gestational-age (SGA) fetus,

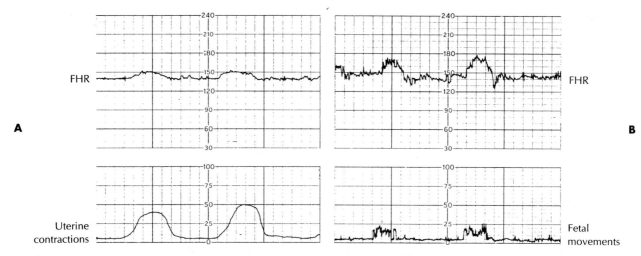

Fig. 14-6 A, Acceleration of FHR with uterine contractions. **B,** Acceleration of FHR with fetal movement. (From Tucker S: *Pocket guide to fetal monitoring and assessment,* ed 3, St Louis, 1996, Mosby.)

maternal diabetes, placenta previa, abruptio placentae, conduction anesthetics (producing maternal hypotension), maternal cardiac disease, and maternal anemia.

Variable deceleration is defined as a visual abrupt decrease in FHR below baseline. The decrease is usually more than 15 beats per minute, lasts at least 15 seconds, and usually returns to baseline in less than 2 minutes from the time of onset (National Institute, 1997). Variable decelerations occur any time during the uterine contracting phase and are caused by compression of the umbilical cord. Table 14-5 contrasts late deceleration with variable deceleration. The appearance of variable deceleration patterns differs from the early and late decelerations, which mirror the uterine contraction. In contrast, variable decelerations are often U or V shaped, characterized by a rapid descent and ascent to and from the nadir (or depth) of the deceleration (see Fig. 14-7). A transitory acceleration of the FHR preceding and following the deceleration is known as "shouldering" and indicates an appropriate compensatory response to the stress of umbilical cord compression.

Variable decelerations may be related to partial, brief compression of the cord. If encountered in the first stage of labor, they can usually be eliminated by changing the woman's position, such as from one side to the other. Oxygen administration to the woman by face mask is sometimes helpful. Variable decelerations most often occur during the second stage of labor as a result of cord compression during fetal descent. Variable decelerations are associated with neonatal depression only when cord compression is severe or prolonged (e.g., tight nuchal cord, short cord, knot in cord, prolapsed cord). Variable decelerations occur in about half of all labors and are usually temporary and correctable by changing the mother's position. A nonreassuring sign is variable deceleration with a slow return to baseline and decreasing variability or deceleration below 70 beats per minute for longer than 60 seconds.

The return to baseline may occur with an "overshoot," a term used to describe an FHR that goes above the baseline and then returns to baseline.

Prolonged decelerations

Prolonged deceleration is a visually apparent decrease in FHR below the baseline 15 beats per minute or more and lasting more than 2 minutes but less than 10 minutes. A deceleration lasting more than 10 minutes is considered a baseline change (National Institute, 1997). Generally, the benign causes are pelvic examination, application of spiral electrode, rapid fetal descent, and sustained maternal Valsalva's maneuver.

Progressive severe variable decelerations, sudden umbilical cord prolapse, and hypotension produced by spinal or epidural anesthesia cause other prolonged decelerations. Paracervical anesthesia, a tetanic contraction, and maternal hypoxia (which may occur during a seizure) often produce prolonged decelerations. When the duration of the deceleration is longer than 1 to 2 minutes, a loss of variability with rebound tachycardia usually occurs. Occasionally, a period of late decelerations follows. These responses normally clear spontaneously. However, when a prolonged deceleration is seen late in the course of severe variable decelerations or during a prolonged series of late decelerations, the prolonged deceleration may occur just before fetal death.

Nurses should notify the physician or nurse midwife immediately and initiate appropriate treatment when they see a prolonged deceleration.

I CARE MANAGEMENT

The care given to women being monitored by EFM or auscultation is the same as that given to the woman experiencing a low-risk labor. Care of the woman being

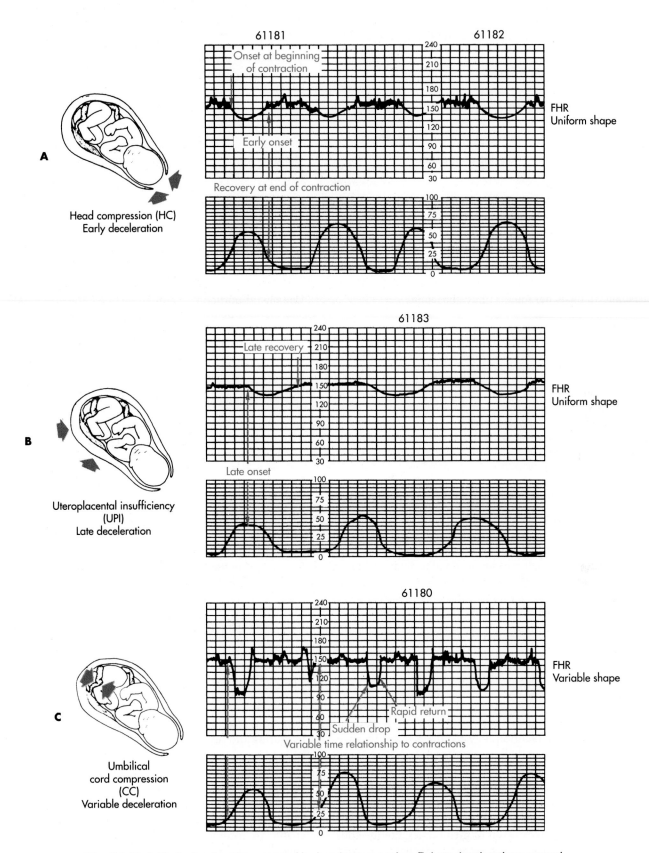

Fig. 14-7 A, Early decelerations caused by head compression. B, Late decelerations caused by uteroplacental insufficiency. C, Variable decelerations caused by cord compression. (From Tucker S: *Pocket guide to fetal monitoring and assessment,* ed 3, St Louis, 1996, Mosby.)

TABLE 14-4 *Acceleration and Early Deceleration*

ACCELERATION	EARLY DECELERATION
DESCRIPTION	
Visually apparent increase of FHR above baseline (see Fig. 14-6)	Transitory decrease of FHR below baseline concurrent with uterine contractions (see Fig. 14-7, *A*)
SHAPE	
May resemble shape of uterine contraction	Uniform shape; mirror image of uterine contraction
ONSET	
Onset to peak <30 sec; often precedes or occurs simultaneously with uterine contraction	In most cases onset is at beginning of contraction
RECOVERY	
Less than 2 minutes from onset	By end of contraction as uterine pressure returns to its resting tone
AMPLITUDE	
Usually 15 beats per minute above baseline	Usually proportional to amplitude of contraction; rarely decelerates below 100 beats per minute
BASELINE	
Usually associated with average baseline variability	Usually associated with average baseline variability
OCCURRENCE	
Variable; may be repetitive with each contraction	Repetitious (occurs with each contraction); usually between 4 and 7 cm dilatation and in second stage of labor
CAUSE	

Spontaneous fetal movement
Vaginal examination
Electrode application
Breech presentation
Occiput posterior position
Uterine contractions
Fundal pressure
Abdominal palpation
	Head compression resulting from following:
	  Uterine contractions
	  Vaginal examination
	  Fundal pressure
	  Placement of internal mode of monitoring

CLINICAL SIGNIFICANCE	
Acceleration with fetal movement signifies fetal well-being representing fetal alertness or arousal states	Reassuring pattern not associated with fetal hypoxemia, acidosis, or low Apgar scores
NURSING INTERVENTION	
None required	None required

monitored by internal methods may vary. FHR pattern recognition and intervention may require a nurse to have additional education and clinical experience.

Assessment and Nursing Diagnoses

The assessment of the patient includes the maternal temperature, pulse, respiratory rate, blood pressure, position, comfort, voiding pattern, status of membranes, uterine contraction pattern, cervical effacement and dilatation, and emotional status. The fetal assessment includes the fetal pre-

sentation, fetal position, FHR, and identification of both reassuring and nonreassuring FHR patterns. A checklist may be used by the nurse to assess the FHR (Box 14-1). All of the assessment information must be documented in the patient's medical record.

Evaluation of the EFM equipment must also be done to ensure that the equipment is working properly and to enable an accurate assessment of the woman and fetus. A checklist for fetal monitoring equipment can be used to evaluate the equipment functions (Box 14-2).

TABLE 14-5 *Late Deceleration versus Variable Deceleration*

	LATE DECELERATION	VARIABLE DECELERATION
Description	Transitory decrease in FHR below baseline rate in contracting phase (see Fig. 14-7, *B*)	Abrupt transitory decrease in FHR that is variable in duration, intensity, and timing related to onset of contractions (Fig. 14-7, *C*)
Shape	Uniform: mirror image of uterine contraction; may be deep or shallow	Variable: characterized by sudden drop in FHR in V, U, or W shape
Onset	Late in contraction phase; after peak of contraction: low point of deceleration occurs well after peak of contraction	Variable times in contracting phase; often preceded by transitory acceleration
Recovery	Well after end of contraction	Return to baseline is rapid, sometimes with transitory acceleration or acceleration immediately preceding and following deceleration (shouldering or "overshoot"); slow return to baseline with severe variable decelerations
Deceleration	Usually proportional to amplitude of contraction; rarely decelerates below 100 beats per minute	*Mild:* decelerates to any level, less than 30 sec with abrupt return to baseline *Moderate:* decelerates above 80 beats per minute, any duration with abrupt return to baseline *Severe:* decelerates below 60 beats per minute for greater than 60 sec, with slow return to baseline
Baseline	Often associated with loss of variability and increasing baseline rate	Mild variables usually associated with average baseline variability; moderate and severe variables often associated with decreasing variability and increasing baseline rate
Occurrence	Occurs with each contraction; may be observed at any time during labor	Variable: commonly observed late in labor with fetal descent and pushing

Cause	Uteroplacental insufficiency caused by the following:
	  Uterine hyperactivity or hypertonicity
	  Maternal supine hypotension
	  Epidural or spinal anesthesia
	  Placenta previa
	  Abruptio placentae
	  Hypertensive disorders
	  Postmaturity
	  Intrauterine growth restriction
	  Diabetes mellitus
	  Intraamniotic infection
		Umbilical cord compression caused by the following:
		  Maternal position with cord between fetus and maternal pelvis
		  Cord around fetal neck, arm, leg, or other body part
		  Short cord
		  Knot in cord
		  Prolapsed cord

Clinical significance	Nonreassuring, worrisome pattern associated with fetal hypoxemia, acidemia, and low Apgar scores: considered ominous if persistent and uncorrected, especially when associated with fetal tachycardia and loss of variability	Variable decelerations occur in about 50% of all labors and usually are transient, correctable, and not associated with low Apgar scores; mild variable decelerations are reassuring: decelerations progressing from moderate to severe are associated with fetal acidemia, hypoxemia, and low Apgar scores; severe variable decelerations with average baseline variability just before birth are usually well tolerated
Nursing intervention	Change maternal position (lateral) Correct maternal hypotension by elevating legs Increase rate of maintenance IV; administer vasopressors Discontinue oxytocin if infusing Administer oxygen at 8 to 10 L/min with tight face mask Fetal scalp or acoustic stimulation Assist with birth (cesarean or vaginal assisted) if pattern cannot be corrected	Change maternal position (side to side); if decelerations are severe, proceed with following measures; Discontinue oxytocin if infusing, consider tocolysis Administer oxygen at 8 to 10 L/min with tight face mask Assist with vaginal or speculum examination If cord is prolapsed, examiner will elevate fetal presenting part with cord between gloved fingers until birth is accomplished Assist with amnioinfusion if ordered Assist with birth (vaginal assisted or cesarean) if pattern cannot be corrected

| BOX 14-1 | *Fetal Heart Rate Assessment Checklist* |

Patient's name _____ Date/time _____

_____

1. What is the baseline fetal heart rate (FHR)?
   _____ Beats per minute
   Check one of the following as observed on the monitor strip:
   _____ Average baseline FHR (110 to 160 beats per minute)
   _____ Tachycardia (>160 beats per minute)
   _____ Bradycardia (<110 beats per minute)
2. What is the baseline variability?
   _____ Moderate variability (6 to 25 beats per minute)
   _____ Minimal variability (> 5 beats per minute)
   _____ Absence of variability
   _____ Marked variability (>25 beats per minute)
3. Are there any periodic or episodic changes in FHR?
   _____ Accelerations with fetal movement
   _____ Repetitive accelerations with each contraction
   _____ Early decelerations (head compression)
   _____ Late decelerations (uteroplacental insufficiency)
   _____ Variable decelerations (cord compression)
   _____ Mild
   _____ Moderate
   _____ Severe
   _____ Prolonged
4. What does the uterine activity panel show?
   _____ Frequency (peak to peak or beginning to beginning)
   _____ Duration (beginning to end)
   _____ Intensity (in mm Hg only with intrauterine catheter)
   _____ Resting time at least 30 seconds
   _____ Resting tone (<15 mm Hg pressure)
COMMENTS: _____
PANEL NUMBER   WHAT CAN BE OR
                      SHOULD HAVE
                      BEEN DONE

Modified from Tucker S: *Pocket Guide to fetal monitoring and assessment,* ed 3, St Louis, 1996, Mosby.

| BOX 14-2 | *Checklist for Fetal Monitoring Equipment* |

PREPARATION OF MONITOR
1. Is the paper inserted correctly?
2. Are transducer cables plugged into the appropriate outlet of the monitor?

ULTRASOUND TRANSDUCER
1. Has ultrasound transmission gel been applied to the transducer?
2. Was the FHR tested and noted on the monitor paper?
3. Does a signal light flash or an audible beep occur with each heartbeat?
4. Is the belt secure and snug but comfortable for the laboring woman?

TOCOTRANSDUCER
1. Is the tocotransducer firmly positioned at the site of the least maternal tissue?
2. Has it been applied without gel or paste?
3. Was the pen-set knob adjusted between the 10- and 20-mm Hg marks and noted on the monitor paper?
4. Was this setting done between contractions?
5. Is the belt secure and snug but comfortable for the laboring woman?

SPIRAL ELECTRODE
1. Are the wires attached firmly to the leg plate?
2. Is the spiral electrode attached to the presenting part of the fetus?
3. Is the inner surface of the leg plate covered with electrode gel, if necessary?
4. Is the leg plate properly secured to the woman's thigh?

INTERNAL CATHETER/STRAIN GAUGE*
1. Is the length line on the catheter visible at the introitus?
2. Is it noted on the monitor paper that a calibration was done?
3. Was the uterine activity tested?

Modified from Tucker S: *Pocket guide to fetal monitoring and assessment,* ed 3, St Louis, 1996, Mosby.
*Some new internal catheters are solid and do not have syringes or stopcocks.

Nursing diagnoses for the woman who is being monitored electronically for fetal status are based on assessment findings. Possible diagnoses are listed in the box.

❙ Nursing Diagnoses_____

Woman Being Monitored Electronically for Fetal Status
Decreased maternal cardiac output related to
- Supine hypotension secondary to maternal position
Ineffective individual coping ability related to
- Lack of knowledge concerning fetal monitoring during labor
- Restriction of mobility or movement during EFM

Impaired fetal gas exchange related to
- Umbilical cord compression
- Placental insufficiency
Risk for fetal injury related to
- Unrecognized hypoxemia and hypoxia or anoxia
- Infection secondary to internal monitoring or blood sampling
Pain related to
- Use of belts to position transducers
- Maternal position
- Application of internal electrode or the obtaining of blood sample

Expected Outcomes of Care

The interventions implemented are determined by the current knowledge of fetal status as revealed by monitoring during labor and by standards for care. The woman's and family's concerns and questions are considered in the planning process. Expected outcomes are set for the pregnant woman, her family, and the fetus and include the following:

- The fetus will not suffer any hypoxemic or hypoxic episodes.
- Should fetal compromise occur, it will be identified promptly (with appropriate nursing interventions such as intrauterine resuscitation initiated), and the physician or nurse-midwife will be notified.
- The pregnant woman and the family will verbalize their understanding of the need for monitoring.
- The pregnant woman and the family will recognize and avoid situations that compromise maternal and fetal circulation.
- The pregnant woman and the family will achieve the type of birth experience that is both physically safe for the mother and fetus/neonate and is emotionally satisfying.

Plan of Care and Interventions

It is the responsibility of the nurse providing care to women in labor to assess FHR patterns, implement independent nursing interventions, document observations and actions according to the established standard of care, and report nonreassuring patterns to the primary care provider (for example, physician, nurse-midwife). (See Box 14-3 for a sample protocol for FHR monitoring.)

Summary guidelines for the care of the woman being monitored electronically for fetal status during labor are listed in Box 14-4 (see also Plan of Care).

It is important to remember that although the use of EFM can be reassuring to many parents, it can be a source of anxiety to some. Therefore the nurse must be particularly sensitive to and respond appropriately to the emotional, informational, and comfort needs of the woman in labor and those of her family (Fig. 14-8).

Electronic fetal monitoring pattern recognition

Nurses must evaluate many factors to determine if an FHR pattern is reassuring or nonreassuring. A complete description of FHR tracings includes both qualitative and quantitative descriptions of baseline rate and variability, presence of accelerations, periodic or episodic decelerations, and changes in the FHR pattern over time (National Institute, 1997). Nurses evaluate these factors based on other obstetric complications, progress in labor, and analgesia or anesthesia. They must also consider the estimated time interval until birth. Interventions are, therefore, based on clinical judgment of a complex, integrated process.

LEGAL TIP   **Fetal Monitoring Standards**

Nurses who care for women during childbirth are legally responsible for correctly interpreting FHR patterns, indicating appropriate nursing interventions based on that pattern, and documenting the outcome of those interventions. Perinatal nurses are responsible for the timely notification of the physician or nurse-midwife in the event of nonreassuring FHR patterns. Perinatal nurses are also responsible for initiating the institutional chain of command should differences in opinion arise among health care providers concerning the interpretation of the FHR pattern and the intervention required.

Other methods of assessment and intervention

Assessment techniques. Other methods of assessment are designed to be used in conjunction with EFM in an effort to identify and intervene on behalf of a fetus that is hypoxemic or acidotic. These methods include fetal blood sampling, FHR response to stimulation, and pulse oximetry monitoring of fetal oxygen saturation. Umbilical cord acid-base determination is an assessment technique that is a useful adjunct to the Apgar score in assessing the immediate condition of the newborn.

Fetal scalp blood sampling. Sampling of the fetal scalp blood was designed to assess the fetal pH, Po_2 and Pco_2. The procedure is performed by obtaining a sample of fetal scalp blood through the dilated cervix after the membranes have ruptured. The scalp is swabbed with a disinfecting solution before making the puncture, and the sample is then collected. However, the blood gas values vary so rapidly with transient circulatory changes that fetal blood sampling is seldom performed. When used, it is usually in tertiary centers with the capability for repetitive sampling and rapid report of results. The circulatory changes that cause the variability and thus undermine the utility of this procedure are maternal acidosis or alkalosis, caput succedaneum, the stage of labor, and the time relationship of scalp sampling to uterine contractions.

Fetal heart rate response to stimulation. Stimulation of the fetus, in order to elicit an acceleration of the FHR of 15 beats per minute for at least 15 seconds, is sometimes used as an alternative to fetal blood sampling (Tucker, 1996). The two methods of fetal stimulation currently in practice include scalp stimulation, using digital pressure during a vaginal examination, and vibroacoustic stimulation, using an artificial larynx or fetal acoustic stimulation device over the fetal head for 1 to 2 seconds. An FHR acceleration usually indicates fetal well-being. If the fetus does not have an acceleration, however, it does not necessarily indicate fetal compromise, but further evaluation of fetal well-being is needed.

BOX 14-3 *Protocol for Fetal Heart Rate Monitoring*

PATIENT/FAMILY TEACHING

Explain purpose of monitoring
Explain procedure
Provide rationale for maternal position other than supine

CARE

Assist woman to a comfortable position other than
 supine
Change maternal position at least every 2 hours
Change placement of external monitor belts every 2
 hours when possible
Provide perineal care as needed when internal
 monitoring is implemented

MATERNAL/FETAL ASSESSMENT

Obtain a 20-minute strip of EFM for all patients admitted
 to labor unit

Low-Risk Patient

Auscultate or assess tracing every 30 minutes in active
 phase of first stage of labor
Auscultate or assess tracing every 15 minutes in second
 stage

High-Risk Patient

Auscultate or assess tracing every 15 minutes in active
 phase and every 5 minutes in second stage

Auscultation—All Patients

Count baseline FHR in between contractions
Assess FHR during the contraction and for at least 30
 seconds after the contraction
Note increases or decreases of FHR
Assess FHR before ambulation
Determine uterine activity by palpation or by external
 and/or internal monitoring
Interpret FHR data, nursing interventions, and patient
 responses
Notify primary health care provider

EFM—All Patients

Assess and interpret baseline FHR, variability of FHR
 (long term for external monitoring; long and short term
 for internal monitoring), and presence or absence of
 decelerations and accelerations

Assessment for All Patients

Assess uterine activity for frequency and duration, the
 intensity of contractions, and uterine resting tone
Assess FHR immediately after rupture of membranes,
 vaginal examinations, and any invasive procedure

REPORTABLE CONDITIONS

Presence of nonreassuring patterns
Worsening of any pattern
Presence of any abnormal FHR rhyhms
Difficulty in obtaining adequate FHR tracing or inadequate
 audible FHR

EMERGENCY MEASURES

Implement the following measures immediately in the
 event of nonreassuring patterns:
Reposition woman in lateral position to increase
 uteroplacental perfusion or relieve cord compression
Administer oxygen at 8 to 10 L/min or per hospital
 protocol via face mask
Discontinue oxytocin if infusing
Correct maternal hypovolemia by increasing IV rate per
 protocol or as ordered
Assess for bleeding or other cause of pattern change,
 such as maternal hypotension
Notify primary health care provider
Anticipate emergency preparation for surgical intervention
 if nonreassuring pattern continues despite interventions

DOCUMENTATION

Patient Record—Auscultation

FHR baseline, rate and rhythm, increases or decreases

Patient Record—EFM

Method of monitoring, change in method, and
 adjustment of equipment
FHR range, variability, presence of decelerations or
 accelerations
Uterine activity as determined by palpation or by external
 and/or internal monitoring
Interpretation of FHR data, nursing interventions, and
 patient responses
Notification of primary health care provider

Monitor Strip

Patient identification data
Assessments, procedures, and interventions
 (medications, etc.)
Notification of primary health care provider
Significant occurrences such as sterile vaginal
 examination, rupture of membranes, etc.
Adjustments of the monitor equipment

BOX 14-4 *Care of Woman Using Electronic Fetal Monitoring*

The following guidelines relate to patient teaching and the functioning of the monitor:

Explain that fetal status can be continuously assessed by FHR, even during contractions.

Explain that the lower tracing on the monitor strip paper shows uterine activity; the upper tracing shows the FHR.

Reassure woman and partner that prepared childbirth techniques can be implemented without difficulty.

Explain that, during external monitoring, effleurage can be performed on sides of abdomen or upper portion of thighs.

Explain that breathing patterns based on the time and intensity of contractions can be enhanced by the observation of uterine activity on the monitor strip paper, which shows the onset of contractions.

Note peak of contraction; knowing that contraction will not get stronger and is half over usually is helpful.

Note diminishing intensity.

Coordinate with appropriate breathing and relaxation techniques.

Reassure woman and partner that the use of internal monitoring does not restrict movement, although she is confined to bed.*

Explain that use of external monitoring usually requires the woman's cooperation during positioning and movement.

Reassure woman and partner that use of monitoring does not imply fetal jeopardy.

Reassure her that the equipment is removed periodically to permit the applicator sites to be washed and other care to be given.

EXTERNAL MONITORING

Ultrasound Transducer

Function

Monitors FHR with high-frequency sound waves.

Nursing Care

Tap transducer before use to ensure sound transmission.

Apply ultrasound transmission gel to transducer, clean abdomen and transducer and reapply gel q2h and prn.

Massage reddened skin areas gently and reposition belt or adhesive device q2h and prn.

Auscultate FHR with stethoscope or fetoscope if in doubt as to validity of tracing.

Position and reposition transducer prn to ensure receipt of clear, interpretable FHR data.

Tocotransducer

Function

Monitors uterine activity via a pressure-sensing device placed on the maternal abdomen.

Nursing Care

Position and reposition qh and prn on the fundus where there is the least maternal tissue.

Keep abdominal strap snug but comfortable for the laboring woman.

Adjust pen-set between contractions to print between 10 and 20 mm Hg on the monitor strip paper.

Palpate fundus every 30 to 60 minutes to assess strength of contraction; only frequency and duration of contractions can be assessed with tocotransducer.

Do not determine woman's need for analgesia based on uterine activity displayed on monitor strip.

Gently massage reddened areas under transducer and belt qh and prn.

INTERNAL MONITORING (SEE FIG. 14-3)

Spiral Electrode

Function

Obtains fetal ECG from presenting part and converts it into FHR.

Nursing Care

Ensure that wires are appropriately attached to leg plate.

Reapply electrode paste to leg plate if needed.

Observe FHR tracing on monitor strip for variability.

Turn electrode counterclockwise to remove; never pull straight out from presenting part.

Administer perineal care after the woman voids during labor and prn.

Intrauterine Catheter

Function

Catheter (may be fluid-filled or solid) that monitors intraamniotic pressure internally.

Nursing Care

Flush open system catheter with sterile water before insertion and prn.

Ensure that the length line on catheter is visible at introitus.

For closed system catheters, set baseline rate between uterine contractions when uterus is relaxed.

For open system catheters, turn stopcock off to woman, then with pressure valve of strain gauge released, flush strain gauge, remove syringe, and set stylus to 0 line of chart paper; test further according to manufacturer's instructions q3h to 4h and prn.

Check proper functioning by tapping catheter, asking woman to cough, or applying fundal pressure; observe appropriate inflection on strip chart.

Keep catheter taped to woman's leg to prevent dislodgement.

Modified from Tucker S et al.: *Patient care standards,* ed 6, St Louis, 1995, Mosby.
*Portable telemetry monitors allow the FHR and uterine contraction patterns to be observed on centrally located electronic display stations. These portable units permit ambulation during electronic monitoring.

≋ **PLAN OF CARE** *EFM During Labor*

NURSING DIAGNOSIS Maternal anxiety related to lack of knowledge about use of electronic monitor

---

Expected Outcomes *The patient will exhibit increased understanding about fetal monitoring and signs of reduced anxiety (i.e., absence of physical indicators, absence of perceived threat, and absence of feelings of dread).*

Nursing Interventions/*Rationales*

Explain and demonstrate to woman and labor support partner how the electronic monitor (internal or external) works in assessing FHR and in detecting and assessing quality of uterine contractions to *remove fear of unknown and ensure that woman can move with the monitor.*

When making adjustment to the monitor, explain to the couple what is being done and why *because information increases understanding and allays anxiety.*

Explain that while a side-lying position or Fowler's position provides for optimum monitoring, position changes decrease discomfort; therefore encourage frequent changes in position (other than supine) and explain any monitoring adjustments that are being made as a result *to reduce discomfort and allay anxiety.*

NURSING DIAGNOSIS Risk for fetal injury related to inaccurate placement of transducers/electrodes, misinterpretation of results or failure to use other assessment techniques to monitor fetal well-being

---

Expected Outcomes *Fetal well-being is adequately assessed, and any fetal compromise is identified immediately.*

Nursing Interventions/*Rationales*

Carefully follow guidelines and checklist for application and initiation of monitoring *to ensure proper placement of monitoring devices and production of accurate output from monitoring device.*

Check placement throughout monitoring process *to ensure that devices remain correctly placed.*

Regularly assess and record results of EFM (FHR and variability, decelerations, accelerations, uterine activity, contractions, uterine resting tone) *to provide consistent and timely evaluation of fetal well-being and progress of labor.*

Auscultate FHR and palpate contractions on a regular basis *to provide a cross-check on the EFM output and ensure fetal well-being.*

From Wong D & Perry S: *Maternal child nursing care,* St Louis, 1998, Mosby.

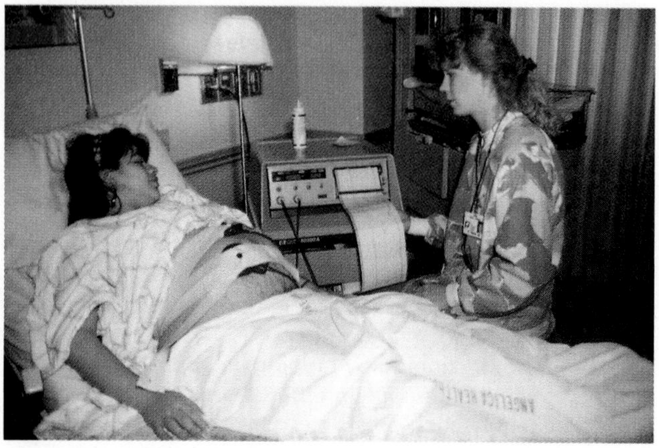

Fig. 14-8 Nurse explains EFM as ultrasound transducer externally monitors the FHR. (Courtesy Marjorie Pyle, RNC, Lifecircle, Costa Mesa, Calif.)

Pulse oximetry monitoring of fetal oxygen saturation. Continuous monitoring of fetal oxygen saturation by pulse oximetry is a method of fetal assessment currently in the clinical investigation stage (Luttkus et al., 1995). The mechanism is the same as for adult and pediatric pulse oximetry, but the method is different in that it requires transcervical insertion of the probe between the fetal presenting part and the uterus, which can only be done after the membranes are ruptured. Multicenter clinical trial testing in the United States and Europe is in process.

Umbilical cord acid-base. In assessing the immediate condition of the newborn after birth, a sample of cord blood is a useful adjunct to the Apgar score. The procedure is generally done by withdrawing blood from the umbilical artery and having the blood tested for pH, Pco_2 and Po_2. Metabolic acidosis can cause a low Apgar score.

Interventions. In addition to the emergency measures for nonreassuring FHR patterns, there are other interventions that may prevent fetal compromise. These are the amnioinfusion and tocolysis.

Amnioinfusion. **Amnioinfusion** is a procedure used during labor to either supplement inadequate amounts of amniotic fluid or dilute meconium-stained amniotic fluid (Schmidt, 1997). The procedure to supplement amniotic fluid is indicated for patients with oligohydramnios, secondary to uteroplacental insufficiency, premature rupture of membranes, or postmaturity, who are at risk for variable decelerations because of umbilical cord compression.

Oligohydramnios is an abnormally small amount of amniotic fluid (< 8 cm) or the absence of amniotic fluid. Without the buffer of amniotic fluid, the umbilical cord can easily become compressed during contractions or fetal movement, diminishing the flow of blood between the fetus and placenta as evidenced by variable decelerations. Amnioinfusion replaces the "cushion" for the cord and relieves both the frequency and intensity of variable decelerations.

Amnioinfusion is also indicated in the presence of moderate to thick meconium to dilute and flush out the meconium with the intent of avoiding meconium aspiration syndrome in the neonate (Strong, 1995).

Risks of amnioinfusion are overdistention of the uterine cavity and increased uterine tone. Techniques of amnioinfusion treatment vary, but usually fluid is administered through an IUPC. The woman's membranes must be ruptured for the IUPC placement. The fluid is administered by attaching plastic (intravenous) tubing to a liter of normal saline or lactated Ringer's solution through a port in the IUPC. Double lumen IUPCs are best because the intrauterine pressure can be monitored without stopping the procedure. The fluid is usually warmed before administration, especially for the preterm or small-for- gestational-age fetus (ACOG, 1995).

The flow rate can be by bolus or continuous flow or by a combination of these two methods (Wenstrom, Andrews & Maher, 1995). The bolus method is useful for treating variable deceleration patterns. About 800 ml of fluid is infused at 10 to 15 ml per minute until the decelerations diminish. Additional boluses are given as needed. A continuous flow rate of about 3 ml per minute is useful for treating oligohydramnios (ACOG, 1995). The combination method is the most common method used. A bolus of 10 to 15 ml per minute is given for 1 hour followed by a maintenance flow rate of 3 ml per minute (Wenstrom, Andrews & Maher, 1995). This method is useful for variable decelerations and for thick meconium-stained fluid.

The time needed to increase the amniotic fluid volume is about 30 minutes (Snell, 1993). Therefore, the treatment for decelerations must be started before the pattern becomes ominous. If the fetal status does not improve or if it worsens, the health care team should be ready for an immediate surgical delivery.

Tocolytic therapy. **Tocolysis** can be achieved through the administration of drugs that inhibit uterine contractions. This therapy can be used as an adjunct to other interventions in the management of fetal compromise when the fetus is exhibiting nonreassuring patterns associated with increased uterine activity. Tocolysis may be considered by the primary health care provider and implemented when other interventions to reduce uterine activity, such as maternal position change and discontinuance of an oxytocin infusion, have no effect on diminishing the uterine contractions. A tocolytic drug such as terbutaline can be administered intravenously to decrease uterine activity. If the FHR pattern improves, the patient may be allowed to continue labor; if there is no improvement, immediate surgical delivery may be needed.

Documentation

Clear and complete documentation on the woman's monitoring strip is started before the initiation of monitoring and consists of identifying information and other relevant data (see later discussion). This documentation is continued and updated according to institutional protocol as monitoring progresses. In some institutions, observations noted and interventions implemented are recorded on the monitor strip to produce a comprehensive document that chronicles the course of labor and the care rendered. In other institutions, this documentation is confined to the labor flow record. Advocates of documenting on both the medical record and the EFM strip cite as advantages of this approach the ease of noting directly on the strip while at the bedside and the improved accuracy in documenting critical events that occur and the interventions implemented. Conversely, others believe that charting on the EFM strip constitutes duplicate documentation of the same information noted in the medical record and thus represents unnecessary additional paperwork for the nurse.

One way to document that frequent maternal-fetal assessments have been done at the bedside is to either initial the EFM strip or depress the "mark" button during these assessments. Data entry devices are now available with some EFM systems; assessments are input and subsequently printed on the strip. A disadvantage of documenting on both the EFM strip and the medical record is that frequently the times noted for events and the interventions on the EFM strip do not correlate with what is later documented in the medical record. These discrepancies can lead those involved in a retrospective review process carried out during litigation to infer that documentation errors have occurred. Therefore, if institutional policy mandates documentation on both the monitor strip and the medical record, it is critically important for the nurse to make sure the times and notations of events and interventions recorded in each place agree. No one method of documentation is right; rather the nurse needs to be aware of and follow individual institutional policies as well as participate in formulating such policies. Many of the aspects of care and events that can be documented on the monitor strip are listed in Box 14-5.

Evaluation

Evaluation of the effectiveness of care for the woman being monitored electronically for fetal status is based on the previously stated outcomes.

BOX 14-5   *Checklist for Reviewing Documentation*

Name: _____

Date: _____

Evaluator: _____

_____

Items to be checked:

_____

DOCUMENTATION

1. Are testing of FHR and UA written on monitor paper at least every 4 hours?
2. Is the monitor paper properly labeled with the following:
   a. Woman's name
   b. Identification number
   c. Date
   d. Time monitor attached and mode
   e. High-risk conditions (pregnancy-induced hypertension, diabetes, etc.)
   f. Membranes intact or ruptured
   g. Gestational age
   h. Dilatation and station
3. Are the following noted?
   a. Maternal position and repositioning in bed
   b. Vaginal examinations
   c. Analgesia or anesthesia
   d. Medications and parenteral fluids given
   e. BP and temperature, pulse, respiration (TPR)
   f. Voidings
   g. O_2 given
   h. Emesis
   I. Pushing
   j. Fetal movement
   k. Notations of baseline or periodic changes
   l. Any change in mode of monitoring
   m. Adjustments of equipment, such as
      (1) Relocation of transducers
      (2) Adjustment of catheter
      (3) Replacement of electrode
      (4) Replacement of catheter
      (5) Time lapse when changing recording paper
   n. Interventions (e.g., amnioinfusion, fetal stimulation, blood sampling)

Modified from Tucker S: *Pocket guide to fetal monitoring and assessment,* ed 3, St Louis, 1996, Mosby.

RESEARCH
Evaluation of a Fetal Monitoring Education Program

For decades electronic fetal monitoring (EFM) has been used to assess fetal well-being during labor and birth in an effort to identify problems that, if uncorrected, can cause short-term or long-term morbidity or even death. For many years, EFM education was practically nonexistent. Gradually, informal programs emerged, providing important basic training for nurses and physicians. However, these programs differed widely in content, clinical application, and format and have not been evaluated. A multicenter study was conducted at twelve hospitals to evaluate the effectiveness of a fetal monitoring education program in increasing nurses' knowledge and clinical skills. One hundred nine registered nurses were randomly assigned within each hospital to an experimental (n = 47) or control (n = 62) group. The nurses in the experimental group were evaluated on a 45-item knowledge test and a 25-item skills checklist during a 1-day fetal monitoring workshop and again at a review session 6 months later. The passing score was at least 75% correct on each test. The percentage of nurses in the experimental group passing both the knowledge and clinical skills test after the workshop was significantly higher (p <0.01) than that of the nurses in the control group: 68.1% versus 6.5%, respectively. A large difference between the groups remained at the 6-month follow-up (experimental, 45%; control, 6.5%). The performance of the nurses in the experimental group improved to an 85% pass rate after they attended the 6-month review session.

CLINICAL APPLICATION OF THE STUDY

With the emphasis of many labor and birth units on competency-based practice, the ability to evaluate the effectiveness of fetal monitoring associated with nurses' knowledge and clinical skills is important. Effective training programs with regular follow-up are essential. A minimum level of competence must be required.

Source: Trepanier M et al.: Evaluation of a fetal monitoring education program, *J Obstet Gynecol Neonatal Nurs* 25(2):137, 1996.

KEY POINTS

- Fetal well-being during labor is gauged by the response of the FHR to uterine contractions.
- FHR characteristics include the baseline FHR and periodic changes in the FHR.
- The monitoring of fetal well-being includes FHR assessment and watching for meconium-stained amniotic fluid.
- It is the responsibility of the nurse to assess FHR patterns, implement independent nursing interventions, and report nonreassuring patterns to the physician or nurse-midwife.
- The emotional, informational, and comfort needs of the woman and her family must be addressed when the mother and her fetus are being monitored.

CRITICAL THINKING EXERCISES

1 *Review three actual or sample fetal monitor strips and determine:*
   a *FHR baseline*
   b *Variability; periodic changes, if any*
   c *Contraction interval, duration, intensity, and resting tone*
   d *What nursing interventions are needed for each example; verify with nursing staff or faculty if actions selected are appropriate*

2 *Role-play a mother in the first stage of labor who is upset and unknowledgeable of the uses of the fetal monitor and a nurse who is using the equipment in an actual case for the first time. Make suggestions concerning actions that would be supportive and reassuring.*

References

American Academy of Pediatrics & American College of Obstetricians and Gynecologists: *Guidelines for perinatal care,* Elk Grove Village, Ill, 1997, AAP/ACOG.

American College of Obstetricians and Gynecologists: *Fetal heart rate patterns: monitoring, interpretation, and management* (ACOG Technical Bulletin No. 207), Washington, DC, 1995, ACOG.

Association of Women's Health, Obstetric, and Neonatal Nurses: *Didactic content and clinical skills verification for professional nurse providers of basic, high-risk, and critical-care intrapartum nursing,* Washington, DC, 1993, AWHONN.

Harvey C: Coming to terms: electronic fetal monitoring update, *Lifelines* 1(3):42, 1997.

Mishell D et al.: *Comprehensive gynecology,* ed 3, St Louis, 1997, Mosby.

National Institute of Child Health and Human Development Research Planning Workshop: Electronic fetal heart rate monitoring: research guidelines for interpretation, *J Obstet Gynecol Neonatal Nurs* 26(6):635, 1997.

Schmidt J: Fluid check: making the case for intrapartum amnioinfusion, *Lifelines* 1(5):46, 1997.

Seidel H et al.: *Mosby's guide to physical assessment,* ed 4, St Louis, 1998, Mosby.

Snell B: The use of amnioinfusion in nurse-midwifery procedures, *J Nurse Midwifery,* 38(2):62S, 1993.

Strong T: Amnioinfusion, *J Reprod Med* 49(2):108, 1995.

Thacker S, Stroup D & Peterson H: Efficacy and safety of intrapartum electronic fetal monitoring: an update, *Obstet Gynecol* 86(4):613, 1995.

Tucker S et al.: *Patient care standards,* ed 6, St Louis, 1995, Mosby.

Tucker S: *Pocket guide to fetal monitoring and assessment,* ed 3, St Louis, 1996, Mosby.

Wenstrom K, Andrews W & Maher J: Amnioinfusion survey: prevalence, protocols, and complications, *Obstet Gynecol* 86(4 Part I):572, 1995.

CHAPTER

15

Nursing Care during Labor and Birth

KAREN A. PIOTROWSKI

LEARNING OBJECTIVES

- *Define the key terms.*
- *Review the factors included in the initial assessment of the woman in labor.*
- *Describe the ongoing assessment of maternal progress during the first, second, and third stages of labor.*
- *State the physical and psychosocial findings indicative of maternal progress during labor.*
- *Discuss aspects of fetal assessment during labor.*
- *Identify signs of developing complications during the first, second, and third stages of labor.*
- *Identify nursing diagnoses and develop a comprehensive plan of care relevant to each stage of labor and birth.*
- *Discuss the nurse's role in managing care for the woman and her significant others (support person[s], family) during each stage of labor and birth.*
- *Describe the influence of cultural and religious beliefs and practices on the process of labor and birth.*
- *Discuss the role of a woman's significant others (support person[s], family) in assisting her during labor and birth.*
- *Outline nursing actions in preparation for birth.*
- *Describe the role and responsibilities of the nurse in an emergency childbirth situation.*
- *Identify the impact of perineal trauma on the woman.*
- *Discuss the nurse's role in reducing the incidence of routine episiotomy.*

KEY TERMS

bloody show
caul
crowning
doula

KEY TERMS—cont'd

duration (of contractions)
episiotomy
Ferguson's reflex
frequency (of contractions)
intensity (of contractions)
Leopold's maneuvers
lithotomy position
nuchal cord
orthostatic hypotension
placental separation
prolapse of the umbilical cord
resting tone (of contractions)
ring of fire
Ritgen maneuver

The labor process is an exciting and anxious time for the woman and her significant others (support persons, family). In a relatively short period of time they experience one of the most profound changes in their lives (Simkin, 1996). For most women, labor begins with the first uterine contraction, continues with hours of hard work during cervical dilatation and birth, and ends as the woman and her significant others begin the attachment process with the newborn. Nursing care focuses on supporting the woman and her significant others throughout the labor process in order to ensure the best possible outcome for all involved.

FIRST STAGE OF LABOR

The first stage of labor begins with the onset of regular uterine contractions and ends with full cervical dilatation. Care begins when the woman reports one or more of the following:

- Onset of progressive, regular uterine contractions that increase in frequency, strength, and duration
- Blood-tinged vaginal discharge (**bloody show**)
- Fluid discharge from the vagina (spontaneous rupture of membranes)

TEACHING GUIDELINES

How to Distinguish True Labor from False Labor

TRUE LABOR

Contractions
  Occur regularly, becoming stronger, lasting longer, and occurring closer together.
  Become more intense with walking.
  Usually felt in lower back, radiating to lower portion of abdomen.
  Continue despite use of comfort measures.
Cervix (by vaginal examination)
  Shows progressive change (softening, effacement, and dilatation signaled by the appearance of bloody show).
  Moves to an increasingly anterior position.
Fetus
  Presenting part usually becomes engaged in the pelvis. This results in increased ease of breathing; at the same time, the presenting part presses downward and compresses the bladder, resulting in urinary frequency.

FALSE LABOR

Contractions
  Occur irregularly or become regular only temporarily.
  Often stop with walking or position change.
  Can be felt in the back or abdomen above the navel.
  Often can be stopped through the use of comfort measures.
Cervix (by vaginal examination)
  May be soft but there is no significant change in effacement or dilatation or evidence of bloody show.
  Is often in a posterior position.
Fetus
  Presenting part is usually not engaged in the pelvis.

I CARE MANAGEMENT

Assessment and Nursing Diagnoses

Assessment begins at the first contact with the woman, whether by telephone or in person. Many women will call the hospital or birthing center first to receive validation that it is all right for them to come to the hospital. The manner in which the nurse communicates with the woman during this first contact can set the tone for a positive birth experience. A caring attitude by the nurse encourages the woman to verbalize questions and concerns. If possible, the nurse needs to have the woman's prenatal record in hand when speaking to her or admitting her for evaluation of labor.

Certain factors are initially assessed to determine if the woman is in true or false labor and whether she should come for further assessment or admission (Varney, 1997) (see Teaching Guidelines box). When a woman calls and there is a question about whether she is in labor (or in labor advanced enough to be admitted), the nurse should suggest

---

| BOX 15-1 | *Telephone Interview with Woman in Latent Phase of Labor* |

The perinatal nurse performs the following steps of the nursing process:

ASSESSMENT
- Gathers data regarding the woman's status, including signs and symptoms indicative of true or false labor.
- Discusses instructions given by the woman's primary health care provider regarding when to come for admission.

PLANNING AND IMPLEMENTATION
- Decides whether the woman will come for labor assessment and admission or be encouraged to stay at home until contractions increase in duration, frequency, and intensity.
- Assures the woman that she is welcome to call the perinatal unit at any time to discuss her labor status.
- Answers questions the woman and her family may have regarding labor or provides instruction as needed (e.g., which entrance of the hospital to enter).
- Suggests a variety of positions she can assume to maximally enhance uteroplacental and renal blood flow (i.e., side-lying position) and enhance the progress of labor (i.e., upright positions and ambulation).
- Suggests diversional activities, such as walking, reading, watching television, talking to friends.
- Suggests measures to maintain comfort, such as a warm bath or shower, back or foot massage.
- Discusses the oral intake of foods and fluids appropriate for early labor (light foods or fluids or clear liquids depending on the preference of her primary health care provider).
- Instructs the woman to come in immediately if membranes rupture, bleeding occurs, or fetal movements change.

EVALUATION
- Evaluates whether instructions and information have been understood by the woman by asking her to verbalize her understanding.

---

that she either call her primary health care provider or come to the hospital (Box 15-1).

The pregnant woman may call the primary health care provider or come to the hospital while in false labor or early in the latent phase of the first stage of labor. It can be discouraging for her and her partner to find out that the contractions that feel so strong and regular to her are not true contractions because they are not causing cervical dilatation or are still not strong or frequent enough for admission.

If the woman lives near the hospital, she may be asked to stay home or return home to allow labor to progress in terms of frequency and intensity of contractions, because the ideal setting for the low-risk woman at this time is the familiar environment of her home. The nurse can use the recommended approach for the telephone interview (see Box 15-1) to assess the woman's status and to give instructions regarding the optimum timing for admission and signs that require immediate notification of the primary health care provider. Measures the woman and her significant others can use to enhance the progress of labor, reduce anxiety, and maintain comfort should be described. The woman is encouraged to ambulate and asked to limit her intake of foods to either light foods and fluids or to clear liquids only, depending on the preferences of her primary health care provider. A warm bath; soothing back, foot, and hand massages; and a warm drink of a preferred liquid such as tea or milk can help the woman to rest and even to sleep, especially if the false or early labor is occurring at night. Diversional activities such as walking outdoors or in the house, reading, watching television, doing needlework, or talking with friends can reduce the perception of early discomfort, help the time pass, and reduce anxiety (Varney, 1997).

The woman who lives at a considerable distance from the hospital may be admitted in early labor. The same measures used by the woman at home should be offered to the hospitalized woman in early labor.

On the woman's arrival at the perinatal unit, assessment is the top priority (Fig. 15-1). The nurse first performs a screening assessment, using the techniques of interview and physical assessment, and reviews the laboratory findings to determine the status of the woman and her fetus and the progress of her labor. The primary health care provider is notified, and if the woman is admitted, a detailed systems assessment is done.

If the woman wishes, her partner is included in the assessment and admission process. Significant others not participating in this process may be directed to the appropriate waiting area, if that is the policy of the unit. In many labor-delivery-recovery (LDR) and labor-delivery-recovery-postpartum (LDRP) rooms, the woman may have anyone she wishes present. The woman is asked to undress and put on her own gown or a hospital gown. Her personal belongings are put away safely. If the woman prefers to wear some items of her own (such as socks), these are noted on her chart.

LEGAL TIP   **Patient's Personal Items**

Most hospitals have a checklist or other way of recording the woman's belongings that becomes part of her permanent record. Both the woman and the admitting nurse must sign this form. Items of value (such as jewelry) should be placed in the safekeeping of a family member.

The nurse orients the woman and her partner to the layout and operation of the unit and room. This includes the use of the call light and telephone system, the location of personal storage areas in the bedside and overbed tables, and how to adjust lighting in the room. An admissions

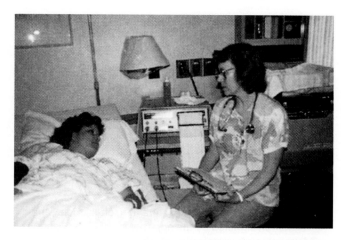

Fig. **15-1** Woman being admitted. (Courtesy Marjorie Pyle, RNC, Lifecircle, Costa Mesa, Calif.)

bracelet is placed on the woman's wrist, as well as an allergy bracelet (usually colored), when relevant. The nurse should reassure the woman that she is in competent, caring hands; that she can ask questions related to her care and status at any time during labor; and that questions will be answered. Anxiety can be minimized if the nurse explains terms commonly used during labor as these come up.

Admission data. Admission forms such as the ones in Fig. 15-2 can provide guidelines for the acquisition of important assessment information when a woman in labor is being evaluated or admitted. Additional sources of data include (1) the prenatal record, (2) the initial interview, (3) physical examination to determine baseline physiologic characteristics, (4) laboratory results, (5) expressed psychosocial and cultural factors, and (6) the clinical evaluation of labor status.

Prenatal data. The screening/triage nurse reviews the prenatal record to identify the woman's individual needs and risks. If the woman has not had any prenatal care, this baseline information needs to be obtained. If the woman is experiencing discomfort, the nurse should ask the questions between contractions, when the woman can concentrate more fully on her answers.

It is important to know the woman's age so that the plan of care can be tailored to her age group needs. Height and weight relationships are important to determine because most women are encouraged by their primary health care provider to gain up to 13.5 kg. A weight gain greater than that recommended may place the woman at a higher risk for cephalopelvic disproportion (CPD) and cesarean birth. This is especially true for women who are petite and have gained 15.75 kg or more. Other factors to consider are the woman's general health status, any current medical conditions or allergies she may have, her respiratory status, and previous surgical procedures she has undergone.

Her past and present obstetric and pregnancy history are carefully noted. The obstetric history includes gravidity (number of pregnancies) and parity (pregnancies carried to

Obstetric Admitting Record — Page 1 of 2

Basic Admission Data

Date ___ / ___ / ___ Time _____

- ☐ Ambulatory
- ☐ Wheelchair
- ☐ Direct admit
- ☐ Transfer from_____
- ☐ Stretcher

G	T	Pt	A	L	L M P / /	E D D / / E D By fetal D assessment / /	Age

Race/Ethnicity_____

Occupation_____ Education_____

Marital status S M Sep D W   Religion_____

MD/CNM _____ Tel no _____ | Support person/Relationship Tel no

Reasons for Admission

- ☐ **Onset of labor**
- ☐ Induction of labor
- ☐ Spontaneous abortion
- ☐ Cesarean section
  - ☐ Primary ☐ Repeat
  - (reason for primary_____)
- ☐ VBAC
- ☐ Tubal ligation
- ☐ Vaginal bleeding
- ☐ PROM
- ☐ Preterm labor

Detail reasons for admission_____

Observation evaluation

- ☐ Fetal status
  - ☐ Ultrasound
  - ☐ Amniocentesis
  - ☐ NST
  - ☐ CST
- ☐ Medical complications _____
- ☐ Obstetric complications _____

Patient Triage Data

Contractions ☐ **None** ☐ Palpation ☐ Tocotransducer

Frequency_____ Duration_____ Intensity_____

Began on___ / ___ / ___Time_____

Membranes ☐ **Intact** ☐ Bulging
  ☐ Ruptured (Date___ / ___ / ___ Time_____)

Fluid ☐ Clear ☐ Bloody ☐ Foul smelling
  ☐ Meconium stained ☐ No foul odor

Vaginal bleeding ☐ **None** ☐ Normal show
  ☐ Bleeding (describe_____)

Cervical Examination

Station_____Effacement_____Dilatation_____cms

Presentation
- ☐ Vertex
- ☐ Face/Brow
- ☐ Breech (type_____)
- ☐ Transverse lie
- ☐ Compound
- ☐ Unknown

Medication allergy/Sensitivity ☐ **None**
  ☐ Identify_____

Other allergy/Sensitivity ☐ **None**
  ☐ Identify_____

Patient Care Data

Personal Effects	Disposition		
Item	With patient	With support person	Other (describe)

Illness (≤ 14 days before admission) ☐ **None**
  ☐ Type/Treatment_____

Recent Exposure to Communicable Disease ☐ **None**
  ☐ Type/Date_____ ___ / ___ / ___

Last Oral Intake
  Fluids___ / ___ / ___ Time_____
  Solids___ / ___ / ___ Time_____

Medications ☐ **None**

Type/Dose	Last taken	With patient		Disposition
		No	Yes	
		☐	☐	
		☐	☐	

Smoker ☐ No ☐ Yes (_____ amt/day)

Alcohol/Drug use ☐ No ☐ Yes

Substances	Amt/Day	Last used
_____	_____	___ / ___ / ___ Time_____
_____	_____	___ / ___ / ___ Time_____

Plans for Birth and Hospital Stay

Support person present in L&D ☐ No ☐ Yes_____
Other family members in L&D ☐ No ☐ Yes_____

Anesthesia ☐ **None**
- ☐ Local ☐ Epidural ☐ Spinal ☐ General

Delivery site
- ☐ DR ☐ Birthing room ☐ LDR ☐ LDRP ☐ OR

Personal requests_____

Adoption ☐ No
  ☐ Yes Contact with infant ☐ No ☐ Yes
  Adoption contact_____

Feeding preference ☐ Breast ☐ Bottle
Room preference ☐ Private ☐ Semi-Private
  ☐ Rooming-In

☐ Tubal ligation Authorization signed ☐ Yes ☐ No
☐ Circumcision Authorization signed ☐ Yes ☐ No

Psychosocial Data

Communication Deficit ☐ **None**
  ☐ Identify_____

Other children ☐ No ☐ Yes Age/Sex_____

_____/_____/_____/

Partner involved ☐ Yes ☐ No
Others involved ☐ No ☐ Identify_____

Admitting signature_____ Time_____

Fig. **15-2** Obstetric admitting record. (Permission to use and/or reproduce this copyrighted material has been granted by the owner, Hollister Incorporated, Libertyville, Ill.) *Continued*

Obstetric Admitting Record	**Page 2 of 2**	

Psychosocial Data (Cont'd.)

Basic needs met   Yes   No   If no, explain

Housing ☐ ☐ _____

Clothing ☐ ☐ _____

Food ☐ ☐ _____

Transportation ☐ ☐ _____

Free from apparent physical/emotional abuse ☐ Yes ☐ No

If no, explain_____

Life Stress   No   Yes   If no, explain

Living ☐ ☐ _____

Working ☐ ☐ _____

Serious illness ☐ ☐ _____

Self Care Needs ☐ None ☐ Needs help with_____

Emotional status   ☐ Happy   ☐ Ambivalent   ☐ Anxious   ☐ Depressed   ☐ Angry

Discharge Planning Data

Discharge planning initiated ☐ **Yes** ☐ No

Discharge needs identified_____

Social service referral ☐ No ☐ Yes ___ / ___ / ___

Planned length of stay_____days

Needs follow-up visit by RN ☐ No ☐ Yes ___ / ___ / ___

Significant Prenatal Data

Prenatal Records Available on Admission

☐ **Yes** ☐ No

Source of prenatal data_____

First prenatal visit___ / ___ / ___

Attended prenatal classes ☐ **Yes** ☐ No

Infant care provider:_____

Lab Findings ☐ **None**

Blood type & Rh _____

Rubella titer _____

Serology _____

HbSAg _____

Fetal Assessment Tests ☐ **None**

Date	Test	Result
/		
/		
/		
/		
/		

Maternal Problems Identified ☐ **None**

	Active	Resolved
1._____	☐	☐
2._____	☐	☐
3._____	☐	☐

Fetal Problems Identified ☐ **None**

	Active	Resolved
1._____	☐	☐
2._____	☐	☐
3._____	☐	☐

Physical Assessment

Detail all abnormal findings

Height	Wt pregrav/grav		
Temp	Pulse	Resp	BP

System	Normal	Abnormal
HEENT	☐	☐
Neurologic	☐	☐
Skin	☐	☐
Breasts	☐	☐
Extremities	☐	☐
Cardiovascular	☐	☐
Respiratory	☐	☐
Abdomen	☐	☐
Gastrointestinal	☐	☐
Urinary	☐	☐
Genitalia	☐	☐

Specimens obtained (check all that apply)

Urine test	Time	Results	Blood test	Time	Results
☐ Urinalysis			☐ Hgb		
☐ C + S			☐ Hct		
☐ Glucose			☐ VDRL/RPR		
☐ Albumin			☐ Type/Screen		
☐ Ketones			☐		
☐ pH			☐		
☐ Blood			☐		

Fetal Evaluation Data

Fundal height_____cms FHR_____

Estimated fetal weight_____

Weeks gestation (est)

By dates_____wks

By ultrasound_____wks

Date___ / ___ / ___

☐ Fetoscope

☐ Doppler

☐ Fetal monitor

☐ Other

Multiple gestation ☐ **No** ☐ Yes

Infant	Presentation	Position
1._____	_____	_____
2._____	_____	_____
3._____	_____	_____

Initial Problems Identified ☐ **None**

1._____

2._____

3._____

Physician/CNM_____

Notified by_____

Date___ / ___ / ___Time_____

_____
Admitting signature

_____
Examiner signature

Date___ / ___ / ___Time_____

Fig. 15-2 cont'd, Obstetric admitting record.

viability). Obstetric problems to consider include a history of vaginal bleeding, pregnancy-induced hypertension (PIH), anemia, gestational diabetes, infections (bacterial or sexually transmitted), and immunodeficiencies.

If this is not the woman's first labor and birth experience, it is important to note the characteristics of her previous experiences. This information includes the duration of previous labors, the type of anesthesia used, and the kind of birth (spontaneous vaginal, forceps-assisted, vacuum-assisted, or cesarean). The woman's perception of her previous labor and birth experiences should be explored because it may influence her attitude toward her current experience. Women can retain long-term memories of their childbirth experiences. The memory of labor and birth events can affect a woman's postpartum emotional adjustment, self-esteem, and ability to parent effectively (DiMatteo et al., 1993; Simkin, 1996).

While reviewing the data on past births, the nurse collects data related to the condition of the babies (i.e., their weight, Apgar scores, and general health at and after birth).

It is important to confirm that the estimated date of birth (EDB) is as accurate as possible. Other data in the prenatal record include patterns of maternal weight gain, physiologic measurements such as maternal vital signs (blood pressure; temperature, pulse, respiration [TPR]), fundal height, baseline fetal heart rate (FHR), and laboratory test results. These tests include determination of the woman's blood type and Rh factor, a complete or partial blood count (CBC or hemoglobin and hematocrit), the 50-g blood glucose test, determination of the rubella titer, serologic tests (Venereal Disease Research Laboratories [VDRL] or rapid plasma reagin [RPR]) test for hepatitis B surface antigen (HBsAG), culture for group B *Streptococcus*, and urinalysis. Additional tests may include a tuberculosis screen with purified protein derivative (PPD), as well as screening for the human immunodeficiency virus (HIV) or the sickle cell trait and other genetic disorders (e.g., maternal serum alpha-fetoprotein [MSAFP]).

Interview. The woman's primary complaint or reason for coming to the hospital is determined in the interview. The primary complaint may be that her bag of waters (BOW, amniotic membranes) ruptured, with or without contractions. The woman may have come in for an obstetric check (which is a period of observation reserved for women who are unsure about the onset of their labor). If used by the hospital and approved by the woman's health insurance plan, this allows time on the unit for the diagnosis of labor without the woman's actual admission to the hospital.

Even the experienced mother may have difficulty determining the onset of labor. The woman is asked to recall the events of the previous days. She is asked to identify as best she can when regular contractions began. She is asked about the following:

- Frequency and duration of contractions.
- Location and character of discomfort from contractions (i.e., back pain, suprapubic discomfort).

- Persistence of contractions despite changes in maternal position when walking or lying down.
- Presence and character of vaginal discharge or show.
- The status of amniotic membranes, such as whether a gush or seepage of fluid has occurred. If there has been a discharge that may be amniotic fluid, she is asked to identify when the fluid was first noted and to describe the fluid (e.g., amount, color, unusual odor). In many instances the findings from a sterile speculum examination and a nitrazine (pH) or fern test can confirm that the membranes are ruptured (see Procedure box).

These descriptions of the contractions and the vaginal discharge help the nurse assess the degree of progress. Bloody/pink show is distinguished from bleeding by the fact that it is pink and feels sticky because of its mucoid nature. It is scant to begin with and increases with effacement and dilatation of the cervix. A woman may report a scant brownish to bloody discharge that may be attributed to cervical trauma resulting from vaginal examination or coitus occurring within the last 48 hours.

In case general anesthesia may be required in an emergency, it is important to assess the woman's respiratory status. The nurse determines this by asking the woman if she has a "cold" or related symptoms: a "stuffy nose," sore throat, or cough. The status of allergies is rechecked, including allergies to drugs routinely used in obstetrics, such as meperidine (Demerol) or lidocaine (Xylocaine). Some allergic responses cause swelling of the mucous membranes of the respiratory tract, which could interfere with breathing and the administration of inhalation anesthesia.

Because vomiting and subsequent aspiration into the respiratory tract can complicate an otherwise normal labor, the nurse records the time of the woman's last oral intake of food and the type of solid food and liquids consumed.

Any information not found in the prenatal record is requested on admission. If the woman has prepared a formal birth plan, a copy will usually be in the prenatal record. The nurse reviews it before the woman arrives in the birthing unit. The nurse uses the information in the birth plan to individualize the care given the woman during labor. The nurse also prepares the woman for the possible need to make changes in her plan as labor progresses and assures her that information will be provided as the need arises so that she can make informed decisions. If no written plan has been made, the nurse discusses the woman's wishes and preferences when she arrives and informs her of any institutional policies that might prevent granting some of the requests. Requests in a birth plan may include choosing her birth companions, wearing her own clothes, bringing her own pillow, using music, videotaping the labor and birth, walking, choosing the mode of fetal monitoring, choosing the position for birth, choosing pain relief methods, having the father cut the umbilical cord, and breastfeeding immediately after birth (Bennett & Brown, 1993; Moore, Hopper & Dip, 1995).

PROCEDURE

Tests for Rupture of Membranes

NITRAZINE TEST FOR pH

Explain procedure to woman/couple.

Wash hands.

Use nitrazine test paper, a dye-impregnated test paper for determining pH. (Differentiates amniotic fluid, which is slightly alkaline, from urine and purulent material [pus], which are acidic.)

Wearing a sterile glove lubricated with water, place a piece of test paper at the cervical os.

OR

Use a sterile, cotton-tipped applicator to dip deep into vagina to pick up fluid; touch applicator to test paper. (Procedure may be done during speculum examination.)

Read results:

Membranes probably intact: identifies vaginal and most body fluids, which are acidic:

Yellow	pH 5.0
Olive-yellow	pH 5.5
Olive-green	pH 6.0

Membranes probably ruptured: identifies amniotic fluid, which is alkaline:

Blue-green	pH 6.5
Blue-gray	pH 7.0
Deep-blue	pH 7.5

Realize that false test results are possible because of presence of bloody show, insufficient amniotic fluid, or semen.

Remove gloves and wash hands.

Document results: positive or negative.

TEST FOR FERNING OR FERN PATTERN

Explain procedure to woman/couple.

Wash hands, put on sterile gloves, obtain specimen of fluid (usually during sterile speculum examination).

Spread a drop of fluid from vagina on a clean glass slide with a sterile, cotton-tipped applicator.

Allow fluid to dry.

Examine slide under microscope: observe for appearance of **ferning** (a frondlike crystalline pattern); do not confuse with cervical mucus test, when high levels of estrogen are responsible for causing the ferning.

Observe for absence of ferning. (Alerts staff to possibility that amount of specimen was inadequate or that specimen was urine, vaginal discharge, or blood.)

Remove gloves and wash hands.

Document results: positive or negative.

●

Psychosocial factors. The woman's general appearance and behavior (and that of her partner) provide valuable clues to the type of supportive care she will need. However, the nurse should keep in mind that general appearance and behavior may vary depending on the stage and phase of labor. Psychosocial factors to assess include the following:

Verbal interactions. Does the woman ask questions? Can she ask for what she needs? Does her partner do all the talking? Does she talk to her support person(s)? Does she talk freely with the nurse or respond only to questions?

Body language. Is she relaxed or tense? What is her anxiety level? What about her partner? How does she react to being touched by the nurse or support person?

Perceptual ability. Is there a language barrier? Can she repeat what she has been told or demonstrate her understanding?

Discomfort level. To what degree does the woman describe what she is experiencing? How does she react to a contraction? Are any nonverbal pain messages seen?

Women with a history of sexual abuse. Memories of sexual abuse can be triggered during labor by intrusive procedures such as vaginal examinations; loss of control; being confined to bed and "restrained" by monitors, intravenous (IV) lines, and epidurals; being watched by students; and experiencing intense sensations in the uterus and genital area.

The nurse can help these women to associate the sensations they are experiencing with the process of childbirth and not their past abuse. The woman's sense of control should be maintained by explaining all procedures and why they are needed, proceeding at the woman's pace by waiting for her to give permission to touch her, accepting her often extreme reactions to labor, and protecting her privacy by limiting the amount of exposure of her body and the number of persons involved in her care. It is recommended that all laboring women be cared for in this manner, since it is not unusual for a woman to decline to reveal a history of sexual abuse. These care measures can help a woman to perceive her childbirth experience in positive terms and to effectively parent her new baby (Burian, 1995; Parratt, 1994; Waymire, 1997).

Stress in labor. The way in which women and their support person or family members approach labor is related to the manner in which they have been socialized to the childbearing process. Their reactions reflect their life experiences regarding childbirth—physical, social, cultural, and religious. Society communicates its expectations regarding acceptable and unacceptable maternal behaviors during labor and birth. These expectations may be used by some women as the basis for evaluating their own actions during childbirth. An idealized perception of labor and birth may be a source of guilt and a sense of failure if the woman finds the process less than joyous, especially when the pregnancy is unplanned or is the product of a shaky or terminated relationship. Often women have heard horror stories or have seen friends or relatives going through labors that appear anything but easy. Multiparous women will often base their expectations of the present labor on their previous childbirth experiences. High expectations for childbirth often result in greater satisfaction and a greater sense of fulfillment with the childbirth experience. On the other hand, women who have lower expectations often have less positive perceptions of their childbirth experience (Nichols, 1996).

GUIDELINES/GUÍAS

What time did the contractions begin?
¿A qué hora le empezaron las contracciones?

How far apart are the contractions?
¿Con qué frecuencia tiene las contracciones?

Have the membranes ruptured? When?
¿Se le rompió la fuente? ¿Cuándo?

What color was the fluid? Red? Pink?
¿Qué color tenía el líquido? ¿Rojo? ¿Rosado?

Have you had bleeding?
¿Ha sangrado?

How much? A cupful? A tablespoon? A teaspoon?
¿Cuánto? ¿Una taza? ¿Una cucharada? ¿Una cucharadita?

When was the last time you ate or drank anything?
¿Cuándo fue la última vez que comió o bebió algo?

Have you had any problems with this pregnancy?
¿Ha tenido algún problema con este embarazo?

Are you taking any medications?
¿Está tomando alguna medicación?

Are you allergic to penicillin or other medicines?
¿Es alérgica a la penicilina u otras medicinas?

Please sign this consent form.
Por favor, firme esta forma de consentimiento.

Usually women in labor have a variety of concerns that they will voice if asked but rarely volunteer. To clear up misinformation, it is important for the nurse to ask the woman what she expects. The following are common concerns that women in labor have: Will my baby be all right? Will I be able to stand labor? Will my labor be long? How will I act? Will I need medication? Will it work for me? Will my partner or someone be there to support me? Do I have to have an IV?

The nurse's responsibility to the woman in labor with regard to these concerns is to answer her questions or find out the answers, to provide support for the woman and her support person or family, to consider the woman and her significant others as partners in the care process, and to serve as their advocate. According to McKay and Smith (1993), women equate emotional support with information giving. Nurses are perceived as supportive when they explain things in detail, use positive terms, and provide accurate information and specific directions. Women feel empowered when they are given information they can understand and that shows support for their efforts. This feeling of empowerment gives women the sense that they have the freedom to participate fully in their labor and birth and fosters a positive perception of the experience. In contrast, a woman's level of anxiety and fear may rise when she does not understand what is being said. The woman who is unfamiliar with expressions such as "bloody show," "the membranes ruptured," "scalp electrode," and "baby's lying on the cord"

could understandably panic. Many such expressions sound violent and could conjure up thoughts of injury or pain.

The woman should understand that she is not expected to act in any particular way and that the process will yield the birth of her baby, which is the only expectation she should have. Nursing support needs to reflect respect for and acceptance of a woman's individuality and behavior. Women need to be able to behave in a manner that is natural for them, to be able to "let go" (Waldenström et al., 1996). The woman's views and expectations regarding the nurse's role as caregiver should be determined. The nurse-patient relationship will become increasingly important as labor progresses (Bryanton, Fraser-Davey & Sullivan, 1994).

The father, coach, or significant other also experiences stress during labor. The nurse can assist and support these people by identifying their needs and expectations and by helping make sure they are met. The nurse can ascertain what role the support person intends to fulfill and whether he or she is prepared for that role by finding out the answers to such questions as: What role does this person expect to play? Is he or she nervous, anxious, aggressive, or hostile? Does he or she look hungry, tired, worried, or confused? Does he or she watch television, sleep, or stay out of the room instead of paying attention to the woman? Does he or she touch the woman? What is the character of the touch? Has the couple attended childbirth classes? The nurse should be sensitive to the needs of support people and provide teaching and support as appropriate. Often the support this person is able to give the laboring woman is in direct proportion to the support he or she receives from the nurses and other health care providers (Nichols, 1993).

Cultural factors. It is important to note the woman's ethnic or cultural and religious background to anticipate nursing interventions that may need to be added or eliminated from the individualized plan of care.

Cultural beliefs and values can influence a woman's reliance on her primary health care provider during labor and her desire to participate in making decisions about the care she receives (Callister, Vehvilainen-Julkunen & Lauri, 1996).

When a nurse is assessing a woman's cultural and religious preferences, Callister (1995) suggests asking questions regarding the following:

- The value and meaning placed on the childbirth experience
- The view of childbirth as a wellness or illness experience and as a private or social event
- The practices regarding diet, medications, activity, and emotional and physical support
- The appropriate maternal and paternal behaviors
- The birth companions—who they should be and what they should do
- The views regarding the newborn and the newborn's care immediately after birth

The woman should be encouraged to request caregiving behaviors and practices that are important to her. If a special request contradicts usual practices in that setting, the woman or the nurse can ask the woman's primary health care provider to write an order to accommodate the special request. For example, in many cultures having a male caregiver examine a pregnant woman is unacceptable. In some cultures it is traditional to take the placenta home; in others the woman is given only certain nourishments during labor. Some women believe that cutting her body, as with an episiotomy, allows her spirit to leave her body and that rupturing the membranes prolongs, not shortens, labor (see Cultural Considerations box).

Within cultures women may have the "right" way to behave in labor instilled in them and to react to the pain experienced in that way. These behaviors can range from total silence to moaning or screaming, but they are not in and of themselves a gauge of the degree of pain. A woman who moans with contractions may not be in as much physical pain as a woman who is silent but winces during contractions (Table 15-1). Some women feel it is shameful to

CULTURAL CONSIDERATIONS
Birth Practices in Different Cultures

South Korea—Stoic response to labor pain; father usually not present.

Japan—Natural childbirth methods practiced; may labor silently; may eat during labor; father may be present.

China—Stoic response to pain; father not present; side-lying position preferred for labor and birth because this position is thought to reduce infant trauma.

India—Natural childbirth methods preferred; father usually not present; female relatives usually present.

Iran—Father not present; prefers female support and female caregivers.

Mexico—May be stoic about discomfort until second stage, then may request pain relief; father and female relatives may be present.

Laos—May use squatting position for birth; father may or may not be present; prefers female attendants.

Geissler E: *Pocket guide to cultural assessment,* St Louis, 1994, Mosby.

TABLE 15-1 *Sociocultural Basis of Pain Experience*	
WOMAN IN LABOR	**NURSE**
PERCEPTION OF MEANING	
Origin: Cultural concept of and personal experience with pain; for example: Pain in childbirth is inevitable, something to be borne. Pain in childbirth can be avoided completely. Pain in childbirth is punishment for sin. Pain in childbirth can be controlled.	Origin: Cultural concept of and personal experience with pain; in addition, nurse becomes accustomed to working with certain "expected" pain trajectories. For example, in obstetrics, pain is expected to increase as labor progresses, be intermittent, and have end point; relief can be derived from medications once labor is well established and fetus or newborn can cope with amount and elimination of medications; relief can also come from woman's knowledge, attitude, and support from family or friends.
COPING MECHANISMS	

Woman may exhibit the following behaviors:
  Be traditionally vocal or nonvocal; crying out or groaning, or both, may be part of her ritual response to pain.
  Use counter stimulation to minimize pain (e.g., rubbing, applying heat, or applying counterpressure).
  Use relaxation, distraction, or autosuggestion as pain-countering techniques.
  Resist any use of "needles" as modes of administering pain relief agents.
	Nurse may respond by:
	  Using self effectively (e.g., using tone of voice, closeness in space, and touch as media for conveying message of interest and caring).
	  Using avoidance, belittling, or other distracting actions as protective device for self.
	  Using pharmacologic resources at hand judiciously.
	  Using comfort measures.
	  Assuming accountability for control and management of pain.

EXPECTATIONS OF OTHERS	
Nurse may be seen as someone who will accept woman's statement of pain and act as her advocate. Medical personnel may be expected to relieve woman of all pain sensations. Nurse may be expected to be interested, gentle, kind, and accepting of behavior exhibited.	Only certain verbal or nonverbal responses to pain may be accepted as appropriate responses. Couple that is prepared for childbirth may be expected to refuse medication and to wish to "do everything on their own." Woman's definition of pain may not be accepted; that is, woman may wish to experience and participate in controlling pain or may not be able to accept any pain as reasonable.

scream or cry out in pain if a man is present (D'Avanzo, 1992). If the woman's support person is her mother, she may perceive the need to "behave" more strongly than if her support person is the father of the baby. She will perceive herself as failing or succeeding on the basis of her ability to adhere to these "standards" of behavior. Conversely, a woman's behavior in response to pain may influence the support received from significant others. In some cultures women who lose control and cry out in pain may be scolded, whereas in other cultures support persons will become more helpful (Weber, 1996).

The non–English-speaking woman in labor. A woman's level of anxiety in labor rises when she does not understand what is happening to her or what is being said (McKay & Smith, 1993). Some misunderstanding may occur with English-speaking women and cause some stress, but the effect of misunderstanding on non–English-speaking women is much more dramatic because they often feel a complete loss of control over their situation if there is no health care provider present who speaks her language. They can panic and withdraw or become physically abusive when someone tries to do something they perceive might harm them or their babies. Sometimes a support person is able to serve as a translator. However, this must be done with caution because the translator may not be able to convey exactly what the nurse or others are saying or what the woman is saying and raise the woman's stress level even more.

Ideally, a bilingual nurse will care for the woman. Alternatively, an employee or volunteer translator may be contacted for assistance. If no one in the hospital is able to translate, a translation service can be called so that a translation can take place over the telephone. For some women, a female translator may be more acceptable. If no translator is available, the labor and birth unit staff can prepare a set of cards with graphic depictions that illustrate common situations that can be used to communicate with non–English-speaking women. Even when the nurse has limited ability to communicate verbally with the woman, in most instances the nurse's efforts to communicate are meaningful and appreciated by the woman. (See Box 2-1 on working with a translator and Guidelines/Guías box on p. 355.)

Physical examination. During the screening/triage process, a quick vaginal examination may be done to rule out imminent birth before proceeding with an initial examination to confirm the onset of true labor. The findings serve as a baseline for assessing the woman's progress from that point. The initial physical examination includes a general systems assessment; performance of Leopold's maneuvers to determine fetal presentation and position and the point of maximum intensity (PMI) for auscultating the FHR; assessment of fetal status; assessment of uterine contractions; and vaginal examination to assess the status of cervical effacement and dilatation, fetal descent, and amniotic membranes and fluid. The most vital aspect of the assessment is the determination of fetal status.

Women often focus on the nature of their contractions as the clearest indicator of how far advanced their labor is. However, the findings from the vaginal examination are actually more valid indicators of the phase of labor, especially for nulliparous women. Rupture of the membranes significantly affects the woman's care plan because, once this occurs, the membranes can no longer protect the intrauterine cavity and fetus from infectious organisms that can travel up the birth canal. The risk of umbilical cord prolapse exists once the membranes have ruptured. Because of the bearing such information has on the care rendered, it is important to obtain as many related pieces of information as possible before planning and implementing care.

The information yielded by a complete and accurate assessment during screening serves as the basis for determining whether the woman should be admitted and what her ongoing care should be. Expected maternal progress and minimum assessment guidelines during the first stage of labor are presented in Table 15-2 and the Care Path.

The assessment procedures described in the following paragraphs can be used as a basis for teaching women and their families. The equipment needed, the nursing actions involved, and the rationale for each procedure can be shared with the woman. The nurse should thoroughly wash her hands before performing any of these procedures. Handwashing is also important after the examinations are completed. Standard Precautions should guide all assessment and care measures. The assessment findings are explained to the woman whenever possible. Throughout labor, accurate documentation is done as soon as possible after a procedure has been performed. This involves the careful noting of the findings and the time the procedure was performed on both the chart and the fetal monitoring strip, which the nurse then initials (Fig. 15-3).

General systems assessment. A brief systems assessment is performed. This includes an assessment of the heart, lungs, and skin; an examination to determine the presence and extent of edema of the legs, face, hands, or sacrum; and testing of deep tendon reflexes and for clonus.

Vital signs (TPR and blood pressure) are assessed on admission, and the initial values are used as the baseline for comparison with subsequent values. If the blood pressure is elevated, it should be reassessed 30 minutes later, between contractions, using a correct-size blood pressure cuff to obtain a reading after the woman has relaxed. To prevent supine hypotension and fetal distress, the woman should be encouraged to lie on her side and not supine (Fig. 15-4). Her temperature is monitored so that infection or a fluid deficit (dehydration associated with inadequate intake of fluids) can be identified. The woman's intake and output should be measured at least every 8 hours. The urinary protein and the ketone levels of each voided specimen should be determined using a dipstick.

TABLE 15-2 *Expected Maternal Progress in First Stage of Labor*

CRITERION	PHASES MARKED BY CERVICAL DILATATION*		
	0-3 CM (LATENT)	4-7 CM (ACTIVE)	8-10 CM (TRANSITION)
Duration†	About 6 to 8 hr	About 3 to 6 hr	About 20 to 40 min
Contractions			
Strength	Mild to moderate	Moderate to strong	Strong to very strong
Rhythm	Irregular	More regular	Regular
Frequency	5 to 30 min apart	3 to 5 min apart	2 to 3 min apart
Duration	30 to 45 sec	40 to 70 sec	45 to 90 sec
Descent			
Station of	Nulliparous: 0	Varies: +1 to +2 cm	Varies: +2 to +3 cm
presenting part	Multiparous: 0 to −2 cm	Varies +1 to +2 cm	Varies: +2 to +3 cm
Show			
Color	Brownish discharge, mucous plug, or pale pink mucus	Pink to bloody mucus	Bloody mucus
Amount	Scant	Scant to moderate	Copious
Behavior and appearance‡	Excited; thoughts center on self, labor, and baby; may be talkative or silent, calm or tense; some apprehension; pain controlled fairly well; alert, follows directions readily; open to instructions	Becomes more serious, doubtful of control of pain, more apprehensive; desires companionship and encouragement; attention more inner directed; fatigue evidenced; malar (cheeks) flush; has some difficulty following directions	Pain described as severe; backache common; frustration, fear of loss of control, and irritability surface; vague in communications; amnesia between contractions; writhing with contractions; nausea and vomiting, especially if hyperventilating; hyperesthesia; circumoral pallor, perspiration of forehead and upper lips; shaking tremor of thighs; feeling of need to defecate, pressure on anus

*In the nullipara, effacement is often complete before dilatation begins; in the multipara, it occurs simultaneously with dilatation. Average total duration: nullipara—10 to 16 hr; multipara—6 to 10 hr.
†Duration of each phase is influenced by such factors as parity, maternal position, and level of activity. For example, the labor of a nullipara tends to last longer, on average, than the labor of a multipara. Women who ambulate and assume upright positions or change positions frequently during labor tend to experience a shorter first stage.
‡Women who have epidural analgesia for pain relief may not demonstrate these behaviors.

Leopold's maneuvers (abdominal palpation). **Leopold's maneuvers** are performed with the woman lying on her back for a brief period (see Procedure box and Fig. 15-5). These maneuvers help identify (1) the number of fetuses; (2) the presenting part, the fetal lie, and the fetal attitude; (3) the degree of the presenting part's descent into the pelvis; and (4) the expected location of the PMI of the FHR on the woman's abdomen.

Assessment of FHR and pattern. It is important for the nurse to understand the relationship between the location of the PMI of the FHR and fetal presentation, lie, and position. A high risk for childbirth complications may be revealed by variations in these findings. The PMI of the FHR is the location on the maternal abdomen where the FHR is heard the loudest. It is usually directly over the fetal back. The PMI is also an aid in determining the fetal presentation and position (Fig. 15-6). In a vertex presentation the FHR is heard below the mother's umbilicus in either the right or left lower quadrant of the abdomen. In a breech presentation the FHR is heard above the mother's umbilicus (Fig. 15-6, *A*). As the fetus descends and rotates internally, the FHR is heard lower and closer to the midline of the maternal abdomen. Diagrams of the PMI for different presentations and positions are presented in Fig. 15-6. The aspects of the assessment recommended for determining fetal status in the low-risk woman during the first stage of labor are summarized in the Care Path. The FHR also must be assessed (1) immediately after rupture of membranes (ROM), because this is the most common time for the umbilical cord to prolapse, (2) after any change in the contraction pattern or maternal status, and (3) before and after medicating the woman or performing a procedure.

Assessment of uterine contractions. A general characteristic of effective labor is regular uterine activity, but uterine activity is not directly related to labor progress. Uterine contractions are the primary powers that act involuntarily to expel the fetus and the placenta from the uterus. There are several ways of evaluating uterine contractions; these

Text continued on p. 364

CARE PATH — Low-Risk Woman in First Stage of Labor

CARE MANAGEMENT	CERVICAL DILATATION		
	0-3 CM (LATENT)	4-7 CM (ACTIVE)	8-10 CM (TRANSITION)
I. ASSESSMENT MEASURES*	**Frequency**	**Frequency**	**Frequency**
• Blood pressure, pulse, respirations	Every 30-60 min	Every 30 min	Every 15-30 min
• Temperature†	Every 4 hr	Every 4 hr	Every 4 hr
• Uterine activity	Every 30-60 min	Every 15-30 min	Every 10-15 min
• Fetal heart rate (FHR)	Every 30-60 min	Every 15-30 min	Every 15-30 min
• Vaginal show	Every 30-60 min	Every 30 min	Every 15 min
• Behavior, appearance, mood, energy level of woman; condition of partner	Every 30 min	Every 15 min	Every 5 min
• Vaginal examination‡	As needed to identify progress	As needed to identify progress	As needed to identify progress
II. PHYSICAL CARE MEASURES§	Stay at home for as long as possible Relaxation measures: rest and sleep if at night Activity—ambulation; emphasize upright positions Diversional activities Nourishment—light foods and full liquids Void every 2 hr Perform basic hygiene measures	Coach breathing techniques Encourage effleurage Assist in using relaxation techniques between contractions Encourage ambulation, upright positions Assist with position changes Use comfort measures desired by woman: massage, hot/cold packs, touch, etc. Initiate hydrotherapy (shower, bath, Jacuzzi) Provide nourishment as desired Encourage voiding every 2 hr Assist with hygiene, perineal care Provide pharmacologic pain relief as indicated Provide relief for partner	Coach breathing techniques Reduce touch if increased sensitivity is noted Help to relax between contractions Assist with position changes Use comfort measures according to acceptance level Continue hydrotherapy if effective Provide clear liquids: sips, ice chips Encourage voiding every 2 hr Provide hygiene measures, emphasizing mouth and perineal care Provide pharmacologic pain relief as indicated Prepare for birth
III. EMOTIONAL SUPPORT	Review birth plan Review process of labor— what to expect, pain management techniques available Redemonstrate breathing techniques Keep informed: progress, procedures	Provide feedback about performance Reduce distractions during contractions Role model comfort measures Reassure, encourage, praise Take charge, talk through contraction until control regained Continue to keep informed	Provide continuous support Reduce distractions Role model care measures to assist partner Continue reassurance, praise, and encouragement Keep informed Take charge as needed

*Full assessment using interview, physical examination, and laboratory testing is performed on admission. Subsequently, frequency of assessment is determined by the risk status of the maternal-fetal unit. More frequent assessment is required in high-risk situations. Frequency of assessment and method of documentation are also determined by agency policy, which is usually based on the recommended care standards of medical and nursing organizations.
†If membranes have ruptured, the temperature should be assessed every 1-2 hr; assess orally or tympanically between contractions.
‡Perform vaginal examination at admission and thereafter only when signs indicate that progress has occurred (e.g., significant increase in frequency, duration, and intensity of contractions; rupture of membranes; perineal pressure); strict aseptic technique should be used. In the presence of vaginal bleeding, the primary health care provider performs the examination under a double setup in a delivery room, or an ultrasonography is performed to determine placental location.
§Physical care measures are performed by the nurse working together with the woman's partner and significant others. The woman is capable of greater independence in the latent phase but needs more assistance during the active and transition phases.

Labor Progress Chart

| Admit date ___ / ___ / ___ | Admit time | Blood type and Rh | Age | G | T | P | A | L | EDB ___ / ___ / ___ LMP ___ / ___ / ___ | | Membranes ☐ **Intact** ☐ Ruptured SROM AROM ☐ Bulging Date ___/___/___ Time _____ | | | | | |

Current date ___ / ___ / ___	**Time →**															
Vital signs Temperature																
Pulse																
Respiration																
Blood pressure																
Maternal Deep tendon reflexes (L/R)	/	/	/	/	/	/	/	/	/	/	/	/	/	/	/	/
Urine (Protein/sugar)	/	/	/	/	/	/	/	/	/	/	/	/	/	/	/	/
Vaginal bleeding																
Uterine activity Monitor mode																
Frequency																
Duration																
Intensity																
Resting tone																
Peak IUP																
MVUs																
Fetal assessment Monitor mode																
Baseline (FHR)																
STV																
LTV																
Accelerations																
Decelerations																
Strip number																
Membranes																
Fluid																
Intake/Output (cc's/Hr) IV																
PO																
Urine																
Emesis																
Cont meds Pitocin mU/min																
MgSO$_4$ gms/hr																
Ritodrine mg/min																
Terbutaline mg/hr																
Intervention Position change																
O$_2$ L/min																
IV bolus																
Initials																

Abbreviations/Key	Vaginal bleeding NS = Normal show ABN = Frank vaginal Bleeding	Monitor mode uterine activity P = Palpation E = External I = Internal	MVUs (montevideo units) The sum of the peak of each uterine contraction minus resting tone, in a 10-minute period.	Monitor mode fetal A = Auscultation (fetoscope) D = Doppler E = External I = Internal	STV (short-term variability) STV + = Present (roughness of tracing line present) STV ∅ = Absent (tracing line is smooth)

Fig. **15-3** Labor in progress chart. (Permission to use and/or reproduce this copyrighted material has been granted by the owner, Hollister Incorporated, Libertyville, Ill.)

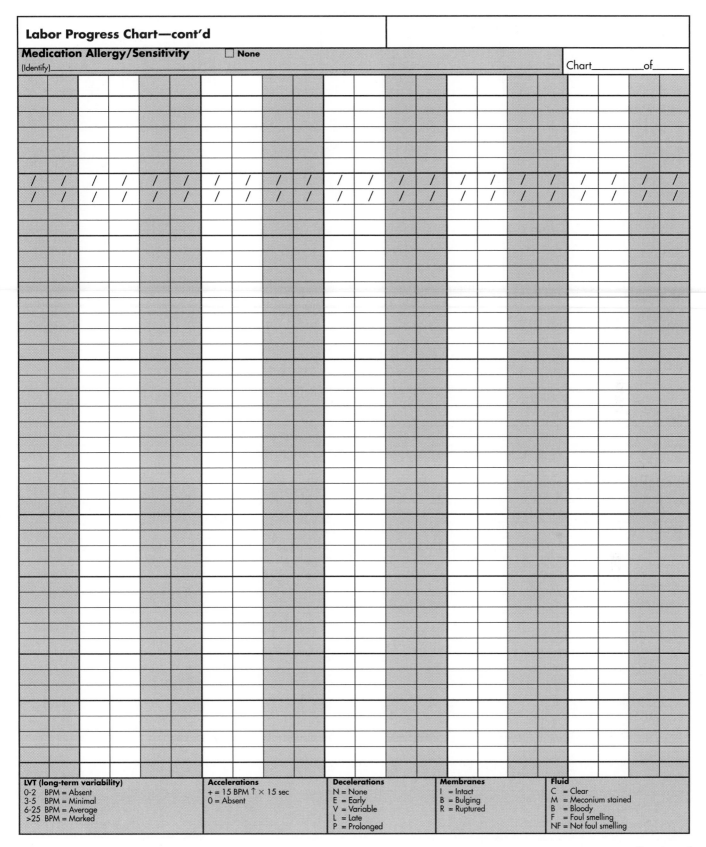

Labor Progress Chart—cont'd

Medication Allergy/Sensitivity ☐ **None**

(Identify)_____

Chart_____of_____

LVT (long-term variability)
0-2 BPM = Absent
3-5 BPM = Minimal
6-25 BPM = Average
>25 BPM = Marked

Accelerations
+ = 15 BPM ↑ × 15 sec
0 = Absent

Decelerations
N = None
E = Early
V = Variable
L = Late
P = Prolonged

Membranes
I = Intact
B = Bulging
R = Ruptured

Fluid
C = Clear
M = Meconium stained
B = Bloody
F = Foul smelling
NF = Not foul smelling

Fig. **15-3 cont'd,** Labor in progress chart.

Continued

Labor Progress Chart—cont'd

Time →					
Mark X	•	10			
-4		9			
-3	**D i l a t a t i o n**	8			
-2		7			
-1		6			
S t a t i o n 0		5			
+1		4			
+2		3			
+3		2			
Effacement % and/or position					
Examined by:					

IV Record

Start date	Time	Solution	Amount (mls)	Medication/Dose added	Initials	Infused date	Time	Amount infused

Teaching

Topic	Date time	Comments
Oriented		
Labor review		
Support person		
Pre-Op		
Safety		

Interval Medications

Date time	Medication/Dose	Route	Site	Initials		Initials	Signature

Progress Notes

Date	Time	

Fig. **15-3 cont'd,** Labor in progress chart.

Labor Progress Chart—cont'd	

Progress Notes (Cont'd.)

Date	Time	

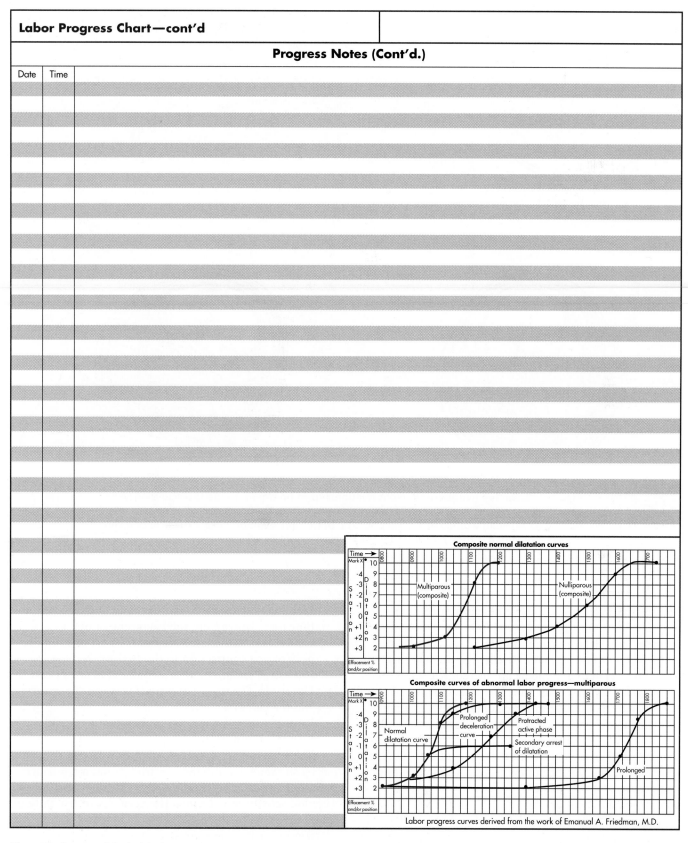

Fig. **15-3 cont'd,** Labor in progress chart.

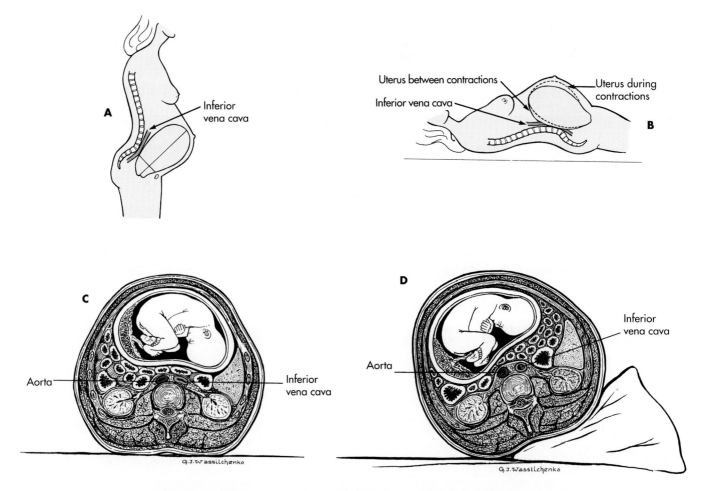

Fig. **15-4** Supine hypotension. Note relationship of pregnant uterus to ascending vena cava in standing position, **A,** and in supine position, **B. C,** Compression of aorta and inferior vena cava with woman in supine position. **D,** Compression of these vessels is relieved by placement of a wedge pillow under the woman's right or left hip.

include the woman's subjective description of them, palpation and timing of the contraction by a health care provider, and electronic monitoring.

Each contraction exhibits a wavelike pattern. It begins with a slow increment (the "building up" of a contraction from its onset), gradually reaches an acme (the peak; intrauterine pressure of 50 to 75 mm Hg), and then diminishes rather rapidly (decrement, the "letting down" of the contraction). An interval of rest follows, during which the intrauterine pressure is 5 to 15 mm Hg); this ends when the next contraction begins. (The outward appearance of the woman's abdomen during and between contractions and the pattern of a typical uterine contraction are shown in Fig. 15-7.)

A uterine contraction is described in terms of the following characteristics:

- **Frequency:** How often uterine contractions occur; the time that elapses from the beginning of one contraction to the beginning of the next or from the peak of one contraction to the peak of the next.
- **Intensity:** The strength of a contraction at its peak.
- **Duration:** The time that elapses between the onset and the end of a contraction.
- **Resting tone:** The tension in the uterine muscle between contractions.

The ways to assess uterine contractions are by palpation or by an external or internal electronic monitor. Frequency and duration can be determined by all three methods of uterine activity monitoring. The accuracy of determining intensity varies by the method used. Palpation is more subjective and may be less precise.

PROCEDURE

Leopold's Maneuvers and Determination of the Points of Maximum Intensity of the FHR

LEOPOLD'S MANEUVERS

Wash hands.

Ask woman to empty bladder.

Position woman supine with one pillow under her head and with her knees slightly flexed.

Place small rolled towel under woman's right hip to displace uterus to left of major blood vessels (prevents supine hypotensive syndrome; see Fig. 15-4).

If right-handed, stand on woman's right, facing her:

1. Identify fetal part that occupies the fundus. The head feels round, firm, freely movable, and palpable by ballottement; the breech feels less regular and softer. This maneuver identifies fetal lie (longitudinal or transverse) and presentation (cephalic or breech) (Fig. 15-5, *A*).

2. Using palmar surface of one hand, locate and palpate the smooth convex contour of the fetal back and the irregularities that identify the small parts (feet, hands, elbows). This maneuver helps identify fetal presentation (Fig. 15-5, *B*).

3. With right hand, determine which fetal part is presenting over the inlet to the true pelvis. Gently grasp the lower pole of the uterus between the thumb and fingers, pressing in slightly (Fig. 15-5, *C*). If the head is presenting and not engaged, determine the attitude of the head (flexed or extended).

4. Turn to face the woman's feet. Using both hands, outline the fetal head (Fig. 15-5, *D*) with the palmar surface of the fingertips. When the presenting part has descended deeply, only a small portion of it may be outlined. Palpation of the cephalic prominence helps identify the attitude of the head. If the cephalic prominence is found on the same side as the small parts, this means that the head must be flexed and the vertex is presenting (Fig. 15-5, *D*). If the cephalic prominence is on the same side as the back, this indicates that the presenting head is extended and the face is presenting (Fig. 15-5, *D*).

Document fetal presentation, position, and lie and whether presenting part is flexed or extended, engaged, or free floating. Use hospital's protocol for documentation (e.g., "Vtx, LOA, floating").

DETERMINATION OF PMI OF FHR

Wash hands.

Perform Leopold's maneuvers.

Auscultate FHR based on fetal presentation identified with Leopold's maneuvers. The PMI is the location where the FHR is heard the loudest, usually over the fetal back (see Fig. 15-6).

Chart PMI of FHR using a two-line figure to indicate the four quadrants of the maternal abdomen, as follows: right upper quadrant (RUQ), left upper quadrant (LUQ), left lower quadrant (LLQ), and right lower quadrant (RLQ):

RUQ	LUQ
RLQ	LLQ

The umbilicus is the reference point for the quadrants (point where the lines cross). The PMI for the fetus in vertex presentation, in general flexion with the back on the mother's right side, commonly is found in the mother's right lower quadrant and is recorded with an "X" or with the FHR, as follows:

$$X \quad \text{or} \quad 140$$

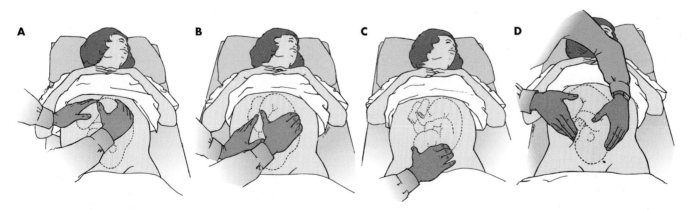

Fig. **15-5** Leopold's maneuvers.

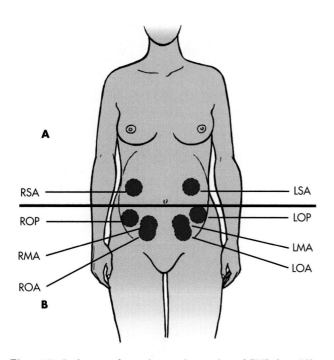

Fig. **15-6** Areas of maximum intensity of FHR for differing positions: *RSA,* right sacrum anterior; *ROP,* right occipitoposterior; *RMA,* right mentum anterior; *ROA,* right occipitoanterior; *LSA,* left sacrum anterior; *LOP,* left occipitoposterior; *LMA,* left mentum anterior; *LOA,* left occipitoanterior. **A,** Presentation is *breech* if FHR is heard *above* umbilicus. **B,** Presentation is *vertex* if FHR is heard *below* umbilicus.

The following terms are used to describe what is felt on palpation:
- *Mild:* Slightly tense fundus that is easy to indent with fingertips (feels like touching finger to tip of nose)
- *Moderate:* Firm fundus that is difficult to indent with fingertips (feels like touching finger to chin)
- *Strong:* Rigid, boardlike fundus that is almost impossible to indent with fingertips (feels like touching finger to forehead)

Women in labor tend to describe the pain of contractions in terms of the sensations they are experiencing in the lower abdomen or back, which may be unrelated to the firmness of the uterine fundus. Thus their assessment of the strength of their contractions can be less valid than that of the health care provider, although the amount of discomfort reported is valid.

External electronic monitoring provides information about the relative strength of the uterine contractions. Internal electronic monitoring using an intrauterine pressure catheter is the most reliable way of assessing the intensity of uterine contractions.

On the woman's admission, a 20- to 30-minute baseline monitoring of uterine contractions and the FHR usually is done (Scott et al., 1994). The minimum assessment times during the various phases of the first stage of labor are given in the Care Path, and the findings expected as labor progresses are summarized in Table 15-2.

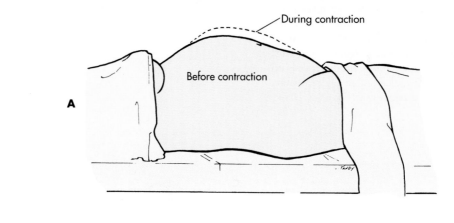

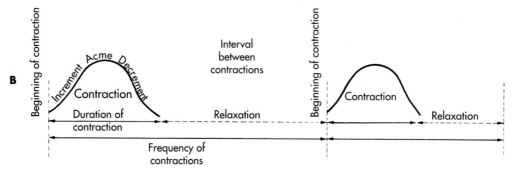

Fig. **15-7** Assessment of uterine contractions. **A,** Abdominal contour before and during uterine contraction. **B,** Wavelike pattern of contractile activity.

The nurse's responsibility in the monitoring of uterine contractions is to ascertain whether they are powerful and frequent enough to accomplish the work of expelling the fetus and the placenta.

Uterine activity must be considered in the context of its effect on cervical effacement and dilatation and on the degree of descent of the presenting part. The effect on the fetus also must be considered. The progress of labor can be effectively verified through the use of graphic charts (partograms) on which cervical dilatation and station (descent) are plotted. This type of graphic charting helps identify early deviations from expected labor pat-terns. Fig. 15-8 shows the expected pattern of cervical dilatation and descent for both nulliparous and multiparous women. Fig. 15-9 provides one example of a partogram; however, hospitals and birthing centers may develop their own graphs for recording assessments. Such graphs may include not only data on dilatation and descent but also on maternal vital signs, FHR, and uterine activity. Regardless of which charting format is used, the nurse is responsible for documenting the findings regarding labor progress and for notifying the primary health care provider of any unexpected or abnormal pattern that emerges.

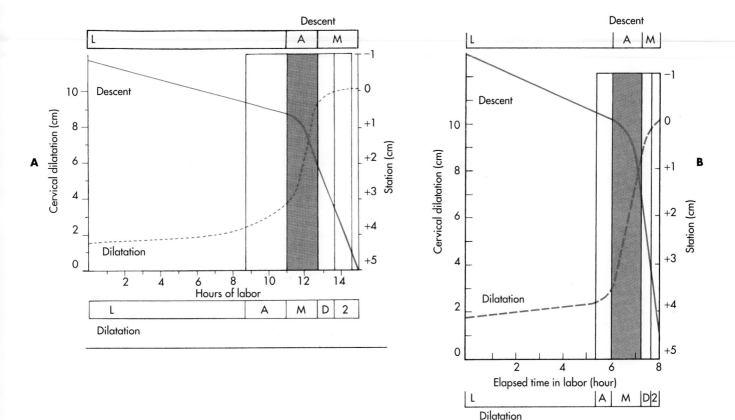

Fig. **15-8** Partograms showing relationship between cervical dilatation and descent of presenting part. **A,** Labor of a nulliparous woman. **B,** Labor of a multiparous woman. The phases of cervical dilatation are identified by the letters *L, A, M,* and *D.* The number *2* refers to the stage of labor. The latent phase *(L)* of the first stage of labor is the time between the onset of labor and the onset of acceleration. The active phase begins with the acceleration phase *(A)* and lasts from the onset of the upward curve of cervical dilatation to the full dilatation of the cervix. Freidman (1978) divides the active phase into three parts: (1) the acceleration phase *(A),* (2) the phase of maximum slope *(M),* and (3) the deceleration phase *(D).* The dotted line denotes cervical dilatation. The phases of descent are identified by the letters *L, A,* and *M,* located at the top of the graph. *L* refers to the latent phase of minimum descent. Active descent *(A)* generally begins when the cervical dilatation curve reaches its phase of maximum slope. The rate of descent reaches its maximum at the beginning of the deceleration phase of cervical dilatation. Maximum descent *(M)* continues in a linear manner until the perineum is reached. The solid line shows the rate of descent.

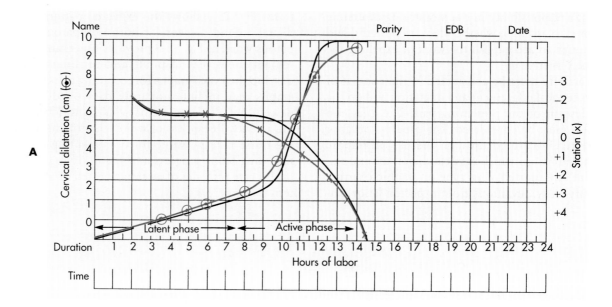

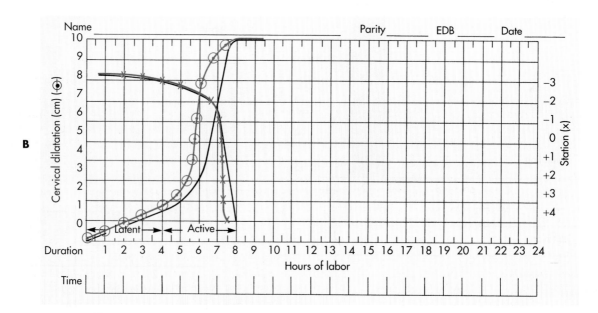

Fig. **15-9** Partogram for assessment of patterns of cervical dilatation and descent. Individual woman's labor patterns *(colored)* superimposed on prepared labor graph *(black)* for comparison. **A,** Labor of a nulliparous woman. **B,** Labor of a multiparous woman. The rate of cervical dilatation is plotted with the circled plot points. A line drawn through these symbols depicts the slope of the curve. Station is plotted with Xs. A line drawn through the Xs reveals the pattern of descent.

It is important for the nurse to recognize that active labor can actually last longer than the expected labor patterns. This finding should not be a cause for concern unless the maternal-fetal unit exhibits signs of distress (Albers, Schiff & Gorwoda, 1996).

Vaginal examination. The vaginal examination reveals whether the woman is in true labor and enables the exam-

iner to determine whether the membranes have ruptured. Because this examination is often stressful and uncomfortable for the woman, it should be performed only when the status of the woman and her fetus indicates the need. For example, a vaginal examination should be performed on admission, when there has been significant progress in uterine activity, on maternal perception of perineal pressure or

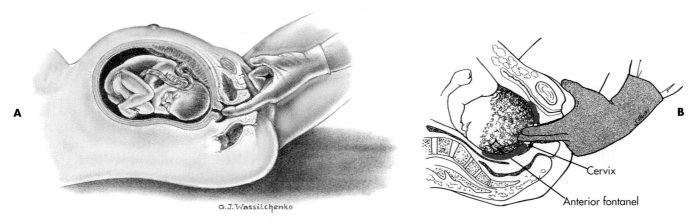

Fig. **15-10** Vaginal examination. **A,** Undilated, uneffaced cervix; membranes intact. **B,** Palpation of sagittal suture line. Cervix effaced and partially dilated.

the urge to bear down, when membranes rupture, or when variable decelerations of the FHR are noted. A full explanation of the examination and support of the woman are important factors in reducing the stress and discomfort associated with the examination.

Vaginal examinations should include the following steps:

1. The nurse assembles all of the equipment needed, including a single sterile glove, antiseptic solution or soluble gel, and a light source. Water should be used for lubrication during the initial examination if rupture of membranes (ROM) is suspected and a nitrazine test is required.

2. The nurse prepares the woman by explaining what will be done, why the examination is being performed, and how it will feel. The woman should be draped to prevent chilling and protect her privacy and positioned to prevent supine hypotension (see Fig. 15-4). The perineum and vulva are cleansed if necessary.

3. The nurse washes his/her hands and puts on the sterile glove using aseptic technique. The nurse explains to the woman that she will feel the nurse inserting the index and middle fingers into the vagina. The nurse should ask the woman for permission to touch her before proceeding (Waymire, 1997). The examination should be performed gently, with concern for the woman's comfort. The nurse acknowledges the woman's expressions of pain or discomfort and anxiety. The woman should be encouraged to breathe slowly and relax her perineum (or gently push her perineal muscles out toward the examining finger).

4. The nurse assesses the status of the following (Fig. 15-10):
    a. Dilatation and effacement of cervix
    b. Presenting part, position, station, and, if vertex, any molding of the head
    c. Membranes—intact, bulging, or ruptured; amniotic fluid—color, clarity, odor, etc.
    d. Presence of stool in rectum

5. The nurse then helps the woman into a comfortable position and discusses the findings of the examination with the woman and support person.

6. The nurse documents all findings and reports them to the primary health care provider.

Laboratory and diagnostic tests. The nurse should anticipate the need for urinalysis, blood tests, and tests for ROM.

Analysis of urine specimen. A clean-catch urine specimen is obtained to acquire further data about the pregnant woman's health. It is a convenient and simple procedure that can provide information about her hydration status (specific gravity, ketones, color, amount), nutritional status (ketones), infection status (e.g., the presence of leukocytes), or the status of possible complications such as PIH, (shown by the finding of protein in the urine). The results can be obtained quickly and help the nurse determine appropriate interventions to implement.

Blood tests. The blood tests performed vary with the hospital protocol and the woman's health status. An example of a minimum assessment is a hematocrit determination, in which the specimen is centrifuged in the perinatal unit. Blood can be obtained by a finger stick or from the hub of a catheter used to start an IV line. More comprehensive blood assessments such as white blood cell count, red blood cell count, the hemoglobin level, hematocrit, and platelet count are included in a CBC. A CBC may be ordered for women with a history of infection, anemia, PIH, and so on.

If the woman's blood type has not been verified, blood is drawn for the purpose of determining the type and Rh factor. If blood typing has already been done, the primary health care provider may choose not to repeat the test. If obvious signs of immunocompromise or substance abuse are present, other diagnostic blood tests may be ordered.

Assessment of amniotic membranes and fluid. Labor is initiated at term by spontaneous rupture of membranes (SROM, SRM) in approximately 25% of pregnant women. A lag period, rarely exceeding 24 hours, may precede the onset of labor. Membranes (the BOW) can also rupture spontaneously any time during labor.

NURSE ALERT *The umbilical cord may prolapse when the membranes rupture. It is the nurse's responsibility to monitor the FHR for several minutes immediately after ROM to ascertain fetal well-being, and then to document the findings.*

Tests for assessing ROM are discussed in the Procedure box. Artificial rupture of membranes (AROM) or amniotomy may be done to augment or induce labor or to facilitate placement of internal monitors when fetal status indicates the need for some form of direct assessment (attachment of a spiral electrode to the presenting part and insertion of an intrauterine pressure catheter). The following routine characteristics of amniotic fluid are assessed.

Color. Amniotic fluid is normally pale and straw colored and may contain white particles (flecks of vernix caseosa). If the amniotic fluid is greenish brown, the fetus has probably experienced a recent hypoxic episode, causing relaxation of the anal sphincter and the passage of meconium, the by-products of fetal ingestion, in utero. Yellow-stained amniotic fluid may indicate fetal hypoxia that occurred 36 hours or more before ROM, fetal hemolytic disease (Rh or ABO incompatibility), or intrauterine infection. Meconium-stained amniotic fluid may be a normal finding in a breech presentation and results from pressure being exerted on the fetal rectum during descent. Although meconium-stained amniotic fluid may be an ominous finding in labor, it is not always associated with fetal hypoxia and must be viewed in the context of the total clinical picture of labor (Scott et al., 1994). Amniotic fluid that is port wine colored may indicate the presence of bleeding associated with premature separation of the placenta (abruptio).

Viscosity and odor. Amniotic fluid normally is watery and lacks a strong odor. Infection is suspected if the fluid is thick, cloudy, or foul smelling, or a combination of these. The presence of considerable meconium can also cause amniotic fluid to have a thick consistency.

Amount. The expected amount of amniotic fluid is 500 to 1200 ml. Most of it originates from the maternal bloodstream, with fetal urine adding to it. *Hydramnios* (>2000 ml of fluid) is the term given an excessively large amount of amniotic fluid and is often associated with congenital anomalies of the fetus, in which the fetus cannot drink the fluid or in which fluid is trapped in the fetal body. *Oligohydramnios* (<500 ml of fluid) is the term given an abnormally small amount of amniotic fluid and can be associated with incomplete formation or absence of the kidneys or obstruction of the urethra. If the fetus is unable to secrete and excrete urine, the volume of amniotic fluid decreases. In some instances, fetal surgical procedures can be performed to relieve some obstructive conditions.

The nurse's responsibility is to report findings promptly to the primary health care provider and to document findings in the labor record and on the monitor strip. If abnormal findings are noted, continuous electronic monitoring usually is implemented and maintained for the duration of labor. The finding of meconium-stained amniotic fluid alerts the nurse to the need to observe fetal status more closely. After birth, the newborn may also be at risk for an alteration in respiratory status if meconium is aspirated into the lungs with the first breath.

Infection. When membranes rupture, microorganisms from the vagina can then ascend into the amniotic sac, causing chorioamnionitis and placentitis to develop. For this reason, maternal temperature and vaginal discharge are assessed frequently (every 1 to 2 hours) so that a developing infection after ROM can be identified early. Even when membranes are intact, however, microorganisms may ascend and cause premature ROM. There is controversy regarding whether prophylactic antibiotic therapy can protect against infection (chorioamnionitis), which involves both the maternal and fetal sides of the membrane.

Signs of potential problems. Assessment findings serve as a baseline for gauging the woman's subsequent progress during the first stage of labor, after she has been admitted. Although some complications of labor are anticipated, others may appear unexpectedly during the clinical course of labor. Knowledge of the physiologic and anatomic changes that occur during pregnancy, careful initial assessment, and follow-up of the woman's progress are necessary in the care of a woman experiencing normal labor and in identifying deviations from normal that could signal potential or actual problems during labor (see Signs of Potential Complications box).

---

signs of POTENTIAL COMPLICATIONS

LABOR

- Intrauterine pressure of more than 75 mm Hg (determined by intrauterine pressure catheter monitoring) or resting tone of more than 15 mm Hg
- Contractions consistently lasting 90 seconds or more
- Contractions consistently occurring 2 minutes or less apart
- Fetal bradycardia, tachycardia, or persistently decreased variability
- Irregular FHR; suspected fetal dysrhythmias
- Appearance of meconium-stained or bloody fluid from the vagina
- Arrest in progress of cervical dilatation or effacement and/or descent of the fetus
- Maternal temperature of 38° C or more
- Foul-smelling vaginal discharge
- Persistent bright or dark red vaginal bleeding

Nursing diagnoses determine the types of nursing actions needed to implement a plan of care. When establishing nursing diagnoses, the nurse should analyze the significance of findings gleaned during the assessment. See Nursing Diagnoses box for a list of selected nursing diagnoses appropriate for the first stage of labor.

Nursing Diagnoses

First Stage of Labor
INITIAL ASSESSMENT

Impaired verbal communication related to:
• Language barrier
Anxiety related to:
• Negative experience with previous childbirth
Knowledge deficit related to:
• Unfamiliar setting and procedures

SUBSEQUENT ASSESSMENTS

Pain related to:
• Intense uterine contractions
Fluid volume deficit related to:
• Decreased fluid intake
Impaired physical mobility related to:
• Fetal monitoring
• Epidural analgesia
Altered patterns of urinary elimination related to:
• Reduced intake of oral fluids
• Bed rest
• Diminished sensation of bladder fullness associated with epidural analgesia
Risk for infection related to:
• Rupture of membranes
• Insertion of internal monitors

ASSESSMENT OF STRESS DURING LABOR

Impaired gas exchange (fetal) related to:
• Maternal position
• Maternal hypotension
• Intense, frequent uterine contractions
• Compression of umbilical cord
Situational low self-esteem (maternal) related to:
• Difficulty in meeting self-expectations
• Loss of control during labor
Fear related to:
• Triggering of memories associated with history of sexual abuse
Situational low self-esteem (father/partner) related to:
• Unrealistic expectations regarding role as labor coach
• Perceived ineffectiveness in meeting needs of laboring woman
Ineffective family coping: compromised, related to:
• Unfamiliarity with comfort measures that can be used for the laboring woman

Expected Outcomes of Care

It is important for the nurse and woman to set and prioritize expected outcomes that focus on the woman, fetus, and couple. Appropriate nursing and patient actions are then determined so that these expected outcomes can be met. This planning with the woman is essential for ensuring the implementation of expected outcomes. Throughout the first stage of labor the woman will:
• Demonstrate expected progression of labor
• Express satisfaction with the assistance of her support person(s)/family and nursing staff
• Verbalize her desires for participating in labor and participate as much as possible throughout labor
• Maintain adequate hydration status through oral and/or IV intake
• Void at least every 2 hours to prevent bladder distention
• Encourage participation of support person by verbalizing discomfort and indicating the need for measures that help reduce discomfort and promote relaxation
• Express satisfaction with her performance during labor

Plan of Care and Interventions

When the woman is admitted, she is moved from the observation area to the labor room, the LDR room, or the LDRP room. If the woman has not already done so, she signs the necessary papers giving permission for care to be given to herself and her newborn.

Standards of care. Standards of care guide the nurse in preparing for and implementing procedures with the expectant mother. Protocols for care based on standards (Box 15-2) include the following tasks:
• Check the primary health care provider's orders.
• Assess the primary health care provider's orders for appropriateness and correctness (e.g., the analgesic to be administered to relieve discomfort).
• Check labels on IV solutions, drugs, and other materials used for nursing care.
• Check expiration date on any packs of supplies used for procedures ordered.
• Ensure that information on the woman's identification band is correct (also check that identification band is accurate; for example, if she has allergies, the band is the appropriate color).
• Employ an empathic approach when giving care:
  −Use words the woman can understand when explaining procedures.
  −Respect the woman's individual needs and behaviors.
  −Establish rapport with the woman and her support person and family.
  −Be kind, caring, and competent when performing necessary procedures.
  −Be aware that pain and discomfort are as the woman describes them.

| BOX 15-2 | *Patient Care Plan Using Protocols and Nursing Standards* |

PATIENT CARE PLAN FOR LABOR   **MARY JAMES**
                                     UNIT NO. 4587024

Date Initiated: _____   Time: _____   RN: _____

OUTCOME STANDARDS:
1. Patient will demonstrate normal labor progress while the fetus tolerates the labor process without demonstrating nonreassuring signs. Date met: _____
2. Patient will participate as desired in decisions about her care. Date met: _____
3. Patient and her partner will verbalize knowledge of labor process and their expectations for the birth experience. Date met: _____

INITIATED Date/RN	PROBLEM	NURSING INTERVENTIONS	DISCONTINUED Date/RN
	Alteration in maternal/ fetal gas exchange	Implement fetal monitoring per protocol or orders from health care provider	
	Risk related to labor progress:	Provide nursing care per hospital procedure manual	
	• Altered pattern of urinary elimination	Implement labor care per protocol or care path	
	• Tissue trauma related to birth	Notify primary health care provider of problems (see Signs of Potential Complications box)	
		Provide care for vaginal birth per hospital procedure manual	
		Provide immediate care for newborn per hospital procedure manual	
		Implement care for fourth stage of labor per protocol or care path	
	Anxiety related to maternal/fetal status	Encourage woman and her partner to express their concerns	
		Keep couple informed of labor progress	
		Involve woman in decision-making regarding her care	
	Knowledge deficit about labor/procedures	Explain procedures in terms woman can understand	
	Pain associated with labor	Promote use of relaxation techniques	
		Provide comfort measures	
		Offer pain medications as ordered	
		Evaluate response to pain relief measures	
	Other problems:		

—Repeat instructions as necessary and ensure that they are understood by the woman. (See Guidelines/Guías box.)

—Carry out appropriate comfort measures such as mouth care and back care and ensure that the support person is coping.

—Recognize that a woman's current childbirth experience and the actions of nurses and other health care providers can have a positive or negative effect on the woman's future childbirth experiences.

• Use Standard Precautions, including precautions appropriate to the performance of invasive procedures.

• Document care according to hospital guidelines and communicate information to the primary health care provider when indicated.

| LEGAL TIP | **Standards of Care for Labor**

1. *Provide explanations of all procedures to woman and family.*
2. *Assess maternal and fetal status, as well as progress of labor.*
   a. *Continue to monitor fetal status until birth.*
   b. *Document all assessment findings.*
   c. *Notify primary health care provider promptly regarding assessment findings, especially those that are unexpected or abnormal.*
   d. *Inform woman and family of maternal and fetal status, as well as progress of labor.*
3. *Intervene based on results of analysis of assessment data.*
   a. *Carry out all orders and protocols for care.*
   b. *Notify primary health care provider regarding outcomes of interventions.*

PLAN OF CARE *First Stage of Labor*

NURSING DIAGNOSIS Anxiety related to labor and the birthing process

Expected outcome *Patient exhibits decreased signs of anxiety.*

Nursing Interventions/*Rationales*

Orient woman to labor and birth unit and explain admission protocol *to allay initial feelings of anxiety.*

Assess woman's knowledge, experience, and expectations of labor; note any signs or expressions of anxiety, nervousness, or fear *to establish a baseline for intervention.*

Discuss the expected progression of labor and describe what to expect during the process *as knowledge can allay anxiety associated with the unknown.*

Actively involve woman in care decisions during labor, interpret sights and sounds of environment (monitor sights and sounds, unit activities), and share information on progression of labor (vital signs, FHR, dilatation, effacement) *to increase her sense of control and allay fears.*

Actively involve significant others in care during labor *to help woman cope with the process.*

NURSING DIAGNOSIS Pain related to increasing frequency and intensity of contractions

Expected Outcome *Patient exhibits signs of decreased discomfort.*

Nursing Interventions/*Rationales*

Assess woman's level of pain and strategies that she has used to cope with pain *to establish a baseline for intervention.*

Encourage significant other to remain as support person during labor process *to assist with support and comfort measures, as measures are often more effective when delivered by a familiar person.*

Instruct woman and support person in use of specific techniques such as conscious relaxation, focused breathing, effleurage, massage, and application of sacral pressure *to increase relaxation, decrease intensity of contractions, and promote use of controlled thought and direction of energy.*

Early in labor, use diversional activities *to provide distractions.*

Encourage regular voiding to decrease chances of distention, *which can increase discomfort during contractions and impede progress of labor.*

Provide comfort measures such as frequent mouth care to prevent dry mouth, application of damp cloth to forehead, and changing of damp gown or bed covers *to relieve discomfort associated with diaphoresis; positioning to reduce stiffness.*

Encourage conscious relaxation between contractions *to prevent fatigue, which contributes to increased pain perceptions.*

Explain what analgesics and anesthesia are available for use during labor and birth *to provide knowledge to help woman make decisions about pain control.*

NURSING DIAGNOSIS Risk for fluid volume deficit related to altered intake during labor.

Expected Outcomes *Fluid balance is maintained, and there are no signs of dehydration.*

Nursing Interventions/*Rationales*

Monitor intake and output, and vital signs and inspect skin turgor and mucous membranes for dryness *to evaluate hydration status.*

Administer oral/parenteral fluids per physician/nurse midwife order *to maintain hydration.*

Monitor any emesis and administer antiemetic per physician/nurse midwife order if necessary *to control emesis and prevent fluid loss.*

NURSING DIAGNOSIS Risk for infection related to rupture of membranes before or during labor.

Expected Outcome *Patient shows no evidence of infection.*

Nursing Interventions/*Rationales*

After rupture of membranes, assess amniotic fluid for alterations in color, odor, amount, and presence of blood and meconium, *which may be indicative of intrauterine infection.*

Monitor vital signs and FHR *to evaluate for signs of infection.*

Maintain Standard Precautions, use good handwashing technique and aseptic technique when indicated, and maintain good perineal hygiene *to prevent spread of microorganisms.*

NURSING DIAGNOSIS Risk for altered pattern of urinary elimination related to sensory impairment secondary to labor.

Expected Outcome *Bladder does not show signs of distention.*

Nursing Interventions/*Rationales*

Palpate the bladder superior to the symphysis on a frequent basis *as distention may occur from increased fluid intake and inability to feel urge to void.*

Encourage frequent voiding and catheterize if necessary *to avoid bladder distention as it impedes progress of fetus down birth canal and may result in trauma to the bladder.*

From Wong D & Perry S: *Maternal child nursing care,* St Louis, 1998, Mosby.

glucose into the bloodstream, which could result in fetal hyperglycemia and fetal hyperinsulinism. After birth, the neonate's high levels of insulin depletes the neonate's glucose stores, and hypoglycemia occurs (Ludka & Roberts, 1993). If maternal ketosis occurs, the primary health care provider may order an IV solution containing a small amount of glucose to provide the calories needed to assist in fatty acid metabolism. Nurses should carefully monitor the intake and output of laboring women receiving IV fluids because they also face an increased danger of hypervolemia as a result of the fluid retention that occurs during pregnancy.

Elimination

Voiding. Voiding every 2 hours should be encouraged by the nurse, especially if the bladder is distended. A distended bladder may impede descent of the presenting part, inhibit uterine contractions, and lead to decreased bladder tone or atony after birth. Women who receive epidural analgesia or anesthesia are especially at risk for the retention of urine, and the need to void should be assessed more frequently in them.

If the woman wants to walk to the bathroom, the nurse should assist her in doing so, unless the primary health care provider has ordered bed rest, the woman is receiving epidural analgesia or anesthesia, or, in the nurse's judgment, ambulation would compromise the status of the laboring woman or her fetus, or both. If external monitoring is being used and the cords will reach, monitoring can continue while the woman uses the bathroom; otherwise, the cords are unplugged from the monitor while the woman is in the bathroom and monitoring is interrupted for that time.

Catheterization. If the woman is unable to void and her bladder is obviously distended, she may need to be catheterized. Most hospitals have protocols that rely on the nurse's judgment concerning the need for catheterization. Before performing the catheterization, the nurse should clean the vulva and perineum because vaginal show and amniotic fluid may be present. If there appears to be an obstacle that prevents advancement of the catheter, this is most likely the presenting part. If the catheter cannot be advanced, the nurse should stop the procedure and notify the primary health care provider of the difficulty.

Bowel evacuation. Most women do not have bowel movements during labor because of decreased intestinal motility. Stool that has formed in the large intestine often is moved downward toward the anorectal area by the pressure exerted by the fetal presenting part as it descends. This stool is often expelled during second-stage pushing and birth. However, the passage of stool with bearing-down efforts increases the risk of infection and may embarrass the woman, thereby reducing the effectiveness of these efforts. To prevent these problems, the nurse should immediately cleanse the perineal area to remove any stool, while at the same time reassuring the woman that the passage of stool at this time is a normal and expected event, since the same muscles used

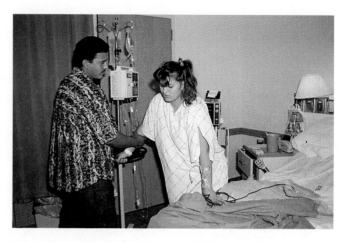

Fig. **15-11** Woman preparing to walk with partner. (Courtesy Marjorie Pyle, RNC, Lifecircle, Costa Mesa, Calif.)

to expel the baby also expel stool. Routine use of an enema to empty the rectum is no longer recommended and is actually considered to be harmful or ineffective and should be eliminated according to the Technical Working Group of the World Health Organization (1997).

If the presenting part is deep in the pelvis, even in the absence of stool in the anorectal area, the woman may feel rectal pressure and think she needs to defecate. The nurse should perform a vaginal examination to assess cervical dilatation and station. When a multiparous woman experiences the urge to defecate, this often means birth will follow quickly.

Ambulation and positioning. The potential advantages of ambulation include enhanced uterine activity, distraction from labor's discomforts, enhanced maternal control, and an opportunity for close interaction with the woman's partner and care provider as they help her to walk. Albers et al. (1997) found that ambulation is associated with a reduced rate of operative delivery (cesarean birth, use of forceps, and vacuum extraction) and less frequent use of narcotic analgesia. Women should be encouraged to labor in any position that is comfortable to them as long as it is not detrimental to the fetus.

Walking, sitting, or standing during labor is more comfortable than lying down and facilitates the progress of labor (Melzak, Belanger & Lacroix, 1991). Ambulation should be encouraged if membranes are intact, if the fetal presenting part is engaged after ROM, and if the woman has not received medication for pain (Fig. 15-11). Ambulation may be contraindicated, however, because of maternal or fetal status.

When the woman lies in bed, she will usually change her position spontaneously as labor progresses (Albers et al., 1997). If she does not change position every 30 to 60 minutes, she should be encouraged to do so. The side-lying (lateral) position is preferred because it promotes optimal uteroplacental and renal blood flow and increases fetal oxygen saturation (Fig. 15-12, *B*). If the woman wants to lie supine,

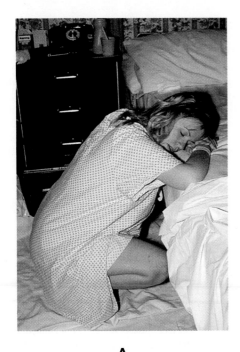

A

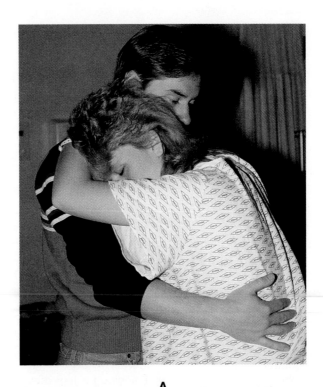

A

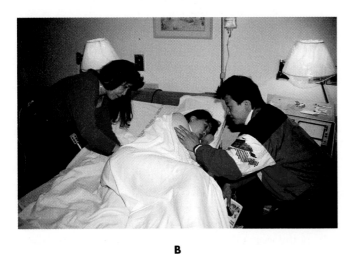

B

Fig. **15-12** Maternal positions for labor. **A,** Squatting. **B,** Lateral position. Support person is applying sacral pressure while partner provides encouragement. (Courtesy Marjorie Pyle, RNC, Lifecircle, Costa Mesa, Calif.)

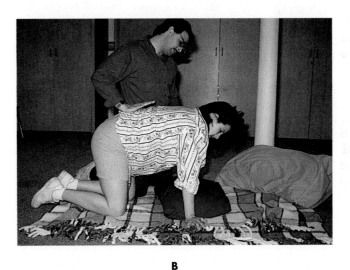

B

Fig. **15-13 A,** Woman standing and leaning forward with support. **B,** Woman in hands-and-knees position. (Courtesy Marjorie Pyle, RNC, Lifecircle, Costa Mesa, Calif.)

the nurse may place a pillow under one hip as a wedge to prevent the uterus from compressing the aorta and vena cava (see Fig. 15-4). Sitting is not contraindicated unless it adversely affects fetal status, which can be determined by checking the FHR. If the fetus is in the occiput posterior position, it may be helpful to encourage the woman to squat during contractions, because this position increases pelvic diameter, allowing the head to rotate to a more anterior position (Fig. 15-12, *A*).

A hands-and-knees position during contractions is also recommended to facilitate the rotation of the fetal occiput from a posterior to an anterior position as gravity pulls the fetus back forward (Fig. 15-13, *B*).

Much research is being directed toward acquiring a better understanding of the physiologic and psychic effects of maternal position in labor. It has been found that fetal presentations and the mechanisms of labor may be helped or hindered by maternal posture (Andrews & Chrzanowski,

---

BOX 15-3 *Some Maternal Positions* during Labor and Birth*

SEMIRECUMBENT POSITION (see Fig. 15-14)
- With woman sitting with her upper body elevated to at least a 30-degree angle, place wedge or small pillow under hip to prevent vena caval compression and reduce likelihood of supine hypotension.
- The greater the angle of elevation, the more gravity or pressure is exerted that promotes fetal descent, the progress of contractions, and the widening of pelvic dimensions.
- Convenient for rendering care measures and for external fetal monitoring.

LATERAL POSITION (see Fig. 15-12 *B*)
- Have woman alternate between left and right side-lying position, and provide abdominal and back support as needed for comfort.
- Removes pressure from the vena cava and back; enhances uteroplacental perfusion and relieves backache.
- Makes it easier to perform back massage or counterpressure.
- Associated with less frequent, but more intense, contractions.
- Obtaining good external fetal monitor tracings may be more difficult.
- May be used as a birthing position.
- Takes pressure off perineum

UPRIGHT POSITION
- The gravity effect enhances the contraction cycle and fetal descent: the weight of the fetus places increasing pressure on the cervix; the cervix is pulled upward, facilitating effacement and dilatation; impulses from the cervix to the pituitary gland increase, causing more oxytocin to be secreted; and contractions are intensified, thereby applying more forceful downward pressure on the fetus, but they are less painful.
- Fetus is aligned with pelvis, and pelvic diameters are widened slightly.
- Effective upright positions include:
  —Ambulation (see Fig. 15-11).
  —Standing and leaning forward with support provided by coach, end of bed, back of chair, or birth ball; relieves backache and facilitates application of counterpressure or back massage (see Fig. 15-13, *A*).
  —Sitting up in bed, chair, birthing chair, or on toilet.
  —Squatting (see Fig. 15-12, *A*).

HANDS-AND-KNEES POSITION—ideal position for posterior positions of the presenting part (see Fig. 15-13, *B*)
- Assume an "all fours" position in bed or on a covered floor; allows for pelvic rocking.
- Relieves backache characteristic of "back labor."
- Facilitates internal rotation of the fetus by increasing mobility of the coccyx, increasing the pelvic diameters, and using gravity to turn the fetal back and rotate the head.

*Assess the effect of each position on the laboring woman's comfort and anxiety level, progress of labor, and FHR pattern. Alternate positions every 30 to 60 minutes.

1990; Biancuzzo, 1993; Carbonne et al., 1996; Simkin, 1995). The variety of positions that are recommended for the laboring woman are described in Box 15-3.

Emergency interventions. Emergency conditions that require immediate nursing intervention can arise with startling speed. A nonreassuring FHR, inadequate uterine relaxation, vaginal bleeding, infection, and prolapse of the cord are highlighted in the Emergency box. Interventions for immediate use are listed.

Support measures. The nurse can alleviate a woman's anxiety by explaining unfamiliar terms, providing information and explanations, and preparing her for sensations she will experience and procedures that will follow. By encouraging the woman or couple to ask questions and by providing honest, understandable answers, the nurse can play an important role in helping the woman achieve a satisfying birth experience (Tomlinson & Bryan, 1996). The learning needs voiced by a woman in labor should be met by the nurse managing her care (Evans & Jeffery, 1995).

Supportive nursing care for a woman in labor includes (1) helping the woman maintain control and participate to the extent she wishes in the birth of her infant; (2) meeting the woman's expected outcomes for her labor; (3) acting as the woman's advocate, supporting her decisions as appropriate and expressing her wishes as needed to other health care providers; (4) helping the woman conserve her energy; (5) helping control the woman's discomfort; and (6) acknowledging the woman's efforts, as well as those of her partner, during labor and providing positive reinforcement.

The nurse serves as a coach to the woman in the absence of other support persons or as an assistant coach to the support persons present. To do this, the nurse must have a thorough knowledge of breathing and relaxation techniques (see Box 13-1).

Couples who have attended childbirth education programs that teach the psychoprophylactic approach will know something about the labor process, coaching techniques, and comfort measures. The nurse should play a supportive role and keep such a couple informed of the progress. Even when expectant parents have not attended such classes, the nurse can teach them various techniques during the early phase of labor. In this case the nurse may provide more of the coaching and supportive care.

Comfort measures vary with the situation (Fig. 15-14). The nurse can draw on the couple's repertoire of comfort measures learned during the pregnancy. Such measures

Interventions for Emergencies

SIGNS

Nonreassuring FHR pattern

- Fetal bradycardia (FHR <110 beats/min for >10 min)†
- Fetal tachycardia (FHR of >160 beats/min for >10 min in term pregnancy)§
- Irregular FHR, abnormal sinus rhythm shown by internal monitor
- Persistent decrease in baseline FHR variability without any identified cause
- Late, severe variable, and prolonged deceleration patterns
- Absence of FHR

INTERVENTIONS*

Notify primary health care provider‡
Change woman to side-lying position
Discontinue oxytocin (Pitocin) infusion, if being infused
Increase IV fluid rate, if fluid being infused per protocol order
Administer oxygen at 8 to 10 L/min by tight face mask
Check maternal temperature for elevation.
Start an IV line if one is not in place
Administer amnioinfusion if ordered
Stimulate fetal scalp or use acoustic stimulation

Inadequate uterine relaxation

- Intrauterine pressure of >75 mm Hg (shown by intrauterine pressure catheter monitoring)
- Contractions consistently lasting >90 sec
- Contraction interval of <2 min

Notify primary health care provider‡
Discontinue oxytocin infusion, if being infused
Change woman to side-lying position
Increase IV fluid rate, if fluid is being infused
Administer oxygen at 8 to 10 L/min by tight face mask
Start an IV line if one is not in place
Palpate and evaluate contractions
Give tocolytics (terbutaline), as ordered

Vaginal bleeding

- Vaginal bleeding (bright red, dark red, or in an amount in excess of that expected during normal cervical dilatation)
- Continuous vaginal bleeding with FHR changes
- Pain; may or may not be present

Notify primary health care provider‡
Anticipate emergency (stat) cesarean birth
DO NOT PERFORM A VAGINAL EXAMINATION

Infection

- Foul-smelling amniotic fluid
- Maternal temperature of >38° C in presence of adequate hydration (straw-colored urine)
- Fetal tachycardia of >160 beats/min for >10 min

Notify primary health care provider‡
Institute cooling measures for laboring woman
Start an IV line if one is not in place
Assist with or perform collection of catheterized urine specimen and amniotic fluid sample and send to the laboratory for urinalysis and cultures

Prolapse of cord (see Fig. 25-18)

- Fetal bradycardia with variable deceleration during uterine contraction
- Woman reports feeling the cord after membranes rupture
- Cord lies alongside or below the presenting part of the fetus; it can be seen or felt in or protruding from the vagina.
- Major predisposing factors are:
  —Rupture of membranes with a gush
  —Loose fit of presenting part in lower uterine segment
  —Presenting part not yet engaged

Call for assistance
Have someone notify the primary health care provider immediately
Glove the examining hand quickly and insert two fingers into the vagina to the cervix; with one finger on either side of the cord or both fingers to one side, exert upward pressure against the presenting part to relieve compression of the cord
Place a rolled towel under the woman's hip
Place woman in extreme Trendelenburg's or modified Sims' position or knee-chest position
Wrap the cord loosely in a sterile towel saturated with warm sterile normal saline if the cord is protruding from the vagina
Administer oxygen at 8 to 10 L/min by face mask until birth is accomplished
Start IV fluids or increase existing drip rate
Continue to monitor FHR by internal fetal scalp electrode, if possible
Do not attempt to replace cord into cervix
Prepare for immediate birth (vaginal or cesarean)

*Because emergency situations are often frightening events, it is important for the nurse to explain to the woman and her support person what is happening and how it is being managed.

†Practice is to intervene within 2 to 30 min of FHR <110 beats/min.

‡In most emergency situations, nurses take immediate action, following a protocol and standards of nursing practice. Another person can notify the primary health care provider, or this can be done by the nurse as soon as possible.

§Nonreassuring sign when associated with late declerations or absence of variability, especially of >180 beats/min.

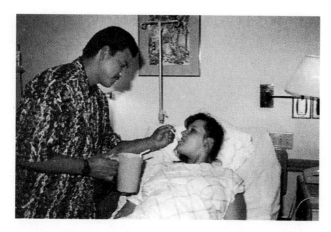

Fig. **15-14** Partner providing comfort measures. (Courtesy Marjorie Pyle, RNC, Lifecircle, Costa Mesa, Calif.)

include maintaining a comfortable, supportive atmosphere in the labor and birth area; using touch therapeutically (e.g., heat or cold applied to the lower back in the event of back labor, a cool cloth applied to the forehead); providing nonpharmacologic measures to relieve discomfort; and administering analgesics when necessary; but most of all, just being there (Table 15-4; see also Care Path).

Labor rooms need to be light and airy, but the bright overhead lights are turned off when not needed. The temperature is controlled to ensure the laboring woman's comfort. The room should be large enough to accommodate a comfortable chair for the woman's partner, the monitoring equipment, and hospital personnel.

Touch. Most women in labor respond positively to touch. They appreciate gentle handling by staff members. Back rubs may be offered, especially if the woman is experiencing back labor. A support person may be taught to exert counterpressure against the mother's sacrum over the occiput of the head of a fetus in a posterior position (see Fig. 15-12, *B*). The back pain is caused by the occiput pressing on spinal nerves, and counterpressure lifts the occiput off these nerves, thereby providing some relief from pain. Once counterpressure is initiated, the woman usually asks her partner to continue doing this for each following contraction. The partner will need to be relieved after a while, however, because exerting counterpressure is hard work. Hand and foot massage can be soothing and relaxing (Simkin, 1995).

The woman's perception of the soothing qualities of touch changes as labor progresses. Many women become more sensitive to touch as labor progresses. They may tell their coach to leave them alone or not to touch them. The partner who is unprepared for this normal response may feel rejected and may react by withdrawing active support. The nurse can reassure them that this response is a positive indication that the first stage is ending and the second stage is approaching. The woman in labor may exhibit a variety of reactions and needs support from her partner and the nurse no matter what her reactions (see Table 15-4).

Relaxation. Relaxation measures for use during labor are often learned in childbirth classes. They include guided imagery, music, and soothing massage. These techniques can provide comfort, prevent fatigue, and help the woman conserve energy for the expulsive work of the second stage of labor. Today, many health care providers advocate the use of warm water (e.g., whirlpool baths or Jacuzzis, showers) for its soothing, relaxing effects, and its ability to reduce discomfort and enhance the progress of labor (Aderhold & Perry, 1991; Rosenthal, 1991; Simkin, 1995). Many new birthing units are installing baths with air jets. The buoyancy of the warm water in a bath, with or without air jets, provides support for tense muscles. The relaxing and soothing effect that the warm water has on muscles yields immediate benefits during labor and also reduces the aftereffects of tense muscles during the immediate postpartum period.

It is recommended that the use of a whirlpool bath or Jacuzzi begin when the woman is in active labor because initiation of this method in the latent phase could slow contractions or stop them temporarily. Showers can also enhance relaxation and reduce pain when warm water is directed over the laboring woman's lower back and abdomen (Simkin, 1995).

The father or partner during labor. Although another woman or a man other than the father may be the woman's partner, the father of the baby is most often the support person during labor. He often is able to provide the comfort measures and touch that the laboring woman needs. When the woman becomes focused on her pain, sometimes the partner can persuade her to try nonpharmacologic variations of comfort measures. In addition, he usually is able to interpret the woman's needs and desires to staff members.

Throughout the past 20 years, childbirth preparation education has been widely available. The ideal father's role was thought to be that of labor coach, and he was expected to actively help the woman cope with labor. However, this expectation may be unrealistic for all men, because some men have concerns about their labor-coaching abilities. Chapman (1992) reported that men assume one of at least three different roles during labor and birth—coach, teammate, or witness. As a coach, the father actively assists the woman during and after contractions. Men who are coaches express a strong need to be in control of themselves and of the labor experience. Women also express a great desire for the father to be physically involved in labor. The father who acts as the teammate assists the woman during labor and birth by responding to such requests for physical or emotional support, or both. Teammates usually adopt the follower or helper role and look to the woman or nurse to tell them what to do. Women express a strong desire to have the father present and willing to help in any way. The father

TABLE 15-4 *Woman's Responses and Support Person's Actions during First Stage of Labor*

WOMAN'S RESPONSES	NURSE/SUPPORT PERSON'S ACTIONS*
DILATATION OF CERVIX 0 TO 3 CM (LATENT) (contractions 10 to 30 sec long, 5 to 30 min apart, mild to moderate)	

Mood: alert, happy, excited, mild anxiety
Settles into labor room; selects focal point
Rests or sleeps, if possible
Uses breathing techniques
Uses effleurage, focusing, and relaxation
  techniques
	Provides encouragement, feedback for relaxation, companionship
	Assists to cope with contractions
	  Encourages use of focusing techniques
	  Helps to concentrate on breathing techniques
	Uses comfort measures
	  Assists woman into comfortable position
	  Informs woman of progress; explains procedures and routines
	  Gives praise
	  Offer fluids, ice chips as ordered

DILATATION OF CERVIX 4 TO 7 CM (ACTIVE) (contractions 30 to 45 sec long, 3 to 5 min apart, moderate to strong)	

Mood: seriously labor oriented, concentration
  and energy needed for contractions, alert,
  more demanding
Continues relaxation, focusing techniques
Uses breathing techniques
	Acts as buffer; limits assessment techniques to between contractions
	Assists with contractions
	  Encourages woman as needed to help her maintain breathing
	   techniques
	Uses comfort measures
	  Assists with frequent position changes, emphasizing side-lying and
	   upright positions
	  Encourages voluntary relaxation of muscles of back, buttocks,
	   thighs, and perineum; effleurage
	  Applies counterpressure to sacrococcygeal area
	  Encourages and praises
	  Keeps woman aware of progress
	  Offers analgesics as ordered
	  Checks bladder; encourages her to void
	  Gives oral care; offers fluids, ice chips as ordered

DILATATION OF CERVIX 8 TO 10 CM (TRANSITION) (contractions 45 to 90 sec long, 2 to 3 min apart, strong)	

Mood: irritable, intense concentration,
  symptoms of transition (e.g., nausea, vomiting)
Continues relaxation, needs greater
  concentration to do this
Uses breathing techniques
  Uses 4:1 breathing pattern if using
   psychoprophylactic techniques
  Uses panting to overcome response to urge
   to push
	Stays with woman; provides constant support
	Assists with contractions
	  Reminds, reassures, and encourages woman to reestablish
	   breathing pattern and concentration as needed
	  Alerts woman to begin breathing pattern before contraction
	   becomes too intense if she is sedated or drowsy
	  Prompts panting respirations if woman begins to push prematurely
	Uses comfort measures
	  Accepts woman's inability to comply with instructions
	  Accepts irritable response to helping, such as counterpressure
	  Supports woman who has nausea and vomiting; gives oral care as
	   needed; gives reassurance regarding signs of end of first stage
	Uses relaxation techniques (effleurage and voluntary relaxation)
	Keeps woman aware of progress

*Provided by nurses and support persons in collaboration with the nurse.

who acts as a witness acts as a companion, giving emotional and moral support. He watches the woman labor and give birth, but he often sleeps, watches television, or leaves the room for long periods. Witnesses believe that there is little they can do to physically help the woman and look to the nurses and health care providers to be in charge of the experience. Women do not expect more of this type of father than to just be present.

Because a father can participate in labor and birth in different ways, nurses need to encourage him to adopt the role most comfortable for him and for the woman, rather than to assume an unnatural role.

The nurse needs to recognize that the feelings of a first-time father change as labor progresses. Often calm at the onset of labor, feelings of fear and helplessness begin to dominate as labor becomes more active and the father realizes that labor is more work than he anticipated. The first-time father may feel excluded as birth preparations begin during the transition phase. Once the second stage begins and birth nears, the father's focus changes from the woman to the baby who is about to be born (Chandler & Field, 1997).

The nurse can support the father in the following ways:

1. Regardless of the degree of involvement desired, explain the layout of the maternity unit; the location of the rest room, cafeteria, waiting room, and nursery; the visiting hours; and the functions of personnel present, and their names. Orient him to the woman's labor room and discuss what he can do there (e.g., sleep, use the telephone).

2. Inform him about the sights and smells he can expect to encounter. Encourage him to leave the room if he needs time to regain his composure, while another person continues to coach until he returns.

3. Respect his or the couple's decisions as to his degree of involvement—whether he is to actively participate in the birthing room or just be kept informed of the progress of labor. When appropriate, provide data on which he or they can base decisions; offer them the freedom to make decisions rather than coerce them one way or another. This is their experience and their baby.

4. Tell him when his presence has been helpful and continue to reinforce this throughout labor.

5. Offer to teach him comfort measures to the extent he wants to know them. Reassure him that he is not assuming the responsibility for observation and management of his partner's labor, rather that his responsibility is to support her as the labor progresses. Suggest alternate comfort measures when the ones he is using are no longer helpful or are rejected by his partner. "Expert watching" or active role modeling can help the partner to learn effective comfort measures (Hodnett, 1996; Tomlinson & Bryan, 1996).

6. Inform him frequently of the woman's progress and her needs. Also keep him informed of procedures to be performed, what the procedures are for, and what is expected of him.

7. Prepare him for changes in the woman's behavior and physical appearance. This is especially true when the mother has just snapped at him and told him to go away. The nurse can reassure the father that this is normal behavior for a woman in transition and that, when he reenters the room after a few minutes, the woman may ask him why he was gone so long (Nichols, 1993).

8. Remind him to eat; offer him snacks and fluids if possible.

9. Relieve him of the job of support person as necessary; offer him blankets if he is to sleep in a chair by the bedside.

10. Acknowledge the stress experienced by each partner during the labor and birth and identify normal responses. The nonjudgmental attitude of staff members helps the father and mother accept their own and each other's behavior.

11. Attempt to modify or eliminate unsettling stimuli, such as extra noise and extra light.

A well-informed father can make an important contribution to the health and well-being of the mother and child, their family interrelationship, and his self-esteem (Queenan, 1990). A significantly lower percentage of women whose partners receive support and assistance from parent education classes, physicians, nurse-midwives, and nurses throughout the childbearing cycle go on to suffer postpartum emotional upsets.

Culture and father participation. A companion is an important source of support, encouragement, and comfort for women during childbirth. The nurse managing the care of pregnant women needs to help these women identify the person, or persons, they wish to be their supportive companions during childbirth. The choice of birth companion is influenced by the woman's cultural and religious background and by trends occurring within the society in which she lives. For example, in Western societies the father is increasingly viewed as the ideal birth companion (Chalmers & Meyer, 1994). For European-American couples, attending childbirth classes together has become a traditional, expected activity—a rite of passage (Finn, 1994). Hmong husbands actively participate in the labor process, often by supporting their wife's position, catching the baby as it emerges, cutting the cord, and burying the placenta (D'Avanzo, 1992). A Mormon woman expects her husband to be present during her labor and to lay his hands on her head in a blessing that imparts strength, comfort, and well-being for safe passage through childbirth (Callister, 1992, 1995). In some cultures the father may be available, but his presence in the labor room with the mother may not be considered appropriate, or he may be present but resist active involvement in her care. Such behavior could be misconstrued by the nursing staff to represent a lack of concern, caring, or interest. Latino women expect their male partner to be present at their bedside during labor, to talk to them, keep them calm, and tell them everything is going to be okay and not to worry. The men are expected to show love and affection by telling the women they love them, by hugging them, and by holding their hand. However, Latino men do not become actively involved in giving their partners care during labor by performing such activities as back rubs and helping with pushing (Khazoyan & Anderson, 1994). Lantican and Corona (1992) have identified the importance of the affectional bond Mexican-American and Filipino women have with their female relatives when it comes to home-related activities such as childbearing. This is also true for the women of many other cultural groups. The presence of another woman or women is highly desired at such occasions. Women who come from some of these cultures and who give birth in the hospital like to have at least one woman present for assistance. Vietnamese and Chinese women prefer a female companion during childbirth and are very concerned about their modesty (D'Avanzo, 1992). Islamic women are also very modest and would not accept the presence of a man during childbirth, even including that of the father (Woods, 1991). The religious beliefs of some Orthodox Jews forbid the father from touching his wife during labor or being present at the birth. Instead, while he prays, the female members of the laboring woman's family act as supportive childbirth companions (Callister, 1995; DeSevo, 1997).

Support of the grandparents. When grandparents act as labor coaches, it is especially important to support and treat them with respect. They may have a way to deal with pain relief based on their experience. They need to be encouraged to help as long as their actions do not compromise the status of the mother or the fetus. Such an acceptable practice would be giving the woman herbal teas during labor. The nurse acknowledges the value of their contributions to supporting the woman, and recognizes the difficulty parents may have in witnessing their child's discomfort or crisis, regardless of the child's age. If they have never witnessed a birth, the nurse may need to provide explanations of what is happening. Many of the activities used to support fathers are also appropriate for grandparents.

Siblings during labor. The preparation of siblings for acceptance of the new child helps promote the attachment process. Such preparation and participation during pregnancy and labor may help the older children accept this change. The older child or children who know themselves to be important to the family become active participants. Rehearsal for the event before labor is essential.

The age and developmental level of children influence their responses; therefore preparation for the children to be present during labor is adjusted to meet each child's needs. The child under 2 years of age shows little interest in pregnancy and labor; for the older child such preparation may reduce fears and misconceptions. Most parents have a "feel" for their children's maturational level and ability to cope. Preparation can include a description of the anticipated sights and sounds, a birth demonstration, a tour of the birthing unit, and an opportunity to be around a real newborn (Jonquil, 1993). The children must learn that their mother will be working hard during labor and birth. She will not be able to talk to them during contractions. She may groan and pant at times. They can be told that labor is uncomfortable but that their mother's body is made for the job. The children should be prepared for the sights, sounds, and smells. Storybooks about the birth process can be read to or by younger children to prepare them for the event. Films for preparing older preschool and school-age children to participate in the birth experience are available. A specific person should be designated to watch over the children who

are participating in their mother's childbirth experience, to provide them with support, explanations, diversions, and comfort as needed.

Doulas. The continuous presence of a trained, experienced woman, called a **doula,** throughout labor has been found not only to reduce the pain and duration of labor, but also to enhance the laboring woman's satisfaction with her experience and to improve outcomes in terms of a decreased rate of operative delivery (cesarean birth, use of forceps, and vacuum extraction) and childbirth complications. In addition, women often demonstrate increased maternal-infant bonding and ability to care for their new baby. The doula focuses on the woman and provides support with soft, reassuring words; by touching, stroking, and hugging; by walking with her; and by helping her to change her position. Support of the woman's partner through encouragement, praise, and role modeling is also an essential activity of the doula (Perez & Herrick, 1998; Simkin, 1996; Zhang et al., 1996). The nurse works with the doula in providing supportive care but retains the overall responsibility for patient care.

Preparation for giving birth. The first stage of labor ends with the complete dilatation of the cervix. For many multiparous women, birth usually occurs within minutes of complete dilatation, perhaps only one push later. Nulliparous women usually push for 1 to 2 hours before giving birth. If the woman has been given epidural anesthesia, pushing can last more than 2 hours. The nurse begins to prepare for birth when a multiparous woman is 6 to 8 cm dilated, because progression during the last few centimeters of dilatation can occur rapidly. Factors that influence the process are fetal position and the size of the baby in relation to previous babies.

Birth setting. Significant changes have occurred in the location where birth takes place. A 1991 survey revealed that more than half of all pregnant women give birth somewhere other than the traditional labor and delivery room (American College of Obstetricians and Gynecologists, 1993). The most common change in birth settings is the LDRP room, where the woman stays during her entire hospitalization (Fig. 15-15). This avoids the necessity of multiple transfers of the woman from the labor room to delivery room to a recovery room and then to a postpartum unit. Another option is the LDR room, where the woman stays during her labor and immediate postpartum recovery period (1 to 2 hours) before her transfer to a "postpartum" room, where she stays for the remainder of her hospitalization. Some hospitals, however, lack birthing rooms, and transfer during second stage is required. If birth is to occur in the delivery room, it is best to transfer the woman early enough to avoid a last-minute rush. For nulliparous women, transfer can take place when the presenting part begins to distend the perineum. For multiparous women, transfer should take place in the first stage, when the cervix is dilated 8 to 9 cm.

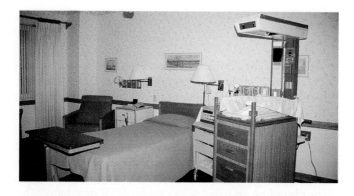

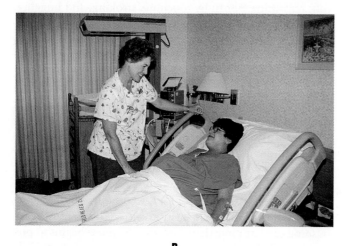

Fig. 15-15 Examples of a labor, delivery, recovery, post-partum (LDRP) room. (A Courtesy Marjorie Pyle, RNC, Lifecircle, Costa Mesa, Calif.)

Birthing centers are a third option. Women give birth in a homelike setting and are discharged after they and their newborn are stable (see Fig. 10-23).

The home is a safe alternative to the hospital or birth center as a site of birth for the motivated low-risk woman. Prior planning is essential to ensure that the birth will be attended by an experienced home birth practitioner and that backup at a hospital is available should complications arise requiring transfer. Research indicates that women who participate in home birth use a greater variety of positions for childbirth, need fewer pharmacologic pain relief measures as a result of feeling more relaxed in their own environment, and experience less severe perineal trauma (Olsen, 1997; Wraight, 1997).

Evaluation

Evaluation of the effectiveness of care of the woman in the first stage of labor is based on the previously stated outcomes.

▌SECOND STAGE OF LABOR

The second stage of labor is the stage in which the fetus is born. It begins at full cervical dilatation (10 cm) and complete effacement (100%) and ends with the baby's birth. The second stage comprises three phases: the latent, descent, and transition phases. Each phase is characterized by maternal verbal and nonverbal behaviors, uterine activity, the urge to bear down, and fetal descent (Table 15-5). The latent phase is a period of rest and relative calm. The woman is quiet and often relaxes with her eyes closed between contractions. The descent phase is characterized by strong urges to bear down as **Ferguson's reflex** is activated when the presenting part presses on the stretch receptors of the pelvic floor. This stimulation causes the release of oxytocin from the posterior pituitary gland, which provokes stronger expulsive uterine contractions. In the *transition phase,* the presenting part is on the perineum and bearing-down efforts are most effective for promoting birth. The woman may be more verbal about the pain she is experiencing; she may scream or swear and may act out of control (Aderhold & Roberts, 1991). The nurse encourages the woman to "listen" to her body as she progresses through the phases of the second stage of labor. When a woman listens to her body to tell her when to bear down, she is using an internal locus of control and often feels more satisfied with her efforts to give birth to her baby. Her sense of self-esteem and accomplishment is enhanced. The woman's trust in her own body and her ability to give birth to her baby should be fostered (Cosner & deJong, 1993; Rothman, 1996; Yeates & Roberts, 1984).

▌CARE MANAGEMENT

Assessment and Nursing Diagnoses

The only certain objective sign that the second stage of labor has begun is the inability to feel the cervix during vaginal examination, indicating that the cervix is fully dilated and effaced (Bennett & Brown, 1993). Other signs that suggest the onset of the second stage include the following:
- Sudden appearance of sweat on upper lip
- An episode of vomiting
- Increased bloody show
- Shaking of extremities
- Increased restlessness; verbalization that "I can't go on"
- Involuntary bearing-down efforts

These signs commonly appear at the time the cervix reaches full dilatation (Bennett & Brown, 1993). However, women with an epidural block may not exhibit such signs. Other indicators for each phase of the second stage are given in Table 15-5.

Assessment is continuous during the second stage of labor. Hospital protocol determines the specific type and timing of assessments, as well as the way in which findings are documented. The Care Path for the second and third

TABLE 15-5	*Expected Maternal Progress in Second Stage of Labor*		
CRITERION	LATENT PHASE (AVERAGE DURATION, 10-30 MIN)	DESCENT PHASE (AVERAGE DURATION VARIES)*	TRANSITION PHASE (AVERAGE DURATION, 5-15 MIN)
Contractions Magnitude (intensity)	Period of physiologic lull for all criteria; period of peace and rest	Significant increase	Overwhelmingly strong Expulsive
Frequency		2 to 2 1/2 min	1 to 2 min
Duration		90 sec	90 sec
Descent, station	0 to +2	Increases and Ferguson's reflex[†] activated, +2 to +4	Rapid, +4 to birth Fetal head visible in introitus; bloody show accompanies birth of head
Show: color and amount		Significant increase in dark red bloody show	
Spontaneous bearing-down efforts	Slight to absent, except during acme of strongest contractions	Increased urge to bear down	Greatly increased
Vocalization	Quiet; concern over progress	Grunting sounds or expiratory vocalization; announces contractions	Grunting sounds and expiratory vocalizations continue; may scream or swear
Maternal behavior	Experiences sense of relief that transition to second stage is finished Feels fatigued and sleepy Feels a sense of accomplishment and optimism, because the "worse is over" Feels in control	Senses increased urge to push Alters respiratory pattern: has short 4- to 5-sec breath-holds with regular breaths in between, 5 to 7 times per contraction Makes grunting sounds or expiratory vocalizations Frequent repositioning	Describes extreme pain Expresses feelings of powerlessness Shows decreased ability to listen or concentrate on anything but giving birth Describes **ring of fire**[‡] Often shows excitement immediately after birth of head

From Anderhold K & Roberts J: Phases of second stage labor: four descriptive case studies, *J Nurse Midwifery* 36(5):267, 1991; Mahan C & McKay S: Are we overmanaging second stage labor? *Contemp OB/GYN* 24:37, 1984.
*Duration of descent phase can vary depending on the following: maternal parity, effectiveness of bearing-down effort, presence of spinal anesthesia or epidural analgesia.
†Pressure of presenting part on stretch receptors of pelvic floor stimulates release of oxytocin from posterior pituitary, resulting in more intense uterine contractions.
‡Burning sensation of acute pain as vagina stretches and fetal head crowns.

stages of labor indicates typical assessments and the recommended frequency for their performance.

Duration of second stage. There is considerable controversy over the precise duration of the second stage of labor and the time limits that should be regarded as normal. Friedman's (Friedman & Sachtleben, 1965) curves for nulliparous and multiparous women are commonly used to determine the progress of the second stage. On the basis of these data the range and average duration of the second stage of labor vary with parity:

Parity	Range (min)	Average (min)
First pregnancy	25-75	57
Subsequent pregnancy	13-17	14.4

A second stage of more than 2 hours in a first pregnancy and of 1 1/2 hours in subsequent pregnancies may be considered prolonged in women without regional analgesia and is reported to the primary health care provider. Using

assessment findings such as the FHR and pattern, the descent of the presenting part, the quality of the uterine contractions, and status of the woman, premature intervention such as the use of episiotomies, forceps, and vacuum extraction can be avoided (Roberts & Woolley, 1996).

The second stage may be prolonged in the woman who has an epidural block, which causes the urge to bear down to be lost or reduced. By allowing the epidural to wear off, the woman's perception of the urge to bear down, and hence her expulsive efforts, can be enhanced (Cosner & deJong, 1993). However, her perception of pain may be intensified.

The method used by a woman to push and the position she assumes during these bearing-down efforts can also affect the duration of the second stage (Aderhold & Roberts, 1991).

Nursing diagnoses give direction to nursing care. The Nursing Diagnoses box lists selected nursing diagnoses for the second stage of labor.

CARE PATH   *Low-Risk Woman in Second and Third Stages of Labor*

CARE MANAGEMENT	SECOND STAGE OF LABOR	THIRD STAGE OF LABOR
I. ASSESSMENT MEASURES*	**FREQUENCY**	**FREQUENCY**
• Blood pressure, pulse, respirations	Every 5-30 min	Every 15 min
• Uterine activity	Assess every contraction	Assess for placental separation
• Bearing-down effort	Assess each effort	
• Fetal heart rate (FHR)	Every 5-15 min	Perform Apgar at 1 and 5 min
• Vaginal show	Every 15 min	Assess bleeding until placental expulsion
• Signs of fetal descent: urge to bear down, perineal bulging, crowning	Every 10-15 min	
• Behavior, appearance, mood, energy level of woman; condition of partner	Every 10-15 min	Assess response to completion of childbirth process, reaction to newborn
II. PHYSICAL CARE MEASURES†	**Latent phase:** Assist to rest in position of comfort Encourage relaxation to conserve energy Promote urge to push; if delayed: ambulation, shower, pelvic rock, position changes **Descent phase:** Assist to bear down effectively Help to use recommended positions that facilitate descent Encourage correct breathing during bearing-down efforts Help to relax between contractions Provide comfort measures as needed Cleanse perineum immediately if fecal material is expelled **Transition phase:** Assist to pant during contraction to avoid rapid birth of head Coach to gently bear down between contractions	Assist to bear down to facilitate delivery of separated placenta Administer oxytocic as ordered Provide pain relief as needed Provide hygiene and comfort measures as needed
III. EMOTIONAL SUPPORT	Keep informed of progress of fetal descent Provide feedback for bearing-down efforts Explain purpose if medications given Role model comfort measures Provide continuous nursing presence Create a quiet, calm environment Reassure, encourage, praise Take charge as needed, until mother regains confidence in ability to birth her baby Offer mirror to watch birth	Keep informed about progress of placental separation Explain purpose if medications given Describe status of perineal tissue and inform if repair is needed Introduce parents to their baby Assess and care for newborn within view of parents; delay eye prophylaxis to facilitate eye contact Provide private time for family to bond with their new baby and help them to create memories Encourage breastfeeding if desired

*Frequency of assessment is determined by the risk status of the maternal-fetal unit. More frequent assessment is required in high-risk situations. Frequency of assessment and method of documentation are also determined by agency policy, which is usually based on the recommended care standards of medical and nursing organizations.

†Physical care measures are performed by the nurse working together with the woman's partner and significant others.

Nursing Diagnoses

Second Stage of Labor

Risk for injury to mother and fetus related to:
- Persistent use of Valsalva's maneuver during bearing-down efforts

Situational low self-esteem related to:
- Lack of knowledge regarding normal, beneficial effects of vocalization during bearing-down efforts
- Inability to carry out birth plan for birth without medication

Ineffective individual coping related to:
- Coaching that contradicts woman's physiologic urge to push

Pain related to:
- Bearing-down efforts and distention of the perineum

Anxiety related to:
- Inability to control defecation with bearing-down efforts
- Lack of knowledge regarding and inexperience with perineal sensations associated with the urge to bear down

Risk for maternal injury related to:
- Inappropriate positioning of mother's legs in stirrups

Risk for infection related to:
- Prolonged rupture of membranes
- Perineal trauma

Situational low self-esteem (partner/father) related to:
- Inability to support mother during final stage of labor

Expected Outcomes of Care

Planning for the second and third stages of labor is done during the first stage of labor. Previously determined expected outcomes may be modified as these stages progress.

Expected outcomes for the woman in the second stage of labor may include that the woman will:
- Actively participate in the labor process
- Sustain no injury during the labor process (nor will the fetus)
- Obtain comfort and support as needed

Plan of Care and Interventions

The nurse implements plans to continuously monitor the second stage and mechanism of birth, the maternal physiologic and emotional responses to the second stage, the partner's response to the second stage, and the fetal response to the stress of the second stage.

The nurse continues to provide comfort measures for the mother, such as positioning; providing mouth care; maintaining clean, dry bedding; and keeping extraneous noise, conversation, and other distractions (e.g., laughing, talking of attending personnel in or outside the labor area) to a minimum. The woman is encouraged to indicate other support measures she would like (see Plan of Care and Table 15-6).

If the mother is to be transferred to another area for birth, the nurse accomplishes the transfer early enough to avoid rushing the woman. The birth area also is readied for the birth.

PLAN OF CARE   *Second Stage of Labor*

> **NURSING DIAGNOSIS** Risk for ineffective individual coping related to birthing process and fatigue of labor

Expected Outcome *Woman actively participates in the birth process with no evidence of injury to her or her fetus.*

Nursing Interventions/*Rationales*

Constantly monitor events of second-stage labor and birth, including physiologic responses of woman and fetus, emotional responses of woman and partner *to ensure maternal, partner, and fetal well-being.*

Provide ongoing feedback to woman and partner *to allay anxiety and enhance participation.*

Continue to provide comfort measures such as positioning; mouth care; clean, dry bedding; cool cloth on forehead; and minimizing distractions *to decrease discomfort and aid in focus on the birth process.*

Encourage woman to experiment with various positions *to assist downward movement of fetus.*

Encourage woman to bear down spontaneously on exhalation *to aid descent and rotation of fetus.*

Teach partner about importance of spontaneous bearing down *to avoid coaching to push, which may contradict or inhibit these spontaneous urges.*

Remind woman not to hold her breath or take short breath-holds while bearing down *as holding breath may trigger a Valsalva's maneuver and increase intrathoracic and cardiovascular pressure and decrease perfusion of placental oxygen, placing the fetus at risk.*

Encourage woman to vocalize as she bears down *to enhance efforts.*

Have woman take deep breaths and relax between contractions *to reduce fatigue and increase effectiveness of pushing efforts.*

If woman seems reluctant to bear down, assess possible contributing factors (e.g., doubts about readiness as a mother; desire for an absent person to be present; fear of the pain of pushing, embarrassment of passing stool while pushing, fear that baby will be in danger when no longer in uterus) and address specific concern *so that woman can participate in labor process effectively.*

Have mother pant as fetal head crowns *to control birth of head.*

From Wong D & Perry S: *Maternal child nursing care,* St Louis, 1998, Mosby.

TABLE 15-6	*Woman's Responses and Support Person's Action during Second Stage of Labor*
WOMAN'S RESPONSES	**NURSE/SUPPORT PERSON'S ACTIONS***
LATENT PHASE Experiences a short period of peace and rest	Encourages woman to "listen" to her body Continues support measures Suggests an upright position to encourage progression of descent if descent phase does not begin after 20 min
DESCENT PHASE Senses increased urgency to bear down as Ferguson's reflex is activated Notes increase in intensity of uterine contractions—alters respiratory pattern: short 4- to 5-sec breath-holds, 5 to 7 times per contraction Makes grunting sounds or expiratory vocalizations	Encourages respiratory pattern of short breath-holds Stresses normality and benefits of grunting sounds and expiratory vocalizations Encourages bearing-down efforts with urge to push Encourages/suggests maternal movement and position changes (upright, if descent is not occurring) Encourages woman to "listen" to her body regarding movement and position change if descent is occurring Discourages long breath-holds If birth is to occur in a delivery room, transfers woman to delivery room early to avoid rushing or, if permitted, offers her option of walking to delivery room Places woman in lateral recumbent position to slow descent if descent is too fast
TRANSITIONAL PHASE Behaves in manner similar to behavior during transition in first stage (8 to 10 cm) Experiences a sense of severe pain and powerlessness Shows decreased ability to listen Concentrates on birth of baby until head is born Experiences contractions as overwhelming in intensity Reports feeling ring of fire as head crowns Maintains respiratory pattern of 3 to 5, 7-sec breath-holds per contraction, followed by forced expiration Eases head out with short expirations Responds with excitement and relief after head is born	Encourages slow, gentle pushing Explains that "blowing away the contraction" facilitates a slower birth of the head Provides mirror to help woman see or touch the emerging fetal head (best to extend over 2 to 3 contractions) to help her understand the perineal sensations Coaches woman to relax mouth, throat, and neck to promote relaxation of pelvic floor Applies warm compress to perineum to promote relaxation

*Provided by nurses and support persons in collaboration with the nurse.

Prebirth considerations

Maternal position. There is no single position for childbirth. Labor is a dynamic, interactive process involving the woman's uterus, pelvis, and voluntary muscles. In addition, angles between the baby and the woman's pelvis constantly change as the infant turns and flexes down the birth canal. The woman may want to assume various positions for childbirth. One position found to be highly effective in facilitating the descent and birth of the fetus is squatting (Andrews & Chrzanowski, 1990; Golay, Vedam & Sorger, 1993; Roberts & Woolley, 1996). A firm surface is required for this position, and the woman will need side support. In a birthing bed a squat bar is available that she can use to help support herself. Another position is the side-lying position, with the upper part of the woman's leg held by the nurse or coach or placed on a pillow (Fig. 15-16, *A*). Some women prefer a semi-sitting position, which can be achieved

with the support of a wedged pillow or with the father or partner supporting the woman (Fig. 15-16, *B*). The hands-and-knees position is an effective position for birth because it enhances placental perfusion, helps rotate the fetus from a posterior to an anterior position, and may facilitate the birth of the shoulders, especially if the fetus is large. Perineal trauma may also be reduced (Biancuzzo, 1991; Gannon, 1992). When a woman uses the standing position for bearing down, her weight is borne on both femoral heads, allowing the pressure in the acetabulum to cause the transverse diameter of the pelvic outlet to increase by up to 1 cm. This can be helpful if descent of the head is delayed because the occiput has not rotated from the lateral (transverse diameter of pelvis) to the anterior position (Biancuzzo, 1993). The nurse should frequently assess the effect of maternal positions on fetal status. If the woman is reluctant or afraid to try different positions, the nurse needs to actively

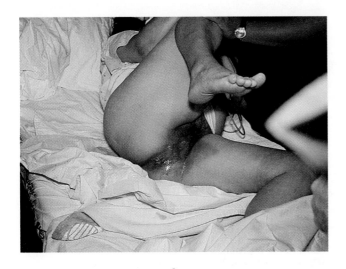

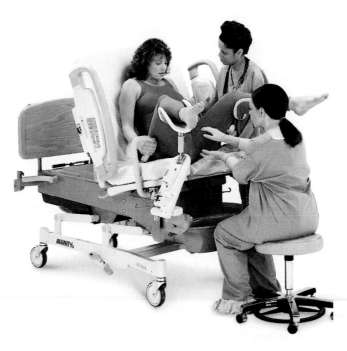

Fig. **15-17** Birth bed. (Courtesy Hill-Rom, Batesville, Ind.)

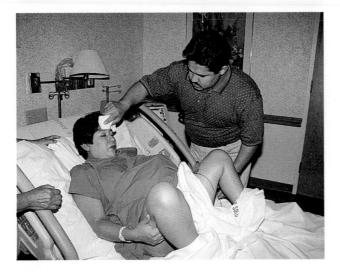

Fig. **15-16 A,** Pushing, side-lying position. Perineal bulging can be seen. **B,** Pushing, semi-sitting position. Partner is wiping woman's face with cool cloth between contractions. (**A,** courtesy Michael S. Clement, MD, Mesa, Ariz; **B,** courtesy Marjorie Pyle, RNC, Lifecircle, Costa Mesa, Calif.)

encourage and help the woman to do so. Information regarding the variety of effective childbirth positions should be an essential component of prepared childbirth classes.

Birthing beds and chairs. The birthing bed (Figs. 15-17 and 15-18) can be set for different positions according to the woman's needs. The woman can squat, kneel, recline, or sit, choosing the position most comfortable for her. At the same time, it affords excellent exposure for the performance of examinations, the placement of internal monitoring devices, and birth. By using the birthing bed, the woman has full control of both seat and back functions and can adjust her position for maximum comfort. The bed also can be

positioned for the administration of anesthesia and can be used for transport to the operating room in the event a cesarean birth proves necessary.

Although birthing beds are more often used today, birthing chairs also may be used and may provide women with a better physiologic position during childbirth, although some women feel restricted by a chair. There is also a potential psychologic advantage to the upright position in that it allows the mother to see the birth as it occurs and also to maintain eye contact with the attendant. Most chairs are designed so that if an emergency occurs, the chair can be adjusted to the horizontal or the Trendelenburg position.

In some hospitals, oversized beanbag chairs are used for both labor and birth. These chairs mold around and support the mother in whatever position she selects. These chairs are of particular value for mothers who wish to be actively involved in the birth process. Birthing stools also can be used to support the woman in an upright position similar to squatting (Waldenström & Gottvall, 1991).

Bearing-down efforts. As the fetal head reaches the pelvic floor, most women experience the urge to bear down. Automatically the woman will begin to exert downward pressure by contracting her abdominal muscles while relaxing her pelvic floor. This bearing down is an involuntary response to Ferguson's reflex, which is activated by the presenting part pressing on stretch receptors of the pelvic musculature. A strong expiratory grunt (vocalization) may accompany the push (McKay & Roberts, 1990). When coaching women to push, the nurse should encourage them

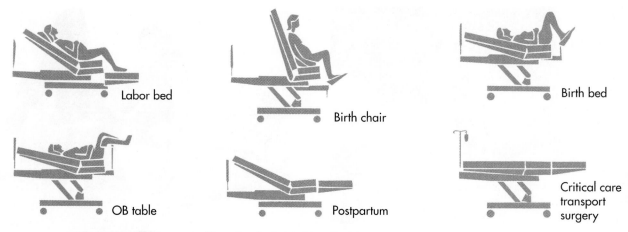

Fig. **15-18** The versatility of today's birthing bed makes it practical in a variety of settings. Note: OB bed used for *lithotomy position.* (Courtesy Hill-Rom, Batesville, Ind.)

to push as they feel like pushing rather than to give a prolonged push on command (Thomson, 1993). The nurse should watch the woman's breathing to make sure she does not hold her breath for more than 5 to 7 seconds at a time (Roberts & Woolley, 1996). Bearing down while exhaling (open-glottis pushing) and taking breaths between bearing-down efforts help to maintain adequate oxygen levels for the mother and fetus. Prolonged breath-holding, which is still a common practice, may trigger Valsalva's maneuver, which occurs when the woman closes the glottis (closed-glottis pushing), thereby increasing intrathoracic and cardiovascular pressure (Metzer & Therrien, 1990). In addition, holding the breath for more than 5 to 7 seconds causes the perfusion of oxygen across the placenta to be diminished, resulting in fetal hypoxia. The nurse should remind the woman to take deep breaths to fully ventilate her lungs before and after each contraction (Hodnett, 1996).

A woman may reach the second stage of labor and then experience a lack of readiness to complete the process and give birth to her child. McKay and Barrows (1991) have identified several factors that may cause a woman to lessen her voluntary bearing-down efforts. These factors can include:

- Doubts about her readiness to be a mother
- Reluctance to care for another baby
- Desire to wait for support person or primary health care provider to arrive
- Fear or anxiety regarding the unfamiliar or painful sensations of the second stage of labor and pushing
- Embarrassment regarding behaviors during pushing, including sounds made and the passage of stool
- Giving up and not wanting to proceed any further toward a vaginal birth
- Fear that the baby will be in danger once it emerges from the protective intrauterine environment

By recognizing that a woman may experience a need to hold back the birth of her baby, the nurse can then address the woman's concerns and effectively coach the woman during this stage of labor.

To ensure the slow birth of the fetal head, the nurse should encourage the woman to control the urge to bear down by coaching her to take panting breaths or to exhale slowly through pursed lips as the baby's head crowns. At this point the woman needs simple, clear directions from one person.

Amnesia between contractions often is pronounced in the second stage, and the woman may have to be roused to get her to cooperate in the bearing-down process. Parents who have attended childbirth education classes may have devised a set of verbal cues for the laboring woman to follow. It is helpful for them to have these cues printed on a card that can be attached to the head of the bed so that the nurse can better substitute as coach if the partner has to leave.

FHR and pattern. As noted previously, the FHR must be checked. If the rate begins to slow or if there is a loss of variability, prompt treatment must be initiated. The woman can be turned on her side to reduce the pressure of the uterus against the ascending vena cava and descending aorta (see Fig. 15-4), and oxygen can be administered by mask at 8 to 10 L/min. This is often all that is necessary to restore the normal rate. If the FHR does not return to normal immediately, the primary health care provider should be notified quickly because medical intervention may be indicated to hasten the birth.

Support of the father or coach. During the second stage the woman needs continuous support and coaching (Table 15-6). Because the coaching process can be physically and emotionally tiring for support persons (Jordan, 1990; Malestic, 1990; Queenan, 1990), the nurse offers them nourishment and fluids and encourages them to take short breaks. The support person who attends the birth in a delivery room is instructed to put on a cover gown or scrub clothes, mask, hat, and shoe covers, as required. The nurse also specifies support measures he or she can use for the laboring woman and points out areas of the room in which the partner can move freely. If birth occurs in an LDR or LDRP room, the partner may be allowed to wear street clothes or be required to wear a clean scrub outfit, cap, and mask (for the birth).

Partners are encouraged to be present at the birth of their infants if this is in keeping with their cultural expectations and beliefs. In this way the psychologic closeness of the family unit is maintained and the partner can continue to provide the supportive care given during labor. The woman and her partner need to have an equal opportunity to initiate the attachment process with the baby.

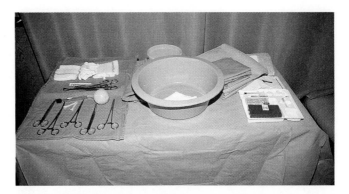

Fig. **15-19** Instrument table. (Courtesy Marjorie Pyle, RNC, Lifecircle, Costa Mesa, Calif.)

LEGAL TIP | **Documentation**

Documentation of all observations (e.g., maternal vital signs, FHR and pattern, progress of labor) and nursing interventions, including patient response, should be done concurrently with care. The course of labor and the maternal-fetal response may change without warning. It is important that all documentation be accurate, complete, and timely. Documentation is done in the labor and delivery record, as well as on the monitor strip.

Supplies, instruments, and equipment. To prepare for birth in any setting, the birthing table or case cart is usually set up during the transition phase for nulliparous women and during the active phase for multiparous women.

The birthing table is prepared, and instruments are arranged on the instrument table (Fig. 15-19). Standard procedures are followed for gloving, identifying and opening sterile packages, adding sterile supplies to the instrument table, and unwrapping and handing sterile instruments to the primary health care provider. The crib and equipment are readied for the support and stabilization of the infant. A radiant warmer for the newborn is turned on when crowning begins to occur in the nulliparous woman and when the multiparous woman is 8 to 9 cm dilated.

The items required in preparation for birth may vary among different facilities; therefore each facility's procedure manual should be consulted to determine the protocols specific to that facility. Following are suggestions for the preparation for birth:
1. The items that follow have to be collected or readied or the following tasks done.
   • Scrubbing items such as scrub brushes, cuticle sticks, and cleaning agent, as well as masks with a shield or protective glasses or goggles.
   • Sterile gowns and gloves for the primary health care provider, sterile drapes and towels for draping the woman, and sterile instruments and other supplies (such as bulb syringes, sutures, and

anesthetic solutions). These are arranged on a sterile, draped table for convenient use.
   • A sterile basin containing water for handwashing during the birth process.
   • Supplies for cleansing the vulva (sterile basin, sterile water, and cleaning solution).
   • Birth area is warmed and free of drafts.
   • Infant identification materials.
   • Infant receiving blankets and heated crib. Also material for prophylactic care of infant's eyes and vitamin K injection.
2. The following equipment should be checked to make sure it is in working order: birthing table (bed or chair), overhead lights, and mirror.
3. Emergency equipment, anesthesia, laryngoscope, and supplies needed for the management of emergency situations such as maternal hemorrhage or fetal respiratory distress should be available and in working order.
4. Additional supplies (anesthetics, oxytocics for injection, obstetric forceps, and vacuum extractor) should be available.
5. The woman's record should be up-to-date and ready for use in the birth area.
6. Specific orders of the primary health care provider regarding labor and birth procedures should be ascertained.

The nurse estimates the time until the birth will occur and notifies the primary health care provider if he or she is not in the patient's room. Even the most experienced nurse can miscalculate the time left before birth occurs, however. Thus every nurse who attends a woman in labor must be prepared to assist with an emergency birth if the primary health care provider is not present (see Box 15-5).

Birth in a delivery room or birthing room. The woman will need assistance if she must move from the labor bed to the delivery table (Fig. 15-20). The woman can help if this is done between contractions, but because of her awkwardness, she cannot be rushed.

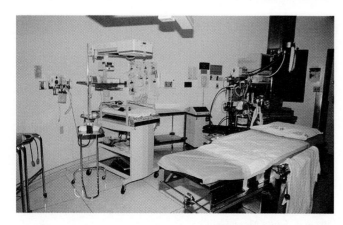

Fig. 15-20 Delivery room. (Courtesy Michael S. Clement, MD, Mesa, Ariz.)

The various positions assumed for birth in a delivery room are Sims' position (if this is the case, the attendant will need to support the upper part of the woman's leg), the dorsal position, and the lithotomy position.

The **lithotomy position** has been the position most commonly used for birth in Western cultures, although this practice is changing slowly. The lithotomy position is a convenient one for the primary health care provider because it enables him or her to deal with any complications that may arise (see Fig. 15-18). To place the woman in this position, her buttocks are brought to the edge of the table and her legs are placed in stirrups. Care must be taken to pad the stirrups, raise and place both legs simultaneously, and adjust the shanks of the stirrups so that the calves of the legs are supported. There should be no pressure on the popliteal space. If the stirrups are not the same height, ligaments in the woman's back can be strained as she bears down, leading to considerable discomfort in the postpartum period. The lower portion of the table may be dropped down and rolled back under the table.

Birth in an LDR or LDRP room. The maternal position for birth varies from a lithotomy position with the woman's legs in stirrups, to one in which her feet rest on foot rests while she holds onto a squat bar, to a side-lying position with the woman's upper leg supported by the coach, nurse, or the squat bar. The foot of the bed can be removed so that the primary health care provider attending the birth can gain better perineal access for performing an episiotomy, delivering a large baby, or getting access to the emerging head to facilitate suctioning. Otherwise the foot of the bed is left in place and lowered slightly to form a ledge that allows access for birth and that also serves as a place to lay the newborn.

Once the woman is positioned for birth, the vulva and perineum are cleansed. Hospital protocols and the preferences of primary health care providers for cleansing may vary and can involve washing the area thoroughly with warm, soapy water or a soapy povidone-iodine (Betadine) solution and then rinsing the area. Next the area may be sprayed with

---

BOX 15-4 **Standard Precautions during Childbirth**

Birth is a time when nurses and other health care providers are exposed to a great deal of maternal and newborn blood and body fluids. Observation of Standard Precautions is necessary to prevent the transmission of infection. Perinatal infections most often are transmitted through contact with body fluids. The Standard Precautions applicable to childbirth include:
- Wash hands before and after putting on gloves and performing procedures.
- Wear gloves (clean or sterile, as appropriate) when performing procedures that require contact with the woman's genitalia and body fluids, including bloody show (e.g., during vaginal examination, amniotomy, hygienic care of the perineum, insertion of an internal scalp electrode and intrauterine pressure monitor, and catheterization).
- Wear cap, a mask that has a shield or protective eyewear, shoe covers, and cover gown during the birth. Gowns worn by the primary health care provider who is attending the birth should have a waterproof front and sleeves and should be sterile.
- Drape the woman with sterile towels and sheets as appropriate. Explain to the woman what can and cannot be touched.
- Help the woman's partner put on appropriate coverings for the birth, such as cap, mask, gown, and shoe covers. Show the partner where to stand and what can and cannot be touched.
- Wear gloves and gown when handling the newborn immediately after birth.
- Use an appropriate method to suction the newborn's airway, such as a bulb syringe, mechanical wall suction, or De Lee oral suction device that prevents the newborn's mucus from getting into the user's airway.

a disinfectant to prevent bacterial contamination (see Box 15-4 for Standard Precautions used during birth).

The circulating nurse (usually the same nurse as the labor nurse) continues to coach and encourage the woman. She auscultates the FHR every 5 to 15 minutes, depending on whether the woman is at low or high risk for problems or per protocol of the birthing facility, or continuously monitors the FHR with electronic monitoring. She keeps the primary health care provider informed of the rate and pattern of the FHR (Tucker, 1996). The equipment for measuring blood pressure should be readied for instant use should signs of shock develop. If blood pressure readings are taken as the woman pushes, the readings will be distorted (increased) by the increase in thoracic and abdominal pressures. A reading is obtained after birth before the woman is transferred to the recovery room. An oxytocic medication such as Pitocin may be prepared so that it is ready to be administered after expulsion of the placenta.

The primary health care provider puts on a cap, a mask that has a shield or protective eyewear, and shoe covers. He

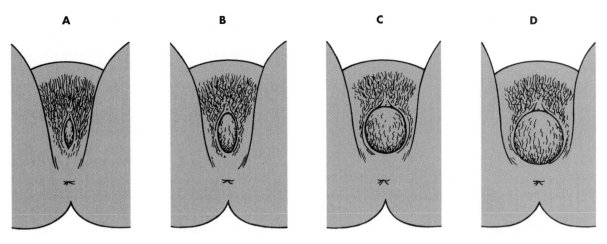

A   **B**   **C**   **D**

Fig. **15-21** Beginning birth with vertex presenting. **A,** Anteroposterior slit. **B,** Oval opening. **C,** Circular shape. **D,** Crowning.

or she must scrub his or her hands and put on a sterile gown (with waterproof front and sleeves) and gloves. Nurses attending the birth may also need to wear caps, protective eyewear, masks, gowns, and gloves. The woman may then be draped with sterile towels and sheets. The partner can help the woman remember not to touch the sterile drapes.

Nursing contact with the parents is maintained by touching, verbal comforting, explaining the reasons for care, and sharing in the parents' joy at the birth of their child.

Mechanism of birth: vertex presentation. Most of the time the birth remains in the hands of the primary health care provider. At times, however, the nurse must assist the woman with giving birth. The nurse's knowledge of the birth process serves as a basis for the way in which she prepares the woman before and during birth. This includes her reviewing with the woman or couple the cardinal movements of labor. That is, once the cervix is fully dilated, descent occurs. The presenting part (usually the vertex) advances with each contraction and recedes slightly as the contraction wanes, but descent is constant. Bulging of the perineum occurs during the descent phase, when the fetal presenting part is distending the perineum but is not yet visible at the introitus. The occiput generally rotates anteriorly, and with voluntary bearing-down efforts, the head appears at the introitus (Fig. 15-21). Although more and more head may be seen with each push, **crowning** occurs when the widest part of the head (the biparietal diameter) distends the vulva just before birth. Immediately before birth, the perineal musculature becomes greatly distended. If an **episiotomy** (incision into the perineum to enlarge vaginal outlet) is necessary, it is done at this time to minimize soft tissue damage.

The three phases of the spontaneous birth of a fetus in a vertex presentation are (1) birth of the head, (2) birth of the shoulders, and (3) birth of the body and extremities.

The speed of the birth of the head must be controlled, because sudden birth of the head may cause severe lacerations that extend through the anal sphincter or even into the woman's rectum. The primary health care provider controls the birth of the head by (1) applying pressure against the rectum, drawing it downward to aid in flexing the head as the back of the neck catches under the symphysis pubis; (2) then applying upward pressure from the coccygeal region (modified **Ritgen maneuver**) (Fig. 15-22) to extend the head during the actual birth, thereby protecting the musculature of the perineum; and (3) assisting the mother with voluntary control of the bearing-down efforts by coaching her to pant while letting uterine forces expel the fetus. Besides protecting the maternal tissues, a gradual birth may prevent fetal intracranial injury.

Occasionally the membranes may not have ruptured before birth. During the birth of the head in this situation, these membranes will look like a hood covering the head. This hood of intact amniotic membranes covering the head during birth is known as a **caul.** In Scotland a child born with a caul is thought to be gifted with "second sight."

The umbilical cord often encircles the neck (**nuchal cord**) but rarely so tightly as to cause hypoxia. After the head is born, gentle palpation is used to feel for the cord. The cord should be slipped gently over the head (see Box 15-6). If the loop is tight or if there is a second loop, the cord is clamped twice, severed between the clamps, and unwound from around the neck before the birth is allowed to continue. Mucus, blood, or meconium in the nasal or oral passages may prevent the newborn from breathing. To eliminate this problem, moist gauze sponges are used to wipe the nose and mouth. A bulb syringe is first inserted into the mouth and oropharynx to aspirate contents and then the nares are cleared in the same fashion while the head is supported.

If meconium has been present in the amniotic fluid during labor, a De Lee suction apparatus is placed on the sterile field and preparations are made for wall suction. Thus when the primary health care provider prepares for birth of the head, the De Lee device is connected to the suction tubing and fluids are withdrawn from the infant's mouth and

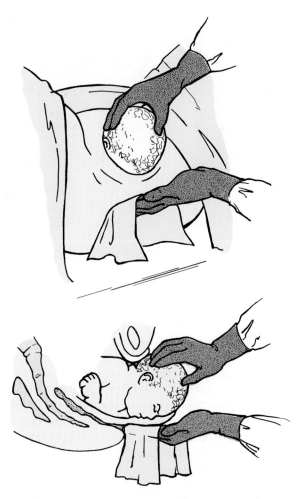

Fig. **15-22** Birth of head using modified Ritgen maneuver. Note control to prevent too rapid birth of head.

nose before the first breath is taken to prevent meconium aspiration. The primary health care provider should refrain from using the De Lee device and oral suction to withdraw fluid from the infant unless the suction device is designed so that it can keep mucus from entering the user's mouth.

Normally the anterior shoulder is delivered with a slight downward traction toward the perineum. The posterior shoulder causes the perineum to distend, and to prevent perineal trauma, the head is lifted toward the symphysis pubis, resulting in the birth of the shoulder over the perineum (Bennett & Brown, 1993; Varney, 1997).

Expulsion of the rest of the body is controlled so that it occurs slowly. While lateral flexion is continued, the primary health care provider supports the weight of the baby to prevent perineal trauma. The body may be rotated slightly to the right or left to facilitate the birth. The time of birth is the precise time when the entire body is out of the woman. This must be recorded on the record.

If the newborn's condition is not compromised, it may be placed on the mother's abdomen immediately after birth and covered with a warm, dry blanket. The cord may be clamped at this time, and the primary health care provider may ask if the woman's partner would like to cut the cord. If so, the primary health care provider provides a sterile pair of scissors and instructs him or her where to cut the cord.

Use of fundal pressure. Fundal pressure is the application of gentle, steady pressure against the fundus of the uterus to facilitate the vaginal birth. Historically it has been used when the administration of analgesia and anesthesia decreased the woman's ability to push during the birth, in cases of shoulder dystocia, and when second-stage fetal bradycardia or other nonreassuring FHR pattern was present. Use of fundal pressure by nurses is not advised because there is no standard technique available for this maneuver, and no current legal, professional, or regulatory standards for its use exist. In cases of shoulder dystocia, suprapubic pressure and maternal position changes (see Chapter 25) are among the recommended interventions (Cosner, 1996; Naif & Morrison, 1994; Piper & McDonald, 1994).

Immediate assessments and care of the newborn. The care given immediately after the birth focuses on assessing and stabilizing the newborn. The nurse's primary responsibility at this time is the infant, because the primary health care provider is involved with the expulsion of the placenta and the care of the mother. The nurse must watch the infant for any signs of distress and initiate appropriate interventions should any appear.

A brief assessment of the newborn can be performed while the mother is holding the infant. This includes checking the infant's airway and Apgar score (see Table 15-3). The nurse dries the infant and covers the infant with a warm blanket. Further examination, identification procedures, and care can be postponed until later in the third stage of labor or early in the fourth stage.

Siblings during the second stage. Parents may wish their other children to be present during the labor and birth process. However, a young child may become frightened by the intensity of the second stage. Sights such as rupture of the membranes and sounds such as their mother's moans, screams, and grunts can be unsettling. It is not uncommon for a woman to say things during the second stage and birth that she would not say otherwise and that might scare her child, such as "I can't take any more. Take this baby out of me" or "This pain is killing me. I'm going to die." The child present during birth therefore needs someone to be close and to give explanations in a simple and calm manner. The child may want to be held.

An alternative to sibling presence at birth is for the sibling to remain in the waiting area with a trusted person until after the birth. At that time the child can be brought into the mother's room and see the baby being held by the mother.

Perineal trauma related to childbirth

Lacerations. Most acute injuries and lacerations of the perineum, vagina, uterus, and their support tissues occur during childbirth, and their management is an obstetric problem. Some injuries to the supporting tissues, whether they were acute or nonacute and whether they were repaired or not, may lead to gynecologic problems later in life (e.g., pelvic relaxation, uterine prolapse, cystocele, rectocele).

The soft tissues of the birth canal and adjacent structures suffer some damage during every birth. Such damage usually is more pronounced in nulliparous women because the tissues are firmer and more resistant than those in multiparous women. Besides this, the perineal skin and vaginal mucosa may appear intact, but numerous small lacerations in underlying muscle and its fascia may be obscured. Damage to pelvic supports usually is readily apparent, however, and thus is repaired after birth.

The tendency to sustain lacerations varies with each woman; that is, the soft tissue in some women may be less distensible. Heredity may be a factor in this. For example, the tissue of light-skinned women, especially those with reddish hair, is not as readily distensible as that of darker-skinned women. In addition, healing may be less efficient in these women.

Immediate repair promotes healing and limits residual damage, as well as decreases the possibility of infection. Immediately after birth the cervix, vagina, and perineum are inspected to look for damage. In addition, during the early postpartum period the nurse and primary health care provider continue to carefully inspect the perineum and to evaluate lochia and symptoms to identify any previously missed damage.

Perineal lacerations. Perineal lacerations usually occur as the fetal head is being born. The extent of the laceration is defined in terms of its depth:

1. First degree. Laceration extends through the skin and structures superficial to muscles.
2. Second degree. Laceration extends through muscles of the perineal body.
3. Third degree. Laceration continues through the anal sphincter muscle.
4. Fourth degree. Laceration also involves the anterior rectal wall.

Perineal injury often is accompanied by small lacerations on the medial surfaces of the labia minora below the pubic rami and to the sides of the urethra and clitoris. Lacerations in this very vascular area often result in profuse bleeding.

Special attention must be paid to third- and fourth-degree lacerations so that the woman retains fecal continence. Measures are then taken to promote soft stools for a few days to increase the woman's comfort and foster healing. Antimicrobial therapy may be instituted in some cases.

Vaginal and urethral lacerations. Vaginal lacerations often occur in conjunction with perineal lacerations. Vaginal lacerations tend to extend up the lateral walls (sulci) and, if deep enough, to involve the levator ani. Additional injury may occur high in the vaginal vault near the level of the ischial spines. Vaginal vault lacerations may be circular

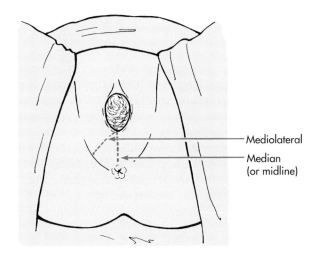

Fig. **15-23** Types of episiotomies.

and may result from forceps rotation, especially in the presence of CPD, rapid fetal descent, or precipitous birth. Lacerations can also occur around the urethra (periurethral) and in the area of the clitoris.

Cervical injuries. Cervical injuries occur when the cervix retracts over the advancing fetal head. These cervical lacerations occur at the lateral angles of the external os; most are shallow, and bleeding is minimal. More extensive lacerations may extend to the vaginal vault or beyond it into the lower uterine segment and may involve serious bleeding. Extensive lacerations may be a consequence of hasty attempts to enlarge the cervical opening artificially or to deliver the fetus before the cervix is fully dilated. Injuries to the cervix can have adverse effects on future pregnancies and childbirths.

Episiotomy. An episiotomy is an incision made in the perineum to enlarge the vaginal outlet. It is performed more commonly in the United States and Canada than in Europe, probably because the side-lying position for birth is used routinely in Europe, whereas the lithotomy position is more commonly used in the United States and Canada. Because the side-lying position causes less tension on the perineum, making it possible for the perineum to stretch gradually, with this position there are fewer indications for the use of episiotomies. The type of episiotomy is designated by the site and direction of the incision (Fig. 15-23).

Midline (median) episiotomy is most commonly used in the United States. It is effective, easily repaired, and generally the least painful. It may extend through the rectal sphincter (third-degree laceration/extension) or even into the anal canal (fourth-degree laceration/extension). Sphincter tone is usually restored following primary healing and a good repair.

Mediolateral episiotomy is used in operative births when the need for posterior extension is likely. Although a fourth-degree laceration may be prevented, a third-degree laceration may occur. Also, the blood loss is greater and the repair more difficult and painful than with midline episiotomies.

Risk factors associated with perineal trauma (episiotomy, lacerations) include nulliparity, occiput posterior position of the fetus, large (macrosomic) infants, use of instruments to facilitate birth, prolonged second stage of labor, and fetal distress. Research has also indicated that the rate of episiotomies is lower when nurse-midwives rather than obstetricians attend births. Socioeconomic factors associated with episiotomies include the Caucasian and Asian races and private insurance and care (Albers et al., 1996; Hueston, 1996; Lydon-Rochelle, Albers & Teaf, 1995).

Alternative measures for perineal management, such as warm compresses, manual support, and massage, have been shown to reduce, to varying degrees, the incidence of episiotomies, but further research is recommended (Albers et al., 1996; Lydon-Rochelle, Albers & Teaf, 1995). Nurses acting as advocates can encourage women to use alternative birthing positions that reduce pressure on the perineum and to use spontaneous bearing-down efforts. In addition, nurses can educate other health care providers about measures to preserve perineal integrity and to be more flexible in defining the maximum limit for the duration of the second stage of labor as long as the maternal-fetal unit is stable (Maier & Maloni, 1997).

Proponents of the use of episiotomy say it serves the following purposes:

- Prevents tearing of the perineum. The clean and properly placed incision heals more properly than does a tear. Some conditions that predispose a woman to perineal tearing and are therefore indications for episiotomy are birth of a large infant, rapid labor in which there is insufficient time for the perineum to stretch, a narrow subpubic arch with a constricted outlet, and malpresentations of the fetus. However, McGuinness, Norr, and Nacion (1991) found that women with episiotomies experienced a longer period of healing than did women without episiotomies. Midline episiotomies are also associated with a higher incidence of third- and fourth-degree lacerations (Labrecque et al., 1997; McGuinness, Norr & Nacion, 1991; Woolley, 1995).
- Possibly minimizes prolonged and severe stretching of the muscles supporting the bladder or rectum, which may later lead to stress incontinence or to prolapse of pelvic organs (uterus, bladder, rectum). Research does not support the claim that pelvic support is protected when episiotomies are performed, however. Episiotomies and the third- and fourth-degree lacerations that can occur actually cut and extend into muscles, thereby prolonging recovery (Paciornik, 1990; Woolley, 1995).
- Reduces duration of the second stage, which may be important for maternal reasons (e.g., a hypertensive state) or fetal reasons (e.g., persistent bradycardia).
- Enlarges the vagina in case manipulation is needed to facilitate the infant's birth (e.g., in a breech presentation or for the application of forceps or a vacuum extractor).

- Shortens the second stage of labor if the well-being of the woman or fetus is in jeopardy, facilitates vacuum-assisted extraction or forceps-assisted birth, prevents cerebral hemorrhage stemming from capillary fragility during the birth of a preterm infant, facilitates the birth of a large infant (more than 4000 g), or facilitates most forceps-assisted breech births. However, research does not support the claims that episiotomies reduce risk for fetal cerebral hemorrhage or distress or shorten the second stage of labor. Further investigation is required to determine if episiotomies are of actual benefit in the instances cited (Woolley, 1995).

Opponents of the routine use of episiotomies say the following:

- The perineum can be prepared for birth through the use of Kegel exercises and massage in the prenatal period. Use of Kegel exercises in the postpartum period improves and restores the tone and strength of the perineal muscles. Health practices, including good nutrition and appropriate hygienic measures, help maintain the integrity and suppleness of the perineal tissue.
- Squatting or lateral positions during childbirth, which encourage women to push as their body tells them to do so, and controlling the emergence of the fetal head while the woman pants and flexion of and counterpressure against the fetal head is accomplished increase the likelihood that the perineum will remain intact or, if lacerations occur, that they will be less severe (Albers et al., 1996; Golay, Vedam & Sorger, 1993).
- Lacerations may occur even with an episiotomy.
- The pain and discomfort resulting from episiotomies is greater than that associated with lacerations and can interfere with mother-infant interactions and the reestablishment of parental sexual intercourse.

Emergency childbirth. Even under the best of circumstances, there probably will come a time when the perinatal nurse will have to assist with the birth of an infant without medical assistance. This situation might arise, for example, in the multiparous woman who arrives at the community hospital fully dilated in the middle of the night. Because it is impossible and unwise to prevent an impending birth, the perinatal nurse needs to be able to function independently and be skilled in the safe birth of a vertex fetus (Box 15-5).

Evaluation

Evaluation of the effectiveness of care of the woman in the second stage of labor is based on the previously stated outcomes.

THIRD STAGE OF LABOR

The third stage of labor lasts from the time the baby is born until the placenta is delivered. The goal in the management of the third stage of labor is the prompt separation

| BOX 15-5 | *Guidelines for Assistance at the Emergency Birth of a Fetus in the Vertex Presentation* |

1. The woman usually assumes the position most comfortable for her. A lateral position is often recommended.
2. Reassure the woman that birth is usually uncomplicated and easy in these situations. Use eye-to-eye contact and a calm, relaxed manner. If there is someone else available, such as the partner, that person could help support the woman in the position, assist with coaching, and compliment her on her efforts.
3. Wash your hands and put gloves on, if possible.
4. Place under woman's buttocks whatever clean material is available.
5. Avoid touching the vaginal area to decrease the possibility of infection.
6. As the head begins to crown, you should do the following:
   a. Tear the amniotic membrane (caul) if it is still intact.
   b. Instruct the woman to pant or pant-blow, thus minimizing the urge to push.
   c. Place the flat side of your hand on the exposed fetal head and apply *gentle* pressure toward the vagina to prevent the head from "popping out." The mother may participate by placing her hand under yours on the emerging head. note: Rapid delivery of the fetal head must be prevented because a rapid change of pressure within the molded fetal skull follows, which may result in dural or subdural tears, and may cause vaginal or perineal lacerations.
7. After the birth of the head, check for an umbilical cord. If the cord is around the baby's neck, try to slip it over the baby's head or pull it *gently* to get some slack so that you can slip it over the shoulders.
8. Support the fetal head as restitution (external rotation) occurs. After restitution, with one hand on each side of the baby's head, exert *gentle* pressure downward so that the anterior shoulder emerges under the symphysis pubis and acts as a fulcrum; then, as *gentle* pressure is exerted in the opposite direction, the posterior shoulder, which has passed over the sacrum and coccyx, emerges.
9. Be alert! Hold the baby securely because the rest of the body may emerge quickly. The baby will be slippery!
10. Cradle the baby's head and back in one hand and the buttocks in the other. Keep the head down to drain away the mucus. Use a bulb syringe, if one is available, to remove mucus from the baby's mouth.
11. Dry the baby quickly to prevent rapid heat loss. Keep the baby at the same level as the mother's uterus until the end of the cord stops pulsating. note: It is important to keep the baby at the same level as the mother's uterus to prevent the baby's blood from flowing to or from the placenta and the resultant hypovolemia or hypervolemia. Also, do not "milk" the cord.
12. Place the baby on the mother's abdomen, cover the baby (remember to keep the head warm, too) with the mother's clothing, and have her cuddle the baby. Compliment her (them) on a job well done, and on the baby, if appropriate.

13. *Wait* for the placenta to separate; *do not* tug on the cord. note: Injudicious traction may tear the cord, separate the placenta, or invert the uterus. Signs of placental separation include a slight gush of dark blood from the introitus, lengthening of the cord, and change in the uterine contour from a discoid to globular shape.
14. Instruct the mother to push to deliver the separated placenta. Gently ease out the placental membranes using an up-and-down motion until the membranes are removed. If birth occurs outside a hospital setting, to minimize complications, do not cut the cord without proper clamps and a sterile cutting tool. Inspect the placenta for intactness. Place the baby on the placenta and wrap the two together for additional warmth.
15. Check the firmness of the uterus. Gently massage the fundus and demonstrate to the mother how she can massage her own fundus properly.
16. If supplies are available, clean the mother's perineal area and apply a peripad.
17. In addition to gentle massage of the fundus, the following measures can be taken to prevent or minimize hemorrhage:
    a. Put the baby to the mother's breast as soon as possible. Sucking or nuzzling and licking the nipple stimulates the release of oxytocin from the posterior pituitary. note: If the baby does not or cannot nurse, manually stimulate the mother's nipples.
    b. Do not allow the mother's bladder to become distended. Assess the bladder for fullness and encourage her to void if fullness is found.
    c. Expel any clots from the mother's uterus.
18. Comfort or reassure the mother and her family or friends. Keep the mother and the baby warm. Give her fluids if available and tolerated.
19. If this is a multifetal birth, identify the infants in order of birth (using letters *A, B,* etc.).
20. Make notations regarding the following aspects of the birth:
    a. Fetal presentation and position
    b. Presence of cord around neck (nuchal cord) or other parts and number of times cord encircled part
    c. Color, character, and amount of amniotic fluid, if rupture of membranes occurs immediately before birth
    d. Time of birth
    e. Estimated time of determination of Apgar score (e.g., 1 and 5 minutes after birth), resuscitation efforts implemented, and ultimate condition of baby
    f. Sex of baby
    g. Time of placental expulsion, as well as the appearance and completeness of the placenta
    h. Maternal condition: affect, amount of bleeding, and status of uterine tonicity
    i. Any unusual occurrences during the birth (e.g., maternal or paternal response, verbalizations, or gestures in response to birth of baby)

and expulsion of the placenta, achieved in the easiest, safest manner.

The placenta is attached to the decidual layer of the basal plate's thin endometrium by numerous fibrous anchor villi—much in the same way as a postage stamp is "attached" to a sheet of postage stamps. After the birth of the fetus, strong uterine contractions occur that cause the placental site to shrink markedly. This causes the anchor villi to break and the placenta to separate from its attachments. Normally the first few strong contractions that occur 5 to 7 minutes after the baby's birth cause the placenta to be sheared away from the basal plate. A placenta cannot be detached from a flaccid (relaxed) uterus because the placental site is not then reduced in size.

▌CARE MANAGEMENT

Assessment and Nursing Diagnoses

Placental separation is indicated by the following signs (Fig. 15-24):

- A firmly contracting fundus

- The uterus changing from a discoid to a globular ovoid shape as the placenta moves into the lower uterine segment
- A sudden gushing of dark blood from the introitus
- Apparent lengthening of the umbilical cord as the placenta gets closer to the introitus
- The finding of a vaginal fullness (the placenta) on vaginal or rectal examination or of fetal membranes at the introitus

Whether the shiny fetal surface of the placenta appears first (Schultze mechanism) or turns so that its dark roughened maternal surface shows first (Duncan mechanism) is of no clinical importance. After the placenta and the amniotic membranes emerge, the primary health care provider examines it for intactness to make sure that no portion remains in the uterine cavity (i.e., no fragments of the placenta or membranes are retained). When indicated, parents should be consulted concerning the disposal of the placenta because some cultures have specific customs regarding the handling and care of the placenta after birth (such as burying the placenta near the home) (D'Avanzo, 1992).

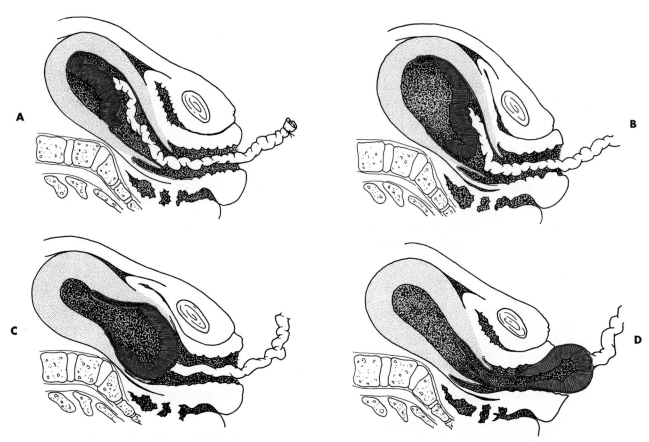

Fig. 15-24 Third stage of labor. **A,** Placenta begins to separate in central portion accompanied by retroplacental bleeding. Uterus changes from discoid to globular shape. **B,** Placenta completes separation and enters lower uterine segment. Uterus is globular in shape. **C,** Placenta enters vagina, cord is seen to lengthen, and there may be an increase in bleeding. **D,** Expulsion (delivery) of placenta and completion of third stage.

Maternal physical status. The physiologic changes in the mother after birth are profound. The cardiac output increases rapidly as maternal circulation to the placenta ceases and the pooled blood from the lower extremities is mobilized. The pulse rate slows in response to the change in cardiac output and tends to remain slightly slower than the prepregnancy rate for about 1 week.

Soon after the birth the woman's blood pressure usually returns to prepregnancy levels. Several factors contribute to an elevated blood pressure at this time: the excitement of the second stage, certain medications, and the time of day (blood pressure is highest during the late afternoon). The effects of analgesics and anesthetics that may have been administered may also cause hypotension to develop in the hour after birth.

Signs of potential problems. Even as the primary health care provider is completing the delivery of the placenta, the nurse is observing the mother for signs of an altered level of consciousness (LOC) or alteration in respirations. Because of the rapid cardiovascular changes taking place (e.g., the increased intracranial pressure during pushing and the rapid increase in cardiac output), this period represents a time when the risk of rupture of a preexisting cerebral aneurysm and the risk of formation of pulmonary emboli are greater than usual. Another dangerous, unpredictable problem that may occur is the formation of an amniotic fluid embolism (AFE) (see Chapter 25).

Nursing diagnoses typical of the third stage of labor are listed in the Nursing Diagnoses box.

I Nursing Diagnoses

Third Stage of Labor
Risk for fluid volume deficit related to:
* Blood loss occurring following placental separation and expulsion
* Inadequate contraction of the uterus
Ineffective individual coping (mother) related to:
* Lack of preparation for sensations that occur during third stage of labor
Anxiety related to:
* Lack of knowledge regarding birth of the placenta
* Occurrence of perineal trauma and the need for repair
Fatigue related to:
* Energy expenditure associated with childbirth and the bearing-down efforts of the second stage
Ineffective family coping related to:
* Unexpected death of fetus before birth or shortly afterwards
* Unexpected birth of an infant with serious congenital anomalies

Expected Outcomes of Care

Planning for this stage of labor focuses on the rapid physiologic changes taking place in the woman and the timely delivery of an intact placenta. At the same time, the emotional environment of the family is also maintained.

Expected outcomes for the third stage of labor may include the following:
* The placenta is expelled, and maternal blood loss is less than 500 ml or less than 1% of body weight.
* The mother is prepared for the sensations she will experience.
* The mother, father or partner, and family initiate the processes of bonding and attachment with the newborn.

Plan of Care and Interventions

To assist the woman in the delivery of the placenta, the nurse or primary health care provider has the woman push when signs of separation have occurred. If possible, the placenta should be expelled by maternal effort during a uterine contraction, but alternate compression and elevation of the fundus, plus minimum, controlled traction on the umbilical cord may be used to facilitate delivery of the placenta and amniotic membranes. If an oxytocic medication is ordered (e.g., 10 to 20 units of Pitocin diluted in an IV solution or 10 units of pitocin given as an intramuscular injection; 0.2 mg of methylergonovine maleate [Methergine] injected intramuscularly), the nurse administers the medication in the dose and by the route indicated by the primary health care provider, after the placenta has been expelled. Oxytocics are administered because they stimulate the uterus to contract, thereby helping to prevent hemorrhage after the placenta is removed. When the third stage is complete and any lacerations are repaired or an episiotomy is sutured, the vulvar area is gently cleansed with warm sterile water or normal saline. The nurse or primary health care provider performs the following:
* Applies a sterile perineal pad/ice pack.
* Removes any drapes and/or places dry linen under the woman's buttocks.
* Repositions the birthing table or bed.
* Lowers the mother's legs simultaneously from the stirrups if she is in a lithotomy position.
* Assists the woman onto her bed if she is to be transferred from the birthing area to the recovery area; assistance is also necessary to move the woman from the birthing table onto a bed if the woman has had anesthesia and does not have full use of her lower extremities.
* Provides the woman with a clean gown and covers her with a warmed blanket.
* Raises the side rails of the bed during the transfer (in some hospitals, the mother is given the baby to hold during the transfer; in other hospitals, the father or partner carries the baby or the nurse or partner transports the baby in a crib, either to the nursery or to the recovery area for the duration of the mother's recovery period).

PLAN OF CARE *Third Stage of Labor*

NURSING DIAGNOSIS Ineffective individual coping related to sense that labor process is over with emergence of neonate and lack of experience with sensations of third stage of labor

Expected outcome *Patient will actively participate in expulsion of the placenta.*

Nursing Interventions/*Rationales*

Explain to woman and labor partner what is expected in the third stage of labor *to enlist cooperation.*

Have woman maintain her position *to facilitate delivery of the placenta.*

Ask mother if she wishes to dispose of the placenta in any specific manner *to comply with certain cultural customs.*

NURSING DIAGNOSIS Fatigue related to energy expenditure required during labor and birth

Expected outcome *Mother's energy levels are restored.*

Nursing Interventions/*Rationales*

Educate mother and partner about need for rest and help them plan strategies (e.g., restricting visitors, increasing role of support systems performing functions associated with daily routines) that allow specific times for rest and sleep *to ensure that woman can restore depleted energy levels in preparation for caring for a new infant.*

Monitor woman's fatigue level and the amount of rest received *to ensure restoration of energy.*

NURSING DIAGNOSIS Risk for fluid volume deficit related to decreased fluid intake and blood loss during the birth

Expected outcomes *Fluid balance is maintained, and there are no signs of dehydration.*

Nursing Interventions/*Rationales*

Monitor fluid loss (i.e., blood, urine, perspiration) and vital signs; inspect skin turgor and mucous membranes for dryness *to evaluate hydration status.*

Administer oral/parenteral fluids per physician/nurse-midwife orders *to maintain hydration.*

Monitor the fundus for firmness after placental separation *to ensure adequate contraction and prevent further blood loss.*

Administer medications per physician/nurse-midwife orders *to aid contraction of the uterus.*

From Wong D & Perry S: *Maternal child nursing care,* St Louis, 1998, Mosby.

If the woman labors, gives birth, and recovers in the same bed and room, she is refreshed following the protocol already described (see Plan of Care). Maternal and neonatal assessments for the fourth stage of labor are instituted (see Chapters 17 and 19). After the woman is transferred or discharged, the birthing area is cleaned as necessary.

Box 15-6 summarizes normal vaginal childbirth.

The family during the third stage. Most parents enjoy being able to handle, hold, explore, and examine the baby immediately after birth. Both parents can assist with the thorough drying of the infant. The infant may be wrapped in a receiving blanket and placed on the woman's abdomen. If skin-to-skin contact is desired, the unwrapped infant may be placed on the woman's abdomen and then covered with a warm blanket.

Holding the newborn next to her skin helps the mother maintain the baby's body heat and provides skin-to-skin contact; care must be taken to keep the head warm. Stockinette caps are sometimes used to cover the newborn's head. It is the nurse's responsibility to make sure the infant stays warm and is in no danger of slipping from the parent's grasp.

Many women wish to begin breastfeeding their newborns at this time to take advantage of the infant's alert state (first period of reactivity) and to stimulate the production of oxytocin that promotes contraction of the uterus. Others prefer to wait until the newborn, parents, and older siblings are together in the recovery area. In some cultures, breastfeeding is not considered acceptable until the milk comes in.

The woman usually feels some discomfort while the primary health care provider carries out the postbirth vaginal examination. Therefore while the process is being completed, the nurse often takes this time to assess the newborn's physical condition; the infant can be weighed and measured, given eye prophylaxis and a vitamin K injection, given an identification bracelet, wrapped in warm blankets, and then given to the partner or back to the mother to hold when she is ready. An in-depth discussion of the care of the newborn after birth is given in Chapters 19 and 20.

Parent-newborn relationships. The woman's reaction to the sight of her newborn may range from excited outbursts of laughing, talking, and even crying to apparent

BOX 15-6   *Normal Vaginal Childbirth*

FIRST STAGE

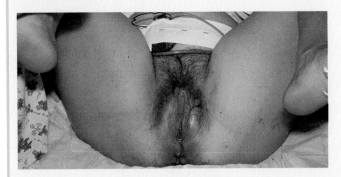

Anteroposterior slit. Vertex visible during contraction.

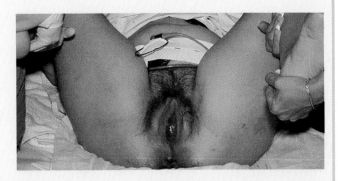

Oval opening. Vertex presenting. Note nurse *(on left)* is wearing gloves but support person *(on right)* is not.

SECOND STAGE

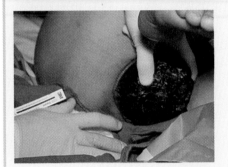

Crowning.

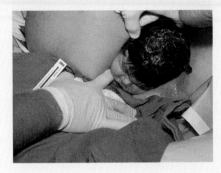

Nurse-midwife using Ritgen maneuver as head is born by extension.

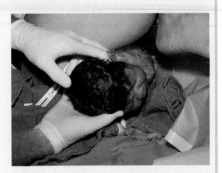

After nurse-midwife checks for nuchal cord, she supports head during external rotation and restitution.

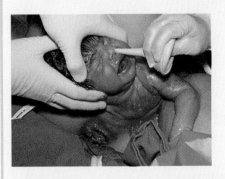

Use of bulb syringe to suction mucus.

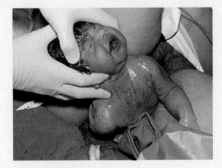

Birth of posterior shoulder.

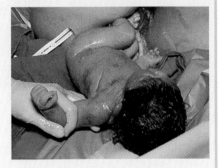

Birth of newborn by slow expulsion.

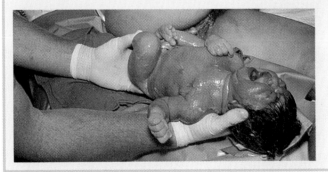

Second stage complete. Note that newborn is not completely pink yet.

Courtesy Michael S. Clement, MD, Mesa, Ariz.

Continued

BOX 15-6 *Normal Vaginal Childbirth–cont'd*

THIRD STAGE

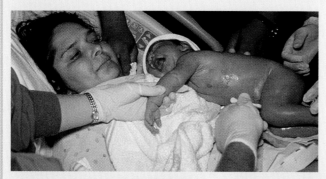

Newborn placed on mother's abdomen while cord is clamped and cut.

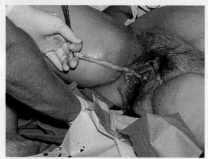

Note increased bleeding as placenta separates.

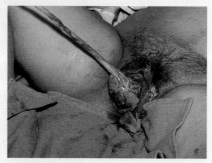

Expulsion of placenta.

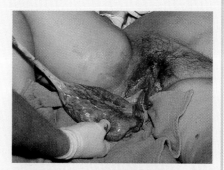

Expulsion is complete, marking the end of the third stage.

THE NEWBORN

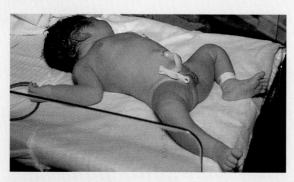

Newborn awaiting assessment. Note color is almost completely pink.

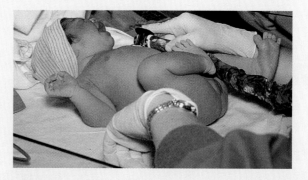

Newborn assessment under radiant warmer.

Parents admiring their newborn.

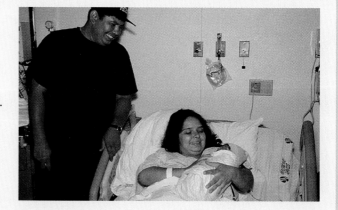

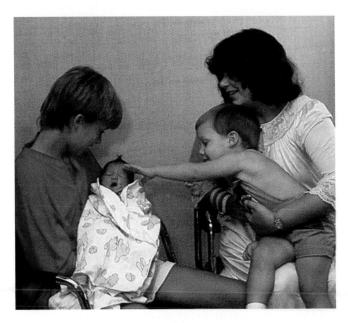

Fig. 15-25 Big brothers become acquainted with new baby sister. (From Wong D: *Whaley & Wong's nursing care of infants and children*, ed 5, St Louis, 1995, Mosby.)

apathy. A polite smile and nod may be her only acknowledgment of the comments of nurses and the primary health care provider. Occasionally the reaction is one of anger or indifference; the woman turns away from the baby, concentrates on her own pain, and sometimes makes hostile comments. These varied reactions can arise from pleasure, exhaustion, or deep disappointment. When evaluating parent-newborn interactions after birth, the nurse should also consider the cultural characteristics of the woman and her family and the expected behaviors of that culture. Whatever the reaction and cause may be, the woman needs continuing acceptance and support from all staff. Notation regarding the parents' reaction to the newborn can be made in the recovery record. Nurses can assess this reaction by asking themselves such questions as: How do the parents look? What do they say? What do they do? The parent-newborn relationship can be further assessed as care is given during the period of recovery. This is especially important if warning signs (e.g., passive or hostile reactions to the newborn, disappointment with gender or appearance of the newborn, absence of eye contact, limited interaction of parents with each other) were noted immediately after birth. The nurse may find it helpful to discuss any warning signs that may have been noted with the woman's primary health care provider.

Siblings, who may have appeared only remotely interested in the final phases of the second stage, tend to experience renewed interest and excitement and can be encouraged to hold the new baby (Fig. 15-25).

Parents usually respond to praise of their newborn. Many need to be reassured that the dusky appearance of their baby's extremities immediately after birth is normal until circulation is well established. If appropriate, the nurse should explain the reason for the molding of the newborn's head. Information about hospital routine can be communicated. It is important, however, for nurses to recognize that the cultural background of the parents may influence their expectations regarding the care and handling of their newborn immediately after birth. For example, some traditional Southeast Asians believe that the head should not be touched because it is the most sacred part of a person's body. They also believe that praise of the baby is dangerous because jealous spirits may then cause the baby harm or take it away (D'Avanzo, 1992). Hospital staff members, by their interest and concern, can provide the environment for making this a satisfying experience for parents, family, and significant others.

Evaluation

Evaluation of the effectiveness of care of the woman in the third stage of labor is based on the previously stated outcomes.

FAMILIES EXPERIENCING LOSS AND GRIEF IN THE INTRAPARTAL PERIOD

Not all labors end with the birth of a healthy, living baby. In some cases the baby is born dead or dies shortly after birth. Women may be admitted to the labor and birth unit already knowing that their baby has died, a fact confirmed in the office of their primary health care provider. For some women, the purpose of admission is to evaluate the health status of a fetus that is exhibiting signs of distress; for example, the mother can no longer perceive fetal movements. Other women may experience a death of a twin or baby in a multifetal gestation. Some women may experience the birth of an infant who is very preterm or has congenital anomalies that are life-threatening.

In these situations women and their significant others will require the empathic support of the nurse who is managing their care. Families should be encouraged to express their feelings to each other and to the nurse and to seek the support of their own spiritual advisor (e.g., priest, minister, rabbi) or one who is assigned to the hospital, if it is appropriate for them to do so. Some hospitals have special support teams specifically available to help patients during times of emotional stress. Women who are laboring when they know that their fetus is in serious jeopardy or has died need continuous emotional support and comfort.

Following the birth of an infant who has died or is dying, it is important that nurses help families to decide about seeing and holding the baby and to be given privacy if they decide to do so. In addition, special memories should be created with the woman and her significant others, including taking photographs, preserving a lock of hair, and taking handprints and footprints. Special memory kits are available to facilitate the process and make it special.

KEY POINTS

- The onset of labor may be difficult to determine for both the nulliparous and multiparous woman.

- The nurse assumes much of the responsibility for assessing the progress of labor and for keeping the primary health care provider informed about progress in labor and deviations from expected findings.

- The fetal heart rate (FHR) and pattern reveal how the fetus is responding to the stress of the labor process.

- Although meconium-stained amniotic fluid may be associated with fetal asphyxia, it is not always an indication of nonreassuring fetal status.

- Assessment of the laboring woman's bladder is critical to ensure her progress and to prevent injury to the bladder.

- Regardless of the actual labor and birth experience, the woman's or couple's perception of the birth experience is most likely to be positive when events and performances are consistent with expectations, especially in terms of maintaining control.

- The woman's level of anxiety may rise when she does not understand what is being said to her about her labor because of the medical terminology used or because of a language barrier.

- Coaching, emotional support, and comfort measures help the woman to use her energy constructively in relaxing and working with the contractions.

- The nurse who is aware of particular sociocultural aspects of helping and coping that pertain to a woman or couple acts as an advocate or protective agent for her or them during labor.

- The quality of the nurse-patient relationship is a factor in the woman's ability to cope with the stressors of the labor process.

- Women with a history of sexual abuse often experience profound stress and anxiety during childbirth.

- The nurse uses professional standards and the nursing process to guide the management of the laboring woman's care.

- When allowed to respond to the rhythmic nature of the second stage of labor, the woman normally changes body positions, bears down spontaneously, and vocalizes when she perceives the urge to push (Ferguson's reflex).

- If any laboring woman states, "The baby is coming!" the baby is coming; an immediate birth should be anticipated.

KEY POINTS—cont'd

- During the second stage, the woman needs continuous monitoring, support, and coaching.

- Episiotomies may be performed and lacerations may occur even during "normal" childbirth, and their appropriate and prompt repair is essential.

- Objective signs indicate that the placenta has separated and is ready to be expelled; excessive traction (pulling) on the umbilical cord before the placenta has separated can result in maternal injury.

- Most parents/families enjoy being able to handle, hold, explore, and examine the baby immediately after the birth.

- Siblings present for labor and birth need preparation and support for the event.

- Women benefit from reviewing their childbirth experiences with the nurse who managed their care during the process of labor and birth.

- When a baby dies or has life-threatening problems, the woman and her family will need emotional support and assistance to work through their grief.

CRITICAL THINKING EXERCISES

1. *A nulliparous woman calls the birthing center and very anxiously tells the nurse, "I am in labor, and I do not know what I am going to do. I have no one to bring me to the center because my husband is on a business trip and will be gone for 2 more days!" Describe the approach the nurse should take in responding to this woman's concerns.*

2. *Today, birth plans are developed by more and more pregnant couples as a method of expressing their wishes and preferences for their childbirth experiences. How should the nurse respond in each of the following situations?*

   a. *A multiparous couple present a birth plan that contains several items that are in conflict with hospital policy. For example, they do not want any electronic fetal monitoring or intravenous therapy, and they want their two children (3 and 5 years old) present for the labor and birth.*

   b. *A nulliparous woman has been admitted in the latent phase of the first stage of labor. The father of her baby will be with her during labor and birth. They have no birth plan and attended no prepared childbirth classes.*

CRITICAL THINKING EXERCISES—cont'd

3 You are the nurse-manager of a birthing center. A group of women approach you about becoming doulas. They have all given birth several times themselves and are active members of the La Leche League (breastfeeding mothers support group) chapter to which you also belong. Describe the approach you would use to help these women meet their goal.

4 You are the nurse-manager of a labor and birth unit of a hospital. After attending a joint statewide medical-nursing educational meeting regarding new approaches to childbirth, you realize that the rate of episiotomy use is higher on your labor and birth unit than on other labor and birth units in your state. At the meeting, several successful measures for reducing the rate of perineal trauma were discussed. Acting as an advocate for your patients, outline the approach you would use to convince the nursing and medical staff that routine use of episiotomies is harmful and can be avoided with changes in childbirth practices.

5 While caring for a woman in the second stage of labor, the nurse observes the woman's partner telling her to hold her breath as long as she can while she pushes with each contraction. How should the nurse respond?

6 Create a management plan for a newly created family-centered birthing unit located in a women's health center. The plan should:

   a Recognize the woman's partner as a member of the team caring for the laboring woman.

   b Appreciate cultural and religious beliefs and practices that influence the manner in which couples and their families approach childbirth.

   c Establish guidelines for the participation of children who will be present during their mother's labor.

References

Aderhold K & Perry L: Jet hydrotherapy for labor and postpartum pain relief, *MCN Am J Matern Child Nurs* 16(2):97, 1991.

Aderhold K & Roberts J: Phases of second stage labor: four descriptive case studies, *J Nurse Midwifery* 36(5):267, 1991.

Albers L, Schiff M & Gorwoda J: The length of active labor in normal pregnancies, *Obstet Gynecol* 87(3):355, 1996.

Albers L et al: Factors related to perineal trauma in childbirth, *J Nurse Midwifery* 41(4):269, 1996.

Albers L et al: The relationship of ambulation in labor to operative delivery, *J Nurse Midwifery* 42(1):4, 1997.

American College of Obstetricians and Gynecologists: More women now deliver in alternative birth sites, *ACOG Newslett* 37 (1):8, 1993.

Andrews C & Chrzanowski M: Maternal position, labor, and comfort, *Appl Nurs Res* 3(1):7, 1990.

Bennett V & Brown L: *Myles textbook for midwives,* ed 12, Edinburgh, 1993, Churchill Livingstone.

Berry L: Realistic expectations of the labor coach, *J Obstet Gynecol Neonatal Nurs* 17(5):354, 1988.

Biancuzzo M: The patient observer: does the hand-and-knees posture during labor help to rotate the occiput posterior fetus? *Birth* 18(1):40, 1991.

Biancuzzo M: Six myths of maternal posture during labor, *MCN Am J Matern Child Nurs* 18(5):264, 1993.

Bryanton J, Fraser-Davey H & Sullivan P: Women's perception of nursing support during labor, *J Obstet Gynecol Neonatal Nurs* 23(8):638, 1994.

Burian J: Helping survivors of sexual abuse through labor, *MCN Am J Matern Child Nurs* 20(5):252, 1995.

Callister L: The meaning of the childbirth experience to the Mormon woman, *J Perinat Educ* 1(1):50, 1992.

Callister L: Cultural meanings of childbirth, *J Obstet Gynecol Neonatal Nurs* 24(4):327, 1995.

Callister L, Vehvilainen-Julkunen K & Lauri S: Cultural perceptions of childbirth, *Holistic Nurs* 14(1):66, 1996.

Carbonne B et al: Maternal position during labor: effects on fetal oxygen saturation measured by pulse oximetry, *Obstet Gynecol* 88(5):797, 1996.

Chalmers B & Meyer D: Companionship in the perinatal period: a cross-cultural survey of women's experiences, *J Nurse Midwifery* 39(4):265, 1994.

Chandler S & Field P: Becoming a father–first-time fathers' experience of labor and delivery, *J Nurse Midwifery* 42(1):17, 1997.

Chapman L: Expectant father's roles during labor and birth, *J Obstet Gynecol Neonatal Nurs* 21(2):114, 1992.

Cosner K: Use of fundal pressure during second-stage labor: a pilot study, *J Nurse Midwifery* 41(4):334, 1996.

Cosner K & deJong E: Physiologic second-stage labor, *MCN Am J Matern Child Nurs* 18(1):38, 1993.

D'Avanzo C: Bridging the cultural gap with Southeast Asians, *MCN Am J Matern Child Nurs* 17(4):204, 1992.

DeSevo M: Keeping the faith: Jewish traditions in pregnancy and childbirth, *Lifelines* 1(4):46, 1997.

DiMatteo M et al: Narratives of birth and the postpartum: analysis of the focus group responses of new mothers, *Birth* 20(4):204, 1993.

Evans S & Jeffery J: Maternal learning needs during labor and delivery, *J Obstet Gynecol Neonatal Nurs* 24(3):235, 1995.

Finn J: Culture care of Euro-American women during childbirth: using Leininger's theory, *J Transcultural Nurs* 5(2):25, 1994.

Friedman E & Sachtleben M: Station of the presenting part, *Am J Obstet Gynecol* 93:522, 1965.

Gannon J: Delivery on the hands and knees: a case study approach, *J Nurse Midwifery* 37(1):48, 1992.

Geissler E: *Pocket guide to cultural assessment,* St Louis, 1994, Mosby.

Golay J, Vedam S & Sorger L: The squatting position for the second stage of labor: effects on labor and on maternal and fetal well-being, *Birth* 20(2):73, 1993.

Hodnett E: Nursing support of the laboring woman, *J Obstet Gynecol Neonatal Nurs* 25(3):257, 1996.

Hueston W: Factors associated with the use of episiotomy during vaginal delivery, *Obstet Gynecol* 87(6):1001, 1996.

Jonquil S: Preparing siblings, *Midwifery Today* 28:34, 1993.

Jordan P: Laboring for relevance: expectant and new fatherhood, *Nurs Res* 39(1):11, 1990.

Khazoyan C & Anderson N: Latina's expectations for their partners during childbirth, *MCN Am J Matern Child Nurs* 19(4):226, 1994.

Labrecque M et al: Association between median episiotomy and severe perineal lacerations in primiparous women, *Can Med Assoc J* 156(6):797, 1997.

Lantican S & Corona D: Comparison of the social support networks of Filipinos and Mexican American primigravidas, *Health Care Women Int* 13:329, 1992.

Ludka L & Roberts C: Eating and drinking in labor, a literature review, *J Nurse Midwifery* 38(4):199, 1993.

Lydon-Rochelle M, Albers L & Teaf D: Perineal outcomes and nurse-midwifery management, *J Nurse Midwifery* 40(1):13, 1995.

Mahan C & McKay S: Are we overmanaging second stage labor? *Contemp OB/GYN* 24:37, 1984.

Maier J & Maloni J: Nurse advocacy for selective versus routine episiotomy, *J Obstet Gynecol Neonatal Nurs J* 26(2):155, 1997.

Malestic S: Fathers need help during labor, too, *RN* 53(7):23, 1990.

McGuinness M, Norr K & Nacion K: Comparison between different perineal outcomes on tissue healing, *J Nurse Midwifery* 36(3):192, 1991.

McKay S & Barrows T: Holding back: maternal readiness to give birth, *MCN Am J Matern Child Nurs* 16(5):251, 1991.

McKay S & Roberts J: Obstetrics by ear: maternal and caregiver perceptions of the meaning of maternal sounds during second stage labor, *J Nurse Midwifery* 35(5):266, 1990.

McKay S & Smith S: "What are they talking about? Is something wrong?" Information sharing during the second stage of labor, *Birth* 20(3):142, 1993.

Melzak R, Belanger E & Lacroix R: Labor pain: effects of maternal position on front and back pain, *J Pain Symptom Manage* 6(8):476, 1991.

Metzer B & Therrien B: Effect of position on cardiovascular response during the Valsalva maneuver, *Nurs Res* 39(4):198, 1990.

Moore M, Hopper U & Dip G: Do birth plans empower women? Evaluation of a hospital birth plan, *Birth* 22(1):29, 1995.

Naef R & Morrison J: Guidelines for the management of shoulder dystocia, *J Perinatol* 14(6):435, 1994.

Nichols F: The meaning of the childbirth experience: a review of the literature, *J Perinat Educ* 5(4):71, 1996.

Nichols M: Paternal perspectives of the childbirth experience, *Matern Child Nurs J* 21(3):99, 1993.

Olsen O: Meta-analysis of the safety of home birth, *Birth* 24(1):4, 1997.

Paciornik M: Commentary: arguments against episiotomy and in favor of squatting for birth, *Birth* 17(2):104, 1990.

Parratt J: The experience of childbirth for survivors of incest, *Midwifery* 10:26, 1994.

Pascoe J: Social support during labor and duration of labor: a community-based study, *Public Health Nurs* 10(2):97, 1993.

Perez P & Herrick L: Doulas: exploring their roles with parents, hospitals, & nurse, *Lifelines*, 2(2):54, 1998.

Piper D & McDonald P: Management of anticipated and actual shoulder dystocia, *J Nurse Midwifery* 39(2 suppl):915, 1994.

Queenan J: Partners in the delivery room: a natural evolution, *Contemp OB/GYN* 35(8):8, 1990.

Roberts J & Woolley D: A second look at the second stage of labor, *J Obstet Gynecol Neonatal Nurs* 25(5):415, 1996.

Rosenthal M: Warm-water immersion in labor and birth, *Female Patient* 16(8):35, 1991.

Rothman B: Women, providers, and control, *J Obstet Gynecol Neonatal Nurs* 25(3):253, 1996.

Scott J et al: *Danforth's obstetrics and gynecology,* ed 7, Philadelphia, 1994, JB Lippincott.

Simkin P: Reducing pain and enhancing progress in labor: a guide to nonpharmacologic methods for maternity caregivers, *Birth* 22(3):161, 1995.

Simkin P: The experience of maternity in a woman's life, *J Obstet Gynecol Neonatal Nurs* 25(3):247, 1996.

Technical Working Group, World Health Organization: Care in normal birth: a practical guide, *Birth* 24(2):121, 1997.

Thomson A: Pushing techniques in the second stage of labour, *J Adv Nurs* 18(2):171, 1993.

Tomlinson P & Bryan A: Family centered intrapartum care: revisiting an old concept, *J Obstet Gynecol Neonatal Nurs* 25(4):331, 1996.

Tucker S: *Pocket guide to fetal monitoring and assessment,* ed 3, St Louis, 1996, Mosby.

Varney H: *Varney's midwifery,* ed 3, Sudberry, Mass, 1997, Jones & Bartlett.

Waldenström U & Gottvall K: A randomized trial of birthing stool or conventional semirecumbent position for second stage labor, *Birth* 18(1):5, 1991.

Waldenström U et al: The childbirth experience: a study of 295 new mothers, *Birth* 23(3):144, 1996.

Waymire V: A triggering time: childbirth may recall sexual abuse memories, *Lifelines* 1(2):47, 1997.

Weber S: Cultural aspects of pain in childbearing women, *J Obstet Gynecol Neonatal Nurs* 25(1):67, 1996.

Wong D: *Whaley and Wong's nursing care of infants and children,* ed 5, St Louis, 1995, Mosby.

Wong D & Perry S: *Maternal child nursing care,* St Louis, 1998, Mosby.

Woods A: Nurse midwifery in rural Pakistan, *J Nurse Midwifery* 36(4):249, 1991.

Woolley R: Benefits and risks of episiotomy: a review of the English-language literature since 1980, parts I and II, *Obstet Gynecol Surv* 50(11):806, 1995.

Wraight A: Home births, *Midwives* 110(1312):104, 1997.

Yeates J & Roberts J: A comparison of two bearing-down techniques during the second stage of labor, *J Nurse Midwifery* 29(1):3, 1984.

Zhang J et al: Continuous labor support from labor attendant for primiparous women: a meta-analysis, *Obstet Gynecol* 88(4):739, 1996.

CHAPTER

16

Physiologic Changes

BETSY STETSON

KEY TERMS

colostrum
diaphoresis
diastasis recti abdominis
diuresis
engorgement (breast)
fourth trimester of pregnancy
hemorrhoids
involution
lochia alba
lochia rubra
lochia serosa
pelvic relaxation
puerperium
subinvolution
thromboembolism

The postpartum period is the 6-week interval between the birth of the newborn and the return of the reproductive organs to their normal nonpregnant state. This period is sometimes referred to as the **puerperium,** or **fourth trimester of pregnancy.** The physiologic changes that occur as the processes of pregnancy are reversed, though distinctive, are considered normal. Many factors, including the mother's energy level and degree of comfort, the health of the newborn, and the care and encouragement given by the health professionals, contribute to the mother's response to her infant during this time. To provide care during the recovery period that is beneficial to the mother, her infant, and her family, the nurse must synthesize knowledge of the following: maternal anatomy and physiology, the newborn's physical and behavioral characteristics, infant care activities, and the family response to the birth of the child. This chapter focuses on anatomic and physiologic changes that occur in the woman during the postpartum period.

REPRODUCTIVE SYSTEM AND ASSOCIATED STRUCTURES

Uterus

Involution process

The process by which the uterus, following birth, returns to a nonpregnant state that is similar to the prepregnant state is called **involution.** This process begins immediately after expulsion of the placenta with contraction of the uterine smooth muscle. It is important to maintain a firmly contracted uterus to prevent excessive blood loss. A boggy (soft, noncontracted) uterus needs to be treated.

At the end of the third stage of labor the uterus is in the midline, about 2 cm *below* the level of the umbilicus, with the fundus resting on the sacral promontory. At this time, the uterus is approximately the size it was at 16 weeks of gestation (about the size of a grapefruit) and weighs about 1,000 g.

Within 12 hours the fundus may be approximately 1 cm *above* the umbilicus (Fig. 16-1). Involution progresses rapidly during the next few days. The fundus descends about 1 to 2 cm every 24 hours. By the sixth postpartum day the fundus is normally located halfway between the symphysis pubis and the umbilicus. A week after childbirth the uterus once again lies in the true pelvis. The uterus should not be palpable abdominally after the ninth postpartum day.

The uterus, which at full term weighs approximately 11 times its prepregnant weight, involutes to about 500 g 1 week after birth and to about 350 g by 2 weeks after birth. At 6 weeks it weighs 50 to 60 g (see Fig. 16-1).

Increased estrogen and progesterone levels are responsible for the massive growth of the uterus during pregnancy. Prenatal uterine growth is the result of both *hyperplasia,* an increase in the number of muscle cells, and *hypertrophy,*

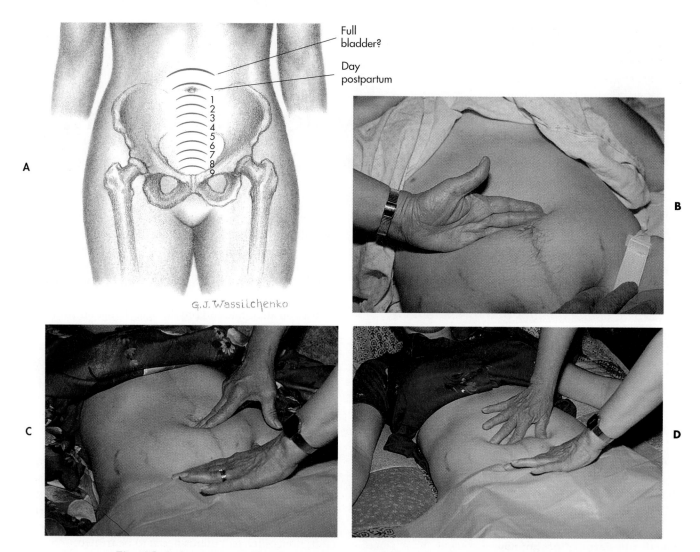

Full bladder?

Day postpartum

1
2
3
4
5
6
7
8
9

G.J. Wassilchenko

A

B

C

D

Fig. **16-1** Assessment of involution of uterus after childbirth. **A,** Normal progress, days 1 through 9. **B,** Size and position of uterus 2 hours after childbirth. **C,** Two days after childbirth. **D,** Four days after childbirth. (*B, C,* and *D* courtesy Marjorie Pyle, RNC, Lifecircle, Costa Mesa, Calif.)

enlargement of the existing cells. Postpartally the decrease in the secretion of these hormones causes *autolysis,* a self-destruction of excess hypertrophied tissue. The additional cells laid down during pregnancy remain, however, and cause a slight increase in uterine size after each pregnancy.

Breastfeeding and fundal massage facilitate involution. **Subinvolution** is the failure of the uterus to return to a nonpregnant state. The most common causes of subinvolution are retained placental fragments and infection.

Contractions

The intensity of uterine contractions increases significantly immediately after birth, presumably in response to the greatly diminished intrauterine volume. Postpartum hemostasis is achieved primarily by compression of intramyometrial blood vessels as the uterine muscle contracts, rather

than by platelet aggregation and clot formation. The hormone oxytocin, which is released from the pituitary gland, strengthens and coordinates the uterine contractions. In turn, this compresses the blood vessels, thus aiding in hemostasis. During the first 1 to 2 postpartum hours, uterine contractions may decrease in intensity and become uncoordinated. Because it is vital that the uterus remain firm and well contracted, exogenous oxytocin (Pitocin) is often administered intravenously or intramuscularly immediately after expulsion of the placenta. Mothers who plan to breastfeed may be encouraged to put the baby to breast immediately after birth because suckling stimulates the release of oxytocin.

Afterpains

In primiparas uterine tone is increased so that the fundus generally remains firm. Periodic relaxation and contraction are more common for multiparas and may cause uncomfortable cramping called *afterpains,* which persist throughout the early puerperium. Afterpains are more noticeable after births in which the uterus was overdistended (e.g., large baby, twins). Breastfeeding and exogenous oxytocic medication usually intensify these afterpains, since both stimulate uterine contractions.

Placental site

Immediately after the placenta and membranes are expelled, vascular constriction and thromboses reduce the placental site to an irregular nodular and elevated area. Upward growth of the endometrium causes sloughing of necrotic tissue and prevents the scar formation that is characteristic of normal wound healing. This unique healing process enables the endometrium to resume its usual cycle of changes and to permit implantation and placentation in future pregnancies.

Endometrial regeneration is completed by the end of the third postpartum week except at the placental site. Regeneration at the placental site usually is not complete until 6 weeks after birth.

Lochia

Postchildbirth uterine discharge, commonly called lochia, is initially bright red, changing later to a pinkish red or reddish brown. It may contain small clots of blood.

For the first 2 hours after birth the amount of uterine discharge should be about that of a heavy menstrual period. After that time, the lochial flow should steadily decrease.

Lochia rubra consists mainly of blood and decidual and trophoblastic debris. The flow pales, becoming pink or brown after 3 to 4 days (lochia serosa). **Lochia serosa** consists of old blood, serum, leukocytes, and tissue debris. About 10 days after childbirth the drainage becomes yellow to white (lochia alba). **Lochia alba** consists of leukocytes, decidua, epithelial cells, mucus, serum, and bacteria. Lochia alba may continue to drain from the vaginal opening for up to and beyond 6 weeks after childbirth (Visness, Kennedy & Ramas, 1997).

It is difficult to judge the amount of lochial flow based only on observation of perineal pads. Luegenbiehl (1990) suggested one method for subjectively estimating postpartal blood loss, which entails gauging the extent of staining on a perineal pad (see Fig. 17-6). Weighing perineal pads before and after use provides a more objective measurement of lochial flow but is not common in practice. Each 1 g increase in weight is roughly equivalent to 1 ml of blood loss. Any estimation of lochial flow is inaccurate and incomplete, however, without considering the time factor. For example, the woman who saturates a peripad in 1 hour or less is bleeding much more than the woman who saturates a peripad in 8 hours.

If the woman receives an oxytocic medication, regardless of the route of administration, the flow of lochia is usually

| TABLE 16-1 | *Lochial and Nonlochial Bleeding* |

LOCHIA	NONLOCHIAL BLEEDING
Lochia usually trickles from the vaginal opening. The steady flow is greater as the uterus contracts.	If the bloody discharge spurts from the vagina, there may be cervical or vaginal tears in addition to the normal lochia.
A gush of lochia may result as the uterus is massaged. If it is dark in color, it has been pooled in the relaxed vagina, and the amount seen lessens to a trickle of bright red lochia (in the early puerperium).	If the amount of bleeding continues to be excessive and bright red, a cervical or vaginal tear may be the source.

scant until the effects of the medication wear off. Also, the amount of lochia is usually less after cesarean births. The flow of lochia usually increases with ambulation and breastfeeding. Lochia tends to pool in the vagina when the woman is lying in bed; the woman may then experience a gush of blood upon standing, a gush which should not be confused with hemorrhage.

Persistence of lochia rubra early in the postpartum period suggests continued bleeding as a result of retained fragments of the placenta or membranes. Recurrence of bleeding about 10 days after birth is from the healing placental site. However, any bleeding occurring 3 to 4 weeks after birth may be caused by infection or subinvolution. The continued flow of lochia serosa or lochia alba may indicate endometritis, particularly if this is accompanied by fever, pain, or abdominal tenderness. Lochia should smell like normal menstrual flow; an offensive odor usually indicates infection.

It is important to remember that all postpartal vaginal bleeding is not necessarily lochia. Another common source of vaginal bleeding after birth is unrepaired vaginal or cervical lacerations. Table 16-1 distinguishes between lochial and nonlochial bleeding.

Cervix

The cervix is soft immediately after birth. By 18 hours postpartum, however, it has shortened, become firm, and regained its form. The cervix up to the lower uterine segment remains edematous, thin, and fragile for several days after birth. The ectocervix (portion of the cervix that protrudes into the vagina) appears bruised and has some small lacerations, constituting an optimal condition for the development of infection. The cervical os, which dilates to 10 cm during labor, closes gradually. It may still be possible to introduce two fingers into the cervical os for the first 4 to 6 days postpartum. By the end of 2 weeks, however, only the smallest curette can be introduced. The external cervical os never regains its prepregnant appearance; it is no longer shaped like a circle but appears as a jagged slit, often described as a fish mouth (see Fig. 9-1). Lactation delays production of cervical and other estrogen-influenced mucus and mucosal characteristics.

Vagina and Perineum

The estrogen deprivation that occurs postpartum is responsible for causing the thinness of the vaginal mucosa and the absence of rugae. The greatly distended, smooth-walled vagina gradually returns to its prepregnant size by 6 to 8 weeks after childbirth. Rugae reappear by about the fourth week, although they are never as prominent as they are in the nulliparous woman. Most rugae may be permanently flattened. The mucosa remains atrophic in the lactating woman, at least until menstruation begins again. Thickening of the vaginal mucosa occurs with the return of ovarian function. The reduced levels of estrogen are responsible for causing a decreased amount of vaginal lubrication. Localized dryness and coital discomfort (dyspareunia) may persist until ovarian function returns and menstruation resumes. Use of a water-soluble lubricant during intercourse is usually recommended to help reduce discomfort.

Initially the *introitus* is erythematous and edematous, especially in the area of the episiotomy or laceration repair. However, it is usually barely distinguishable from that of a nulliparous woman if lacerations and an episiotomy have been carefully repaired, if hematomas are prevented or treated early, and if the woman observes good hygiene during the first 2 weeks after birth.

Most *episiotomies* are visible only if the woman is lying on her side with her buttock raised or if she is placed in the lithotomy position. A good light source is essential for visualization of some episiotomies. An episiotomy heals the same way as any surgical incision. Signs of infection (pain, redness, warmth, swelling, or discharge) or the loss of approximation (separation of the incision edges) may occur. Healing should occur within 2 to 3 weeks.

Hemorrhoids (anal varicosities) are commonly seen (see Fig. 9-9). Women often experience associated symptoms such as itching, discomfort, and bright red bleeding with defecation. Hemorrhoids usually decrease in size within 6 weeks of childbirth.

Pelvic Muscular Support

The supporting structure of the uterus and vagina may be injured during childbirth and may contribute to gynecologic problems later. The supportive tissues of the pelvic floor that are torn or stretched during childbirth may require up to 6 months to regain tone. Women are often encouraged to do Kegel exercises after birth to help strengthen perineal muscles and promote healing (see Chapter 4). The term **pelvic relaxation** refers to the lengthening and weakening of the fascial supports of pelvic structures. These structures include the uterus, upper posterior vaginal wall, urethra, bladder, and rectum. Although pelvic relaxation can occur in any woman, it is usually a direct but delayed complication of childbirth.

ENDOCRINE SYSTEM

Placental Hormones

Significant hormonal changes occur during the postpartal period. Expulsion of the placenta results in dramatic decreases of the hormones produced by that organ. Decreases in human placental lactogen (hPL), estrogens, cortisol, and the placental enzyme insulinase cause the diabetogenic effects of pregnancy to be reversed, resulting in significantly lower blood sugar levels in the immediate puerperium. Mothers with type 1 diabetes will thus be likely to require much less insulin for several days after birth. Because these normal hormonal changes make the puerperium a transitional period for carbohydrate metabolism, it is more difficult to interpret the results of glucose tolerance tests at this time.

Estrogen and progesterone levels drop markedly following expulsion of the placenta, reaching their lowest levels 1 week into the postpartum period. Decreased estrogen levels are associated with breast engorgement and with the diuresis of excess extracellular fluid that has accumulated during pregnancy. The estrogen levels in nonlactating women begin to rise by 2 weeks after birth and are higher by postpartum day 17 than in women who breastfeed (Bowes, 1996).

Pituitary Hormones and Ovarian Function

Lactating and nonlactating women differ considerably in the time when the first ovulation occurs and when menstruation is reestablished. The persistence of elevated serum prolactin levels in breastfeeding women appears to be responsible for suppressing ovulation. Because levels of follicle-stimulating hormone (FSH) have been shown to be identical in lactating and nonlactating women, it is thought that ovulation is suppressed in lactating women because the ovary does not respond to FSH stimulation when increased prolactin levels are present (Bowes, 1996). Another theory is that endogenous opiate levels play an important role in regulating the hormone levels of lactating women (Gordon et al., 1993).

Prolactin levels in blood rise progressively throughout pregnancy. In women who breastfeed, however, prolactin levels remain elevated into the sixth week after birth (Bowes, 1996). Serum prolactin levels are influenced by the frequency of breastfeeding, the duration of each feeding, and the degree to which supplementary feedings are used. The individual differences in the strength of the infant's sucking stimulus probably also affect prolactin levels. This emphasizes the fact that breastfeeding is not a reliable form of birth control. After birth, prolactin levels decline in nonlactating women, reaching the prepregnant range within 2 weeks.

Ovulation occurs as early as 27 days after birth in non-lactating women, with a mean time of about 70 to 75 days. Ovulation resumes by 2 months postpartum in most non-breastfeeding women (Bowes, 1996; Gordon et al., 1993). About 90% of nonbreastfeeding women resume menstruating by 3 months after birth (Gordon et al., 1993). The mean time to ovulation in women who breastfeed is about 190 days (Bowes, 1996). In lactating women, both the resumption of ovulation and the return of menses are determined in large part by breastfeeding patterns (Gordon et al., 1993). The fact that 25% of breastfeeding women ovulate before their first postpartum menstrual period occurs reemphasizes the need for discussion of contraceptive options early in the puerperium (Zlatnik, 1994).

The first menstrual flow after childbirth is usually heavier than normal. Within three to four cycles the amount of menstrual flow has returned to the woman's prepregnant volume.

ABDOMEN

When the woman stands up during the first days after birth, her abdominal muscles protrude and give her a still-pregnant appearance. During the first 2 weeks after birth the abdominal wall is relaxed. It takes approximately 6 weeks for the abdominal wall to return almost to its prepregnancy state. The skin regains most of its previous elasticity, but some striae may persist. The return of muscle tone depends on previous tone, proper exercise, and the amount of adipose tissue. On occasion, with or without overdistention because of a large fetus or multiple fetuses, the abdominal wall muscles separate, a condition termed **diastasis recti abdominis** (see Fig. 9-13). Persistence of this defect may be disturbing to the woman, but surgical correction is rarely necessary. With time, the defect becomes less apparent.

URINARY SYSTEM

The hormonal changes of pregnancy (high steroid levels) may be partly responsible for causing an increase in renal function, whereas the diminishing steroid levels after birth may partly explain the reduced renal function that occurs during the puerperium. Kidney function returns to normal within a month after birth. About 2 to 8 weeks are required for the pregnancy-induced hypotonia and dilatation of the ureters and renal pelves to return to the prepregnant state (Cunningham et al., 1997). In a small percentage of women, dilatation of the urinary tract may persist for 3 months, which increases the chance for the development of a urinary tract infection.

Urine Components

The renal glycosuria induced by pregnancy disappears, but lactosuria may occur in lactating women. The blood urea nitrogen (BUN) level increases during the puerperium as *autolysis* of the involuting uterus occurs. This breakdown of excess protein in the uterine muscle cells also results in a mild (+1) proteinuria for 1 to 2 days after childbirth in about 50% of women (Simpson & Creehan, 1996). Ketonuria may occur in women with an uncomplicated birth or after a prolonged labor with dehydration.

Postpartal Diuresis

Within 12 hours of birth, women begin to lose the excess tissue fluid that has accumulated during pregnancy. One mechanism responsible for reducing these retained fluids of pregnancy is the profuse **diaphoresis** that often occurs, especially at night, for the first 2 or 3 days after childbirth. Postpartal **diuresis,** caused by decreased estrogen levels, removal of increased venous pressure in the lower extremities, and loss of the remaining pregnancy-induced increase in blood volume, is another mechanism by which the body rids itself of excess fluid. The fluid loss through perspiration and the increased urinary output accounts for a weight loss of approximately 2.25 kg during the puerperium. This elimination of excess fluid accumulated during pregnancy is sometimes referred to as *reversal of the water metabolism of pregnancy.*

Urethra and Bladder

Trauma to the urethra and bladder may occur during the birth process as the infant passes through the pelvis. As a result the bladder wall may be hyperemic and edematous, often with small areas of hemorrhage. Clean-catch or catheterized urine specimens after birth often reveal hematuria from bladder trauma. The urethra and urinary meatus may also be edematous.

Birth-induced trauma, increased bladder capacity following childbirth, and the effects of conduction anesthesia combine to cause a decrease in the urge to void. In addition, pelvic soreness from the forces of labor, vaginal lacerations, or the episiotomy reduces or alters the voiding reflex. Decreased voiding, along with postpartal diuresis, may result in bladder distention. Immediately after birth, excessive bleeding can occur if the bladder becomes distended because this pushes the uterus up and to the side and prevents the uterus from firmly contracting. Later in the puerperium overdistention can make the bladder more susceptible to infection and impede the resumption of normal voiding (Cunningham et al., 1997). With adequate emptying of the bladder, bladder tone is usually restored 5 to 7 days after childbirth.

GASTROINTESTINAL SYSTEM

Appetite

The mother is usually hungry shortly after giving birth and can tolerate a light diet. Most new mothers are ravenously hungry after full recovery from analgesia, anesthesia, and fatigue. Requests for extra portions of food and frequent snacks are not uncommon.

Motility

Typically, decreased muscle tone and motility of the gastrointestinal tract persist for only a short time after childbirth. Analgesia and anesthesia may delay a return to normal tonicity and motility, however.

Bowel Evacuation

A spontaneous bowel evacuation may be delayed until 2 to 3 days after childbirth. This can be explained by decreased muscle tone in the intestines during labor and the immediate puerperium, prelabor diarrhea, lack of food, or dehydration. The mother often anticipates discomfort during the bowel movement because of perineal tenderness as a result of episiotomy, lacerations, or hemorrhoids and therefore resists the urge to defecate. Regular bowel habits need to be reestablished when bowel tone returns.

Obstetric trauma (e.g., direct injury to the sphincter muscle, damage to the innervation of the pelvic floor) is perhaps the leading cause of anal incontinence in otherwise healthy women (Toglia, 1996). Third-degree and fourth-degree lacerations occur in 17% to 25% of midline episiotomies (Crawford et al., 1993). Crawford et al. (1993) compared differences in symptoms reported by 35 women with these types of lacerations and 35 women without injury to the sphincter. Data were collected by chart review and by telephone interview 9 to 12 months after the women gave birth. More women (17%) with sphincter injury reported incontinence of gas than women (3%) without injury. Nurses need to prepare women in prenatal classes regarding episiotomy and the possible sequelae. Also pelvic floor (Kegel) exercises should be encouraged.

▌ BREASTS

Promptly after childbirth there is a reduction in the concentrations of hormones that stimulated breast development during pregnancy (estrogen, progesterone, human chorionic gonadotropin, prolactin, cortisol, and insulin). The time it takes for these hormones to return to prepregnancy levels is determined in part by whether the mother breastfeeds her infant.

Breastfeeding Mothers

As lactation is established, a mass (lump) may be felt in the breast. Unlike the lumps associated with fibrocystic breast changes or cancer (which may be consistently palpated in the same location), a filled milk sac will shift position from day to day. Before lactation begins, the breasts feel soft, and a yellowish fluid, **colostrum,** can be expressed from the nipples. Colostrum is rich in antibodies and high in protein. After lactation begins, the breasts feel warm and firm. Tenderness may persist for about 48 hours after the start of lactation. Bluish white milk (having a skim milk appearance) can be expressed from the nipples. The nipples are examined for erectility

and signs of irritation (e.g., cracks, blisters, or reddening). See Chapter 17 for measures to prevent irritation.

Nonbreastfeeding Mothers

Generally the breasts feel nodular (in nonpregnant women they feel granular). The nodularity is bilateral and diffuse.

Prolactin levels drop rapidly. Colostrum is excreted for the first few days after childbirth. Palpation of the breast on the second or third day, as milk production begins, may reveal tissue tenderness in some women. On the third or fourth postpartum day, **engorgement** may occur. The breasts become distended (swollen), firm, tender, and warm to the touch (caused by vasocongestion). Breast distention is primarily caused by the temporary congestion of veins and lymphatics rather than from an accumulation of milk. Milk is present but should not be expressed. Axillary breast tissue (the tail of Spence) and any accessory breast or nipple tissue along the milk line may also be involved. Engorgement resolves spontaneously, and discomfort usually decreases within 24 to 36 hours. A breast binder or tight bra, ice packs, and/or mild analgesics may be used to relieve discomfort. Nipple stimulation is avoided. If suckling is never begun (or is discontinued), lactation ceases within a few days to a week.

▌ CARDIOVASCULAR SYSTEM

Blood Volume

The changes in blood volume after birth depend on several factors, such as blood loss during childbirth and the amount of extravascular water (physiologic edema) mobilized and subsequently excreted. Blood loss results in an immediate but limited decrease in total blood volume. Thereafter most of the blood volume increase during pregnancy (1,000 to 1,500 ml) is eliminated within the first 2 weeks after birth, with return to nonpregnant values by 6 months postpartum (Simpson & Creehan, 1996).

Pregnancy-induced hypervolemia (an increase in blood volume of at least 40% more than prepregnancy values near term) allows most women to tolerate a considerable blood loss during childbirth. Many women lose approximately 300 to 400 ml of blood during vaginal birth of a single fetus and about twice this amount during cesarean birth.

The readjustments in the maternal vasculature after childbirth are dramatic and rapid. The woman's response to blood loss during the early puerperium differs from that in a nonpregnant woman. Three postpartum physiologic changes help to protect the woman from excessive blood loss: (1) elimination of uteroplacental circulation reduces the size of the maternal vascular bed by 10% to 15%, (2) loss of placental endocrine function removes the stimulus for vasodilation, and (3) mobilization of extravascular water stored during pregnancy increases blood volume. Thus hypovolemic shock usually does not occur in women who experience a normal blood loss during the early puerperium.

TABLE 16-2 *Vital Signs After Childbirth*	
NORMAL FINDINGS	**DEVIATIONS FROM NORMAL FINDINGS AND PROBABLE CAUSES**
TEMPERATURE During first 24 hours may rise to 38° C as a result of dehydrating effects of labor. After 24 hours the woman should be afebrile.	A diagnosis of puerperal sepsis is suggested if a rise in maternal temperature to 38° C is noted after the first 23 hours after childbirth and recurs or persists for 2 days. Other possibilities are mastitis, endometritis, urinary tract infections, and other systemic infections.
PULSE Pulse, along with stroke volume and cardiac output, remains elevated for the first hour or so after childbirth. It then begins to decrease at an unknown rate. By 8 to 10 weeks after childbirth the pulse has returned to a prepregnant rate.	A rapid pulse rate or one that is increasing may indicate hypovolemia as a result of hemorrhage.
RESPIRATIONS The respiration rate should decrease to within the woman's normal prebirth range by 6 to 8 weeks after childbirth.	Hypoventilation may occur after an unusually high subarachnoid (spinal) block.
BLOOD PRESSURE Blood pressure is altered *slightly* if at all. Orthostatic hypotension, as indicated by feelings of faintness or dizziness immediately after standing up, can develop in the first 48 hours as a result of the splanchnic engorgement that may occur after birth.	A low or decreasing blood pressure may indicate the existence of hypovolemia secondary to hemorrhage. However, it is a late sign, and other symptoms of hemorrhage usually alert the staff. An increased reading may result from excessive use of vasopressor or oxytocic medications. Since pregnancy-induced hypertension (PIH) can persist into or occur first in the postpartum period, routine evaluation of blood pressure is needed. If a woman complains of headache, hypertension must be ruled out as a cause before analgesics are administered.

Cardiac Output

The pulse rate, stroke volume, and cardiac output increase throughout pregnancy. Immediately after the birth, they remain elevated or rise even higher for 30 to 60 minutes as the blood that was shunted through the uteroplacental circuit suddenly returns to the maternal systemic venous circulation. These values increase regardless of the type of birth or use of conduction anesthesia (Bowes, 1996). Data regarding the exact return of cardiac hemodynamic levels to normal are not available, but cardiac output values remain elevated for at least 48 hours after birth, decrease rapidly in the first 2 weeks postpartum, and return to prepregnancy level by 24 weeks postpartum (Simpson & Creehan, 1996).

Vital Signs

Few alterations in vital signs are seen under normal circumstances. There may be a small, transient rise in both systolic and diastolic blood pressure lasting about four days after the birth (Bowes, 1996) (Table 16-2). Respiratory function returns to prepregnancy state by 6 to 8 weeks after birth. After the uterus is emptied, the diaphragm descends, the normal cardiac axis is restored, and the point of maximum impulse (PMI) and the electrocardiogram (ECG) are normalized.

Blood Components

Hematocrit and hemoglobin

During the first 72 hours after childbirth there is a greater loss in plasma volume than in the number of blood cells. This results in a rise in the hematocrit and hemoglobin levels by the seventh day after birth. There is no accelerated red blood cell (RBC) destruction during the puerperium, but any excess will disappear gradually in accordance with the life span of the RBC. The exact time when the RBC volume returns to prepregnancy values is not known, but it is within normal limits when measured 8 weeks after childbirth (Bowes, 1996).

White blood cell count

Normal leukocytosis of pregnancy averages about 12,000/mm^3. During the first 10 to 12 days after childbirth, values between 20,000 and 25,000/mm^3 are common. Neutrophils are the most numerous white blood cells (WBCs).

This leukocytosis, coupled with the normal increase in the erythrocyte sedimentation rate that occurs, may obscure the diagnosis of acute infections at this time.

Coagulation factors

Clotting factors and fibrinogen levels are normally increased during pregnancy and remain elevated in the immediate puerperium. This hypercoagulable state, when combined with the vessel damage that occurs during childbirth and the immobility of the woman during recovery, increases the risk of **thromboembolism** (blood clots), especially after cesarean birth. Fibrinolytic activity also increases during the first few days after childbirth (Bowes, 1996). Levels of factors I, II, VIII, IX, and X decrease to prepregnant levels within a few days. Fibrin split products, probably released from the placental site, can also be found in maternal blood.

Varicosities

Varicosities (varices) of the legs and around the anus (hemorrhoids) are common during pregnancy. Varices, even the less common vulvar varices, regress (empty) rapidly immediately after childbirth. Surgical repair of varicosities is not considered during pregnancy. Total or near total regression of the varices is expected after childbirth.

NEUROLOGIC SYSTEM

Neurologic changes during the puerperium are those resulting from a reversal of maternal adaptations to pregnancy and those resulting from trauma during labor and childbirth.

Pregnancy-induced neurologic discomforts abate after birth. The elimination of physiologic edema through the diuresis that occurs after childbirth relieves carpal tunnel syndrome by easing the compression of the median nerve. The periodic numbness and tingling of fingers that afflict 5% of pregnant women usually disappear after childbirth unless lifting and carrying the baby aggravates the condition. Headache requires careful assessment. Postpartum headaches may be caused by various conditions, including pregnancy-induced hypertension (PIH), stress, and the leakage of cerebrospinal fluid into the extradural space during placement of the needle for administration of epidural or spinal anesthesia. Headaches last from 1 to 3 days to several weeks, depending on the cause and effectiveness of the treatment.

MUSCULOSKELETAL SYSTEM

Adaptations in the mother's musculoskeletal system that occur during pregnancy are reversed in the puerperium. These adaptations include the relaxation and subsequent hypermobility of the joints and the change in the mother's center of gravity because of the enlarging uterus. Stabi-

RESEARCH

Factors Related to Postpartum Weight Gain and Body Image

After giving birth, women express concerns about returning to prepregnancy weight. There are many reasons why maternal weight gain remains after childbirth. These reasons may include lifestyle factors, the amount of weight gained during the pregnancy, and the body image attitudes of women. Lactation specialists claim that breastfeeding may increase the amount of weight loss or decrease the time it takes to lose weight. In this study, the relationship of lifestyle variables to postpartum weight gain and body image attitudes of bottle- and breastfeeding women was examined. One hundred one bottle-feeding women and 106 breastfeeding women returned an eight-page questionnaire that measured body image, aerobic exercise, dietary fat intake, overall lifestyle, and psychologic skill in managing distress and problem solving. No significant differences were found for prepregnancy body mass index, gestational weight gain, time since delivery, or social variable. The method of feeding (bottle versus breast) was not associated with significant differences in postpartum weight gain or body image. Bottle-feeding mothers with higher postpartum weight gains exercised less and had higher fat intake and were dissatisfied with body image more than mothers who had gained less during their pregnancy.

CLINICAL APPLICATION OF THE STUDY

When nurses assist women in deciding to breastfeed or bottle feed their newborns, postpartum weight reduction related to method of feeding should not be emphasized. Counseling of women struggling with weight gain must include changes in dietary fat habits and physical activity. Nurses must recognize the interaction of a healthy diet, lifestyle modification, and exercise to be effective in counseling women about weight management.

Source: Walker L & Freeland-Graves J: Lifestyle factors related to postpartum weight gain and body image in bottle- and breastfeeding women, *J Obstet Gynecol Neonatal Nurs* 27(2):151, 1998.

lization of joints is complete by 6 to 8 weeks after birth. However, although all other joints return to their normal prepregnant state, those in the parous woman's feet do not. The new mother may notice a permanent increase in shoe size.

INTEGUMENTARY SYSTEM

Chloasma of pregnancy usually disappears at the end of pregnancy. Hyperpigmentation of the areolae and linea nigra may not regress completely after childbirth. These changes in pigmentation may be permanent in some women. Stretch marks on breasts, abdomen, hips, and thighs may fade but usually do not disappear.

Vascular abnormalities such as spider angiomas (nevi), palmar erythema, and epulis generally regress in response to the rapid decline in estrogens after the end of pregnancy. For some women, spider nevi persist indefinitely.

The abundance of fine hair seen during pregnancy usually disappears after birth; however, any coarse or bristly hair that appears during pregnancy usually remains. Fingernails return to their prepregnancy consistency and strength.

The profuse diaphoresis that occurs in the immediate postpartum period is the most noticeable change in the integumentary system.

IMMUNE SYSTEM

No significant changes in the maternal immune system occur during the postpartum period. The mother's need for rubella vaccination or for prevention of Rh isoimmunization is determined.

KEY POINTS

- The uterus involutes rapidly after birth, returning to the true pelvis within 1 week.
- The rapid drop in estrogen and progesterone after expulsion of the placenta is responsible for triggering many of the anatomic and physiologic changes in the puerperium.
- Assessment of lochia and fundal height is essential to monitor the progress of normal involution and to identify potential problems.
- Breastfeeding is *not* a reliable form of birth control.
- Under normal circumstances, few alterations in vital signs are seen after childbirth.
- Activation of blood-clotting factors, immobility, and sepsis predispose the woman to thromboembolism.
- Marked diuresis, decreased bladder sensitivity, and overdistention of the bladder can lead to problems with urinary elimination.
- Postpartum physiologic changes allow the woman to tolerate considerable blood loss at birth.

CRITICAL THINKING EXERCISES

1 *What aspects of the normal postpartum physiologic changes would you explain to a new mother who is going home in 24 hours after birth?*
   a *How would your explanation be different if the woman had given birth to other children?*
   b *How would you explain these changes to a woman who doesn't speak English?*
2 *Assess the accuracy of subjective estimates of blood loss.*
   a *Pour measured amounts of a red fluid on perineal pads or on plastic-backed underpads.*
   b *Ask nursing students, maternity nurses, medical students, obstetricians, nurse midwives, and anesthesiologists to make independent assessments of the volume.*
   c *Calculate percentage of correct responses among the total group and within each category of observer.*
   d *Compare the results. Do profession, area of specialization, or years of experience correlate with more reliable estimates? Were people more likely to overestimate or underestimate the amount? Were the estimates for perineal pads or for underpads different? Were the errors in judgment large enough to raise concern about the accuracy of estimates of blood loss?*

References

Bowes W: Postpartum care. In Gabbe S, Niebyl J & Simpson J, editors: *Obstetrics: normal and problem pregnancies,* ed 3, New York, 1996, Churchill Livingstone.

Crawford L et al.: Incontinence following rupture of the anal sphincter during delivery, *Obstet Gynecol* 82(4Pt1):527, 1993.

Cunningham F et al.: *Williams obstetrics,* ed 20, Stamford, Conn, 1997, Appleton & Lange.

Gordon K et al.: Physiologic and psychologic adaptations in the puerperium. In Moore T et al., editors: *Gynecology and obstetrics: a longitudinal approach,* New York, 1993, Churchill Livingstone.

Henly S et al.: Anemia and insufficient milk in first-time mothers, *Birth* 22(2):87, 1995

Luegenbiehl D et al.: Standardized assessment of blood loss, *MCN Am J Matern Child Nurs* 15(4):241, 1990.

Simpson K & Creehan P: *AWHONN'S Perinatal nursing,* Philadelphia, 1996, Lippincott.

Toglia M: Anal incontinence: an underrecognized, undertreated problem, *The Female Patient* 21:27, 1996.

Visness C, Kennedy K & Ramos R: The duration and character of postpartum bleeding among breast-feeding women, *Obstet Gynecol* 89(2):159, 1997.

Zlatnik F: The normal and abnormal puerperium. In Scott J et al., editors: *Danforth's obstetrics and gynecology,* ed 7, Philadelphia, 1994, Lippincott.

CHAPTER

17

Assessment and Care during the Fourth Trimester

BETSY STETSON

LEARNING OBJECTIVES

- *Define the key terms.*
- *Identify the priorities of maternal care given during the fourth stage of labor.*
- *Identify common selection criteria for safe early postpartum discharge.*
- *List the pros and cons of early postpartum discharge.*
- *Give examples of physical and psychosocial nursing diagnoses pertaining to women in the postpartum period.*
- *Identify expected outcomes for postpartum physical and psychosocial care.*
- *Summarize nursing interventions to prevent infection and excessive bleeding.*
- *Summarize nursing interventions to promote normal bladder and bowel patterns and care for the breasts of women who are breastfeeding or bottle-feeding.*
- *Explain the influence of cultural expectations on postpartum adjustment.*
- *Discuss the nurse's responsibilities related to discharge teaching and preparation for home care.*
- *Describe the nurse's role in these postpartum follow-up strategies: home visits, telephone follow-up, warm lines and help lines, support groups, referrals, and community resources.*

KEY TERMS

afterbirth pains
couplet care
early postpartum discharge
engorgement
fourth stage of labor
Homans' sign
Kegel exercises
Kleihauer-Betke test
oxytocic medications
postpartum support group
referral process
Rh immune globulin
rubella vaccine

KEY TERMS—cont'd

sitz bath
splanchnic engorgement
suppression of lactation
thrombus
uterine atony
warm lines

The goal of nursing care in the immediate postpartum period is to assist women and their partners during their initial transition to parenting. The approach to the care of women after birth has changed from one modeled on sick care to one that is wellness oriented. Consequently, in the United States most women remain hospitalized as few as 1 or 2 days after giving birth and some for as few as 6 hours. Because there is so much important information to be shared with these women in a very short time, it is vital that their care be thoughtfully planned and provided. The nurse provides care that focuses on the woman's physiologic recovery, her psychologic well-being, and her ability to care for herself and her new baby. In addition, the nurse considers the needs of other family members and includes strategies in the plan of care to assist the family in adjusting to the new baby.

To provide quality care, the nurse must be knowledgeable about physical changes in the mother and psychosocial and emotional changes in the entire family. This chapter focuses on using the nursing process to meet both the mother's and the family's needs during this crucial time.

THE FOURTH STAGE OF LABOR

The first 1 to 2 hours after birth, sometimes referred to as the **fourth stage of labor,** is a crucial time for the mother and newborn. Both are not only recovering from the physical process of birth but are also becoming acquainted with each other and with additional family members. During this time, maternal organs start to undergo readjustment to the nonpregnant state, and the functions of body systems begin to stabilize. Meanwhile, the newborn continues to make the transition from an intrauterine to extrauterine existence.

> **NURSE ALERT** *The nurse's role during the fourth stage of labor is to monitor the recovery of the new mother and infant and to promptly identify and manage any deviations from the normal processes that may occur.*

The fourth stage of labor is an excellent time to begin breastfeeding because the infant is in an alert state and ready to nurse. Breastfeeding at this time also promotes the contraction of the uterus and thereby the prevention of maternal hemorrhage. Getting breastfeeding off to a good start is not just encouraging for the mother; it is also physiologically vital for the infant. Colostrum loosens mucus and acts as a laxative, thus promoting the rapid elimination of meconium. It also decreases the likelihood of hypoglycemia, reduces the severity of physiologic hyperbilirubinemia, and provides important immunologic benefits.

In most centers, the mother remains in the labor and birth area during this recovery time. In an institution where labor, delivery, and recovery (LDR) rooms are used, the woman stays in the same room where she gave birth. In traditional settings, women are taken from the delivery room to a separate recovery area for observation. Arrangements for the care of the newborn vary during the fourth stage of labor. In many settings, the baby remains at the mother's bedside and the labor or birth nurse cares for both of them. In other institutions, the baby is taken to the nursery for several hours of observation after an initial bonding period with the parents (Fig. 17-1).

Assessment

If the recovery nurse has not previously cared for the new mother, her assessment begins with an oral report from the nurse who attended the woman during labor and birth

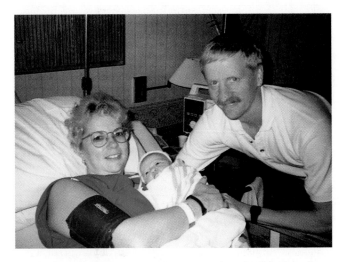

Fig. **17-1** Parents becoming acquainted with daughter. (Courtesy Jan Harmon, St Louis.)

and a review of the prenatal, labor, and birth records. Of primary importance are conditions that could predispose the mother to hemorrhage, such as precipitous labor, a large baby, grand multiparity, or induced labor. For healthy women, hemorrhage is probably the most dangerous potential complication that can occur.

To help the nurse provide comprehensive care, use of a worksheet or recovery record is suggested. Fig. 17-2 illustrates an easy-to-use flow sheet that has the essential immediate postpartum and anesthesia recovery assessments. During the first hour in the recovery room, physical assessments of the mother are frequent. All factors except temperature are assessed every 15 minutes for 1 hour. Temperature is assessed every 4 to 8 hours. After the fourth 15-minute assessment, if all parameters have stabilized within the normal range, the process is usually repeated every 30 minutes during the second hour. Box 17-1 describes the physical assessment of the mother during the fourth stage.

During the fourth stage of labor, many postpartum patients experience intense tremors that resemble shivering from a chill. They are commonly seen after birth and are not related to infection. Several theories have been offered to explain these tremors or shivering, such as their being the result of a sudden release of pressure on pelvic nerves after birth, a response from a fetus-to-mother transfusion that occurred during placental separation, a reaction to maternal adrenaline production during labor and birth, or a reaction to epidural anesthesia. The nurse can help women who experience these chills by providing warm blankets and reassurance that the chills or tremors are common, self-limiting, and last only a short while.

The nutritional status of the woman is assessed. Restriction of food and fluid intake and the loss of fluids (blood, perspiration, or emesis) during labor cause many women to express a strong desire to eat or drink soon after birth. In the absence of complications, a woman who has given birth vaginally, has recovered from the effects of the anesthetic, and has stable vital signs, a firm uterus, and small to moderate lochial flow may have fluids and a regular diet as desired (American Academy of Pediatrics & American College of Obstetricians and Gynecologists, 1997).

Postanesthesia Recovery

The woman who has given birth by cesarean or has received regional anesthesia for a vaginal birth requires special attention during the recovery period. In fact, obstetric recovery areas are held to the same standard of care that would be expected of any other postanesthesia recovery room. A recovery from anesthesia requires the nurse to have available cardiopulmonary support and emergency supplies (e.g., resuscitation bag, face mask) (Johnson & Johnson, 1996). A postanesthesia recovery (PAR) score is determined for each patient upon her arrival and is

Procedure: _____

Diagnosis: _____

Physician: _____

Anesthesia: _____

Anesthetist: _____

Armbands: _____ mother _____ infant

Clothing: _____ c̄ family _____ c̄ patient

Maternity Recovery Room Record

Admission note:

Activity		
Able to move 4 extremities voluntarily or on command		2
Able to move 2 extremities voluntarily or on command		1
Able to move 0 extremities voluntarily or on command		0
Respiration		
Able to deep breathe and cough freely		2
Dyspnea or limited breathing		1
Apneic		0
Blood pressure		
BP ± mm Hg of preanesthetic level		2
BP ± 25-50 mm Hg of preanesthetic level		1
BP ± Greater than 50 mm Hg of preanesthetic level		0
Conscious level		
Fully aware		2
Arousable on calling		1
Not responding		0
Color		
Pink		2
Pale, dusky, blotchy, jaundiced, other		1
Cyanotic		0

Par score: ADM: _____ DC: _____   Homan's Sign   Pos ☐   Neg ☐

				Bonding	Teaching
Activity				☐ Appropriate	☐ Fundal massage
Respiration				☐ Inappropriate	☐ TC & DB
Blood pressure				☐ NA (explain)	☐ Breastfeeding
Conscious level					☐ Assistance on 1st ambulation
Color					
Total				☐ _____	

Vital signs: Initial hour: q 15 min then Routine: q 4 h other per protocol Tox*: q 1 h	Time									Meds / IV / Rate	Time / Initial
	BP										
	Pulse										
	Resp / O₂ Sat										
Fundus FB-Fingerbreath B-Boggy FM-Firm MD-Midline	Fundus										
Lochia CL-Clots MOD-Moderate SM-Small LG-Large	Lochia										
Bladder D-Distended F-Foley ND-Nondistended	Bladder										
Episiotomy/Incision NL-Normal D-Dry ABNL-Abnormal I-Intact	Epis / Inc										
q 4°	Temp										
Clear CL Wheezing W Diminished D	Breath sounds										
q 1° / q 4°	DTR / Protein										
Admission intake Total											
Admission output Total									Intake total Shift 7A 3P 11P	Signature	
Initials									Output total Shift 7A 3P 11P		

Discharge note

Report called to: _____

Anesthesia D/C:

Epidural catheter: In   Out   NA

IV _____ cc LTC†

@ D/C

*Toxemia (preeclampsia).

†LTC, Left to count.

Fig. 17-2 An example of a maternity recovery room record. (Courtesy The Regional Medical Center at Memphis [The Med], Memphis, Tenn.)

| BOX 17-1 | *Assessment During Fourth Stage of Labor* |

Before beginning the assessment, wash hands thoroughly, assemble necessary equipment, and explain the procedure to the patient.

BLOOD PRESSURE
Measure blood pressure per assessment schedule.

PULSE
Assess rate and regularity.

TEMPERATURE
Determine temperature.

FUNDUS
Put on clean examination gloves.

Position woman with knees flexed and head flat.

Just below the umbilicus, cup hand and press firmly into abdomen. At the same time, stabilize the uterus at the symphysis with the opposite hand.

If fundus is firm (and bladder is empty), with uterus in midline, measure its position relative to woman's umbilicus. Lay fingers flat on abdomen under umbilicus; measure how many fingerbreadths (fb) or centimeters (cm) fit between the umbilicus and top of fundus. If the fundus is above the umbilicus, this is recorded as plus fb or cm; if below, as minus fb or cm.

If the fundus is *not* firm, massage it gently to help it contract and expel any clots before measuring the distance from the umbilicus.

Place hands appropriately; massage gently *only until firm.*

Expel clots while keeping hands placed as shown in Fig. 17-3. With upper hand, apply firm pressure downward toward vagina; observe perineum for amount and size of expelled clots.

BLADDER
Assess distention by noting location and firmness of uterine fundus and by observing and palpating bladder. A distended bladder is seen as a rounded suprapubic bulge that is dull to percussion and fluctuates like a water-filled balloon. When the bladder is distended, the uterus is usually *boggy* in consistency, well above the umbilicus, and to the woman's right side.

Assist woman to void spontaneously. *Measure amount of urine voided.*

Catheterize as necessary.

Reassess after voiding or catheterization to make sure the bladder is not palpable and the fundus is firm and in the midline.

LOCHIA
Observe lochia on perineal pads and on linen under the mother's buttocks. Determine amount and color; note size and number of clots and odor.

Observe perineum for source of bleeding (e.g., episiotomy, lacerations).

PERINEUM
Ask or assist woman to turn on her side and flex upper leg on hip.

Lift upper buttock.

Observe perineum in good lighting.

Assess episiotomy site or laceration repair for intactness, hematoma, edema, bruising, redness, and drainage.

Assess for presence of hemorrhoids.

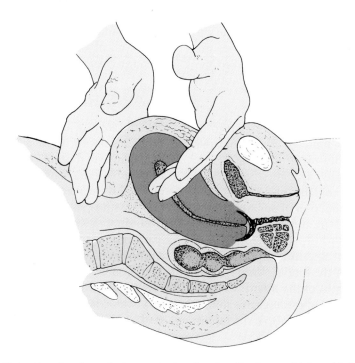

Fig. **17-3** Palpating fundus of uterus during the fourth stage of labor. Note that upper hand is cupped over fundus: lower hand dips in above symphysis pubis and supports uterus while it is massaged gently.

updated as part of every 15-minute assessment. Components of the PAR score include activity, respirations, blood pressure, level of consciousness, and color.

> **NURSE ALERT** *Regardless of her obstetric status, no woman should be discharged from the recovery area until she has completely recovered from the effects of anesthesia.*

If the woman received general anesthesia, she should be awake and alert and oriented to time, place, and person. Her respiratory rate should be within normal limits and her oxygen saturation levels at least 95%, as measured by a pulse oximeter; she should be encouraged to deep breathe. If the woman received epidural or spinal anesthesia, she should be able to raise her legs (extended at the knees, off the bed) or flex her knees, place her feet flat on the bed, and raise her buttocks well off the bed. The numb or tingling prickly sensation should be entirely gone from her legs. Often it takes 1 1/2 to 2 hours for these anesthetic effects to disappear.

Transfer from the recovery area

After the initial recovery period of 1 to 2 hours has been completed, the woman may be transferred to a postpartum room in the same or another nursing unit. In facilities where labor, delivery, recovery, postpartum (LDRP) rooms are used, the nurse who provides care during the recovery period usually continues the care for the woman. In an LDR room or traditional setting, the woman is transferred to a separate unit where the postpartum nursing staff assumes her care. Women who have received general or regional anesthesia must be cleared for transfer from the recovery area by a member of the anesthesia care team. In some settings, the baby will remain with the mother wherever she goes. In other institutions, the baby may be taken to the nursery for several hours of observation during the mother's initial recovery period.

In preparing the transfer report, the recovery nurse uses information from the records of admission, birth record, and recovery. Information that must be communicated to the postpartum nurse includes identity of the health care provider; gravidity and parity; age; anesthetic used; any medications given; duration of labor and time of rupture of membranes; oxytocin induction or augmentation; type of birth and repair; blood type and Rh status; status of rubella immunity; syphilis and hepatitis serology test results; intravenous infusion of any fluids; physiologic status since birth; description of the fundus, lochia, bladder, and perineum; sex and weight of the infant; time of birth; pediatrician; chosen method of feeding; any abnormalities noted; and assessment of initial parent-infant interaction.

This information is also documented for the nursing staff in the newborn nursery. In addition, specific information should be provided regarding the infant's Apgar scores, weight, voiding and whether fed since birth. Nursing interventions that have been completed (e.g., eye prophylaxis, vitamin K injection) must also be recorded.

Table 17-1 gives examples for documenting this information before the transfer of the woman from the recovery area.

Women who give birth in birthing centers may go home within a few hours after the woman's and infant's conditions are stable.

DISCHARGE—BEFORE 24 HOURS AND AFTER 48 HOURS

Postpartum home care has been an area of significant growth and interest because of the shortening hospital stay and the need of women, newborns, and family for ongoing care in the home. **Early postpartum discharge,** *shortened hospital stay,* and *one-day maternity stays* are all terms for the decreasing hospital stays of mothers and their babies after a low-risk birth.

In years past it was common for maternity stays to be set at a predetermined duration (usually counted in days) after birth. For example, the usual length of stay was 3 days after a vaginal birth and 5 days after a cesarean birth. Knowing the number of days enabled the health care team and family to plan care accordingly. Then for several years, it was common for the length of stay to be 24 hours or less for women who experienced a normal vaginal birth and approximately 72 hours for women who experienced a cesarean birth.

This trend of shortened hospital stay was based largely on efforts to reduce health care costs (economic factors) coupled with consumer demands to have less medical intervention and more family-centered experiences (Wilkerson, 1996), all of which has increasingly affected numbers of maternity patients and the nurses who provide their care.

LAWS RELATING TO DISCHARGE

Health care providers expressed concern that some medical problems do not show up in the first 24 hours after birth and that new mothers have not sufficiently learned how to care for their newborns and identify newborn health problems such as jaundice and dehydration related to breastfeeding difficulties (Havens & Hannan, 1996). According to Rubin, the first day after birth is a time when women need to rest and be physically cared for and is not a time conducive to learning (Evans, 1995). There has also been concern that shortened hospital stays will increase maternal hospital readmission for infection, hypertension, and hemorrhage of women who delivered vaginally (Bragg et al., 1997).

Parents are experiencing a major life transition during the immediate days and weeks of the fourth trimester. They are recovering from the events surrounding birth, adjusting

TABLE 17-1	*Recovery Nurse's Report*	
ITEM	EXAMPLE OF DOCUMENTATION OF MOTHER	EXAMPLE OF DOCUMENTATION OF NEWBORN
Type of labor and birth: unusual observations, if any, of the placenta	Spontaneous or assisted (forceps) vaginal birth; vertex presentation	Spontaneous or assisted (forceps, vacuum extractor) vaginal birth in vertex presentation
Gravidity and parity, age	G1, P1, 22 years old	G1, P1, 22 years old
Anesthesia and analgesia used	None; epidural, low spinal, local	None; epidural, low spinal, or local
Condition of perineum	Episiotomy; repair of lacerations	
Events since birth	Vital signs, BP, fundus, lochia, intake and output, medications (dosage, time of administration, and results), response to newborn, observation of family interactions, including siblings, if present	Nursed at breast; took nipple well Voided × 1; meconium × 1 Eye prophylaxis given Vitamin K injection given Held by siblings who are happy (or have other response) to newborn
Condition and sex of newborn; other information	Apgar at 1 and 5 min; time of birth; eye prophylaxis given; weight; whether breastfeeding or bottle feeding; if breastfeeding, whether newborn was at breast; name of pediatrician; sex of the baby	Apgar scores at 1 and 5 min Male; 3400, name of pediatrician; breastfeeding or bottle feeding; mother's hepatitis B status and GBS status
Relevant information from prenatal record	Need for rubella vaccination; presence of infections; hepatitis B status; blood type; Rh status; GBS status and treatment if positive	Unremarkable pregnancy
Miscellaneous information IV drip	If IV drip is infusing, rate of infusion, medications added (e.g., Pitocin), whether to keep open or discontinue after completion of bag that is hung	
Social factors	If woman is releasing baby for adoption, whether she wants to see baby, breastfeed, allow visitors, or other preferences she may have	Baby up for adoption; to stay in NBN until discharge

BP, Blood pressure; *GBS*, group Beta *Streptococcus*; *NBN*, newborn nursery.

to the demands of a newborn, parenting, applying their post-discharge instructions, shifting priorities, and realigning some roles while assuming new ones. An additional challenge occurs when there are other children at home who must be helped to adjust in sharing their home and parents with the newborn. The stress inherent in such profound transitions is the source of a tremendous potential for crisis and growth during the early postpartum period.

The widespread concern for the potential increase in adverse maternal-child outcomes from hospital early discharge practices led the American College of Obstetricians and Gynecologists (ACOG), the American Academy of Pediatrics (AAP), and other professional health care organizations to promote the enactment of federal and various state maternity length of stay bills to ensure adequate care for both the mother and the newborn. The landmark passage of the Newborns' and Mothers' Health Protection Act

of 1996 provides minimum federal standards for health plan coverage for mothers and their newborns (Ferguson & Engelhard, 1996). Under the Act, all health plans are required to allow the new mother and newborn to remain in the hospital for a minimum of 48 hours after a normal vaginal birth and for 96 hours after a cesarean birth unless the attending provider, in consultation with the mother, decides upon early discharge.

Recent research studies to determine the appropriate length of hospital stay for newborns seem to support this legislation. One large study (Liu et al., 1997) found that newborns discharged early (less than 30 hours after birth) were more likely to be rehospitalized for jaundice, dehydration, and infection within one month of life than newborns discharged later (30 to 72 hours after birth). Edmonson, Stoddard, and Owens (1997) were unable to find any significant reason for newborn readmission; however, they concluded that readmission was more likely among babies who were first born, breastfed, or born to unmarried and poorly educated women.

Several early postpartum hospital discharge programs that provided extensive prenatal preparation and postpartum follow-up found it generally safe for mothers who gave birth vaginally and their newborns to be discharged less than 48 hours after birth (Carty & Bradley, 1990; Welt et al., 1993; Williams & Cooper, 1996).

Proponents of early postpartum discharge cite the following advantages of the practice:
- Reinforces the concept of childbirth as a normal physiologic event.
- Allows shorter separations between mothers and other children.
- Extends a couple's sense of control and participation beyond the birth itself.
- Capitalizes on the security of the home environment during the stressors of early parenting.
- Decreases unnecessary exposure to the pathogens in the hospital environment (Harrison, 1990).
- Allows beds on the maternity service to be used more effectively (that is, quick turnover in patients or greater availability for patients with a complication).
- Allows more time for mother/father/partner/infant and other family members to bond (Fig. 17-4).
- Creates less disruption in the daily life of the family.
- Promotes active family involvement of family and support persons in assisting the mother and newborn.

Opponents of early postpartum discharge cite the following disadvantages of the practice:
- Complications (maternal or newborn) may go unrecognized.
- Families may be or feel unprepared for the reality they face once the baby is at home.
- The mother is fatigued from the labor and childbirth process.
- The mother is experiencing postpartum pain or discomfort.
- The length of time for learning after the birth in the hospital setting is decreased.
- A vulnerability and crisis potential exists for both patients and families.

The protest against early discharge becomes more cogent in the conventional health care arena in which care does not include a home care visit and there is a long interval between discharge and the first follow-up examination.

The future of early postpartum discharge

Currently there is much debate about the best practice for women, newborns, and their families in terms of the length of hospitalization. All components of health care systems (that is, hospitals, physicians, nurses, nurse-midwives, home

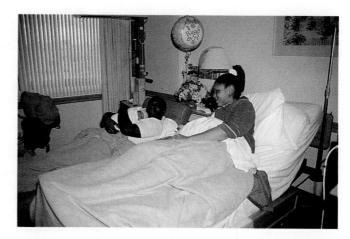

Fig. 17-4 Bonding and attachment begun early after birth are fostered in the postpartum period. (Courtesy Marjorie Pyle, RNC, Lifecircle, Costa Mesa, Calif.)

health care, managed care, and HMOs) are exploring models that ensure the delivery of safe, effective care.

The specialty of postpartum home care has emerged as increased numbers of patients are being referred for home follow-up after a short maternity stay or for follow-up after a cesarean birth (Brooten, 1995). With this trend, new and existing home care programs are likely to extend their services and service area to a greater number of patients. In addition, common problems such as maternal infection and infant hyperbilirubinemia, identified after discharge, can be treated in the home.

Criteria for Discharge

Early discharge and postpartum home care can be a safe and satisfying option for women and their families when it is comprehensive and based on individual needs (Wilkerson, 1996). However, early discharge is not appropriate for every mother and newborn (AAP & ACOG, 1997). Hospital stays need to be long enough to identify problems and to ensure that the woman is sufficiently recovered and prepared to care for herself and the baby at home.

It is essential that nurses consider the medical needs of the woman and her baby and provide care that is coordinated to meet those needs in order to provide timely physiologic interventions and treatment to prevent morbidity and hospital readmission. With predetermined criteria for identifying low risk in the mothers and newborns (Box 17-2), the length of hospitalization can be based on the medical need for care in an acute care setting or in consideration of the ongoing care needed in the home environment (AAP & ACOG, 1997; Britton, Britton & Beebe, 1994).

In conjunction with the attending physician or nurse-midwife and family, the hospital-based maternity nurse is

Criteria for Early Discharge

MOTHER

Uncomplicated pregnancy, labor, vaginal birth, and postpartum course

No evidence of premature rupture of membranes

Blood pressure, temperature stable and within normal limits

Ambulating unassisted

Voiding adequate amounts without difficulty

Hemoglobin >10 g

No significant vaginal bleeding; perineum intact or no more than second-degree episiotomy or laceration repair; uterus is firm

Received instructions on postpartum self-care

INFANT

Term infant (38 to 42 weeks) with weight appropriate for gestational age of 2,500 g (5 lb, 8 oz)

Normal findings on physical assessment

Temperature, respirations, and heart rate within normal limits and stable

At least two successful feedings completed (normal sucking and swallowing)

Urination and stooling have occurred at least once

No evidence of significant jaundice in the first 24 hours after the birth

No excessive bleeding at the circumcision site for at least 2 hours

Screening tests performed according to state regulations; tests to be repeated at follow-up visit if done before the infant is 24 hours old

Initial Hepatitis B vaccine given or scheduled for first follow-up visit

Laboratory data reviewed: maternal syphilis and Hepatitis B status; infant or cord blood type and Coombs' test results if indicated

GENERAL

No social, family, or environmental risk factors identified

Family or support person available to assist mother and infant at home

Follow-up scheduled within 1 week if discharged before 48 hours after the birth

Documentation of skill of mother in feeding (breast or bottle), cord care, skin care, perineal care, infant safety (use of car seat, sleeping positions), and recognizing signs of illness and common infant problems

Source: American Academy of Pediatrics: Hospital stay for healthy term infants, *Pediatrics* 96(1): 788, 1995; Britton J, Britton H & Beebe S: Early discharge of the term newborn: a continued dilemma, *Pediatrics* 94(1): 3, 1994.

instrumental in determining the readiness of a woman for home care and in preparing the woman and the family for the home care plan of treatment. An example of a care path for the progression of postpartum physical, psychosocial, and self-care changes and for the teaching needs of women

after uncomplicated, vaginal birth within a 24-hour time frame is found on page 424. A similar format can be used for a cesarean birth care path with time frame adjustments accounting for a longer hospital stay (e.g., 3 to 4 days) (Simpson & Creehan, 1996).

Care paths provide the nurse with an organized approach toward meeting essential maternal-newborn care and teaching goals within a limited time frame. Other methods such as postpartum order sets and maternal-newborn teaching checklists (Fig. 17-5) can also be used to accomplish designated patient care and educational outcomes. By determining what is most appropriate for the individual woman and newborn, the length of stay and care coordinated by the health care team can be adjusted to ensure the delivery of safe and effective care.

Hospital-based maternity nurses continue to play invaluable roles as caregivers, teachers, and patient and family advocates in developing and implementing effective home care strategies. It is imperative that nurses adapt their care to meet the needs of their patients and families in the acute care setting (Lukacs, 1991). In collaboration with other health care providers, the nurse is instrumental in determining whether the mother and newborn meet the criteria for early discharge. With coordination, clinical care and education can be planned and provided throughout pregnancy, during the hospital stay, and in the home after discharge to ensure the family's continued well-being.

CARE MANAGEMENT— PHYSICAL NEEDS

Assessment and Nursing Diagnoses

After completion of the initial 1- to 2-hour recovery period following childbirth, mothers are usually transferred by wheelchair or gurney from the labor and birth unit to a postpartum unit. At this time the nurse who was present for the birth may continue to provide care, or a postpartum nurse may assume this responsibility. In hospitals using the labor, delivery, recovery, postpartum (LDRP) concept, however, the woman remains in the same room where she labored and gave birth.

A complete physical assessment, including measurement of vital signs, is performed upon admission to the postpartum unit. If the woman's vital signs are within normal limits, they will likely be assessed every 4 to 8 hours for the remainder of her hospitalization. Other components of the initial assessment include the mother's emotional status, energy level, degree of physical discomfort, hunger, and thirst. Intake and output assessments should always be done if an intravenous infusion or a urinary catheter is in place. If the woman gave birth by cesarean, the incisional dressing should be assessed as well. To some degree, her knowledge level concerning self-care and infant care can also be determined at this time.

Text continues on p. 427

Date of Birth: _____

Hour of Birth: _____

The uncomplicated vaginal birth patient's admission/discharge is based on a 24-hour length of stay post-birth based on individual needs.

*IHSP denotes a test done to determine if follow-up needed in Infant Hearing Screening Program (IHSP).

Time:

		RECOVERY	Adm. TO PP UNIT-8 HOURS	9-16 HOURS	17-24 HOURS/DISCHARGE
PRIMARY PHYSIOLOGIC FOCUS		Patient will have normal vital signs as documented on flowsheet.	Patient will have normal VS and moderate lochia rubra.	Patient will have normal VS and minimal lochia rubra.	Patient will have normal VS and minimal lochia rubra.
		NA MET VARIANCE	NA MET VARIANCE	NA MET VARIANCE	NA MET VARIANCE
		Vital signs every 15 min. × one hr, then every 4 hours. Assess perineum/episiotomy. Ice pack prn. Assess lochia.	Vital signs every 4 hours. Assess perineum/episiotomy. Ice pack prn. Assess lochia.	Vital signs every shift. Assess perineum/episiotomy. Ice pack prn. Assess lochia.	Vital signs every shift. Assess perineum/episiotomy. Ice pack prn. Assess lochia.
IVs/LABWORK/ MEDICATIONS		RECOVERY	Adm. TO PP UNIT-8 HOURS	9-16 HOURS	17-24 HOURS/DISCHARGE
		Patient will have appropriate lab work done and medication given by time of transfer to Mother/Baby Unit.	Patient will begin to verbalize understanding of hepatitis status and medication requirements.	Patient will have appropriate lab work done by 16 hours PP.	Patient will have appropriate lab work done and appropriate meds initiated.
		NA MET VARIANCE	NA MET VARIANCE	NA MET VARIANCE	NA MET VARIANCE
		CBC, if not done prior to birth. Urine drug screen if ordered. U/A—dipstick (Send to lab, if abnormal).	Review hepatitis B status. Medication regimen initiated.	CBC. Review Rubella status. Review Hgb & Hct.	Fe Tab. Prenatal Vitamin. Rubella vaccine, if appropriate. RhoGAM, if indicated. Laxative.
NUTRITION/ ELIMINATION		RECOVERY	Adm. TO PP UNIT -8 HOURS	9-16 HOURS	17-24 HOURS/DISCHARGE
		Patient will be up to bathroom prior to transfer.	Patient will resume normal nutritional status and bladder function.	Patient will resume normal nutritional status and bladder function.	Patient will have normal bowel and bladder function.
		NA MET VARIANCE	NA MET VARIANCE	NA MET VARIANCE	NA MET VARIANCE
		Assess bladder fullness. Assist to bathroom. Assess for tolerance of P.O. intake.	Encourage ambulation. Encourage P.O. fluids. Assist to bathroom as needed. Assess bladder function. Encourage P.O. intake.	Encourage ambulation. Encourage P.O. fluids Assist to bathroom as needed Assess bladder function. Encourage P.O. intake.	Encourage ambulation. Encourage P.O. fluids. Assist to bathroom as needed. Laxative prn.
PSYCHOSOCIAL		RECOVERY	Adm.-PP UNIT-8 HOURS	9-16 HOURS	17-24 HOURS/DISCHARGE
		Patient/family will begin attachment behaviors with newborn.	Patient/family will demonstrate appropriate attachment behaviors.	Family will verbalize comfort with new infant.	Family will verbalize comfort with new infant.
		NA MET VARIANCE	NA MET VARIANCE	NA MET VARIANCE	NA MET VARIANCE
		Encourage mother/family members to hold and touch infant. Provide skin-to-skin contact of mother/infant. Provide mother the opportunity to breastfeed, if applicable.	Offer flexible rooming-in with infant. Allow for verbalization of patient's feelings. Assess discharge needs and need for Social Service consult.	Reinforce interventions.	Reinforce interventions. Completion of birth certificate. Arrange for home visit.

Miami Valley Hospital
Dayton, Ohio 45409

CARE PATH *24-Hour Vaginal Birth Without Complications—cont'd*

<table>
<tr><td rowspan="7">SELF-CARE ACTIVITY</td><td>RECOVERY</td><td>Adm. TO PP UNIT 8 HOURS</td><td>9-16 HOURS</td><td>17-24 HOURS/DISCHARGE</td></tr>
<tr><td>Patient will begin self-care activities as tolerated.</td><td>Patient will be up to bathroom/shower with assistance.</td><td>Patient will be up to bathroom/shower independently.</td><td>Patient will be up to bathroom/shower independently.</td></tr>
<tr><td>NA MET VARIANCE</td><td>NA MET VARIANCE</td><td>NA MET VARIANCE</td><td>NA MET VARIANCE</td></tr>
<tr><td>Instruct patient in pericare and pad changes.</td><td>Reinforce proper pericare. Instruct on use of Sitz bath. Encourage patient to shower.</td><td>Reinforce proper pericare. Reinforce use of Sitz bath.</td><td>Reinforce proper pericare. Reinforce use of Sitz bath.</td></tr>
<tr><td>RECOVERY</td><td>Adm. TO PP UNIT 8 HOURS</td><td>9-16 HOURS</td><td>17-24 HOURS/DISCHARGE</td></tr>
<tr><td>Patient will begin to verbalize and/or demonstrate self-care and infant care activities.</td><td>Patient will begin to verbalize and/or demonstrate self- and infant care activities.</td><td>Patient/family will demonstrate appropriate infant care activities.</td><td>Patient/family will demonstrate appropriate infant care activities.</td></tr>
<tr><td>NA MET VARIANCE</td><td>NA MET VARIANCE</td><td>NA MET VARIANCE</td><td>NA MET VARIANCE</td></tr>
<tr><td rowspan="9">TEACHING/ DISCHARGE PLANNING</td><td colspan="4">DATE</td></tr>
<tr><td colspan="4">INITIALS</td></tr>
<tr><td>Teaching to include: Breastfeeding latch-on and positioning, if applicable. Appropriate handwashing techniques. Cough and deep breathing exercises. Instruct in pain relief techniques/medication.</td><td>Teaching to include: Breastfeeding/formula initial feeding information. Breast care. Perineal care. Proper nutrition. Safety issues reviewed.</td><td>Teaching to include: Attendance at mother/baby care class. Breast care or formula information. Newborn channel. Lactation consult prn. Appropriate hand-washing techniques.</td><td>Teaching to include: Reinforcement of teaching from mother/baby class. Plans for self/infant follow-up. Review IHSP.* Review Baby Net program. Telephone # for follow-up questions. Home-going meds and purposes.</td></tr>
<tr><td>1.</td><td>1.</td><td>1.</td><td>1.</td></tr>
<tr><td>2.</td><td>2.</td><td>2.</td><td>2.</td></tr>
<tr><td>3.</td><td>3.</td><td>3.</td><td>3.</td></tr>
<tr><td>4.</td><td>4.</td><td>4.</td><td>4.</td></tr>
</table>

Variance Documentation: _____

_____

_____

_____

_____

_____

Miami Valley Hospital
Dayton, Ohio 45409

Abbott Northwestern Hospital
A HealthSpan™ Organization
SELF/FAMILY LEARNING CHECKLIST

Patient Name, Social Security #, Date of Birth

I learn best by: ☐ Group classes   ☐ Individual instruction   ☐ Video instruction   ☐ Reading it myself

Please indicate your desired learning needs by placing a check in one of the columns next to each topic.

| KEY | 1 = Most important to learn before I go home |
| | 2 = I already know |

(Please DATE when learning need is met.)

CARING FOR YOURSELF	1	2	DATE	CARING FOR BABY	1	2	DATE
Episiotomy and perineal care				Diapering			
Vaginal discharge				Baby bath, skin and cord care			
Hemorrhoids/Constipation				Circumcised/uncircumcised care			
Breast care				Burping			
Nutrition				Bowel movements/wet diapers			
Activity				Sleeping habits			
Postpartal exercises				Newborn behavior			
Return of menstruation				Jaundice			
Family planning				Signs of illness			
Blood clots				Car seat safety			
Postpartum emotions				General infant safety/poison control			
Postpartum warning signs				Signs/symptoms of dehydration			
				Bulb syringe			
Cesarean Birth							
Incisional care				**BREASTFEEDING**			
				Sore nipples			
				Positioning			
				Frequency of feedings			
AFTER DISCHARGE				Expressing/storing milk			
When to call health care provider				Engorgement			
				Feeding water			
				Nursing while working			
OTHER				Weaning			
Working mothers							
Day care				**BOTTLE FEEDING**			
Sibling adjustment				Types of formula			
Single parent support				Preparing formula			
Time out for parents				Frequency of feedings			
Infant safety and security							
Infant As A Person Class							
New Parent Connection							

MEDICATIONS AT HOME

MEDICATIONS	STRENGTH	DOSAGE	FREQUENCY	PURPOSE/SPECIAL INSTRUCTIONS
			times per day	
			times per day	
			times per day	

RESOURCES REFERRALS
☐ Physician Discharge Instructions _____
☐ Home Care Agency _____
☐ Other Referrals _____

VALUABLES: ☐ Returned ☐ None   **MEDICATIONS:** ☐ Returned ☐ None   ☐ Room checked for belongings
Patient verbalized understanding of discharge information received.

PATIENT OR SUPPORT PERSON _____   NURSE'S SIGNATURE _____   DATE _____

SELF/FAMILY LEARNING CHECKLIST

(sidebar) SELF/FAMILY LEARNING CHECKLIST

Fig. **17-5** Self/family learning checklist. (Copyright Abbott Northwestern Hospital of Allina Health System, Minneapolis and St. Paul, Minn.)

GUIDELINES/GUÍAS

Are you planning to breastfeed or bottle feed?
¿Piensa darle pecho o biberón al bebé?

Lie down.
Acuéstese.

I am going to take your vital signs.
Le voy a tomar sus signos vitales.

I need to take your blood pressure.
Necesito tomarle la presión arterial.

Do you need to use the bathroom?
¿Necesita usar el baño?

I need to examine you.
Le voy a hacer un examen.

Spread your knees and legs apart.
Separe las piernas, por favor.

Roll over on your side.
Póngase al lado.

Would you like some pain medication?
¿Desea medicina para calmar el dolor?

Would you like to take a sitz bath?
¿Desea tomar un baño de asiento?

signs of POTENTIAL COMPLICATIONS

PHYSIOLOGIC PROBLEMS

Temperature	More than 38° C after the first 24 hours
Pulse	Tachycardia, marked bradycardia
Blood pressure	Hypotension or hypertension
Energy level	Lethargy, extreme fatigue
Uterus	Deviated from the midline, boggy, remains above the umbilicus after 24 hours
Lochia	Heavy, foul odor; bright red bleeding that is not lochia
Perineum	Pronounced edema, not intact, signs of infection, marked discomfort
Legs	Homans' sign positive; painful, reddened area; warmth on posterior aspect of calf
Breasts	Redness, heat, pain, cracked and fissured nipples, inverted nipples, palpable mass
Appetite	Lack of appetite
Elimination	*Urine:* inability to void, urgency, frequency, dysuria; *bowel:* constipation, diarrhea
Rest	Inability to rest or sleep

Ongoing physical assessment

The postpartum woman should be evaluated thoroughly during each nursing shift throughout hospitalization (see Guidelines box). Physical assessments include evaluation of the breasts, uterine fundus, lochia, perineum, bladder and bowel function, vital signs, and legs. If a patient has an intravenous (IV) line in place, her fluid and hematologic status should be evaluated before it is removed. Signs of potential problems that may be identified during the assessment process are listed in the Signs of Potential Complications box.

Routine laboratory tests

Several laboratory tests may be performed in the immediate postpartum period. Hemoglobin and hematocrit values are often requested on the first postpartum day to assess blood loss during childbirth. In some hospitals a clean-catch or catheterized urine specimen may be obtained and sent for routine urinalysis or culture and sensitivity, especially if an indwelling urinary catheter was inserted during the intrapartum period.

Although all women experience similar physiologic changes during the postpartum period, certain factors act to make each woman's experience unique. From a physiologic standpoint, the length and difficulty of the labor, type of birth (vaginal or cesarean), presence of episiotomy or lacerations, and whether the mother plans to breastfeed or bottle feed are important factors to be investigated with each woman. After analyzing the data obtained during the assessment process, the nurse establishes nursing diagnoses that will guide the plan of care. Examples of nursing diagnoses frequently established for the postpartum patient are listed in the box.

Nursing Diagnoses

The Postpartum Patient
Risk for infection related to
• Childbirth trauma to tissues
Constipation or urinary retention related to
• Postchildbirth discomfort
• Childbirth trauma to tissues
Sleep pattern disturbance related to
• Discomforts of postpartum period
• Long labor process
• Infant care and hospital routine
Pain related to
• Involution of uterus
• Trauma to perineum
• Episiotomy
• Hemorrhoids
• Engorged breasts
Risk for injury related to
• Postpartum hemorrhage
• Effects of anesthesia
Ineffective breastfeeding related to
• Maternal discomfort
• Infant positioning

Expected Outcomes of Care

The nursing plan of care includes both the postpartum woman and her infant, even if the nursery nurse retains primary responsibility for the infant. In many hospitals, **couplet care** (also called mother and baby care or single room maternity care) is practiced. Nurses in these settings have been educated in both mother and infant care and function as the primary nurse for both mother and infant, even if the infant is kept in the nursery. This approach is a variation of rooming-in, in which the mother and child room together and mother and nurse share the care of the infant. The organization of the mother's care must take the newborn into consideration. The day actually revolves around the baby's feeding and care times.

Once the nursing diagnoses are formulated, the nurse plans with the patient what nursing measures will be appropriate and which are to be given priority. During her hospital stay the mother is encouraged to assume increasing responsibility for her self-care and her infant's care. As the patient and her partner provide more care for herself and the baby, the nurse's role changes from one of providing direct care to one of teaching, encouragement, and support.

The nursing plan of care will include periodic assessments to detect deviations from normal physical changes, measures to relieve discomfort or pain, safety measures to prevent injury or infection, and teaching and counseling measures designed to promote the patient's feelings of competence in self-care and baby care. Family members are included in the teaching. The nurse evaluates continuously and is ready to change the plan if indicated. Almost all hospitals use standardized care plans as a base. The nurse's ability to adapt the standardized plan to specific medical and nursing diagnoses results in individualized patient care. Caution is advised against total reliance on a standardized plan; by doing so the uniqueness of the individual may be overlooked.

Expected outcomes for the postpartum period are based on the nursing diagnoses identified for the individual patient. Examples of common expected outcomes for physiologic needs are that the woman will:
- Remain free from infection
- Demonstrate normal involution and lochial characteristics
- Remain comfortable and injury free
- Demonstrate normal bladder and bowel patterns
- Demonstrate knowledge of breast care for breastfeeding and bottle feeding, as appropriate
- Protect the health of future pregnancies and children
- Integrate the newborn into the family

Plan of Care and Interventions

Nurses assume many roles while implementing the nursing plan of care. They provide direct physical care, teach mother and baby care, and provide anticipatory guidance and counseling. Perhaps most important of all they nurture the patient by providing encouragement and support as the woman begins to assume the many tasks of motherhood. Nurses who take the time to "mother the mother" do much to increase feelings of self-confidence in new mothers.

The first step in providing individualized care is to confirm the patient's identity by checking her wristband. At the same time, the infant's identification number is matched with the corresponding band on the mother's and, in some instances, the father's wrist. The nurse demonstrates caring and respect by determining how the mother wishes to be addressed and then notes her preference in her record and in her nursing plan of care.

The woman and her family are oriented to their surroundings. Familiarity with the unit, routines, resources, and personnel reduces one potential source of anxiety—the unknown. The mother is reassured by knowing whom and how she can call for assistance and what she can expect in the way of supplies and services. If the woman's usual daily routine before admission differs from the facility's routine, the nurse works with the woman to develop a mutually acceptable routine.

Infant abduction from hospitals in the United States has increased in the past few years. The mother should be taught to check the identity of any person who comes to remove the baby from her room. Hospital personnel usually wear picture identification badges. On some units, all staff members wear matching scrubs or special badges. Other units use closed circuit television or computer monitoring systems. As a rule, the baby is never carried in a staff member's arms between the mother's room and the nursery but is always wheeled in a bassinet, which also contains baby care supplies. Patients and nurses must work together to ensure the safety of newborns in the hospital environment.

Implementation of the nursing plan of care involves putting into practice specific activities that should result in achieving the expected outcomes planned for each individual patient (see Plan of Care).

Prevention of infection

One important means of preventing infection is maintenance of a clean environment. Bed linens should be changed as needed. Disposable pads and draw sheets may need to be changed frequently. Patients should avoid walking about barefoot to avoid contaminating bed linens when they return to bed. Supervision of use of equipment to prevent cross-contamination is also necessary. For example, a common **sitz bath** or heat lamp must be scrubbed after each woman's use. Staff members are another important part of the hospital environment. Personnel must be conscientious about their handwashing

PLAN OF CARE *Postpartum Care—Vaginal Birth*

> **NURSING DIAGNOSIS** Risk for fluid volume deficit related to uterine atony/hemorrhage

Expected Outcomes *Fundus is firm, lochia is moderate, and there is no evidence of hemorrhage.*

Nursing Interventions/*Rationales*

Monitor lochia (color, amount, consistency) and count and weigh sanitary pads if lochia is heavy *to evaluate amount of bleeding.*

Monitor and palpate fundus for location and tone *to determine status of uterus and dictate further interventions because atonic uterus is most common cause of postpartum hemorrhage.*

Monitor intake and output, assess for bladder fullness, and encourage voiding *because a full bladder interferes with involution of the uterus.*

Monitor vital signs (increased pulse and respirations, decreased blood pressure) and skin temperature and color *to detect signs of hemorrhage/shock.*

Monitor postpartum hematology studies *to assess effects of blood loss.*

If fundus is boggy, apply gentle massage and assess tone response *to promote uterine contractions and increase uterine tone.* (Do not overstimulate because doing so can cause fundal relaxation.)

Express uterine clots *to promote uterine contraction.*

Explain to the woman the process of involution and teach her to assess and massage the fundus and to report any persistent bogginess *to involve her in self-care and increase sense of self-control.*

Administer oxytocic agents per physician/nurse-midwife order and evaluate effectiveness *to promote continuing uterine contraction.*

Administer fluids, blood, blood products, or plasma expanders as ordered *to replace lost fluid and lost blood volume.*

> **NURSING DIAGNOSIS** Pain related to postpartum physiologic changes (hemorrhoids, episiotomy, breast engorgement, cracked/sore nipples)

Expected Outcome *Patient exhibits signs of decreased discomfort.*

Nursing Interventions/*Rationales*

Assess location, type, and quality of pain *to direct intervention.*

Explain to the woman the source and reasons for the pain, its expected duration, and treatments *to decrease anxiety and increase sense of control.*

Administer prescribed pain medications *to provide pain relief.*

If pain is perineal (episiotomy, hemorrhoids), apply ice packs in the first 24 hours *to reduce edema and vulvar irritation and reduce discomfort;* encourage sitz baths using cool water first 24 hours *to reduce edema* and warm water thereafter *to promote circulation;* apply witch hazel compresses *to reduce edema;* teach woman to use prescribed perineal creams, sprays, or ointments *to depress response of peripheral nerves;* teach woman to tighten buttocks before sitting and to sit on flat, hard surfaces *to compress buttocks and reduce pressure on the perineum.* (Avoid donuts and soft pillows as they separate the buttocks and decrease venous blood flow, increasing pain.)

If pain is from breasts and woman is breastfeeding, encourage use of a supportive bra *to increase comfort;* ascertain that infant has latched on correctly *to prevent sore nipples;* vary infant position during feeding *to prevent sore nipples.*

If breasts are engorged, have woman use warm compresses or take a warm shower before breastfeeding *to stimulate milk flow and relieve stasis.*

If nipples are sore, have woman air-dry nipples after feeding *to toughen nipples,* apply breast creams as prescribed *to soften nipples and relieve irritation and wear breast shields in her bra to relieve irritation.*

If pain is from breast and woman is not breastfeeding, encourage use of a tight supportive bra or breast binder and application of ice packs *to reduce lactation and decrease heaviness.*

> **NURSING DIAGNOSIS** Sleep pattern disturbance related to excitement, discomfort, and environmental interruptions

Expected Outcome *Patient sleeps for uninterrupted periods of time and feels rested after waking.*

Nursing Interventions/*Rationales*

Establish woman's routine sleep patterns and compare with current sleep pattern, exploring things that interfere with sleep, *to determine scope of problem and direct interventions.*

Individualize nursing routines to fit woman's natural body rhythms (i.e., wake/sleep cycles), provide a sleep-promoting environment (i.e., darkness, quiet, adequate ventilation, appropriate room temperature), prepare for sleep using woman's usual routines (i.e., back rub, soothing music, warm milk), teach use of guided imagery and relaxation techniques *to promote optimum conditions for sleep.*

Avoid things or routines (i.e., caffeine, foods that induce heartburn, fluids, strenuous mental/physical activity) *that may interfere with sleep.*

Administer sedation or pain medication as prescribed *to enhance quality of sleep.*

Advise woman/partner to limit visitors and activities *to avoid further taxation and fatigue.*

Teach woman to use infant nap time as a time for her also to nap *to replenish energy and decrease fatigue.*

Continued

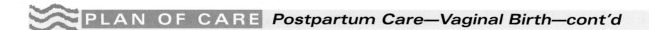

> **NURSING DIAGNOSIS** Risk for infection related to altered primary defenses in the postpartum period

Expected Outcome *Patient shows no evidence of infection.*

Nursing Interventions/*Rationales*

Maintain Standard Precautions and use good handwashing technique when providing care *to prevent spread of infection.*

Use strict aseptic technique when performing invasive procedures such as urinary catheterization or insertion of intravenous lines *to reduce risk of nosocomial infection.*

Monitor vital signs *because elevated temperature, pulse, respiratory rate, and blood pressure may indicate infection.*

Monitor for pallor, fatigue, malaise, chills, and loss of appetite, *which may indicate infection.*

Monitor lochia for foul smell *indicative of infection.*

Monitor IV site and episiotomy site for signs such as pain, redness, edema, heat, and drainage, *which are indicative of infection.*

Monitor urine for color, concentration, odor, clouding, casts, and sediment, *which may indicate a urinary tract infection.*

Monitor breasts for infected nipple fissures, hot engorged tissue, or obstruction of milk flow, *which are indicative of mastitis.*

Monitor laboratory values (i.e., white blood cell count, cultures) *for indicators of infection.*

Assist woman to maintain good personal hygiene habits (i.e., wiping perineal region from front to back, keeping area dry, frequent change of peripads, proper use of sitz bath, and perineal irrigation) *to reduce introduction of bacteria.*

Ensure adequate nutritional intake (high protein, iron, vitamin C) *to promote healing.*

From Wong D & Perry S: *Maternal child nursing care,* St Louis, 1998, Mosby.

---

techniques to prevent cross infection. Standard Precautions must be practiced. Staff members with colds, coughs, or skin infections (e.g., a cold sore on the lip [herpes simplex virus, type 1]) must follow hospital protocol when in contact with postpartum patients. In many hospitals, staff with open herpetic lesions, strep throat, conjunctivitis, upper respiratory infections or diarrhea are encouraged to avoid contact with mothers and infants by staying home until the condition is no longer contagious.

Proper care of the episiotomy site and any perineal lacerations prevents infection in the genitourinary area and aids the healing process. Educating the woman to wipe from front to back (urethra to anus) after voiding or defecating is a simple first step. In many hospitals a squeeze bottle filled with warm water or other antiseptic solutions is used after each voiding to cleanse the perineal area (Box 17-3). The patient should also be taught to change her perineal pad from front to back each time she voids or defecates and to wash her hands thoroughly before and after doing so.

Prevention of excessive bleeding

The most frequent cause of excessive bleeding following childbirth is **uterine atony,** failure of the uterine muscle to contract firmly. The two most important interventions for preventing excessive bleeding, therefore, are maintaining good uterine tone and preventing bladder distention.

> NURSE ALERT *If uterine atony occurs, the relaxed uterus distends with blood and clots, and blood vessels in the placental site are not clamped off, thus excessive bleeding results.*

Excessive blood loss following childbirth may also be caused by vaginal or vulvar hematomas, unrepaired lacerations of the vagina or cervix, and retained placental fragments.

A perineal pad saturated in 15 minutes or less or pooling of blood under the buttocks are indications of excessive blood loss, requiring immediate notification of the primary health care provider. A perineal pad that is soaked through from end to end contains approximately 68 to 80 ml of blood (Luegenbiehl et al., 1990). Blood loss is usually described subjectively as scant, light, moderate, or heavy (profuse). Fig. 17-6 shows examples of perineal pad saturation corresponding to each of these descriptions. More reliable estimates of blood loss include weighing blood clots and items saturated with blood (1 ml of blood equals 1 g), using devices that catch and measure blood flowing from the vagina, and establishing the ml of blood it takes to saturate perineal pads being used (Johnson & Johnson, 1996).

> NURSE ALERT *The nurse always checks under the mother's buttocks as well as on the perineal pad. Blood may flow between the buttocks onto the linens under the mother while the amount on the perineal pad is slight and thus excessive bleeding goes undetected.*

Blood pressure is not a reliable indicator of impending shock from early hemorrhage. More sensitive means of identifying shock are provided by respirations, pulse, skin condition, urinary output, and level of consciousness (Johnson & Johnson, 1996). The frequent physical assessments performed during the fourth stage of labor are designed to provide prompt identification of excessive bleeding (see Emergency box.)

| BOX 17-3 | *Interventions for Episiotomy, Lacerations, and Hemorrhoids* |

Explain both procedure and rationale before implementation.

CLEANSING

Wash hands before and after cleansing perineum and changing pads.

Wash perineum with mild soap and warm water at least once daily.

Cleanse from symphysis pubis to anal area.

Apply peripad from front to back, protecting inner surface of pad from contamination.

Wrap soiled pad and place in covered waste container.

Change pad with each void or defecation or at least 4 times per day.

Assess amount and character of lochia with each pad change.

ICE PACK

Apply a covered ice pack to perineum from front to back.

1. During first 2 hours to decrease edema formation and increase comfort
2. After the first 2 hours following the birth to provide anesthetic effect

SQUEEZE BOTTLE

Demonstrate for and assist woman; explain rationale.

Fill bottle with tap water warmed to approximately 38° C (comfortably warm on the wrist).

Instruct woman to position nozzle between her legs so that squirts of water reach perineum as she sits on toilet seat. Explain that it will take whole bottle of water to cleanse perineum.

Remind her to blot dry with toilet paper or clean wipes.

Remind her to avoid contamination from anal area.

Apply clean pad.

SITZ BATH

Built-in type:

Prepare bath by thoroughly scrubbing with cleaning agent and rinsing.

Pad with towel before filling.

Fill one-half to one-third full with water of correct temperature: 38° to 40.6° C. Some women prefer cool sitz baths. Ice is added to water to lower the temperature to the level comfortable for the woman.

Encourage woman to use at least twice a day for 20 minutes.

Place call bell within easy reach.

Teach woman to enter bath by tightening gluteal muscles and keeping them tightened and then relaxing them after she is in the bath.

Place dry towels within reach.

Ensure privacy.

Check woman in 15 minutes; assess pulse as needed.

Disposable type:

Clamp tubing and fill bag with warm water.

Raise toilet seat, place bath in bowl with overflow opening directed toward back of toilet.

Place container above toilet bowl.

Attach tube into groove at front of bath.

Loosen tube clamp to regulate rate of flow: fill bath to about one-half full; continue as above for built-in sitz bath.

SURGI-GATOR

Assemble Surgi-Gator (Fig. 17-7).

Instruct woman regarding use and rationale.

Follow package directions.

Instruct woman to sit on toilet with legs apart and to put nozzle so tip is just past the perineum, adjusting placement as needed.

Remind her to return her applicator to her bedside stand.

DRY HEAT

Inspect lamp for defects.

Cover lamp with towels.

Position lamp 50 cm from perineum; use 3 times a day for 20-minute periods.

Teach regarding use of 40-W bulb at home.

Provide draping over woman.

If same lamp is being used by several women, clean it carefully between uses.

TOPICAL APPLICATIONS

Apply anesthetic cream or spray: use sparingly 3 to 4 times per day.

Offer witch hazel pads (Tucks) after voiding or defecating; woman pats perineum dry from front to back, then applies witch hazel pads.

Fig. **17-6** Blood loss after birth is assessed by the extent of perineal pad saturation as (from left to right) scant (<2.5 cm); light (<10 cm); moderate (<15 cm); or heavy (one pad saturated within 2 hours).

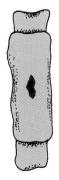
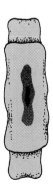
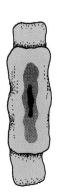
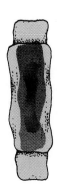

EMERGENCY

Hypovolemic Shock

SIGNS AND SYMPTOMS

Persistent significant bleeding—perineal pad soaked within 15 minutes; **may not be accompanied by a change in vital signs or maternal color or behavior.**

Woman states she feels weak, light-headed, "funny," "sick to my stomach," or "sees stars."

Woman begins to act anxious or exhibits air hunger.

Woman's skin turns ashen or grayish.

Skin feels cool and clammy.

Pulse rate increases.

Blood pressure declines.

INTERVENTIONS

Notify primary health care provider.

If uterus is atonic, massage gently and expel clots to cause uterus to contract; compress uterus manually, as needed, using two hands. Add oxytocic agent to IV drip, as ordered.

Give oxygen by face mask or nasal prongs at 8 to 10 L/min.

Tilt the woman to her side or elevate the right hip; elevate her legs to at least a 30-degree angle.

Provide additional or maintain existing IV infusion of lactated Ringer's solution or normal saline solution to restore circulatory volume.

Administer blood or blood products, as ordered.

Monitor vital signs.

Insert an indwelling urinary catheter to monitor perfusion of kidneys.

Administer emergency medications, as ordered.

Prepare for possible surgery or other emergency treatments or procedures.

Chart incident, medical and nursing interventions instituted, and results of treatments.

Maintenance of uterine tone. A major intervention to restore good tone is stimulation by gently massaging the uterine fundus until firm (see Fig. 17-3). Fundal massage may cause a temporary increase in the amount of vaginal bleeding seen as pooled blood leaves the uterus. Clots may also be expelled. Patient education is extremely important in maintaining uterine tone. Fundal massage can be a very uncomfortable procedure. Understanding the causes and dangers of uterine atony and the purpose of fundal massage can help the woman to be more cooperative. Teaching the woman to do self-fundal massage enables her to maintain some control and decreases her anxiety. The uterus may remain boggy even after massage and expulsion of clots. If this occurs, it is a major warning sign of uterine atony. The nurse must remain with the patient and summon help, including notifying the primary health care provider immediately. Additional interventions likely to be employed are administration of intravenous fluids and **oxytocic medications** (drugs that stimulate contraction of the uterine smooth muscle). Table 26-1 contains information about common oxytocic medications.

LEGAL TIP | **Patient Abandonment**

In an emergency situation the nurse must remain with the patient and call for help. Leaving the patient can lead to a charge of patient abandonment.

Prevention of Bladder Distention. A full bladder causes the uterus to be displaced above the umbilicus and well to one side of midline in the abdomen. It also prevents the uterus from contracting normally. Nursing interventions focus on helping the woman spontaneously empty her bladder as soon as possible. The first priority is to assist the woman to the bathroom or onto a bedpan if she is unable to ambulate. Having the woman listen to running water, placing her hands in warm water, or pouring water from a squeeze bottle over her perineum may stimulate voiding. Other techniques include assisting the woman into the shower or sitz bath and encouraging her to void or placing spirits of peppermint in a bedpan under the woman. The vapors may relax the urinary meatus and trigger spontaneous voiding. Administering analgesics, if ordered, may be indicated because some women may fear voiding because of the anticipated pain. If these measures are unsuccessful, a sterile catheter may be inserted to drain the urine.

Evaluation of the woman's responses to intervention is an ongoing part of the nursing process. All responses to interventions should be carefully recorded. If the expected outcomes are not met or new needs emerge, the plan of care is modified accordingly. For example, if the uterus is firm and the bladder empty, something other than uterine atony is causing the excessive bleeding. Further assessment is necessary to determine the cause and correct the problem. See Chapter 26 for further discussion of postpartum hemorrhage.

Promotion of comfort, rest, ambulation, and exercise

Comfort. Most women experience some degree of discomfort during the immediate postpartum period. Common causes of discomfort include afterbirth pains, episiotomy or perineal lacerations, hemorrhoids, and breast engorgement. The woman's description of the type and severity of her pain is the nurse's best guide in choosing an appropriate intervention. To confirm the location and extent of discomfort, the nurse inspects and palpates areas of pain as appropriate for redness, swelling, discharge, and heat and observes for body tension, guarded movements, and facial tension. Blood pressure, pulse, and respirations may be elevated in response to acute pain. Diaphoresis may accompany severe pain. A lack of objective symptoms does not necessarily mean there is no pain because there may also be a cultural component to the expression of pain. Nursing interventions are intended to eliminate the pain sensation

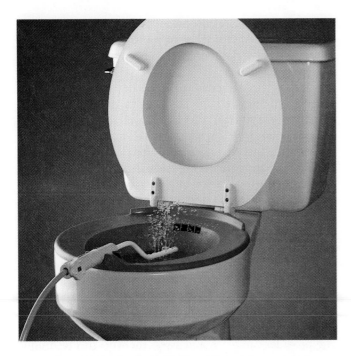

Fig. **17-7** Hygienic sitz bath (SurgiGator) for perineal care. (Courtesy Andermac, Inc., Yuba City, Calif.)

entirely or reduce it to a tolerable level that allows the woman to care for herself and her baby. Nurses may employ both nonpharmacologic and pharmacologic interventions to promote comfort. Depending on reported severity, nonpharmacologic measures should be employed either alone or in combination with pharmacologic interventions. Pain relief is enhanced by using more than one method or route.

Nonpharmacologic interventions. **Afterbirth pains** are the menstrual-like cramps experienced by many women as the uterus contracts following childbirth. Warmth, distraction, deep breathing, imagery, therapeutic touch, relaxation, and interaction with the infant may decrease the discomfort associated with these uterine contractions.

Simple interventions that can decrease the discomfort associated with an episiotomy or perineal lacerations include encouraging the woman to lie on her side whenever possible and to use a pillow when sitting. Other interventions include application of an ice pack, topical applications (if ordered), dry heat, cleansing with a squeeze bottle or SurgiGator (Fig. 17-7), and a cleansing shower, tub bath, or sitz bath. Many of these interventions are also effective for hemorrhoids, especially ice packs, sitz baths, and topical applications (such as witch hazel pads). Box 17-3 gives more specific information about these interventions.

Pharmacologic interventions. Most primary health care providers routinely order a variety of analgesics to be administered as needed, including both narcotic and nonnarcotic

(nonsteroidal antiinflammatory medications) choices, with their dosage and time frequency ranges. Topical application of antiseptic or anesthetic ointment or sprays is a common pharmacologic intervention. Patient-controlled analgesia (PCA) pumps and continuous epidural analgesia infusions are two newer technologies now frequently used to provide postpartum pain relief after ceserean birth. The nurse should carefully monitor all patients receiving opioids because respiratory depression and decreased intestinal motility are side effects. Many women want to participate in decisions about analgesia. Severe pain, however, may interfere with active participation in choosing pain relief measures. If an analgesic is to be given, the nurse must make a clinical judgment of the type, dosage, and frequency from the medications ordered. The woman is informed of the prescribed analgesic and its common side effects; this teaching is documented.

Breastfeeding mothers often have concerns about the effects on the infant of taking an analgesic. Although nearly all drugs present in maternal circulation are also found in breast milk, many analgesics commonly used during the postpartum period are considered relatively safe for breastfeeding mothers (see Appendix C). Often the timing of medications can be adjusted to minimize infant exposure. A mother may be given pain medication immediately after breastfeeding, for example, so that the interval between medication administration and the next nursing period is as long as possible. The decision to administer medications of any kind to a breastfeeding mother must always be made by carefully weighing the woman's need for the medication against actual or potential risks to the infant.

If acceptable pain relief has not been obtained in 1 hour and there has been no change in the initial assessment, the nurse may need to contact the primary care provider for additional pain relief orders or further directions. Unrelieved pain results in fatigue, anxiety, and a worsening perception of the pain. It might also indicate the presence of a previously unknown or untreated problem. Further assessment and treatment will likely be necessary to determine the cause of the pain and correct it.

Rest. The excitement and exhilaration experienced after the birth of the infant may make rest difficult. The new mother, who is often anxious about her ability to care for her infant or is uncomfortable, may also have difficulty sleeping. In the days that follow, the demands of the infant, along with the influence of the hospital environment and routines, contribute to alterations in her sleep pattern.

Fatigue. Fatigue is common in the postpartum period (Pugh & Milligan, 1995) and involves both physiologic components associated with long labors, cesarean birth, anemia, and breastfeeding and psychologic components related to depression and anxiety. Infant behavior can also be related to fatigue, particularly with mothers of more difficult infants.

Interventions must be planned to meet the woman's individual needs for sleep and rest. Backrubs, other comfort measures, and medication for sleep for the first few nights may be necessary. Support and encouragement in mothering behaviors help to reduce anxiety. Hospital and nursing routines may also be adjusted to meet individual needs. In addition, the nurse can help the family limit visitors and provide a comfortable chair or bed for the partner.

Ambulation. Early ambulation is successful in reducing the incidence of thromboembolism and in promoting the woman's more rapid recovery of strength. Confinement to bed is not required for the woman who had general anesthesia, epidural or spinal anesthesia, or local anesthesia such as pudendal block. Free movement is permitted once the anesthetic wears off unless an analgesic has been administered. After the initial recovery period is over, the mother is encouraged to ambulate frequently.

> **NURSE ALERT** *Having a hospital staff or family member present the first time the woman gets out of bed after childbirth is a wise idea because she may feel weak, dizzy, faint, or light-headed.*

The rapid decrease in intraabdominal pressure after birth results in a dilation of blood vessels supplying the intestines, which is known as **splanchnic engorgement,** and causes blood to pool in the viscera. This condition contributes to the development of orthostatic hypotension and may occur when the woman who has recently given birth sits or stands up, first ambulates, or takes a warm shower or sitz bath (Johnson & Johnson, 1996). The nurse needs to also consider several factors, such as the baseline blood pressure, amount of blood loss, and type, amount, and timing of analgesic or anesthetic medications administered when assisting a woman to ambulate.

Prevention of **thrombus** (clot formation) is part of the nursing plan of care. Women who must remain in bed after giving birth are at an increased risk for the development of thrombus. If a woman remains in bed longer than 8 hours (e.g., after cesarean birth), exercise to promote circulation in the legs is indicated using the following routine:
1. Alternate flexion and extension of feet.
2. Rotate ankle in circular motion.
3. Alternate flexion and extension of legs.
4. Press back of knee to bed surface; relax.

If the woman is susceptible to thromboembolism, she is encouraged to walk about actively and discouraged from sitting immobile in a chair. Women with varicosities are encouraged to wear support hose. If a thrombus is suspected—as evidenced by a positive **Homans' sign** (complaint of pain in calf muscles when the foot is dorsiflexed) or warmth, redness, or tenderness in the suspected leg—the primary health care provider should be notified immediately; meanwhile the woman should be confined to bed, with the affected limb elevated on pillows.

Exercise. Most women who have just given birth are extremely interested in regaining their nonpregnant figure. Postpartum exercise can begin soon after birth, although

the woman should be encouraged to start with simple exercises and gradually progress to more strenuous ones. Fig. 17-8 illustrates a number of exercises appropriate for the new mother.

Kegel pelvic exercises to strengthen muscle tone are extremely important, particularly after vaginal birth. To perform them, the woman consciously contracts and relaxes the muscles around the vagina. **Kegel exercises** help women to regain the muscle tone that is often lost as pelvic tissues are stretched and torn during pregnancy and birth. Women who maintain muscle strength may benefit years later by experiencing less stress urinary incontinence.

However, it is essential that women learn to perform the Kegel exercises correctly (see Teaching Guidelines box in Chapter 4). Studies have shown that approximately one fourth of all women who learn Kegel exercises are doing them incorrectly and may increase their risk of incontinence (Sampselle & Miller, 1996). This may occur when women inadvertently bear down on the pelvic floor muscles (Valsalva effort), thrusting the perineum outward. The health care provider can teach and assess the woman's technique during the pelvic examination at the 6-week check-up, inserting two fingers intravaginally and checking whether the pelvic floor muscles correctly contract and relax.

Promotion of nutrition

During the hospital stay, most women display a good appetite and eat well; nutritional snacks are usually welcomed. Women may request that family members bring to the hospital favorite or culturally appropriate foods. Cultural dietary preferences must be respected. This interest in food presents an ideal opportunity for nutritional counseling on dietary needs after pregnancy, such as for breastfeeding, preventing constipation and anemia, weight loss, and promoting healing and well-being (see Chapter 11). Prenatal vitamins and iron supplements are often continued until 6 weeks postpartum or the ordered supply has been used.

Promotion of normal bladder and bowel patterns

Bladder. After giving birth the mother should void spontaneously within 6 to 8 hours. The first several voidings should be measured to document adequate emptying of the bladder. A volume of at least 150 ml is expected for each voiding. Some women experience difficulty in emptying the bladder, possibly as a result of diminished bladder tone, edema from trauma, or fear of discomfort. Nursing interventions for inability to void and bladder distention are discussed on p. 432.

Bowel. Nursing interventions to promote normal bowel elimination include educating the woman about measures to avoid constipation. These interventions include ensuring adequate roughage and fluid intake and promoting exercise. Alerting the woman to side effects of medications such

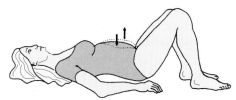

Abdominal Breathing. Lie on back with knees bent. Inhale deeply through nose. Keep ribs stationary and allow abdomen to expand upward. Exhale slowly but forcefully while contracting the abdominal muscles; hold for 3 to 5 seconds while exhaling. Relax.

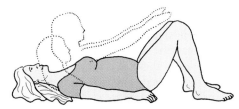

Reach for the Knees. Lie on back with knees bent. While inhaling, deeply lower chin onto chest. While exhaling, raise head and shoulders slowly and smoothly and reach for knees with arms outstretched. The body should only rise as far as the back will naturally bend while waist remains on floor or bed (about 6 to 8 inches). Slowly and smoothly lower head and shoulders back to starting position. Relax.

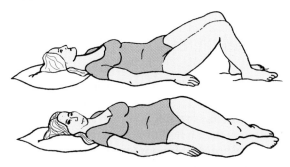

Double Knee Roll. Lie on back with knees bent. Keeping shoulders flat and feet stationary, slowly and smoothly roll knees over to the left to touch floor or bed. Maintaining a smooth motion, roll knees back over to the right until they touch floor or bed. Return to starting position and relax.

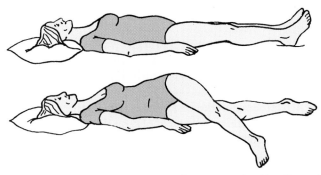

Leg Roll. Lie on back with legs straight. Keeping shoulders flat and legs straight, slowly and smoothly lift left leg and roll it over to touch the right side of floor or bed and return to starting position. Repeat, rolling right leg over to touch left side of floor or bed. Relax.

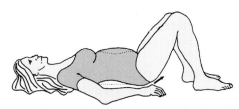

Combined Abdominal Breathing and Supine Pelvic Tilt (Pelvic Rock). Lie on back with knees bent. While inhaling deeply, roll pelvis back by flattening lower back on floor or bed. Exhale slowly but forcefully while contracting abdominal muscles and tightening buttocks. Hold for 3 to 5 seconds while exhaling. Relax.

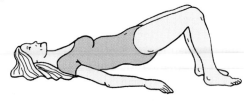

Buttocks Lift. Lie on back with arms at sides, knees bent, and feet flat. Slowly raise buttocks and arch back. Return slowly to starting position.

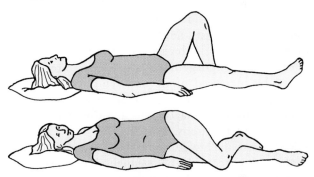

Single Knee Roll. Lie on back with right leg straight and left leg bent at the knee. Keeping shoulders flat, slowly and smoothly roll left knee over to the right to touch floor or bed and then back to starting position. Reverse position of legs. Roll right knee over to the left to touch floor or bed and return to starting position. Relax.

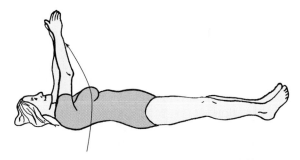

Arm Raises. Lie on back with arms extended at 90 degree-angle from body. Raise arms so they are perpendicular and hands touch. Lower slowly.

Fig. 17-8 Postpartum exercise should begin as soon as possible. The woman should start with simple exercises and gradually progress to more strenuous ones.

as narcotic analgesics (i.e., decreased gastrointestinal tract motility) may encourage her to implement measures to reduce the risk of constipation. Stool softeners or laxatives are often routinely ordered and may be necessary during the early postpartum period. With early discharge, a new mother is often home before having a bowel movement.

Breastfeeding promotion and lactation suppression

Breastfeeding promotion. The first 2 hours after birth are an excellent time to encourage the mother to breastfeed. The infant is in an alert state and ready to breastfeed. Breastfeeding aids in the contraction of the uterus and prevention of maternal hemorrhage. This is a wonderful opportunity for the nurse to instruct the mother in breastfeeding and to assess the physical appearance of the breasts. (See Chapter 21 for further information on assisting the breastfeeding woman.)

Lactation suppression. Suppression of lactation is necessary when the woman has decided not to breastfeed or in the event of neonatal death. One very important nonpharmacologic intervention is wearing a well-fitted support bra or breast binder continuously for at least the first 72 hours after giving birth. Women should also avoid any breast stimulation, including running warm water over the breasts, newborn suckling, or pumping of the breasts. A few nonbreastfeeding mothers experience severe breast **engorgement** (swelling of breast tissue caused by increased blood and lymph supply to the breasts preceding lactation). If breast engorgement occurs, it can usually be managed satisfactorily with nonpharmacologic interventions.

Ice packs to the breasts are helpful in decreasing the discomfort associated with engorgement. The woman should use a 15 minutes on, 45 minutes off schedule to prevent the rebound swelling that can occur if ice is used continuously, or she should place fresh cabbage leaves inside her bra. Cabbage leaves have been used to treat swelling in other cultures for years (Roberts, 1995). The exact mechanism of action is not known, but it is thought that naturally occurring plant estrogens or salicylates may be responsible for the effects. The leaves are replaced each time they wilt. A mild analgesic may also be necessary to help the mother through this uncomfortable time. Medications that were once prescribed for lactation suppression (estrogen, estrogen and testosterone, and bromocriptine) are no longer used to suppress lactation.

Health promotion of future pregnancies and children

If the assessment data indicate the need, rubella vaccination and Rh immune globulin (RhoGAM) are administered during the puerperium. Failure to administer these products to women at risk of contracting rubella or developing Rh

isoimmunization can seriously jeopardize the health of any future pregnancies and children.

Rubella vaccination. For women who have not had rubella (10% to 20% of all women) or women who are serologically negative (i.e., titer of 1:8), a subcutaneous injection of **rubella vaccine** is recommended in the immediate post-birth period to prevent fetal anomalies in future pregnancies. Sero-conversion occurs in approximately 90% of women vaccinated after birth. The live attenuated rubella virus is not communicable; therefore breastfeeding mothers can be vaccinated. However, because the virus is shed in urine and other body fluids, the vaccine should not be given if the mother or other household members are immunocompromised. Rubella vaccine is made from duck eggs, so women who have allergies to these eggs may develop a hypersensitivity reaction to the vaccine for which they will need adrenaline. A transient arthralgia or rash is common in vaccinated women but is benign. Because the vaccine may be teratogenic, the patient must be informed about the vaccine (see Legal Tip).

LEGAL TIP | **Rubella Vaccination**

Informed consent for rubella vaccination in the postpartum period includes information about the possible side effects and the risk of teratogenic effects. Women must understand that they must practice contraception to avoid pregnancy for 2 to 3 months after being vaccinated.

Prevention of Rh isoimmunization. Injection of **Rh immune globulin** (a solution of gamma globulin that contains Rh antibodies) within 72 hours after birth prevents sensitization in the Rh-negative woman who has had a fetomaternal transfusion of Rh-positive red blood cells (RBCs). The Rh immune globulin promotes lysis of the fetal Rh-positive blood cells before the mother forms her own antibodies against them.

NURSE ALERT | *Postpartally, Rh immune globulin is administered to all Rh-negative, antibody (Coombs')-negative women who give birth to Rh-positive infants.*

The administration of 300 µg (1 vial) of Rh immune globulin is usually sufficient to prevent maternal sensitization. If a large fetomaternal transfusion is suspected, however, the dosage needed should be determined by performing a **Kleihauer-Betke test,** which detects the amount of fetal blood in the maternal circulation. If more than 15 ml of fetal blood is present in maternal circulation, the dosage of Rh immune globulin must be increased.

A 1:1,000 dilution of Rh immune globulin is crossmatched to the mother's RBCs to ensure compatibility. Because Rh immune globulin is a blood product, precautions similar to those used for transfusing blood are necessary when it is given. The identification number on the patient's hospital wristband should correspond to the identification number found on the laboratory slip. The nurse must also check to see that the lot number on the laboratory slip corresponds to the lot number on the vial. Finally, the expiration date on the vial should be checked to ensure a usable product.

NURSE ALERT *Rh immune globulin is administered to the mother intramuscularly. It should never be given to an infant.*

Rh immune globulin suppresses the immune response. Therefore the woman who receives both Rh immune globulin and rubella vaccine must be tested at 3 months to see if she has developed rubella immunity. If not, the woman will need another dose of rubella vaccine.

There is some disagreement about whether Rh immune globulin should be considered a blood product. Health care providers need to discuss the most current information about this issue with women whose religious beliefs conflict with having blood products administered to them.

Evaluation

The nurse can be reasonably assured that care was effective when the expected outcomes of care for physical needs have been achieved.

I CARE MANAGEMENT— PSYCHOSOCIAL NEEDS

Meeting the psychosocial needs of new mothers involves planning care that considers the composition and functioning of the entire family. Nurses assess the parents' reactions to the birth experience, feelings about themselves, and interactions with the new baby and other family members. Specific interventions are then planned to increase the parents' knowledge and self-confidence as they assume the care and responsibility of the new baby and integrate a new member into their existing family structure in a way that meets their cultural expectations.

Assessment and Nursing Diagnoses

Impact of the birth experience

Many women indicate a need to examine the birth process itself and look at their own intrapartal behavior in retrospect. Their partners may express similar desires. During pregnancy the woman and her partner may have developed a specific birth plan that included a vaginal birth and very little medical intervention. If their birth experience was quite different (e.g., labor induction, epidural anesthesia, cesarean birth), both partners may need to mourn the loss of their expectations before they can adjust to the reality of their birth experience. Inviting them to review the events and describe how they feel helps the nurse to assess how well they understand what happened and how well they have been able to put their childbirth experience into perspective.

Feelings about giving birth can affect both partners' adaptation to parenting.

Impact of cultural diversity

The final component of a complete psychosocial assessment is the patient's cultural beliefs and values. Much of a woman's behavior during the postpartum period is strongly influenced by her cultural background. In today's world, where travel is commonplace, nurses are likely to come in contact with women from many different countries and cultures. The nurse must remember that all cultures have developed safe and satisfying methods of caring for new mothers and babies. Only by understanding and respecting the values and beliefs of each woman can the nurse design a plan of care to meet her individual needs.

Following is an example of one "clash of cultures." The nurse in this case was able to take this information and modify her plan of care to make it culturally relevant, and therefore more satisfying, for the patient.

A Vietnamese woman who had been in the United States for 4 years requested rooming-in facilities following childbirth. Instead of participating in the care of her infant, she refused to do so, remained in bed, wore a woolen cap, and appeared distressed and angry. The staff were puzzled and upset by her behavior. One nurse decided to put newly learned concepts concerning cross-cultural nursing into effect. She began by praising the woman's ability to speak English and, after eliciting a smile, remarked, "Every country has developed good ways to look after mothers and babies. Would you tell me about the care in Vietnam?" There was an immediate response. The woman explained that in her country women remained in bed for 10 days after birth, and the biggest danger to their health was getting a cold. The baby was kept in the room with his mother, but either a grandmother or nurse took complete charge of the care.

Maternal self-image

An important assessment concerns the woman's self-concept, body image, and sexuality. How this new mother feels about herself and her body during the puerperium may affect her behavior and adaptation to parenting. The woman's self-concept and body image may also affect her sexuality.

Feelings related to sexual adjustment after childbirth are often a cause of concern for new parents. Women who have recently given birth may be reluctant to resume sexual intercourse for fear of pain or may worry that coitus could damage healing perineal tissue. Because many new parents are anxious for information but reluctant to bring up the subject, postpartum nurses should matter-of-factly include the topic of postpartum sexuality during their routine physical assessment. While examining the episiotomy site, for example, the nurse can say, "I know you're sore right now, but it probably won't be long until you (or you and your partner) are ready to make love again. Have you thought about what that might be like? Would you like to ask me questions?" This approach assures the woman and her partner that resuming sexual activity is a legitimate concern for new parents and indicates the nurse's willingness to answer questions and share information.

Maternal adjustment

After analyzing the data obtained during the assessment process, the nurse establishes nursing diagnoses to provide a guide for planning care. Examples of nursing diagnoses related to psychosocial issues that are frequently established for the postpartum patient are listed in the box.

| Nursing Diagnoses_____

Psychosocial Issues
Altered family processes related to
- Unexpected birth of twins

Impaired verbal communication related to
- Patient's deafness
- Patient's language not the same as nurse's

Altered parenting related to
- Long, difficult labor
- Unmet expectations of labor and the birth

Anxiety related to
- Newness of parenting role

Risk for situational low self-esteem related to
- Body image changes

Expected Outcomes of Care

The psychosocial plan of care for the postpartum woman includes all family members. The postnatal period is a crucial one for the family because it contains the potential for crisis in family adjustment. Developing a plan of care that recognizes family strengths and provides support for family weaknesses does much to help family members take on new tasks and responsibilities.

Expected psychosocial outcomes during the postpartum period are based on the nursing diagnoses identified for the individual patient and her family. Examples of common expected outcomes include that the patient (family) will:
- Identify measures that promote a healthy personal adjustment in the postpartum period.
- Maintain healthy family functioning based on cultural norms and personal expectations.

Plan of Care and Interventions

Cultural issues must also be considered when planning care. In contrast with Allopathic medicine, there are many traditional health beliefs and practices among the different cultures within the American population. Traditional health practices that are used to maintain health or to avoid illnesses deal with the whole person (body, mind, and spirit)

and tend to be culturally based. There is increasing scientific information about the effect of these traditional health practices on maintaining a person's health (Spector, 1995).

Women from various cultures may view health as a balance between opposing forces (e.g., yin vs. yang), being in harmony with nature, or just "feeling good." Traditional practices may include the observance of certain dietary restrictions, clothing, or taboos for balancing the body; participation in certain activities such as sports and art for maintaining mental health; and use of silence, prayer, or meditation for developing spiritually. Practices (e.g., using religious objects, eating garlic) are used to protect oneself from illness and may involve avoiding people who are believed to create hexes, spells, or who have an evil eye. Restoration of health may involve a person taking folk medicines (e.g., herbs, animal substances) or using a traditional healer.

Childbirth occurs within this sociocultural context. Rest, seclusion, dietary restraints, and ceremonies honoring the mother are all common traditional practices that are followed for the promotion of the health and well-being of the mother and baby (D'Avanzo, 1992; Horn, 1990; Jambunathan, 1995; Jiménez, 1995; Lipson et al., 1996; Schneiderman, 1996; Spector, 1995).

There are several common traditional health practices used and beliefs held by women and their families during the postpartum period. In Asia, for example, pregnancy is considered to be a hot (yang) condition, then childbirth results in a sudden loss of yang forces. Therefore balance needs to be restored by increasing the return of yang forces present in hot food, hot water, and warm air (Jambunathan, 1995). Hmong women reported that if they did not follow the traditional diet after childbirth, they would not be able to bear another child and would have "sagging and shaking legs" in old age (Jambunathan, 1995).

Another common belief is that the mother and baby remain in a weak and vulnerable state for a period of several weeks following birth (Jambunathan, 1995; Jiménez, 1995; Schneiderman, 1996). During this time the mother may remain in a passive role, not take baths or showers, and stay in bed to prevent cold air from entering her body.

Women who have immigrated to the United States or other Western nations without their extended family may not have much help at home, thus making it extremely difficult for them to observe these activity restrictions (Park & Peterson, 1991). Box 17-4 lists some common cultural beliefs about the postpartum period.

It is important that nurses consider all cultural aspects when planning care and not use their own cultural beliefs as the framework for that care. A nursing diagnosis of noncompliance is not appropriate for a patient who has a language barrier or behaves culturally different than what is generally expected by nurses during postpartum care. Although the beliefs and behaviors of other cultures may

Some Cultural Beliefs about the Postpartum Period and Contraception

POSTPARTUM CARE

Chinese, Mexican, Korean, and Southeast Asian women may wish to eat only warm foods and drink hot drinks to replace blood loss and to restore the balance of hot and cold in their bodies. These women may also wish to stay warm and avoid bathing, exercises, and hair washing for 7 to 30 days after childbirth. Self-care may not be a priority; care by family members is preferred. The woman has respect for elders and authority. These women may wear abdominal binders. They may prefer not to give their babies colostrum.

Haitian women may request to take the placenta home to bury or burn.

Muslim women follow strict religious laws on modesty and diet. A Muslim woman must keep her hair, body, arms to the wrist, and legs to the ankles covered at all times. She cannot be alone in the presence of a man other than her husband or a male relative. Observant Muslims will not eat pork or pork products and are obligated to eat meat slaughtered according to Islamic laws (halal meat). Kosher meat, seafood, or a vegetarian diet if halal meat is not available is usually accepted.

CONTRACEPTION

Birth control is government mandated in mainland *China*. Most *Chinese women* will have an IUD inserted after the birth of their first child. Women do not want hormonal methods of contraception because they fear putting these medications in their bodies.

Saudi Arabian and Hispanic women will likely choose the rhythm method because most are Catholic.

(East) Indian men are encouraged to have voluntary sterilization by vasectomy.

Muslim couples may practice contraception by mutual consent as long as its use is not harmful to the woman. Acceptable contraceptive methods include foam and condoms, the diaphragm, and natural family planning.

Hmong women highly value and desire large families, which limits birth control practices.

seem different or strange, they should be encouraged as long as the mother wants to conform to them and she and the baby suffer no ill effects. The nurse needs to determine if a woman is using any folk medicine during the postpartum period because active ingredients in folk medicine may have adverse physiologic effects on the patient when ingested with prescribed medicines (Lea, 1994). Also, the nurse should not assume that a mother desires to use traditional health practices that represent a particular cultural group merely because she is a member of that culture. Many young women who are first-generation or second-generation Americans follow their cultural traditions only when older family members are present or not at all.

Nursing needs to be culturally relevant. As in planning care to meet physiologic needs, standardized care plans must be adapted to meet the specific needs of the individual families. The nurse needs to be open and to continue to learn about how best to meet the health needs of childbearing women with diverse cultural backgrounds.

The nurse functions in the roles of teacher, encourager, and supporter rather than doer while implementing the psychosocial plan of care for a postpartum patient. Implementation of the psychosocial care plan involves carrying out specific activities to achieve the expected outcomes of care planned for each individual patient.

Promoting parental acquaintance, bonding and attachment, and parenting skills are discussed in Chapter 18.

Evaluation

The nurse can be reasonably assured that care was effective if expected outcomes for care for psychosocial needs have been met.

▌DISCHARGE TEACHING

Self-Care, Signs of Complications

Bridging the gap between hospital and home care requires sensitive and knowledgeable nursing care. Discharge planning begins at the time of admission to the unit and should be reflected in the plan of care developed for each individual patient. For example, a great deal of time during the hospital stay is usually spent in teaching about maternal and newborn care because all women must be capable of providing basic care for themselves and their infants at the time of discharge. It is also crucial that every woman be taught to recognize physical signs and symptoms that might indicate problems and how to obtain advice and assistance quickly if these signs appear. The Signs of Potential Complications box on p. 427 lists several common indications of maternal physical problems in the postpartum period. Before discharge, women also need basic instruction regarding the resumption of intercourse, prescribed medications, routine mother-baby checkups, and contraception.

Just before the time of discharge, the nurse reviews the woman's chart (audits the chart) to see that laboratory reports, medications, signatures, and so on are in order. Some hospitals have a checklist to follow before the woman's discharge. The nurse verifies that medications, if ordered, have arrived on the unit, that any valuables kept secured during the woman's stay have been returned to her and that she has signed a receipt for them, and that the infant is ready to be discharged.

The nurse is careful not to administer any medication that would make the mother sleepy if she is the one who will be holding the baby on the way out of the hospital. In most instances the woman is seated in a wheelchair and is usually given the baby to hold. Some families leave unescorted and ambulatory, depending on hospital protocol. The woman's possessions are gathered and taken out with her and her family; usually they are placed on some type of cart or carried by family members. *The woman's and the baby's identification bands are carefully checked.* As the woman and the baby are assisted into the car, the nurse should make sure that there is a car seat in which to secure the baby.

| LEGAL TIP | Early Discharge

> *Whether or not the woman and her family have chosen early discharge, the nurse and the primary care provider are held responsible if the woman is discharged before her condition has stabilized within normal limits. If complications occur, the medical and nursing staff could be sued for abandonment.*

Sexual Activity

Many couples resume sexual activity before the traditional postpartum checkup 6 weeks after childbirth. Risk of hemorrhage and infection are minimal approximately 2 weeks postpartum. Couples may be anxious about the topic but feel uncomfortable and unwilling to bring it up. It is important that the nurse discuss the physical and psychologic effects that giving birth can have on lovemaking. The Home Care box contains helpful information about the resumption of sexual intercourse. Current contraceptive options are discussed in detail in Chapter 7.

Prescribed Medications

Most patients have at least one medication prescribed for their use after discharge. Many health care providers routinely have women continue to take their prenatal vitamins and iron during the 6-week postpartum period. It is especially important that women who are breastfeeding or who are discharged with a lower than normal hematocrit level take these medications as ordered. Women with extensive episiotomies (third or fourth degree) or vaginal lacerations are usually given stool softeners to take at home. Pain relief medications (analgesics or nonsteroidal antiinflammatory medications) may be prescribed, especially for women who had cesarean birth. The nurse should make certain that the patient knows the route, dosage, and frequency of all ordered medications and the common side effects.

Routine Mother and Baby Checkups

Women who have experienced uncomplicated vaginal births are still commonly scheduled for the traditional 6-week postpartum examination. Patients who have had a cesarean birth are often seen in the health care provider's office or clinic 2 weeks after hospital discharge. The date and time for the follow-up appointment should be included in the discharge orders. If an appointment has not been made before the patient leaves the hospital, she should be encouraged to call the health care provider's office or clinic immediately and schedule an appointment herself.

HOME CARE *Patient Instructions for Self-Care*
Resumption of Sexual Intercourse

- You can safely resume sexual intercourse by the second to fourth week after birth when bleeding has stopped and the episiotomy has healed. For the first 6 weeks to 6 months, the vagina does not lubricate well.
- Your physiologic reactions to sexual stimulation for the first 3 months after birth will be slower and less intense. The strength of the orgasm is reduced.
- A water-soluble gel, cocoa butter, or a contraceptive cream or jelly might be recommended for lubrication. If some vaginal tenderness is present, your partner can be instructed to insert one or more clean, lubricated fingers into the vagina and rotate them within the vagina to help relax it and to identify possible areas of discomfort. A position in which you have control of the depth of the insertion of the penis also is useful. The side-by-side or female-on-top position may be more comfortable.
- The presence of the baby influences postbirth lovemaking. Parents hear every sound made by the baby; conversely you may be concerned that the baby hears every sound you make. In either case, any phase of the sexual response cycle may be interrupted by hearing the baby cry or move, leaving both of you frustrated and unsatisfied. In addition, the amount of psychologic energy expended by you in child care activities may lead to fatigue. Newborns require a great deal of attention and time.
- Some women have reported feeling sexual stimulation and orgasms when nursing their babies. Nursing mothers often are interested in returning to sexual activity before nonnursing mothers.
- You should be instructed to correctly perform the Kegel exercises to strengthen your pubococcygeal muscle. This muscle is associated with bowel and bladder function and with vaginal feeling during intercourse.

Parents who have not already done so need to make plans for newborn follow-up at the time of discharge. Most offices and clinics like to see newborns for an initial examination within the first week or by 2 weeks of age. Again, if an appointment for a specific date and time was not made for the infant before leaving the hospital, the parents should be encouraged to call the office or clinic right away.

Follow-up after Discharge

Increasingly, postpartum care is being rendered in the home setting as postbirth hospital stays have become shorter. Maternity nurses play a key role in ensuring ongoing safe and effective care for the mother and her baby until the infant is 1 year old (Perinatal Health: Strategies for the 21st Century, 1992).

Home care is one delivery component available along the perinatal continuum of care (see Fig. 3-2). This continuum begins with family planning and preconception, then prenatal, intrapartum, postpartum, and newborn care, and finally interconceptional and infant care. This perspective of perinatal care provides a basis for analyzing the quality of care, maternal-newborn outcomes, cost, and use of health care resources over the long term. Because the health care status of pregnant women can change at any point on this continuum, regular or high-technologic home health care may be required at some time during the prenatal or postpartum periods. The need for home care can occur at any time on the perinatal care continuum, not merely following hospitalization (although this may be the case for many conditions).

As maternity care continues to consist of frequent and brief contact with health care providers throughout the prenatal and postpartum periods, nurses are developing innovative nursing delivery methods and innovative ways to communicate that care is provided. The Association of Women's Health, Obstetric, and Neonatal Nurses (AWHONN) (1994) published guidelines for postpartum home care that has helped design comprehensive perinatal home care follow-up services.

Bakewell-Sachs and Persily (1995) and Brooten (1995) discussed the need for the development of a variety of services linking maternity patients throughout the perinatal continuum of care, especially for postpartum families discharged early (in the fourth trimester) when rapid physiologic and psychosocial transitions are occurring. Programs offering a variety of postpartum follow-up services include the following:

- Early discharge preparatory classes
- Telephone follow-up
- Warm lines and help lines
- Home visiting programs
- Parent support groups
- Infant feeding resource centers
- Perinatal home care

Although postpartum follow-up services may be offered by hospitals, maternity centers, home care agencies, public health agencies, private physicians, or entrepreneurs, it is the nursing profession that is a constant presence in this care. The common goal of these services is to ensure that the mother, newborn, and family have an optimal opportunity to prepare for and enjoy safe, comprehensive, and quality perinatal care.

Telephone follow-up

As part of the routine follow-up of a woman and her infant after discharge from the hospital, many providers are implementing one or more postpartum telephone follow-up calls to their patients for assessment, health teaching, identification of complications to effect timely intervention, and referrals. Telephone follow-up may be part of the services offered by the hospital, private physician or clinic, or a private agency and may be either a separate service or combined with other strategies for extending postpartum care. If no home care follow-up is provided, then telephone follow-up may take its place. If the family has a home care visit, this follow-up is incorporated into that care.

The purpose of the telephone follow-up calls should be explained to the family before discharge from the hospital. A mutually agreeable time is scheduled for the initial call. The ideal time for a telephone call varies according to family needs (Wilkerson, 1996). In some cases the most appropriate time for the initial call might be within the first few hours after discharge to ascertain that the homecoming has not been a problem. In other situations, 1 to 3 days after discharge might be the most appropriate time for the call (Evans, 1995). The number of calls and the time intervals between calls will vary based on the family's assessed need and other strategies being provided.

All therapeutic dialogue between nurse and patient, including that by telephone, is purposeful and goal directed. This is not a social call even though there may be some small talk when reestablishing rapport between the nurse and patient. During the telephone follow-up, the nurse will ask questions with the following goals (Fig. 17-9):

- To obtain evidence of the mother's physiologic recovery, comfort, and rest
- To determine evidence of psychologic well-being of the mother, including the presence of crisis-preventing balancing factors
- To obtain selected evidence of physiologic adaptation in the newborn
- To establish the perceived level of parental adjustment to parenthood and the stresses inherent in the early fourth trimester
- To identify learning needs of the family
- To determine the extent to which a relationship is being formed between the newborn, siblings, parents, and grandparents
- To explore areas that are sources of special concerns or challenges, as well as place unsettling demands on family members

In opening the conversation, the nurse should reintroduce herself to family members and reinforce the reason for the telephone call. The nurse should ask if the call has been made at a convenient time; otherwise, the effectiveness of the call is questionable. For example, a mother who has just settled a fussy baby and is attempting to relax herself would not be well served by a follow-up call at this time. Furthermore, mone common courtesy dictates that nurses determine whether the call is an unwelcome interruption, for whatever reason. If so, a more suitable time should be mutually set.

The focus and content of a follow-up call is determined in the discharge summary or records from the postpartum hospital stay. Use of discharge notes to guide the assessment ensures that an area of particular concern is not overlooked. An additional advantage is in the personalization and sense of warmth and regard such an approach communicates. For example, rather than asking how other children are reacting to the new baby, the nurse can ask specifically, "How is

Doctors Medical Center
1441 Florida Ave.
Modesto, CA 95350

48-HR TELEPHONE FOLLOW-UP

Address _____

P.O. Box _____ City _____ Zip _____

Telephone [HOME _____ | MESSAGE _____]

Support Person _____

Primary Language _____

Delivery Date _____ Discharge Date _____

Childbirth Educator _____

Obstetrician _____ Cty Clinic ☐ Cty FP ☐

Pediatrician _____ Cty Clinic ☐ Cty FP ☐

MATERNAL HISTORY	NEWBORN HISTORY

Grav____ Para____ Ab____ Still-birth____ Living Child____

Del: Vag ☐ Epis ☐ Cesarean ☐ VBAC ☐

Miscarriage ☐ Stillbirth ☐ Neonatal Death ☐

Discharge Medications _____

Low Hgb ☐ Diabetic ☐ ↑ BP ☐ Infection ☐ BTL ☐

CONCERNS:

Newborn's Legal Name _____ Sex: F M
(FIRST) (LAST)

Birth Weight _____ Breastfeeding ☐ Bottle Feeding ☐

Newborn Nursery ☐ ICN/CCN ☐ Diagnosis _____

Newborn discharge with mother Yes ☐ No ☐

DISCHARGE NURSE: _____

Checklists

MATERNAL
Breasts
Engorgement
Nipples
Perineum
Sitz baths
Cleansing
Vaginal Discharge
Hemorrhoids
Voiding/Bowel Mvmt.
Fluids/Nutrition
Abd Incision
Pain
Medications
Rest/Sleep
Psychosocial
Birth Control
NEWBORN
Feeding
Breast
Bottle
Frequency
Tolerance
Sleep Patterns
Voiding/Stooling
Circumcision
Cord Care
Skin
Rashes
Jaundice
Infant Care
Infant CPR Referral

How do you feel? _____

Call Made   Date/Time/Initial _____

_____ ☐ Postcard Sent Date _____

Problems Identified _____

_____
_____
_____
_____
_____
_____

Follow-up Plan/Appointments _____

_____
_____
_____
_____
_____
_____
_____
_____
_____
_____

C.C.   Nurse Calling

1. _____   2. _____

CHART

Fig. **17-9** Postpartum telephone follow-up form. (Courtesy Doctors Medical Center, Modesto, Calif.)

Leslie responding to his new brother?" or, "Is your Mom still with you or has she gone back to South Carolina?" The latter question shows more interest than "Who is helping you at home?"

The nurse allows the conversation to develop as naturally as possible so that the woman does not feel rushed or interrupted as rapport is established. This will be particularly important if the telephone caller is not the nurse who cared for the family in the health care facility. A natural progression has the additional advantage of revealing cues, such as the topic the mother chooses to address first, which often indicates her area of greatest concern. Open-ended questions facilitate the telephone interaction most effectively, such as, "How are things going since you left the hospital? You mentioned frequent headaches since you got home. Tell me more about those." Or "How are you and Peter collaborating on the baby's care?" Because specific assessment data about the mother, infant, and family are necessary, the nurse eventually will guide the assessment to these areas so that the aforementioned goals for the call can be met.

An effective postpartum telephone follow-up should assess the physiologic and psychologic well-being of mother and infant and the transitions each family member is making to the new lifestyle and changes in the family configuration. To determine the crisis potential in the family, the nurse is careful to address each of the balancing factors. Consider, for example, the nurse making a return call to check on the status of a new mother who has been experiencing sore nipples. At an earlier call, the nurse had reinforced teaching about varying the infant's position on the breast to minimize stress to the nipple and had referred the mother to La Leche League. Today the nurse moves quickly to an assessment of the balancing factors, starting with "How have things been going since we spoke last?" Depending on the answer, the nurse may address a second factor by asking, "What have you been able to try?" After hearing the answer, the nurse might follow up by asking, "And how is that working?" The nurse would determine if the mother has called La Leche and how productive this intervention has been. Additional teaching or referral, possibly to the primary caregiver, may be necessary at this time.

The primary interventions available to providers extending care by telephone include patient advocacy, education, reassurance and positive feedback, corrective feedback, supportive counseling, anticipatory guidance, and referral. Interventions are selected on the basis of the findings yielded by a careful assessment and are provided in collaboration with the family.

Both the assessment data elicited and interventions employed during the postpartum follow-up call are recorded. Documentation serves both legal and reimbursement purposes.

Advantages and limitations. Telephone follow-up affords contact with the postpartum family during the vulnerable time when support and intervention may be particularly effective. Most patients can be reached by telephone. Although calls are more cost-effective than home visits, they are limited by the indirect nature of the assessment. If the mother's perception of her well-being (or that of the newborn or family) is inaccurate or falsely reported, problems may be missed, and intervention will not be based on relevant data. Also, visual aids and hands on demonstrations cannot be used for clarifying and reinforcing information (Evans, 1995). This disadvantage can be overcome by combining both strategies: telephone calls and home visits.

Planning and documentation plus the conversation can take 20 to 30 minutes per call. Consequently, there is a limit to the number of calls that can be handled each day. In addition, the effectiveness of telephone calls to postpartum women is limited by the telephone skills and listening ability of the caller and by the comfort the mother experiences in providing personal data to the faceless caller.

This service is further dependent on families having access to a phone. If the family does not have a phone, other services need to be implemented to meet the needs of the family.

Warm lines and help lines

The **warm line** represents another type of telephone link between the new family and concerned caregivers or experienced parent volunteers. Warm line services sometimes are best understood in contrast to hot lines, which may be more familiar to new parents. For example, they might have seen advertisements of hot lines in their area that provide emergency help to prevent suicide or child abuse.

In contrast, a **warm line** is a helpline or consultation service, not a crisis intervention line. The warm line is appropriately used for dealing with less extreme concerns that may seem urgent at the time the call is placed but are not actual emergencies. Calls to warm lines commonly relate to infant feeding, prolonged crying, or sibling rivalry. One new mother called because she noticed a drop of blood on her daughter's diaper. Once given the reason for the blood and informed that its presence was normal, she was appropriately reassured. Another mother called to talk about how it felt when her 4-year-old son screamed out, "I hate you and I hate that baby." Warm line services may extend beyond the fourth trimester. Even parents with adolescent children may profit from the helping relationship of a warm line. Families need to call when concerns arise and be given phone numbers for easy access for answers to their questions.

People who answer warm line calls need to be good listeners who are empathic and able to use techniques such as open-ended questions, restating, and reflecting to encourage the caller to communicate. The caller is given an unhurried opportunity to share feelings or concerns. It is her story, and she is allowed to tell it in her own way. Questions are often used to clarify what the caller is saying.

The person answering the line assesses the caller for evidence of impending crisis by tactfully asking such questions as the following: "What is the situation or concern?" and "What has already been tried in order to cope? What resources are available?" Advice is not given; rather callers are helped to explore options available to them. Referrals may be made to support groups or to community agencies. When medical problems are identified, referrals are made to the appropriate physician. Williams and Cooper (1996) found that some of the major concerns of callers were about infant care and feeding, followed by need for pain management and reduction of anxiety for the mother.

Advantages and limitations. The primary advantage of the warm line is quick access to a good listener, whether nurse or trained volunteer, 24 hours a day, 365 days a year. Because it is an advertised helpline, couples may feel more comfortable and less intimidated about making the call.

Inasmuch as the warm line offers round-the-clock service, there are potential difficulties in staffing. When a limited staffing necessitates use of an answering machine or message service, the resource is less effective. Having to leave a message negates the advantage of immediate access. Although some people welcome the anonymity of a faceless listener, they may be less willing to leave a recorded message.

The cost of the warm line is minimal if volunteers are used; the only costs are the telephone service itself and advertisement. The financial commitment obviously increases when any of the staff members are salaried.

For some nurses who staff such phone lines, the inability to evaluate the effectiveness of their interventions is frustrating. There are generally no provisions for follow-up with the caller to determine the extent to which the problem has been resolved, if at all (Evans, 1995).

Home follow-up

Many discharge programs are making postpartum home visits a standard part of perinatal care (Williams & Cooper, 1996), and they are a vital component of such care. The referral form for the home care agency is completed by the hospital and submitted to the agency on the day of the woman's discharge (Fig. 17-10). This ensures that there is no delay in the follow-up services. The hospital also gives the family the name of the agency and its phone number as part of the list of resources to contact in the event certain needs arise.

Upon receipt of the referral form, the home care agency verifies the manner of reimbursement for the home visit (unless payment for the visit is bundled with a pregnancy or labor/birth reimbursement package). This information is communicated to the family.

The day after discharge, the home care agency contacts the mother to screen for maternal and newborn complica-

tions. This phone interview also helps the mother and nurse determine the most appropriate day to schedule the home visit.

The home visit is most commonly scheduled on the woman's second day home from the hospital, but it may be scheduled on the first, third, or fourth day home, depending on the individual family's situation and needs. Additional visits are planned throughout the first week, as needed. The home visits may be extended beyond that time if the family's needs warrant it and if a home visit is the most appropriate option for carrying out the follow-up care required to meet the specific needs identified.

A home visit progresses more effectively if it is pre-planned and well organized. In advance, the nurse reviews the hospital's discharge summary, teaching plan, and any other records, including the physician's orders; this serves to structure the interview and physical assessment and hence provide continuity of care. Before the visit, the nurse also obtains directions to the family's home and gets a map, if necessary. The protocol for a postpartum home visit is summarized in Box 3-2.

Support groups

Humans are inherently social beings, involved on a daily basis in some kind of group—groups of family members, classmates, co-workers, and friends. Education, work, worship, and leisure time often take place in groups. Thus at times of difficult transitions, it seems reasonable for people to turn to groups for support. Nurses are generally familiar with the benefits of support groups for such diverse groups as the newly divorced or widowed people, those recently diagnosed with acquired immunodeficiency syndrome (AIDS) or cancer, and those undergoing mastectomy, colostomy or recovering from heart attack. In obstetrics, those who have experienced a miscarriage or early infant death may also seek out support groups.

A special group experience is sometimes sought by the woman adjusting to motherhood. On occasion, postpartum women who have met earlier in prenatal clinics or on the hospital unit may begin to associate for mutual support. Members of Lamaze classes who attend a postpartum reunion may decide to extend their relationship during the fourth trimester. Realizing the value of group support, nurses may wish to make postpartum support groups available as a strategy for bridging the hospital and home experience.

A **postpartum support group** enables parents to share in and support each other as they adjust to parenting. For example, new parents often report surprise at the amount of fatigue they initially experience. Schedules must be readjusted and priorities realigned to accommodate infant care and interruptions in sleep. It is not uncommon for the new mother to find it difficult even to schedule time for her own shower. One first-time mother told of being amazed when her husband returned home from work and she realized

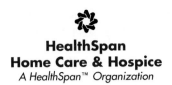

**HealthSpan
Home Care & Hospice**
A HealthSpan™ Organization

**POSTPARTUM
HOME CARE REFERRAL**

Mother's Name: _____

Address/phone where mother will be staying:

Address: _____

City: _____

Phone #: _____

Language spoken: ☐ English ☐ Other: _____

Understands English: ☐ Well ☐ Poor

☐ Mother Needs Interpreter ☐ Hearing Impaired

Who interpreted in hospital: _____

Mom agrees to this referral: ☐ Yes ☐ No

Currently being seen by PHN: ☐ Yes ☐ No

Mom's M.D./Midwife: _____

Phone #: _____

Next Appt: _____

MOTHER:

Gravida_____ T_____ P_____ A_____ L_____

Marital Status: S M W D Sep

Normal Maternal Exam: ☐ Yes ☐ No (explain below)

Epis/Incision: _____

Hgb pp: _____

Meds: _____

Allergies: _____

OTHER ISSUES:

Diabetic: _____

Other: _____

Psycho/Social Issues:

☐ Parent/Child Interaction ☐ Adolescent Mother

☐ Mental Health Status ☐ Drug Use/Dependency

☐ Previous Losses ☐ Hx of Family Abuse

☐ Developmentally Delayed Parents ☐ Limited Support System

☐ Other: _____

Husband/Significant Other: _____

Baby's Name: _____ ☐ M ☐ F

DOB/Time: _____

Mother's Discharge Date/Time: _____

Newborn Discharge Date (if different from mother's): _____

Baby's M.D. (Full Name): _____

Phone #: _____

Next Appt: _____

BABY:

Gestation: _____ Weeks ☐ Fetal Loss

Birth Weight: _____ Discharge Weight: _____

Apgars: 1" _____ 5" _____

Feeding Issues: _____

Feedings: Breast _____ Bottle _____

Normal Infant Exam: ☐ Yes ☐ No (explain below)

Circumcised: ☐ Yes ☐ No

Cord Clamp Off: ☐ Yes ☐ No

Voidings: ☐ Yes ☐ No

Stooling: ☐ Yes ☐ No

☐ Newborn screen was done in hospital—after baby 24 hours of age.

☐ Newborn screen to be drawn at clinic.

☐ Newborn screen to be drawn at home.

   ☐ Lab slip sent home with family.

ADDITIONAL COMMENTS or ABNORMAL FINDINGS FOR MOTHER OR BABY: _____

_____

_____

Faxed to Home Care ☐ Facesheet ☐ Referral *Referral Completed By:* _____

Fig. **17-10** Referral form. (Copyright HealthSpan Home Care and Hospice of Allina Health System, St. Paul, Minn.)

that she had not found time to change out of her night-gown and robe that day. A father expressed his fatigue in this way: "It never ceases to amaze me that an 8-pound baby girl can wear down a 200-pound father and a 136-pound mother."

Often in a postpartum support group, an experienced mother can impart concrete information that can be valuable to other group members. For example, one new mother shared the use of her husband's socks with the toe cut out. Sliding the sock over her left arm provided enough traction to keep the wet, soapy baby from slipping off the supporting arm while she gave the infant his bath. Another new mother shared her nurse-midwife's advice to place warm (not hot), newly brewed tea bags on sore nipples. The warmth and the tannic acid in the tea promote comfort and healing, respectively. An inexperienced mother may find herself imitating the behavior of someone in the group whom she perceives as particularly capable. She may imitate someone's way of positioning a baby or find herself folding her daughter's diapers differently after watching someone else's technique.

Referrals

The **referral process** is an essential part of comprehensive, continuous patient care and community health nursing.

Nurses who care for postpartum women are in a unique position to assess a woman's appropriateness for home health care.

The focus of nursing assessment includes the woman's physical and psychologic status, her level of knowledge about self-care activities, her willingness to learn, the availability of caregivers and social support in the home, and her level of comfort with home care. If the referral is for a mother and infant home care visit, then the nursing assessment should include newborn data. The content of the newborn assessment includes physical status, physiologic adjustment to extrauterine environment, normalcy of physical and behavioral findings, and ability of the parents to meet the infant's needs. These data provide baseline information at the time of the home care nurse referral.

Community resources

To develop an effective referral system, it is important that the nurse have an understanding of the needs of the patient and family and of the organization and community resources that are available for meeting those needs. Locating and compiling information about available community services contributes to the development of a referral system. It is important for the nurse to develop his or her own resource file of services that are frequently used by health care providers.

The nurse can begin by gathering existing information from community resources such as the local health department, library, or church; local resource agencies such as Planned Parenthood, HAND, or La Leche League; and major service organizations such as March of Dimes, American Red Cross, and WIC Supplemental Nutrition Program. Also, national perinatal organizations such as Nursing Mothers Counsel, Depression After Delivery-National, Postpartum Support, International, Positive Pregnancy and Parenting Fitness, National Perinatal Association, and Child Welfare League of America can be helpful. These services can provide published resource guides and lists of community service agencies specific to the group or condition that they represent (McGuire, Gerber, & Clemen-Stone, 1996; Perinatal Resources, 1997).

RESEARCH
Postpartum Teaching Priorities

Health education is an important part of maternal-child nursing care. During the postpartum period, nurses educate mothers about health behaviors that enhance positive maternal-infant outcomes, especially those related to self and infant care. Nurses and patients set goals together and plan the process of implementation to maximize goal achievement and mutual satisfaction. Mothers tend to be eager learners who can identify their own learning needs. This often results in misalignment of teaching priorities. Literature suggests that perceptions of maternal learning needs differ between mothers and nurses. In this study, mothers' and nurses' perceptions of postpartum learning needs and effective teaching modalities were compared. A convenience sample of 236 mothers and 82 nurses were asked to complete a 44-item questionnaire to assess perceived learning needs of mother and infant care topics. Mothers were given a questionnaire during their postpartum stay before discharge and nurses rated similar items on the basis of their perception of what is most important for mothers to learn during their postpartum stay. Mothers and nurses agreed that topics related to immediate physical health needs were most important. Unmarried mothers considered topics related to personal care and mobility as most important. First-time mothers rated more topics as important than did experienced mothers. Individual teaching was rated most effective by both groups. The study supports postpartum education that focuses on the physical needs of mothers and infants, as well as individual teaching models.

CLINICAL APPLICATION OF THE STUDY

Nurses cannot teach mothers about every topic of interest during the postpartum hospital stay. The immediate physical health needs of mothers and infants, as well as signs of illness, need to be addressed first. Nurses should assess individual learning needs of different groups of mothers and accommodate these needs whenever possible.

Source: Berger D & Loveland Cook C: Postpartum teaching priorities: the viewpoints of nurses and mothers, *J Obstet Gynecol Neonatal Nurs* 27(2):161, 1998.

KEY POINTS

- Postpartum care is modeled on the concept of health.
- Cultural beliefs and practices affect the patient's response to the puerperium.
- The nursing plan of care includes assessments to detect deviations from normal, comfort measures to relieve discomfort or pain and safety measures to prevent injury or infection.
- The nurse provides teaching and counseling measures designed to promote the patient's feelings of competence in self-care and baby care.
- The nurse must exhibit both clinical and decision-making skills to provide safe and effective physical care. Common nursing interventions include evaluating and treating the boggy uterus and the full urinary bladder, providing for pharmacologic and nonpharmacologic relief of pain and discomfort associated with the episiotomy or lacerations, and instituting measures to promote or suppress lactation.
- Nurses can help to promote the health of the patient's future pregnancies and children by administering rubella vaccine and Rh immune globulin if indicated.
- Meeting the psychosocial needs of new mothers involves planning care that takes into consideration the composition and functioning of the entire family.
- Early postpartum discharge will continue to be the trend as a result of consumer demand, medical necessity, discharge criteria for low-risk childbirth, and cost-containment measures.
- The short-stay option in perinatal care is safer when selection criteria are used to determine a woman's eligibility for early discharge and when home care follow-up is available.
- Early discharge classes, postpartum telephone follow-up, home visits, warm lines and help lines, support groups, referrals, and community resources—used either individually or in combination—are effective means of preventing crisis and facilitating physiologic and psychologic adjustments in the postpartum period.
- Postpartum follow-up programs are most effective when planned on the basis of needs assessment and when revised on the basis of the access to the program and the cost and quality of the program.

CRITICAL THINKING EXERCISES

1 *Tina is a primigravida, 15 years old, and she gave birth to an 8 pound girl 24 hours ago. Physically, she is meeting all expected outcomes. However, Tina is having difficulty breastfeeding and is uncertain about how to bathe and care for the baby. She seems to have difficulty recognizing the baby's cues. Tina is also in need of baby clothes and equipment (e.g., car seat). Tina plans to stay with her parents while she continues her high school education and is eager to go home as soon as possible to see her friends.*

  a *Determine if Tina would be eligible for early home discharge and explain why.*

  b *Develop a home care discharge plan for Tina.*

  c *Discuss the type of follow-up postpartum home care services needed to ensure a continuum of comprehensive postpartum care for Tina.*

  d *Identify existing community resources that you would suggest to Tina and explain your rationale.*

  e *What does the nurse need to consider in order to make the referral with Tina more successful?*

2 *Mrs. Chow is a Chinese primipara who has a temperature of 37.8° C 12 hours after birth. The nurse noticed that Mrs. Chow has not gotten up, is covered with several blankets and a robe, and has not taken any liquids or eaten much food on her food tray. The nursing staff members tell you to make her follow the physician's order for activity, that is, to get out of bed as needed and to perform self-care activities.*

  a *Identify five cultural issues that are in conflict in this situation.*

  b *List several culturally sensitive nursing diagnoses.*

  c *Discuss how the nurse could approach and communicate with Mrs. Chow to facilitate understanding and modification of care.*

  d *List several nursing interventions that incorporate Mrs. Chow's cultural practices and promote safe, postpartum recovery.*

3 *You made a follow-up telephone call 48 hours after Mrs. Lamada has been discharged from the hospital. In addition to the new baby boy, Mrs. Lamada has a 2-year-old daughter. Your telephone assessment reveals the following findings: Mrs. Lamada reports the following:*

  —The 2-year-old is "clinging" to her all of the time and has wet her underpants several times.

Continued

CRITICAL THINKING EXERCISES—cont'd

—*The infant looks yellowish and is not breastfeeding well.*

—*She is not sure how to care for the baby's circumcision.*

—*She is not getting any rest and is very tired.*

—*Her husband is unable to help.*

For each of the identified problems, do the following:

a *Formulate and prioritize several nursing diagnoses.*

b *Plan and prioritize patient-centered goals and expected outcomes.*

c *Choose interventions that include appropriate referrals and community resources and indicate rationales for them.*

d *Discuss how a nurse could evaluate the effectiveness of her telephone care plan.*

References

American Academy of Pediatrics & American College of Obstetricians and Gynecologists: *Guidelines for Perinatal Care,* ed 3, Elk Grove Village, Ill, 1997, American Academy of Pediatrics.

Association of Women's Health, Obstetric, and Neonatal Nurses (AWHONN): *Didactic content and clinical skills verification for professional nurse providers of perinatal home care,* Washington, DC, 1994, AWHONN.

Bakewell-Sachs S & Persily C: Perinatal partnerships in practice: a conceptual framework for giving care across the childbearing continuum, *J Perinat Neonat Nurs* 9(1):31, 1995.

Bragg E et al.: The effect of an early postpartum discharge program on maternal readmission rate in a tertiary medical center, *J Perinatol* 17(3):254, 1997.

Britton J, Britton H & Beebe S: Early discharge of the term newborn: a continued dilemma, *Pediatrics* 94(1):3, 1994.

Brooten D: Perinatal care across the continuum: early discharge and nursing home follow-up, *J Perinat Neonat Nurs* 9(1):38, 1995.

Carty E & Bradley C: A randomized, controlled evaluation of early postpartum hospital discharge, *Birth* 17(4):100, 1990.

D'Avanzo C: Bridging the cultural gap with Southeast Asians, *MCN Am J Matern Child Nurs* 17(4):204, 1992.

Edmonson M, Stoddard J & Owens L: Hospital readmission with feeding-related problems after early postpartum discharge of normal newborns, *JAMA* 278(4):299, 1997.

Edwards M: The crisis of the fourth trimester, *Birth Fam J* 1:19, 1974.

Evans C: Postpartum home care in the United States, *J Obstet Gynecol Neonatal Nurs* 24(2):180, 1995.

Ferguson S & Engelhard C: Maternity length of stay and public policy: issues and implications, *J Pediatr Nurs* 11(6):392, 1996.

Harrison L: Patient education in early postpartum discharge programs, *MCN Am J Matern Child Nurs* 15(1):39, 1990.

Havens D & Hannan C: Legislation to mandate maternal and newborn length of stay, *J Pediatr Health Care* 10(3):141, 1996.

Horn B: Cultural concepts and postpartal care, *J Transcult Nurs* 2(1):48, 1990.

Jambunathan J: Hmong cultural practices and beliefs: the postpartum period, *Clin Nurs Res* 4(3):335, 1995.

Jiménez S: The Hispanic culture, folklore, and perinatal health, *J Perinatal Educ* 4(1):9, 1995.

Johnson & Johnson: *Compendium of postpartum care,* Skillman, NJ, 1996, Johnson & Johnson Consumer Products, Inc.

Lea A: Nursing in today's multicultural society: a transcultural perspective, *J Adv Nurs* 20(2):307, 1994.

Lipson J, Dibble S & Minarik P: *Culture & nursing care: a pocket guide,* San Francisco, 1996, UCSF Nursing Press.

Liu L et al.: The safety of newborn early discharge, *JAMA* 278(4):293, 1997.

Luengenbiehl D: Standardized assessment of blood loss, *MCN Am J Matern Child Nurs* 15(4):241, 1990.

Lukacs A: Issues surrounding early postpartum discharge: effects on the caregiver, *J Perinat Neonat Nurs* 5(1):33, 1991.

Park K & Peterson L: Beliefs, practices, and experiences of Korean women in relation to childbirth, *Health Care Women Int* 12:261, 1991.

Perinatal health: strategies for the 21st century, Maternal and Child Health Bureau, Washington, DC, 1992.

Perinatal resources: publications and organizations, *J Perinatal Educ* 6(2):61, 1997.

Pugh L & Milligan R: Patterns of fatigue during childbearing, *Appl Nurs Res* 8(3):140, 1995.

Roberts K: A comparison of chilled cabbage leaves and chilled gel-paks in reducing breast engorgement. *J Hum Lact* 11(1):17, 1995.

Sampselle C & Miller J: Pelvic muscle exercise: effective patient teaching, *The Female Patient,* 21:29, 1996.

Schneiderman J: Postpartum nursing for Korean mothers, *MCN Am J Matern Child Nurs* 21(3):155, 1996.

Simpson K & Creehan P: *AWHONN's perinatal nursing,* Philadelphia, 1996, Lippincott.

Spector R: Cultural concepts of women's health and health-promoting behaviors, *J Obstet Gynecol Neonatal Nurs* 24(3):241, 1995.

Welt S et al.: Feasibility of postpartum rapid hospital discharge: a study from a community hospital population, *Am J Perinatol* 10(5):384, 1993.

Wilkerson N: Appraisal of early discharge programs, *J Perinatal Educ* 5(2):1, 1996.

Williams L & Cooper M: A new paradigm for postpartum care, *J Obstet Gynecol Neonatal Nurs* 25(9):745, 1996.

CHAPTER

18

Adaptation to Parenthood

LIENNE D. EDWARDS

LEARNING OBJECTIVES

- *Define the key terms.*
- *Describe the two components of the parenting process.*
- *Discuss five preconditions that influence attachment.*
- *Describe the sensual responses that strengthen attachment.*
- *Differentiate the three periods in parental role change after childbirth.*
- *Identify infant behaviors that facilitate and inhibit parental attachment.*
- *Identify behaviors of the three phases of maternal adjustment.*
- *Explain paternal adjustment.*
- *Discuss three ways to facilitate parent-infant adjustment.*
- *Discuss maternal age (adolescence and over 35) as a factor influencing parental response.*
- *Describe sibling adaptation.*
- *Describe grandparent adaptation.*
- *Discuss nursing care management for assisting adaptation to parenthood.*

KEY TERMS

acquaintance
attachment
biorhythmicity
bonding
claiming process
en face
engrossment
entrainment
fourth trimester
infant-parent interaction
 rhythm
  repertoire of behaviors
  responsivity
letting-go phase
maternal adjustment
paternal adjustment
postpartum blues
reciprocity
sibling rivalry
synchrony
taking-hold phase
taking-in phase
transition to parenthood

Becoming a parent creates a period of change and instability for all men and women who decide to have children. This holds true whether parenthood is biologic or adoptive and whether the parents are married husband-wife couples, cohabiting couples, single mothers, single fathers, lesbian couples with one woman as biologic mother, or gay male couples who adopt a child. To promote adaptation to parenthood, parents need behaviors and skills to deal with the changes and disequilibrium caused by parenthood. Parents must explore their relationship with the infant and redefine the relationship between themselves. Parents must adjust their own lives to include the infant, while older siblings must adjust to the infant's claim on parental time and love. A thorough understanding of the process parents go through during their transition to parenthood guides the nurse in helping family members adapt.

PARENTING PROCESS

During pregnancy the mother provides an environment in which her unborn child develops and grows. This close, symbiotic union ends with birth. At this point, other people assume partial or complete involvement in the infant's care. Whoever assumes the parental role—woman or man, biologic or adoptive—enters into a crucial relationship with the child that persists throughout the life of each. Parenthood is optional. For children, however, parenthood is all important; their continued existence depends on the quality of care they receive.

Sank (1991) describes parenting as a process of role attainment and role transition that begins during pregnancy. The transition ends when the parent develops a sense of comfort and confidence in performing the parental role. The parenting process has two components.

449

The first component in the process of parenting includes knowledge of and skill in child care activities such as feeding, holding, clothing, and bathing the infant and protecting the infant from harm. The ability to competently and confidently perform these task-oriented activities does not appear automatically with the birth of a child. Many parents must learn to do these tasks, and this learning process can be difficult. However, almost all parents become adept in caregiving activities when they have the desire to learn and the support of others.

The second component, valuing and comfort, includes an attitude of tenderness, awareness, and concern for the infant's needs and desires. This component of parenting profoundly affects the manner in which the practical aspects of child care are performed and the emotional response of the child to the care. A positive parent-child relationship is mutually rewarding.

Nurses can enable inexperienced parents to feel confident and competent in their new roles. They can provide opportunities for parents to practice child care tasks in the hospital, birth setting, or in the home, where assistance and feedback are available. Nursing approaches and strategies can enhance parents' self-concept by helping them feel more comfortable and confident in their parenting skills.

▌ PARENTAL ATTACHMENT, BONDING, AND ACQUAINTANCE

Although much research has been directed toward unraveling the process by which a parent comes to love and accept a child and a child comes to love and accept a parent, researchers still do not know what motivates and commits parents and children to decades of supportive and nurturing care of each other. This process is referred to as **attachment.**

Using the terms *attachment* and *bonding*, Klaus and Kennell initially proposed that the period shortly after birth was important to mother-infant attachment (Klaus et al., 1972). They defined the phenomenon of **bonding** as a sensitive period in the first minutes and hours after birth when mothers and fathers must have close contact with their infants for optimum later development (Klaus & Kennell, 1976). Subsequently, Klaus and Kennell (1982) revised their theory of parent-infant bonding and acknowledged the adaptability of human parents, stating it took longer than minutes or hours for parents to form an emotional relationship with their infants. The terms *attachment* and *bonding* continue to be used interchangeably.

The process of attachment has been described as linear—beginning during pregnancy, intensifying during the early postpartum period, having developmental periods of progress and regression, and being constant and consistent once established.

Researchers have documented that, for the attachment process to begin favorably, several conditions must exist. Parents need to be emotionally healthy to have compe-

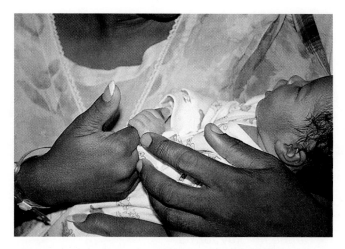

Fig. 18-1 Hands. (Courtesy Majorie Pyle, RNC, Lifecircle, Costa Mesa, Calif.)

tent communication and caregiving skills and to perceive social support from their partner, family, and friends. A parent-infant fit, relative to infant state, temperament, and gender, is also helpful. When any of these conditions are absent or distorted, nurses must intervene to facilitate the attachment process.

Attachment is developed and maintained by proximity and interaction with the infant, through which the parent becomes acquainted with the infant, identifies the infant as an individual, and claims the infant as a member of the family. Attachment is facilitated by positive feedback (i.e., social, verbal, and nonverbal responses, whether real or perceived, that indicate acceptance of one partner by the other). Attachment occurs through a mutually satisfying experience. A mother commented on her son's grasp reflex, "I put my finger in his hand, and he grabbed right on. It is just a reflex, I know, but it felt good anyway" (Fig. 18-1).

A list of infant behaviors affecting parental attachment that continues to be a classic comprehensive reference is presented in Table 18-1. A corresponding list of parental behaviors that affect infant attachment is presented in Table 18-2.

An important part of attachment is **acquaintance** (Klaus & Kennell, 1983). Parents use eye contact (Fig. 18-2), touching, talking, and exploring to become acquainted with their infant during the immediate postpartum period. Adoptive parents undergo the same process when they first meet their new child. During this period, families engage in the **claiming process,** which is the identification of the new baby (Fig. 18-3). The child is first identified in terms of "likeness" to other family members, then in terms of "differences," and finally in terms of "uniqueness." The unique newcomer is thus incorporated into the family. Mothers and fathers scrutinize their infant carefully and point out characteristics that the child shares with other family members and that are indicative of a relationship between them.

TABLE 18-1 *Infant Behaviors Affecting Parental Attachment*

FACILITATING BEHAVIORS	INHIBITING BEHAVIORS
Visually alert; eye contact; tracking or following of parent's face	Sleepy; eyes closed most of the time; gaze aversion
Appealing facial appearance; randomness of body movements reflecting helplessness	Resemblance to person parent dislikes; hyperirritability or jerky body movements when touched
Smiles	Bland facial expression; infrequent smiles
Vocalization; crying only when hungry or wet	Crying for hours on end; colicky
Grasp reflex	Exaggerated motor reflex
Anticipatory approach behaviors for feedings; sucks well; feeds easily	Feeds poorly; regurgitates; vomits often
Enjoys being cuddled, held	Resists holding and cuddling by crying, stiffening body
Easily consolable	Inconsolable; unresponsive to parenting, caretaking tasks
Activity and regularity somewhat predictable	Unpredictable feeding and sleeping schedule
Attention span sufficient to focus on parents	Inability to attend to parent's face or offered stimulation
Differential crying, smiling, and vocalizing; recognizes and prefers parents	Shows no preference for parents over others
Approaches through locomotion	Unresponsive to parent's approaches
Clings to parent; puts arms around parent's neck	Seeks attention from any adult in room
Lifts arms to parents in greeting	Ignores parents

From Gerson E: *Infant behavior in the first year of life,* New York, 1973, Raven Press.

TABLE 18-2 *Parental Behaviors Affecting Infant Attachment*

FACILITATING BEHAVIORS	INHIBITING BEHAVIORS
Looks; gazes; takes in physical characteristics of infant; assumes *en face* position; eye contact	Turns away from infant; ignores infant's presence
Hovers; maintains proximity; directs attention to, points to infant	Avoids infant; does not seek proximity; refuses to hold infant when given opportunity
Identifies infant as unique individual	Identifies infant with someone parent dislikes; fails to discern any of infant's unique features
Claims infant as family member; names infant	Fails to place infant in family context or identify infant with family member; has difficulty naming
Touches; progresses from fingertip to fingers to palms to encompassing contact	Fails to move from fingertip touch to palmar contact and holding
Smiles at infant	Maintains bland countenance or frowns at infant
Talks to, coos, or sings to infant	Wakes infant when infant is sleeping; handles roughly; hurries feeding by moving nipple continuously
Expresses pride in infant	Expresses disappointment, displeasure in infant
Relates infant's behavior to familiar events	Does not incorporate infant into life
Assigns meaning to infant's actions and sensitively interprets infant's needs	Makes no effort to interpret infant's actions or needs
Views infant's behaviors and appearance in positive light	Views infant's behavior as exploiting, deliberately uncooperative; views appearance as distasteful, ugly

From Mercer R: Parent-infant attachment. In Sonstegard L et al, editors: *Women's health,* vol 2, *Childbearing,* New York, 1983, Grune & Stratton.

The claiming process is revealed by maternal comments such as the following: "Russ held him close and said, 'He's the image of his father,' but I found one part like me—his toes are shaped like mine."

On the other hand, some parents react negatively. They "claim" the infant in terms of the discomfort or pain the baby causes. They interpret the infant's normal responses as being negative toward them and react to the child with dislike or indifference. They do not hold the infant close or touch the infant for comforting.

Nurses play an important role in facilitating parental attachment (Fig. 18-4). They can enhance positive parent-infant contacts by heightening parental awareness of an infant's responses and ability to communicate. As parents attempt to become competent and loving in their role, nurses can bolster the parents' self-confidence and egos.

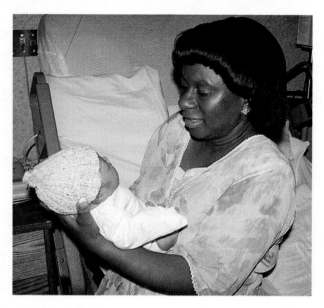

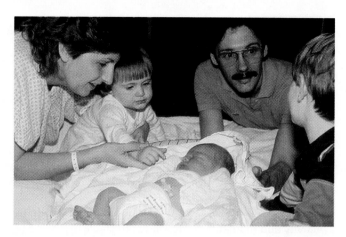

Fig. **18-3** Family members examine the new baby. They discuss how she resembles them and other family members. (Courtesy Marjorie Pyle, RNC, Lifecircle, Costa Mesa, Calif.)

Fig. **18-2** Mother and baby make eye contact in *en face* position. (Courtesy Marjorie Pyle, RNC, Lifecircle, Costa Mesa, Calif.)

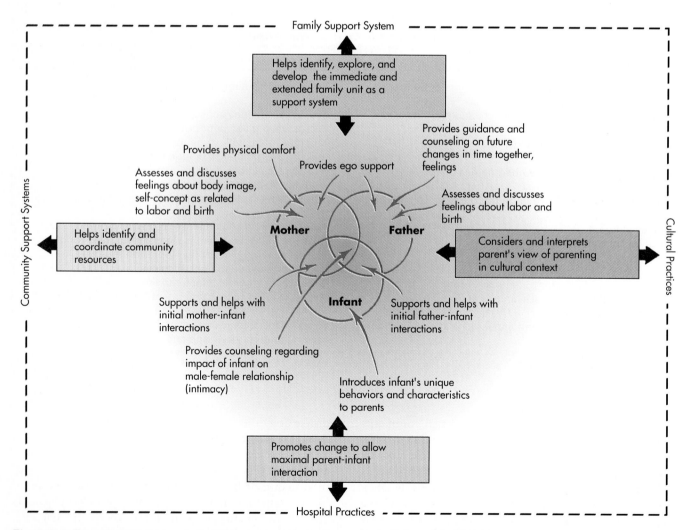

Family Support System

Helps identify, explore, and develop the immediate and extended family unit as a support system

Provides physical comfort

Provides ego support

Provides guidance and counseling on future changes in time together, feelings

Assesses and discusses feelings about body image, self-concept as related to labor and birth

Assesses and discusses feelings about labor and birth

Community Support Systems

Helps identify and coordinate community resources

Mother

Father

Cultural Practices

Considers and interprets parent's view of parenting in cultural context

Infant

Supports and helps with initial mother-infant interactions

Supports and helps with initial father-infant interactions

Provides counseling regarding impact of infant on male-female relationship (intimacy)

Introduces infant's unique behaviors and characteristics to parents

Promotes change to allow maximal parent-infant interaction

Hospital Practices

Fig. **18-4** The role of the nurse in facilitating parental attachment to the infant. (Modified from Mercer R: Parent-infant attachment. In Sonstegard L et al, editors: *Women's health*, vol 2, *Childbearing*, New York, 1983, Grune & Stratton.)

TABLE 18-3 *Examples of Parent-Infant Attachment Interventions*

INTERVENTION LABEL/ DEFINITION	CRITICAL ACTIVITIES	SUPPORTING ACTIVITIES
ATTACHMENT PROMOTION		
Facilitation of development of parent-infant relationship	Give parents opportunity to hold infant soon after birth Keep infant with parents after birth when possible	Provide rooming-in in hospital Provide pain relief for mother Provide opportunity for parents to see, hold, and examine newborn immediately after birth
ENVIRONMENTAL MANAGEMENT: ATTACHMENT PROCESS		
Manipulation of environment that facilitates development of parent-infant relationship	Allow for family visitation as desired Create environment that fosters privacy	Permit father/significant other to sleep in room with mother Provide rocking chair
FAMILY INTEGRITY PROMOTION: CHILDBEARING FAMILY		
Facilitation of growth of individuals or families who are adding infant to family	Convey accepting attitude (for nonthreatening environment for family to express feelings) Reinforce parenting behaviors	Offer to be listener for significant other Discuss sibling's reaction to newborn, as appropriate
LACTATION COUNSELING		
Use of interactive helping process to assist in maintenance of successful breastfeeding	Educate parents about infant feeding for informed decision making Give parents recommended education material, as needed	Provide information about advantages and disadvantages of breastfeeding Inform parents about appropriate classes or groups for breastfeeding
PARENT EDUCATION: CHILDBEARING FAMILY		
Preparation of individuals to perform their role as parents	Reinforce skills parent does well in caring for infant to promote confidence Assist parents in interpreting infant cues	Monitor learning needs of family Appraise parents' learning styles (how they learn best)
RISK IDENTIFICATION: CHILDBEARING FAMILY		
Identification of individuals or families who are likely to have difficulties in parenting and prioritization of strategies to prevent parenting problems	Review maternal history of chemical dependency, noting duration, type of drug(s), and time and strength of last dose before birth Monitor behaviors indicative of problem with attachment	Determine parents' feelings about unplanned pregnancy Determine economic, marital, and educational status of parents

From McCloskey J & Bulechek G: *Nursing interventions classification,* ed 2, St Louis, 1996, Mosby.

Nursing interventions related to the promotion of parent-infant attachment are numerous and varied. Six attachment-promotion intervention labels with critical and supporting nursing activities are presented in Table 18-3.

Nursing considerations for fostering parent-infant attachment among special populations may vary (Geissler, 1994; Symanski, 1992; Tedder, 1991). For example, economically disadvantaged mothers, especially adolescents, are not as likely to be aware of the benefits of bonding or to be knowledgeable of normal infant behaviors. These women may not be aware of maternity care options such as rooming-in, or they may be less assertive in asking for such options. The nurse needs to be a patient educator and advocate, explaining the choices and the potential benefits. The nurse should ensure a supportive, encouraging environment that will help mothers engage in positive interactions with their infants. The nurse can capture the mother's attention with a mother-infant interactional experience using the Brazelton Neonatal Behavioral Assessment Scale and, at the same time, increase the mother's knowledge of infant behavior. Written material can be provided after the assessment to reinforce the behavioral concepts.

Low-income mothers may have to contend with stressors that distract them from developing a relationship with their babies. Inability to pay for infant supplies or child care, chaotic home situations, and worry over eligibility for social and health care services deplete these women's psychologic energy.

Nurses need to conduct nonjudgmental, individual assessments of resources and social networks to avoid inaccurate and stereotypic assumptions. Nurses can help economically disadvantaged mothers access social services, such as the Women, Infants, and Children (WIC) program and Medicaid. For mothers whose home environments provide little or no support and multiple stressors, early discharge may not be optimal. Nurses can advocate for longer hospital stays for these mothers when the hospital environment is more conducive to bonding.

Childbearing practices and rituals of other cultures may not be congruent with standard practices associated with bonding in the Anglo-American culture. For example, Chinese families traditionally use extended family members to care for the newborn so that the mother can rest and recover, especially after a cesarean birth. Some Native American, Asian, and Hispanic women do not initiate breast-feeding until their breast milk comes in. Haitian families do not name their babies until after the confinement month. The amount of eye contact also varies among cultures. Yup'ik Eskimo mothers almost always position their babies so that eye contact can be made (Geissler, 1994).

Nurses should become knowledgeable of the childbearing beliefs and practices of diverse cultural and ethnic groups. Because individual cultural variations exist within groups, nurses need to clarify with the patient and family members or friends what cultural norms the patient follows. Incorrect judgments may be made about mother-infant bonding if nurses do not practice culturally sensitive care.

PARENT-INFANT CONTACT

Since the early 1970s consumers have strived for childbirth practices that promote the family as the focus of care. The alternatives of home birth, birthing centers, and family-centered maternity care units reflect parents' desires to share in the birth process and have more contact with their infants.

Early Contact

Research with mammals other than humans indicates that early contact between the mother and her offspring is important in developing future relationships. The first hours or days after birth may be a sensitive time for parent-infant interaction. Early close contact during the first hours or days after birth may facilitate the attachment process between parent and child. This does not mean that a delay will inhibit this process (humans are too resilient for that), but additional psychologic energy may be needed to achieve the same effect. To date, no scientific evidence has demonstrated that immediate contact after birth is essential for the human parent-child relationship. In fact, research evidence is conflicting.

In the 1980s Siegel (1982) documented the positive effect of early contact on early maternal affectional behavior. In the 1990s Mercer and Ferketich (1990) found that, for low-risk, as well as high-risk, mothers and fathers, early contact was not predictive of parent-infant attachment during the first postpartum day. More recently Prodromidis et al. (1995) studied early and extended contact for young,

unmarried, predominantly African-American, low socioeconomic mothers. They found that mothers who had early and extended contact (rooming-in) with their infants during the first 18 hours after birth looked at, talked to, and touched their newborns more than did mothers who had minimal contact (infant feedings only).

Women who have had a long, difficult labor are often too exhausted to respond other than in a superficial way to the newborn. They may welcome the attention of others and be grateful that the infant is healthy, but their primary need centers on recovery from the physical and emotional aspects of pregnancy and childbirth. Infants born at risk as a result of either fetal or maternal disabilities are usually transferred to the intensive care nursery as quickly as possible. Concerns for their need for intensive medical and nursing interventions take priority over the need for close contact with the parents. Opportunities for parents to be with the infant in the intensive care nursery, to touch or hold the baby if at all possible, and to receive reports of the infant's progress must be part of the nursing plan of care.

Parents who desire but are unable to have early contact with their newborn can be reassured that such contact is not essential for optimal parent-infant interactions. Otherwise, adopted infants would not form the usual affectional ties with their parents. Nor does the mode of infant-mother contact after birth (skin-to-skin versus wrapped) appear to have any important effect. Nurses need to counsel parents to assure them that the emotional bond to the infant is not necessarily weaker because they missed early contact or the contact was not skin-to-skin. Nurses need to stress that the parent-infant relationship is a process that occurs over time.

Extended Contact

The provision of rooming-in facilities for the mother and her baby is a prevalent aspect of family-centered care. The infant is transferred to the area from the transitional nursery (if the facility uses one) after showing satisfactory extrauterine adjustment. The father is encouraged to visit and to participate in the infant's care, and siblings and grandparents are encouraged to visit and become acquainted with the infant. Many hospitals have established family birth units such as labor-delivery-recovery (LDR) rooms, labor-delivery-recovery-postpartum (LDRP) rooms, and single-room maternity care (SRMC). The mother is accompanied by the father or partner during the birth of the infant, and all three may remain together until discharged around 48 hours after birth. Whether rooming-in or a family birth unit is the method of family-centered care, mothers and their partners are considered equal and integral members of the developing family (Fig. 18-5). Some hospitals arrange for the discharge of mother and infant any time from 2 to 24 hours after birth if the condition of the mother and that of the infant warrants it. Follow-up care with nursing personnel from a home health care agency is often part of this plan.

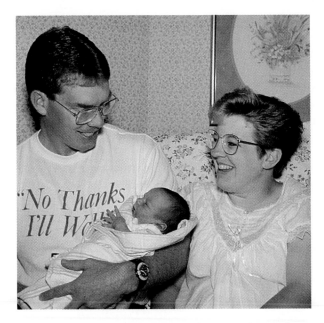

Fig. **18-5** Mother, father, and newborn are integral members of the developing family. (Courtesy Michael S. Clement, MD, Mesa, Ariz.)

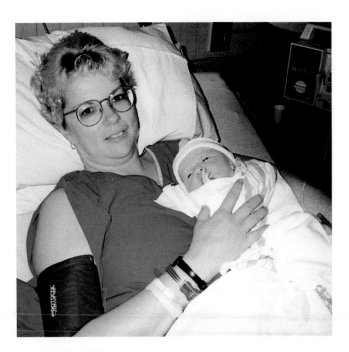

Fig. **18-6** Mother enfolding newborn daughter in her arms. (Courtesy Jan Harmon, St Louis.)

Mother-baby care is another form of family-centered care. Care for the mother and infant is provided by a primary nurse, fostering family unity. Parents are more likely to be more self-confident in care, and maternal attachment and maternal role attainment are promoted.

Extended contact with the infant should be available for all parents, but especially for those assessed to be at risk for parenting inadequacies. Any activity that optimizes family-centered care is worthy of serious consideration by postpartum nurses.

COMMUNICATION BETWEEN PARENT AND INFANT

Each interaction of parent and infant strengthens the parent-infant relationship through the use of sensual responses or abilities (touch, eye contact, voice, and odor). The nurse should keep in mind that there may be cultural variations in these interactive behaviors used in communications between parent and infant.

The Senses

Touch

Touch is used extensively by parents and other caregivers as a means of becoming acquainted with the newborn. Many mothers reach out for their infants as soon as they are born and the cord is cut. They lift them to their breasts, enfold them in their arms, and cradle them (Fig. 18-6). Once the child is close to them, they begin the exploration process with their fingertips, one of the most touch-sensitive areas of the body. Studies have depicted a predictable pattern of

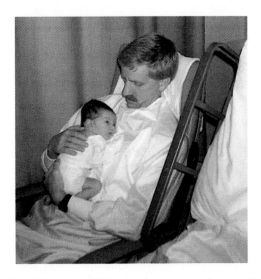

Fig. **18-7** Father holding newborn son. (Courtesy Jan Harmon, St Louis.)

touch behavior (Klaus & Kennell, 1982; Rubin, 1963; Tulman, 1985). The caregiver begins with a fingertip exploration of the infant's head and extremities. Within a short time the caregiver uses the palm to caress the infant's trunk and eventually enfolds the infant. Gentle stroking motions are used to soothe and quiet the infant: patting or gently rubbing the back is a comfort to the infant after feedings. Infants also pat the mother's breast as they nurse. Both seem to enjoy sharing each other's body warmth. There is a desire in parents to touch, pick up, and hold their baby (Fig. 18-7). They comment on the softness of the infant's skin and are aware of milia and rashes. As parents become increasingly sensitive to the infant's like or dislike of different types of touch, they draw closer to their baby.

Variations in touching behaviors have been noted in mothers from different cultural groups (Galanti, 1991; Inman, 1996; Jambunathan & Stewart, 1995; Jiménez, 1995). For example, minimal touching and cuddling is a traditional Southeast Asian practice thought to protect the child from evil spirits. Because of tradition and spiritual beliefs, women in India and Bali have practiced infant massage since ancient times.

Eye contact

Parents repeatedly make eye contact with their new baby. Some mothers remark that once their babies have looked at them, they feel much closer to them. Parents spend much time getting their babies to open their eyes and look at them. In American culture, eye contact appears to have a cementing effect on the development of a beginning and trusting relationship and is an important factor in human relationships at all ages. In other cultures, eye contact may be perceived differently. For example, in Mexican culture, sustained direct eye contact is considered to be rude, immodest, and dangerous for some. This danger may arise from the *mal ojo* (evil eye), resulting from excessive admiration. Women and children are thought to be more susceptible to the *mal ojo* (Geissler, 1994).

As newborns become functionally able to sustain eye contact with their parents, time is spent in mutual gazing, often in the *en face* position (see Fig. 18-2). *En face,* "face-to-face," is a position in which the parent's face and the infant's face are approximately 20 cm apart on the same plane. Nursing and medical practices need to be implemented that encourage this interaction. Immediately after birth, for example, the infant can be positioned on the mother's abdomen or breasts with the mother's and the infant's faces on the same plane so that they can easily make eye contact. Lights can be dimmed so that the infant's eyes will open. Instillation of prophylactic antibiotic ointment in the infant's eyes can be delayed until the infant and parents have had some time together in the first hour after birth.

Voice

The shared response of parents and infants to each other's voices is remarkable. Parents wait tensely for the first cry. Once that cry has reassured them of their new baby's well-being, they begin comforting behaviors. As the parents talk in high-pitched voices, the infant usually calms, alerts, and turns toward them.

Infants respond to higher-pitched voices and can distinguish their mother's voice from others soon after birth. Infants use their cries to signal hunger, pain, boredom, and tiredness. With experience, parents learn to distinguish such cries.

Odor

Another behavior shared by parents and infants is a response to each other's odor. Mothers comment on the smell of their babies when first born and can distinguish the smell of their own baby from other babies. Infants learn rapidly to distinguish the odor of their mother's breast milk.

Entrainment

Newborns move in time with the structure of adult speech. They wave their arms, lift their heads, and kick their legs, seemingly "dancing in tune" to a parent's voice. This means that culturally determined rhythms of speech have been ingrained in the infant long before spoken language is used to communicate. Carryover, or **entrainment,** is evident once the child begins to talk. This shared rhythm also gives the parent positive feedback and establishes a positive setting for effective communication.

Biorhythmicity

The fetus is in tune with the mother's natural rhythms, such as heartbeats. After birth a crying infant may be soothed by being held in a position where the mother's heartbeat can be heard or by hearing a recording of a heartbeat. One of the newborn's tasks is to establish a personal rhythm, or **biorhythmicity.** Parents can help in this process by giving consistent loving care and using their infant's alert state to develop responsive behavior and thereby increase social interactions and opportunities for learning. The more quickly parents become competent in child care activities, the more quickly their psychologic energy can be directed toward observing and responding to the communication cues the infant gives them.

Reciprocity and Synchrony

Reciprocity is a type of body movement or behavior that provides the observer with cues. The observer or receiver interprets those cues and responds to them. Reciprocity often takes several weeks to develop with a new baby. For example, when the newborn fusses and cries, the mother responds by picking up and cradling the child; the child becomes quiet and alert and establishes eye contact; the mother verbalizes, sings, and coos while the child maintains eye contact. The child then averts the eyes and yawns; the mother decreases her active response. If the parent continues to stimulate the infant, the child may become fussy.

Synchrony refers to the "fit" between the infant's cues and the parent's response. When parent and child experience a synchronous interaction, it is mutually rewarding (Fig. 18-8). Parents need time to interpret the infant's cues correctly. For example, after a certain time the infant develops a different cry in response to situations such as boredom, loneliness, hunger, and discomfort. The parent may

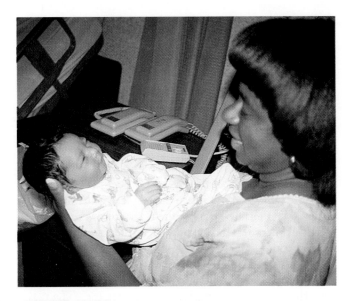

Fig **18-8** Sharing a smile: example of synchrony. (Courtesy Marjorie Pyle, RNC, Lifecircle, Costa Mesa, Calif.)

need assistance in deciphering these cries, along with trial-and-error interventions, before synchrony develops.

PARENTAL ROLE AFTER CHILDBIRTH

The care and nurturing of a child are initiated well before birth. The mother who carries out the dictates of health (e.g., diet, rest, and exercise) for the "good of her baby," the partner who supports and nurtures her, and the parents who become aware of and attach to their unborn child are already functioning in the parental role.

The 6 weeks after birth form what is called the **fourth trimester.** During the postpartum period, new tasks and responsibilities arise, and old behaviors need to be modified or new ones added. The responses of mothers and their partners to the parental role change over time and tend to follow a predictable course. During the first 3 to 4 weeks after birth, parents have to reorganize their relationship with the newborn. What was accomplished through the biologic process of pregnancy now requires an array of caregiving activities. The infant's needs for shelter, nourishment, protection, and socializing must be met. These early weeks are characterized by intense learning and the need for nurturing.

The weeks after represent a time of drawing together and uniting the family unit. This period of consolidation involves negotiations as to roles (wife-husband, mother-father, mother-partner, parent-child, sibling-sibling). Successful role negotiation promotes family adaptation and integrity.

Adaptation involves a stabilizing of tasks, a coming to terms with commitments. Parents demonstrate growing

competence in child care activities and are more attuned to their infant's behavior. Typically, the period from the decision to conceive through the first months of having a child is termed the **transition to parenthood.**

Transition to Parenthood

The transition to parenthood is frequently described as a time of disorder and disequilibrium, as well as satisfaction, for mothers and their partners. Usual methods of coping often seem ineffective. For example, some parents can be so distressed that they are unable to be supportive of each other. Men typically identify their spouses as their primary or only source of support. The transition can be harder for fathers who feel deprived because the mothers, who are also experiencing stress, cannot provide the usual level of support. Strong emotions such as helplessness, inadequacy, and anger that arise when dealing with a crying infant catch many parents unprepared. On the other hand, parenthood allows adults to develop and display a selfless, warm, and caring side of themselves, which may not be expressed in other adult roles.

Historically, the transition to parenthood was viewed as a crisis (Dyer, 1963; LeMasters, 1957). The current perspective is that parenthood is a developmental transition (Demick, Bursik & Dibiase, 1993) rather than a major life crisis for the majority of families. A concept that is derived from the developmental crisis perspective but that has relevance for the developmental transition theory is that, at the point of crisis, a moment occurs when a person is mentally and physically prepared for, the culture is pushing for, and the person is reaching out to achieve some developmental change. Because of this, the person is motivated for change. For the majority of mothers and their partners, the transition to parenthood represents such a period and is viewed as an opportunity rather than a time of danger. Parents are stimulated to try new coping strategies as they work to master their new roles and reach new developmental levels.

Parental Tasks and Responsibilities

Parents need to reconcile the actual child with the fantasy and dream child. This means coming to terms with the infant's physical appearance, sex, innate temperament, and physical status. If the real child differs greatly from the fantasy child, parents may delay acceptance of the child. In some instances, they may never accept the child.

Some parents are startled by the appearance of the neonate—size, color, molding of the head, or bowed appearance of the legs. Many fathers have commented that they thought the odd shape of the child's head (molding) meant the child would be mentally retarded.

Although many parents know the sex of the infant before birth because of the use of ultrasound assessments, for those who do not have this information, disappointment over the sex of the infant can take time to resolve. The parents may provide adequate physical care but find it difficult to be sincerely involved with the infant until this internal conflict has been resolved. As one mother remarked, "I really wanted a boy. I know it is silly and irrational, but when they said, 'She's a lovely little girl,' I was so disappointed and angry—yes, angry—I could hardly look at her. Oh, I looked after her okay, her feedings and baths and things, but I couldn't feel excited. To tell the truth, I felt like a monster not liking my child. Then one day she was lying there and she turned her head and looked right at me. I felt a flooding of love for her come over me, and we looked at each other a long time. It's okay now. I wouldn't change her for all the boys in the world."

Nursing care plans need to include discussion about reconciliation of the real versus the fantasy child. Nurses need to provide opportunities for parents to discuss their lack of parental feelings without fear of censure or ridicule. Often the expression of doubts and concerns provides relief and makes it easier for parents to deal with and resolve such feelings.

Parents need to establish the newborn as a person separate from themselves, that is, as someone having many dependency needs and requiring much nurturing. Nurses can discuss with parents that this acceptance of the infant as a separate being with many needs evolves over time. Parents who see the baby by ultrasound assessments during pregnancy may begin to appreciate earlier that the baby is a real—and separate—human being.

Parents need to become adept in the care of the infant, noting the communication cues given by the infant to indicate needs and responding appropriately to those needs.

Parents need to establish reasonable evaluative criteria for assessing the success or failure of the care given to the infant. Parents are surprisingly sensitive to infant responses. One father spoke about his first attempt to give his child a kiss. At that moment the child turned her head. The father felt hurt, although he understood that the baby was totally unaware of her own movements. The infant's response to the parental care and attention may be interpreted by the parent as a comment on the quality of that care. Examples of infant behaviors that are interpreted by parents as positive responses to their care include being consoled easily, enjoying being cuddled, and making eye contact. Spitting frequently after feedings, crying, and being unpredictable may be perceived as negative responses to parental care. Continuation of these infant responses that are viewed as negative by the parent can result in alienation of parent and child to the detriment of the infant.

Self-esteem grows with competence. Mothers of preterm infants have noted that their own efforts appear inadequate after the skillful handling of their infants by nurses. Breastfeeding makes many mothers feel they are contributing in a unique way to the welfare of the infant.

Assistance, including advice by husbands, partners, wives, mothers, mothers-in-law, and professional workers, can either be seen as supportive or an indication of how inept these people have judged the new parents to be. Criticism, real or imagined, of the new parents' ability to provide adequate physical care, nutrition, or social stimulation for the infant can prove devastating. By providing encouragement and praise for parenting efforts, nurses can bolster the new parents' confidence. Parents should feel safe discussing concerns about other peoples' criticisms with the nurses, who can help them practice assertiveness techniques to use with unwanted "critics." The nurses, as patient advocates, can also use positive, nonjudgmental approaches to help critics direct their advice constructively.

The newborn must assume a place within the family group. Whether the infant is the firstborn or the last born, all family members must adjust their roles to accommodate the newcomer. The firstborn child needs support to accept a rival for parental affections. An older child needs help dealing with losing a favored position in the family hierarchy. The parents are expected to negotiate these changes.

Parents need to establish the primacy of their adult relationships to maintain the family as a group. Because this includes reorganizing many roles (e.g., sexual, child care, career, and community roles), time and energy must be provided for this vital task.

Maternal Adjustment

Three phases are evident as the mother adjusts to her parental role. These phases of **maternal adjustment** are characterized by dependent behavior, dependent-independent behavior, and interdependent behavior (Table 18-4).

Dependent phase

During the first 24 to 48 hours after childbirth the mother's dependency needs predominate. To the extent that these needs are met by others, the mother is able to divert her psychologic energy to her child rather than focus them on herself. She needs "mothering" herself to "mother." Rubin (1961) aptly described these few days as the **taking-in phase**, a time when nurturing and protective care are required by the new mother. In Rubin's classic description the taking-in phase lasts 2 to 3 days. More recent studies by Ament (1990) and Wrasper (1996) support the direction of postpartum behavioral charges reported by Rubin, but found that women now move more rapidly through the taking-in phase. A strong taking-in phase was noted only in the first 24 hours after birth (Ament, 1990).

For 24 hours after the birth, mature and apparently healthy women appear to suspend their involvement in everyday responsibilities. They rely on others to satisfy their needs for comfort, rest, nourishment, and closeness to their families and newborn.

This dependent phase is a time of great excitement during which parents need to verbalize their experience of pregnancy and birth. Focusing on, analyzing, and accepting these experiences help the parents move on to the next phase. Some parents use staff members or other mothers

TABLE 18-4	*Phases of Maternal Postpartum Adjustment*
PHASE	**CHARACTERISTICS**
Dependent: taking-in*	• First 24 hours (range of 1 to 2 days) • Focus: self and meeting of basic needs • Reliance on others to meet needs for comfort, rest, closeness, and nourishment • Excited and talkative • Desire to review birth experience
Dependent-independent: taking-hold*	• Starts second or third day; lasts 10 days to several weeks • Focus: care of baby and competent mothering • Desire to take charge • Still need for nurturing and acceptance by others • Eagerness to learn and practice—optimal period for teaching by nurses • Handling of physical discomforts and emotional changes • Possible experience with "blues"
Interdependent: letting go*	• Focus: forward movement of family as unit with interacting members • Reassertion of relationship with partner • Resumption of sexual intimacy • Resolution of individual roles

*From Rubin R: Maternal touch at first contact with the newborn infant, *Nurs Outlook,* 11:828, 1963.

as an "audience," whereas others are more comfortable talking with family and friends about the pregnancy and birth experience.

Because anxiety and preoccupation with her new role often narrow a mother's perceptions, information may have to be repeated. The new mother may require reminders to rest or, conversely, to ambulate enough to promote recovery. Hospital or birth center routines may not necessarily be an important priority to the new mother; she may take showers when examinations are scheduled and be involved in a telephone conversation rather than "being ready" for the baby. Regulations seem cumbersome, and sometimes mothers and their families have difficulty accepting rules that interfere with their need to share reactions about their child.

Physical discomfort from an episiotomy, sore nipples, hemorrhoids, afterpains, and occasionally a sprained coccygeal joint can interfere with the mother's need for rest and relaxation. The selective use of comfort measures and medication depends on the nurse. Many women hesitate to ask for medication, believing that any pain they experience is normal and to be expected; breastfeeding mothers may fear the effects of the medication on the infant; few have a knowledge of the use of heat or cold to relieve local pain.

Dependent-independent phase

If the mother has received adequate nurturing in the first few hours or days, by the second or third day, her desire for independent action reasserts itself. In the dependent-independent phase, the mother alternates between a need for extensive nurturing and acceptance by others and the desire to "take charge" once again. She responds enthusiastically to opportunities to learn and practice baby care or, if she is an accomplished mother, to carry out or direct this care. Rubin (1961) describes this phase as the **taking-hold phase,** noting that it lasts approximately 10 days. Several studies (Ament, 1990; Martell, 1996; Wrasper, 1996) have found that contemporary women exhibit taking-hold behaviors sooner than did the women in Rubin's study; however, the peak and duration of the taking-hold phase were not determined. In a study by Martell (1996) women exhibited some taking-in and taking-hold behaviors but not in the sequence of postpartum phases described originally by Rubin.

Childbirth preparation classes, current obstetric pain management, early contact with the newborn, rooming-in, and early discharge are some of the current obstetric practices that seem to enhance taking-hold behaviors (Martell, 1996; Wrasper, 1996). Given these changes in health care and in women's lives, more research is needed to evaluate the effect of such changes on patterns of women's behaviors during the postpartum period.

Most mothers are discharged home during this dependent-independent phase. Contemporary mothers have short hospital stays, ranging from 6 to 48 hours for low-risk, uncomplicated births and from 48 to 96 hours for a cesarean birth. Once home, mothers must continue to cope with physical adaptations and psychologic adjustments.

In a study of the experience of low-risk mothers (25 multiparas and 25 primiparas) during the first 2 weeks postpartum, the majority of mothers identified fatigue as their major physical concern (Ruchala & Halstead, 1994; Smith-Hanrahan & Deblois, 1995). This fatigue affected various aspects of their lives, such as their relationships with their husbands and other family members and household responsibilities. Other physical concerns were loss of weight or figure, pain from the episiotomy or cesarean incision, sexual relations, and hemorrhoids. Most women described the early postpartum period as hectic and a time of adjustment. Several also said it was an enjoyable time. Primiparas reported feeling uncertain, trapped, and overwhelmed by fatigue and lack of experience in infant care. Many of the multiparas described their experience as being better than with previous births, primarily because of their comfort with caring for an infant.

Emotional concerns were a recurring theme, with mothers reporting feeling "down," being tense and irritable, and being depressed. All who reported feeling depressed said that it was transient, lasting less than a week. Crying was the most frequently reported emotional symptom. A primipara said, "It bothers me being so easily depressed . . . when

I cry so easily. . . . It goes with the territory, though, I guess. It won't last forever" (Ruchala & Halstead, 1994). All mothers said that they realized the emotional changes were normal and ascribed them to fatigue, physical discomfort, the condition of their bodies, the infants' temperaments, and the impact of the infant on their freedom. Those mothers who reported feeling confident in caring for their infants identified someone, usually their own mothers, who had influenced them or been a role model for infant care.

These findings have implications for nursing care. Prenatally and postnatally, nurses can discuss the usual postpartum concerns that mothers experience and provide anticipatory guidance on coping strategies, such as resting when the infant sleeps and planning with an extended family member or friend to do the housework for the first week or two after the baby is born. Once a mother is home, periodic phone calls from a nurse who cared for her in the birth setting can provide the mother with an opportunity to vent her concerns and get support and advice from "her nurse." Nurses should plan additional supportive counseling for first-time mothers inexperienced in child care, women whose careers had provided outside stimulation, women who lack friends or family members with whom to share delights and concerns, and adolescent mothers. When possible, postpartum home visits are included in the plan of care.

Postpartum "blues"

The "pink" period surrounding the first day or two after birth, characterized by heightened joy and feelings of well-being, is often followed by a "blue" period. Up to 80% of women experience the **postpartum blues,** or "baby blues," (Albright, 1993) that occur in women of all ethnic and racial groups (Campbell, 1992). During the blues, women are emotionally labile, often crying easily and for no apparent reason. This lability seems to peak around the fifth day, subsiding by the tenth day. Other symptoms of postpartum blues include depression, a let-down feeling, restlessness, fatigue, insomnia, headache, anxiety, sadness, and anger. Biochemical, psychologic, social, and cultural factors have been explored as possible causes of the postpartum depressive state; however, the etiology remains unknown. Whatever the cause, the early postpartum period appears to be one of emotional and physical vulnerability for new mothers, who may be psychologically overwhelmed by the reality of parental responsibilities. The mother may feel deprived of the supportive care she received from family members and friends during pregnancy. Some mothers regret the loss of the mother-unborn child relationship and mourn its passing. Still others experience a let-down feeling when labor and birth are complete. Fatigue after childbirth is compounded by the around-the-clock demands of the new baby and can accentuate the feelings of depression. A lowered level of circulating glucocorticoids or a subclinical hypothyroidism may

HOME CARE *Patient Instructions for Self-Care*
Coping with Postpartum Blues
- Remember that the "blues" are normal.
- Get plenty of rest; nap when the baby does if possible. Go to bed early, and let friends know when to visit.
- Use relaxation techniques learned in childbirth classes (or ask the nurse to teach you and your partner some techniques).
- Do something for yourself. Take advantage of the time your partner or family members care for the baby—soak in the tub or go for a walk.
- Plan a day out of the house—go to the mall with the baby, being sure to take a stroller or carriage, or go out to eat with friends without the baby. Many communities have churches or other agencies that provide child care programs such as Mothers' Morning Out.
- Talk to your partner about the way you feel—for example, about feeling tied down, how the birth met your expectations, and things that will help you.
- If you are breastfeeding, give yourself and your baby time to learn.
- Seek out and use community resources such as La Leche League or community mental health centers. Some nationally recognized resources are as follows:

  Postpartum Support International
  927 N. Kellogg Avenue
  Santa Barbara, CA 93111 (805) 967-7636

  Depression After Delivery (DAD) Support Network
  P.O. Box 1282
  Morrisville, PA 19067 (215) 295-3994 telephone "warm line" and (800) 944-4773

exist during the puerperium. To help mothers cope with postpartum blues, nurses can suggest various strategies (see Home Care box).

"Am I Blue?" (Johnson & Johnson, 1996), a self-administered questionnaire, can help mothers to assess their level of "blues" and to decide when to seek advice from their nurse, nurse-midwife, or physician (Fig. 18-9). Nurse home visits and telephone follow-up calls to assess the mother's pattern of "blue" feelings and behavior over time are important.

Although the postpartum blues are usually mild and short-lived, approximately 12% of women experience a more severe syndrome called postpartum depression (PPD) (Albright, 1993). PPD is considered to be a type of mental illness that is placed on a continuum of postpartum emotional reactions ranging from the baby blues to postpartum psychoses (Fig. 18-10). It can occur within days of the birth or appear gradually, up to a year later. (See Chapter 26 for a discussion of PPD.)

Am I Blue?

Many new mothers feel anxious, sad, or angry about the changes in their lives after the birth of their new baby. It is perfectly normal to feel this way, but sometimes the feelings grow so strong that they make life difficult. This quiz lists many feelings and experiences of "blue" or depressed mothers. Mark how strong each of these feelings or experiences is for you, compared with what is normal for you. For example: Do you feel no anger [0]; mild (very little) anger [1]; moderate (some) anger [2]; or severe (very strong) anger [3] compared with the way you usually feel? Add up your total score when you are finished, and discuss the results with your health care provider.

0 = Not there at all 1 = Mild 2 = Moderate 3 = Severe	0	1	2	3
Anger				
Anxiety attacks: periods of very strong fear, shortness of breath, rapid heartbeat				
Increased or decreased appetite and/or weight gain or loss that doesn't seem normal				
Strong feeling that you need to get away, need more time for your own interests				
Problems in a relationship with a family member, lover, close friend, etc.				
Crying spells				
Less interest in your personal appearance				
Less motivation—less energy or interest in accomplishing goals				
Depression				
Fatigue—feeling tired or exhausted				
Fear of harming yourself or your baby				
Loss of your sense of humor				
Nervousness, feeling tense or edgy				
Feelings of guilt				
Feelings of panic				
Feeling alone or lonely; without the support of others				
Feeling no love, or not enough love, for your baby				
Feeling forgetful, distracted, absent-minded—having trouble concentrating				
Frustration				
Hopelessness				
Insomnia				
Feeling irritable, bad-tempered				
Loss of sexual desire and/or pleasure in sex				
Loss of self-respect or confidence—feeling like you don't count or can't do anything right				
Feeling confused, uncertain				
Mood swings—your moods and emotions change all the time				
Obsessive thoughts—ideas or feelings you can't stop from repeating in your mind				
Odd or frightening thoughts—thoughts or images that scare you or that you can't control				
Thoughts of suicide, feeling like you want to die				
Feeling sad, unhappy				
				TOTAL

SCORE:

0 – 31 = MILD BLUES

This will probably pass, but pay attention to your feelings and needs.

32 – 64 = MODERATE BLUES

You may want to ask for help from a close friend or family member, or ask the advice of your health care provider.

65 – 98 = SEVERE BLUES

You could be depressed; see your health care provider for a check-up and advice as soon as possible.

If you are afraid you might harm yourself or your baby—ask a health care provider you trust for help—you don't have to be alone!

Fig. **18-9** Am I Blue? (Courtesy Johnson & Johnson Consumer Products. Skillman, NJ.)

Lesser Severity ◄   ► **Greater Severity**

"Maternity Blues" ("baby blues")	Postnatal Depression (mild-moderate postpartum depression) (Postpartum Panic Disorder)*	Major Postpartum Depression (severe postpartum depression)	Postpartum Psychosis (puerperal psychosis)	Postpartum Psychotic Depression (Pauliekhoff's amentia)
Affects 50%-85%	Affects 10%-20%	Affects 0.1%-0.2% (Affects 1 in 3 or 4 with a history of a previous episode)		
Minimal dysfunction	Moderate dysfunction	Maximal dysfunction		
Self-limiting				
Onset day 3-10	Insidious development	Slow onset	Early onset (may be confused with "baby blues")	Combined qualities of both postpartum psychosis and major postpartum depression
	Numerous physical signs and symptoms	Numerous physical signs and symptoms	Vivid hallucinations and delusions	
	Often unrecognized	Rapid improvement may be followed by relapse	Mercurial changeability	Episodes of hallucinations and delusions (often concealed) alternate with periods of apparent lucidity
	Deleterious effect on maternal-child relationship, marriage, and family life	Grave suicidal concerns		
	Hangs on interminably			
Enlightened support of family and friends effective		Skilled professional intervention vital		
Help-seeking behavior discouraged by social pressure	Help-seeking behavior often discouraged and trivialized	Help-seeking behavior discouraged by stigma of mental illness and severe dysfunction		
Potential for violence low		Potential for violence high (suicide and infanticide)		
Excellent prognosis	Excellent prognosis with recognition and treatment	Excellent prognosis with recognition and treatment		
Self-limiting				

*Postpartum panic disorder is atypical in that symptoms are primarily anxiety and fear rather than depression. Development may not be insidious, and the incidence is unknown.

Fig. 18-10 Continuum of postpartum emotional reactions. (From Harberger P, Berchtold N & Honikman J: Cries for help. In Hamilton J & Harberger P, editors: *Postpartum psychiatric illness: a picture puzzle*, Philadelphia, 1992, University of Pennsylvania Press.)

Interdependent phase

In this phase, interdependent behavior reasserts itself, and the mother and her family move forward as a unit with interacting members. The relationship of the partners, although altered by the introduction of a child, resumes many of its former characteristics. A primary need is to establish a lifestyle that includes, but in some respects also excludes, the child. The couple must share interests and activities that are adult in scope.

Even without a postpartum physical examination and physician/nurse-midwife recommendation, the couple may begin to engage in sexual intercourse by the fourth week after the child is born. Some couples begin earlier, as soon as it can be accomplished without discomfort, depending on factors such as timing, amount of vaginal dryness, and breastfeeding status. Sexual intimacy enhances the adult aspect of the family, and the adult pair share a closeness denied to other family members. Many new fathers speak of the alienation experienced when they observe the intimate mother-child relationship, and some are frank in expressing feelings of jealousy toward the infant. The resumption of sexual intimacy seems to bring the parents' relationship back into focus.

The interdependent phase, termed the **letting-go phase,** is often stressful for the parental pair. Interests and needs often diverge during this time. Women and their partners must resolve the effects on their relationship of their individual roles related to child rearing, homemaking, and careers. Mothers (and partners) may take a more traditional role in an effort to adapt to parenthood. A special continuing effort has to be undertaken to strengthen the adult-adult relationship as a basis for the family unit.

Little is known about postpartum maternal adjustment in the lesbian couple.

Relationship satisfaction in first-time lesbian parent couples appears related to egalitarianism, commitment, sexual compatibility, and communication skills, as well as the birth mother's decision for insemination by an anonymous sperm donor (Osterwell, 1991). Similar to heterosexual parent couples, most lesbian parent couples voice concern about less time and energy for their relationship after the arrival of the baby (Gartrell et al., 1996). Both partners consider themselves to be equal parents of the baby who share actively in child rearing (Brewaeys et al., 1995).

Lesbian couples face strong social sanctions regarding pregnancy and parenting. Their families may not have resolved the initial dismay and guilt over learning of their daughters' homosexuality, or they may disagree with the lesbian couple's decision to parent. In situations where family support is limited or absent, the nurse can help the couple locate more supportive social groups, lesbian or heterosexual.

Paternal Adjustment

Research on **paternal adjustment** to parenthood indicates that fathers go through a predictable three-stage process during the first 3 weeks of their transition to parenthood (Henderson & Brouse, 1991) (Table 18-5). During this period, fathers experience intense emotions. Stage 1 (expectations) involves approaching the experience with preconceptions about what it will be like when the baby is home. In stage 2 (reality) some fathers realize that their expectations are not based on fact. Many fathers acknowledge that their expectations were of limited value once they were immersed in the reality of parenthood. Feelings that often accompany this reality are sadness, ambivalence, jealousy, frustration at not being able to participate in breastfeeding, and an overwhelming desire to be more involved, most of which are different from the feelings mothers report. On the other hand, some fathers are pleasantly surprised at the ease and fun of parenting. Stage 3 (transition to mastery) involves a conscious decision to take control and to become more actively involved in the infant's life.

First-time fathers perceive the first 4 to 10 weeks of parenthood in much the same way mothers do, that is, as a period characterized by uncertainty, increased responsibility, disruption of sleep, and inability to control time needed to care for the infant and reestablish the marital dyad. Fathers express concern about (1) decreased attention from their partners relative to their personal relationship, (2) mother's lack of recognition of the father's desire to participate in decision making for the infant, and (3) limited time available to establish a relationship with their infants. These concerns can precipitate feelings of jealousy of the infant. Discussing their needs with the partner and becoming more involved with their infants and partner can help alleviate such feelings of jealousy. A consistent finding in the literature is that fathers who feel affection and support in the relationships with their partners or mates are more involved with infant care and their involvement

STAGES	CHARACTERISTICS
Stage 1: Expectations	Father has preconceptions about what life will be like after baby comes home
Stage 2: Reality	Father realizes that expectations are not always based on fact
	Common feelings experienced are as follows:
	Sadness
	Ambivalence
	Jealousy
	Frustration
	Overwhelming desire to be more involved
	Some fathers are pleasantly surprised at ease and fun of parenting
Stage 3: Transition to mastery	Father makes conscious decision to take control and become more actively involved with infant

TABLE 18-5   *Transition to Fatherhood: A Three-Stage Process*

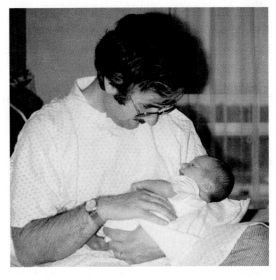

Fig. **18-11** Engrossment. Father absorbed in looking at his newborn. (Courtesy Lienne Edwards, Charlotte, NC.)

is more responsive, affectionate, and developmentally stimulating (Broom, 1994; Edwards, 1990; Ferketich & Mercer, 1995; Nugent, 1991).

Father-infant relationship

In American culture, neonates have a powerful impact on their fathers, who become intensely involved with their babies (Fig. 18-11). The term used for the father's absorption, preoccupation, and interest in the infant is **engrossment**.

Characteristics of engrossment include sensual responses relating to touch and eye contact and the father's keen awareness of features both unique and similar to himself that validate his claim to the infant. An outstanding response is one of strong attraction to the newborn. Fathers spend considerable time "communicating" with the infant and taking delight in the infant's response to them. A sense of increased self-esteem and a sense of being proud, bigger, more mature, and older are all experienced by fathers after seeing their baby for the first time.

Jordan (1990) found that the infant held the key to the recognition of the father as a parent. The ability of the infant to communicate to the father that he was a special person (e.g., by turning to the father's voice or smiling at the father) was a powerful stimulus to making the father feel important and competent.

Much has to be learned about the relationships between fathers and their offspring. The majority of studies on fathers of infants have focused on the amount of time fathers spend with their infants and what they do when they are with their infants. Two consistent findings are that (1) fathers spend less time than mothers with infants and (2) fathers' interactions with infants tend to be characterized by stimulating social play rather than caretaking. In the United States, fathers tend to take the lead in initiating play and to play in a rougher manner, whereas mothers tend to take the lead in caregiving activities. In India, fathers are not characterized as vigorous, playful partners. They appear to use more affectional display than very rough play with infants (Roopnarine et al., 1990). The subtle and more open differences in stimulation from two sources, mother and father, provide a wider social experience for the infant.

Research has demonstrated that fathers can be sensitive and competent in caring for infants (Broom, 1994; Edwards, 1990; McBride, 1992), yet few studies have tried to identify factors that influence fathers' parental competence with infants. Some of the factors identified that are associated with fathers' parental competence are family functioning, partner relationships, and a sense of mastery (Ferketich & Mercer, 1995) plus knowledge of infant development and an infant with an "easier" temperament (Edwards, 1990).

One way nurses can help fathers to feel more competent in the parental role is to teach and provide information. Men entering parenthood with knowledge and realistic expectations may cope more successfully with the demands of a young infant and develop nurturing relationships with their infants. For nurses, dissemination of information can be a cost-effective intervention. Use of videos on infant cognitive and social capabilities, early infant care and stimulation, and direct parent teaching methods, such as exposure to newborn assessments, has been successful (Koniak-Griffin, Verzemmnieks & Cahill, 1992; McBride, 1992; Tedder, 1991; Wolfson, Lacks & Futteman, 1992).

Impact of fatherhood

The impact of first-time fatherhood on men has been investigated by Drobeck (1990). For white, middle-class American husbands, first-time fatherhood is seen as a maturing event during which increased responsibility is assumed. Fathers report taking their work more seriously while at the same time trying to balance work and family demands. These men experience an identity change, developing an image of themselves as a father. Over time, they develop strong bonds with their infants and feel a sense of fulfillment and purpose in life.

Studies investigating the impact of fatherhood on African-American men are sparse. One study on parental role attainment by African-American parents (Sank, 1991) provides nurses with some understanding of the father's experience. Self-concept was found to be the best predictor of these fathers' parental role attainment during the postpartum period. Fathers felt less competent with the skill and knowledge component of parenting than did the mothers but were at ease with the valuing and comfort component. Although these fathers did not see themselves as skillful as their partners in caring for infants, they valued parenthood and felt comfortable in the father role.

Despite their active involvement in the perinatal period, fathers tend to gravitate toward a more traditional division of family responsibilities. One reason for this return to more traditional roles may be the new father's concerns about his ability to support his new family financially. As a first-time father explained: "The cost of child care was amazing. I would have never guessed how much of a drain child care could put on our income" (Leventhal-Belfer, Cowan & Cowan, 1992).

Fathers can benefit from nursing interventions during the postpartum period just as mothers can. Nurses can arrange to teach infant care when the father is present and provide anticipatory guidance for fathers about the transition to parenthood. Separate prenatal and parenting classes and parenting support groups for fathers can provide them with an opportunity to discuss their concerns and have some of their needs met. Postpartum phone calls and home visits by the nurse need to include time for assessment of the father's adjustment and needs.

INFANT-PARENT INTERACTION

It has long been recognized that newborns participate actively in shaping their parents' reaction to them. Research has demonstrated that the behavioral characteristics of the infant influence parenting behaviors (Edwards, 1990; Jones & Heerman, 1992). The infant and the parents each have unique rhythms, behaviors, and response styles that are brought to every interaction. **Infant-parent interactions** can be facilitated in any of three ways: (1) modulation of rhythm, (2) modification of behavioral repertoires, and (3) mutual responsivity. Nurses can teach parents about

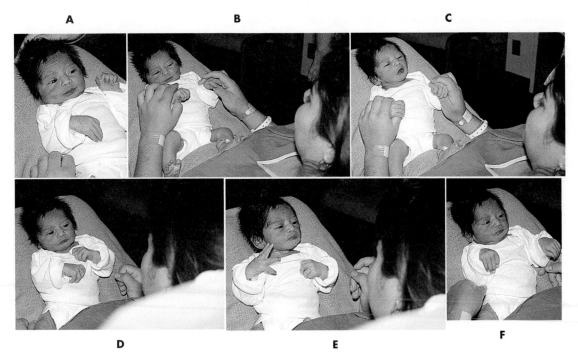

Fig. 18-12 Holding newborn in *en face* position, mother works to alert her daughter, 6 hours old. **A,** Infant is quiet and alert. **B,** Mother begins talking to daughter. **C,** Infant responds, opens mouth like her mother. **D,** Infant gazes at her mother. **E,** Infant waves hand. **F,** Infant glances away, resting. Hand relaxes. (Courtesy Marjorie Pyle, RNC, Lifecircle, Costa Mesa, Calif.)

these three aspects of infant-parent interaction through discussions, written materials, and videotapes on infant capabilities (e.g., *The Amazing Newborn*). A creative approach is to videotape the parent-infant pair during an interaction and then use the individualized tape to discuss the pair's rhythm, behavioral repertoire, and responsivity.

Rhythm

To modulate **rhythm,** both parent and infant must be able to interact. Therefore the infant must be in the alert state, one of the most difficult of the sleep-wake states to maintain. The alert state occurs most often during a feeding or in face-to-face play (Fig. 18-12, *A*). The parent must work hard to help the infant maintain the alert state long enough and often enough for interactions to take place. The *en face* position (the parent's face is positioned in the same plane as that of the newborn) is usually assumed (see Fig. 18-12, *D*). Multiparous mothers in particular are very sensitive and responsive to the infant's feeding rhythms. Mothers learn to reserve stimulation for pauses in sucking activity and not to talk or smile excessively while the infant is sucking because the infant will stop feeding to interact with her. With maturity the infant can sustain longer interactions by modulating activity rhythms, that is, limb movement, sucking, gaze alternation, and habituation (Fig. 18-13). Meanwhile, the parent becomes more attuned to the infant's rhythms and learns to modulate the rhythms, facilitating a rhythmic turn-taking interaction.

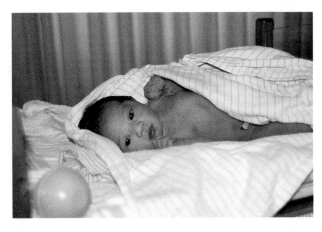

Fig. 18-13 Infant in alert state. (Courtesy Marjorie Pyle, RNC, Lifecircle, Costa Mesa, Calif.)

Repertoire of Behaviors

The infant and both parents have a **repertoire of behaviors** they can use to facilitate interactions. Parents engage in these behaviors depending on the extent of contact and caregiving of the infant.

The infant's behavioral repertoire includes gazing, vocalizing, and facial expressions. The infant is able to focus and follow the human face from birth and is also able to alternate the gaze voluntarily, looking away from the parent's face when understimulated or overstimulated (see Fig. 18-12, *F*). One of the key responses for the parents to learn is to be sensitive to the infant's capacity for attention and inattention. Developing this sensitivity is especially important when interacting with preterm infants.

Body gestures form a part of the infant's "early language." Babies greet parents with waving hands (see Fig. 18-12, *E*) or a reaching out of hands. They can raise an eyebrow or soften their expression to elicit loving attention. Game playing can stimulate them to smile or laugh. Pouting or crying, arching of the back, and general squirming usually signal the end of an interaction.

The parents' repertoire includes various types of interactive behaviors, such as constantly looking at the infant and noting the infant's response. New parents often remark that they are exhausted from looking at the baby and smiling. Adults also "infantilize" their speech to help the infant "listen." They do this by slowing the tempo, speaking loudly and rhythmically, and emphasizing key words. Phrases are repeated frequently. Infantilizing does not mean using "baby talk," which involves distortion of sounds.

Facial expressions such as slow and exaggerated looks of surprise, happiness, and confusion are often used by parents to communicate these emotions to the infant. Games such as "peek-a-boo" and imitation of the infant's behaviors are other means of interaction. For example, if the baby smiles, so does the parent; if the baby frowns, the parent responds in kind.

Responsivity

Contingent responses (**responsivity**) are those that occur within a specific time and are similar in form to a stimulus behavior. The adult has the feeling of having an influence on the interaction. Infant behaviors such as smiling, cooing, and sustained eye contact, usually in the *en face* position, are viewed as contingent responses. The infant's responses act as rewards to the initiator and encourage the adult to continue with the game when the infant responds positively. When the adult imitates the infant, the infant appears to enjoy it. In turn, soon after birth, the infant imitates behaviors of adults. There is a progression in the types of behaviors that parents present for the baby to imitate; for example, in early interactions the parent will grimace rather than laugh, which is in keeping with the infant's developmental level. Such "turnabout" behaviors sustain interactions and promote harmony in the relationship.

▌FACTORS INFLUENCING PARENTAL RESPONSES

How parents respond to the birth of their child is influenced by various factors, including age, social networks, socioeconomic conditions, and personal aspirations for the future.

Age

Maternal age has a definite effect on the outcome of pregnancy. The mother and fetus are both at highest risk when the mother is an adolescent or is more than 35 years old.

The adolescent mother

Although it is biologically possible for the adolescent female to become a parent, her egocentricity and concrete thinking interfere with her ability to parent effectively. The very young adolescent mother is inexperienced and unprepared to recognize the early signs of illness, potential danger, or household hazards. She may inadvertently neglect her child. The higher mortality rates among the infants of adolescent mothers are attributed to the inexperience, lack of knowledge, and immaturity of the mothers, causing them to be unable to recognize a problem and obtain the necessary resources to rectify the situation. Nevertheless, in most instances, with adequate support and developmentally appropriate teaching, adolescents can learn effective parenting skills.

The developmental tasks of parenthood include (1) reconciling the imagined infant with the actual infant, (2) becoming adept at caregiving activities, (3) being aware of the infant's needs, and (4) establishing oneself and one's infant as a family.

The transition to parenthood may be difficult for adolescent parents. Coping with the developmental tasks of parenthood is often complicated by the unmet developmental needs and tasks of adolescence. These young parents may experience difficulty accepting a changing self-image and adjusting to new roles related to the responsibilities of infant care. They may feel "different" from their peers, excluded from "fun" activities, and prematurely forced to enter an adult social role. The conflict between their own desires and the infant's demands, in addition to the low tolerance for frustration that is typical of adolescence, further contribute to the normal psychosocial stress of childbirth. Maintaining a relationship with the baby's father is beneficial for the mother and the infant. The involvement of the father is related to appropriate maternal behaviors (Ruff, 1990).

Some differences between adolescent and adult mothers have been observed. For example, adolescent mothers provide warm and attentive physical care; however, they use less verbal interaction than do older parents, and adolescents tend to be less responsive to their infants than older mothers. Thompson et al. (1995) found that adolescent mothers were at-risk for non-nurturing behaviors with their infant. Interventions emphasizing verbal and nonverbal communication skills between mother and child are important. Such intervention strategies must be concrete and specific because of the cognitive level of adolescents. Although some observers suggest that some adolescents may use more aggressive behaviors, a higher incidence of child abuse has not been documented. In comparison with adult mothers, teenage mothers have a limited knowledge of child development. They tend to expect too much of their children too soon and often characterize their infants as being fussy. This limited knowledge may cause teenagers to respond to their infants inappropriately.

Many young mothers pattern their maternal role on what they themselves experienced. Therefore nurses need to determine the kind of support that people close to the young mother are able and prepared to give, as well as the kinds of community aid available to supplement this support. The majority of adolescent mothers can identify at least one source of social support, with their own mother being their predominant source of support (Thompson et al., 1995).

The need for continued assessment of the new mother's parenting abilities during this postbirth period is essential. In addition, continued support should also be provided by involving the grandparents (Fig. 18-14) and other family members, as well as through home visits and group sessions for discussion of infant care and parenting problems. Outreach programs concerned with self-care, parent-child interactions, child injuries, and failure to thrive, in addition to programs that provide prompt and effective community intervention, prevent more serious problems from occurring. As the adolescent performs her mothering role within the framework of her family, she may need to address dependency versus independency issues. The adolescent's family members may also need help adapting to their new roles.

The adolescent father

As with the adolescent mother, the nurse must be aware of the male adolescent's cognitive-developmental levels, values, and culture. The more successful outreach programs also address cultural diversity in teenage fathers.

The adolescent father and mother face immediate developmental crises, which include completing the developmental tasks of adolescence, making a transition to parenthood, and sometimes adapting to marriage. These transitions can be stressful. The nurse may initiate interaction with the adolescent father by asking him to be present when postpartum home visits are made and to accompany the mother and the baby to well-baby checks at the clinic or pediatrician's office. With the adolescent mother's agreement, the nurse may contact the father directly. The decision to include the young father in all aspects of the care is based on assessment in the following four areas: (1) the couple's relationship; (2) levels of stress, concern, and coping; (3) educational and vocational goals; and (4) the level of health education knowledge. Adolescent fathers, as do all fathers, need support to discuss their emotional responses to the pregnancy. The nurse's nonjudgmental attitude is essential for open communication. The father's feelings of guilt, powerlessness,

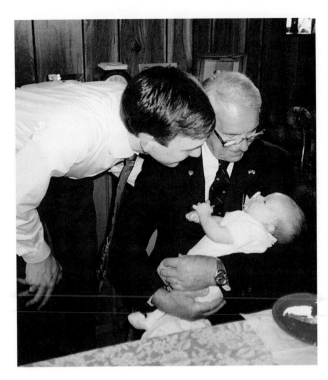

Fig. **18-14** Father, grandfather, and new grandson get acquainted. (Courtesy Eric Schult.)

or bravado should be recognized because of their negative consequences for both the parents and the child. Counseling of adolescent fathers needs to be reality oriented. Topics such as finances, child care, parenting skills, and the father's role in the birth experience need to be discussed. Teenage fathers also need to know about reproductive physiology and birth control options.

The adolescent father may continue to be involved in an ongoing relationship with the young mother and his baby. In many instances he also plays an important role in the decisions about child care and raising the child. The nurse supports the young father by helping him develop realistic perceptions of his role as "father to a child." The nurse encourages him to use coping mechanisms that are not detrimental to his own, his partner's, or his child's well-being. The nurse enlists support systems, parents, and professional agencies on his behalf. The father is encouraged to be involved in decisions regarding future contraception and safer sex practices.

Maternal age greater than 35 years

Issues and concerns related to women with a maternal age over 35 years have become increasingly more prominent in the last decade. There have always been women older than 35 years who have continued their childbearing either by choice or because of a lack or failure of contraception during the perimenopausal years. Added to this group are women who have postponed pregnancy because of careers or other reasons and women with infertility problems who have become pregnant because of technologic advances that have increased the alternatives for couples desiring children.

Older mothers have unique needs related to increased biologic risk. Higher rates of gestational diabetes, pregnancy-induced hypertension, gestational bleeding, abruptio placentae, and intrapartal fetal distress have been reported (Berkowitz et al., 1990). Many of these mothers, because they are less physically resilient than younger women, may need to stay in the hospital longer rather than be forced into an early discharge.

Researchers have examined the adjustment of midlife mothers to parenthood. Many older mothers reported having a hard time coping, especially with irregular sleep patterns and the fussy periods babies have in the late afternoon and early evening. Mothers admitted to unrealistic preconceptions about parenting. As one mother said, "I was surviving, not living, for the first 3 months. I couldn't get over how dramatically my life changed. I had thought the baby would adjust to our lifestyle. I didn't understand that *everyone* had to adapt" (Cain, 1994).

Adjusting to the enormity of the change was a pervading theme. A factor that helped these older mothers adjust and see themselves as competent parents was support from their partners. Support from other family members was also important for positive self-evaluation of parenting and help in dealing with stress (Reece, 1993).

Older mothers reported having to adjust to changes in the relationships with their partners. Some women regarded the changes as negative (e.g., having less time together), whereas others saw the changes as positive (e.g., feeling closer to their partners). Because many of these couples had been together for many years before the baby was born, the loss of the "just-the-two-of-us" aspect of the relationship was stressful (Cain, 1994). One mother stated, "We were by ourselves for so long, it was a hard adjustment—very, very difficult."

Changes in the sexual aspect of a relationship can be a stressor for new midlife parents. Mothers reported that finding time and energy for a romantic rendezvous was more difficult. They attributed much of this to the reality of caring for an infant but also mentioned the decreasing libido that normally accompanies getting older. Many of today's midlife mothers spent their late adolescence and early adulthood in the late 1960s and early 1970s, when youth spoke openly about sex and participated actively in the sexual revolution (Cain, 1994). As one woman so aptly expressed it, having no sex life along with a decreased libido was "more than an adjustment. It's practically an identity crisis. Now that our mid-life conservatism has taken over, there seems to be no one with whom to discuss our fears and changes. We're all seemingly back in the closet."

New mothers who are also perimenopausal may find it hard to distinguish fatigue, loss of sleep, decreased libido,

---

BOX 18-1	*Resources for Older Parents*
Parentage (for the new parent more than 35 years old) 19 West 21st Street New York, NY 10010 (800) 299-4818	Mothers at Home 301A Old Courthouse Road Vienna, VA 22182 (703) 827-5903
FEMALE (Formerly Employed Mother at the Leading Edge) P.O. Box 31 Elmhurst, IL 60126 (708) 941-3553	National Adoptive Hotline (202) 328-8072

or other physiologic symptoms as the cause of the changes in their sex lives. Although many women view menopause as a natural stage of life, for midlife mothers this cessation of menstruation coincides with the state of parenthood. The changes of midlife and menopause can add more emotional and physical stress to older mothers' lives because of the time- and energy-consuming aspects of raising a young child (Cain, 1994). Resources that older parents may find helpful are listed in Box 18-1.

Paternal age greater than 35 years

Literature on the experiences of first-time fathers with a paternal age over 35 years is sparse. However, in the available literature, older fathers described their experience of midlife parenting as wonderful but not without drawbacks. What they saw as positive aspects of parenthood in older years included increased love and commitment between the spouses, a reinforcement of why one married in the first place, a feeling of being complete, experiencing of "the child" again in oneself, more financial stability than in younger years, and more freedom to focus on parenting rather than on career. A common theme expressed was sharing: sharing joy, sharing in raising the child, sharing as a family. The main drawback of midlife parenting that these men reported was the change that it made in the relationships with their partners. They missed the deeper and more selfish couple relationship and looked forward to the time when they could have that again (Cain, 1994). Some fathers mentioned age as a disadvantage: "Sometimes I think I'm the oldest father in [the group]. I can't do quite as many physical things as I used to when I was younger." All fathers seemed to qualify statements about the less desirable side of parenting with positive statements such as "... but, I would not change it for the world!" or "I can't imagine life not being a parent now."

Social Support

Social support is strongly related to positive adaptation by new parents during the transition to parenthood (Gjerdingen,

Froberg & Fontaine, 1991). Social support is multidimensional and includes the number of members in a person's social network, types of support, perceived general support, actual support received, and satisfaction with support available and received. The type and satisfaction of support seem to be more important than the total number of support network members.

Across cultural groups, families and friends of new parents form an important dimension of the parent's social network. For example, the extended family unit is the single strongest unit in the lives of most Asians (Manio & Hall, 1987). Extended family are also relied on heavily after childbirth by Jordanians (Geissler, 1994). Social networks provide a support system on which parents can rely for assistance (Reece, 1993), but they can also be a source of conflict. Sometimes a large network can cause problems because it results in conflicting advice from numerous people. Grandparents or in-laws are most appreciated when they assist with household responsibilities and do not intrude into the parents' privacy or judge them critically (Hansen & Jacob, 1992).

Women who have given birth before may have different support needs than first-time mothers. First-time mothers may need more follow-up for parenting skills, including referral to community resources. Women with other children may be more realistic in anticipating physical limitations and the changes in roles and relationships. However, these experienced mothers express concerns over separation from their firstborn, loss of the exclusive relationship with the older child or children, and the challenge of caring for two or more children.

Because of the extent of restructuring and reorganization that occurs in a family with the birth of another child, the mother's moods and fatigue in the postpartum period can be helped more by situation-specific support from family and friends than from general support (Gottlieb & Mendelson, 1995). General support addresses feeling loved, respected, and valued. Situation-specific support relates to practical concerns such as physical needs and child care. For example, the practical support of a grandparent bathing the infant can help lessen a second-time mother's feelings of loss by providing her time to be with her firstborn child. Second-time mothers report that practical support is the most useful and desirable type of support during the postpartum period (Jordan, 1989).

Nurses need to be aware that not all types of support are equally beneficial to mothers postpartally and therefore need to assess the presence and types of practical help available to new mothers. The assumption that second-time (experienced) mothers are "old pros" and therefore do not need help should be avoided. Because second-time mothers may expect this of themselves, nurses can help these mothers explore the differences associated with adding another child to the family and identify the types of support that they need the most. As Gottlieb and Mendelson (1995) suggest, there must be a "fit" between the availability of support and a parent's needs for the support to be effective, and support may change with changing situations.

Culture

Cultural beliefs and practices are important determinants of parenting behaviors. They influence the interactions with the infant, as well as the parent's or family's caregiving style. For example, the provision for a period of rest and recuperation for the mother after birth is prominent in several cultures. Asian mothers must remain at home with the baby for at least 30 days after birth and are not supposed to engage in household chores, including care of the infant. Many times the grandmother takes over the baby's care immediately, even before discharge from the hospital (Geissler, 1994; Manio & Hall, 1987). Likewise, Jordanian mothers have a 40-day lying-in after birth during which their mothers or sisters care for the baby (Geissler, 1994). Hispanics practice the *cuarentena,* a 40-day period after birth during which the mother is expected to recuperate and get acquainted with her infant. Traditionally this involves many restrictions concerning food (spicy or cold foods, fish, pork, and citrus are avoided; tortillas and chicken soup are encouraged), exercise, and activities, including sexual intercourse. Abdominal binding is a traditional practice, and many women avoid tub bathing and washing their hair. Traditional Hispanic husbands do not expect to see their wives or infants until both have been cleaned and dressed after birth (Geissler, 1994).

Desire for and valuing of children is salient in all cultures (Hammer & Turner, 1990). In Asian families, children are valued as a source of family strength and stability, are perceived as wealth, and are objects of parental love and affection. Infants almost always are given an affectionate "cradle" name that is used during the first years of life; for example, a Filipino girl might be called "Ling-Ling" and a boy "Bong-Bong" (Manio & Hall, 1987). In the Yup'ik culture of the Alaskan Eskimos, where sharing has been necessary for survival throughout their history, children are looked on as security. There is no concept of illegitimacy; whether parents are married does not matter. Every child is welcomed and loved. Adoption is common and is usually within the extended family (e.g., by grandparents) (MacDonald-Clark & Boffman, 1995).

Differing cultural values can influence parents' interactions with health care professionals; for example, Asians are taught to be humble and obedient; to be outspoken is frowned on. They are brought up not to question authority figures (such as a nurse), to avoid confrontation, and to respect the yin-yang balance in nature. Because of these learned values, an Asian mother might not confront the nurse about the length of time it has taken to receive the medication requested for her episiotomy pain. A mother may nod and say, "Yes" in response to the nurse's directions for using an iced sitz bath but then will not use the sitz bath. The "yes," in this case, is a gesture of courtesy, meaning "I'm listening"; it is not an indication of agreement to comply. The mother does not use the iced sitz bath because of her traditional avoidance of bathing and cold in the puerperium. Because all members of a cultural group do not necessarily adhere to traditional practices, validating which cultural practices are important to individual parents is important. (A thorough discussion of parenting in diverse cultures, especially in African-American families, is presented by Hammer and Turner [1990]. Also refer to Table 2-2 for various examples of some traditional cultural beliefs that may be important to parents from various cultures.)

Knowledge of cultural beliefs can help the nurse make more accurate assessments and diagnoses of observed parenting behaviors. For example, nurses may become concerned when they observe cultural practices that appear to reflect poor maternal-infant bonding (Galanti, 1991). Algerian mothers may not unwrap and explore their infants as part of the acquaintance process because in Algeria, babies are wrapped tightly in swaddling clothes to protect them physically and psychologically (Geissler, 1994). The nurse may observe a Vietnamese woman who gives care to her infant but refuses to cuddle or further interact with her child. This apparent lack of interest in the newborn is this cultural group's attempt to ward off "evil spirits" and actually reflects an intense love and concern for the child (Galanti, 1991). An Asian mother might be criticized for almost immediately relinquishing the care of the infant to the grandmother and not even attempting to hold her baby when it is brought to her room. However, in Asian extended families, members show their support for a new mother's rest and recuperation by assisting with the care of the baby (Manio & Hall, 1987). Contrary to the guidance given to mothers in the United States about "nipple confusion," a mix of breastfeeding and bottle feeding is standard practice for Japanese mothers. This is out of concern for the mother's rest during the first 2 to 3 months and does not lead to any problems with lactation; breastfeeding is widespread and successful among Japanese women (Sharts-Hopko, 1995).

Discontinuities of culture and related traditions may be problematic for some families during the transition to parenthood. Hansen and Jacob (1992) found that when the couples' backgrounds diverged in ethnicity, religion, or socioeconomics, the differences had a major impact on intergenerational relationships. Some couples were unable to integrate the differences and chose either the maternal or the paternal family for support, thus magnifying the conflict between generations. Some couples broke completely with both families.

In helping new families adjust to parenthood, nurses must provide culturally sensitive care by following principles that facilitate nursing practice within transcultural situations (Box 18-2).

| BOX 18-2 | *Principles for Facilitating Nursing Practice Within Transcultural Situations* |

- *The stress of new parenthood overlies the stressors of transcultural migration.* It is exacerbated to the extent that patients do not speak the dominant language. Because of emigration, the patient may also be experiencing altered socioeconomic status and isolation from loved ones, and it may have resulted from war, famine, or other great suffering.
- *Nurses may be able to foster connections with networks of specific cultural groups, although with the awareness that intracultural differences, like religion, can create important barriers.* Bilingual volunteers can be a great help in easing hospital stays for non–English-speaking patients and their families.
- *Nurses can enhance their ability to care for large immigrant populations by learning about those cultures* through reading, talking with representatives of the groups, attending educational programs, or viewing films.
- *Nurses will serve as more effective interpreters of the childbearing experience to transcultural patients if they operate on the assumptions that patients (1) do not know what will be done to them, (2) may not convey their needs or may express them differently, and (3) may not know how they are expected to respond in the situation.* Caring behaviors are culture specific. For example, informed consent is an American issue that has no meaning in some other cultures. Withholding food from a Japanese woman in labor, to her, undermines her energy for effective pushing. Expecting new mothers to assume child care within a day after birth can seem callous to people in cultures who place a high value on recuperation. Devaluing traditional practices of the mother's cultural group devalues her as a person.
- *Differing practices must be evaluated from the standpoint of safety as understood by health care professionals in the United States, but a healthy measure of humility is warranted.*

Socioeconomic Conditions

Socioeconomic conditions often determine access to available resources. Parents whose economic condition is made worse with the birth of each child and who are unable to use an effective method of fertility management may find childbirth complicated by concern for their own health and a sense of helplessness. Mothers who are single, separated, or divorced from their husbands or without a partner, family, and friends for whatever reason may view the birth of a child with dread. Serious financial problems may override any desire for mothering the infant. Nurses need to be sensitive to the stressors that economically disadvantaged mothers have to contend with and consider these in efforts to foster mother-infant bonding (Sharts-Hopko, 1995). Nursing measures designed to help mothers in trying socioeconomic circumstances involve referral to social and economic community service agencies, as well as health care agencies. A satisfactory outcome for such problems often requires long-term commitments from both the woman or couple and the community. Adequate situational supports need to be instituted in the prenatal period.

Personal Aspirations

For some women, parenthood interferes with or blocks their plans for personal freedom or advancement in their career. Resentment concerning this loss may not have been resolved during the prenatal period, and if it remains unresolved, it will spill over into caregiving activities and may result in indifference and neglect of the infant. Conversely, it may result in excessive concern and the setting of impossibly high standards by the mother for her own behavior or the infant's behavior.

Nursing intervention includes providing opportunities for parents to express their feelings freely to an objective listener; to discuss measures to permit personal growth of the parent (e.g., by part-time employment, volunteer work, and the use of agencies that provide babysitting care or mother-substitutes during parents' vacations); and to learn about the care of their child.

I PARENTAL SENSORY IMPAIRMENT

In the early dialogue between the parent and child, all senses—sight, hearing, touch, taste, and smell—are used by each to initiate and sustain the attachment process. A parent who has an impairment of one of the senses needs to maximize use of the remaining senses.

Visually Impaired Parent

Although parents who are visually impaired need the presence and the support of another responsible person, they can become adept in many child care activities, as the following report indicates:

> We had always planned to have a child. My family and Dick's both wanted us to have the happiness of children and were willing to help us with the baby care. First I bathed and changed a doll; then I practiced caring for my sister's baby. I would feel in all the creases with my finger to see if they were clean and dry. We used disposable diapers that do not need pins. My mother made baby clothes with fastenings of press cloth (Velcro) so I would not have to fiddle with buttons. I feel really confident now. I know I can't do everything for her, but I can do enough to feel like a mother, and I know she will have all the love she needs.

A strength that visually impaired people have is a heightened sensitivity to other sensory outputs. A blind mother

---

BOX 18-3   *Nursing Approaches for Working with Visually Impaired Parents*

- Parents who are blind need oral teaching by health care providers because maternity information is not accessible to blind people.
- A visually impaired parent needs an orientation to the hospital room that allows the parent to move about the room independently. For example, "Go to the left of the bed and trail the wall until you feel the first door. That is the bathroom."
- Parents who are blind need explanations of routines.
- Parents who are blind need to feel devices (e.g., monitors, pelvic models) and to hear descriptions of the devices.
- Visually impaired parents need a chance to ask questions.
- Visually impaired parents need the opportunity to hold and touch the baby after birth.
- Nurses need to demonstrate baby care by touch and to follow with, "Now let me see you do it."
- Nurses need to give instructions such as, "I'm going to give you the baby. The head is to your left side."

---

can tell when her infant is facing her because she can feel the baby's breath on her face.

One of the major difficulties that visually impaired parents experience is the skepticism, open or hidden, of health care professionals. Blind people sense a reluctance on the part of others to acknowledge that they have a right to be parents. All too often, nurses and doctors lack the experience to deal with the childbearing and childrearing needs of visually impaired mothers, as well as mothers with other disabilities (such as hearing impaired, physically impaired, and mentally challenged). Shyness, fear, or reluctance on the part of nurses can result in visually impaired parents being left alone or being involved in awkward conversations. The best approach by the nurse is to assess the mother's capabilities. From that basis, the nurse can make plans to assist the woman, often in much the same way as for a mother with sight. Visually impaired mothers have made suggestions for providing care for women such as themselves during childbearing (Box 18-3). Such approaches by the nurse can help avoid a sense of increased vulnerability on the mother's part.

Eye contact is considered important in American culture. With a parent who is visually impaired, this critical factor in the parent-child attachment process is obviously missing. However, the blind parent, who may never have experienced this method of strengthening relationships, does not miss it. The infant will need other sensory input from that parent. An infant looking into the eyes of a mother who is blind may not be aware that the eyes are unseeing. Other people in the newborn's environment can also participate in active eye contact to supply this need. A problem may arise, however, if the visually impaired parent has an impassive facial expression. Her infant, making repeated unsuccessful attempts to engage in face play with the mother, will abandon the behavior with her and intensify it with the father or other people in the household. Nurses can provide anticipatory guidance regarding this situation and help the mother learn to nod and smile while talking and cooing to the infant.

Hearing-Impaired Parent

The parent who has a hearing impairment faces another set of problems, particularly if the deafness dates from birth or early childhood. The mother and her partner are likely to have established an independent household. A number of devices that transform sound into light flashes are now marketed and can be fitted into the infant's room to permit immediate detection of crying. Even if the parent is not speech trained, vocalizing can serve as both a stimulus and a response to the infant's early vocalizing. Deaf parents can provide additional vocal training by use of records and television so that from birth the child is aware of the full range of the human voice. Sign language is acquired readily by young children, and the first sign used is as varied as the first word.

Section 504 of the Rehabilitation Act of 1973 requires that hospitals and other institutions receiving funds from the U.S. Department of Health and Human Services use various communication techniques and resources with the deaf, including having staff members or certified interpreters who are proficient in sign language. For example, provision of written materials with demonstrations and having nurses stand where the parent can read their lips (if the parent practices lipreading) are two techniques that can be used. A creative approach is for the nursing unit to develop videotapes in which information on postpartum care, infant care, and parenting issues is signed by an interpreter and spoken by a nurse. A videotape in which a nurse signs while speaking would be ideal.

▌ SIBLING ADAPTATION

Because the family is an interactive, open unit, the addition of a new family member affects everyone in the family. Siblings are no exception. Older children have to assume new positions within the family hierarchy. The older child's goal is to maintain the lead position. Parents are faced with the task of caring for a new child while not neglecting the others. Parents need to distribute their attention in an equitable manner.

Reactions of siblings may result from temporary separation from the mother, changes in the mother's or father's behavior, or the siblings' response to the infant's coming home. Sibling reactions are manifested in behavioral

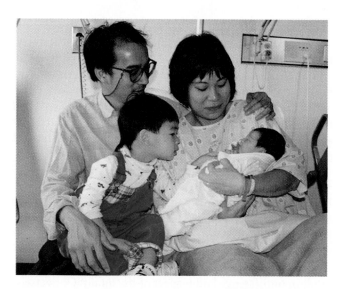

Fig. 18-15 Parents introducing "big" brother to infant daughter. (Courtesy Kim Molloy, San Jose, Calif.)

changes. Positive behavioral changes include interest in and concern for the baby and increased independence. Regression in toileting and sleep habits, aggression toward the baby, and increased seeking of attention and whining are examples of negative behaviors.

The introduction of a baby into a family with one or more children challenges parents to promote acceptance of the baby by siblings (Fig. 18-15). The parents' attitudes toward the arrival of the baby can set the stage for the other children's reactions. In some families, parental support promotes sibling adjustment; in others the needs of the sibling shapes the parental support.

Because the baby absorbs the time and attention of the important people in the other children's lives, jealousy is to be expected once the initial excitement of having a new baby in the home is over. However, more recent research suggests that the expectation of **sibling rivalry,** or negative behaviors in siblings, may have been overemphasized. Guillicks and Crase (1993) studied the difference between parental expectations for sibling behavior and actual sibling behavior 4 weeks after the birth of a second child. They found that parents expected more negative behaviors toward the infant than they observed. The firstborn children continued their usual routines, were more pleased with the newborns, and were more understanding of the infants' need for care than the parents predicted. Parents also reported that the levels of developmentally appropriate behaviors in siblings were similar prenatally and postnatally.

Parents, especially mothers, spend much time and energy promoting sibling acceptance of a new baby. Participating in sibling preparation classes makes a difference in the ability of mothers to cope with sibling behavior (Fortier et al., 1991). Older children are actively involved in preparing for

Strategies for Facilitating Sibling Acceptance of a New Baby

- Take your firstborn child on a tour of your hospital room and point out similarities to his or her birth. "This is like the room I was in with you, and the baby is in the same kind of bassinet that you were in."
- Have a small gift from the baby to give to your older child each day.
- Give the older child a T-shirt that says, "I'm a big brother" (or sister).
- Arrange for your children to be in the first group (grandparents, sister) to see the newborn. Let them hold the baby in the hospital. One mother and father arranged for their firstborn son to be present at the births of his three brothers and to be the first one to hold them.
- Plan time for both children. "When I get home, I'll arrange my day so that I can have the baby's care done in the morning while Sam (first child) is at school. Maybe the baby will sleep part of the afternoon, and I can spend some time with Sam."
- Fathers can spend time with the older sibling while mothers are taking care of the baby and vice versa. Siblings like to have time and attention from both parents.
- Give preschool and early school-aged siblings a newborn doll as "their baby" to care for. Give sibling a photograph of the new baby to take to school to show off "his" or "her" baby. Older siblings may enjoy the responsibility of helping care for the newborn, such as learning how to give the baby a bottle or change a diaper. One mother let her preschooler help burp the new baby by patting on the baby's back. She figured her son could pat the baby fairly firmly without harming him and at the same time get out some pent-up aggressive feelings.

the infant, and this involvement intensifies after the birth of the infant. Parents face a number of tasks related to sibling rivalry and adjustment. For example, parents have to manage the feeling of guilt that the older children are being deprived of parental time and attention. They also have to monitor the behavior of older children toward the more vulnerable infant and divert aggressive behavior. Strategies that parents have used to facilitate acceptance of a new baby by siblings are presented in Box 18-4.

Siblings demonstrate acquaintance behaviors with the newborn. The acquaintance process depends on the information given to the child before the baby is born and on the child's cognitive development level. The initial behaviors of siblings with the newborn include looking at the infant and touching the head. The initial adjustment of older children to a newborn takes time, and children should be allowed to interact at their own pace rather than being forced to do so (Fig. 18-16). To expect a young child to

accept and love a rival for the parents' affection assumes an unrealistic level of maturity. Sibling love grows as does other love, that is, by being with another person and sharing experiences. The relationship that develops between siblings has been conceptualized as sibling attachment (Teti & Ablard, 1989). This bond between siblings involves a secure base in which one child provides support for the other, is missed when absent, and is looked to for comfort and security.

Direct sibling contact does not place healthy newborns at risk for exposure to pathogenic organisms. Therefore separation of newborns and older siblings does not appear to be justified.

GRANDPARENT ADAPTATION

Grandparents are unique. They contribute to a sense of family continuity and provide maintenance of cultural traditions. They can educate their grandchildren about their roots and relate anecdotes about their parents. In turn, the presence of grandchildren often helps relieve the grandparents' loneliness and boredom. Grandparents who are free to love the grandchild can have a significant positive influence on the child's life.

Just as the new parents go through a transition to parenthood, grandparents experience a transition to grandparenthood (see Fig. 18-14). Intergenerational relationships shift, and grandparents must deal with changes in practices and attitudes toward childbirth, child rearing, and men's and women's roles at home and in the workplace. The degree to which grandparents understand and accept current practices can influence how supportive they are perceived to be by their adult children (Hansen & Jacob, 1992).

At the same time that they are adjusting to grandparenthood, the majority of grandparents are experiencing normative middle- and old-age life transition issues, such as retirement, a move to smaller housing, and need support from their adult children. Some may feel regret about their limited involvement because of poor health or geographic distance. Maternal grandmothers, more so than the other three grandparents, may have high expectations of themselves that cause them to be very self-critical (Hansen & Jacob, 1992).

The extent of involvement of grandparents in the care of the newborn depends on many factors (e.g., the willingness of the grandparents to become involved, the proximity of the grandparents, and ethnic and cultural expectations of the grandparents' role) (Hansen & Jacob, 1992). If the new parents live in the United States, Asian grandparents, for example, typically are asked to come to the United States to care for the baby and the mother after birth and to care for the children once the parents return to work (Manio & Hall, 1987). In the United States, paternal grandparents, in contrast to those in other cultures, frequently consider themselves

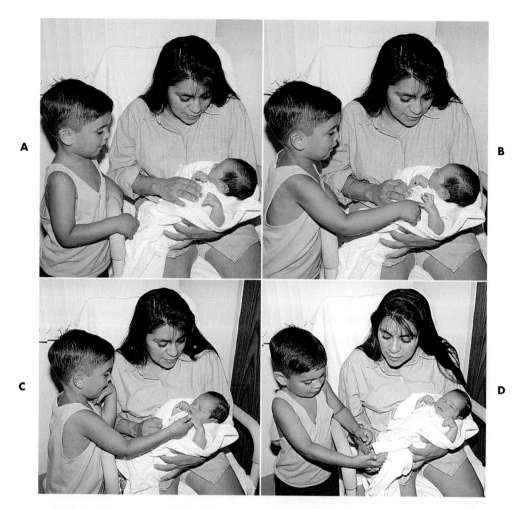

Fig. 18-16 First meeting. **A,** Boy with mother during first meeting with new sibling. **B,** First tentative touch. **C,** Testing with fingertip. **D,** Relationship more secure; it is now okay to hold with whole hand. (Courtesy Marjorie Pyle, RNC, Lifecircle, Costa Mesa, Calif.)

secondary to the maternal grandparents. Less seems expected of them, and they are initially less involved. Nevertheless, these grandparents are eager to help and express great pleasure in their son's fatherhood and his involvement with the baby. Support that they provide for their son has been shown to be positively related to his support of the new mother and to a smoother parental adjustment for the new parents (Hansen & Jacob, 1992).

For first-time parents, pregnancy and parenthood can reawaken old issues related to dependence versus independence. From interviews with expectant parents, Hansen and Jacob (1992) found that the couples did not desire their parents' help immediately after the baby arrived. They wanted time "to be a family," inferring a couple-baby unit, not the intergenerational family network. Intergenerational help was perceived to be interference. Contrary to their expectations, however, these new parents did call on their parents for help. The majority of maternal grandmothers were present soon after the birth, being called in on short notice by the parents after several nights with a crying infant. Grandparents,

respecting their children's wishes for autonomy while remaining available, provided most of the support.

As parents are assisted in working through differing opinions and unresolved conflicts (e.g., feelings of dependency and control) between themselves and their parents, they can move toward mastery of the developmental tasks of adulthood. The support of grandparents can be a stabilizing influence for families undergoing developmental transitions such as childbearing and new parenthood (Hansen & Jacob, 1992; Strom et al., 1992-1993). Grandparents can foster the learning of parental skills and preserve tradition. The maternal grandmother is an important model for childrearing practices, a source of knowledge, and a support person. In the case of teenage mothers, the regular assistance of grandparents with child care has allowed these young mothers to continue their education (Unger & Cooley, 1992).

Nurses should be aware that the transition to parenthood and grandparenthood offers and demands new intergenerational adaptations. Rather than taking for granted intergenerational support between adult children and their parents, nurses must acknowledge the wide range of dynamic issues that enhance or mitigate experiences of intergenerational support. Early in pregnancy, a family assessment that includes an intergenerational perspective can identify whether grandparents are included in the couple's social support network and whether their support is wanted and helpful.

One simple technique to help people span the generation gap is through a printed "letter to new parents" (written from the grandparents' perspective), which can be included in prenatal kits distributed in childbirth preparation classes and made available to all family members on the postpartum unit. Another way to help grandparents bridge the generation gap and understand their adult children's parenting concepts is to offer classes. Included in these classes would be information about up-to-date childbearing practices (especially family-centered care), infant care, feeding, and safety (car seats), as well as exploration of roles that grandparents play in the family unit. Both techniques can foster open discussion between the generations about the feelings and needs of parents and grandparents.

CARE MANAGEMENT: PRACTICAL SUGGESTIONS FOR THE FIRST WEEKS AT HOME

Numerous changes occur during the first weeks of parenthood. Care management should be directed toward helping parents cope with infant care, role changes, altered lifestyle, and change in family structure resulting from the addition of a new baby. Parents may have inadequate or incorrect understanding of what to expect in the early postpartum weeks. Developing skill and confidence in caring for an infant can be especially anxiety provoking.

Nurses, especially those making postpartum visits to parents' homes, are in a prime position to help new families. The nurse's role becomes primarily one of teacher-supporter, focusing on enabling new parents to become capable of self-care and infant care and of meeting the needs of the family unit.

Assessment and Nursing Diagnoses

Assessment should include a psychosocial assessment focusing on parent-infant attachment, adjustment to the parental role, sibling adjustment, social support, and education needs, as well as mother's and baby's physical adaptation. Early home visits are an excellent opportunity for the nurse to assess beginnings of successful or harmful parenting behaviors. Parents demonstrating loving and nurturing behaviors with their infant need to be given positive reinforcement. Parents who interact in inappropriate or abusive ways with their infant should be followed more closely, and an appropriate mental health practitioner or professional social worker should be notified (Johnson & Johnson, 1996).

Home visits often offer an opportunity to involve all family members. The mother, father, siblings, and even grandparents may ask questions and express concerns. The nurse can share her assessments and observations and develop a plan of care collaboratively with the family. Nursing diagnoses pertinent to the period of adaptation to parenthood are presented in the Nursing Diagnoses box.

Nursing Diagnoses

Adaptation to Parenthood
Family coping: potential for growth related to:
- Positive attitude and realistic expectations for newborn and adapting to parenthood
- Nurturing behaviors with newborn
- Verbalizing positive, joyous factors in lifestyle change; perceived strong and satisfying social support system

Ineffective family coping
Ineffective individual coping related to:
- Disorganization and role change during assumption of parent role and adaptation to parenthood
- Unrealistic expectations of newborn/infant and family life changes
- Lack of social support system or perceived dissatisfaction with social support system
- Fatigue and interrupted sleep

Risk for altered parenting related to:
- Lack of knowledge of infant care
- Feelings of incompetence and/or lack of confidence
- Unrealistic expectations of newborn/infant
- Lack of satisfying social support systems
- Fatigue from interrupted sleep

Parental role conflict related to:
- Role transition and role attainment
- Unwanted pregnancy
- Lack of resources to support parenting (e.g., hourly wage earner without paid leave)
- Unplanned pregnancy interfering with professional career

Altered parent-infant attachment
Risk for altered parent-infant attachment related to:
- Difficult labor and birth
- Postpartum complications
- Neonatal complications/anomalies
- Unrealistic expectations of newborn
- Lack of knowledge
- Lack of satisfying social support system

Expected Outcomes of Care

A plan of care is formulated in collaboration with the family, incorporating their priorities and preferences, to meet their specific needs. Goals are set and prioritized. Expected outcomes for effective adaptation to parenthood include that the parents will do the following:

- Interact with the newborn in a loving and nurturing way
- Demonstrate behaviors that reflect appreciation of sensory and behavioral capacities of the infant
- Respond appropriately to infant cues
- Verbalize increasing confidence and competence in feeding, diapering, dressing, and sensory stimulation of the infant
- Identify deviations from normal in the infant that should be brought to the immediate attention of the primary health care provider
- Relate not only stressful or challenging factors in lifestyle change, but also positive and joyous ones
- Describe or demonstrate emergency procedures and verbalize ways of getting emergency help
- Interact in a supportive manner
- Collaborate effectively with each other in caring for the newborn and other children
- Relate effectively to the newborn's grandparents and siblings

Plan of Care and Interventions

Instructions for the first days at home

Parents, especially first-time parents, must be helped to anticipate what the transition from hospital to home will be like. Anticipatory guidance can help prevent a shock of reality that might negate the parents' joy or cause them undue stress. Even the simplest strategies can provide enormous support. Written information reinforcing education topics is helpful to provide to parents, as is a list of available community resources, both local and national (Box 18-5). An excellent resource for the nurse is the *Compendium of Postpartum Care,* developed by Johnson and Johnson Products, Inc., in association with the Association of Women's Health, Obstetric, and Neonatal Nurses (1996). Postpartum nurses will find the "Patient Handouts" section especially useful. It includes handouts on topics such as rest and exercise, emotional well-being during adaptation to parenthood, understanding the blues, and what to expect and do regarding the infant's health. Classes in the prenatal period or during the postpartum stay are helpful. Instructions for the first days at home should at a minimum include activities of daily living, dealing with visitors, and activity and rest.

Activities of daily living. Given the demands of a newborn, the mother's discomfort or fatigue associated with giving birth, and a busy homecoming day, even small details of daily life can become stressful. Such things as using disposable diapers, preparing frozen and/or microwave dinners, or getting takeout meals, can decrease stress by eliminating at least one or two parental responsibilities during the first few days at home.

Visitors. New parents are often inadequately prepared for the reality of bringing a new infant home because they

---

BOX 18-5 *Resources for New Parents*

The Fatherhood Project at the Families and Work Institute
330 Seventh Avenue
New York, NY 10001   (212) 465-2044

The Institute for Responsible Fatherhood and Family Revitalization
1090 Vermont Avenue NW
Suite 1100
Washington, DC 20005-4961   (202) 789-6376
or (800) 7-FATHER

At-Home Dad (newsletter for fathers who stay at home)
61 Brightwood Avenue
North Andover, MA 01845-1702 (E-mail: athomedad@aol.com

Postpartum Support International
927 N. Kellogg Avenue
Santa Barbara, CA 93111 (805) 967-7636

La Leche League International
9616 Minneapolis Avenue
P.O. Box 1209
Franklin Park, IL 60131 (708) 455-7730
(Local La Leche League groups are usually listed in city and town phone books)

Motherhood Maternity Health and Fitness Program
SBI Corporation
1106 Stratford Drive
Carlisle, PA 17013 (800) MOM-WELL
 (Fax: (717) 258-4641)

Single Parent Resource Center
141 W. 28th Street
Suite 302
New York, NY 10001 (212) 947-0221

Parent Effectiveness Training
120 Woodbine Street
Bergenfield, NJ 07621 (201) 387-0600
(Book and parenting guide)

Pink Inc.! Publishing
P.O. Box 866
Atlantic Beach, FL 32233-0866 (904) 731-7120

---

romanticize the homecoming. One mother stated, "By the time we drove an hour through traffic, my stitches were hurting and all I wanted was a warm sitz bath and some private time with Bill and the baby, in that order. Instead, a carload of visitors pulled into the driveway as we were unbuckling the baby from his car seat. I thought I would surely cry."

The nurse can help parents explore ways, in advance, to assert their need to limit visitors. When family and friends ask what they can do to help, new parents can suggest they prepare and bring them a meal or pick up items at the store. Parents can work out a signal for alerting the partner that the mother is getting tired or uncomfortable and needs the partner to invite the visitors to another room or to leave. Some mothers find that wearing a robe and not appearing ready for company leads visitors to stay a shorter time. A sign on the front door saying, "Mother and baby resting. . . . Please do not disturb" may be useful.

Activity and rest. Since mothers have reported fatigue as a major problem during the first few weeks after giving birth, mothers need to be encouraged to limit their activities and be realistic about their level of fatigue. Activities should not be sustained for long periods of time. Family, friends, and neighbors can be solicited for support and help with meals, housecleaning, picking up other children, etc. Rest periods throughout the day are important. Mothers can nap when the baby sleeps. Adequate nutrition is also important for postpartum recovery and in dealing with fatigue.

On postpartum days 1 through 3, mothers can begin a regimen of light exercise, especially Kegel and isometric abdominal muscle–toning exercises. Many new mothers have concerns about body image. The nurse can help new mothers develop realistic expectations of how quickly and to what extent their bodies will return to the nonpregnant state.

New parents also need to develop realistic expectations about resumption of their sexual life. Nurses need to let couples know that it is normal to feel that their sex life is somewhat limited by fatigue, the baby's needs, and the woman's physical recovery and emotional changes. It is helpful for the nurse to bring up the subject, since many couples are reluctant to do so.

Infant care

Providing practical suggestions for infant care can help parents adjust to parenthood. Mothers and fathers want to feel capable and confident in the physical care of their infant. The nurse should assess each parent's need for instruction on care such as bathing, clothing, and safety.

Infant bathing. The infant bath time provides a wonderful opportunity for parent-infant social interaction. Some fathers consider this their own special time with their babies. While bathing their baby, parents can talk to the infant, caress and cuddle the infant, and engage in arousal and imitation of facial expressions and smiling.

Sponge baths are used until the infant's umbilical cord falls off and the umbilicus is healed (see Chapter 20 for the Home Care box on sponge baths). At about 10 to 14 days, tub baths can be started (Box 18-6). Newborns do not need a bath every day. The diaper area and creases under the arms and neck need more attention. Parents can pick a time that is easy for them and when the baby is awake, usually before a feeding.

Questions have arisen about some routine practices: use of soap, lotion, oil, and powder. An important consideration in skin cleansing is preservation of the skin's acid mantle. The acid mantle is formed from the uppermost horny layer of the epidermis, sweat, superficial fat, metabolic products, and external substances such as amniotic fluid,

---

| BOX 18-6 | *Tub Bathing* |

See guidelines for sponge bathing (Chapter 20).
Place liner on bottom of tub to prevent infant from slipping.
Add 3 inches of comfortably warm water (36.6° to 37.2° C—pleasantly warm to your inner wrist).
Wash face and shampoo hair as for sponge bath.
Undress baby. Lower infant slowly into water.
Hold baby safely with fingers under the baby's armpit, with your thumb around the shoulder. The other hand supports the baby's bottom and legs.

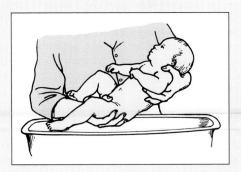

Wash the front of the baby.
Go from front to back between the legs. Rinse with a wet washcloth.

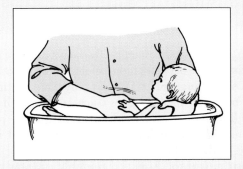

Wash the baby's back with your free hand lathered with soap.
Rinse well with the wet washcloth.

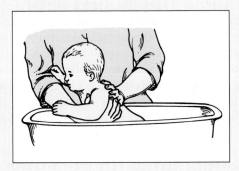

Remove infant from the water and gently pat dry.

| BOX 18-7 | *Tips for Keeping Your Baby Safe* |

- Never leave your baby alone on a bed, couch, or table. Even newborns can move enough to eventually reach the edge and fall off.
- Never put your baby on a cushion, pillow, beanbag, or waterbed to sleep. Your baby may suffocate. Also, do not keep pillows, large floppy toys, or loose plastic sheeting in the crib.
- Do not place your infant on his or her stomach to sleep during the first few months of life. The American Academy of Pediatrics advises against this prone position because it has been associated with an increased incidence of sudden infant death syndrome (SIDS). The side-lying or back-lying position is preferable.
- When using an infant carrier, stay within arm's reach when the carrier is on a high place, such as a table, sofa, or store counter. If at all possible, place the carrier on the floor near you.
- Infant carriers do not keep your baby safe in a car. Always place your baby in an approved car safety seat when traveling in a motor vehicle (car, truck, bus, or van). Car safety seats are recommended for travel on trains and airplanes as well. Use the car seat for *every* ride. Your baby should be in a rear-facing infant car seat from birth to 20 pounds, and the car seat should be in the back seat of the car (see Fig. 18-17). This is especially important in vehicles with front passenger air bags, since air bags, when they inflate, can be fatal for infants and toddlers.

- When bathing your baby, never leave him or her alone. Newborns and infants can drown in 1 to 2 inches of water.
- Be sure that your hot water heater is set at 49° C or less. Always check bathwater temperature with your elbow before putting your baby in the bath.
- Do not tie anything around your baby's neck. Pacifiers, for example, tied around the neck with a ribbon or string may strangle your baby.
- Check your baby's crib for safety. Slats should be no more than 2½ inches apart. The space between the mattress and sides should be less than 2 finger widths. There should be no decorative knobs on the bedposts.
- Keep crib or play pen away from window blind and drapery cords; your baby could strangle on them.
- Keep crib and play pen well away from radiators, heat vents, and portable heaters. Linens in crib or playpen could catch fire if in contact with these heat sources.
- Install smoke detectors on every floor of your home. Check them once a month to be sure they work. Change batteries once a year.
- Avoid exposing your baby to cigarette or cigar smoke in your home or other places. Passive exposure to tobacco smoke greatly increases the likelihood that your infant will have respiratory symptoms and illnesses.
- Be gentle with your baby. Do not pick your baby up or swing your baby by the arms or throw him or her up in the air.

microorganisms, and cosmetics. By 4 days of age, the newborn skin surface becomes more acidic, falling to within the bacteriostatic range (pH <5). Thus only plain, warm water should be used. Alkaline soaps (such as Ivory), oils, powders, and many lotions alter the acid mantle and provide a medium for bacterial growth. Powders are not recommended, because the infant can inhale powder.

Infant clothing. Parents commonly ask how warmly they should dress their infant. A simple rule of thumb is to dress the child as the parents would dress themselves, adding or subtracting clothes and wraps for the infant as necessary. A shirt and diaper may be sufficient clothing for the young infant. A bonnet is needed to protect the scalp and to minimize heat loss if it is cool or to protect against sunburn and to shade the infant's eyes if it is sunny and hot. Wrapping the infant snugly in a blanket maintains body temperature and promotes a feeling of security. Overdressing in warm temperatures can cause discomfort and prickly heat rash. Underdressing in cold weather also can cause discomfort; cheeks, fingers, and toes can easily become frostbitten.

Infants have sensitive skin; therefore new clothes should be washed before putting them on the infant. Baby clothes should be washed with a mild detergent and hot water. A double rinse usually removes traces of the potentially irritating cleansing agent or acid residue from urine or stool. If possible, the clothing and bed linens are dried in the sun to neutralize residue. Parents who have to use coin-operated machines in laundromats to wash and dry clothes may find it expensive or impossible to wash and rinse the baby's clothes well.

Bedding requires frequent changing. The top of a plastic-coated mattress should be washed frequently, and the crib or bassinet should be dusted with a damp cloth. The infant's toilet articles may be kept convenient for use in a box, basket, or plastic carrier.

Infant safety. Providing for the safety of an infant is not a matter of common sense. There are many things new parents may not be aware of that are potential dangers to their infant (e.g., window blind cords near the crib or a parent throwing an infant in the air during play). Nurses should provide parents with concrete instructions on infant safety (Box 18-7). An excellent resource for the nurse is *Protecting Your Newborn, Video and Instructor's Guide,* produced in 1997 by the Ford Motor Company and the U.S. Department of Transportation National Highway Traffic Safety Administration (NHTSA). This guide includes a pamphlet with color pictures demonstrating the correct use of infant and child car seats and a set of handouts on child passenger safety tips (Fig. 18-17). The NHTSA also has a toll-free Auto Safety Hotline (800-424-9393) and a Web page (www.nhtsa.dot.gov) for parents to use.

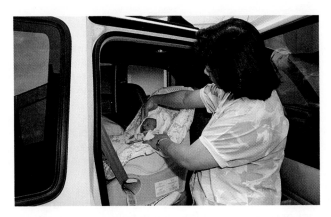

Fig. **18-17** Mother places new baby in rear-facing infant seat in rear seat of car. (Courtesy Marjorie Pyle, RNC, Lifecircle, Costa Mesa, Calif.)

Anticipatory guidance regarding the newborn

Anticipatory guidance helps prepare new parents for what to expect as their newborn grows and develops. Parents with realistic expectations of infant needs and behavior are prepared better to adjust to the demands of a new baby and to parenthood itself.

In giving anticipatory guidance, the nurse should not try to cover all content at one time. New parents can be overwhelmed by a large volume of information and become anxious. Printed materials and audiotapes and/or videotapes for parents to take home are helpful as well. These resources (1) reinforce content discussed in the hospital, (2) allow parents another chance to review the material in private and at their own pace, and (3) provide new information not covered in the hospital. Anticipatory guidance needs to include the following: newborn sleep-wake cycles, interpretation of crying and quieting techniques, infant developmental milestones, sensory enrichment/infant stimulation, recognizing signs of illness, and well-baby follow-up and immunizations.

Development of day-night routines. Nurses can help prepare new parents for the fact that most newborns cannot tell the difference between night and day and must learn the rhythm of day-night routines. Nurses should provide basic suggestions for settling a newborn and for helping him or her develop a predictable routine. Examples of such suggestions include:

1. In the late afternoon, bring the baby out to the center of family activity. Keep the baby there for the rest of the evening. If the baby falls asleep, let the baby do so in the infant seat or in someone's arms. Save the crib or bassinet for nighttime sleep.
2. Give the baby a bath right before bedtime. This soothes the baby and helps him or her expend energy.
3. Feed the baby for the last evening time around 11 PM and put him or her to bed in the crib or bassinet.

4. For nighttime feedings and diaper changes, keep a small night-light on to avoid turning on bright lights. Talk in soft whispers (if at all) and handle the baby gently and only as absolutely necessary to feed and diaper. Nighttime feedings should be all business and no play! Babies usually go back to sleep if the room is quiet and dark.

A predictable, stable routine gradually develops for most babies; however, there will be some babies who never develop one. New parents will find it easier if they are willing to be flexible and to give up some control during those early weeks.

Interpretation of crying and quieting techniques. Crying is an infant's first social communication. Some babies cry more than others, but all babies cry. They cry to communicate that they are hungry, uncomfortable, wet, ill, or bored, and sometimes for no apparent reason at all. The longer parents are around their infants, the easier it becomes to interpret what a cry means. Many infants have a fussy period during the day, often in the late afternoon or early evening when everyone is naturally tired. Environmental tension adds to the length and intensity of crying spells. Babies also have periods of vigorous crying where no comforting can help. These periods of crying may last for long stretches until the infants seem to cry themselves to sleep. Possibly the infants are trying to discharge enough energy so that they can settle themselves down. The nurse needs to reinforce for new parents that time and infant maturation will take care of these types of cries.

Crying because of colic is a common concern of new parents. Babies with colic cry inconsolably for several hours, pull their legs up to their stomach, and pass large amounts of gas. No one really knows what colic is or why babies get it. Parents can be encouraged to contact their nurse-practitioner or pediatrician if they are concerned that their baby has colic.

Developmentalists studying the roots of human behavior have long recognized that certain types of sensory stimulation can calm and quiet infants and help them get to sleep. Important characteristics of this sensory stimulation—whether tactile, vestibular, auditory, or visual—appear to be that the stimulation is mild, slow, and rhythmic, and consistently and regularly presented. Tactile stimulation can include warmth, patting, back rubbing, and covering the skin with textured cloth. Swaddling to keep arms and legs close to the body (as in utero) provides widespread and constant tactile stimulation and a sense of security. Vestibular stimulation is especially effective and can be accomplished by mild rhythmic movement such as rocking or by holding the infant upright, as on the parent's shoulder.

The nurse can teach parents a number of strategies that help to quiet a fussy baby, to prevent crying, and to induce quiet attention or sleep (Box 18-8).

Developmental milestones. Knowledge of infant growth and development helps parents have realistic

BOX 18-8	*Infant Quieting Techniques*

- Many newborns feel insecure in the center of a large crib. They prefer a small, warm, soft space that reminds them of intrauterine life. Try a smaller bed, such as a bassinet, portable crib, buggy, or cradle, or use a rolled-up blanket to turn a corner of the big crib into a smaller place.
- Carry your baby in a frontpack or backpack.
- Swaddle your newborn snugly in a receiving blanket. Swaddling keeps your newborn's arms and legs close to his or her body, similar to the intrauterine position. It makes the newborn feel more secure.
- Prewarm the crib sheets with a hot water bottle or heating pad that you remove before putting your baby to bed. Some babies startle when placed on a cold sheet.
- Some newborns need extra sucking to soothe themselves to sleep. Breastfeeding mothers may prefer to let their infant suckle at the breast as a soothing technique. Other mothers choose to use a pacifier. Stroke the pacifier against the roof of the baby's mouth to encourage him or her to suck it during the first 2 weeks. Around 3 months of age, infants become able to consistently find and suck their thumbs as a way of self-consoling.
- A rhythmic, monotonous noise simulating the intrauterine sounds of your heartbeat and blood flow may help your infant settle down. Some parents have found that putting the baby in a portable crib beside the dishwasher or washing machine helps settle a fussy baby.
- Movement often helps quiet a baby. Take your baby for a ride in the car, or take your baby for an outing in a stroller or carriage. Rock your baby in a rocking chair or cradle.
- Place your baby on his or her stomach across your lap; pat and rub his or her back while gently bouncing your legs or swaying them from left to right.
- Babies enjoy close skin-to-skin contact. A combination of this and warm water often helps soothe a fussy baby. Fill your tub with warm water. Get in and let the baby lie on your chest so that the baby is immersed in the water up to his or her neck. Cuddle the baby close.
- Let your baby see your face. Talk to your baby in a soothing voice.
- Your baby may simply be bored. Bring him or her into the room where you and the rest of the family are. Change your baby's position; many babies like to be upright, such as being held up on your shoulder.

expectations of what an infant can do. When parents understand and appreciate the limitations and developing abilities of their infant, adjustment to parenthood can go more smoothly. Emphasizing the individuality of the infant enhances the capacity of the family to offer their infant an optimally nurturing environment (Brazelton, 1995).

Nurses can play a crucial role in the success of a family system through efforts to enable new parents to understand and enhance their baby's development. For this role, Brazelton (1995) suggests the concept of "touchpoints" for intervention, that is, points at which a change in the system (baby, parent, and family) is brought about by the baby's spurts in development (cognitive, motor, or emotional).

Immediately before each spurt in development, there is a predictable short period of disorganization in the baby. Parents are likely to feel disorganized and stressed as well. Because these periods of disorganization are predictable, nurses can offer parents anticipatory guidance to help them understand what happens with infant development and to prepare them for the subsequent spurts in development.

Two touchpoints occur during the early postpartum-newborn period: one soon after birth and another at 2 to 3 weeks (Brazelton, 1995). In the hospital or at a home visit during the first week, the nurse can use Brazelton's Neonatal Behavioral Assessment Scale (Brazelton & Nugent, 1996) to demonstrate to parents their baby's amazing repertoire of abilities. In this way, parents begin to appreciate their baby's individuality and become more sensitive to their baby's

behavioral cues. At 2 to 3 weeks, the home care nurse or pediatric office nurse should assess for the regular end-of-the-day fussy period that most infants have between 3 and 12 weeks of age. Helpful topics to include in the anticipatory guidance are (1) the normalcy and positive value of the fussy period, (2) how to settle a fussy baby, and (3) ways to help a baby develop a predictable schedule.

It is also helpful for nurses to provide parents with information on month-by-month infant growth and development. Written information that parents can refer to later is especially helpful. See Table 18-6 for a summary of infant growth and development during the first 2 to 3 months.

Infant stimulation. Interacting with their parents is an important way in which infants learn about themselves and their environment. Nurses can teach parents a variety of ways to stimulate their infant's development and to enrich the infant's learning environment. Home health nurses are in a prime position to evaluate the home environment and to make suggestions to parents for promotion of their baby's physical, cognitive, and emotional development. Suggestions for teaching infants during the first few months are presented in Boxes 18-9 and 18-10. Table 18-7 presents suggestions for visual, auditory, tactile, and kinetic stimulation.

Another method of sensory enrichment that parents can learn to use is infant massage. This type of nurturing touch can help create a loving bond between the infant and parent and has been shown to contribute to the physical and emotional well-being of the massage giver and receiver

TABLE 18-6 *Growth and Development During Infancy*

1 MONTH	2 MONTHS	3 MONTHS
PHYSICAL		
Weight gain of 150 to 210 g weekly for first 6 months Height gain of 2.5 cm monthly for first 6 months Head circumference increases by 1.5 cm monthly for first 6 months Primitive reflexes present and strong Doll's eye reflex and dance reflex fading Preferential nose breathing (most infants)	Posterior fontanel closed Crawling reflex disappears	Primitive reflexes fading
GROSS MOTOR		
• Assumes flexed position with pelvis high but knees not under abdomen when prone (at birth, knees flexed under abdomen) • Can turn head from side to side when prone, lifts head momentarily from bed Has marked head lag, especially when pulled from lying to sitting position Holds head momentarily parallel and in midline when suspended in prone position Assumes asymmetric tonic neck reflex position when supine When held in standing position, body limp at knees and hips In sitting position back is uniformly rounded, absence of head control	• Assumes less flexed position when prone—hips flat, legs extended, arms flexed, head to side Less head lag when pulled to sitting position Can maintain head in same plane as rest of body when held in ventral suspension When prone, can lift head almost 45 degrees off table When held in sitting position, head is held up but bobs forward Assumes asymmetric tonic neck reflex position intermittently	Able to hold head more erect when sitting, but still bobs forward Has only slight head lag when pulled to sitting position Assumes symmetric body positioning Able to raise head and shoulders from prone position to a 45- to 90-degree angle from table; bears weight on forearms When held in standing position, able to bear slight fraction of weight on legs Regards own hand
FINE MOTOR		
Hands predominantly closed Grasp reflex strong Hand clenches on contact with rattle	Hands frequently open Grasp reflex fading	• Actively holds rattle but will not reach for it Grasp reflex absent Hands kept loosely open Clutches own hand; pulls at blanket and clothes
SENSORY		
• Able to fixate on moving object in range of 45 degrees when held at a distance of 20-25 cm Visual acuity approaches 20/100* Follows light to midline Quiets when hears a voice	Binocular fixation and convergence to near objects beginning When supine, follows dangling toy from side to point beyond midline Visually searches to locate sounds Turns head to side when sound is made at level of ear	• Follows object to periphery (180 degrees) • Locates sound by turning head to side and looking in same direction Begins to have ability to coordinate stimuli from various sense organs
VOCALIZATION		
Cries to express displeasure Makes small throaty sounds Makes comfort sounds during feeding	• Vocalizes, distinct from crying Crying becomes differentiated Coos Vocalizes to familiar voice	• Squeals aloud to show pleasure Coos, babbles, chuckles Vocalizes when smiling "Talks" a great deal when spoken to Less crying during periods of wakefulness
SOCIALIZATION/COGNITION		
Is in sensorimotor phase—stage I, use of reflexes (birth-1 month), and stage II, primary circular reactions (1-4 months) Watches parent's face intently as she or he talks to infant	• Demonstrates social smile in response to various stimuli	Displays considerable interest in surroundings Ceases crying when parent enters room Can recognize familiar faces and objects, such as feeding bottle Shows awareness of strange situations

From Wong D: *Whaley & Wong's nursing care of infants and children,* ed 5, St Louis, 1995, Mosby.
• Milestones that represent essential integrative aspects of development that lay the foundation for the achievement of more advanced skills.
*Degree of visual acuity varies according to vision measurement procedure used.

BOX 18-9   *Teaching Your Newborn*

- Newborns learn things every day. You can teach your newborn by playing with him or her and giving your newborn toys that help him or her to learn.
- Talk to your baby a lot. Tell your baby what is going on in the room ("Listen to the dog barking."). Label objects that you see or use ("Here's the washcloth.") and describe things you are doing ("Let's put the shirt over Kerry's head!").
- Look at your baby's face and make eye contact. Play face-making games: smile, stick out your tongue, open your eyes wide. As your baby gets older, he or she will try to imitate these facial expressions.
- Babies like music and rhythmic movement. Rock or swing your baby as you sing to him or her in a gentle voice.
- Acknowledge your baby's attempts to "answer" your talking and singing. He or she will respond to you by looking in your direction, making eye contact, moving his or her arms and legs, and/or making sounds.
- Babies like bright colors and vivid contrasts. Show your baby pictures and objects that are black and white, bright primary colors (red, blue, yellow, green), and/or large patterns. Keep colorful mobiles and toys where your baby can see them.
- Babies like to be held upright. Holding your newborn on your shoulder lets your baby look around his or her world and provides vestibular stimulation. Let your baby lift his or her head for a few seconds. Keep your hand ready to support your baby's head.

BOX 18-10   *Teaching Your 1- to 2-Month-Old Infant*

At 1-2 months of age, your infant is gaining more control of his or her movements: more head control, even holding an object briefly in his or her hand. Your baby also is becoming more social. He or she demonstrates behaviors to engage you in interaction: smiling, cooing, making longer eye contact, and following you with his or her eyes.
During these months you can help your baby learn if you:

- Put your baby on his or her stomach on a blanket on the floor. Lie on your stomach facing your baby. Talk to your baby to get him or her to raise his or her head to see you.
- Roll your baby onto his or her back and play with your baby's legs. Move the legs in a bicycle-riding motion. Try to get your baby to kick his or her legs.
- Play hand games, such as pat-a-cake, with your baby; kiss your baby's fingers; place your baby's hands on your face. Bring your baby's hands in front of his or her eyes as you play; get your baby to look at his or her hands.
- Encourage your baby to watch and follow things with his or her eyes. Use a noise-making toy, such as a rattle or a chime, or a brightly colored object about 12 inches from his or her eyes; move it slowly to one side and then the other. Objects hanging from a play frame are good for your baby to watch while he or she is on his or her back or sitting in an infant seat.
- Continue to talk and sing a lot to your baby. Continue to tell your baby what you are doing with him or her and what is going on in the immediate environment.
- Keep your baby near you during times when the family usually is together, such as at mealtimes. Infant seats, especially ones that bounce or rock, and infant swings are good to use at these times.

(Schneider, 1997). Infant massage is not manipulative, but a gentle, warm communication. It is done *with* the infant, not *to* the infant, the focus being on reciprocal interaction between infant and parent. The parent talks to the infant, asks permission to start the massage, questions the infant, and facilitates dialogue.

Schneider (1997) outlines the many benefits of infant massage (Box 18-11), one of the most important for the parents being improved ability to read their infant's cues. Positive cues include eye contact, smiling, looking at the parent's face, babbling or cooing, and smooth movements of arms and legs. Negative cues from the infant include pulling away, frowning, grimacing, turning the head away, arching the back, crying, squirming, and flailing the arms and legs. Increased ability to read their infant's cues can increase parental confidence and self-esteem, thereby assisting adaptation to parenthood.

Optimally, parents can learn infant massage from a certified infant massage instructor (CIMI). Nurses can provide parents with names, addresses, and phone numbers of CIMIs in their community, as well as contact information for the International Association of Infant Massage

(IAIM; 800-248-5432). Parents may find helpful the book *Infant Massage: A Handbook for Loving Parents* by Vimala McClure. Also, nurses can consider becoming CIMIs via the certification program offered by IAIM and thus provide this service to their community.

Well-baby follow-up and immunizations. Parents should be advised to plan for their infant's health follow-up care at the following ages: 2 to 4 weeks of age, then every 2 months until 6 to 7 months, then every 3 months until 18 months, at 2 years, at 3 years, at preschool, and every 2 years thereafter. These well-baby follow-up visits with a nurse-practitioner or pediatrician are important for the parents, as well as the infant. They provide a time for parents to have questions answered, to get reassurance about their adaptation to parenthood, and to receive anticipatory guidance for the ensuing weeks before the next well-baby visit.

TABLE 18-7 *Infant Sensory Stimulation: From Birth Through 3 Months*

AGE (MONTHS)	VISUAL STIMULATION	AUDITORY STIMULATION	TACTILE STIMULATION	KINETIC STIMULATION
SUGGESTED ACTIVITIES				
Birth-1	Look at infant at close range Hang bright, shiny object within 20-25 cm of infant's face and in midline Hang mobiles with black-and-white contrast designs	Talk to infant, sing in soft voice Play music box, radio, television Have ticking clock or metronome nearby	Hold, caress, cuddle Keep infant warm May like to be swaddled	Rock infant, place in cradle Use carriage for walks
2-3	Provide bright objects Make room bright with pictures or mirrors on walls Take infant to various rooms while doing chores Place infant in infant seat for vertical view of environment	Talk to infant Include in family gatherings Expose to various environmental noises other than those of home Use rattles, wind chimes	Caress infant while bathing, at diaper change Comb hair with a soft brush	Use infant swing Take in car for rides Exercise body by moving extremities in swimming motion Use cradle gym

From Wong D: *Whaley & Wong's nursing care of infants and children*, ed 5, St Louis, 1995, Mosby.

BOX 18-11 *Benefits of Infant Massage*

IN THE PSYCHOSOCIAL DOMAIN

Benefits to the Infant of Receiving Massage
- Promotes bonding and attachment
- Promotes body/mind/spirit connection
- Increases self-esteem
- Increases sense of love, acceptance, respect, and trust
- Enhances communication

Benefits to the Parent of Giving Massage
- Improves ability to read infant cues
- Improves synchrony between caregiver and infant
- Promotes bonding
- Increases confidence in parenting
- Increases communication—verbal and nonverbal
- Improves relaxation
- Provides time to share and quality time
- Promotes parenting skills

IN THE PHYSIOLOGIC/PHYSICAL GROWTH DOMAIN

Benefits to the Infant of Receiving Massage
- Improves relaxation and release of accumulated stress
- Stimulates circulation
- Strengthens digestive, circulatory, and gastrointestinal systems, which can lead to weight gain
- Reduces discomfort from teething, congestion, gas, colic, and emotional stress
- Improves muscle tone coordination
- Increases elimination, circulation, and respiration
- Improves sleep patterns
- Increases hormonal function

Benefits to the Parent of Giving Massage
- Improves sense of well-being
- Reduces blood pressure
- Reduces stress
- Improves overall health

From Schneider E: Touch communication: the power of infant massage, *Massage Magazine* 68:40, 1997.

The schedule for immunizations should be reviewed with parents (Table 18-8). An infant's ability to protect himself or herself against antigens by the formation of antibodies develops sequentially; therefore the infant must be developmentally capable of responding to these antibodies. This is the reason for planning sequential immunizations for infants.

A form of passive immunity is already present in colostrum and breast milk. However, these antibodies are specific for microbes present in the mother's gastrointestinal tract and protect against overgrowth as fresh colonization occurs in the newborn.

The active ingredients in immunizations for diphtheria-pertussis-tetanus (DPT), hepatitis B, rubella, measles, and

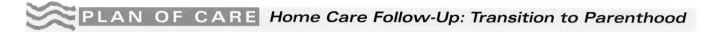

PLAN OF CARE   *Home Care Follow-Up: Transition to Parenthood*

NURSING DIAGNOSIS Risk for ineffective breastfeeding related to frustration with the process

Expected Outcomes *Woman expresses physical and psychologic comfort with the feeding process, and infant feeds successfully and appears satisfied for at least 1 hour after feeding.*

Nursing Interventions/*Rationales*

Explore woman's knowledge of breastfeeding, assess for presence of flat or inverted nipples, determine level of ambivalence and anxiety tied to breastfeeding, and observe the technique being used *to evaluate the process and direct nursing interventions.*

If a problem area is identified, refer to the nursing care plan in Chapter 21 on breastfeeding.

NURSING DIAGNOSIS Risk for infant care deficit related to lack of experience/lack of support

Expected Outcomes *Infant care routines are adequate, and infant appears healthy.*

Nursing Interventions/*Rationales*

Observe infant care routines (bathing, diapering, feeding, play) *to evaluate parental ease with care and adequacy of techniques.*

Discuss parental concerns about care issues and infant response *to assess for possible problem areas.*

Observe infant appearance (height-weight ratio, head circumference, fontanels, skin tone and turgor); assess infant's vital

signs, overall tone, reflexes, and age-appropriate developmental skills *to evaluate for signs indicative of inadequate care.*

Explore available support systems for infant care *to determine adequacy of existing system.*

Help parents identify and address areas of care that need improvement *to ensure infant safety and health.*

Demonstrate troublesome care routines and have involved family members return demonstration *to facilitate improvements in care.*

Provide ongoing follow-up as needed *to ensure amelioration of identified potential and actual care deficits.*

NURSING DIAGNOSIS Sleep pattern disturbance related to infant demands and environmental interruptions

Expected Outcome *Woman sleeps for uninterrupted periods and feels rested on waking.*

Nursing Interventions/*Rationales*

Discuss woman's routine and specify things that interfere with sleep *to determine scope of problem and direct interventions.*

Explore ways woman and significant others can make environment more conducive to sleep (i.e., privacy, darkness, quiet, back rubs, soothing music, warm milk); teach use of guided imagery and relaxation techniques *to promote optimal conditions for sleep.*

Avoid things or routines (i.e., caffeine, foods that induce heartburn, strenuous mental/physical activity) *that may interfere with sleep.*

Advise family to limit visitors and activities *to avoid further taxation and fatigue.*

TABLE 18-8 *Immunizations*	
IMMUNIZATION	**AGE OF ORIGINAL IMMUNIZATION**
DTP (diphtheria, tetanus, pertussis)	2, 4, 6 mo
HIB (*Haemophilus influenzae* b conjugate vaccine)	2, 4, 6 mo (HIBTITER vaccine); 2, 4 mo (PedvaxHIB vaccine)
TOPV (trivalent oral poliovirus vaccine)	2, 4 mo
MMR (measles, mumps, rubella)	15 mo (12 mo if community outbreak)
HBV (hepatitis B)	Before hospital discharge, 1-2 mo, 6-18 mo, or 1-2 mo, 4 mo, 6-18 mo
Tuberculin skin test (not an immunization)	12-15 mo

mumps, as well as the oral poliovirus vaccine (OPV), do not appear to be altered by breast milk and should be given according to the regular recommended schedule (Lawrence, 1994).

Recognizing signs of illness. As well as explaining the need for well-baby follow-up visits, the nurse should discuss with parents the signs of illness in newborns (Box 18-12). Parents should be advised to call their nurse-practitioner or pediatrician immediately if they notice such signs and to ask about over-the-counter medications, such as Tylenol for infants, to keep at home. (See Plan of Care.)

Evaluation

Evaluation is based on the expected outcomes of care. The plan is revised as needed based on the evaluation findings.

≋ **PLAN OF CARE** *Home Care Follow-Up—cont'd*

Have family plan specific times to care for the newborn to allow mother time to sleep; have mother learn to use infant nap time as a time for her to nap as well *to replenish energy and decrease fatigue.*

> **NURSING DIAGNOSIS** Risk for impaired home maintenance management related to addition of new family member/inadequate resources/inadequate support systems

Expected Outcome *Home exhibits signs of safe and functional environment.*

Nursing Interventions/*Rationales*

Observe the home environment (i.e., available living space and sleeping arrangements; adequacy of facilities for food preparation and storage, hygiene and toileting; overall state of repair; cleanliness; presence of safety hazards) *to determine adequacy and effective use of resources.*

Observe arrangements for the newborn, such as sleeping space, care equipment and supplies (bathing, changing, feeding, transportation) *to determine adequacy of resources.*

Explore who is responsible for cooking, cleaning, child care, and newborn care and determine whether the mother seems adequately rested *to determine adequacy of support systems.*

Collaborate with family to remedy identified safety issues immediately *to prevent physical injury.*

Identify and arrange referrals to needed social agencies (i.e., Aid to Families with Dependent Children [AFDC], Women, Infants, and Children [WIC] program, food pantries) *to ameliorate resource deficits (finances, supplies, equipment).*

Identify and arrange referrals if needed for additional support (i.e., housekeeper, child care, postpartum support groups, "warm lines") *to supplement existing support systems.*

Continue home visitation as needed and provide coordination with referral services *to facilitate successful adaptation of environment.*

> **NURSING DIAGNOSIS** Risk for altered family processes related to inclusion of new family member

Expected Outcome *Infant is successfully assimilated into family structure.*

Nursing Interventions/*Rationales*

Explore with family the ways that the birth and neonate have changed family structure and function *to evaluate functional and role adjustment.*

Observe family interaction with the newborn and note degree of bonding, evidence of sibling rivalry, and involvement in newborn care *to evaluate acceptance of newest family member.*

Assist family in reframing any perceived negative outcomes in a more positive light *to promote constructive interaction.*

Clarify identified misinformation and misperceptions *to promote clear communication.*

Assist family to explore options for solutions to identified problems *to promote effective problem resolution.*

Support family efforts as they move toward adjusting and incorporating the new member *to reinforce new functions and roles.*

If needed, make referrals to appropriate social services or community agencies *to ensure ongoing support and care.*

From Wong D & Perry S: *Maternal child nursing care,* St Louis, 1998, Mosby.

| BOX 18-12 | *Signs of Illness to Report Immediately* |

- Fever: temperature above 38° C axillary (under arm for 3 to 4 minutes); also, a continual rise in temperature
- Hypothermia: temperature below 36.6° C axillary
- Poor feeding or little interest in food: refusal to eat for two feedings in a row
- Vomiting: more than one episode of forceful vomiting or frequent vomiting (over a 6-hour period)
- Diarrhea: two consecutive green, watery stools (NOTE: Stools of breastfed infants are normally looser than stools of formula-fed infants. Diarrhea will leave a water ring around the stool, whereas breastfed stools will not.)
- Decreased bowel movement: less than two soiled diapers/day after 48 hours or less than three soiled diapers by the fifth day of life
- Decreased urination: no wet diapers for 18 to 24 hours or less than six to eight wet diapers per day

- Breathing difficulties: labored breathing with flared nostrils or absence of breathing for more than 15 seconds (NOTE: A newborn's breathing is normally irregular and between 30 to 40 breaths per minute. Count the breaths for a full minute.)
- Cyanosis whether accompanying a feeding or not
- Lethargy: sleepiness, difficulty waking, or periods of sleep longer than 6 hours (Most newborns sleep for short periods, usually from 1 to 4 hours, and wake to be fed.)
- Inconsolable crying (attempts to quiet not effective) or continuous high-pitched cry
- Bleeding or purulent drainage from umbilical cord or circumcision
- Drainage developing in the eyes

RESEARCH

The Changing Self-Concept of Pregnant and Parenting Teens

The variable of self-concept associated with adolescent pregnancy has a long history of investigation. The majority of the studies suggest that adolescent pregnancy is both a cause and a result of low self-concept. The majority of studies found differences in self-concept between pregnant and parenting teens and nonpregnant teens, with pregnant and parenting teens having a significantly lower self-concept than their nonpregnant peers. The purpose of this study was to reinvestigate the self-concept of pregnant and parenting teens and to compare these with the published adolescent norms of the Tennessee Self-Concept Scales and sociodemographics. In this descriptive study, 126 adolescent women 14 to 19 years of age who were either pregnant with their first child or had delivered their first child within the past 9 months were surveyed. Pregnant and parenting teens had higher self-concepts than the reported normative group. There were also relevant variations in self-concept in relation to sociodemographics. The older sample of pregnant and parenting teens (mean age of 17.83 years) had a self-concept similar to the junior high school normative sample than to their senior high school-age counterparts. Self-concept varies in relation to the pregnant and parenting teens' age, years of schooling, types of schools attended, income sources, and receipt of public assistance.

Clinical Application of the Study: This study has implications for nurses in terms of program development and evaluation, health marketing, and development of primary prevention strategies. If pregnancy or parenting experience elevates self-concept, how long does this elevation of self-concept last? It is important for nurses to have in place throughout their programs occasional checkpoints to reassess what may be a very changeable state.

Source: Alpers R: The changing self-concept of pregnant and parenting teens, *J Prof Nurs* 14(2):111, 1998

KEY POINTS

- The birth of a child necessitates changes in the existing interactional structure of a family.
- Either parent may exhibit "motherliness."
- Attachment is the process by which the parent and child come to love and accept each other.
- Attachment is strengthened through the use of sensual responses or interactions by both partners in the parent-child interaction.

KEY POINTS—cont'd

- Early contact with the newborn is not essential for attachment to occur.
- For the biologic parent, the parental role does not begin at birth but rather enlarges and intensifies from the preconception decision to have a child.
- The father is considered an equal and integral part of the developing family.
- In adjusting to the parental role, the mother moves from a dependent state (taking in) to an interdependent state (letting go).
- Mothers may exhibit signs of postpartum blues (baby blues).
- Fathers experience emotions and adjustments during the transition to parenthood that are similar to, and also distinctly different from, those of mothers.
- Modulation of rhythm, modification of behavioral repertoires, and mutual responsivity facilitate infant-parent adjustment.
- A primary need of parents is to establish a lifestyle that includes, but in some respects excludes, the child.
- Many factors influence adaptation to parenthood (e.g., age, culture, socioeconomic level, and expectations of what the child will be like).
- Parents face a number of tasks related to sibling adjustment that require creative parental interventions.
- Grandparents can be a source of knowledge and support and can have a positive influence on the postpartum family.
- Anticipatory guidance helps prepare new parents for what to expect.

CRITICAL THINKING EXERCISES

1 *You are the nurse in a neighborhood health clinic that has a partnership with three communities: two whose residents are blue collar and one whose residents are of a low socioeconomic level, living in subsidized housing. At a regular meeting with the neighborhood advisory group, a priority identified is the need for a support group and parenting classes for the young fathers. These young men have children between the ages of 2 weeks and 2 years.*

   a *What are the common concerns/needs of these fathers of newborns and young children?*

CRITICAL THINKING EXERCISES—cont'd

b *How will you determine what content to include in the classes? Outline the content for the parenting classes; state a rationale to justify each area of content.*

c *How will you design the support group? What should be the goal/purpose of the support group?*

d *Identify community resources you will use for the support group and the parenting classes.*

e *How will the demographic characteristics of the residents of these communities influence the design and content of the support group and the parenting classes?*

2 *Kim Huong, from Southeast Asia, has been in the United States for 19 months. She gave birth to a 6-pound 12-ounce daughter by cesarean 48 hours ago. Over the last 2 days Kim has exhibited minimal touching and cuddling of her daughter. Kim's mother, who has come to the United States to stay with Kim for a year, usually changes the baby's diapers and feeds the baby her formula. One of the nurses voices concern that Kim is not bonding appropriately with her daughter.*

a *List maternal behaviors indicative of bonding/attachment.*

b *Describe standard childbearing practices and beliefs associated with bonding in the United States.*

c *What are possible reasons for Kim's behavior with her daughter?*

d *What are possible reasons for the grandmother's involvement?*

e *Describe the approach you will take with Kim to provide culturally sensitive care for her, her newborn, and her family.*

f *Respond to the nurse's concern that Kim is not bonding appropriately.*

References

Albright A: Postpartum depression: an overview, *J Counseling Dev* 71(3):316, 1993.

Alpers R: The changing self-concept of pregnant and parenting teens, *J Prof Nurs* 14(2):111, 1998.

Ament L: Maternal tasks of the puerperium reidentified, *J Obstet Gynecol Neonatal Nurs* 19(4):330, 1990.

Berkowitz G et al: Delayed childbearing and the outcome of pregnancy, *N Engl J Med* 322(10):659, 1990.

Brazelton T: Working with families: opportunities for early intervention, *Pediatr Clin North Am* 42(1): 1, 1995.

Brazelton T & Nugent J: *Neonatal behavioural assessment scale*, ed 3, London, 1996, MacKeith.

Brewaeys A et al: Lesbian mothers who conceived after donor insemination: a follow-up study, *Hum Reprod* 10(10):2731, 1995.

Broom B: Impact of marital quality and psychological well-being on parental sensitivity, *Nurs Res* 43(3):138, 1994.

Cain M: *First time mothers, last chance babies: parenting at 35+*, Far Hills, NJ, 1994, New Horizon Press.

Campbell L: Maternity blues: a model for biological research. In Hamilton J & Harberger P, editors: *Postpartum psychiatric illness: a picture puzzle*, Philadelphia, 1992, University of Pennsylvania Press.

Demick J, Bursik K & Dibiase R, editors: *Parental development*, Hillsdale, NJ, 1993, Lawrence Erlbaum.

Drobeck B: *The impact on men of the transition to fatherhood: a phenomenological investigation*, doctoral dissertation, 1990, Texas Women's University.

Dyer F: Parenthood as crisis: a re-study, *Marriage Fam Living* 25:196, 1963.

Edwards L: *Paternal, infant, and social contextual characteristics as determinants of competent parental functioning by fathers with young infants*, doctoral dissertation, Greensboro, NC, 1990, University of North Carolina at Greensboro.

Ferketich S & Mercer R: Predictors of role competence for experienced and inexperienced fathers, *Nurs Res* 44(2):89, 1995.

Fortier J et al: Adjustment to a newborn: sibling preparation makes a difference, *J Obstet Gynecol Neonatal Nurs* 20(1):73, 1991.

Galanti G: *Caring for patients from different cultures*, Philadelphia, 1991, University of Pennsylvania Press.

Gartrell N et al: The National Lesbian Family Study: interview with prospective mothers, *Am J Orthopsychiatry* 66(2):272, 1996.

Geissler E: *Pocket guide to cultural assessment*, St Louis, 1994, Mosby.

Gerson E: *Infant behavior in the first year of life*, New York, 1973, Raven Press.

Gjerdingen D, Froberg D & Fontaine P: The effects of social support on women's health during pregnancy, labor and delivery, and the postpartum period, *Fam Med* 23:370, 1991.

Gottlieb L & Mendelson M: Mothers' moods and social support when a second child is born, *Matern Child Nurs J* 23(3):3, 1995.

Gullicks J & Crase S: Sibling behavior with a newborn: parents' expectations and observations, *J Obstet Gynecol Neonatal Nurs* 22(5):438, 1993.

Hammer T & Turner P: *Parenting in contemporary society*, ed 2, Englewood Cliffs, NJ, 1990, Prentice Hall.

Hansen L & Jacob E: Intergenerational support during the transition to parenthood: issues for new parents and grandparents, *Fam Soc J Contemp Hum Serv* 73(8):471, 1992.

Harberger P, Berchtold N & Honikman J: Cries for help. In Hamilton J & Harberger P, editors: *Postpartum psychiatric illness: a picture puzzle*, Philadelphia, 1992, University of Pennsylvania Press.

Henderson A & Brouse A: The experiences of new fathers during the first three weeks of life, *J Adv Nurs* 16(3):293, 1991.

Inman M: The power of touch: infant massage therapy, *Childbirth Instructor Magazine*, 4th quarter, 1996.

Jambunathan J & Stewart S: Hmong women in Wisconsin: what are their concerns in pregnancy and childbirth? *Birth* 22(4): 204, 1995.

Jiménez S: The Hispanic culture, folklore, and perinatal health, *J Perinat Educ* 4(1):9, 1995.

Johnson & Johnson: *Compendium of postpartum care*, Skillman, NJ, 1996, Johnson & Johnson Consumer Products.

Jones O & Heerman J: Parental division of infant care: contextual influences and infant characteristics, *Nurs Res* 41(4):228, 1992.

Jordan P: Support behaviors identified as supportful and desired by second-time parents over the perinatal period, *Matern Child Nurs J* 18:133, 1989.

Jordan P: Laboring for relevance: expectant and new fatherhood, *Nurs Res* 39(1):11, 1990.

Klaus M & Kennell J, editors: *Maternal-infant bonding,* St Louis, 1976, Mosby.

Klaus M & Kennell J: *Parent-infant bonding,* ed 2, St Louis, 1982, Mosby.

Klaus M & Kennell J: *Bonding: the beginnings of parent-infant attachment,* St Louis, 1983, Mosby.

Klaus M et al.: Maternal attachment: importance of the first post-partum days, *New Engl J Med* 286:460, 1972.

Koniak-Griffin D, Verzemmnieks I & Cahill D: Using videotape instruction and feedback to improve adolescents' mothering behaviors, *J Adolesc Health* 13(7):570, 1992.

Lawrence R: *Breastfeeding: a guide for the medical profession,* ed 4, St Louis, 1994, Mosby.

LeMasters E: Parenthood as crisis, *Marriage Fam Living* 19:352, 1957.

Leventhal-Belfer L, Cowan D & Cowan C: Satisfaction with child care arrangements: effects on adaptation to parenthood, *J Orthopsychol* 62(2):165, 1992.

MacDonald-Clark N & Boffman J: Mother-child interaction among the Alaskan Eskimos, *J Obstet Gynecol Neonatal Nurs* 24(5):450, 1995.

Manio E & Hall R: Asian family traditions and their influence in transcultural health care delivery, *Children's Health Care* 15(3):172, 1987.

Martell L: Is Rubin's "taking-in" and "taking-hold" a useful paradigm? *Health Care Women Int* 17(1):1, 1996.

McBride B: Parent education and support programs for fathers: outcome effects on paternal involvement, *Early Childhood Dev Care* 67 (Feb):73, 1992.

McCloskey J & Bulechek G: *Nursing interventions classification,* ed 2, St Louis, 1996, Mosby.

Mercer R: Parent-infant attachment. In Sonstegard L et al, editors: *Women's health,* vol 2, *Childbearing,* New York, 1983, Grune & Stratton.

Mercer R & Ferketich S: Predictors of parental attachment during early parenthood, *J Adv Nurs* 15(3):268, 1990.

Nugent J: Cultural and psychological influences on the father's role in infant development, *J Marriage Fam* 53:475, 1991.

Osterwell D: *Correlates of relationship satisfaction in lesbian couples who are parenting their first child together,* doctoral dissertation, Berkeley, 1991, California School of Professional Psychology.

Prodromidis M et al: Mothers touching newborns: a comparison of rooming-in versus minimal contact, *Birth* 22(4):196, 1995.

Reece J: Social support and the early maternal experience of primiparas over 35, *Matern Child Nurs J* 21(3):91, 1993.

Roopnarine J et al: Characteristics of holding, patterns of play, and social behaviors between parents and infants in New Delhi, India, *Dev Psychol* 26(4):667, 1990.

Rubin R: Maternal behavior, *Nurs Outlook* 9:682, 1961.

Rubin R: Maternal touch at first contact with the newborn infant, *Nurs Outlook* 11:828, 1963.

Ruchala P & Halstead L: The postpartum experience of low-risk women: a time of adjustment and change, *Matern Child Nurs J* 22(3):83, 1994.

Ruff C: Adolescent mothering: assessing their parenting capabilities and their health education needs, *J Natl Black Nurses Assoc* 4(1):55, 1990.

Sank J: *Factors in the prenatal period that affect parental role attainment during the postpartum period in Black American mothers and fathers,* doctoral dissertation, Austin, Texas, 1991, University of Texas at Austin.

Schneider E: Touch communication: the power of infant massage, *Massage Magazine,* 68:40, 1997.

Sharts-Hopko N: Birth in the Japanese context, *J Obstet Gynecol Neonatal Nurs* 24(14):343, 1995.

Siegel E: A critical examination of studies of parent-infant bonding. In Klaus M & Robertson M, editors: *Birth interaction and attachment,* Evansville, Ind, 1982, Johnson & Johnson Baby Products.

Smith-Hanrahan C & Deblois D: Postpartum early discharge, *Clin Nurs Res* 4(1):50, 1995.

Strom R et al: Strengths and needs of Black grandparents, *Int J Aging Hum Dev* 36(4):255, 1992-1993.

Symanski M: Maternal-infant bonding, *J Nurse Midwifery* 37:675, 1992.

Tedder J: Using the Brazelton Neonatal Assessment Scale to facilitate the parent-infant relationship in a primary care setting, *Nurse Pract* 16(3):26, 1991.

Teti D & Ablard K: Security of attachment and infant-sibling relationships: a laboratory study, *Child Dev* 60:1519, 1989.

Thompson P et al: Adolescent parenting: outcomes and maternal perceptions, *J Obstet Gynecol Neonatal Nurs* 24(8):713, 1995.

Tulman L: Mothers and unrelated persons' initial handling of newborn infants, *Nurs Res* 34(4):205, 1985.

Unger D & Cooley M: Partner and grandmother contact in Black and White teen parent families, *J Adolesc Health* 13(7):546, 1992.

Wolfson A, Lacks P & Futteman A: Effects of parent training on infant sleep patterns, parents' stress, and perceived parental competence, *J Consult Clin Psychol* 60(1):41, 1992.

Wong D: *Whaley and Wong's nursing care of infants and children,* ed 5, St Louis, 1995, Mosby.

Wong D & Perry S: *Maternal child nursing care,* St Louis, 1998, Mosby.

Wrasper C: Discharge and timing and Rubin's concept of puerperal change, *J Perinat Educ* 5(2):13, 1996.

CHAPTER

19

Immediate Care of the Newborn

BETTE B. HAMMOND

KEY TERMS

Apgar score
brown fat
cold stress
hyperbilirubinemia
hypothermia
ophthalmia neonatorum
sleep-wake states
surfactant
thermoregulation
transition period

TRANSITION TO EXTRAUTERINE LIFE

The neonatal period is the time from birth through the twenty-eighth day of life. During this time the newborn must accomplish a number of physiologic and behavioral adjustments in order to establish and maintain an extrauterine life. Many of the physiologic adjustments occur shortly after birth and set the stage for future growth and development. The term infant (between 38 and 42 weeks of gestation) normally makes this adjustment without difficulty.

Nurses play a vital role during this transition period. They help the newborn infant make a safe transition to extrauterine life and assist the mother and her significant others throughout their transition to parenthood. Nurses perform the initial assessment of the newborn infant, provide a physical environment conducive to adaptation, and monitor the newborn infant's condition during the early adaptation phases.

Physiologic Adjustments

The neonate undergoes rapid and complex physiologic changes after birth. All systems either become functional or adapt to extrauterine life during the neonatal period (Lowe & Reiss, 1996).

Respiratory system

The most critical adjustment a newborn must make at birth is the establishment of respirations. At term the lungs hold approximately 20 ml fluid/kg (Blackburn & Loper, 1992). Air must be substituted for the fluid that filled the respiratory tract. During normal vaginal birth some lung fluid is squeezed or drained from the newborn's trachea and lungs. With the first breath of air, the newborn begins a sequence of cardiopulmonary changes.

Maintaining a clear airway. *Initial breathing* is probably the result of a reflex triggered by pressure changes, chilling, noise, light, and other sensations related to the birth process. In addition, the chemoreceptors in the aorta and carotid bodies initiate neurologic reflexes when arterial oxygen pressure (Po_2) falls from 80 to 15 mm Hg, arterial carbon dioxide pressure (Pco_2) rises from 40 to 70 mm Hg, and arterial pH falls below 7.35. When these changes are extreme, respiratory depression can occur. In most cases an exaggerated respiratory reaction follows within 1 minute of birth, and the infant takes a first gasping breath and cries.

Certain respiratory patterns are characteristic of the normal term newborn. After respirations are established, breaths are shallow and irregular, ranging from 30 to 60 breaths/min, with short periods of apnea (less than 15 seconds). These short periods of apnea occur most often during the active (rapid eye movement [REM]) sleep cycle and decrease in frequency and duration with age. Apneic periods over 15 seconds in duration should be evaluated.

> **NURSE ALERT** *Newborn infants are preferential nose breathers. The reflex response to nasal obstruction is to open the mouth to maintain an airway. This response is not present in most infants until 3 weeks after birth. Therefore cyanosis or asphyxia may occur with nasal blockage.*

Maintaining adequate oxygen supply. During the first hour of life the pulmonary lymphatics continue to remove large amounts of fluid. Removal of fluid is also a result of the pressure gradient from alveoli to interstitial tissue to blood capillary. Reduced vascular resistance accommodates this flow of lung fluid.

Abnormal respiration and failure to completely expand the lungs retard the movement of fetal lung fluid from alveoli and interstices into the pulmonary circulation. Retention of fluid interferes with the infant's ability to maintain adequate oxygenation.

The chest circumference is approximately 30 to 33 cm at birth. Auscultation of the chest of a newborn infant reveals loud, clear breath sounds that seem very near, because little chest tissue intervenes. The ribs of the infant articulate with the spine at a horizontal rather than a downward slope; consequently, the rib cage cannot expand with inspiration as readily as an adult's. Neonatal respiratory function is largely a matter of diaphragmatic contraction. The negative intrathoracic pressure is created by the descent of the diaphragm, much like negative pressure is created in the barrel of a syringe when medication is drawn up by retracting the plunger. The newborn infant's chest and abdomen rise simultaneously with inspiration. Seesaw respirations are not normal (Fig. 19-1).

The alveoli of the infant's lungs are lined with **surfactant**. Lung expansion augments surfactant secretion. Surfactant functions (1) to lower surface tension, therefore requiring less pressure to keep the alveolus open, and (2) to maintain alveolar stability by changing surface tension as the size of the alveolus changes. The surfactant system develops as the infant develops in utero. Fetal pulmonary maturity can be determined by examining amniotic fluid for lecithin/sphingomyelin ratio (L/S) and other phospholipid levels. Phosphatidylglycerol appears at 35 to 36 weeks; its presence is a more predictable indicator of lung maturity.

The ratio of lecithin to sphingomyelin increases with gestational age. Mature fetal lungs have an L/S ratio greater than 2:1. Infants born before the L/S ratio is 2:1 will have varying degrees of respiratory distress. Characteristics of the respiratory system of the neonate and the effects of these characteristics on respiratory function are listed in Table 19-1.

Respiratory distress. Most term infants breathe spontaneously and continue to have normal respirations. However, infants can manifest other problems through respiratory distress. Signs of respiratory distress may include nasal flaring, retractions (indrawing of tissue between the ribs, below the rib cage, or above the sternum and clavicles), or grunting with expirations. Any increased use of the intercostal muscles may be a sign of distress. Seesaw respirations instead of normal abdominal respirations are not normal and should be reported (Fig. 19-1, *B*). A respiratory rate that is less than 30 or greater than 60 breaths/min with the infant at rest needs to be reported to the pediatrician. The respiratory rate of the infant is negatively influenced (slowed or depressed) by the analgesics or anesthetics administered to the mother during labor and birth. Apneic episodes also can be related to rapid warming or cooling of the infant, whereas tachypnea may result from aspiration or a diaphragmatic hernia. Apneic periods longer than 15 seconds must be reported to the pediatrician for evaluation. Even a normal-appearing infant requires close observation because changes in the respiratory system can occur very rapidly.

Circulatory system

The circulatory system changes markedly after birth. The foramen ovale, ductus arteriosus, and ductus venosus close. The umbilical arteries, umbilical vein, and hepatic arteries become ligaments (see Fig. 8-9).

The infant's first breath inflates the lungs and reduces pulmonary vascular resistance to the pulmonary blood flow.

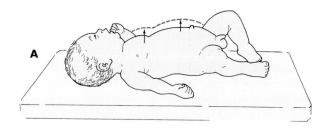
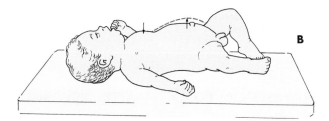

Fig. 19-1 Comparison of normal and seesaw respirations. **A,** Normal respiration. Chest and abdomen rise with inspiration. **B,** Seesaw respiration. Chest wall retracts and abdomen rises with inspiration. (Courtesy Mead Johnson & Co, Evansville, Ind.)

The pulmonary artery pressure drops. This sequence is the major mechanism by which pressure in the *right atrium declines*. The increased pulmonary blood flow returned to the left side of the heart *increases* the pressure in the *left atrium*. This change in pressures causes a functional closure of the foramen ovale. During the first few days of life, crying may reverse the flow through the foramen ovale temporarily and lead to mild cyanosis.

When the Po_2 level in the arterial blood approximates 50 mm Hg, the ductus arteriosus constricts (fetal $Po_2 \cong 27$ mm Hg). Later, the ductus arteriosus occludes and becomes a ligament. With the clamping and severing of the cord, the umbilical arteries, umbilical vein, and ductus venosus close immediately and are converted into ligaments. The hypogastric arteries also occlude and become ligaments.

Heart rate. The heart rate averages 140 beats/min at birth, with variations from 120 to 160 beats/min noted during sleeping and waking states.

Heart sounds after birth reflect the series action of the heart pump. They are described as the familiar "lub, dub, lub, dub" sound. The "lub" is associated with closure of the mitral and tricuspid valves at the beginning of systole and the "dub" with closure of the aortic and pulmonic valves at the end of systole. The "lub" is the first heart sound, and the "dub" is the second heart sound. The normal cycle of the heart starts with the beginning of systole. Heart sounds during the neonatal period are higher pitched, shorter in duration, and of greater intensity than those of adults. The first sound is typically louder and duller than the second sound, which is sharp in quality. Most heart murmurs heard during the neonatal period have no pathologic significance, and more than half disappear by 6 months.

By term gestation the infant's heart lies midway between the crown of the head and the buttocks. The point of maximum impulse (PMI) in the newborn infant is at the fourth intercostal space and to the left of the midclavicular line. The PMI is often visible.

Blood pressure and volume. The newborn infant's average systolic blood pressure is 78, and the average diastolic pressure is 42. The blood pressure varies from day to day during the first month of life. A drop in systolic blood pressure (about 15 mm Hg) the first hour after birth is common. Crying and moving usually cause increases in the systolic blood pressure.

Blood volume in the newborn ranges from 80 to 110 ml/kg during the first several days and doubles by the end of the first year. Proportionately, the newborn has approximately 10% greater blood volume and nearly 20% greater red blood cell (RBC) mass than the adult. However, the newborn's blood has about 20% less plasma volume when compared by kilogram of body weight with the adult. The infant born prematurely has a relatively greater blood volume than the term newborn. This is because the preterm infant has a proportionately greater plasma volume, not a greater RBC mass.

Early or late clamping of the cord changes circulatory dynamics of the newborn. Late clamping expands the blood volume from the so-called placental transfusion. This, in turn, causes an increase in the heart's size, increased systolic blood pressure, and a higher respiratory rate.

Thermoregulation

Heat regulation is second to the establishment of respirations and circulation as a factor critical to an infant's survival. **Thermoregulation** is the maintenance of balance between heat loss and heat production (Shurhan, 1996). Newborns are homeothermic; that is, they attempt to stabilize their internal body temperatures within a narrow range. Hypothermia from excessive heat loss is a common and dangerous problem in neonates. The infant's ability to produce heat often approaches the capacity of the adult. However, the tendency toward rapid heat loss in a cold environment is increased in the newborn and poses a hazard.

Heat production. Heat production is often referred to as *thermogenesis* (*thermo*, "heat"; *genesis*, "origin"). The shivering mechanism of heat production is rarely operable in the newborn. Nonshivering thermogenesis is accomplished primarily by **brown fat,** which is unique to the newborn (Fanaroff & Martin, 1997), and secondarily by increased metabolic activity in the brain, heart, and liver. Brown fat is located in superficial deposits in the interscapular region

TABLE 19-1	*Characteristics of the Respiratory System of the Neonate*

CHARACTERISTIC	EFFECT ON FUNCTION
Lung elastic tissue and recoil is decreased	Lung compliance is decreased; more work and higher pressure are required to expand; risk of atelectasis
Limited movement of diaphragm	Respiratory movement less effective; risk of atelectasis
Preferential nose breather; larynx and epiglottis high	Can breathe and swallow at the same time; risk of airway obstruction; difficulty intubating
Airway passages small and compliant; high airway resistance; weak cough reflex	Risk of obstruction of airway and apnea
Surfactant system altered in immature infants	Atelectatic areas; work of breathing increased; risk of respiratory distress syndrome (RDS)
Respiratory control immature	Respirations irregular; unable to increase rate and depth of respirations rapidly

From Blackburn S: Alterations of the respiratory system in the neonate: implications for clinical practice, *J Perinat Neonat Nurs* 6(2):46, 1992.

and axillae, as well as in deep deposits at the thoracic inlet, along the vertebral column, and around the kidneys. Brown fat has a richer vascular and nerve supply than ordinary fat. Heat produced by intense lipid metabolic activity in brown fat can warm the newborn by increasing heat production as much as 100%. Reserves of brown fat, usually present for several weeks after birth, are rapidly depleted with cold stress. The less mature the infant, the less reserve of this essential fat is available at birth.

Heat loss. Heat loss in the newborn occurs by four modes:

1. *Convection* is the flow of heat from the body surface to cooler ambient air. Because of heat loss by convection, the ambient temperatures in the nursery are kept at 24° C, and newborns are wrapped to protect them from the cold.
2. *Radiation* is the loss of heat from the body surface to a cooler solid surface not in direct contact but in relative proximity. Nursery cribs and examining tables are placed away from outside windows to prevent this type of heat loss.
3. *Evaporation* is the loss of heat that occurs when a liquid is converted to a vapor. In the newborn, heat loss by evaporation occurs as a result of vaporization of moisture from the skin. This heat loss can be intensified by failure to dry the newborn directly after birth or by too slow drying of the infant after a bath.
4. *Conduction* is the loss of heat from the body surface to cooler surfaces in direct contact. When admitted to the nursery, the newborn is placed in a warmed crib to minimize heat loss. Loss of heat must be controlled to protect the infant.

As already noted, control of such modes of heat loss is the basis of caregiving policies and techniques (Table 19-2).

Effects of cold stress. **Cold stress** imposes metabolic and physiologic demands on all newborn infants, regardless of gestational age and condition (Fig. 19-2). The respiratory rate increases as a response to the increased need for oxygen when the oxygen consumption increases significantly in cold stress. Oxygen consumption and energy in the cold-stressed newborn are diverted from maintaining normal brain cell and cardiac function and growth to thermogenesis for survival.

If the newborn infant cannot maintain an adequate oxygen tension, vasoconstriction follows and jeopardizes pulmonary perfusion. As a consequence, arterial blood gas levels of Po_2 decrease, and the blood pH drops. These changes may cause respiratory distress or aggravate existing respiratory distress syndrome (RDS). Moreover, decreased pulmonary perfusion and oxygen tension may maintain or reopen the right-to-left shunt across the patent ductus arteriosus.

The basal metabolism rate increases with cold stress. If cold stress is prolonged, anaerobic glycolysis occurs, resulting in increased production of acids. Metabolic acidosis develops, and if there is a defect in respiratory function,

TABLE 19-2	*Mechanisms of Heat Loss in the Newborn*	
DEFINITION	**NURSING IMPLICATION**	
CONVECTION		
Flow of heat from body surface to cooler ambient air	Maintain nursery ambient temperature at 24° C. Wrap newborn to protect from the cold.	
RADIATION		
Loss of heat from body surface to cooler solid surfaces that are not in direct contact with each other, but in relative proximity to each other	Place nursery cribs and examining tables away from outside windows.	
EVAPORATION		
Loss of heat that occurs when a liquid is converted to a vapor (e.g., vaporization of moisture from the skin); invisible vapor, also known as insensible water loss (IWL)	Dry infant after birth. Bathe and dry infant rapidly in a warm environment.	
CONDUCTION		
Loss of heat from body surface to cooler surfaces that are in direct contact with each other	At birth, wrap newborn in a warmed blanket. Place infant in a warmed bed.	

respiratory acidosis also develops. Excessive fatty acids displace the bilirubin from the albumin-binding sites. The resulting increased level of circulating unbound bilirubin increases the risk of kernicterus even at serum bilirubin levels of 10 mg/dl or less.

Hematopoietic system

Hematopoietic characteristics of the newborn include certain variations from the hematopoietic system of the adult. There are differences in RBCs and leukocytes and relatively few differences in platelets.

At birth the average values of hemoglobin, hematocrit, and RBCs are higher than those values found in adults. Newborn hemoglobin ranges from 14.5 to 22.5 g/dl, the hematocrit ranges from 44% to 72%, and the RBC count ranges from 5 to 7.5 million/mm^3. The hemoglobin and RBC count fall and reach the average levels of 11 to 17 g/dl and 4.2 to 5.2 million/mm^3, respectively, by the end of the first month.

The newborn infant's blood contains about 80% fetal hemoglobin. The percentage of fetal hemoglobin falls to 55% by 5 weeks and falls to 5% by 20 weeks of age. The fall

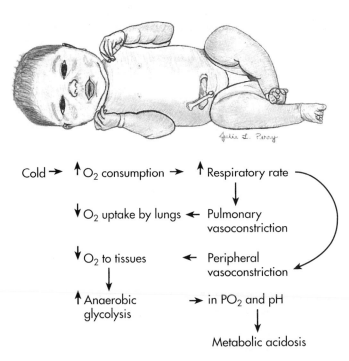

Fig. **19-2** Effects of cold stress. When an infant is stressed by cold, oxygen consumption increases and pulmonary and peripheral vasoconstriction occurs, thereby decreasing oxygen uptake by the lungs and oxygen to the tissues; anaerobic glycolysis increases; and there is an increase in P_{O_2} and pH, leading to metabolic acidosis.

occurs because of the shorter life span of the cells containing fetal hemoglobin. Iron stores generally are sufficient to sustain normal RBC production for 5 months, and as a result the slight, brief anemia is not serious.

The values may be affected by several factors. Delayed clamping of the cord causes a rise in hemoglobin, hematocrit, and RBC count. Samples of capillary blood will give higher values than venous blood. The time after birth when the blood sample is obtained is important; there is a slight rise in RBCs after birth, followed by a substantial drop.

Leukocytosis, with the white blood cell (WBC) count approximately 18,000/mm^3, is normal at birth. The number, largely polymorphs, increases to between 23,000 and 24,000/mm^3 during the first day after birth. A level of 11,500/mm^3 normally is maintained during the neonatal period. In contrast to adults, the WBC count of the newborn does not increase markedly in infections. In most instances sepsis is accompanied by a decline in WBCs, particularly in neutrophils.

Platelet count and aggregation are essentially the same in newborn infants as in adults. Bleeding tendencies in the newborn are rare, and unless there is a marked vitamin K deficiency, clotting is sufficient to prevent hemorrhage.

The infant's blood group is established early in fetal life. However, during the neonatal period there is a gradual increase in the strength of the agglutinogens present in the RBC membrane.

Renal system

By the fourth month of fetal life the kidneys are formed. In utero, urine forms in the kidneys and is excreted into the amniotic fluid.

At term gestation the kidneys occupy a large portion of the posterior abdominal wall. The bladder lies close to the anterior abdominal wall and is partially an abdominal, as well as a pelvic, organ. In the newborn almost all palpable masses in the abdomen are renal in origin.

Kidney function similar to that of an adult is not approached until the second year of life. The newborn has a narrow range of chemical balance and safety. Diarrhea, infection, or improper feeding can lead rapidly to acidosis and fluid imbalances such as dehydration or edema. Renal immaturity also limits the newborn infant's ability to excrete drugs.

Small amounts of urine are usually present in the bladder at birth; however, the newborn may not void for 12 to 24 hours. Voiding after this period is frequent. About 6 to 10 voidings a day of pale, straw-colored urine are indicative of adequate fluid intake. Generally, term infants void 15 to 60 ml of urine per kilogram per day (Fanaroff & Martin, 1997). Sometimes pink-tinged stains ("brick dust") appear on the diaper. These stains are caused by urate crystals and are normal.

Differences in the newborn's fluid and electrolyte balance from adult physiologic response include the following:

- Distribution of extracellular and intracellular fluid. About 40% of the body weight of the newborn is extracellular fluid, whereas in the adult it is 20%.
- Rate of exchange of extracellular fluid. Each day the newborn takes in and excretes 600 to 700 ml of water, which is 20% of the total body fluid, or 50% of the extracellular fluid. In comparison, the adult exchanges 2000 ml of water, which is 5% of the total body fluid and 14% of the extracellular fluid.
- Composition of body fluids. There is a higher concentration of sodium, phosphates, chloride, and organic acids and a lower concentration of bicarbonate ions in the newborn. These findings mean that the newborn is in a compensated acidotic state.
- The glomerular filtration rate is about 30% in the newborn, compared with 50% in the adult. This results in a decreased ability to remove nitrogenous and other waste products from the blood. However, the newborn's ingested protein is almost totally metabolized for growth.
- The decreased ability to excrete excessive sodium results in hypotonic urine, compared with plasma.
- The sodium reabsorption decreases as a result of lowered sodium-potassium–activated adenosine-triphosphatase (ATPase) activity.

- The newborn can dilute urine down to 50 milliosmols (mOsm). The capacity to dilute urine exceeds the capacity to concentrate it. There is some limitation in the ability to increase urinary volume.
- The newborn can concentrate urine from 600 to 700 mOsm, compared with the adult's capacity of 1400 mOsm. The inability to concentrate urine is not absolute, but in terms of adult function, it is somewhat limited. The newborn's specific gravity ranges from 1.005 to 1.015.
- The newborn has a higher renal threshold for glucose.

Laboratory values for newborns appear in Appendix B.

Gastrointestinal system

The term newborn is capable of swallowing, digesting, metabolizing, and absorbing proteins and simple carbohydrates, and emulsifying fats. With the exception of pancreatic amylase, the characteristic enzymes and digestive juices are present even in low-birth-weight infants.

In the adequately hydrated newborn infant the mucous membrane of the mouth is moist and pink. Pallor and cyanosis of the mucous membrane are normally not present. Drooling of mucus is common in the first few hours after birth. Retention cysts, small whitish areas (Epstein's pearls), may be found on the gum margins and at the juncture of the hard and soft palate. The hard and soft palates are intact. The cheeks are full because of well-developed sucking pads. These, like the labial tubercles (sucking calluses) on the upper lip, disappear when the sucking period is over. Occasionally an infant may be born with one or more teeth; this occurs more often among Native American infants.

A special mechanism, present in normal newborns weighing more than 1500 g, coordinates the breathing, sucking, and swallowing reflexes necessary for oral feeding. Sucking in the newborn takes place in small bursts of three or four sucks at a time. In the term newborn, longer and more efficient sucking attempts occur after only a few hours. The newborn infant is unable to move food from the lips to the pharynx, making it necessary to place the nipple (breast or bottle) well inside the infant's mouth. Peristaltic activity in the esophagus is uncoordinated in the first few days of life. It quickly becomes a coordinated pattern in normal infants, and they swallow easily.

Bacteria are not present in the infant's gastrointestinal (GI) tract at birth. Soon after birth, oral and anal orifices permit entrance of bacteria and air. Bowel sounds can be heard 1 hour after birth. Generally, the highest bacterial concentration is found in the lower portion of the intestine, particularly in the large intestine. The normal intestinal flora help synthesize vitamin K, folic acid, and biotin.

The capacity of the stomach varies from 30 to 90 ml depending on the size of the infant. Emptying time for the stomach varies greatly. Several factors, such as time and volume of feedings, type and temperature of food, and psychic stress, may affect the emptying time. This can range from 1 to 24 hours. Regurgitation may be noted during the neonatal period. The cardiac sphincter and nervous control of the stomach are still immature.

Digestion. The infant's gastric acidity at birth normally equals the adult level but is reduced within a week and may remain reduced for 2 to 3 months. The reduction in gastric acidity may lead to "colic." Infants with colic usually remain awake, crying in apparent distress between feedings, often between the same two feedings every day. Nothing seems to appease them. They appear to "grow out" of this behavior by 3 months of age.

Further digestion and absorption of nutrients occur in the small intestine. Pancreatic secretions, secretions from the liver through the common bile duct, and secretions from the duodenal portion of the small intestine make this complex process possible.

The newborn infant's ability to digest carbohydrates, fats, and proteins is regulated by the presence of certain enzymes. Most of these enzymes are functional at birth. One exception is *amylase*, produced by the salivary glands after about 6 months and by the pancreas at about 6 months of age. This enzyme is necessary to convert starch into maltose. The other exception is *lipase*, also secreted by the pancreas, which is necessary for the digestion of fat. Thus the normal newborn is capable of digesting simple carbohydrates and proteins but has a limited ability to digest fats.

Stools. At birth the lower intestine is filled with *meconium*. Meconium is formed during fetal life from the amniotic fluid and its constituents, intestinal secretions, and cells shed from the mucosa. Meconium is greenish black and viscous, and it contains occult blood. The first meconium passed is sterile, but within hours all meconium passed contains bacteria. About 69% of normal term infants pass meconium within 12 hours of life, 94% by 24 hours, and 99.8% in 48 hours.

Distention of the stomach muscles causes a corresponding relaxation and contraction of the muscles of the colon. As a result, infants often have bowel movements during or just after a feeding. Stooling at these times has been attributed to the gastrocolic reflex.

Feeding behaviors. Variations occur among infants regarding interest in food, symptoms of hunger, and amount ingested at any one time. The amount that the infant takes at any one feeding depends, of course, on the size of the infant, but other factors seem to play a part as well. For example, if put to breast, some infants nurse immediately, whereas others require a learning period of up to 48 hours before nursing can be said to be effective. Random hand-to-mouth movement and sucking of fingers have been seen in utero. These actions are well developed at birth and intensify with hunger.

Hepatic system

The liver and gallbladder are formed by the fourth week of gestation. In the newborn the liver can be palpated about

1 cm below the right costal margin, because it is enlarged and occupies about 40% of the abdominal cavity.

Iron storage. The fetal liver (which serves as the site for production of hemoglobin after birth) begins storing iron in utero. If the mother had adequate iron intake during pregnancy, the infant will have an iron store that will last until the fifth month of life.

Conjugation of bilirubin. Bilirubin is a yellow pigment derived from the hemoglobin released with the breakdown of RBCs and the myoglobin in muscle cells. The hemoglobin is phagocytized by the reticuloendothelial cells, converted to bilirubin, and released in an unconjugated form. Unconjugated bilirubin, termed *indirect bilirubin,* is relatively insoluble in water and is almost entirely bound to circulating albumin, a plasma protein. The unbound bilirubin can leave the vascular system and permeate other extravascular tissues (e.g., the skin, sclera, and oral mucous membranes). The resultant yellow coloring is termed *jaundice.*

The liver controls the amount of circulating unbound bilirubin. In the liver the unbound bilirubin is conjugated with glucuronide in the presence of the enzyme glucuronyl transferase. The conjugated form of bilirubin is excreted from liver cells as a constituent of bile. It is termed *direct bilirubin* and is soluble in water. Along with other components of bile, direct bilirubin is excreted into the biliary tract system that carries the bile into the duodenum. Bilirubin is converted to urobilinogen and stercobilin within the duodenum through the action of the bacterial flora. Urobilinogen is excreted in urine and feces; stercobilin is only excreted in the feces (Fig. 19-3). Total serum bilirubin is the sum of conjugated (direct) and unconjugated (indirect) bilirubin.

Adequate serum albumin-binding sites are available unless the infant experiences asphyxia neonatorum, cold stress, or hypoglycemia. Maternal prebirth ingestion of drugs, such as sulfa drugs and aspirin, can reduce the amount of serum albumin-binding sites in the newborn. Although the newborn has the functional capacity to convert bilirubin, physiologic hyperbilirubinemia occurs in most infants.

Physiologic jaundice. Physiologic jaundice, or neonatal **hyperbilirubinemia,** is a normal occurrence in 50% of term and in 80% of preterm newborns. Neonatal jaundice occurs because the newborn has a higher rate of bilirubin production. The number of fetal RBCs per kilogram of weight is greater than in the adult. The fetal RBCs have a shorter survival time—40 to 90 days, compared with 120 days in the adult. In addition, there is considerable reabsorption of bilirubin from the neonatal small intestine. The incidence and severity of physiologic jaundice is increased in Native Americans, Asians, and Eskimos (Merenstein & Gardner, 1998). Although neonatal jaundice is considered benign, bilirubin may accumulate to hazardous levels and become pathologic.

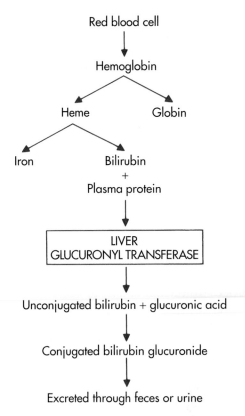

Fig. 19-3 Formation and excretion of bilirubin. (From Wong D: *Whaley & Wong's nursing care of infants and children,* ed 5, St Louis, 1995, Mosby.)

Physiologic jaundice fulfills the following specific criteria (Korones, 1995):

(1) The infant is otherwise well; (2) in term infants, jaundice first appears after 24 hours and disappears by the end of the seventh day; (3) in premature infants, jaundice is first evident after 48 hours and disappears by the ninth or tenth day; (4) serum unconjugated bilirubin concentration does not exceed 12 mg/100 ml, either in term or preterm infants; (5) hyperbilirubinemia is almost exclusively of the unconjugated variety, and conjugated (direct) bilirubin should not exceed 1 to 1.5 mg/100 ml; (6) daily increments of bilirubin concentration should not surpass 5 mg/100 ml. Bilirubin levels in excess of 12 mg/100 ml may indicate either an exaggeration of the physiologic handicap or the presence of disease.

| NURSE ALERT | *At any serum bilirubin level, the appearance of jaundice during the first day of life or persistence beyond the ages previously delineated usually indicates a pathologic process.* |

Jaundice is generally first noticed in the head, especially the sclera and mucous membranes, and then progresses gradually to the thorax, abdomen, and extremities.

Several hospital practices may influence the appearance and degree of physiologic hyperbilirubinemia. *Early feeding* tends to keep the serum bilirubin level low by stimulating intestinal activity and the passage of meconium and stool. Removal of intestinal contents prevents the reabsorption (and recycling) of bilirubin from the gut. The risk of hyperbilirubinemia increases with delayed clamping of the cord.

Cold stress of the newborn may result in acidosis and raise the level of free fatty acids. In the presence of acidosis, albumin binding of bilirubin is weakened and bilirubin is freed. Kernicterus, the most serious complication of neonatal hyperbilirubinemia, is caused by the precipitation of bilirubin in neuronal cells, resulting in their destruction. Cerebral palsy, mental retardation, or other neurologic problems may occur in survivors.

In cases where the infant is discharged from the hospital before 48 hours after birth or the infant is born at home, a professional attendant may not be available to assess pathologic rises in circulating unbound bilirubin. Therefore all parents need instruction in how to assess jaundice and to whom to report the findings.

Jaundice associated with breastfeeding. Two types of jaundice are associated with breastfeeding: breast-*feeding* jaundice and breast *milk* jaundice. Breastfeeding jaundice is associated with the breastfeeding pattern and occurs earlier than breast milk jaundice. Breast milk jaundice is thought to be caused by the presence of an enzyme in the milk and lasts longer than breastfeeding jaundice.

Breastfeeding jaundice. Breastfeeding jaundice usually becomes apparent about the third day of life. There is no other clinical cause. Dehydration, lack of fluid, and weight loss are not causes (Lawrence, 1994). Research has documented that the number of breastfeedings during the first 3 days of life relates to bilirubin levels. The greater the number of feedings, the lower the bilirubin level (Lawrence, 1994). The newborn should be fed eight or more times per day. The mother is encouraged to feed her infant around the clock. Colostrum (a precursor to milk) is a natural laxative that helps promote passage of meconium. Consequently, early, frequent nursings will enhance meconium excretion and decrease bilirubin levels (Lawrence, 1994).

Breast milk jaundice. Breast milk jaundice is defined as increasing indirect hyperbilirubinemia after the first week of life. (See Chapter 21 for a discussion of this topic.)

Immune system adaptations

The cells that supply the infant with immunity develop early in fetal life; however, they are not activated for several months. For the first 3 months of life, the infant is protected by passive immunity received from the mother. Natural barriers such as the stomach's acidity or the production of pepsin and trypsin, which maintain sterility of the small intestine, do not fully develop until 3 to 4 weeks of age. The membrane-protective IgA is missing from the respiratory and urinary tracts, and unless the newborn is breastfed, it is absent from the GI tract as well. The infant begins to synthesize IgG, and about 40% of

adult levels are reached by 1 year of age. Significant amounts of IgM are produced at birth, and adult levels are reached by 9 months of age. The production of IgA, IgD, and IgE is much more gradual, and maximum levels are not attained until early childhood. The infant who is breastfed receives passive immunity through the colostrum and the breast milk. The protection provided varies with the infant's age and maturity, as well as the mother's own immune system (Lawrence, 1994).

Integumentary system

All of the skin structures are present at birth. The epidermis and dermis are loosely bound and very thin. *Vernix caseosa,* a whitish cheeselike substance, is fused with the epidermis and serves as a protective covering. The infant's skin is very sensitive and can be easily damaged. The term infant has an erythematous skin (beefy red) for a few hours after birth, after which the skin fades to its normal color. The skin often appears blotchy or mottled, especially over the extremities. The hands and feet appear slightly cyanotic. This bluish discoloration, *acrocyanosis,* is caused by vasomotor instability, capillary stasis, and a high hemoglobin level. This is normal, is transient in occurrence, and persists over the first 7 to 10 days, especially with exposure to the cold.

The healthy term newborn is plump. Subcutaneous fat accumulated during the last trimester acts to insulate the infant. The skin may be slightly tight, suggesting fluid retention. Fine *lanugo hair* may be seen on the face, shoulders, and back. Actual edema of the face and *ecchymosis* (bruising) may have resulted from face presentation or forceps birth. Petechiae may be present if increased pressure was applied to an area. Petechiae scattered over the infant's body should be reported to the pediatrician because their presence may indicate a problem such as low platelet count or infection.

Caput succedaneum. Caput succedaneum is an easily identifiable edematous area of the scalp (Fig. 19-4, *A*). The sustained pressure of the presenting vertex against the cervix results in compression of local vessels, thus slowing venous return. The slower venous return causes an increase in tissue fluids within the skin of the scalp, and an edematous swelling develops. This boggy edematous swelling, present at birth, extends across suture lines of the skull and disappears spontaneously within 3 to 4 days.

Cephalhematoma. Cephalhematoma is a collection of blood between a skull bone and its periosteum. Therefore a cephalhematoma never crosses a cranial suture line (Fig. 19-4, *B*). Bleeding may occur with spontaneous birth from pressure against the maternal bony pelvis. Low-forceps birth, as well as difficult forceps rotation and extraction, may also cause bleeding. This soft, fluctuating, irreducible fullness does not pulsate or bulge when the infant cries. It appears several hours after birth or the day after

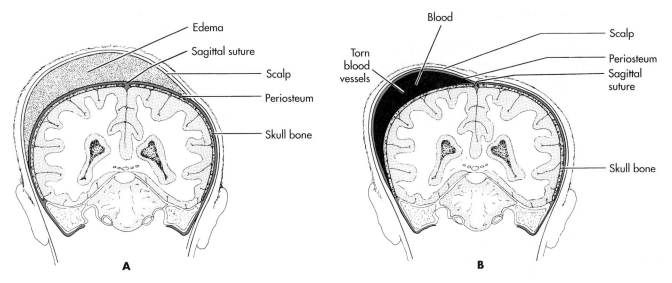

Fig. **19-4** Differences between caput succedaneum and cephalhematoma. **A,** Caput succedaneum: edema of scalp noted at birth; crosses suture line. **B,** Cephalhematoma: bleeding between periosteum and skull bone appearing within first 2 days; does not cross suture lines.

birth, or it becomes apparent after absorption of a caput succedaneum. It is usually largest on the second or third day, by which time the bleeding stops. The fullness of cephalhematoma spontaneously resolves in 3 to 6 weeks. It is not aspirated because infection may develop if the skin is punctured.

As the hematoma resolves, the hemolysis of RBCs occurs. Hyperbilirubinemia may result after the newborn is home. Therefore the parents are instructed to observe the newborn for jaundice and may be asked to bring the infant back to the clinic or doctor's office to be rechecked before the usual 2- to 4-week visit.

Desquamation. Desquamation (peeling) of the infant's skin does not occur until a few days after birth. Its presence at birth is an indication of postmaturity.

Sweat and oil glands. Sweat glands are present at birth but do not respond to increases in ambient or body temperature. There is some fetal *sebaceous* (oil) *gland* hyperplasia and secretion of sebum as a result of the hormonal influences of pregnancy. Vernix caseosa is a product of the sebaceous glands. Distended sebaceous glands, noticeable in the newborn, particularly on the chin and nose, are known as *milia*. Although sebaceous glands are well developed at birth, they are only minimally active during childhood. They become more active as androgen production increases before puberty.

Mongolian spots. Mongolian spots, bluish-black areas of pigmentation, may appear over any part of the body's surface, including the extremities. They are more commonly noted on the back and buttocks. These pigmented areas are noted in infants whose ethnic origins are in the Mediterranean area, Latin America, Asia, or Africa. They are more

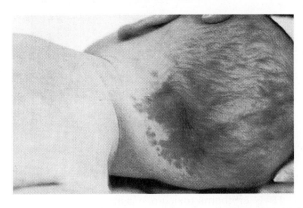

Fig. **19-5** Telangiectatic nevi (stork bite). (Courtesy Mead Johnson & Co, Evansville, Ind.)

common in dark-skinned individuals regardless of race. They fade gradually over a period of months or years.

Nevi. Known as "stork bites," telangiectatic nevi are pink and easily blanched (Fig. 19-5). They appear on the upper eyelids, nose, upper lip, lower occiput bone, and nape of the neck. They have no clinical significance and fade between the first and second years.

The strawberry mark, or nevus vasculosus, is the second most common type of capillary hemangioma. It consists of dilated, newly formed capillaries occupying the entire dermal and subdermal layers with associated connective tissue hypertrophy. The typical lesion is a raised, sharply demarcated, bright or dark red, rough-surfaced swelling that resembles a strawberry. Lesions are usually single but may be multiple; 75% occur in the head region. These lesions can remain until the child is of school age or sometimes even longer.

A port-wine stain, or nevus flammeus, is usually observed at birth and is composed of a plexus of newly formed capillaries in the papillary layer of the corium. It is red to purple; varies in size, shape, and location; and is not elevated. True port-wine stains do not blanch on pressure and do not disappear spontaneously. They are most often found on the face.

Erythema toxicum. A transient rash, erythema toxicum is also called *erythema neonatorum,* or "flea-bite" dermatitis (Fig. 19-6). It has lesions in different stages, erythematous macules, papules, or small vesicles, and it may appear suddenly anywhere on the body. The rash is thought to be an inflammatory response. Eosinophils, which help decrease inflammation, are found in the vesicles. The rash is found only in term infants during the first 3 weeks after birth (Seidel et al., 1998). Although the appearance is alarming, it has no clinical significance and requires no treatment.

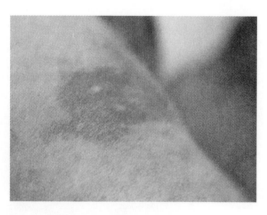

Fig. **19-6** Erythema toxicum. (Courtesy Mead Johnson & Co, Evansville, Ind.)

Reproductive system

Female. At birth the ovaries contain thousands of primitive germ cells. These represent the full complement of potential ova, since no oogonia form after birth in term infants. The ovarian cortex, which is primarily made up of primordial follicles, forms a thicker portion of the ovary in the newborn than it does in the adult. The number of ova decrease from birth to maturity by approximately 90%.

An increase of estrogen during pregnancy followed by a drop after birth results in a mucoid vaginal discharge and even some slight bloody spotting (pseudomenstruation). External genitals are usually edematous with increased pigmentation. In term newborn infants the labia majora and minora cover the vestibule (Fig. 19-7, *A*). In preterm infants the clitoris is prominent and the labia majora are small and widely separated. Vaginal or hymenal tags are common findings and have no clinical significance. Vernix caseosa may be present between the labia.

Male. The testes descend into the scrotum in 90% of newborn boys. Although this percentage drops with preterm birth, by 1 year of age the incidence of undescended testes in all boys is less than 1%. Spermatogenesis does not occur until puberty.

A tight prepuce (foreskin) is common in newborns. The urethral opening may be completely covered by the prepuce, which may not be retractable for 3 to 4 years. Smegma, a white, cheesy substance, is commonly found under the foreskin.

In response to maternal estrogen, external genitals in the term newborn may be increased in size and pigmentation. Rugae cover the scrotal sac (Fig. 19-7, *B*). Hydroceles (accumulation of fluid around the testes) are common and usually decrease in size without treatment.

Swelling of breast tissue. Swelling of the breast tissue in newborn infants of both sexes is caused by the

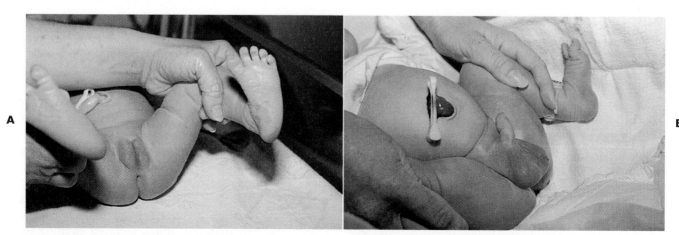

A   B

Fig. **19-7** External genitalia. **A,** Genitals in female term infant. Note mucoid vaginal discharge. **B,** Genitals in male infant. Uncircumcised penis. Rugae cover scrotum, indicating term gestation. Cord has been swabbed with ethylene blue to prevent infection. (Courtesy Marjorie Pyle, RNC, Lifecircle, Costa Mesa, Calif.)

increase in estrogen during pregnancy. In a few newborns a thin discharge from the nipple ("witch's milk") can be seen. The finding has no clinical significance, requires no treatment, and will subside as the maternal hormones are eliminated from the newborn infant's body. Breast tissue and areola size increase with gestation.

Skeletal system

The cephalocaudal direction of development is evident in total body growth. The head at term is one fourth of the body length. The arms are slightly longer than the legs.

The face is small in relation to the skull, which is comparatively larger and heavier. Cranial size and shape can be distorted by molding (shaping of the fetal head by overlapping of the cranial bones; Fig. 19-8).

There are two curvatures in the vertebral column: thoracic and sacral. When the infant gains head control, another curvature occurs in the cervical region. The base of the spine should be checked for a dimple. A dimple may be associated with spina bifida occulta.

In newborn infants there is a significant separation of the knees when the ankles are held together, which results in an appearance of bowlegs. At birth, there is no apparent arch to the foot. The extremities should be symmetric and of equal length. The hips should be checked for dysplasia, using Ortolani's maneuver (see Chapter 20). Fingernails and toenails should be present. There are creases on the palms of the hand. Creases cover the soles of term infant's feet (Alexander & Kuo, 1997).

Neuromuscular system

The term newborn is a vital, responsive, and reactive being with a remarkable capacity for social interaction and self-organization (Fanaroff & Martin, 1997).

Growth of the brain after birth follows a predictable pattern of rapid growth during infancy and early childhood. This growth becomes more gradual during the remainder of the first decade and minimal during adolescence. The cerebellum ends its growth spurt, which began at about 30 weeks of gestation, by the end of the first year. Perhaps this is why the brain is vulnerable to nutritional trauma or other trauma during early infancy.

The brain requires glucose as a source of energy and a large supply of oxygen for adequate metabolism. Such requirements signal a need for careful assessment of the newborn's ability to maintain an open airway and assessment of respiratory conditions requiring oxygen therapy. The necessity for glucose requires careful monitoring of those newborn infants who may have hypoglycemic episodes.

Spontaneous motor activity may be seen in transient tremors of the mouth and chin, especially when crying, and of extremities, notably the arms and hands. These tremors are normal. Persistent tremors or tremors involving the total body, however, may be indicative of pathologic conditions. Marked tonicity, clonicity, and twitching of facial muscles are signs of convulsions. There is a need to distinguish normal tremors from tremors of hypoglycemia and central nervous system (CNS) disorders so that corrective care can be initiated as necessary (Carey, 1996).

Neuromuscular control in the newborn, although still very limited, can be noted. If newborns are placed face-down on a firm surface, they will turn their heads to the side to maintain an airway. They attempt to hold their heads in line with their bodies if they are raised by their arms.

Newborn reflexes. The normal infant has many primitive reflexes. The times at which these newborn reflexes appear and disappear reflect the maturity and intactness of the developing nervous system.

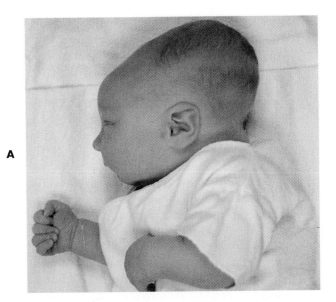

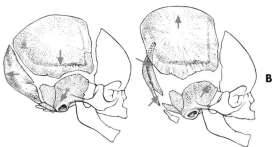

Fig. **19-8** Molding. **A,** Significant molding, soon after birth. **B,** Schematic of bones of skull when molding is present. (*A,* Courtesy Kim Malloy, San Jose, Calif.)

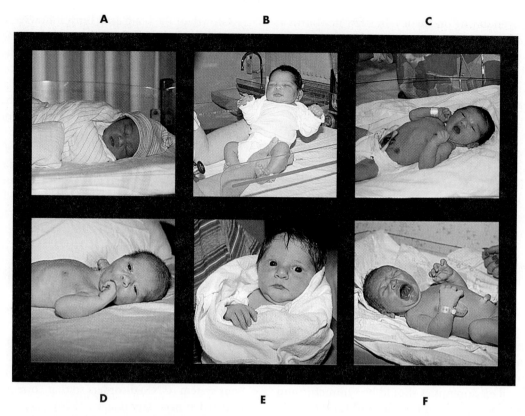

Fig. 19-9 Summary of newborn sleep-wake states. States of consciousness: **A**, Deep sleep. **B**, Light sleep. **C**, Drowsy. **D**, Quiet alert. **E**, Active alert. **F**, Crying. (Courtesy Marjorie Pyle, RNC, Lifecircle, Costa Mesa, Calif.)

The most common reflexes found in the normal newborn are described in Chapter 20.

Behavioral Adaptations

The behavioral adaptations of the neonate form the basis of the infant's social capabilities. The behavioral characteristics of the infant play a major role in the ultimate relationship between the infant and the parents. Normal newborns differ in their activity levels, feeding patterns, sleeping patterns, and responsiveness. Parents' reactions to their newborns are often determined by these differences. Behavioral characteristics, as well as physical characteristics, change during the period of transition. Knowledge of these characteristics and changes can help promote parent-infant bonding (see also Chapter 18).

Transition period

The neonate undergoes phases of instability during the first several hours of life. This **transition period** from intrauterine to extrauterine life involves both physiologic and behavioral characteristics. The first phase lasts up to 30 to 60 minutes after birth and is called the first period of reactivity. The infant's heart rate increases to 160 to 180 beats/min followed by a gradual fall to 100 to 120 beats/min. Respirations are irregular with a rate of 60 to 80 breaths/min. Crackles, grunting, nasal flaring, and chest retractions may be noted, as

well as periods of apnea up to 15 seconds in length. The infant is alert with head movement, startle reaction, tremors, and crying. There is also a decrease in body temperature, increase in motor activity, and increase in muscle tone. During this time bowel sounds may become present, meconium may be passed, and saliva is produced. This is a good time for the infant to interact with the parents.

After the first period of reactivity the infant sleeps, with decreased motor activity and heart rate. The second period of reactivity occurs 4 to 8 hours after birth. This period may last up to several hours, with periods of tachypnea and tachycardia, increased muscle tone and mucus production, and passage of meconium. All newborns experience this transition period, regardless of gestational age or type of birth.

Sleep-wake states

Variations in the state of consciousness of infants are called **sleep-wake states** (Brazelton & Nugent, 1996). The six states form a continuum from deep sleep to extreme irritability (Fig. 19-9). There are two sleep states—deep sleep and light sleep—and four wake states—drowsy, quiet alert, active alert, and crying. Each state has specific characteristics and state-related behaviors. The optimum state of arousal is the quiet alert state. During this state infants may be seen as smiling, vocalizing, moving in synchrony with

TABLE 19-3 *Apgar Score*

SIGN	SCORE		
	0	1	2
Heart rate	Absent	Slow (<100)	Over 100
Respiratory rate	Absent	Slow, weak cry	Good cry
Muscle tone	Flaccid	Some flexion of extremities	Well flexed
Reflex irritability	No response	Grimace	Cry
Color	Blue, pale	Body pink, extremities blue	Completely pink

speech, watching their parents' faces, and responding to people speaking to them. The infants' reaction to internal and external stimuli and ability to control their responses while in these sleep-wake states reflect their ability to organize behavior.

CARE MANAGEMENT FROM BIRTH THROUGH THE FIRST 2 HOURS

Initial Assessment and Nursing Diagnoses

The initial assessment of the neonate is done at birth and uses the Apgar score (Letko, 1996) (Table 19-3) and a brief physical examination (Box 19-1). A gestational age assessment is done within 2 hours of birth (see Fig. 20-1), and a more comprehensive physical assessment may be completed within 24 hours of birth (Tappero & Honeyfield, 1996) (see Table 20-1).

Apgar score

The **Apgar score** permits a rapid assessment of the need for resuscitation based on five signs that indicate the physiologic state of the neonate (see Table 19-3): *heart rate,* based on auscultation with a stethoscope; *respiration,* based on observed movement of the chest wall; *muscle tone,* based on degree of flexion and movement of the extremities; *reflex irritability,* based on response to gentle slaps on the soles of the feet; and *color,* described as pallid, cyanotic, or pink. Each item is scored as a 0, 1, or 2. Evaluations are made 1 and 5 minutes after birth. Scores of 0 to 3 indicate severe distress, scores of 4 to 6 indicate moderate difficulty, and scores of 7 to 10 indicate that the infant will have no difficulty adjusting to extrauterine life. Apgar scores do not predict future neurologic outcome.

Initial physical assessment

The *initial physical assessment* includes a brief review of systems (see Box 19-1). For this initial brief examination, the nurse assesses the following:
1. *External:* notes skin color, staining, peeling, or wasting (dysmaturity); notes length of nails and creases on soles of feet; checks for presence of breast tissue; assesses nasal patency by covering one nostril at a time while observing respirations and color; notes

BOX 19-1 *Initial Physical Assessment by Body System*

CNS [ ] moves extremities, muscle tone good
[ ] symmetric features, movement
[ ] suck, rooting, Moro response, grasp reflexes good
[ ] anterior fontanel soft and flat
CV [ ] heart auscultation, strong and regular
[ ] no murmurs heard
[ ] pulses strong/equal bilaterally
RESP [ ] lungs auscultated, clear bilaterally
[ ] respiratory rate <60 breaths/min
[ ] chest expansion symmetric
[ ] no upper airway congestion
GU [ ] male: urethral opening at tip of penis
testes descended bilaterally
female: vaginal opening apparent
GI [ ] abdomen soft, no distention
[ ] cord attached and clamped
[ ] anus appears patent
ENT [ ] eyes clear
[ ] palates intact
[ ] nares patent
SKIN Color [ ] pink [ ] acrocyanotic
[ ] no lesions or abrasions
[ ] no peeling
[ ] birthmarks _____
[ ] caput/molding
[ ] vacuum "cap"
[ ] forceps marks
[ ] other
Comments: _____
_____
_____
_____
_____

meconium staining of cord, skin, fingernails, or amniotic fluid (staining may indicate fetal hypoxia; offensive odor may indicate intrauterine infection)
2. *Chest:* palpates for site of PMI and auscultates for rate and quality of heart tones and murmurs; notes character of respirations and presence of crackles or rhonchi; notes equality of breath sounds on each side of chest by holding stethoscope in each axilla

---

BOX 19-2 *Routine Admission Orders*

Vital signs: on admission and q30min × 2, q1h × 2, then q8h

Weight, length, and head and chest circumference on admission; then weigh daily

Tetracycline or erythromycin ophthalmic ointment 5 mg/g 1½ to 2 cm line in lower conjuctiva of each eye (ou)

Vitamin K 1 mg IM

Hematocrit by warm heel stick within 3 to 8 hours of age; call health care provider if <44 or >72

Dextrostix prn; notify health care provider if <40 mg/dl; offer early D5W p.o.

Feedings: sterile water × 1 by nurse within first 4 hours of life; if tolerated, begin formula q3-4h on demand (Breastfeeding on demand may be initiated immediately after birth without initial sterile water feeding.)

Rooming-in as desired and infant's condition permits

Newborn screen for phenylketonuria (PKU), thyroxine (T₄), and galactosemia or other screening tests as ordered at least 24 hours after first feeding

---

3. *Abdomen:* verifies presence of a domed abdomen and absence of anomalies; notes number of vessels in cord
4. *Neurologic:* checks muscle tone and reflex reaction; assesses Moro reflex; palpates anterior fontanel for fullness or bulge; notes by palpation the presence and size of the fontanels and sutures
5. *Other observations:* notes gross structural malformations obvious at birth

The nurse responsible for the care of the newborn immediately after birth verifies that respirations have been established, dries the infant, assesses temperature, and places identical identification bracelets on the infant and the mother. In some settings, the father also wears an identification bracelet. The infant may be wrapped in a warm blanket and placed in the arms of the mother, given to the father to hold, or kept undressed under a radiant warmer. In some settings, immediately after birth the infant is placed on the mother's abdomen to allow skin-to-skin contact, which contributes to maintenance of the infant's optimum temperature and parental bonding. The infant may be admitted to a nursery or remain with the parents throughout the hospital stay.

The initial examination of the newborn can occur while the nurse is drying and wrapping the infant, or observations can be made while the infant is lying on the mother's abdomen or in her arms immediately after birth. Efforts should be directed to minimizing interference in the initial parent-infant acquaintance process. If the infant is breathing easily, has good color, and is normal in appearance, then further examination can be delayed until after the parents have had an opportunity to interact with the infant.

Routine procedures and the admission process can be carried out in the mother's room or in a separate nursery. Box 19-2 shows an example of newborn routine orders.

Nursing diagnoses are established after analysis of the findings of the physical assessment. Examples of nursing diagnoses for the newborn are found in the Nursing Diagnoses box.

❙ Nursing Diagnoses

The Newborn

Ineffective airway clearance related to:
• Airway obstruction with mucus

Impaired gas exchange related to:
• Hypothermia

Ineffective thermoregulation related to:
• Heat loss to the environment

Risk for infection related to:
• Umbilical cord stump

Risk for injury related to:
• Helplessness

Risk for pain related to:
• Circumcision without anesthesia

Expected Outcomes of Care

The expected outcomes for newborn care apply both to the infant and to the caregiver. The expected outcomes for the infant include that the infant will achieve the following:
• Maintain effective breathing patterns
• Maintain effective thermoregulation
• Remain free from infection
• Receive the necessary nutrition for growth
• Establish adequate elimination patterns
• Experience minimal pain related to circumcision (if performed)

Expected outcomes for the parents include that they will do the following:
• Attain knowledge, skill, and confidence relevant to infant-care activities
• State understanding of biologic and behavioral characteristics of the newborn
• Have opportunities to intensify relationships with their newborn
• Begin to integrate the infant into the family
• Demonstrate behavior and lifestyle changes that reduce the potential for problems to develop

Plan of Care and Interventions

Events can occur rapidly in newborns immediately after birth. Assessment must therefore be followed quickly by the implementation of appropriate care.

Stabilization and resuscitation

Maintaining a patent airway. Generally, the normal term infant born vaginally has little difficulty clearing the air passages. Most secretions are moved by gravity and brought to the oropharynx by the cough reflex to be drained or swallowed. The infant is maintained in a side-lying position with a rolled blanket at the back to facilitate drainage (Fig. 19-10). If excessive mucus is present, the foot of the crib may be slightly elevated, and the oropharynx is suctioned with a bulb syringe (Fig. 19-11) or a DeLee mucus-trap suction catheter (Fig. 19-12). The nurse may perform gentle percussion over the chest wall using a soft circular mask or a percussion cup to aid in loosening secretions before suctioning (Fig. 19-13). "Milking" the trachea is ineffective, may injure cartilage, and often delays effective suctioning.

Suctioning of upper airway. If the infant has excess mucus in the respiratory tract, the mouth and nasal passages may be suctioned with a bulb syringe. The infant who is coughing and choking on the secretions should be supported with the head downward. The infant should never be suspended by the ankles. First, suction the mouth. This prevents the infant from inhaling pharyngeal secretions by gasping as the nares are touched. The bulb is compressed and inserted into one side of the mouth. The center of the infant's mouth is avoided because this could stimulate the gag reflex. The nasal passages are suctioned one nostril at a time. When the infant's cry does not sound as though it is through mucus or a bubble, suctioning can be stopped. The bulb syringe should always be kept in the infant's crib. The parents should be given demonstrations on how to use the bulb syringe and asked to perform a return demonstration.

The DeLee mucus-trap suction apparatus is used most commonly during the birth process. The isolated DeLee suction method (Busse bac/shield) provides safe oral or mechanical suctioning of newborns while preventing the transmission of bacteria, viruses, and other infectious material from the newborn to the user.

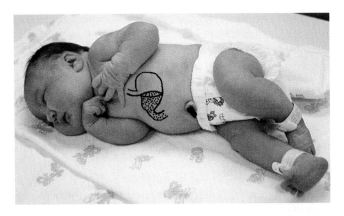

Fig. **19-10** Side-lying position. Infant is turned to right side and supported in this position to facilitate drainage from mouth and promote emptying of stomach contents into the small intestine. (From Wong D: *Whaley and Wong's nursing care of infants and children,* ed 5, St Louis, 1995, Mosby.)

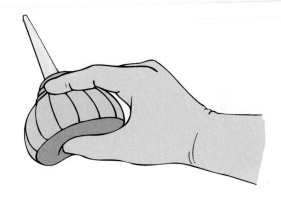

Fig. **19-11** Bulb syringe. Bulb must be compressed before insertion.

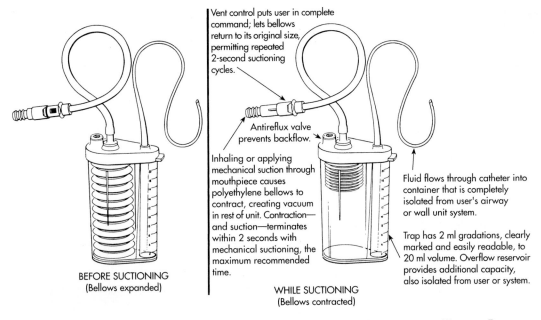

Vent control puts user in complete command; lets bellows return to its original size, permitting repeated 2-second suctioning cycles.

Antireflux valve prevents backflow.

Inhaling or applying mechanical suction through mouthpiece causes polyethylene bellows to contract, creating vacuum in rest of unit. Contraction—and suction—terminates within 2 seconds with mechanical suctioning, the maximum recommended time.

Fluid flows through catheter into container that is completely isolated from user's airway or wall unit system.

Trap has 2 ml gradations, clearly marked and easily readable, to 20 ml volume. Overflow reservoir provides additional capacity, also isolated from user or system.

BEFORE SUCTIONING
(Bellows expanded)

WHILE SUCTIONING
(Bellows contracted)

Fig. **19-12** Isolated DeLee suction method with catheter and mucus trap. (Courtesy Busse Hospital Disposables, Hauppauge, NY.)

Use of a nasopharyngeal catheter with mechanical suction apparatus. Deeper suctioning may be necessary to remove excessive or tenacious mucus from the infant's nasopharynx. Proper tube insertion and suctioning for 10 seconds or less per tube insertion will help prevent laryngospasms and oxygen depletion. If wall suction is used, the pressure should be adjusted to less than 80 mm Hg. The catheter is lubricated in sterile water. The catheter is inserted either orally along the base of the tongue or horizontally through the nose into the nares. Then it is raised to advance it beyond the bend at the back of nares. After the catheter is properly placed, suction is created by placing a thumb over the control as the catheter is carefully rotated and gently withdrawn. This procedure may need to be repeated until the infant's cry sounds clear and air entry into the lungs is heard by stethoscope.

Relieving airway obstruction. A choking infant needs immediate attention. Often, simply repositioning the infant and suctioning the mouth and nose with the bulb syringe

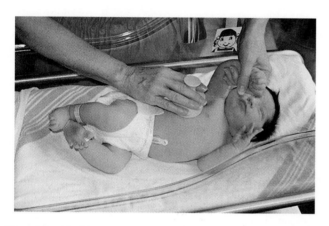

Fig. 19-13 Chest percussion. Nurse performs gentle percussion over the chest wall using a percussion cup to aid in loosening secretions before suctioning.

EMERGENCY

Relieving Airway Obstruction

Back blow and chest thrusts are used to clear an airway obstructed by a foreign body.

BACK BLOWS (FIG. 19-14, A)
Position the infant prone over forearm with the head down and the infant's jaw firmly supported.
Rest the supporting arm on the thigh.
Deliver four back blows forcefully between the infant's shoulder blades with the heel of the free hand.

TURN INFANT
Place the free hand on the infant's back to sandwich the baby between both hands; one hand supports the neck, jaw, and chest while the other supports the back.
Turn the infant over and place the head lower than the chest, supporting the head and neck.
Alternative position: Place the infant face down on your lap with the head lower than the trunk; firmly support the head. Apply back blows and then turn the infant as a unit.

CHEST THRUSTS (FIG. 19-14, B)
Provide four downward chest thrusts on the lower third of the sternum.
Remove foreign body, if it is visible.

OPEN AIRWAY
Open airway with the head-tilt/chin-lift maneuver and attempt to ventilate.
Repeat the sequence of back blows, turning, and chest thrusts.
Continue these emergency procedures until signs of recovery occur:
  Palpable peripheral pulses return.
  The pupils become normal in size and are responsive to light.
  Mottling and cyanosis disappear.
Record the time and duration of the procedure and the effects of this intervention.

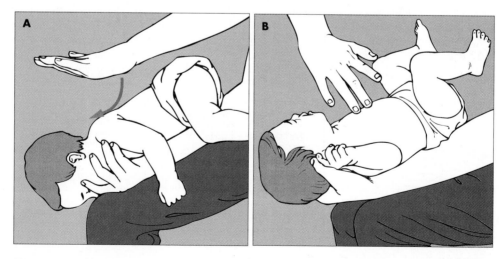

Fig. 19-14 Back blows and chest thrust in infant to clear airway obstruction. **A,** Back blow. **B,** Chest thrust.

eliminates the problem. The infant should be positioned with the head slightly lower than the body to facilitate gravity drainage. The nurse should also listen to the infant's respiration and lung sounds with a stethoscope to determine whether there are crackles and wheezes. If the lungs are clear, the bulb syringe is used to clear the mouth and nose. If the bulb syringe does not provide relief, mechanical suction can be used.

If these measures do not relieve the obstruction, the nurse gives the infant back blows and chest thrusts (see Emergency box at left). To do this, the nurse places the infant face down over the arm with the head lower than the trunk and supported. The nurse can additionally support the infant by supporting his or her own arm firmly against his or her own thigh. The nurse then delivers four quick, sharp back blows between the infant's shoulder blades with the heel of the hand (Fig. 19-14, *A*). After this, the nurse places his or her free hand on the infant's back so that the infant is "sandwiched" between the nurse's two hands, making certain that the neck and chin are well supported. While the nurse maintains support with the infant's head lower than the trunk, the nurse turns the infant and places the infant supine on his or her thigh, and then applies four chest thrusts in rapid succession in the same way as the external chest compressions are performed for cardiopulmonary resuscitation (see Emergency box and Figs. 19-14, *B*, and 19-17).

All personnel working with infants must have current infant CPR certification. Many institutions offer infant CPR courses to new parents (Donaher-Wagner & Braun, 1992). Because cardiac and respiratory arrest can occur in infants, careful monitoring is necessary so that rapid treatment can be instituted.

Maintaining an adequate oxygen supply. Four conditions are essential for maintaining an adequate oxygen supply:
- A clear airway
- Respiratory efforts
- A functioning cardiopulmonary system
- Heat support (exposure to cold stress increases oxygen needs)

Signs of potential complications related to abnormal breathing are shown in the Signs of Potential Complications box.

signs of POTENTIAL COMPLICATIONS

ABNORMAL NEWBORN BREATHING
- Bradypnea: respirations (≤25/min)
- Tachypnea: respirations (≥60/min)
- Abnormal breath sounds: crackles, rhonchi, wheezes, expiratory grunt
- Respiratory distress: nasal flaring, retractions, chin tug, labored breathing

Maintenance of body temperature

Effective neonatal care is based on the maintenance of an optimal thermal environment. Cold stress is detrimental to the newborn. It increases the need for oxygen and can upset the acid-base balance. The infant may react by increasing his or her respiratory rate and may become cyanotic. There are several ways to stabilize the newborn's body temperature: by placing the infant directly on the mother's abdomen and covering the infant with a warm blanket; by drying and wrapping the newborn in warmed blankets immediately after birth, taking care to keep the head well covered while the parent is holding the newborn; and by keeping the ambient temperature of the nursery at 24° C.

If the infant does not remain with the parents during the first 1 to 2 hours after birth, the thoroughly dried, unclothed infant can be placed under a radiant heat panel or warmer until the body temperature stabilizes. The infant's skin temperature is used as the point of control when using a warmer with a servocontrol mechanism. The control panel usually is maintained between 36° and 37° C. This setting should maintain the infant's skin temperature around 36.5° C. A thermistor probe (automatic sensor) is taped to the right upper quadrant of the abdomen immediately below the right intercostal margin, never over a bone. This will ensure detection of minor changes resulting from peripheral vasoconstriction, vasodilation, or increased metabolism long before a change in deep (core) body temperature develops. The other end of the probe cord is attached to the control panel. The sensor needs to be checked periodically to make sure it is securely attached to the infant's skin. An axillary temperature should be taken every hour until the newborn's temperature stabilizes. Initial temperatures as low as 36° C are not uncommon. By the twelfth hour, the newborn's temperature should stabilize within the normal range.

During all procedures, heat loss must be avoided or minimized for the newborn; therefore examinations and activities are performed with the newborn under a heat panel. The initial bath is postponed until the newborn's skin temperature reaches 37° C (see Research box).

Warming infant with hypothermia. Even a normal term infant in good health can become hypothermic. Birth in a car on the way to the hospital, a cold birthing room, or inadequate drying and wrapping immediately after birth may cause the infant's temperature to fall below the normal range (**hypothermia**). Warming the hypothermic infant is accomplished with care. Rapid warming or cooling may cause apneic spells and acidosis in an infant. Therefore the warming process is monitored to progress slowly over a period of 2 to 4 hours.

Immediate interventions

It is the nurse's responsibility to perform certain interventions immediately after birth to provide for the safety of the newborn.

Cardiopulmonary Resuscitation

Wash hands before and after touching infant and
equipment. Wear gloves, if possible.

ASSESS RESPONSIVENESS

Observe color; tap or gently shake shoulders.
Yell for help; if alone, perform CPR for 1 min before
calling for help again.

POSITION INFANT

Turn the infant onto back, supporting the head and neck.
Place the infant on firm, flat surface.

AIRWAY

Open the airway with the head tilt-chin lift method
(Fig. 19-15).
Place one hand on the infant's forehead and tilt the head
back.
Place the fingers of other hand under the bone of the
lower jar at the chin.

BREATHING

Assess for evidence of breathing:
  Observe for chest movement.
  Listen for exhaled air.
  Feel for exhaled air flow.
To breathe for infant:
  Take a breath.
  Place mouth over the infant's nose and mouth to create
  a seal.
NOTE: When available, a mask with a one-way valve
  should be used.
Give two slow breaths (1 to 1.5 sec/breath), pausing to
inhale between breaths.
NOTE: Gently puff the volume of air in your cheeks into
infant. Do not force air.
The infant's chest should rise slightly with each puff; keep
fingers on the chest wall to sense air entry.

CIRCULATION

Assess circulation:
Check pulse of the brachial artery (Fig. 19-16) while
maintaining the head tilt.
If the pulse is present, initiate rescue breathing. Continue
doing once every 3 seconds or 20 times/min until
spontaneous breathing resumes.
If the pulse is absent, initiate chest compressions and
coordinate them with breathing.
Chest compression. There are two systems of chest
compression. Nurses should know both methods.
Maintain the head tilt and:
  1. Place thumbs side-by-side in the middle third of the
     sternum with fingers around the chest and
     supporting the back (Fig. 19-17).
     —Compress the sternum 1.25 to 2 cm.
  2. Place index finger of hand just under an imaginary
     line drawn between the nipples. Place the middle
     and ring fingers on the sternum adjacent to the index
     finger.
     —Using the middle and ring fingers, compress the
     sternum approximately 1.25 to 2.5 cm.
Avoid compressing the xiphoid process.
Release the pressure without moving the thumbs/fingers
form the chest.
Repeat at least 100 times/min, doing five compressions in
3 seconds or less.
Perform 10 cycles of five compressions and one
ventilation.
After the cycles, check the brachial artery to determine
whether there is a pulse.
Discontinue compressions when the infant's spontaneous
heart rate reaches or exceeds 80 beats/min.
Record the time and duration of the procedure and the
effects of intervention.

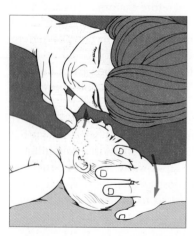

Fig. **19-15** Opening airway with
head tilt–chin lift method.

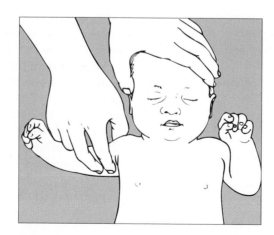

Fig. **19-16** Checking pulse of brachial
artery.

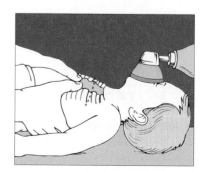

Fig. **19-17** Side-by-side thumb
placement for chest compressions
in newborns.

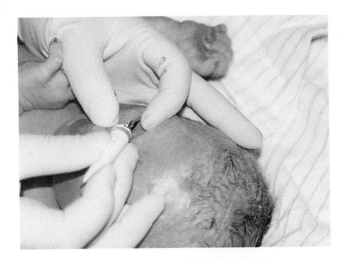

Fig. **19-18** Instillation of medication into eye of newborn. Thumb and forefinger are used to open the eye; medication is placed in the lower conjunctiva from the inner to the outer canthus. (Courtesy Marjorie Pyle, RNC, Lifecircle, Costa Mesa, Calif.)

Identification.

The nurse applies matching identification bracelets to the newborn and mother immediately after birth. Information on the bracelets should include name, sex, date and time of birth, and identification number, according to hospital protocol. In some institutions the father or significant other also wears a matching identification bracelet. Infants are also foot printed using a form that includes the mother's fingerprints, name, and date and time of birth. These identification procedures must be performed before the mother and infant are separated.

Prophylactic care

Vitamin K administration. Administering vitamin K intramuscularly is routine in the newborn period. A single parenteral dose of 0.5 to 1 mg of vitamin K is given soon after birth to prevent hemorrhagic disorders (Snapp, 1996). Vitamin K is produced in the GI tract starting soon after microorganisms are introduced. By day 8, normal newborns are able to produce their own vitamin K.

Eye prophylaxis. The instillation of a prophylactic agent in the eyes of all neonates is mandatory in the United States as a precaution against **ophthalmia neonatorum** (Fig. 19-18). This is an inflammation of the eyes resulting from gonorrheal or chlamydial infection contracted as the newborn passes through the mother's infected birth canal. In some Canadian institutions the parents may sign a form refusing such eye prophylaxis. In the United States, if the family objects to this treatment, the primary care provider asks the parents to sign an informed consent form, and their refusal is noted in the neonate's record. The agent used for prophylaxis varies according to hospital protocols, but the usual agents are forms of erythromycin and tetracycline. Canadian hospitals have not recommended the use of silver nitrate since 1986. Its use in the United States is minimal because silver nitrate does not protect against chlamydial infection and can cause chemical conjunctivitis. In some institutions, eye prophylaxis is delayed until an hour or so after birth so that eye contact and parent-infant attachment and bonding are facilitated. The Centers for Disease Control and Prevention specify that a delay of up to 2 hours is safe.

Umbilical cord care. The care of the umbilical cord is the same as that for any surgical wound (Krebs, 1998). The goal of care is prevention and early identification of hemorrhage or infection. The umbilical cord stump is an excellent medium for bacterial growth and can easily become infected.

NURSE ALERT *If bleeding from the blood vessels of the cord is noted, the nurse checks the clamp (or tie) and applies a second clamp next to the first one. If bleeding is not stopped immediately, the nurse calls for assistance.*

Hospital protocol directs the time and technique for routine cord care. The stump and base of the cord should be assessed for edema, redness, and purulent drainage with each diaper change. The nurse cleanses the cord and skin area around the cord with the prescribed preparation (e.g., erythromycin solution, triple blue dye, or alcohol). The cord clamp is removed after 24 hours when the cord is dry.

Promote parent-infant bonding.

Today's childbirth practices strive to promote the family as the focus of care. Parents generally desire to share in the birth process and have early contact with their infants. Early contact between mother and newborn can be important in developing future relationships. It also has a positive effect on the duration of breastfeeding. There are physiologic benefits of early mother-infant contact. Oxytocin and prolactin levels rise in the mother while sucking reflexes are activated early in the infant. The process of developing active immunity begins as the infant ingests flora from the mother's skin. The nurse should encourage early contact between the newborn and the parents if the condition of both mother and infant allow it. The infant is often placed on the mother's abdomen or at breast. During the first 30 to 60 minutes after birth, when the newborn is in the first period of reactivity, the family unit should be provided privacy to allow for development of the parent-infant relationship.

Evaluation

Evaluation of the effectiveness of care of the newborn is based on the previously stated outcomes.

RESEARCH

A Newborn's First Bath: When?

Blood, once thought to be sterile body fluid, is now recognized as a dangerous substance. All newborns must be considered contaminated with blood-borne pathogens until they are cleansed of blood and amniotic fluids. Present practice, which is based on thermoregulatory theory, dictates that newborn bathing be delayed until normal body temperature is achieved and maintained. There is no evidence to indicate when the thermoregulation of the newborn is complete, nor is there any evidence that supports delaying the bathing of newborns until normal body temperature is sustained. This randomized, comparative study was conducted to determine the effects of early admission bathing on thermoregulation in newborns. One hundred healthy term newborns admitted within a 3-month period were included in the study. Newborns in the experimental group with a minimum rectal temperature of 36.5° C were bathed after the newborn admission assessment examination was completed (M = 61.5 minutes of age), whereas newborns in the control group were bathed at the standard of 4 hours of age (M = 252.12 minutes of age). There were no significant differences ($p < .05$) in rectal temperatures between the groups during the admission assessment examination, before bathing, immediately after bathing, 1 hour after bathing, or 2 hours after bathing. No significant differences were found between the groups in type of birth, time of birth, birth weight, gestational age, Apgar scores at 1 and 5 minutes, air temperature, apical health rate, or respiratory rate.

CLINICAL APPLICATION OF THE STUDY

Healthy term newborns whose rectal temperatures are greater than 36.5° C can be bathed immediately after the admission assessment examination, thus reducing the risk of spreading blood-borne pathogens to health care staff. This also provides the opportunity for skin-to-skin touching earlier than traditional bathing would allow.

Source: Penny-MacGillivary T: A newborn's first bath: when? *J Obstet Gynecol Neonatal Nurs* 25(6):481, 1996.

KEY POINTS

- By term the infant's various anatomic and physiologic systems have reached a level of development and functioning that permit a physical existence apart from the mother.
- There are several significant differences between the respiratory, renal, and thermogenic systems in the newborn and those of an adult.

KEY POINTS—cont'd

- At any serum bilirubin level, the appearance of jaundice during the first day of life usually indicates a pathologic process.
- Chilling (cold stress) of a newborn, even a healthy term newborn, may result in acidosis and raise the level of free fatty acids.
- Many reflex behaviors are important for the newborn's survival.
- Maintenance of adequate ventilation includes ensuring an adequate airway and body temperature.
- Each nurse must develop skill in relieving airway obstruction.
- A major role for the nurse includes implementing identification and prophylactic care interventions, such as cord care, eye prophylaxis, and vitamin K administration.
- The individual personalities and behavioral characteristics of infants play a major role in the ultimate relationship between infants and their parents.
- Sleep-wake cycles and other factors influence the newborn's behavior.

CRITICAL THINKING EXERCISES

1 *Observe a normal newborn immediately after birth. Record physiologic and behavioral observations. Note any deviations from normal. Observe again at 2 hours of age and note any changes. Explain how findings can be used to plan care of the newborn.*

2 *Design teaching materials that can be used to teach new parents who don't speak English how to treat choking in the newborn. Include use of a bulb syringe and back blows/chest thrusts.*

References

Alexander M & Kuo K: Musculoskeletal assessment of the newborn, *Orthop Nurs* 16(1):21, 1997.

Blackburn S: Alterations of the respiratory system in the neonate: implications for clinical practice, *J Perinat Neonat Nurs* 6(2):46, 1992.

Blackburn S & Loper D: *Maternal, fetal and neonatal physiology: a clinical perspective,* Philadelphia, 1992, WB Saunders.

Brazelton T & Nugent K: *Neonatal behavioral assessment scale,* ed 3, London, 1996, MacKeith.

Carey B: Physical assessment of the newborn: a comprehensive approach to the art of physical assessment—neurologic assessment, *Mother Baby J* 1(3):33, 1996.

Dohaner-Wagner BM & Braun DH: Infant cardiopulmonary resuscitation for expectant and new parents, *MCN Am J Matern Child Nurs* 17(1):27, 1992.

Fanaroff A & Martin R: *Neonatal-perinatal medicine: diseases of the fetus and infant,* ed 6, St Louis, 1997, Mosby.

Korones S: *High-risk newborn infants: the basis for intensive care,* ed 5, St Louis, 1995, Mosby.

Krebs T: Cord care: is it necessary? *Mother Baby J* 3:5, 1998.

Lawrence R: *Breastfeeding: a guide for the medical profession,* ed 4, St Louis, 1994, Mosby.

Letko M: Understanding the Apgar score, *J Obstet Gynecol Neonatal Nurs* 25(4):299, 1996.

Lowe N & Reiss R: Parturition and fetal adaptation, *J Obstet Gynecol Neonatal Nurs* 25(4): 339, 1996.

Merenstein G & Gardner S: *Handbook of neonatal intensive care,* ed 4, St Louis, 1998, Mosby.

Seidel H et al: *Mosby's guide to physical examination,* ed 4, St Louis, 1998, Mosby.

Sheeran M: Thermoregulation in neonates: obtaining an accurate axillary temperature measurement, *J Neonatal Nurs* 2(4):6, 1996.

Snapp B: Hemorrhagic disease of the newborn and vitamin K, *Mother Baby J* 1(4):17, 1996.

Tappero E & Honeyfield M: Physical assessment of the newborn: a comprehensive approach to the art of physical examination, *Mother Baby J* 1(1):39, 1996.

Wong D: *Whaley and Wong's nursing care of infants and children,* ed 5, St Louis, 1995, Mosby.

CHAPTER

Assessment and Care of the Newborn

CECILIA TILLER AND SHANNON E. PERRY

LEARNING OBJECTIVES

- *Define the key terms.*
- *Gather appropriate health history information from the prenatal and intrapartal periods.*
- *Identify the sequence to follow in the physical assessment of a neonate.*
- *Explain what is meant by a safe environment.*
- *Compare gestational age of newborns following examinations.*
- *Discuss factors that influence the behavior of the newborn.*
- *Describe precautions to observe whenever administering an intramuscular injection to a newborn.*
- *Discuss phototherapy and the guidelines for teaching parents about this treatment.*
- *Explain the purposes for and methods of circumcision, the postoperative care of the circumcised infant, and parent teaching information regarding circumcision.*
- *Review procedures for doing a heel stick, collecting urine specimens, assisting with venipuncture, and restraining the newborn.*
- *Review the anticipatory guidance nurses provide for parents before discharge.*

KEY TERMS

acid mantle
acrocyanosis
Brazelton Neonatal Behavioral Assessment Scale (BNBAS)
circumcision
habituation
hyperbilirubinemia
inborn error of metabolism
phimosis
phototherapy
protective environment

The numerous biologic changes the neonate makes during the transition to extrauterine life were discussed in the preceding chapter. The first 24 hours of life are critical because respiratory distress and circulatory failure can occur rapidly and with little warning.

Although most infants make the necessary biopsychosocial adjustment to extrauterine existence without undue difficulty, their well-being depends on the care they receive from others. The nursing care described in this chapter is based on careful assessment of the infant's biologic and behavioral responses and the subsequent formulation of nursing diagnoses.

I CARE MANAGEMENT

From Birth through the First 2 Hours

Care begins immediately after the birth and focuses on assessing and stabilizing the newborn's condition. This care was discussed in Chapter 19. Care management focuses on assessment and care after the initial evaluation and immediate care.

From 2 Hours after Birth until Discharge

The infant's admission to the nursery may be delayed, or it may never actually occur. Depending on the routine of the hospital, the infant commonly remains with the mother in the birthing area or is transferred to either the nursery or to the postpartum unit with the mother. Many hospitals have adopted variations of single-room maternity care (SRMC) in which one nurse provides care for the mother and newborn. SRMC allows the infant to remain with the parents after the birth. Many of the procedures, such as weighing and measuring the infant, instilling eye medications, administering the intramuscular (IM) injection of vitamin K, and physically assessing the infant, may be carried out in the labor and birth unit. Nurses who work in an SRMC unit; labor, delivery, and recovery (LDR) room; or labor, delivery, recovery, and postpartum (LDRP) room need to be educated in obstetric, neonatal, and postpartum nursing care and be competent in providing it.

Regardless of the way in which care is physically organized, many hospitals still have a small holding nursery, which is available for the performance of procedures or on the request of the mother who wishes her infant to be placed

510

there. This setup promotes parent-infant bonding while still allowing the new parents some time to be alone.

Assessment and Nursing Diagnoses

Even with the changing placement of nursery care, the routine procedures and admission processes are still necessary. All these procedures can be carried out in any LDR, LDRP, SRMC, or separate-nursery setting. If an infant is transferred to the nursery, the infant's identification is verified by the nurse receiving the infant, who places the baby in a warm environment and begins the admission process (see Box 19-1).

Assessment of clinical gestational age

Assessment of gestational age is important because perinatal morbidity and mortality are related to gestational age and birth weight. A commonly used method of determining gestational age is the simplified *Assessment of Gestational Age* by Ballard, Novak, and Driver (1979). The Ballard scale can be used to measure gestational ages of infants between 35 and 42 weeks. It assesses six external physical and six neuromuscular signs. Each sign has a number score, and the cumulative score correlates with a maturity rating of 26 to 44 weeks of gestation. The score is accurate to plus or minus 2 weeks and is accurate for infants of all races (Stevens-Simon et al, 1989).

The *New Ballard Scale,* a revision of the original scale, can be used with newborns as young as 20 weeks' gestation. The tool has the same physical and neuromuscular sections but includes -1 to -2 scores that reflect signs of extremely premature infants, such as fused eyelids; imperceptible breast tissue; sticky, friable, transparent skin; no lanugo; and square-window (flexion of wrist) angle greater than 90 degrees (Fig. 20-1, *A*). The examination of infants with a gestational age of 20 weeks or less should be performed at a postnatal age of less than 12 hours. For infants with a gestational age of at least 26 weeks, the examination can be performed up to 96 hours after birth. The scale overestimates gestational age by 2 to 4 days in infants younger than 37 weeks' gestation, especially at gestational ages of 32 to 37 weeks (Ballard et al., 1991).

Weight related to gestational age. The weight of the infant at birth also correlates with the incidence of perinatal morbidity and mortality. Because many infants who weigh less than 2,500 gm are not preterm by gestational age, there is often confusion between the preterm and the small-for-gestational-age infants. Fetal growth, gestational age, and fetal maturity are closely related but are not synonymous. Maturity implies functional capacity—the degree to which the neonate's organ systems are able to adapt to the requirements of extrauterine life. Therefore gestational age is more closely related to fetal maturity than is birth weight. Because heredity influences size at birth, it is important to note the size of other family members as part of the assessment process.

Classification of infants at birth by both weight and gestational age provides a more satisfactory method than weight or gestational age alone for predicting mortality risks and providing guidelines for management of the neonate. The infant's birth weight, length, and head circumference are plotted on standardized graphs that identify normal values for gestational age (Fig. 20-1, *B*). The infant whose weight is *appropriate for gestational age (AGA)* (between 10th and 90th percentile) can be presumed to have grown at a normal rate regardless of the time of birth—preterm, term, or postterm. The infant who is *large for gestational age (LGA)* (above 90th percentile) can be presumed to have grown at an accelerated rate during fetal life; the *small-for gestational-age (SGA)* infant (below 10th percentile) can be presumed to have grown at a restricted rate during intrauterine life. Birth weight and gestational age influence mortality: the lower the birth weight and gestational age, the higher the risk of mortality.

Physical assessment

A complete physical examination should be done within 24 hours of birth, after the newborn's temperature stabilizes or under a radiant warmer.

Maternal record review. Inclusion of the maternal history and the prenatal and intrapartal records provides a background for the recognition of any potential problems. By knowing the type of analgesia and anesthesia the mother received in labor, the nurse may then be able to understand the reasons for the infant's current status. Pertinent information from the mother's prenatal record and her labor and birth record may be recorded on a form similar to the one shown in Fig. 20-2. The nurse can use these data to plan care for the newborn.

The parents' presence during this examination encourages discussion of parental concerns and actively involves the parents in the health care of their infant from birth. It also affords an opportunity for the nurse to observe parental interactions with the infant. This in turn aids in the early identification of learning needs and the diagnosis of areas of concern in the parent-infant relationship.

The area used for the examination should be well lighted, warm, and free from drafts. The infant is undressed as needed and placed on a firm, warmed flat surface or under a radiant warmer. The infant may need to be picked up and cuddled at times for reassurance.

Data are either recorded as descriptive notes or summarized on standard forms. Data may include name; hospital number; birth date; type of delivery; estimated date of birth (EDB); weight, length, chest and head circumferences; race; sex; mother's and infant's blood type and Rh factor; Coombs' test results; and time of examination.

Physical examination

The assessment of the newborn should progress systematically from head to toe, with evaluation of each

NEUROMUSCULAR MATURITY

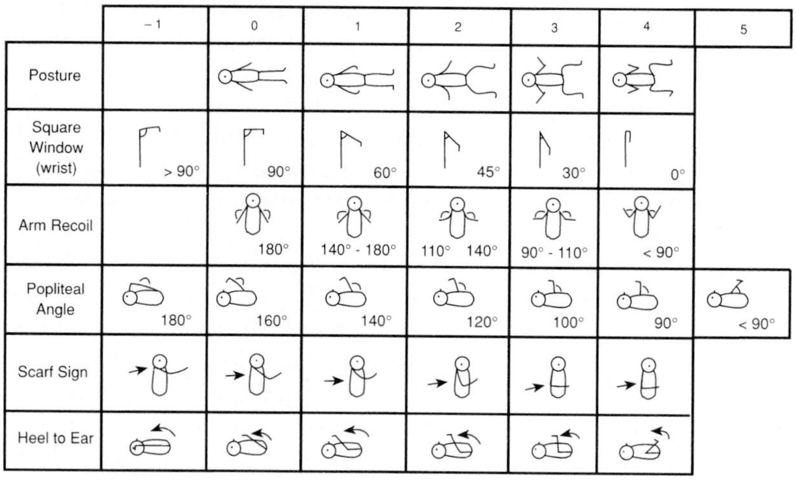

	−1	0	1	2	3	4	5
Posture							
Square Window (wrist)	> 90°	90°	60°	45°	30°	0°	
Arm Recoil		180°	140° - 180°	110° 140°	90° - 110°	< 90°	
Popliteal Angle	180°	160°	140°	120°	100°	90°	< 90°
Scarf Sign							
Heel to Ear							

A PHYSICAL MATURITY

								MATURITY RATING	
								score	weeks
Skin	sticky friable transparent	gelatinous red, translucent	smooth pink, visible veins	superficial peeling or rash, few veins	cracking pale areas rare veins	parchment deep cracking no vessels	leathery cracked wrinkled	-10	20
								-5	22
Lanugo	none	sparse	abundant	thinning	bald areas	mostly bald		0	24
								5	26
Plantar Surface	heel-toe 40-50 mm: -1 <40 mm: -2	>50 mm no crease	faint red marks	anterior transverse crease only	creases ant. 2/3	creases over entire sole		10	28
								15	30
Breast	imperceptible	barely perceptible	flat areola no bud	stippled areola 1-2 mm bud	raised areola 3-4 mm bud	full areola 5-10 mm bud		20	32
Eye/Ear	lids fused loosely: -1 tightly: -2	lids open pinna flat stays folded	sl. curved pinna; soft; slow recoil	well-curved pinna; soft but ready recoil	formed & firm instant recoil	thick cartilage ear stiff		25	34
								30	36
Genitals (male)	scrotum flat, smooth	scrotum empty faint rugae	testes in upper canal rare rugae	testes descending few rugae	testes down good rugae	testes pendulous deep rugae		35	38
								40	40
Genitals (female)	clitoris prominent labia flat	prominent clitoris small labia minora	prominent clitoris enlarging minora	majora & minora equally prominent	majora large minora small	majora cover clitoris & minora		45	42
								50	44

Fig. 20-1 Estimation of gestational age. **A,** New Ballard Scale for newborn maturity rating. Expanded scale includes extremely premature infants and has been refined to improve accuracy in more mature infants. (**A** from Ballard J et al.: New Ballard Score, expanded to include extremely premature infants, *J Pediatr* 119(3):417, 1991.)

system, that is, cardiovascular, respiratory, and so on. Descriptions of any variations from normal and all abnormal findings are included. (Table 20-1 summarizes the newborn assessment.)

General appearance. Features to assess in the general survey include posture, head size, lanugo, vernix caseosa, breast tissue, sole creases, cry, and state of alertness. The normal resting position of the neonate is one of general flexion. The umbilicus is the center of the newborn's body. The neck is short and the abdomen rounded.

Vital signs. The temperature, heart rate, and respiratory rate are always obtained. Blood pressure (BP) may not be routinely assessed unless cardiac problems are suspected. An irregular, very slow, or very fast heart rate may indicate a need for BP measurements.

Temperature. The axillary temperature is a safe, accurate substitute for the rectal temperature (Yetman et al., 1993). Rectal and axillary temperatures differ by only 0.1° C (Yetman et al., 1993). Temperature should therefore be measured by the axillary route. Electronic

CLASSIFICATION OF NEWBORNS—
BASED ON MATURITY AND INTRAUTERINE GROWTH
Symbols: X - 1st Examination O - 2nd Examination

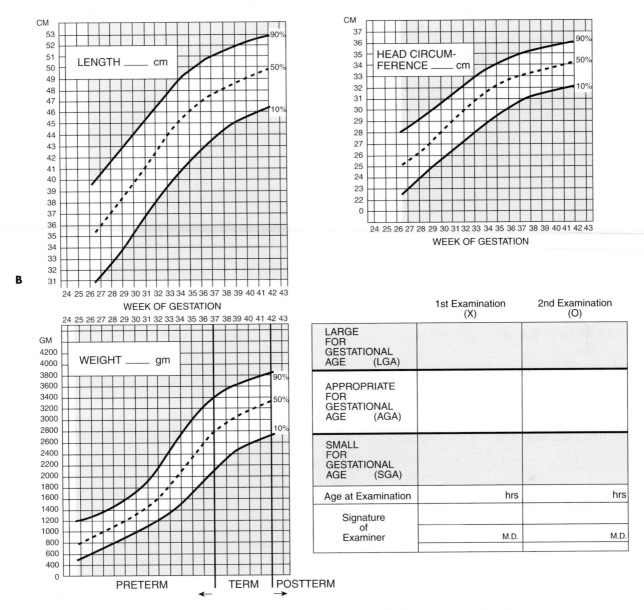

Fig. 20-1 cont'd, Estimation of gestational age. **B,** Newborn classification based on maturity and intrauterine growth. (**B** modified from Lubchenco L, Hansman C & Boyd E: Intrauterine growth in length and head circumference as estimated from live births at gestational ages from 26 to 42 weeks, *J Pediatr* 37(3):403, 1966; and Battaglia F & Lubchenco L: A practical classification of newborn infants by weight and gestational age, *J Pediatr* 71(2):159, 1967.)

thermometers have expedited measurement of temperature and provide a reading within 1 minute. If standard mercury thermometers are used, they should be held in place for at least 3 minutes. Taking an infant's temperature may cause the infant to cry and struggle against the placement of the thermometer in the axilla. Tympanic thermometers may be used after the newborn's ear canals are free of vernix. Before taking the temperature, the examiner may want to determine the heart and respiratory rates while the infant is quiet and at rest. The normal axillary temperature averages 37° C with a range from 36.5° to 37.2° C.

Neonatal Health History

Date _____   Name of infant _____
Sex _____ Time and date of delivery _____ Type_____

PRENATAL DATA
Maternal age _____ Blood type and Rh (Indirect Coombs') _____
EDC* via dates _____ EDC via ultrasound _____

PREVIOUS OBSTETRIC HISTORY
Parity (explain all items) _____
Prior pregnancies: Date _____ Gestational age_____ Sex _____ Weight_____ Delivery_____

COMPLICATIONS OF THIS PREGNANCY
Preeclampsia _____ Hypertension_____ Diabetes (class) _____ Bleeding _____ Viral/bacterial infection _____

DRUG USE
Over the counter_____ Prescription _____

OTHER DRUGS
Alcohol_____ Cocaine _____ Heroin_____ Methadone_____ Other _____

FETAL TESTING AND RESULTS
AFP assay _____ Ultrasound_____ Amniocentesis _____ NST _____ BPS† _____

INTRAPARTUM DATA
Onset of contractions _____ Rupture of membranes (ROM) When?_____
Any abnormalities?_____ Maternal vital signs _____ Any elevations?_____
Medications during labor: Anesthesia/analgesia_____Time last administered _____
Length of stages of labor: First _____ Second_____
Fetal monitoring (external/internal)_____ Fetal distress?_____ Fetal pH?_____

IMMEDIATE CONDITION
Apgar score: 1 min _____ 5 min _____ 10min _____
Any resuscitation?_____ Whiffs O₂ _____ Suction _____ Other_____
Spontaneous breathing established _____ Medications_____

OTHER OBSERVATIONS
Voided_____ Stool_____ Breastfed _____ Bonding time _____
First Temperature _____ Eye prophylaxis with_____Vitamin K IM?_____ Time _____

Fig. **20-2** Neonatal health history. (From Dickason E, Silverman B & Kaplan J: *Maternal-infant nursing care,* ed 3, St Louis, 1998, Mosby.)
*Estimated Date of Confinement (birth).
†Biophysical Profile Score.

Respiration. The respiratory rate varies with the state of alertness after birth. The average respiratory rate is 40 breaths/min but will vary between 30 and 60 breaths/min and may be higher than 60 breaths/min if the newborn is very active or crying. Respirations are abdominal in nature and can be counted by observing or by lightly feeling the rise and fall of the abdomen or by listening with a stethoscope. Neonatal respirations are shallow and irregular. It is important to count the respirations for a full minute to obtain an accurate count because of normal short periods of apnea. The examiner should also observe for symmetry of chest movement.

Most term infants establish respirations spontaneously and continue to have adequate respirations. However, infants can manifest other problems through respiratory distress. Signs of respiratory distress may include nasal

Text continues on p. 519

TABLE 20-1 *Summary of Physical Assessment of the Newborn*

USUAL FINDINGS	COMMON VARIATIONS/MINOR ABNORMALITIES	POTENTIAL SIGNS OF DISTRESS/ MAJOR ABNORMALITIES
GENERAL MEASUREMENTS		
Head circumference—33-35 cm; about 2-3 cm larger than chest circumference (Fig. 20-3, *A*) *Chest circumference*—30.5-33 cm (Fig. 20-3, *B*) *Crown-to-rump length*—31-35 cm; approximately equal to head circumference (Fig. 20-3, *D*) *Head-to-heel length*—48-53 cm	Molding after birth may decrease head circumference Head and chest circumference may be equal for first 1-2 days after birth	Head circumference <10th or >90th percentile
Birth weight—2,500-4,000 gm (see Fig. 20-5)	Loss of 10% of birth weight in first week; regained in 10-14 days	Birth weight <10th or >90th percentile
VITAL SIGNS		
Temperature		
Axillary—36.5°-37.2° C	Crying may increase body temperature slightly Radiant warmer will falsely increase axillary temperature	Hypothermia Hyperthermia
Heart rate		
Apical—120-140 beats/min	Crying will increase heart rate; sleep will decrease heart rate During first period of reactivity (6-8 hr), rate can reach 180 beats/min	Bradycardia—Resting rate below 80-100 beats/min Tachycardia—Rate above 160-180 beats/min Irregular rhythm
Respirations		
30-60 breaths/min	Crying will increase respiratory rate; sleep will decrease respiratory rate During first period of reactivity (6-8 hr), rate can reach 80 breaths/min	Tachypnea—Rate above 60 breaths/min Apnea >20 seconds
Blood pressure		
Oscillometric—65/41 mm Hg in arm and calf	Crying and activity will increase BP Placing cuff on thigh may agitate infant; thigh (BP) may be higher than arm or calf BP by 4-8 mm Hg	Oscillometric systolic pressure in calf 6-9 mm Hg less than in upper extremity (sign of coarctation of aorta)
GENERAL APPEARANCE		
Posture—Flexion of head and extremities, which rest on chest and abdomen	*Frank breech*—Extended legs, abducted and fully rotated thighs, flattened occiput, extended neck	Limp posture, extension of extremities
SKIN		
At birth, bright red, puffy, smooth Second to third day, pink, flaky, dry Vernix caseosa Lanugo Edema around eyes, face, legs, dorsa of hands, feet, and scrotum or labia *Acrocyanosis*—Cyanosis of hands and feet *Cutis marmorata*—Transient mottling when infant is exposed to decreased temperature	Neonatal jaundice after first 24 hr Ecchymoses or petechiae caused by birth trauma *Milia*—Distended sebaceous glands that appear as tiny white papules on cheeks, chin, and nose *Miliaria or sudamina*—Distended sweat (eccrine) glands that appear as minute vesicles, especially on face *Erythema toxicum*—Pink papular rash with vesicles superimposed on thorax, back, buttocks, and abdomen; may appear in 24-48 hr and resolve after several days (Fig. 19-6)	Progressive jaundice, especially in first 24 hr Cracked or peeling skin Generalized cyanosis Pallor Mottling Grayness Plethora Hemorrhage, ecchymoses, or petechiae that persist *Sclerema*—Subcutaneous fat necrosis Poor skin turgor Rashes, pustules, or blisters *Café-au-lait spots*—Light brown spots

Continued

TABLE 20-1 *Summary of Physical Assessment of the Newborn—cont'd*

USUAL FINDINGS	COMMON VARIATIONS/MINOR ABNORMALITIES	POTENTIAL SIGNS OF DISTRESS/ MAJOR ABNORMALITIES
SKIN—cont'd		
	Harlequin color change—Clearly outlined color change as infant lies on side; lower half of body becomes pink, and upper half is pale *Mongolian spots*—Irregular areas of deep blue pigmentation, usually in sacral and gluteal regions; seen predominantly in newborns of African, Native American, Asian, or Hispanic descent *Telangiectatic nevi ("stork bites")*—Flat, deep pink localized areas usually seen in back of neck (see Fig. 19-5)	*Nevus flammeus*—Port-wine stain *Nevus vasculosus*—Strawberry mark
HEAD		
Anterior fontanel—Diamond shaped, 2.5-4 cm *Posterior fontanel*—Triangular, 0.5-1 cm Fontanels should be flat, soft, and firm Widest part of fontanel measured from bone to bone, not suture to suture	Molding after vaginal birth (see Fig. 19-8) Third sagittal (parietal) fontanel Bulging fontanel because of crying or coughing *Caput succedaneum*—Edema of soft scalp tissue *Cephalhematoma (uncomplicated)*—Hematoma between periosteum and skull bone	Fused sutures Bulging or depressed fontanels when quiet Widened sutures and fontanels *Craniotabes*—Snapping sensation along lambdoid suture that resembles indentation of ping-pong ball
EYES		
Lids usually edematous Color—Slate gray, dark blue, brown Absence of tears Presence of red reflex Corneal reflex in response to touch Pupillary reflex in response to light Blink reflex in response to light or touch Rudimentary fixation on objects and ability to follow to midline	Epicanthal folds in Asian infants Searching nystagmus or strabismus (Fig. 20-4) *Subconjunctival (scleral) hemorrhages*—Ruptured capillaries, usually at limbus	Pink color of iris Purulent discharge Upward slant in non-Asians Hypertelorism (3 cm or greater) Hypotelorism Congenital cataracts Constricted or dilated fixed pupil Absence of red reflex Absence of pupillary or corneal reflex Inability to follow object or bright light to midline Blue sclera Yellow sclera
EARS		
Position—Top of pinna on horizontal line with outer canthus of eye Startle reflex elicited by a loud, sudden noise Pinna flexible, cartilage present	Inability to visualize tympanic membrane because of filled aural canals Pinna flat against head Irregular shape or size Pits or skin tags	Low placement of ears Absence of startle reflex in response to loud noise Minor abnormalities may be signs of various syndromes, especially renal
NOSE		
Nasal patency Nasal discharge—thin white mucus Sneezing	Flattened and bruised	Nonpatent canals Thick, bloody nasal discharge Flaring of nares (alae nasi) Copious nasal secretions or stuffiness (may be minor)
MOUTH AND THROAT		
Intact, high-arched palate Uvula in midline Frenulum of tongue Frenum of upper lip Sucking reflex—Strong and coordinated	*Natal teeth*—Teeth present at birth; benign but may be associated with congenital defects *Epstein pearls*—Small, white epithelial cysts along midline of hard palate	Cleft lip Cleft palate Large, protruding tongue or posterior displacement of tongue Profuse salivation or drooling

TABLE 20-1 *Summary of Physical Assessment of the Newborn—cont'd*

USUAL FINDINGS	COMMON VARIATIONS/MINOR ABNORMALITIES	POTENTIAL SIGNS OF DISTRESS/ MAJOR ABNORMALITIES
MOUTH AND THROAT—cont'd		
Rooting reflex		*Candidiasis (thrush)*—White, adherent patches on tongue, palate, and buccal surfaces
Gag reflex		
Extrusion reflex		
Absent or minimal salivation		Inability to pass nasogastric tube
Vigorous cry		Hoarse, high-pitched, weak, absent, or other abnormal cry
NECK		
Short, thick, usually surrounded by skinfolds	*Torticollis* (wry neck)—Head held to one side with chin pointing to opposite side	Excessive skinfolds
		Resistant to flexion
Tonic neck reflex		Absence of tonic neck reflex
		Fractured clavicle
CHEST		
Anteroposterior and lateral diameters equal	Funnel chest (pectus excavatum)	Depressed sternum
Slight sternal retractions evident during inspiration	Pigeon chest (pectus carinatum)	Marked retractions of chest and intercostal spaces during respiration
Xiphoid process evident	Supernumerary nipples	Asymmetric chest expansion
Breast enlargement	Secretion of milky substance from breasts ("witch's milk")	Redness and firmness around nipples
		Wide-spaced nipples
LUNGS		
Respirations chiefly abdominal	Rate and depth of respirations may be irregular; periodic breathing	Inspiratory stridor
Cough reflex absent at birth, present by 1-2 days	Crackles shortly after birth	Expiratory grunt
		Retractions
Bilateral equal bronchial breath sounds		Persistent irregular breathing
		Periodic breathing with repeated apneic spells
		Seesaw respirations (paradoxical)
		Unequal breath sounds
		Persistent fine crackles
		Wheezing
		Diminished breath sounds
		Peristaltic sounds on one side, with diminished breath sounds on same side
HEART		
Apex—Fourth to fifth intercostal space, lateral to left sternal border	*Sinus arrhythmia*—Heart rate increases with inspiration and decreases with expiration	*Dextrocardia*—Heart on right side
S_2 slightly sharper and higher in pitch than S_1	Transient cyanosis on crying or straining	Displacement of apex, muffled
		Cardiomegaly
		Abdominal shunts
		Murmurs
		Thrills
		Persistent cyanosis
		Hyperactive precordium
ABDOMEN		
Cylindric in shape (Fig. 20-3)	Umbilical hernia	Abdominal distention
Liver—Palpable 2-3 cm below right costal margin	*Diastasis recti*—Midline gap between recti muscles	Localized bulging
Spleen—Tip palpable at end of first week of age	*Wharton's jelly*—unusually thick umbilical cord	Distended veins
		Absent bowel sounds
Kidneys—Palpable 1-2 cm above umbilicus		Enlarged liver and spleen
		Visible peristaltic waves
Umbilical cord—Bluish white at birth with two arteries and one vein		Scaphoid or concave abdomen
		Ascites
		Green umbilical cord

Continued

TABLE 20-1 *Summary of Physical Assessment of the Newborn—cont'd*

USUAL FINDINGS	COMMON VARIATIONS/MINOR ABNORMALITIES	POTENTIAL SIGNS OF DISTRESS/ MAJOR ABNORMALITIES
ABDOMEN—cont'd		
Femoral pulses—Equal bilaterally		Presence of only one artery in cord
		Urine or stool leaking from cord
		Palpable bladder distention following scanty voiding
		Absent femoral pulses
		Cord bleeding or hematoma
FEMALE GENITALIA (FIG. 19-17, *A*)		
Labia and clitoris usually edematous	*Pseudomenstruation*—Blood-tinged or mucoid discharge	Enlarged clitoris with urethral meatus at tip
Urethral meatus behind clitoris	Hymenal tag	Fused labia
Vernix caseosa between labia		Absence of vaginal opening
Urination within 24 hr		Meconium from vaginal opening
		No urination within 24 hr
		Masses in labia
		Ambiguous genitalia
MALE GENITALIA (FIG. 19-17, *B*)		
Urethral opening at tip of glans penis	Urethral opening covered by prepuce	*Hypospadias*—Urethral opening on ventral surface of penis
Testes palpable in scrotum	Inability to retract foreskin	*Epispadias*—Urethral opening on dorsal surface of penis
Scrotum usually large, edematous, pendulous, and covered with rugae; usually deeply pigmented in dark-skinned ethnic groups	*Epithelial pearls*—Small, firm, white lesions at tip of prepuce	*Chordee*—Ventral curvature of penis
Smegma	Erection or priapism	Testes not palpable in scrotum or inguinal canal
Urination within 24 hr	Testes palpable in inguinal canal	No urination within 24 hr
		Inguinal hernia
	Scrotum small	Hypoplastic scrotum
	Hydrocele—Fluid in scrotum	Masses in scrotum
		Meconium from scrotum
		Discoloration of testes
		Ambiguous genitalia
BACK AND RECTUM		
Spine intact, no openings, masses, or prominent curves	Green liquid stools in infant under phototherapy	Anal fissures or fistulas
Trunk incurvation reflex	Delayed passage of meconium in very low-birth-weight neonates	Imperforate anus
Anal reflex		Absence of anal reflex
Patent anal opening		No meconium within 36 hr
Passage of meconium within 48 hr		Pilonidal cyst or sinus
		Tuft of hair along spine
		Spina bifida (any degree)
EXTREMITIES		
Ten fingers and toes	Partial syndactyly between second and third toes	*Polydactyly*—Extra digits
Full range of motion	Second toe overlapping into third toe	*Syndactyly*—Fused or webbed digits
Nail beds pink, with transient cyanosis immediately after birth	Wide gap between first (hallux) and second toes	*Phocomelia*—Hands or feet attached close to trunk
Creases on anterior two thirds of sole	Deep crease on plantar surface of foot between first and second toes	*Hemimelia*—Absence of distal part of extremity
Sole usually flat	Asymmetric length of toes	Hyperflexibility of joints
Symmetry of extremities	Dorsiflexion and shortness of hallux	Persistent cyanosis of nail beds
Equal muscle tone bilaterally, especially resistance to opposing flexion		Yellowing of nail beds
Equal bilateral brachial pulses		Sole covered with creases
		Transverse palmar (simian) crease
		Fractures
		Decreased or absent range of motion

TABLE 20-1	*Summary of Physical Assessment of the Newborn—cont'd*	
USUAL FINDINGS	**COMMON VARIATIONS/MINOR ABNORMALITIES**	**POTENTIAL SIGNS OF DISTRESS/ MAJOR ABNORMALITIES**
EXTREMITIES—cont'd		*Dislocated or subluxated hip* Limitation in hip abduction Unequal gluteal or leg folds Unequal knee height Audible click on abduction (Ortolani's sign) Asymmetry of extremities Unequal muscle tone or range of motion

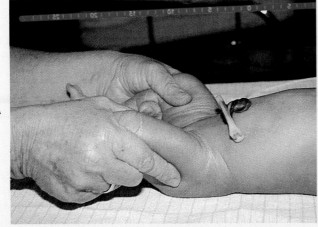 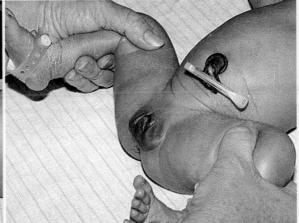

Method of assessing for hip dysplasia or dislocation using Ortolani's maneuver. **A,** Examiner's middle fingers are placed over greater trochanter and thumbs over inner thigh opposite lesser trochanter. **B,** Gentle pressure is exerted to further flex thigh on hip, and thighs are rotated outward. If hip dysplasia is present, head of femur can be felt to slip forward in acetabulum and flip back when pressure is released and legs returned to their original position. A click is sometimes heard *(Ortolani's sign)*. (Courtesy Marjorie Pyle, RNC, Lifecircle, Costa Mesa, Calif.)

NEUROMUSCULAR SYSTEM		
Extremities usually maintain some degree of flexion Extension of an extremity followed by previous position of flexion Head lag while sitting, but momentary ability to hold head erect Able to turn head from side to side when prone Able to hold head in horizontal line with back when held prone	Quivering or momentary tremors	*Hypotonia*—Floppy, poor head control, extremities limp *Hypertonia*—Jittery, arms and hands tightly flexed, legs stiffly extended, startles easily Asymmetric posturing (except tonic neck reflex) *Opisthotonic posturing*—Arched back Signs of paralysis Tremors, twitches, and myoclonic jerks Marked head lag in all positions

From Wong D & Perry S: *Maternal child nursing care,* St Louis, 1998, Mosby.

flaring, retractions (indrawing of tissue between ribs, below rib cage, or above sternum and clavicles), or audible grunting with expirations. Any increased use of intercostal muscles may be a sign of distress. A respiratory rate that is less than 30 or greater than 60 breaths/min, with the infant at rest, must be evaluated further. The respiratory rate of the infant may be influenced (slowed/depressed) by the analgesics or anesthetics the mother received during labor and birth. Apneic periods longer than 15 seconds must be reported to the primary health care provider for evaluation.

Heart rate. Apical pulse rates should be obtained on all infants. Auscultation should be for a full minute, preferably when the infant is asleep. The infant may need to be held and comforted during assessment. Heart rate may range

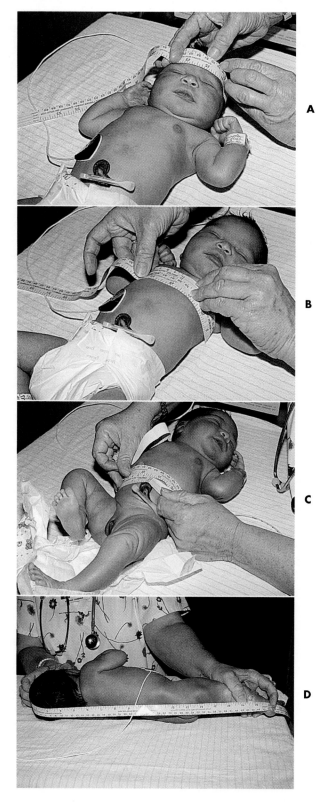

Fig. **20-3** Measurements. **A,** Circumference of head. **B,** Circumference of chest. **C,** Abdominal circumference. **D,** Length, crown to heel. If measurements are taken before infant's initial bath, the nurse must wear gloves. (Courtesy Marjorie Pyle, RNC, Lifecircle, Costa Mesa, Calif.)

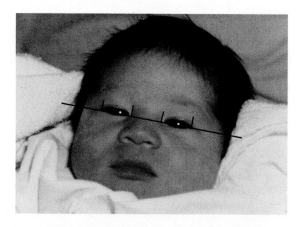

Fig. **20-4** Eyes. Pseudostrabismus: inner epicanthal folds cause the eyes to appear misaligned; however, corneal light reflexes are perfectly symmetric. Eyes are symmetric in size and shape and are well placed.

from 100 to 180 beats/min shortly after birth and, when the infant's condition has stabilized, from 120 to 140 beats/min.

Auscultation of the specific components of the *heart sounds* is difficult because of the rapid rate and effective transmission of respiratory sounds. However, the *first (S₁)* and *second (S₂) sounds* should be clear and well defined; the second sound is somewhat higher in pitch and sharper than the first. *Murmurs* are often heard in the newborn, especially over the base of the heart or at the left sternal border in the third or fourth interspace. Ordinarily they are not associated with specific cardiac defects because they commonly represent the incomplete functional closure of fetal shunts. However, any murmur or other unusual sounds should always be recorded and reported.

| NURSE ALERT | *Because auscultation of neonatal breath sounds and heart tones is often difficult for the novice untrained ear, practice auscultating one parameter at a time. Close your eyes and mentally block out the extraneous sounds heard, such as room noise or neonatal movement; offer the newborn a pacifier. Auscultation of a murmur and decreased air movement in specific lung fields requires patience and practice; it may require auscultating the heart tones or breath sounds for 1 to 3 minutes each.* |

Blood pressure. If BP is measured, a Doppler (electronic) monitor facilitates this procedure. It is important to use the correct size BP cuff. Neonatal BP usually is highest immediately after birth and falls to a minimum by 3 hours after birth. It then begins to rise steadily and reaches a plateau between 4 and 6 days after birth. This measurement is usually equal to that of the immediate postbirth BP. The BP reading varies with the neonate's activity but averages 65/41 mm Hg at 1 to 3 days of age.

BP may be measured in both arms and legs to detect any discrepancy between the two sides or between the upper

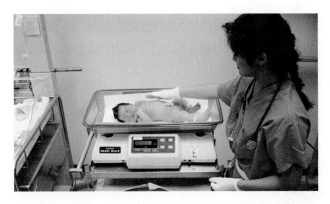

Fig. 20-5 Weighing the infant. Note that a hand is held over infant as a safety measure. The scale is covered to protect against cross infection. (Courtesy Kim Molloy, San Jose, Calif.)

and lower body. A discrepancy of 10 mm Hg or more between the arms and legs may signal a cardiac defect such as coarctation of the aorta.

Baseline measurements of physical growth. The examiner takes and records baseline measurements to help assess the progress of the neonate. Measurements are used to determine the neonate's growth patterns. These may be recorded on growth charts. The following measurements are made when the neonate is assessed.

Weight. The birth weight of a term infant ranges from 2,500 to 4,000 g (Fig. 20-5). The infant is commonly weighed at the same time every day during the hospital stay. Normally, neonates lose 10% or less of their birth weight after birth. This is caused by the excretion of fluids through the lungs, urinary bladder, and bowels, and the low level of intake during the first few days of life. They usually regain their birth weight by 10 to 14 days of age.

Circumferences and length. The circumferences of the head and chest, and sometimes the abdomen, are measured during the initial assessment and are usually not repeated unless there is an indication for need (i.e., severe molding, hydrocephaly, distended abdomen). Length is measured at birth and usually not again until the infant is seen by the health care provider for routine well-baby care (see Fig. 20-3).

Skin texture, color, opacity. Observations should include color and color changes during activity, familial and racial features, rashes, milia, anomalies or deformities, birthmarks, jaundice, petechiae, forceps marks, tone, and turgor (hydration status). Any of these characteristics should be noted and recorded.

Color varies with racial background, pigmentation, and physiologic changes. **Acrocyanosis** is characterized by bluish discoloration of the hands and feet. This normal condition is caused by vasomotor instability and poor peripheral circulation.

The newborn's skin often appears mottled, which is a response to temperature changes. Harlequin color changes may be seen. This occurs when one side of the body

develops a deep red color. Harlequin color is a response to a normal vasomotor disturbance causing the blood vessels on one side of the body to constrict while those on the other side dilate. Although a common occurrence, it should be recorded and reported.

The skin is inspected for any signs of lesions or birthmarks. Location, size, color, characteristics, and distribution should be noted and recorded. The examiner inspects the scalp for any sign of a lesion from an internal scalp electrode. Forceps or vacuum cup marks should also be noted and recorded.

Head and neck. Molding may give the neonate's head an asymmetric appearance (see Fig. 19-8). Parents should be reassured that this will go away and that nothing need be done to the head. With each assessment the fontanels are palpated. They should be open, feel soft, and may pulsate. The posterior fontanel is frequently not palpable. The examiner inspects the neonate's face for symmetry and provides reassurance to parents as needed for any asymmetry that is noted.

If subconjunctival hemorrhage occurred during birth, the eyes should be carefully inspected for resolution of the hemorrhage. Tears are not usually produced until 2 months of age.

Any problems with the tongue or mouth should have been identified during the initial assessment. The nurse should be alert constantly for feeding problems, regurgitation, or aspiration. The infant may become congested and have problems breathing. The physician should be notified if this occurs.

The ears are inspected for symmetric shape and size. The top of the ear should align with the inner and outer canthi of the eyes (see Fig. 20-4). Skin tags, pinpoint holes, and sinus tracts along the helix or preauricular surface may represent minor abnormalities. Hearing can be checked by watching the neonate respond to voices or other sounds.

Chest. The thoracic cavity should be cylindric and symmetric. In the SGA or preterm neonate a smaller chest circumference is to be expected. Normally, chest wall excursion is equal bilaterally.

The ribs should be flexible and symmetric, with no palpable masses. The xiphoid process may be palpable at the bottom of the sternum. In a thin neonate, it may be visible.

Breast size. The examiner assesses breast tissue through observation and palpation. There are two methods to measure breast tissue. In the first method, the nipple is palpated gently with one finger. In the second method, the second and third fingers are placed on either side of the nipple. Measurement is taken between the two fingers to determine the amount of breast tissue.

Breast tissue and areola size increase with gestation. Increased breast tissue may indicate subcutaneous fat accumulation from accelerated intrauterine growth (as occurs in the LGA neonate). In contrast, the SGA or postterm neonate may have decreased breast tissue from inadequate fetal growth or lost fetal weight. The nipples are inspected for spacing and number. Supernumerary nipples may appear as darkened spots just below or beside natural nipples (Tappero & Honeyfield, 1996). Any discharge is noted.

Abdomen. The abdomen should have a symmetric, slightly rounded contour. Peristaltic waves normally are not visible; however, the abdomen should move visibly during breathing. The umbilical cord remnant should appear black (or purple if triple dye was used).

The umbilical cord begins to dry, shrivel, and blacken by the second or third day of life. The umbilicus should be inspected frequently for signs of infection (foul odor, redness, and purulent drainage), granuloma (small, red, raw-appearing polyp where the umbilical cord separates), bleeding, and discharge. The cord normally falls off by 2 weeks after birth. By the time the neonate is 1 month old, the umbilicus should be healed.

In the hospital, the umbilical cord is usually cleaned with alcohol or other designated solution with each assessment and with diaper changes if the cord is moist. This ritual reduces the colonization with *Staphylococcus aureus* but does not decrease the infection rate (Krebs, 1998). The cord clamp is removed when the cord is dry, in about 24 hours. (See Home Care box.)

The abdomen is palpated gently to determine softness. Masses and abnormalities should have been identified at the initial assessment. When the abdomen is distended, it feels tight and looks large and full. Abdominal circumference should be measured if the abdomen appears distended. The primary health care provider should be notified of the findings.

Genitalia. The genitalia should be kept clean and dry. The number of voidings and type and number of stools are recorded and described as necessary. If the male neonate is circumcised, he must be observed for signs of bleeding and ability to void. Any discharge or abnormalities should be recorded and reported.

Back and anus. To assess the back the examiner positions the neonate prone and inspects for spinal alignment, enlargement, and masses. The back should be straight. The sacrum is examined for dimpling, a tuft of hair, or bulges. The vertebral column is palpated for enlargement and signs of pain (Kenner, Brueggmeyer & Gunderson, 1993).

The perineum should be smooth and without dimpling or extra orifices. The anus should be midline and patent. The anal sphincter is assessed by lightly stroking the anus with a cotton-tipped applicator and observing anal constriction—a reaction called the anal wink (Mass et al., 1991). Passage of meconium indicates patency of the rectum, which should be noted.

Extremities. The extremities are inspected for length, symmetry relative to each other and to the body as a whole, equality, muscle tone, and range of motion. Normally, the term neonate has a full range of motion, which can be tested either actively or passively. The preterm neonate has limited flexion, especially of the arms. The examiner inspects the hands and feet for the number of digits, palmar and

---

HOME CARE *Patient Instructions for Self-Care*

Cord Care

1. Wash hands thoroughly with an antibacterial soap before touching the cord.
2. Handle the cord minimally until the cord separates.
3. Fold diapers under the umbilical cord to prevent soiling of the cord and to keep the cord dry.
4. When the cord is soiled, clean the area with warm water and dry thoroughly.
5. Apply an antimicrobial agent to the base of the cord only if your health care provider recommends one. Compared to dry care, antimicrobials do not reduce the infection rate.
6. Use low-alkaline or nonalkaline soap to bathe the infant and wash around the cord stump.
7. Do not immerse the baby for bathing until the cord detaches.
8. If redness or discharge appears around the cord stump, notify your physician or nurse practitioner.

Krebs T: Cord care: is it necessary? *Mother Baby J* 3(2):5, 1998.

---

plantar creases, and abnormalities such as webbing (Tappero & Honeyfield, 1996).

Movement of the arms should be assessed. Trauma to the brachial plexus during a difficult delivery may result in brachial palsy. The most common type, Duchenne-Erb paralysis, involves the fifth and sixth cervical nerve roots. The affected arm is held in a position of tight adduction and internal rotation at the shoulder. The grasp reflex on the affected side may be intact; however, Moro's reflex is absent on that side. With treatment, most neonates have complete recovery.

To assess leg length, the examiner extends the legs simultaneously. The legs should be equal length, with symmetric skin folds. The examiner inspects the legs in both the prone and supine positions.

Plantar (sole) creases should be assessed immediately after birth because the drying effect of environmental exposure causes additional creases to form.

Neurologic assessment. The physical assessment includes a neurologic assessment of the newborn's reflexes (Table 20-2). This provides useful information about the infant's nervous system and state of neurologic maturation. Many reflex behaviors, such as sucking and rooting, are important for survival. Other reflexes, such as gagging, coughing, and sneezing, act as safety mechanisms. The assessment needs to be carried out within 48 hours because abnormal signs present in the early neonatal period may disappear. They may reappear months or years later as abnormal functions.

Behavioral characteristics

The healthy infant must achieve behavioral and biologic tasks to develop normally. Behavioral characteristics form

Text continues on p. 527

| TABLE 20-2 | Assessment of Newborn's Reflexes |

REFLEX	ELICITING THE REFLEX	CHARACTERISTIC RESPONSE	COMMENTS
Sucking and rooting	Touch infant's lip, cheek, or corner of mouth with nipple	Infant turns head toward stimulus, opens mouth, takes hold, and sucks	Response is difficult if not impossible to elicit after infant has been fed; if response weak or absent, consider prematurity or neurologic defect Parental guidance: Avoid trying to turn head toward breast or nipple, allow infant to root; response disappears after 3-4* mo but may persist up to 1 yr
Swallowing	Feed infant; swallowing usually follows sucking and obtaining fluids	Swallowing is usually coordinated with sucking and usually occurs without gagging, coughing, or vomiting	If response is weak or absent, this may indicate prematurity or neurologic defect Sucking and swallowing are often uncoordinated in preterm infant

Grasp
  Palmar
  Plantar
	Place finger in palm of hand
	Place finger at base of toes
		Infant's fingers curl around examiner's fingers, toes curl downward	Palmar response lessens by 3-4 mo; parents enjoy this contact with infant; plantar response lessens by 8 mo

Extrusion	Touch or depress tip of tongue	Newborn forces tongue outward	Response disappears at approximately 4 mo
Glabellar (Myerson's)	Tap over forehead, bridge of nose, or maxilla of newborn whose eyes are open	Newborn blinks for first four or five taps	Continued blinking with repeated taps is consistent with extrapyramidal disorder
Tonic neck or "fencing"	With infant falling asleep or sleeping, turn head quickly to one side	With infant facing left side, arm and leg on that side extend; opposite arm and leg flex (turn head to right, and extremities assume opposite postures)	Responses in leg are more consistent Complete response disappears by 3-4 mo; incomplete response may be seen until third or fourth year After 6 wk, persistent response is sign of possible cerebral palsy

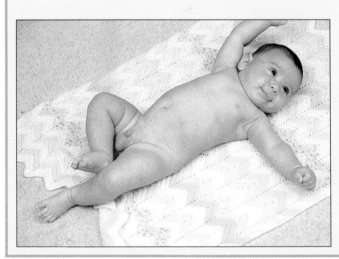

Classic pose in spontaneous tonic neck reflex. (Courtesy Marjorie Pyle, RNC, Lifecircle, Costa Mesa, Calif.)

*All durations for persistence of reflexes are based on time elapsed after 40 weeks of gestation; that is, if this newborn was born at 36 weeks of gestation, add 1 month to all time limits given.

Continued

TABLE 20-2 *Assessment of Newborn's Reflexes—cont'd*

REFLEX	ELICITING THE REFLEX	CHARACTERISTIC RESPONSE	COMMENTS
Moro's	Hold infant in semisitting position, allow head and trunk to fall backward to an angle of at least 30 degrees Place infant on flat surface, strike surface to startle infant	Symmetric abduction and extension of arms are seen; fingers fan out and form a C with thumb and forefinger; slight tremor may be noted; arms are adducted in embracing motion and return to relaxed flexion and movement Legs may follow similar pattern of response Preterm infant does not complete "embrace"; instead, arms fall backward because of weakness	Response is present at birth; complete response may be seen until 8 wk; body jerk only is seen between 8 and 18 wk; response is absent by 6 mo if neurologic maturation is not delayed; response may be incomplete if infant is deeply asleep; give parental guidance about normal response Asymmetric response may connote injury to brachial plexus, clavicle or humerus Persistent response after 6 mo indicates possible brain damage

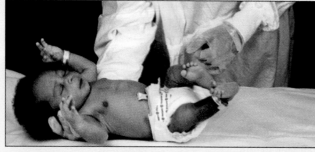

A, Moro's reflex.

REFLEX	ELICITING THE REFLEX	CHARACTERISTIC RESPONSE	COMMENTS
Stepping or "walking"	Hold infant vertically, allowing one foot to touch table surface	Infant will simulate walking, alternating flexion and extension of feet; term infants walk on soles of their feet, and preterm infants walk on their toes	Response is normally present for 3 to 4 wk

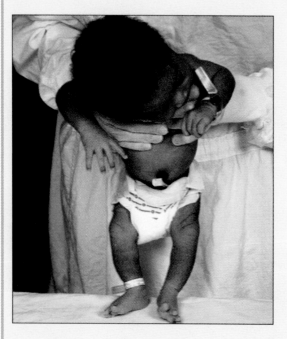

B, Stepping reflex. (From Dickason E, Silverman B & Kaplan J: *Maternal-infant nursing care,* ed 3, St Louis, 1998, Mosby.)

TABLE 20-2	*Assessment of Newborn's Reflexes—cont'd*

REFLEX	ELICITING THE REFLEX	CHARACTERISTIC RESPONSE	COMMENTS
Crawling	Place newborn on abdomen	Newborn makes crawling movements with arms and legs	Response should disappear at approximately 6 wk
Deep tendon	Use finger instead of percussion hammer to elicit patellar, or knee jerk, reflex; newborn must be relaxed	Reflex jerk is present; even with newborn relaxed, nonselective overall reaction may occur	
Crossed extension	Infant should be supine; extend one leg, press knee downward, stimulate bottom of foot; observe opposite leg	Opposite leg flexes, adducts, and then extends	Absence suggests spinal cord lesion; weak response suggests peripheral nerve damage

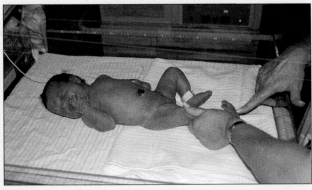

Crossed extension reflex. With the infant in supine position, examiner extends one leg of the infant and presses the knee down. Stimulation of sole of foot of fixated limb should cause free leg to flex, adduct, and extend as if attempting to push away stimulating agent. This reflex should be present during newborn period. (Courtesy Marjorie Pyle, RNC, Lifecircle, Costa Mesa, Calif.)

Startle	Perform sharp hand clap; best elicited if newborn is 24-36 hr old or older	Arms abduct with flexion of elbows, hands stay clenched	Response should disappear by 4 mo Response is elicited more readily in preterm newborn (inform parents of this characteristic)
Babinski's sign (plantar)	On sole of foot, beginning at heel, stroke upward along lateral aspect of sole, then move finger across ball of foot	All toes hyperextend, with dorsiflexion of big toe—recorded as a positive sign	Absence requires neurologic evaluation, should disappear after 1 yr

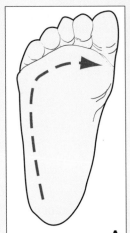
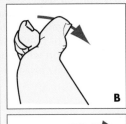
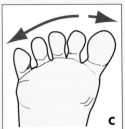

Babinski's reflex. **A**, Direction of stroke. **B**, Dorsiflexion of big toe. **C**, Fanning of toes. (From Wong D: *Whaley and Wong's nursing care of infants and children*, ed 5, St Louis, 1995, Mosby.)

Pull-to-sit (traction)	Pull infant up by wrists from supine position with head in midline	Head will lag until infant is in upright position, then head will be held in same plane with chest and shoulder momentarily before falling forward; infant will attempt to right head	Response depends on general muscle tone and maturity and condition of infant

Continued

TABLE 20-2 *Assessment of Newborn's Reflexes—cont'd*

REFLEX	ELICITING THE REFLEX	CHARACTERISTIC RESPONSE	COMMENTS
Trunk incurvation (Galant)	Place infant prone on flat surface; run finger down back about 4-5 cm (1-1/2 to 2 in) lateral to spine, first on one side and then down other	Trunk is flexed and pelvis is swung toward stimulated side	Response disappears by fourth week Absence suggests general depression of nervous system abnormality

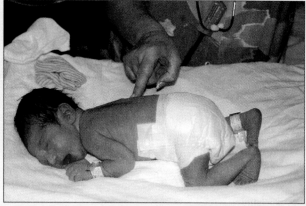

Trunk incurvation reflex. In prone position, infant responds to linear skin stimulus (blunt end of pin or finger) along paravertebral area by flexing the trunk and swinging the pelvis toward stimulus. With transverse lesions of cord, no response below the level of the lesion is present. Response may vary but should be obtainable in all infants, including preterm ones. If not seen in the first few days, it is usually apparent by 5 to 6 days. (Courtesy Marjorie Pyle, RNC, Lifecircle, Costa Mesa, Calif.)

REFLEX	ELICITING THE REFLEX	CHARACTERISTIC RESPONSE	COMMENTS
Magnet	Place infant in supine position; partially flex both lower extremities and apply pressure to soles of feet	Both lower limbs should extend against examiner's pressure	Absence suggests damage to spinal cord or malformation. Reflex may be weak or exaggerated after breech birth.

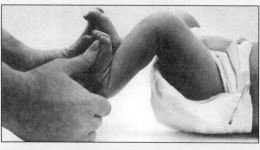

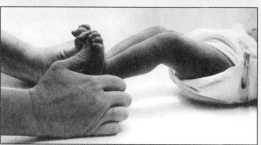

Magnet reflex. With child in supine position and lower limbs semiflexed, light pressure is applied with fingers to both feet. Normally, while examiner's fingers maintain contact with soles of feet, the lower limbs extend. Weak reflex may be seen after breech presentation *without* extended legs or may indicate sciatic nerve stretch syndrome. Breech presentation *with* extended legs may evoke exaggerated response. (Courtesy Mead Johnson & Co, Evansville, Ind.)

REFLEX	ELICITING THE REFLEX	CHARACTERISTIC RESPONSE	COMMENTS
Additional newborn responses Yawn, stretch, burp, hiccup, sneeze	These are spontaneous behaviors	May be slightly depressed temporarily because of maternal analgesia or anesthesia, fetal hypoxia, or infection	Parental guidance: Most of these behaviors are pleasurable to parents Parents need to be assured that behaviors are normal Sneeze is usually response to lint, etc., in nose and not an indicator of a cold No treatment is needed for hiccups, sucking may help

the basis of the social capabilities of the infant. The behavioral characteristics of the newborn represent a continuing phase in human development that began in utero. Individual personalities and behavioral characteristics of infants play a major role in the ultimate relationship between infants and their parents.

Assessment of infant behavior. The **Brazelton Neonatal Behavioral Assessment Scale (BNBAS)** can be used to systematically assess the infant's behavior (Brazelton & Nugent, 1996). The BNBAS is an interactive examination that assesses the infant's response to 28 areas organized according to the clusters in Box 20-1. It is generally used as a research or diagnostic tool and requires special training.

The Mother's Assessment of the Behavior of her Infant (MABI) (Field et al., 1978) is based on the BNBAS and provides more parental interaction in the assessment of infant behavior.

In addition to use as initial and ongoing tools to assess neurologic and behavioral responses, the scales can be used to assess initial parent-infant relationships and as a guide for parents to help them focus on their infant's individuality and to develop a deeper attachment to their child. Showing parents the unique characteristics of their infant assists parents to develop a more positive perception of the infant with increased interaction between infant and parent.

Assessment of attachment behaviors. One of the most important areas of assessment is careful observation of those behaviors thought to indicate the formation of emotional bonds between the newborn and family, especially the mother. Although the words "bonding" and "attachment" are sometimes referred to as separate phenomena, with *bonding* representing the development of emotional ties from parent to infant and *attachment* representing the emotional ties from infant to parent, in this discussion the words are used interchangeably to denote both processes.

Unlike physical assessment of the neonate, which has concrete guidelines to follow, assessment of parent-infant attachment requires much more skill in terms of observation and interviewing. Rooming-in of mother and infant and liberal visiting privileges for father, siblings, and grandparents facilitate recognition of behaviors that demonstrate positive or negative attachment. Guidelines for assessment of bonding behaviors are presented in the accompanying Teaching Guidelines box.

Talking to the parents uncovers many variables that can affect the development of attachment and parenting. What expectations do they have for this child? In other words, how similar are their predictions of the fantasy child and their realizations about the real child? Encourage them to talk about their relationship with their own parents, since the type of parenting that parents received as a child influences their child-rearing practices. Was this a planned pregnancy? How do they see the addition of a dependent family member affecting their lifestyle? What arrangements have they made in terms of such changes in lifestyle? What sup-

---

BOX 20-1 | *Clusters of Neonatal Behaviors in BNBAS*

Habituation—ability to respond to and then inhibit responding to discrete stimulus (light, rattle, bell, pinprick) while asleep
Orientation—quality of alert states and ability to attend to visual and auditory stimuli while alert
Motor performance—quality of movement and tone
Range of state—measure of general arousal level or arousability of infant
Regulation of state—how infant responds when aroused
Autonomic stability—signs of stress (tremors, startles, skin color) related to homeostatic (self-regulator) adjustment of the nervous system
Reflexes—assessment of several neonatal reflexes

TEACHING GUIDELINES
Assessing Attachment Behavior

When the infant is brought to the parents do they reach out for the infant and call the infant by name? (Recognize that in some cultures, parents may not name the infant in early newborn period.)
Do the parents speak about the infant in terms of identification—whom the infant looks like; what appears special about their infant over other infants?
When parents are holding the infant what kind of body contact is there—do parents feel at ease in changing the infant's position; are fingertips or whole hands used; are there parts of the body they avoid touching or parts of the body they investigate and scrutinize?
When the infant is awake, what kinds of stimulation do the parents provide—do they talk to the infant, to each other, or to no one; how do they look at the infant—direct visual contact, avoidance of eye contact, or looking at other people or objects?
How comfortable do the parents appear in terms of caring for the infant? Do they express any concern regarding their ability or disgust for certain activities, such as changing diapers?
What type of affection do they demonstrate to the newborn, such as smiling, stroking, kissing, or rocking?
If the infant is fussy, what kinds of comforting techniques do the parents use, such as rocking, swaddling, talking, or stroking?

---

port system or significant others are available for assistance? What are their views regarding childrearing?

The labor process also significantly affects the immediate attachment of mothers to their newborn children. Factors such as a long labor, feeling tired or "drugged" after birth, and problems with breastfeeding can delay the development of initial positive feelings toward the newborn.

During pregnancy, and often even before conception occurs, parents develop an image of the "ideal" or "fantasy" infant. At birth the fantasy infant becomes the real infant. How closely the dream child resembles the real child influences the bonding process. Assessing such expectations during pregnancy and at the time of the infant's birth allows identification of discrepancies in the parents' view of the fantasy child versus the real child.

Because attachment involves a mutually reciprocal interchange, observing the interaction between parent and infant is very important. An excellent opportunity exists during feeding. A useful instrument for systematically describing the parent's and infant's behaviors is the *Nursing Child Assessment Feeding Scale (NCAFS)* (Barnard, 1994). It consists of 76 behavioral items; 50 items describe the parent's behavior regarding sensitivity to cues, response to child's distress, social-emotional growth fosterings, and cognitive growth fostering. Twenty-six items focus on the child's behavior in terms of clarity of cues and responsiveness to parent. The results can also be shared with the parent to encourage discussion of feelings about the infant and to highlight behaviors of the dyad that foster successful interaction (Fuller, 1990). The NCAFS is appropriate for use with infants during the first year.

State-related behaviors. Infants use purposeful behavior to maintain the quiet alert state, the optimal arousal state. They actively withdraw by increasing physical distance, reject by pushing away with hands and feet, decrease sensitivity by falling asleep or breaking eye contact by turning head, or use signaling behaviors, such as fussing and crying (Brazelton & Nugent, 1996). These behaviors permit infants to quiet themselves and reinstate readiness to interact.

The first 6 weeks of life involve a steady decrease in the proportion of active REM sleep to total sleep. A steady increase in the proportion of quiet sleep to total sleep also occurs. Periods of wakefulness increase 25% over the first 3 or 4 weeks of life. For the first few weeks the wakeful periods seem dictated by hunger, but soon thereafter a need for socializing appears as well. The newborn sleeps approximately 17 hours a day, with periods of wakefulness gradually increasing. By the fourth week of life, some infants stay awake from one feeding to the next. Children do not achieve the adult sleeping pattern until 4 to 5 years of age.

Other factors influencing behavior of newborns. A number of variables affect the newborn's responses. Several factors are discussed below.

Gestational age. The gestational age of the infant and level of central nervous system (CNS) maturity affect the observed behavior. In an infant with an immature CNS the entire body responds to a pinprick of the foot. The mature infant withdraws only the foot. CNS immaturity is reflected in reflex development and sleep-wake cycles. Preterm infants have brief periods of alertness but have difficulty maintaining this state. Premature or sick infants show fatigue or stress sooner than full-term, healthy infants (Tappero & Honeyfield, 1996).

Time. The time it takes for infants to recuperate from labor and birth affects the behavior of infants as they initially attempt to become oriented. Time elapsed since the previous feeding and time of day may also influence infants' responses.

Stimuli. Environmental events and stimuli affect the behavioral responses of infants. Nurses in intensive care nurseries observe that infants respond to loud noises, bright lights, monitor alarms, and tension in the unit. If a mother is tense and has a fast heartbeat while feeding an infant, the infant will have an increase in heart rate that is similar to the mother's. In addition, the newborn responds differently to animate and inanimate stimulation.

Medication. Controversy surrounds the effects of maternal medication (analgesia, anesthesia) during labor on infant behavior. Some researchers note that infants of mothers given medications may continue to demonstrate poor state organization after the fifth day. Others maintain that the effect can be beneficial or nonexistent (Dixon & Stein, 1992).

Ethnicity. Some of the most interesting research findings have been regarding the ethnic differences in infant behavior (Chitty & Winter, 1989; Freedman, 1979). Freedman (1979) found that Chinese-American infants had more self-quieting activities, fewer state changes, and more rapid responses to consoling activities than white American infants. The results from a study of Navajo newborns reinforced the stereotype of the stoic, impassive Native American (Freedman, 1979). Among Navajo babies, crying was rare and limb movements reduced, and calming was almost immediate after tests for Moro's reflex. In Freedman's study (1979), Japanese newborns were more sensitive and irritable than either Chinese or Navajo newborns. Mexican mothers use tactile stimulation more often than vocalizations to quiet their newborns (Garcia-Coll, 1990). These studies suggest that neonatal behavior represents a behavioral phenotype, which expresses a complex relationship among genetic endowment, intrauterine environment, and maternal obstetric history (Garcia-Coll, 1990). Because these studies occurred 10 to 20 years ago, they need to be replicated.

Sensory behaviors. From birth, infants possess sensory capabilities that indicate a state of readiness for social interaction. Infants effectively use behavioral responses in establishing their first dialogues. These responses, coupled with the newborns' "baby appearance" (with the face being proportioned such that the forehead and eyes are larger than the lower portion of the face) and their smallness and helplessness, rouse feelings of wanting to hold, protect, and interact with them.

Vision. At birth the eye is structurally incomplete and the muscles are immature. The pupils react to light, the blink reflex is easily stimulated, and the corneal reflex is activated by light touch. The clearest visual distance is 17 to 20 cm, which is about the distance the infant's face is from the mother's face as she breastfeeds or cuddles. Infants are sensitive to light. They will frown if a bright light is flashed in their eyes and will turn toward a soft, red light. If the room is darkened, they will open their eyes wide and look about. This is noticeable when the birthing area is darkened after birth. By 2 months of age, infants can detect color but seem more attracted by black-and-white patterns at 5 days of age and younger (Kenner, Brueggemeyer & Gunderson, 1993).

Response to movement is noticeable. If a bright object is shown to newborns (even at 15 minutes of age), they will follow it visually and some will even turn their heads to do so. Because human eyes are bright, shiny objects, newborns will track their parents' eyes. Parents often comment on how exciting this behavior is.

Visual acuity is surprising; even at 2 weeks of age, infants can distinguish patterns with stripes 3 mm (1/8 inch) apart. By 6 months their vision is as acute as that of an adult. They prefer to look at patterns rather than plain surfaces, even if the latter are brightly colored. They prefer more complex patterns to simple ones. They prefer novelty (changes in pattern) by 2 months of age. The infant of a few weeks of age is therefore capable of responding actively to an enriched environment.

From birth onward, infants are able to fix their eyes and gaze intently at objects. They gaze at their parents' faces and respond to changes in them with apparent imitative effect. This ability permits parents and infants to gaze into each other's eyes, and a subtle communication pattern is thereby formed. The development of eye-to-eye contact is very important for parent-infant attachment. Children of visually impaired parents and parents who have visually impaired children must circumvent this obstacle for the formation of a relationship.

Hearing. As soon as the amniotic fluid drains from the ear, the infant's hearing is similar to an adult's. This may occur as early as 1 minute of age. Loud sounds of about 90 decibels cause the infant to respond with a startle reflex. The newborn responds to low-frequency sounds such as a heartbeat or lullaby by decreasing motor activity or stopping crying. The response to a high-frequency sound elicits an alerting reaction (Barr, 1990). Screening for hearing impairment can occur in the newborn using an auditory brainstem response (Letko, 1992).

The infant responds readily to the mother's voice. This may be a response to having heard or felt sound waves from the mother's voice while in utero.

This selective listening to maternal voice sounds and rhythms during intrauterine life prepares newborns for recognition and interaction with their primary caregivers—their mothers. Newborns are accustomed in the uterus to hearing the regular rhythm of the mother's heartbeat. As a result, they respond by relaxing and ceasing to fuss and cry if a regular heartbeat simulator is placed in their cribs.

The acute sensitivity of infants to the human voice has been tested experimentally. In observations of the responses of quiet, alert newborns to computer-simulated cries and the cries of human newborns, more restlessness and crying occurred in response to the genuine cry. Newborns less than 35 hours old typically began to cry when subjected to the cry of other newborns but quieted at the sound of their own cry (Barr, 1990).

The internal and middle portions of the ear are larger at birth, but the external canal is small. The mastoid process and bony parts of the external canal have not developed. Therefore the tympanic membrane and facial nerve are very close to the surface and can be easily damaged.

Touch. The infant is responsive to touch on all parts of the body. The face (especially the mouth), the hands, and the soles of the feet appear to be the most sensitive. Reflexes can be elicited by stroking the infant. The newborn's responses to touch suggest this sensory system is well prepared to receive and process tactile messages. Touch and motion are essential to normal growth and development (Gunzenhauser, 1990). However, each infant is unique, and variations can be seen in newborns' responses to touch.

The new mother uses touch as one of the first interaction behaviors: fingertip touch, soft stroking of the face, and gentle massage of the back. Because touch between strangers is avoided in some cultures, this automatic maternal touching behavior seems to evidence an already intimate relationship. Birth trauma or stress and depressant drugs taken by the mother during labor decrease the infant's sensitivity to touch or painful stimuli.

Taste. The newborn has a well-developed taste system, and different solutions elicit different facial expressions. A tasteless solution produces no response, whereas a sweet solution causes eager sucking. A sour solution results in puckering of the lips, and a bitter solution causes a grimace. Newborns prefer glucose water over plain water (Lawrence, 1994). The taste response is independent from cortical levels of the nervous system.

Young infants are particularly oriented toward the use of their mouths, both for meeting their nutritional needs for rapid growth and releasing tension through sucking. The early development of circumoral sensation, muscle activity, and taste would seem to be preparation for survival in the extrauterine environment.

Smell. The newborn's sense of smell appears to be well developed at birth. Newborns react similarly to adults when exposed to strong or pleasant odors. Breastfed infants are able to smell breast milk and can differentiate their mother from other lactating women (Lawrence, 1994). These maternal odors are believed to influence bonding and adequate feeding.

The significance of smell in the maternal identification of her offspring and vice versa in the animal world is well documented. Mothers and fathers can identify their newborns by smell (Porter, Cernoch & Perry, 1983). Mothers report that from the time of birth, their infant had a unique smell (Field et al., 1978).

Response to environmental stimuli. Infants respond to the environment in a number of ways. Classic studies have identified individual variations in the primary reaction pattern of newborns and described them as temperament (Dixon & Stein, 1992; Thomas et al., 1961, 1970). Their style of behavioral response to stimuli is guided by the temperament affecting the newborn's sensory threshold, ability to habituate, and response to maternal behaviors.

The human newborn possesses sensory receptors capable of responding selectively to various stimuli present in the internal and external environment. The infant also possesses individual characteristics that affect the response. The range of responses may impress the parent with the newborn's formidable neurologic capacity.

Habituation. **Habituation** is a protective mechanism that allows the infant to become accustomed to environmental stimuli. Habituation is a psychologic and physiologic phenomenon whereby the response to a constant or repetitive stimulus is decreased. In the term newborn this can be demonstrated in several ways. Shining a bright light into a newborn's eyes will cause a startle or squinting the first two to three times. The third or fourth flash will elicit a diminished response, and by the fifth or sixth flash, the infant ceases to respond (Brazelton & Nugent, 1996). The same response pattern holds true for the sounds of a rattle or a pinprick to the heel. A newborn presented with new stimuli becomes wide eyed and alters its gaze for a time but will eventually show a diminished interest.

The ability to habituate also allows the newborn to select stimuli that promote continued learning about the social world, thus avoiding overload. The intrauterine experience seems to have programmed the newborn to be especially responsive to human voices, soft lights, soft sounds, and sweet tastes (Dixon & Stein, 1992).

The newborn quickly learns the sounds in a newborn nursery and the home and is able to sleep in their midst. The selective responses of the newborn indicate cerebral organization capable of remembering and making choices. The ability to habituate depends on state of consciousness, hunger, fatigue, and temperament. These factors also affect consolability, cuddliness, irritability, and crying.

Consolability. Barr (1990) described variations in the ability of newborns to console themselves or to be consoled. In the crying state, most newborns initiate one of several ways to reduce their distress. Hand-to-mouth movements are common, with or without sucking, as well as alerting to voices, noises, or visual stimuli.

Cuddliness. Cuddliness is especially important to parents because they often gauge their ability to care for the child by the child's responses to their actions. The degree to which newborns will mold into the contours of the persons holding them varies. Barr (1990) tested the effect of body contact and vestibular stimulation in both soothing babies and creating alertness. The vestibular stimulation of being picked up and moved had the greater effect.

Irritability. Some newborns cry longer and harder than others. For some the sensory threshold seems low. They are readily upset by unusual noises, hunger, wetness, or new experiences, and thus respond intensely. Others with a high sensory threshold require a great deal more stimulation and variation to reach the active, alert state (Barr, 1990).

Crying. Crying in an infant may signal hunger, pain, desire for attention, or fussiness. Some mothers state that they are eventually able to distinguish the reasons for crying. This is a means of communication.

Barr (1990) reported five characteristics of crying. (1) Crying progressively increases to a peak in the second month and then gradually decreases. (2) A diurnal rhythm is present, with more crying occurring in the evening hours. (3) Babies vary considerably in the amount and timing of crying. (4) Individual day-to-day variations seem to occur. (5) The crying does not seem to differ with different caretakers.

Analyses of the physical and behavioral assessment findings lead to nursing diagnoses for the newborn and for the parent(s) of the newborn. Possible nursing diagnoses are listed in the accompanying box.

▍Nursing Diagnoses

The Newborn
Ineffective breathing pattern related to:
- Obstructed airway

Impaired gas exchange related to:
- Hypothermia (cold stress)

Risk for ineffective thermoregulation related to:
- Heat loss to environment

Risk for infection related to:
- Environmental factors

Risk for pain related to:
- Circumcision

Possible nursing diagnoses *for the parent or parents* are as follows:

Potential for growth in family coping related to:
- Knowledge of newborn's social capabilities
- Knowledge of newborn's dependency needs
- Knowledge of biologic characteristics of the newborn

Situational low self-esteem related to:
- Misinterpretation of newborn's responses

Expected Outcomes of Care

The expected outcomes for newborn care relate to the infant and parents. The expected outcomes for the infant include that the infant will:

- Make the transition from intrauterine to extrauterine life
- Maintain effective breathing patterns
- Maintain effective thermoregulation
- Remain free from infection

For the parents, expected outcomes will include:

- Attain knowledge, skill, and confidence relevant to infant-care activities
- State understanding of biologic and behavioral characteristics of their newborn
- Demonstrate interactional/lifestyle behaviors that promote healthy family functioning

- Have opportunities to intensify their relationship with the infant
- Begin to integrate the infant into the family

Plan of Care and Interventions
Protective Environment

The provision of a **protective environment** is basic to the care of the newborn. The construction, maintenance, and operation of nurseries in accredited hospitals are monitored by national professional organizations such as the American Academy of Pediatrics and local or state governing bodies. In addition, hospital personnel develop their own policies and procedures for protecting the newborns under their care. Prescribed standards cover areas such as the following:

1. *Environmental factors:* Adequate lighting, elimination of potential fire hazards, safety of electrical appliances, adequate ventilation, and controlled temperature (warm and free of drafts) and humidity (lower than 50%).
2. *Measures to control infection:* Adequate floor space to permit the positioning of bassinets at least 60 cm apart, handwashing facilities, and areas for the cleaning and storage of equipment and supplies.

Only those personnel directly involved in the care of mothers and infants are allowed in this area, thereby reducing the opportunities for the transmission of pathogenic organisms.

NURSE ALERT *Personnel are instructed to use good handwashing techniques, with handwashing between each infant handling being the single most important measure in the prevention of neonatal infection.*

Health care personnel must wear gloves when handling the infant until blood and amniotic fluid have been removed from its skin, when drawing blood (e.g., heel stick), when caring for a fresh wound (e.g., circumcision), and when changing diapers.

Visitors and health care providers such as nurses, physicians, parents, brothers and sisters, department supervisors, electricians, and housekeepers are expected to wash their hands before coming in contact with infants or equipment. Cover gowns are not necessary (Rush et al., 1990).

Persons with infectious conditions are excluded from contact with newborns, or the infected persons must take special precautions when working with the infants. This includes persons with upper respiratory tract infections, gastrointestinal tract infections, and infectious skin conditions. Most agencies have now coupled this day-to-day self-screening of personnel with yearly health examinations.

3. *Safety factors.* Security measures have been implemented in many agencies in response to the infant abductions from nurseries that have been occurring with greater frequency. Some examples of the measures that have been instituted are the placement of identical identification bracelets on

BOX 20-2	*Standard Laboratory Values in a Term Infant**
Hematocrit	40% to 65%
Glucose	45-90 mg/dl
Bilirubin, direct	At 3-4 days: 4-6 mg/dl
	May rise to 12 mg/dl

*Heel stick capillary blood

infants and their parents, and infants are footprinted or have identification pictures taken after birth before they leave the mother's side.

Personnel wear picture identification badges or other badges that identify them as newborn personnel. There may be infant tracking systems in mother-baby units that set off an alarm if a baby is left alone or is with unauthorized personnel. Mothers are also instructed to be certain they know the identity of anyone who cares for the infant and never to release the infant to anyone who is not wearing the appropriate identification.

Laboratory and diagnostic tests

The measurement of blood glucose levels and urinalysis are commonly performed in newborns. Other tests may be performed as needed, including the measurement of bilirubin levels, newborn screening tests (e.g., phenylketonuria [PKU]), hematocrits, and drug tests. Standard laboratory values for a term newborn are given in Box 20-2.

Some states require that newborns be tested for up to nine disorders. Information about the tests required in a particular state can be obtained from state health departments. About 30 states require testing for sickle cell anemia and some states now require testing for cystic fibrosis (March of Dimes, 1994). Some of the major disorders for which infants are screened are described in Table 20-3. A blood sample is collected for most of these tests using a heel stick.

Newborn screening tests. The most widespread use of postnatal testing for genetic disease is the routine screening of newborns for inborn errors of metabolism such as phenylketonuria (PKU), which is mandatory in most states in the United States. An **inborn error of metabolism** is the term applied to a large group of disorders caused by a metabolic defect that results from the absence of or change in a protein, usually an enzyme, and mediated by the action of a certain gene. These defects can involve any substrate produced from protein, carbohydrate, or fat metabolism. Inborn errors of metabolism are recessive disorders, and for them to occur, a person must receive a defective gene from each parent. The parents usually are unaffected because their normal dominant gene directs the synthesis of sufficient protein to meet their metabolic needs under normal circumstances. With the advent of new biochemical techniques, it is now possible to detect the abnormal gene responsible for causing an increasing number of these disorders.

TABLE 20-3   *Newborn Screening Summary*

DISORDER/EVIDENCE	SYMPTOMS	SCREENING INCIDENCE	TREATMENT
PKU (classic) Elevated phenylalanine	Severe mental retardation, eczema, seizures, behavior disorders, decreased pigmentation, distinctive "mousey" odor	1:10,000 to 1:15,000 More common in Caucasians	Lifelong dietary management with low-phenylalanine diet; possible tyrosine supplementation
Congenital hypothyroidism (primary) Low T_4, elevated TSH	Mental and motor retardation, short stature, coarse, dry skin and hair, hoarse cry, constipation	Overall 1:4,000 with ethnic variation 1:12,000 African-American 1:1,000 Native American	Maintain l-thyroxine levels in upper half of normal range; periodic bone age to monitor growth
Galactosemia (transferase deficiency) Elevated galactose; low or absent fluorescence	Neonatal death from severe dehydration, sepsis, or liver pathology; mental retardation, jaundice, blindness, cataracts	1:10,000 to 1:90,000	Eliminate galactose and lactose from the diet; soy formulas in infancy; lactose-free solid foods
Maple syrup urine disease (MSUD) Elevated leucine	Acidosis; hypertonicity and seizures, vomiting, drowsiness, apnea, coma; infant death or severe mental retardation and neurologic impairment; behavioral disorders	1:90,000 to 1:200,000	Diet low in leucine, isoleucine, and valine; thiamine supplement if responsive
Homocystinuria Elevated methionine	Mental retardation, seizures, behavioral disorders, early-onset thromboses, dislocated lenses, tall lanky body habitus	1:200,000	Methionine-restricted diet; cystine supplement; vitamin B_6 supplement if responsive
Congenital adrenal hyperplasia (CAH) Elevated 17-hydroxyprogesterone; abnormal electrolytes	Hyponatremia, hypokalemia, hypoglycemia, dehydration, and early death; ambiguous genitalia in females; progressive virilization in both sexes	1:15,000 to 1:3,000 native Eskimos	Replace corticosteroids; plastic surgery to correct ambiguous genitalia
Biotinidase deficiency Deficient or absent activity of biotinidase on colorimetric assay	Mental retardation, seizures, ataxia, skin rash, hearing loss, alopecia, optic nerve atrophy, coma, and death	1:60,000 to 1:100,000	10 mg biotin daily

Data from Wright L, Brown A & Davidson-Mundt A: Newborn screening: the miracle and the challenge, *J Pediatr Nurs* 7(1):26, 1992.

PKU results from a deficiency of the enzyme phenylalanine dehydrogenase. The test for PKU is not reliable until the newborn has ingested an ample amount of the amino acid phenylalanine, a constituent of both human and cow milk. The nurse must document the initial ingestion of milk and perform the test at least 24 hours after that time. If the infant is found to have PKU, a diet low in phenylalanine is begun soon after birth. Breastfeeding or partial breastfeeding may be possible for some infants if the phenylalanine levels are monitored carefully and remain within acceptable limits (Lawrence, 1994). Although severe mental retardation is seen less in affected children living in countries where there is neonatal screening for PKU, many affected children have some intellectual impairment.

Galactosemia, caused by a deficiency of the enzyme galactose 1-phosphate uridyl transferase, results in the inability to convert galactose to glucose. Galactosemia can be detected by measuring the blood levels of galactose in the urine of newborns suspected of having the disease who have ingested formula containing galactose. Early symptoms are vomiting, weight loss, and CNS symptoms, including poor feeding, drowsiness, and seizures. If the disorder goes untreated, the galactose levels will continue to increase and the affected infant will show failure to thrive, mental retardation, cataracts, jaundice, hepatomegaly, and cirrhosis of the liver, with death possibly occurring in the first month of life. Therapy consists of eliminating galactose from the diet.

Routine screening for hypothyroidism is mandated. This involves the measurement of thyroxine (T_4) in a drop of blood obtained from a heel stick at 2 to 5 days of age. At this time the normally expected increase in T_4 would be lacking in newborns with hypothyroidism. *Cretinism* develops in

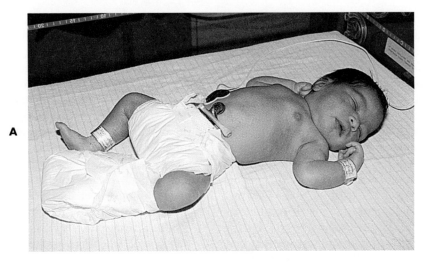

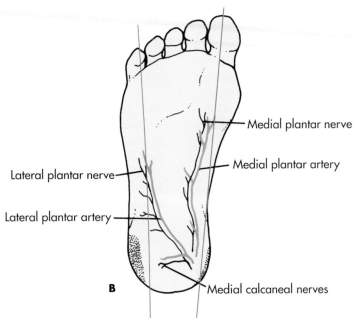

Fig. **20-6** Heel stick. **A,** Newborn with foot wrapped for warmth to increase blood flow to extremity before heel stick. **B,** Heel stick sites (*shaded areas*) on infant's foot for obtaining samples of capillary blood. (**A** Courtesy Marjorie Pyle, RNC, Lifecircle, Costa Mesa, Calif.)

untreated affected people. The same blood sample can be used to test for all three of these metabolic disorders—PKU, galactosemia, and hypothyroidism.

Urine or meconium screening may be used to identify substances abused by the mother. Initially costly and of limited availability, tests of meconium collected on day 1 or 2 of life have been shown to be both sensitive and reliable in detecting the metabolites of several street drugs, including cocaine (Bibb et al., 1995).

Collection of specimens

The ongoing evaluation of a newborn often requires the acquisition of blood by the heel stick or venipuncture method or the collection of a urine specimen.

Heel stick. Most blood specimens are drawn by laboratory technicians. Nurses, however, may be required to perform heel sticks to obtain blood for glucose monitoring and to measure hematocrit levels. The same technique is needed to complete the PKU form or to test for galactosemia and hypothyroidism or other inborn errors of metabolism.

It is helpful to warm the heel before the sample is taken, because the application of heat for 5 to 10 minutes helps dilate the vessels in the area. However, second- and third-degree thermal burns have been reported to result from inappropriate heel-warming techniques. A cloth soaked with warm water and wrapped loosely around the foot can effectively warm the foot (Fig. 20-6, *A*). Disposable heel warmers are also available from a variety of companies but should be used with care to prevent burns. Nurses should wear gloves when collecting any specimen. The nurse first cleanses the area with alcohol, restrains the infant's foot with her free hand, and then punctures the site with an appropriate device.

The most serious complication of an infant heel stick is necrotizing osteochondritis resulting from lancet penetration of the bone. To prevent this, the stick should penetrate no deeper than 2.4 mm. To identify the appropriate puncture site, the nurse should draw an imaginary line from between the fourth and fifth toes that runs parallel to the lateral aspect of the heel, where the stick should be made; a line can also be drawn from the great toe to the heel that runs parallel to the medial aspect of the heel, another site for a stick (Fig. 20-6, *B*). Repeated trauma to the walking surface of the heel can cause fibrosis and scarring that may lead to problems with walking (Reiner, Meltes & Hayes, 1990; Wong, 1995), so care must be taken to minimize such trauma.

After the specimen has been collected, pressure should be applied with a dry gauze square but no further alcohol should be applied because this will cause the site to continue to bleed. The site is then covered with an adhesive bandage. The nurse makes sure the equipment used is properly disposed of, reviews the laboratory slip for correct identification, and checks the specimen to make sure the labeling and routing information is adequate.

A heel stick can be traumatic for the infant and, because pain pathways are present and functional in the infant, can cause pain. After several heel sticks, infants have been observed to withdraw their feet when they are touched. Therefore, to reassure the infant and promote feelings of safety, the neonate should be cuddled and comforted when the procedure is complete. Rocking the infant or giving him or her a pacifier is also an effective comforting measure (Campos, 1994).

Venipuncture. Venous blood samples can be drawn from radial veins, jugular veins, or femoral veins, or they can be drawn through peripheral lock devices. However, use of such a device may shorten the use of the device as an IV site (Wong, 1995). If an IV site is used to obtain a blood specimen, it is important to consider the type of fluid being infused, because contamination of the blood with the fluid can alter the results.

When venipuncture is required, positioning of the needle is extremely important. Although regular venipuncture needles may be used for this purpose, some personnel prefer to use scalp vein needles. It is necessary to be very patient during the procedure, because the blood return in small veins is slow, meaning also that the small needle must remain in place longer. If the radial vein is used, the infant's arm is exposed and held securely in place.

If venipuncture or arterial puncture is being performed for blood gas studies, crying, fear, and agitation will affect the values. Therefore every effort must be made to keep the infant quiet during the procedure. For blood gas studies the

blood sample tubes are packed in ice to reduce blood cell metabolism and are taken immediately to the laboratory for analysis (Wong, 1995).

Pressure must be maintained over an arterial or femoral vein puncture for at least 5 minutes to prevent bleeding from the site. The nurse should then observe the infant frequently for evidence of bleeding or hematoma formation at the puncture site for an hour after any venipuncture. The infant's tolerance of the procedure should also be noted and recorded. The infant should be cuddled and comforted (e.g., rocked, given a pacifier) when the procedure is completed (Van Cleve et al., 1995).

Obtaining urine specimen. Examination of urine is a valuable laboratory tool for infant assessment, but the way in which the urine specimen is collected may influence the results. In addition, the urine sample should be fresh and examined within 1 hour of collection.

A variety of urine collection bags are available, including the Hollister U-Bag (Fig. 20-7). These are clear plastic, single-use bags with an adhesive material around the opening at the point of attachment.

To prepare the infant, the nurse removes the diaper and places the infant supine. The genitalia, perineum, and surrounding skin are washed and thoroughly dried because the adhesive on the bag will not stick to moist, powdered, or oily skin surfaces. The protective paper is removed to expose the adhesive (see Fig. 20-7, *A*). In female infants the perineum is first stretched to flatten skin folds and then the adhesive area on the bag pressed firmly onto the skin all around the urinary meatus and vagina. (NOTE: Start with the narrow portion of the butterfly-shaped adhesive patch.) The nurse must be sure to start at the bridge of skin separating the rectum from the vagina and work upward (see Fig. 20-7, *B*). In male infants the penis and scrotum are tucked through the opening into the collection bag before the nurse removes the protective paper from the adhesive and presses it firmly onto the perineum, making sure the entire adhesive is firmly attached to skin and the edges of the opening do not pucker (see Fig. 20-7, *C*). This helps ensure a leak-proof seal and decreases the chance of contamination from stool. Cutting a slit in the diaper and pulling the bag through the slit may also help prevent leaking.

The diaper is carefully replaced, and the bag is checked frequently. The bag is removed when 1 to 2 ml of urine has been obtained. The infant's skin is observed for signs of irritation while the bag is in place. The specimen can be aspirated with a syringe or drained directly from the bag. To drain the bag, the bag is held in the one hand and tilted to keep urine away from the tab. The tab is then removed and the urine drained into a clean receptacle (see Fig. 20-7, *D*).

Collection of a 24-hour specimen can be a challenge. To do this the infant may need to be restrained. The 24-hour U-Bag is applied in the same manner as that just described, and the urine collected is drained into a receptacle. The

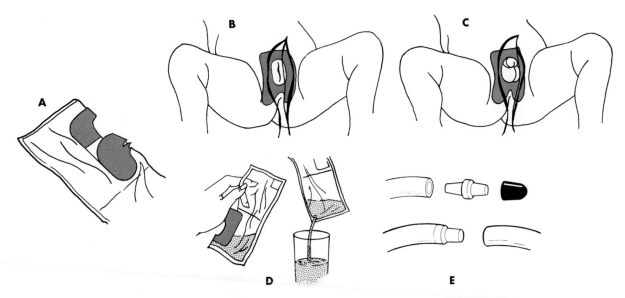

Fig. **20-7** Collection of urine specimen. **A,** Protective paper is being removed from the adhesive surface. **B,** Applied to girls. **C,** Applied to boys. **D,** Cut to drain urine. **E,** Collection tube. (Permission to use and/or reproduce this copyrighted material has been granted by the owner, Hollister, Incorporated, Libertyville, Ill.)

collection tube can be shortened or capped (see Fig. 20-7, *E*). During the collection the infant's skin is watched closely for signs of irritation and lack of a proper seal.

For some types of urine tests, urine can be aspirated directly from the diaper by means of a syringe without a needle. If the diaper has absorbent gelling material that traps urine, a small gauze dressing or some cotton balls can be placed inside the diaper and the urine aspirated from them (Wong, 1995).

Therapeutic interventions

Intramuscular injection. It is routine to administer a single parenteral dose of 0.5 to 1 mg of vitamin K intramuscularly to an infant soon after birth to prevent hemorrhagic disorders because normal newborns are not able to produce their own vitamin K until about 8 days after birth. Vitamin K is produced in the gastrointestinal tract starting soon after microorganisms are introduced.

Hepatitis B vaccination (HBV) is recommended for all infants. Infants at highest risk of contracting hepatitis B are those born to women who come from Asia, Africa, South America, the South Pacific, or southern or eastern Europe. If the infant is born to an infected mother or to a mother who is a chronic carrier, hepatitis vaccine and hepatitis B immune globulin (HBIG) should be administered within 12 hours of birth. The hepatitis vaccine is given in one site and the HBIG in another. The first dose of the vaccine for infants born to healthy women may be given at birth or at 1 or 2 months of age. Parental consent should be obtained before administering these medications.

In most cases a 25-gauge, ⅝-inch needle should be used for the vitamin K and hepatitis vaccine injections.

A 22-gauge needle may be necessary if thicker medications such as some penicillins are to be given.

Selection of the injection site is important. Injections must be given in muscles large enough to accommodate the medication, but major nerves and blood vessels avoided. The muscles of newborns may not tolerate more than a 0.5-ml IM injection. The preferred site for newborns is the vastus lateralis (Fig. 20-8) although the rectus femoris muscle can also be used. Except for the femoral artery on the medial aspect of the thigh, these two muscles are free of important nerves and blood vessels. The vastus lateralis muscle is the larger of the two and is well developed in the newborn. The posterior gluteal muscle is very small and poorly developed in infants; it is also dangerously close to the sciatic nerve, which occupies a proportionately larger space in infants than in older children. Therefore it is not recommended that it be used as an injection site until the child has been walking for at least 1 year.

Newborn infants offer little, if any, resistance to injections. Although they squirm and may be difficult to hold in position if they are awake, they can usually be restrained without the need for assistance from a second person if the nurse is experienced.

The neonate's leg should be stabilized, and gloves should be worn by the person giving the injection. The nurse cleanses the injection site with alcohol and then stabilizes the infant's muscle between her thumb and first finger. The needle is inserted into the vastus lateralis at a 90-degree angle. The muscle is then released and the plunger of the syringe gently withdrawn. If no blood is aspirated, the medication is injected. If blood is aspirated, the needle is withdrawn and the injection is given in another site. After the

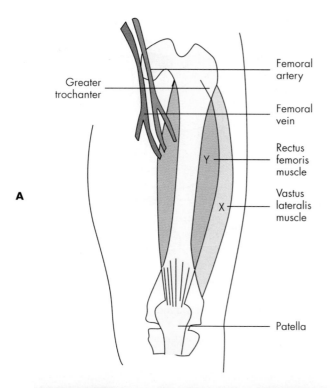

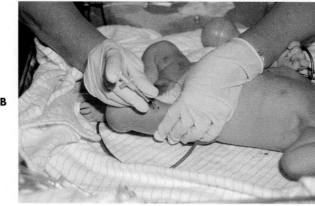

Fig. **20-8** Intramuscular injection sites. **A,** Acceptable intramuscular injection site for children. *X,* Preferred injection site; *Y,* alternate injection site. **B,** Infant's leg stabilized for intramuscular injection. Nurse is wearing gloves to give injection. (**B** courtesy Marjorie Pyle, RNC, Lifecircle, Costa Mesa, Calif.)

injection has been given, the needle is withdrawn quickly and the site massaged with a dry gauze square. It is not uncommon for blood to ooze from the injection site, but it is not necessary to cover the site with an adhesive bandage. Pressure should be applied until oozing stops.

The nurse should always remember to comfort the infant after an injection and to properly discard equipment. It is important to record the name of the medication, the date and time of administration, the amount, the route, the site of injection, and the infant's tolerance of injection.

Therapy for hyperbilirubinemia. The best therapy for hyperbilirubinemia is prevention. This is done by feed-

ing the newborn soon after birth because this stimulates the gastrocolic reflex and the passage of meconium in which bilirubin is excreted. However, even despite this, the term infant may have trouble conjugating the amount of bilirubin derived from disintegrating fetal red blood cells. As a result, the serum levels of unconjugated bilirubin may rise beyond normal limits, causing **hyperbilirubinemia** (see Chapter 19). If this goes untreated, the levels can continue to rise, and with this increase the risk of kernicterus. The goal of hyperbilirubinemia treatment therefore is to help reduce the newborn's serum levels of unconjugated bilirubin. There are two principal ways of doing this: phototherapy and exchange blood transfusion. Exchange transfusion is used to treat those infants whose raised bilirubin levels cannot be controlled by phototherapy.

Phototherapy. During **phototherapy** the unclothed infant is placed approximately 45 to 50 cm away from a bank of lights. The distance may vary based on unit protocol and type of light used. The infant is turned every 2 hours to expose all body surfaces to the light. This is done for several hours or days until the infant's serum bilirubin level decreases to within an acceptable range. The decision to discontinue therapy is based on the observation of a definite downward trend in the bilirubin values. After therapy has been terminated, the infant may have a rebound in the bilirubin levels, which is usually harmless.

Several precautions must be taken while the infant is undergoing phototherapy. The lamp energy output should be monitored routinely during treatment with a photometer (Fanaroff & Martin, 1997). The infant's eyes must be protected by an opaque mask to prevent overexposure to the light, and the eye shield should completely cover the eyes but not occlude the nares. In addition, before the mask is applied, the infant's eyes should be closed gently to prevent excoriation of the corneas. The mask should be removed during infant feedings so that the eyes can be checked and the parents can have visual contact with the infant (Fig. 20-9, *A* and *B*).

To promote optimal skin exposure, yet sufficient protection of the genitals and bedding, often a "string bikini" made from a disposable face mask is used instead of a diaper. Before its application, the metal strip must be removed from the mask so that the infant is not burned. Lotions and ointments should not be applied to the infant because they absorb heat and this can cause burns.

Phototherapy may cause the infant to sleep for longer than the usual 4-hour periods, but the infant needs to be kept on a regular feeding schedule. The number and consistency of stools are monitored. Because bilirubin breakdown increases gastric motility, which results in the formation of loose stools that can cause skin excoriation and breakdown, the infant's buttocks are cleaned after each stool to help maintain skin integrity.

Because the infant is unclothed and the lights produce heat, the infant's temperature may become elevated, and

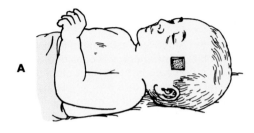

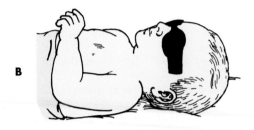

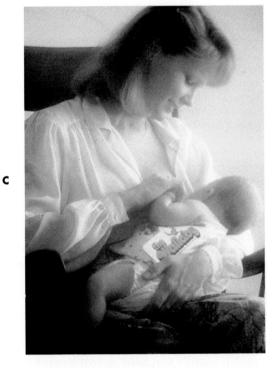

Fig. 20-9 Eye patches for newborn receiving phototherapy. **A,** Small Velcro patch stuck to both sides of head. **B,** Eye cover sticks to Velcro patch, which reduces movement of eye cover and facilitates removal for feedings. **C,** A mother can nurse her baby without interrupting phototherapy. (Courtesy Respironics, Inc., Marietta, Ga.)

for this reason needs to be monitored at least every 4 hours. The lights also accelerate the rate of insensible water loss, making it possible for fluid loss and dehydration to occur. Therefore it is important that the infant be adequately hydrated. All aspects of the phototherapy rendered should be accurately recorded in the infant's chart.

An alternative device for phototherapy that is as safe and effective as traditional phototherapy is a fiberoptic panel attached to an illuminator. This fiberoptic blanket, which essentially wraps light around the newborn's torso, delivers continuous phototherapy. While wearing it the newborn can remain in the mother's room in an open crib or in her arms; follow unit protocol for the use of eye patches (see Fig. 20-9, *C*). The blanket may also be used for home phototherapy.

Parent education. Serum levels of bilirubin in the newborn continue to rise until the fifth day of life. However, because most parents leave the hospital within 48 hours and some as early as 6 hours after birth, parents must be able to assess the newborn's degree of jaundice. They should therefore have written instructions for assessing the infant's condition that include the name of the person they should contact to report their findings. Some hospitals have a nurse make a home visit to evaluate the infant's condition. If it proves necessary to measure the infant's bilirubin levels after discharge from the hospital, either the home care nurse may draw the blood specimen or the parents may take the baby to a laboratory for the determination (see the Teaching Guidelines box).

Circumcision. Circumcision is commonly performed in the United States, although there is controversy over its value. A properly performed newborn circumcision prevents **phimosis** (a rare condition that can interfere with or impede the flow of urine and predispose males to the development of infection between the foreskin and glans penis) and may reduce the risk of urinary tract infections. In addition, the incidence of penile cancer has been found to be lower in American men who are circumcised. However, there is still conflicting evidence regarding the association between circumcision and sexually transmitted diseases. Because there are potential medical benefits and advantages, as well as disadvantages and risks, to newborn circumcision, and because of the continuing controversy about these advantages and disadvantages, the decision to perform this elective surgical procedure is left to the parents.

Circumcision is a matter of personal parental choice. Parents usually decide to have their newborn circumcised for one or more of the following reasons: hygiene, religious conviction, tradition, culture, or social norms. Regardless of the reason for the decision, it should be made only after parents have been given the available facts and have sufficient time to review their options.

Expectant parents need to begin learning about circumcision during the prenatal period, but circumcision often is not discussed with the parents before labor. In many instances, it is only when the mother is being admitted to the hospital or birth unit that she is first confronted with the decision regarding circumcision. Because the stress of the intrapartal period makes this a difficult time for parental decision making, this is not an ideal time to broach the topic of circumcision and expect a well-thought-out decision. The mother may be asked to sign a circumcision permit form

TEACHING GUIDELINES

Hyperbilirubinemia

DEFINITIONS

Hyperbilirubinemia: higher levels of bilirubin than normal.
Bilirubin: end product of RBCs when they mature and break down.
RBCs: red blood cells.
Jaundice: yellow skin, sclerae, and mucous membranes caused by circulating bilirubin.
Phototherapy: the use of fluorescent light to break down the bilirubin in the skin into substances that can be excreted in the feces (stool) and urine.
Bililites: fluorescent lights used for phototherapy.

HOW JAUNDICE HAPPENS

When RBCs break down, they release bilirubin, which then circulates in the blood. The bilirubin combines with another substance in the liver. This combined substance moves through the blood to the kidneys and the intestines, where it is eliminated in the urine and the stool. The bilirubin gives the yellow color to urine and the brown color to the stool.

Before birth, babies have more RBCs in each ounce of blood than adults have. The RBCs of the unborn infant also have a shorter life span (70 to 90 days) than RBCs formed after birth (120 days). When the RBCs of a fetus break down, the bilirubin produced by this is carried by the fetus's blood, through the placenta, and to the mother's liver to be excreted.

After birth, the infant's liver must get rid of the bilirubin. Even though a baby's liver functions well, it may not be able to get rid of all the bilirubin produced by breakdown of RBCs. Bilirubin then seeps out of the blood and into the tissues, coloring them yellow (jaundice). The blood level of bilirubin rises quickly up to the fifth day and then it declines; the jaundice usually clears up by the end of the week.

THE DANGER OF EXCESS BILIRUBIN

Some newborns seem to have extra bilirubin to excrete. High levels of bilirubin may cause damage to the brain.

According to the American Academy of Pediatrics guidelines (1994), phototherapy is considered in a healthy term infant who is 1 to 2 days old if the total bilirubin level is 12 mg/dl or more, or it is instituted if the bilirubin level is 15 mg/dl or more. The infant is placed under phototherapy lights or on a bili blanket. This helps the infant eliminate the extra bilirubin and prevents damage to the brain.

CARING FOR THE INFANT

The newborn is placed in an incubator under phototherapy lights so that it can be kept warm and the nurse can observe it.

The infant wears an eye mask to keep the light out of the eyes.

The baby is undressed so that as much light as possible can reach the skin.

The newborn may wear a "string bikini" as a small diaper, which is made out of a paper diaper or a face mask.

The baby's temperature is taken often so that any changes in temperature can be noted and the infant is not allowed to become too hot or too cold.

The baby may be given extra water to drink or extra breastfeedings because infants have watery, green stools resulting from the excretion of the extra bilirubin and this can lead to dehydration.

The newborn is taken out from under the lights for feedings and cuddling unless a bili blanket is being used. There is no need to remove the bili blanket for feeding.

Blood is taken from the heel to check the amount of bilirubin still in the newborn's blood and the nurse updates the parents about the results.

AFTER THE NEWBORN GOES HOME

The parents should be encouraged to ask any questions that they might have. The nurse gives them a telephone number to call at any hour with their questions. If therapy is continued at home, referral is made to home care.

---

during the admission process, but usually this request is made after the birth. Some hospitals require parents to sign a different form stating they do not wish their male infant to be circumcised, if that is their desire.

Procedure. **Circumcision** involves removing the prepuce (foreskin) of the glans. The procedure is usually not done immediately after birth because of the danger of cold stress but is performed in the hospital before the infant's discharge. The circumcision of a Jewish male is performed on the eighth day after birth and is done at home, unless the infant is unwell. This is logical from a physiologic standpoint because clotting factors drop somewhat immediately after birth and do not return to prebirth levels until the end of the first week.

Feedings are usually withheld up to 4 hours before the circumcision to prevent vomiting and aspiration. To prepare the infant for the circumcision, he is positioned on a plastic restraint form (Fig. 20-10) and his penis is cleansed with soap and water or a preparatory solution such as povidone-iodine. The infant is draped to provide warmth and a sterile field, and the sterile equipment is readied for use.

Although some circumcision procedures require no special equipment or appliances, (Fig. 20-11), numerous instruments have been designed for this purpose. Use of the Yellen or Mogen clamp (Fig. 20-12) may make this an almost bloodless operation. The procedure itself takes only a few minutes to perform. After it is completed, a small petrolatum gauze dressing or a generous amount of

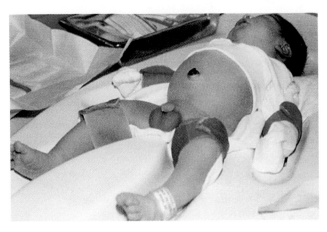

Fig. 20-10 "Circ board" restrains infant during circumcision. (Courtesy Marjorie Pyle, RNC, Lifecircle, Costa Mesa, Calif.)

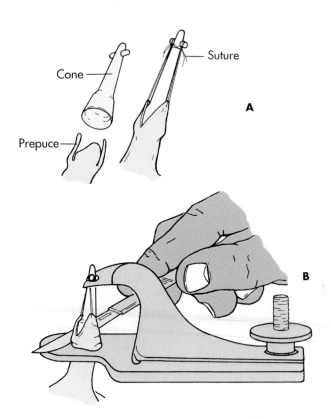

Fig. 20-12 Circumcision with Yellen clamp. A, Prepuce drawn over cone. B, Yellen clamp is applied, hemostasis occurs, then prepuce (over cone) is cut away.

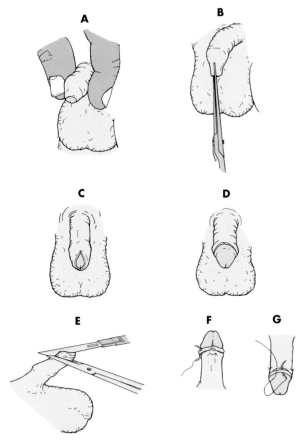

Fig. 20-11 Technique of circumcision. A to D, Prepuce is stripped and slit to facilitate its retraction behind glans penis. E, Prepuce is now clamped and excessive prepuce cut off. F and G, Suture material used is plain 00 or 000 catgut in a very small needle; some physicians prefer silk suture.

petrolatum may be applied for the first day to keep a diaper from adhering to the site. A Plastibell may also be used for the circumcision. The advantages to its use are that it applies constant direct pressure to prevent hemorrhage during the procedure, and afterwards protects against infection, keeps the site from sticking to the diaper, and prevents pain with urination. When using the bell for circumcision, it is first fitted over the glans, the suture is tied around the rim of the bell, and excess prepuce is then cut away. The plastic rim remains in place for about a week until it falls off, after healing has taken place (Fig. 20-13). Petrolatum does not need to be applied when the bell is used.

Discomfort. Circumcision is painful, and the pain is manifested by both physiologic and behavioral changes in the infant. Local anesthesia (dorsal penile nerve block) may be used to reduce the physiologic response to the pain.

A eutectic (easily melted) mixture of local anesthetics (EMLA) may be used to control the pain of circumcision (Lander et al., 1997). EMLA, 5% lidocaine-prilocaine cream, is applied to the penis for 60 to 90 minutes before the procedure. A transparent occlusive dressing is applied over a thick layer of the cream (Wong, 1995).

In the Jewish ritual the newborn is given a few drops of wine to relax him in preparation for the procedure. The

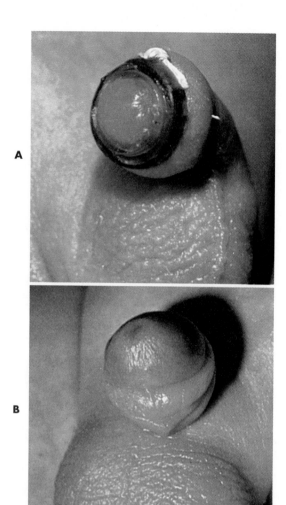

A

B

Fig. **20-13** Circumcision using Hollister plastibel. **A,** Suture around rim of plastibel controls bleeding. **B,** Plastic rim and suture drop off in 7 to 10 days. (Permission to use and/or reproduce this copyrighted material has been granted by the owner, Hollister, Incorporated, Libertyville, Ill.)

HOME CARE *Patient Instructions for Self-Care*
Circumcision
Wash hands before touching newly circumcised penis.

CHECK FOR BLEEDING
- Check circumcision for bleeding every hour for the first 12 hours after the procedure.
- If bleeding occurs, apply gentle pressure with a folded sterile gauze square. If bleeding does not stop with pressure, notify primary health care provider.

OBSERVE FOR URINATION
- Check to see that infant urinates after being circumcised.
- Infant should have a wet diaper 6 to 10 times per 24 hours.

KEEP AREA CLEAN
- Change diaper and inspect circumcision at least every 4 hours.
- Wash penis gently with warm water to remove urine and feces. Apply petrolatum to the glans with each diaper change (omit petrolatum if Plastibell was used).
- Use soap only after circumcision is healed.
- Fanfold diaper to prevent pressure on the circumcised area.

CHECK FOR INFECTION
- Glans penis is dark red after circumcision, then becomes covered with a yellow exudate in 24 hours. This is normal and will persist for 2 to 3 days. Do not attempt to remove it.
- Redness, swelling, or discharge indicate infection. Notify primary health care provider if you think the circumcision area is infected.

PROVIDE COMFORT
- Circumcision is painful. Handle the area gently.
- Provide extra holding, feeding, and opportunities for nonnutritive sucking for a day or two.

pain may not end when the operation is over, however, because the wound takes as long as a week to heal.

If the infant has undergone circumcision without anesthesia, he is comforted until he is quieted (Marchette et al., 1991), then he is returned to his mother. These infants usually are fussy for about 2 to 3 hours afterwards and may refuse a feeding. It is not uncommon for the infant to have a loose, green stool after the circumcision.

Care of the newly circumcised penis. The nurse checks the penis hourly for the next 12 hours to make sure no bleeding is occurring and voiding is normal. If bleeding is noted from the circumcision, the nurse applies gentle pressure to the site of bleeding with a folded sterile 4 × 4-in (10 × 10-cm) gauze pad or sprinkles powdered gel foam on it. If bleeding is not easily controlled, a blood vessel may need to be ligated. In this event, one nurse notifies the physician and prepares the necessary equipment (circumcision

tray and suture material), while another nurse maintains *intermittent* pressure until the physician arrives. If the parents take the baby home before the end of the 12-hour observation period, they have to be taught proper care (see Home Care box). Before the infant is discharged, the nurse checks to see that the parents have the physician's telephone number.

Nursing actions are planned and implemented to prevent infection. Prepackaged wipes for cleaning the diaper area should not be used because they contain alcohol, which delays healing and causes discomfort. Instead the nurse washes the penis gently with water to remove urine and feces and reapplies fresh petrolatum around the glans after each diaper change. The glans penis, which is normally dark red during healing, becomes covered with a yellow exudate in 24 hours. This is part of normal healing, not an infective process. No attempt is made to remove the exudate, which persists for 2 to 3 days. Parents should be taught to fanfold the diaper so that it does not press on the circumcised area. They should also be encouraged to change the diaper at least every 4 hours to prevent it from sticking to the penis.

Discharge planning and teaching—anticipatory guidance

Infant care activities can cause much anxiety for the new parent (see the Plan of Care box, p. 546). The kind of support given by the nursing staff members can be an important factor in determining whether new mothers seek and accept help in the future. Whether this is the woman's or parents' first baby, an adolescent whose mother will be the primary caregiver, and whether they attended parenthood preparation classes, parents appreciate anticipatory guidance in the care of their infant. The nurse should not try to cover all the content at one time because the parents can be overwhelmed by too much information and become anxious. However, because of the early discharge of new mothers that is currently common practice (see Box 17-2 for the criteria for infant discharge), it may be a problem for the nurse to impart all of the information necessary. As a result, many institutions have developed home visitation programs that take the necessary teaching to the new parents (see Chapter 18), although the hospital nurse still provides most of the essential information for newborn care. In the inpatient setting, priorities of care must be established and a systematic teaching plan for infant care devised. One way to accomplish this is to use critical path case management. A care path may also be developed that covers the changes expected in the infant during the first several days. Such a care path is shown on p. 542. When variations from the care path occur, further assessment and intervention may be necessary.

The care of the newborn is shared by the nurse and the parents, with the nurse acting as teacher and support person. As soon as the mother feels physically able, she is encouraged to participate in her infant's care. The care given the infant is supervised, and the parents are encouraged to ask questions. The mother's need for knowledge and the factors that may hinder her learning are determined through questioning and observation. The content taught and teaching aids used should be in keeping with the mother's level of understanding. Films and tapes can be valuable time-savers as teaching tools. Most hospitals also provide parents with written instructions for infant care.

To set priorities for teaching, the nurse follows parental cues. Knowledge deficits should be identified before teaching begins. Normal growth and development and the changing needs of the infant (e.g., for stimulation, exercise, and social contacts), as well as the following topics should be included during the discharge planning session with parents.

Positioning and holding. Positioning the infant on the right side after feeding promotes gastric emptying into the small intestine (see Fig. 19-10). Placing the infant in the crib in a side-lying position also promotes the drainage of mucus from the mouth and applies no pressure to the umbilical cord or the sensitive circumcised penis. The American Academy of Pediatrics advises against placing an infant in the prone position during the first few months of life and suggests that the side-lying or back-lying position is preferable. The placement of infants in prone positions has been associated with an increased incidence of sudden infant death syndrome (SIDS) (Havens & Zink, 1994).

Anatomically the infant's shape—barrel chest and flat, curveless spine—makes it easy for the child to roll when startled. The placement of a folded or rolled blanket against the infant's spine will keep him or her from rolling to the supine position and promote a feeling of security. Care must be taken to prevent the infant from rolling off of flat, unguarded surfaces. When an infant is on such a surface, the parent or nurse who must turn away from the infant even for a moment should always keep one hand placed securely on the infant.

The infant is always held securely with its head supported because newborns are unable to maintain an erect head posture for more than a few moments. Fig. 20-14 illustrates various positions for holding an infant with adequate support.

Using the bulb syringe. The parents should be shown the way to use the bulb syringe and asked to demonstrate the technique back to the nurse. If the infant has excess mucus in the respiratory tract, the nurse or parent may need to aspirate the mouth and nasal passages with a bulb syringe. The infant who is coughing and choking on the secretions should be supported with its head downward. The mouth is suctioned first because, if the nasal passages are suctioned first, the infant may inhale the pharyngeal secretions by gasping when the nares are touched. The bulb is compressed and inserted into one side of the mouth (see Fig. 19-11). The center of the infant's mouth should be avoided, however, because this could stimulate the gag reflex. The nasal passages are then suctioned one nostril at a time. When the infant's cry does not sound as though it were coming through mucus or a bubble, suctioning can be stopped. It is current practice to keep the bulb syringe in the infant's crib.

Temperature. The following topics should be reviewed:

- The causes of an elevated body temperature (such as exercise, cold stress with resultant vasoconstriction, minimum response to infection) and the body's response to extremes in environmental temperature.
- Signs to be reported, such as high or low temperatures with accompanying fussiness, stuffy nose, lethargy, irritability, poor feeding, and crying.
- Ways to promote normal body temperature, such as giving a warm tub bath, dressing the infant appropriately for the air temperature, and protecting the infant from long exposure to sunlight.
- The method for taking the baby's axillary temperature.

CARE PATH *Neonatal Adaptation to Extrauterine Life*

	DAY 1	DAY 2	DAY 3	DAY 4	DAY 7	DAY 14
WEIGHT		Loss of 5% to 10% of birth weight	Gain of 150 to 300 gm per day			Birth weight regained
TEMPERATURE	Stabilized at 37° C					
FEEDINGS						
VOLUME						
FORMULA	15 to 60 ml	60 to 90 ml	60 to 90 ml	60 to 90 ml	60 to 90 ml	60 to 90 ml
BREAST		Softening of at least one breast at each feeding				
FREQUENCY						
FORMULA	6 to 10 times/24 hr		6 to 10 times/24 hr		6 to 10 times/24 hr	
BREAST	8 to 12 times/24 hr		8 to 12 times/24 hr		8 to 12 times/24 hr	
VOIDING	At least 1 time in first 24 hr	2 to 6 times/24 hr	6 to 10 times/24 hr			6 to 10 times/24 hr
STOOLS		Meconium; at least 1 time in first 48 hours	Transitional stool; 1 to 5/day	Yellow stool; 1 to 5/day		Yellow stool; 1 to 2/day
SLEEP	16 to 20 hr/24 hr					16 to 20 hr/24 hr
UMBILICAL CORD	Moist; clamped	Dry; clamp removed				Cord off
CIRCUMCISION	Red; sore	Yellow exudate covers glans	Healing	Healing		Healed
COLOR	Pink; acrocyanosis	Pink; slight jaundice	Peak of jaundice		Pink	
BILIRUBIN LEVEL	0 to 6 mg/dl	≤8 mg/dl	≤12mg/dl		≤2 mg/dl	
LABORATORY TESTS	Glucose when required; HCT	PKU, T₄, galactose				Repeat PKU, if needed
MEDICATIONS	Eye prophylaxis and vitamin K within 2 hours of birth; HBV within 12 hours of birth					

HBV, Hepatitis B vaccination.

Elimination. A review includes the following reminders:
- Changes to be expected in the color of the stool (meconium to transitional to soft yellow/golden yellow) and the number of bowel evacuations, plus the odor of stools for breastfed and bottle-fed infants (see Chapter 21).
- The color of normal urine and the number of voidings (six to ten) to expect each day.

Bathing. Bathing serves a number of purposes. It provides opportunities for (1) completely cleansing the infant, (2) observing the infant's condition, (3) promoting comfort, and (4) parent-child-family socializing.

An important consideration in skin cleansing is the preservation of the skin's **acid mantle,** which is formed from the uppermost horny layer of the epidermis, sweat, superficial fat, metabolic products, and external substances such as amniotic fluid, and microorganisms. At birth the skin

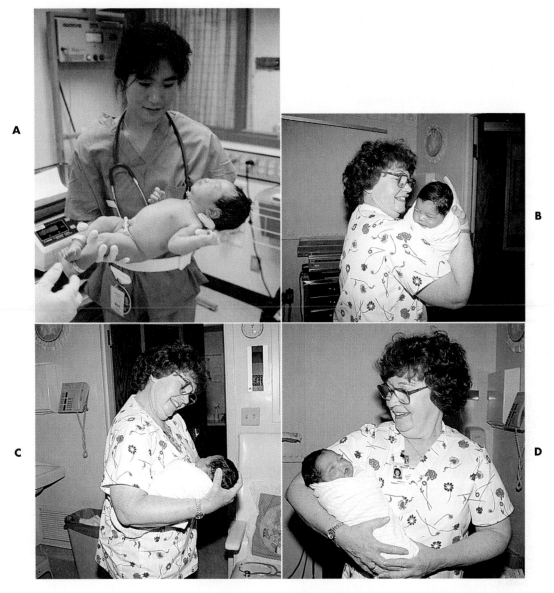

Fig. **20-14** Holding baby securely with support for head. **A,** Holding infant while moving infant from one place to another. Baby is undressed to show posture. **B,** Holding baby upright in "burping" position. **C,** "Football" hold. **D,** Cradling hold. (**A** courtesy Kim Molloy, San Jose, Calif.; **B, C,** and **D** courtesy Marjorie Pyle, RNC, Lifecircle, Costa Mesa, Calif.)

has a pH of 6.34. Within 4 days, however, the pH of the newborn's skin surface falls to within the bacteriostatic range (pH <5) (Krebs, 1998). Consequently, only plain warm water should be used for the bath during that 4-day period. Alkaline soaps such as Ivory, oils, powder, and lotions should not be used during this time because they alter the acid mantle, thus creating a medium for bacterial growth. Although the sponging technique is generally used, bathing the newborn by immersion has been found to allow less

heat loss and provoke less crying but is not advised until the umbilical cord falls off (about 10 days to 2 weeks after birth).

See the accompanying Home Care box for information regarding sponge bathing, skin care, cord care, cutting nails, and dressing the infant and Chapter 18 for information on infant clothing.

Infant feeding. The infant may be put to breast shortly after birth, preferably within 1 hour of birth. If the infant is to be bottle fed, a nurse may first offer it a few sips

HOME CARE *Patient Instructions for Self-Care*

Sponge Bathing

FITTING BATHS INTO FAMILY'S SCHEDULE

Give a bath at any time convenient to you but not immediately after a feeding period because the increased handling may cause regurgitation.

PREVENTING HEAT LOSS

The temperature of the room should be 24° C, and the bathing area should be free of drafts.

Control heat loss during the bath to conserve the infant's energy. Bathing the infant quickly, exposing only a portion of the body at a time, and thorough drying are all parts of the bathing technique.

GATHERING SUPPLIES AND CLOTHING BEFORE STARTING

Clothing suitable for wearing indoors: diaper, shirt; stretch suit or nightgown optional.

Unscented, mild soap.

Pins, if needed for diaper, closed and placed well out of baby's reach.

Cotton balls.

Towels for drying infant and a clean washcloth.

Receiving blanket.

Tub for water or use a sink.

BATHING THE BABY

Bring infant to bathing area when all supplies are ready. *Never leave the infant alone on bath table or in bath water, not even for a second!* If you have to leave, take the infant with you or put back into crib.

Test temperature of the water. It should feel pleasantly warm to the inner wrist 36.6° to 37.2° C.

Do not hold infant under running water—water temperature may change, and infant may be scalded or chilled rapidly.

Wash infant's head before unwrapping and undressing to prevent heat loss.

Cleanse the eyes from the inner canthus outward, using separate parts of a clean washcloth for each eye. For the first 2 to 3 days there may be a discharge resulting from the reaction of the conjunctiva to the substance (erythromycin) used as a prophylactic measure against infection. Any discharge should be considered abnormal and reported to the health care provider.

Wash the scalp with water and mild soap; rinse well and dry thoroughly. Scalp desquamation, called *cradle cap*, often can be prevented by removing any scales with a fine-toothed comb or brush after washing. If condition persists, the health care provider may prescribe an ointment to massage into the scalp.

Creases under the chin and arms and in the groin may need daily cleansing. The crease under the chin may be exposed by elevating the infant's shoulders 5 cm and letting the head drop back.

Cleanse ears and nose with twists of moistened cotton or a corner of the washcloth. Do not use cotton-tipped swabs because these may cause injury.

Undress baby and wash body and arms and legs. Pat dry gently. Baby may be tub bathed after the cord drops off and umbilicus and circumcised penis are completely healed.

PREVENTING SKIN TRAUMA

The fragile skin can be injured by too vigorous cleansing. If stool or other debris has dried and caked on the skin, soak the area to remove it. Do not attempt to rub it off, because abrasion may result. Gentleness, patting dry rather than rubbing, and use of a mild soap without perfumes or coloring are recommended. Chemicals in the coloring and perfume can cause rashes on sensitive skin.

CARE OF THE CORD

Use a cotton swab. Dip swab in solution the health care provider has ordered and cleanse around base of the cord, where it joins the skin. Notify the health care provider of any odor, discharge, or skin inflammation around the cord. The clamp is removed when the cord is dry (approximately 24 hours). The diaper should not cover the cord because a wet or soiled diaper will slow or prevent drying of the cord and foster infection. When the cord drops off after a week to 10 days, small drops of blood may be seen when the baby cries. This will heal itself. It is not dangerous.

CARE OF HANDS AND FEET

Wash and dry between the fingers and toes.

Do not cut fingernails and toenails immediately after birth. The nails have to grow out far enough from the skin so that the skin is not cut by mistake. If the baby scratches himself or herself, apply loosely fitted mitts over each of the baby's hands. Do so as a last resort, however, because it interferes with the baby's ability for self-consolation sucking on thumb or finger. When the nails have grown, the fingernails and toenails can be cut more easily with manicure scissors (preferably scissors with rounded tips) when the infant is asleep. Nails should be kept short.

CLEANSING GENITALS

Cleanse the genitals of infants daily and after voiding and defecating. For girls, the genitals may be cleansed by separating the labia and gently washing from the pubic area to the anus. For uncircumcised boys, gently pull back (retract) the foreskin. Stop when resistance is felt. Wash and rinse the tip (glans) with soap and warm water and replace the foreskin. The foreskin must be returned to its original position to prevent constriction and swelling. In most newborns the inner layer of the foreskin adheres to the glans and the foreskin cannot be retracted. By the age of 3 years in 90% of boys, the foreskin can be retracted easily without causing pain or trauma. For others, the foreskin is not retractable until adolescence. As soon as the foreskin is partly retractable, and the child is old enough, he can be taught self-care.

DRESSING THE INFANT

When dressing the infant, bunch up the shirt in both hands and expand the neck opening before placing the neck opening over the face; then slip the shirt over the rest of the head. Do not pull shirts roughly over the face or catch fingers in shirt sleeves.

If cloth diapers are used, their absorbency can be increased by placing the bulk of the diaper in the front for a boy and in the back for a girl. In this way, more urine can be absorbed and the skin better protected. The diaper between the infant's legs should not be bulky because this can outwardly displace the hips. A soaker pad can be placed under the infant so that it and not the blanket absorbs the overflow urine. The continual use of plastic or rubber pants may lead to diaper rash.

When possible, store infant's towels, washcloths, and supplies separate from those of the family for 2 to 4 months to prevent infection.

---

of sterile water to make certain its sucking and swallowing reflexes are intact and that there are no anomalies such as a tracheoesophageal fistula. Most infants are on demand-feeding schedules and are allowed to feed when they awaken. Ordinarily, mothers are encouraged to feed their infants every 3 to 4 hours during the day and only when the infant awakens during the night in the first few days after birth. Breastfed babies nurse more often than bottle-fed babies because breast milk is digested faster than formulas made from cow's milk and the stomach empties sooner as a result. Water supplements are usually not recommended. For a thorough discussion of infant feeding, see Chapter 21.

Nonnutritive sucking. Sucking is the infant's chief pleasure. However, sucking may not be satisfied by breast-feeding or formula feeding alone. In fact, it is such a strong need that infants who are deprived of sucking, such as those with a cleft lip, will suck on their tongue. Some newborns are born with sucking pads on their fingers that developed during in utero sucking. Several benefits of non-nutritive sucking have been documented, such as an increased weight gain in premature infants and decreased crying (Treloar, 1994).

Problems arise when parents are concerned about the sucking of fingers, thumb, or pacifier and try to restrain this natural tendency. Before giving advice, nurses should investigate the parents' feelings and base the guidance they give on the information elicited. For example, some parents may see no problem with the use of a finger but may find the use of a pacifier objectionable. In general there is no need to restrain either practice, unless thumb sucking persists past 4 years of age or past the time when the permanent teeth erupt (approximately 6 years of age). Parents are advised to consult with their pediatrician and pediatric nurse practitioner about this topic.

To decrease an infant's dependence on nonnutritive sucking, the feeding time can be prolonged. One way of doing this in bottle-fed infants is to use a small-holed, firm nipple because this necessitates stronger sucking and slows the feeding. A parent's excessive use of the pacifier to calm the child should also be explored, however. It is not unusual for parents to place a pacifier in their infant's mouth as soon as it begins to cry, thus only reinforcing a pattern of distress-relief.

If parents choose to let their child use a pacifier, they need to be made aware of certain safety considerations before purchasing one. A homemade or poorly designed pacifier can be dangerous because the entire object may be aspirated if it is small or a portion may become lodged in the pharynx. Improvised pacifiers, such as those commonly made in hospitals from a padded nipple, also pose dangers because the nipple may separate from the plastic collar and be aspirated. In addition, parents may continue to offer this pacifier to the infant at home rather than obtaining a more appropriate one. Safe pacifiers are made of one piece that includes a shield or flange that is large enough to prevent entry into the mouth and a handle that can be grasped (Fig. 20-15).

Evaluation

Evaluation is based on the expected outcomes. The Plan of Care is revised as needed based on the evaluation (see Plan of Care).

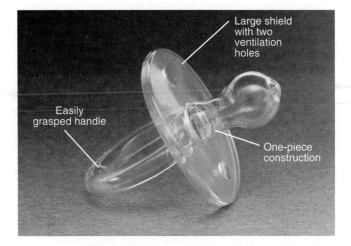

Fig. 20-15 Design of safe pacifier. (From Wong D: *Whaley & Wong's nursing care of infants and children*, ed 5, St Louis, 1995, Mosby.)

Large shield with two ventilation holes

Easily grasped handle

One-piece construction

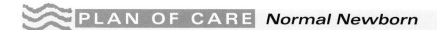

PLAN OF CARE *Normal Newborn*

NURSING DIAGNOSIS Risk for ineffective airway clearance related to excess mucus/improper positioning

Expected Outcome *Infant's airway remains patent; breathing is regular and unlabored.*

Nursing Interventions/*Rationales*

Suction mouth and nasopharynx with bulb syringe as needed; clean nares of crusted secretions *to clear airway and prevent aspiration.*

Position neonate on right side after feeding *to prevent aspiration* and on back or side when sleeping *to prevent suffocation.*

Keep diapers, clothing, and covers loose enough *to allow for maximum lung expansion.*

Teach parents how to hold, suction, and position the infant with return demonstration *to ensure parental skill at airway clearance and maintenance.*

Teach parents that gagging, coughing, and sneezing are normal infant responses *that aid the infant in clearing airways.*

Teach parents feeding techniques that prevent overfeeding and distention of abdomen and teach them to burp infant frequently *to prevent regurgitation and aspiration.*

NURSING DIAGNOSIS Risk for ineffective thermoregulation related to immature regulatory system changes in environment

Expected Outcome *Infant temperature remains at optimum level 36.5° C to 37.2° C.*

Nursing Interventions/*Rationales*

Keep infant adequately covered with clothing and blankets *to ensure sufficient warmth to maintain temperature.* (Do not overdress.)

Maintain room temperature between 24° to 25.6° C with 40% to 50% humidity *to optimize environment.*

Keep infant away from drafts, fans, air-conditioning vents; avoid environmental temperature extremes and rapid changes in temperature *to prevent temperature alteration.*

Use warm water for bathing in room with stable temperature, wrap in towel, and dry immediately after bath *to prevent chilling.*

NURSING DIAGNOSIS Risk for infection related to immature immunologic defenses/environmental exposure

Expected Outcome *No evidence of infection of eyes, respiratory system, genital area, umbilical cord.*

Nursing Interventions/*Rationales*

Have all care providers use good handwashing technique before and after handling the infant *to prevent spread of infection.*

Keep eyes and eyelashes clean and free of mucus; provide prescribed eye prophylaxis *to prevent infection.*

Keep genital area clean and dry using proper cleansing techniques *to prevent skin irritation, cross-contamination, and infection.*

Keep umbilical stump clean and dry and place diapers below the stump *to minimize chance of infection.*

If circumcised, keep site clean, glans dressed with sterile petrolatum, and diaper applied loosely *to prevent trauma and infection* and *to promote healing.*

Monitor eyes, respiratory system, skin, genitalia, umbilical cord, circumcision site for signs of infection; monitor vital signs; monitor ordered laboratory values *to detect infection early to promote rapid treatment and healing.*

Administer topical, oral, and parenteral antibiotics per physician order *to eradicate pathogens.*

Teach parents to avoid smoke-filled environments, people with respiratory infections, substances that can induce aspiration pneumonia such as baby powder *to protect infant from respiratory compromise.*

Teach parents to avoid prolonged public outings, touching and holding by large numbers of people, people with infectious diseases, and contaminated food sources *to reduce potential sources of infection.*

NURSING DIAGNOSIS Risk for trauma related to physical helplessness

Expected Outcome *Infant remains free of physical injury.*

Nursing Interventions/*Rationales*

Employ appropriate methods of handling, holding (i.e., protect head, avoid picking up by extremities), and transporting infant (i.e., use appropriate car seat with proper technique) *to prevent injury.*

Monitor environment *to prevent injury* (i.e., avoid use of pointed or sharp objects around infant, supervise infant and sibling/pet interactions, supervise infant on raised surfaces with no sides).

Modify environment *to prevent injury* (i.e., place potentially harmful objects out of reach; keep caretaker and infant fingernails trimmed, avoid jewelry that may scratch infant, check width of slats in infant crib, keep crib rails up when infant is in crib).

From Wong D & Perry S: *Maternal child nursing care,* St Louis, 1998, Mosby.

RESEARCH

Sudden Infant Death Syndrome and Infant Sleep Positions

Sudden infant death syndrome (SIDS) is the primary cause of infant death outside the neonatal period. The etiology of SIDS has been studied extensively but remains unclear. Recommendations for different sleeping positions have caused some confusion about the best positioning for infants. This study explored the evolution of the various recommendations regarding infant positioning. Lockridge examined the American Academy of Pediatrics (AAP) recommendations from 1992 international research that suggested an association between SIDS and prone sleeping patterns. Controversial guidelines on infant sleep position were issued that advocate supine or sidelying positions. In 1996 the initial guidelines were modified to recommend supine as the preferred sleep position during infancy. The AAP stressed that both sidelying and supine positions place the infant at less risk for SIDS than the prone position but that the supine position offered the lowest risk of SIDS for healthy newborns.

CLINICAL APPLICATION OF STUDY

Nurses providing parent education regarding the safest infant sleeping positions should be aware of the current AAP recommendations and provide parents with the most updated information.

Source: Lockridge T: Now I lay me down to sleep: SIDS and infant sleep positions, *Neonatal Netw* 16(6):25 1997.

KEY POINTS

- Assessment of the newborn requires data from the prenatal, intrapartal, and postpartal periods.
- The newborn assessment should proceed systematically so that each system is thoroughly evaluated.
- Many reflex behaviors are important for the newborn's survival.
- Individual personalities and behavioral characteristics of infants play a major role in their ultimate relationships with their parents.
- The development of parent-child love does not occur without feedback.
- State and other factors influence the newborn's behavior.
- Each newborn has a predisposed capacity to handle the multitude of stimuli in the external world.
- Providing a protective environment is a key responsibility of the nurse and includes such measures as careful identification

KEY POINTS—cont'd

procedures, restraining techniques, ways to prevent infection, and support of physiologic functions.
- Parent education is a major responsibility of the nurse and includes the involvement of parents in all phases of the nursing process.
- Circumcision is an elective surgical procedure.
- Whether or not this is the mother's or parents' first baby, parents appreciate being given anticipatory guidance in the care of their child.

CRITICAL THINKING EXERCISES

1 *Observe and record findings of normal newborns of at least two ethnic groups immediately after birth and in a follow-up period. Include both physiologic and behavioral data and compare findings. Explain the way this information can be used in planning care.*

2 *Prepare and conduct one 20-minute class in infant care for parents. Before the class, prepare a written teaching plan that includes an assessment of patients' learning needs; a teaching-learning diagnosis; a plan with prioritized patient-centered goals; content and teaching methods with rationale; and evaluative criteria. If possible, several students can present their teaching plans to the group for debate, critique, and suggestions for modification. After the class, critique the total experience. What insights have you achieved?*

3 *Discuss changes in attitude and expectations toward the newborn and the way these might affect treatment and care of the newborn. Discuss how this new information can be used to update grandparents (or older pregnant women).*

4 *Use the newborn's sensory abilities and social responses to design a nursery for the new baby (in the home). Incorporate these abilities into a list of suggestions for appropriate parent-infant interactions.*

References

American Academy of Pediatrics Provisional Committee for quality improvement and subcommittee on hyperbilirubinemia: Practice parameter: management of hyperbilirubinemia in the healthy term newborn, *Pediatrics* 94(4 Pt 1):558, 1994.

Ballard J et al.: New Ballard Score, expanded to include extremely premature infants, *J Pediatr* 119(3):417, 1991.

Ballard J, Novak D & Driver M: A simplified score for assessment of fetal maturation of newly born infants, *J Pediatr* 95(5):769, 1979.

Barnard K: *NCAST feeding manual* , Seattle, 1994, University of Washington.

Barr R: The normal crying curve: what do we really know? *Dev Med Child Neurol* 32(4):356, 1990.

Battaglia F & Lubchenco L: A practical classification of newborn infants by weight and gestational age, *J Pediatr* 71(2):159, 1967.

Bibb K et al.: Drug screening in mothers using meconium samples, paired urine samples and interviews, *J Perinatol* 15(3):199, 1995.

Brazelton T & Nugent K: *Neonatal behavioural assessment scale,* ed 3, London, 1996, MacKeith.

Campos R: Rocking and pacifiers: two comforting interventions for heelstick pain, *Res Nurs Health* 17(5):321, 1994.

Chitty L & Winter R: Perinatal mortality in different ethnic groups, *Arch Dis Child* 64(7):1036, 1989.

Dickason E, Silverman B & Kaplan J: *Maternal-infant nursing care,* ed 3, St Louis, 1998, Mosby.

Dixon S & Stein M: *Encounters with children: pediatric behavior and development,* ed 2, St Louis, 1992, Mosby.

Fanaroff A & Martin R: *Neonatal-perinatal medicine, diseases of the fetus and infant,* ed 6, St Louis, 1997, Mosby.

Field T et al.: Mothers' assessments of the behavior of their infants, *Infant Beh Dev* 1:156, 1978.

Freedman D: Ethnic differences in babies, *Hum Nature* Jan: 36, 1979.

Fuller J: Early patterns of maternal attachment, *Health Care Women Int* 11(4):433, 1990.

Garcia-Coll C: Developmental outcome of minority infants: a process-oriented look into our beginning, *Child Dev* 61(2):270, 1990.

Gunzenhauser N, editor: *Advances in touch; new implications in human development,* Skillman, NJ 1990, Johnson & Johnson Consumer Products.

Havens D & Zink R: The "back to sleep" campaign, *J Pediatr Health Care* 8(5):240, 1994.

Kenner C, Brueggemeyer A & Gunderson L: *Comprehensive neonatal nursing,* Philadelphia, 1993, WB Saunders.

Krebs T: Cord care: is it necessary? *Mother Baby J* 3(2):5, 1998.

Lander J et al.: Comparison of ring block, dorsal penile nerve block, and topical anesthesia for neonatal circumcision: a randomized controlled trial, *JAMA* 278(24):2157, 1997.

Lawrence R: *Breastfeeding: a guide for the medical profession,* ed 4, St Louis, 1994, Mosby.

Letko M: Detecting and preventing infant hearing loss, *Neonat Netw* 11(5):33, 1992.

Lubchenco L, Hansman C & Boyd E: Intrauterine growth in length and head circumference as estimated from live births at gestational ages from 26 to 42 weeks, *J Pediatr* 37(3):403, 1966.

March of Dimes: *Public health information sheet: newborn screening tests,* White Plains, NY, 1994, March of Dimes.

Marchette L et al.: Pain reduction interventions during neonatal circumcision, *Nurs Res* 40(4):241, 1991.

Mass G et al.: Routine examination in the neonatal period, *Br Med J* 302 (6781):878, 1991.

Porter R, Cernoch J & Perry S: The importance of odors in mother-infant interactions, *Matern Child Nurs J* 12(3):147, 1983.

Reiner C, Meltes S & Hayes J: Optimal sites and depths for skin puncture of infants and children as assessed from anatomical measurements, *Clin Chem* 36(3):547, 1990.

Rush J et al.: A randomized trial of a nursery ritual: wearing cover gowns to care for healthy newborns, *Birth* 17(1):25, 1990.

Stevens–Simon C et al.: Effects of race on validity of clinical estimates of gestational age, *J Pediatr* 115(6):1000, 1989.

Tappero E & Honeyfield M, editors: *Physical assessment of the newborn,* Petaluma, Calif, 1996, NICU.

Thomas A et al.: Individuality in responses of children to similar environmental situations, *Am J Psychiatr* 117:798, 1961.

Thomas A et al.: The origin of personality, *Sci Am* 223(2):102, 1970.

Treloar D: The effect of nonnutritive sucking on oxygenation in healthy, crying full-term infants, *Appl Nurs Res* 7(2):52, 1994.

Van Cleve I et al.: Pain responses of hospitalized neonates to venipuncture, *Neonat Netw* 14(6):31, 1995.

Wong D: *Whaley & Wong's nursing care of infants and children,* ed 5, St Louis, 1995, Mosby.

Wong D & Perry S: *Maternal child nursing care,* St Louis, 1998, Mosby.

Wright L, Brown A & Davidson-Mundt A: Newborn screening: the miracle and the challenge, *J Pediatr Nurs* 7(1):26, 1992.

Yetman R et al.: Comparison of temperature measurements by an aural infrared thermometer with measurements by traditional rectal and axillary techniques, *J Pediatr* 122(5):769, 1993.

CHAPTER

Newborn Nutrition and Feeding

KATHRYN RHODES ALDEN

In the minds of many, nutrition and nurturing are synonymous. One's effectiveness as a parent is often judged on the growth and development of the infant, which is largely dependent on proper nutrition. Infant feeding is more than the provision of nutrition; it represents opportunity for social, psychologic, and even educational interaction between parent and infant. Thus the selection of an infant feeding method is an emotion-laden decision for most prospective parents who are seeking optimal health and well-being for their offspring.

Through preconception and prenatal education and counseling, nurses play an instrumental role in assisting parents with the selection of an infant feeding method. They should be aware that this decision is influenced by a variety of physical, psychologic, social, cultural, and economic factors. In addition, nurses must be knowledgeable about the advantages and disadvantages of breastfeeding and formula feeding as they provide information to expectant parents. Whether the parents choose to breastfeed or formula feed, nurses provide support and ongoing education. Education of parents is necessarily based on current research findings and standards of practice.

Skillful health supervision of infants requires that the nurse be knowledgeable about nutritional needs and expectations for normal growth and development. This chapter focuses on infant nutrition during the first 6 months of life with emphasis on the neonatal period, when feeding practices and patterns are being established.

RECOMMENDED INFANT NUTRITION

The American Academy of Pediatrics (AAP) recommends breast milk as the optimum nutrition for infants and recommends that breastfeeding continue through the first year and beyond (AAP, 1997). While formula is considered a safe alternative for most infants, it is the responsibility of all health care providers, including nurses, to encourage parents to breastfeed their infants.

BREASTFEEDING RATES

Based on the recommendation by the AAP, it is surprising that just over half of the babies born in the United States are breastfed. We are currently experiencing a resurgence in breastfeeding initiation rates, as well as in continuance of breastfeeding through the first 6 months. This increase has been gradual, but certain. After a low of 26.5% in 1970, breastfeeding initiation rates climbed to 58% in 1985, only to gradually decline to 51.5% in 1990. Since that time, breastfeeding rates have steadily risen to 59.4% in 1995. Likewise, the number of infants still breastfeeding at 6 months has increased from 14.1% in 1970 to 20.8% in 1995 (Ryan, 1997).

Breastfeeding rates have increased across all demographic groups, although the most significant increases are seen among women who have historically been less likely to breastfeed. These individuals are typically young (less than 25 years old), lower-income, African-American primiparas with grade school education or less, employed full time outside the home, residing in the South Atlantic region of the United States, mothers of low-birth-weight infants, and enrolled in the Women, Infants, and Children (WIC) program (Ryan, 1997).

The characteristics of women most likely to breastfeed has remained consistent over the years. These women are multiparas, college educated, with higher incomes, not employed outside the home, residents of western states, not participating in the WIC program, and mothers of newborns with normal birth weights (Ryan, 1997).

BENEFITS OF BREASTFEEDING

Human milk is designed exclusively for human infants and is nutritionally superior to any alternative. Breast milk is considered a living tissue because it contains almost as many live cells as blood. It is bacteriologically safe and always fresh. The nutrients in breast milk are more easily absorbed than those in formula (Worthington-Roberts & Williams, 1993).

Numerous research studies have identified the beneficial effects of human milk for infants during the first year of life. Long-term epidemiologic studies have shown that these benefits do not cease when the infant is weaned, but instead extend into childhood and beyond. Breastfeeding has many advantages for mothers, for families, and for society in general. In discussing the benefits of breastfeeding with parents, it is critical that nurses and other health care providers have a thorough understanding of these benefits from both a physiologic and a psychosocial perspective.

Advantages for the infant include:

- Breast milk enhances maturation of the infant gastrointestinal (GI) tract and contains immune factors that contribute to a lower incidence of diarrheal illness, celiac disease, and Crohn's disease (Barnard, 1997; Dewey, Heinig & Nommsen-Rivers, 1995; Fuchs, Victoria & Martines, 1996; Howie et al., 1990; Lopez-Alarcon, Villalpando & Fajardo, 1997).
- Breastfed infants receive specific antibodies and cell-mediated immunologic factors that protect against otitis media and respiratory illnesses such as respiratory syncytial virus (RSV) and pneumonia (Dewey, Heinig & Nommsen-Rivers, 1995; Lopez-Alarcon, Villalpando & Fajardo, 1997; Sassen, Brand & Grote, 1994).
- Human milk provides protective effects against allergies in infants from families at high risk. Allergic manifestations occur at a greater rate and are more severe in formula-fed infants (Halken & Host, 1996; Saarinen & Kajosaari, 1995).
- There is a lower risk of sudden infant death syndrome (SIDS) among breastfed infants (Ford et al., 1993).
- Infants who are breastfed have a lower incidence of childhood cancers such as lymphoma and leukemia and type 1 diabetes (Lawrence, 1997; Shu et al., 1995).
- Antibody responses to parenteral and oral vaccines are greater in breastfed infants (Hahn-Zoric et al., 1990).
- Children who were breastfed as infants show improved performance on tests of development or cognition, have improved verbal ability, and show improved school performance (Florey, Leech & Blackhall, 1995; Lucas & Morley, 1991; Lucas et al., 1994).

Maternal benefits include:

- Women who breastfeed have a decreased risk of ovarian, uterine, and premenopausal breast cancer (Hirose et al., 1995; Rosenblatt et al., 1995).
- Breastfeeding promotes uterine involution and is associated with decreased incidence of postpartum hemorrhage (Lawrence, 1994).
- Breastfeeding women tend to return to prepregnancy weight more quickly and have a lower incidence of obesity later in life (Lawrence, 1997).
- Women who breastfeed are less likely to develop osteoporosis in later life (Melton et al., 1993).
- Breastfeeding provides a unique bonding experience and increases maternal role attainment (Lawrence, 1997).

Benefits to families and society include:
- Breastfeeding represents lower cost to families. The cost of formula is twice that of extra food for the lactating mother. Breastfeeding is convenient; there are no bottles to purchase or clean. Less time is lost from work because of the need to stay home with a sick infant (Riordan, 1997).
- Lower health care costs for families and society directly related to breastfeeding could save federal, state, and local governments billions of dollars each year. The amount of money spent on WIC programs could be significantly reduced if more women chose to breastfeed (Riordan, 1997; Tuttle & Dewey, 1996).
- Intangible benefits for families and society include increased quality of life through psychologic benefits for mothers and infants, increased mothering behaviors, and more free time for interaction with family and friends, along with less worry associated with ill infants (Montgomery & Splett, 1997).

CHOOSING AN INFANT FEEDING METHOD

Women who elect to breastfeed their infants most often do so because they are aware of the benefits to the infant. Many are seeking the unique bonding experience between mother and infant that is characteristic of breastfeeding. The support of the partner and family is a major factor in the mother's decision to breastfeed and in her ability to do so successfully. Prenatal preparation ideally includes the father of the baby, with information about benefits of breastfeeding and how he can participate in infant care and nurturing (Bar-Yam & Darby, 1997).

Parents who elect to formula feed often make this decision without complete information and understanding of the benefits of breastfeeding and the potential hazards of formula feeding (Walker, 1993). Numerous myths and misconceptions about breastfeeding influence women's decision making. Many women see bottle feeding as more convenient or less embarrassing than breastfeeding. Some lack confidence in their ability to produce an adequate quantity or quality of breast milk. Breastfeeding is seen by some women as incompatible with an active social life, or they think that it will prevent them from going back to work. There are significant societal barriers against breastfeeding in public. A major barrier for many women is the influence of family and friends; this is especially true for lower-income mothers, where bottle feeding is the norm.

To make an informed decision about an infant feeding method, parents must be presented with factual information about the nutritional and immunologic needs of the infant that *are* met by human milk, the potential benefits to the infant and the mother, and the inherent risks associated with infant formulas. The nurse must provide this information to parents in a nonjudgmental manner and respect their decision. Some health care professionals may attempt to avoid this responsibility with the rationalization that they do not want parents to feel guilty if they choose not to breastfeed. However, the nurse is required to give complete information about infant feeding to parents and to document having done so.

The key to encouraging mothers to breastfeed is education, beginning as early as possible during pregnancy and even before pregnancy. Prenatal breastfeeding classes are an excellent vehicle to relay important information to expectant parents. Each encounter with an expectant mother is an opportunity to dispel myths, clarify misinformation, and address personal concerns. Connecting expectant mothers with women who are breastfeeding or have successfully breastfed and are from similar backgrounds may be helpful. Peer counseling programs, such as those instituted by WIC programs, are beneficial, particularly in lower socioeconomic groups, where bottle feeding is common.

The postnatal period is not too late to educate parents about the benefits of breastfeeding. For those women with limited access to health care, the postpartum period may provide the first opportunity for education about breastfeeding. Even women who have indicated the desire to bottle feed may benefit from information about the differences in formula and breast milk for their infants. Offering these women the chance to try breastfeeding with the assistance of a nurse may influence a change in infant feeding practices.

It is the responsibility of the nurse and other health care professionals to promote feelings of competence and confidence in the breastfeeding mother and to reinforce the unequaled contribution she is making toward the health and well-being of her infant. To provide effective support for the mother, health care professionals must necessarily be knowledgeable about benefits of breastfeeding, the basic process of breastfeeding, breastfeeding management, and interventions for common problems (Box 21-1).

CULTURAL INFLUENCES ON INFANT FEEDING

Cultural beliefs and practices are significant influences on infant feeding methods. While there are recognized cultural norms, one cannot assume that generalized observations about any cultural group hold true for all members of that group. Within the United States there are many regional and ethnic cultures. Dealing effectively with these groups requires that the nurse be knowledgeable about and sensitive to the cultural factors influencing infant feeding practices.

Persons who have immigrated to the United States from poorer countries often choose to formula feed their infants because they believe it is a better, more "modern" method.

BOX 21-1 **AWHONN's Guidelines for Breastfeeding Support**

- During pregnancy a breast assessment is performed that includes a breastfeeding history, a breast examination, and a medication use history.
- A prenatal plan of care is developed to prepare the woman for lactation.
- Immediately after birth, the newborn is kept with the mother when possible so that breastfeeding can be initiated when the newborn is most receptive.
- After birth:
  —Assistance with latch-on and positioning are given as needed.
  —Encouragement of frequent feedings is reinforced.
  —Discharge instructions for knowing criteria for successful breastfeeding are given.
  —Information about community resources for breastfeeding are given.
- Especially for premature and low-birth-weight infants, encouragement is given to breastfeed.

Source: AWHONN: *Standards and guidelines for professional nursing practice in the care of women and newborns,* ed 5, Washington, DC, 1998, The Association.

Others adopt formula feeding because they want to adapt to American culture and perceive that it is the custom to bottle feed (Rassin et al., 1994).

As many as 50 of 120 cultures studied by Morse, Jehle, and Gamble (1990) typically do not give colostrum to newborns and begin breastfeeding after the milk has "come in." This is true for some Filipinas, Mexican-Americans, Vietnamese, Hmong, Koreans, and Nigerians. When breastfeeding is delayed until the milk is in, babies are given prelacteal food. In India, infants may be fed such liquids as honey, tea, water, or sugar water before the initiation of breastfeeding (Choudhry, 1997). Other cultures begin breastfeeding immediately and offer the breast each time the infant cries. Cultural attitudes regarding modesty and breastfeeding are important considerations.

Some cultures have specific beliefs and practices related to the mother's intake of foods that foster milk production. Korean mothers often eat seaweed soup and rice to enhance milk production. Hmong women believe that boiled chicken, rice, and hot water is the only appropriate nourishment during the first postpartum month. The balance between energy forces, hot and cold, or yin and yang is integral to the diet of the lactating mother. Hispanics, Vietnamese, Chinese, East Indians, and Arabs often use this belief in choosing foods. "Hot" foods are considered best for new mothers; this does not necessarily relate to the temperature or spiciness of foods. For example, chicken and broccoli are considered "hot," whereas many fresh fruits and vegetables are considered "cold." Families often bring desired foods into the health care setting.

In Kenya, mothers feed preterm infants only by breast and often begin feeding earlier than the practice in other countries. Kenyans never use gavage tubes. Preterm babies are cup fed until they are able to suck.

FEEDING READINESS

Term neonates are born with reflexes that facilitate feeding: rooting, sucking, and swallowing. Healthy newborns have experience with sucking on fingers and swallowing amniotic fluid for several weeks in utero but have made no connection between sucking and satiation. Neither have they needed to suck, swallow, and breathe before they emerged from the uterus. While the majority of newborns do not experience hunger or thirst in the first hours after birth, they will suckle when given the opportunity. Newborns of mothers who experienced an unmedicated labor have been noted to crawl to the breast when laid on the mother's abdomen, seek out the nipple, and begin to suckle (Widstrom, Ransjo-Arvidsson & Christensson, 1993).

Physical assessment of the newborn reveals signs that the baby is physiologically ready to begin feeding:
- Vital signs (temperature, respirations, heart rate) within normal limits
- Unlabored respirations; nares patent
- Active bowel sounds
- No abdominal distention

When newborns experience hunger, they usually cry vigorously until their needs are met. Some infants, however, will withdraw into sleep because of discomfort associated with hunger. Babies exhibit **feeding-readiness cues** that can be recognized by a knowledgeable caregiver. Instead of waiting to feed until the infant is crying distraughtly or withdraws into sleep, it is better to begin a feeding when the baby exhibits some of these cues (even during light sleep):
- Hand-to-mouth or hand-to-hand movements
- Sucking motions
- Rooting
- Mouthing

Babies normally consume small amounts of milk during the first 3 days of life. The breastfed infant receives colostrum, which is very concentrated and high in protein. Similarly, bottle-fed infants initially require small feedings. However, as the baby adjusts to extrauterine life and the digestive tract is cleared of meconium, milk intake increases from 15 to 30 ml per feeding in the first 24 hours to 60 to 90 ml or more per feeding thereafter.

At birth and for several months thereafter, all of the secretions of the infant's digestive tract contain enzymes especially suited to the digestion of human milk. The ability to digest foods other than milk depends on the physiologic development of the infant. The capacities for salivary, gastric, pancreatic, and intestinal digestion increase with age, indicating that the natural time for introduction of solid foods may be around 6 months of age.

Babies are born with a tongue extrusion reflex that causes them to push out of the mouth anything placed on the tongue. This reflex disappears by 6 months—another indication of physiologic readiness for solids.

Early introduction of solids may make the infant more prone to food allergies. Regular feeding of solids can lead to decreased intake of breast milk or formula and has been associated with early cessation of breastfeeding (Grossman et al., 1990).

NUTRIENT NEEDS

Fluids

The fluid requirement for normal infants is about 150 ml/kg/24 hr. This amount of fluid will produce about 100 ml of urine per 24 hours. This need is easily met in the infant who is breastfeeding or consuming properly prepared formula.

Neither breastfed nor formula-fed infants need to be fed water, not even those living in very hot climates (Lawrence, 1994). Indeed, feeding infants water may only decrease the caloric consumption at a time when infants need to be growing rapidly. Water intoxication can result from feeding infants excessive amounts of water (Naylor et al., 1992; Newman, 1992). Symptoms of water intoxication include hyponatremia, weakness, restlessness, nausea, vomiting, diarrhea, polyuria or oliguria, and convulsions.

Energy

Infants require adequate caloric intake to provide energy for growth, digestion, physical activity, and maintenance of organ metabolic function. For the first 6 months of life, the recommended daily dietary allowance (RDA) for energy is approximately 108 kcal/kg of body weight. This decreases to 98 kcal/kg for the second 6 months (Food & Nutrition Board, 1989). Human milk and infant formula provide approximately 67 kcal/dl.

Carbohydrate

Because newborns have only small hepatic glycogen stores, carbohydrates should provide at least 40% to 45% of the total calories in the diet. Moreover, newborns may have a limited ability to carry out gluconeogenesis (the formation of glucose from amino acids and other substrates) and ketogenesis (the formation of ketone bodies from fat), which are mechanisms that provide alternative sources of energy.

As the primary carbohydrate in human milk, lactose is the most abundant carbohydrate in the diet of infants up to 6 months of age. It provides calories in an easily available form. Its slow breakdown and absorption probably also increase calcium absorption. Corn syrup solids or glucose polymers have been added to infant formulas to supplement the lactose in the cow's milk and thereby provide sufficient carbohydrates.

Fat

For infants to acquire adequate calories from the limited amount of human milk or formula they are able to consume, at least 15% of the calories provided must come from fat (triglycerides). This fat must therefore be easily digestible. The fat in human milk is easier to digest and absorb than that in cow's milk because of the arrangement of the fatty acids on the glycerol molecule. Fat absorption is also related to the natural lipase activity present in human milk.

Cow's milk is used in most infant formulas, but the milk fat is removed, and another fat source such as corn oil, which can be digested and absorbed by the infant, is added in its place. If whole milk or evaporated milk without added carbohydrate is fed to infants, the resulting fecal loss of fat and therefore loss of energy may be excessive because the milk moves through the infant's intestines too quickly for adequate absorption to take place. This can lead to poor weight gain.

In addition to its energy contributions, fat also furnishes essential fatty acids (EFAs), which are required for growth and tissue maintenance. EFAs are components of cell membranes and precursors of some hormones. An inadequate intake of EFAs results in eczema and growth failure. The lack of EFAs in skim and low-fat milk is another reason for not feeding these products to infants.

Protein

The protein requirement per unit of body weight is greater in the newborn than at any other time of life. The RDA for protein during the first 6 months is 2.2 gm/kg.

The protein content of human milk, which is lower than that of unmodified cow's milk, is ideal for the newborn. Human milk contains far more lactalbumin in relation to casein, and lactalbumin is more easily digested than casein. In addition, the amino acid composition of human milk is suited to the newborn's metabolic capabilities. For example, the phenylalanine and methionine levels are low, and cystine and taurine levels are high. The protein in some commercial formulas is modified so that the amount of lactalbumin, or whey, protein is increased and the relative proportion of casein is decreased to more closely approximate the protein composition of human milk.

Vitamins

Human milk contains all of the vitamins required for infant nutrition, with individual variations based on maternal diet and genetic differences. Vitamins are added to cow's milk formulas to resemble levels found in breast milk. While cow's milk contains adequate amounts of vitamin A and vitamin B complex, vitamin C (ascorbic acid) and vitamin E must be added.

Vitamin D is also added to commercial infant formulas. While human milk may be somewhat deficient in vitamin D, supplementation may not be necessary provided that the infant is exposed to sunlight for 30 minutes per week wearing only a diaper, or for 2 hours per week fully clothed but without a hat. To prevent rickets, supplementation may be recommended for preterm or dark-skinned infants with limited exposure to the sun, as well as infants whose mothers eat vegetarian diets that exclude meat, fish, and dairy products.

Vitamin K, required for blood coagulation, is produced by intestinal bacteria. However, the gut is sterile at birth, and a few days are needed for intestinal flora to become established and produce vitamin K. To prevent hemorrhagic problems in the newborn, an injection of vitamin K is given at birth.

Minerals

The mineral content of commercial infant formula is designed to reflect that of breast milk. Unmodified cow's milk is much higher in mineral content than human milk, providing evidence of its unsuitability for infants during the first year of life. Minerals are typically highest in human milk during the first few days after birth and decrease slightly throughout lactation.

The ratio of calcium to phosphorus in human milk is 2:1, a proportion optimal for bone mineralization. While cow's milk is high in calcium, the calcium-to-phosphorus ratio is low, resulting in decreased calcium absorption. Consequently, young infants fed unmodified cow's milk are at risk for hypocalcemia, seizures, and tetany. The calcium-to-phosphorus ratio in commercial infant formula is between that of human milk and cow's milk.

Iron levels are low in all types of milk; however, iron from human milk is better absorbed (50%) than from cow's milk, iron-fortified formula, or infant cereals. Breast-fed infants draw on iron reserves deposited in utero and benefit from the high lactose and vitamin C levels in human milk that facilitate iron absorption. The infant who is entirely breastfed normally maintains adequate hemoglobin levels for the first 6 months. After that time, iron-fortified cereals and other iron-rich foods are added to the diet. Infants who are weaned from the breast before 6 months of age and all formula-fed infants should receive an iron-fortified commercial infant formula until 12 months of age.

Fluoride levels in human milk and commercial formulas are low. This mineral, which is important in the prevention of dental caries, may cause spotting of the permanent teeth (fluorosis) in excess amounts. It is recommended that a fluoride supplement be given only to those infants not receiving fluoridated water after the age of 6 months (AAP, 1997).

I OVERVIEW OF LACTATION

Milk Production

Each female breast is composed of approximately 15 to 20 segments (lobes) embedded in fat and connective tissues and lavishly supplied with blood vessels, lymphatic vessels,

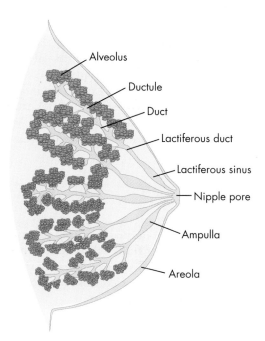

Fig. **21-1** Detailed structural features of human mammary gland.

and nerves (Fig. 21-1). Within each lobe are alveoli, the milk-producing cells, surrounded by myoepithelial cells, which contract to send the milk forward into the ductules. Each ductule enlarges into **lactiferous ducts** and **sinuses** where milk collects just behind the nipple. Each nipple has 15 to 20 pores through which milk is transferred to the suckling infant. The size of the breast is not an accurate indicator of its ability to produce milk. Because of the effects of estrogen and progesterone during pregnancy, the lobular components of the breast enlarge while the ductal system proliferates and differentiates. The nipples become more erect, and pigmentation of the areola increases. The breasts increase in size and sensitivity and exhibit more prominent veins. Around the sixteenth week of gestation the alveoli begin producing **colostrum** (early milk) in response to human placental lactogen.

After birth of the neonate, there is a precipitous drop in the mother's estrogen and progesterone levels, which triggers the release of **prolactin** from the anterior pituitary. During pregnancy, prolactin prepares the breasts to secrete milk and, during lactation, to synthesize and secrete milk (Lawrence, 1994). Prolactin, one of the two hormones necessary for milk production, is subsequently produced in response to infant suckling and emptying of the breasts (note that lactating breasts are never completely empty; milk is constantly being produced by the alveoli as the infant feeds) (Fig. 21-2, *A*). Milk production is a **supply-meets-demand system;** that is, as milk is removed from the breast, more is produced. Incomplete emptying of the breasts with feedings can lead to a decreased milk supply.

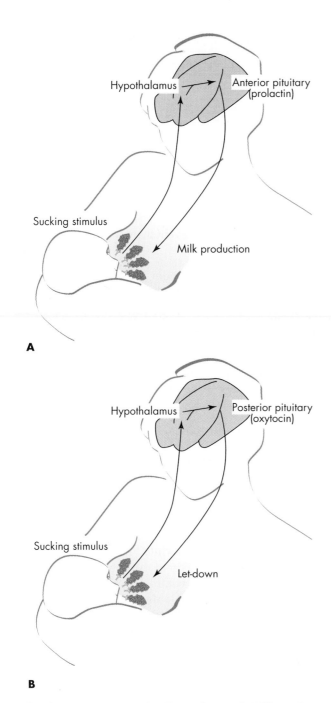

Fig. **21-2** Maternal breastfeeding reflexes. **A,** Milk production. **B,** Let-down.

Prolactin levels are highest during the first 10 days after birth, gradually declining over time, but remaining above baseline levels for the duration of lactation.

Oxytocin is the other hormone essential to lactation. As the nipple is stimulated by the suckling infant, the posterior pituitary is prompted by the hypothalamus to produce oxytocin. This hormone is responsible for the **milk ejection reflex (MER),** or **let-down reflex** (Fig. 21-2, *B*). The myoepithelial cells surrounding the alveoli respond to

oxytocin by contracting and sending the milk forward through the ducts to the nipple. Many "let-downs" can occur with each feeding session. The milk ejection reflex can be triggered by thoughts, sights, sounds, or odors that the mother associates with her baby (or other babies), such as hearing the baby cry. Many women report a tingling "pins and needles" sensation in the breasts as let-down occurs, although some mothers can detect milk ejection only by observing the sucking and swallowing of the infant. Let-down may also occur during sexual activity, since oxytocin is released during orgasm.

Oxytocin is the same hormone that stimulates uterine contractions during labor. Consequently, the laboring woman can experience let-downs that may be evidenced by leakage of colostrum. This readies the breast for immediate feeding by the infant after birth. Oxytocin has the important function of contracting the mother's uterus after birth to control postpartum bleeding and promote uterine involution. Thus mothers who breastfeed are at decreased risk for postpartum hemorrhage. These uterine contractions that occur with breastfeeding can be painful during and after the feeding, particularly in multiparas. The "afterpains" usually subside within 3 to 5 days after giving birth.

Prolactin and oxytocin have been referred to as the "mothering hormones," since they are known to affect the postpartum woman's physical state, as well as her emotions. Many women report feeling thirsty or very relaxed during breastfeeding, probably as a result of these hormones.

The **nipple erection reflex** is an integral part of lactation. When the infant cries, suckles, or rubs against the breast, the nipple becomes erect. This assists in the propulsion of milk through the lactiferous sinuses to the nipple pores. Nipple sizes, shapes, and ability to become erect vary with individuals. Some women have flat or **inverted nipples** that do not become erect with stimulation. Babies are usually able to learn to successfully breastfeed with any nipple. It is important that these infants are not offered bottles or pacifiers until breastfeeding is well established.

Uniqueness of Human Milk

Human milk is a highly complex species-specific fluid uniquely designed to meet the needs of the human infant. It is a dynamic substance whose composition changes to meet the changing nutritional and immunologic needs of the infant. It is specific to the needs of each newborn; for example, the milk of preterm mothers differs in composition from that of mothers who give birth at term.

The components of human milk are continually being investigated. Human milk contains antimicrobial factors (antibodies) that provide protection against a broad spectrum of bacterial, viral, and protozoan infections. Secretory IgA is the major antibody in human milk. Other factors in human milk that protect against infection include lactoferrin, the bifidus factor, oligosaccharides, milk lipids,

TABLE 21-1   *Summary of Immune Properties of Breast Milk*

COMPONENT	ACTION
WHITE BLOOD CELLS	
B lymphocytes	Give rise to antibodies targeted against specific microbes.
Macrophages	Kill microbes outright in baby's gut, produce lysozyme, and activate other components of the immune system.
Neutrophils	May act as phagocytes, ingesting bacteria in baby's digestive system.
T lymphocytes	Kill infected cells directly or send out chemical messages to mobilize other defenses. They proliferate in the presence of organisms that cause serious illness in infants. They also manufacture compounds that can strengthen an infant's own immune response.
MOLECULES	
Antibodies of secretory IgA class	Bind to microbes in infant's digestive tract and thereby prevent them from passing through walls of the gut into body's tissues.
B_{12}-binding protein	Reduces amount of vitamin B_{12}, which bacteria need in order to grow.
Bifidus factor	Promotes growth of *Lactobacillus bifidus,* a harmless bacterium, in infant's gut. Growth of such nonpathogenic bacteria helps to crowd out dangerous varieties.
Fatty acids	Disrupt membranes surrounding certain viruses and destroy them.
Fibronectin	Increases antimicrobial activity of macrophages; helps to repair tissues that have been damaged by immune reactions in infant's gut.
Gamma-interferon	Enhances antimicrobial activity of immune cells.
Hormones and growth factors	Stimulate infant's digestive tract to mature more quickly. Once the initially "leaky" membranes lining the gut mature, infants become less vulnerable to microorganisms.
Lactoferrin	Binds to iron, a mineral many bacteria need to survive. By reducing the available amount of iron, lactoferrin thwarts growth of pathogenic bacteria.
Lysozyme	Kills bacteria by disrupting their cell walls.
Mucins	Adhere to bacteria and viruses, thus keeping such microorganisms from attaching to mucosal surfaces.
Oligosaccharides	Bind to microorganisms and bar them from attaching to mucosal surfaces.

From Newman J: How breast milk protects newborns, *Sci Am* 273(6):76, 1995.

and milk leukocytes. There are antiinflammatory agents, growth factors, hormones, and enzymes in human milk, many of which contribute to the maturation of the infant's intestine. Immunomodulating agents found in human milk are instrumental in preventing disease after infancy (Goldman, 1993; Newman, 1992) (Table 21-1).

Human milk composition and volumes vary according to the stage of lactation. In **lactogenesis** stage I, beginning in pregnancy, the breasts are preparing for milk production. Colostrum is present in the breasts at this time. Colostrum, a clear yellowish fluid, is more concentrated than mature milk and is extremely rich in immunoglobulins. It has higher concentrations of protein and minerals, but less fat than mature milk. The high protein level of colostrum facilitates binding of bilirubin, and the laxative action of colostrum promotes early passage of meconium. Colostrum gradually changes to mature milk; this is referred to as "the milk coming in" or as lactogenesis stage II. By the third to fifth day after birth, most women have experienced this onset of copious milk secretion. Breast milk continues to change in composition for approximately 10 days, when the mature milk is established. This is considered stage III of lactogenesis (Lawrence, 1994; Riordan & Auerbach, 1993).

The composition of mature milk changes during each feeding. Initially, a bluish-white foremilk is released that is part skim milk (about 60% of the volume) and part whole milk (about 35% of the volume). It provides primarily lactose, protein, and water-soluble vitamins. The hindmilk, or cream (about 5%), is usually let down 10 to 20 minutes into the feeding, although it may occur sooner. It contains the denser calories from fat necessary for ensuring optimal growth and contentment between feedings. Because of this changing composition of human milk during each feeding, it is important to breastfeed the infant long enough to supply a balanced feeding.

Milk production gradually increases, so that by the time her infant is 2 weeks old, the mother produces 720 to 900 ml of milk every 24 hours. Babies experience fairly predictable **growth spurts** (at about 10 days, 6 weeks, 3 months, and 4 to 6 months), when more frequent feedings stimulate increased milk production. These growth spurts usually last 24 to 48 hours, and then the infants resume their usual feeding pattern.

Although nearly every woman can lactate, there are some mothers who have insufficient glandular development to exclusively breastfeed their infants. These women often have immature-appearing breasts and experienced little or no

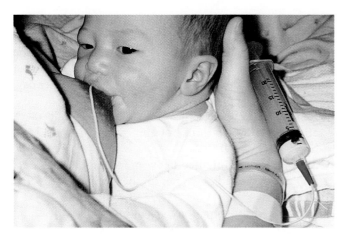

Fig. 21-3 Mother using supplementer made from a large syringe with a shortened 5-French gavage feeding tube attached. (From Lowdermilk D, Perry S & Bobak I: *Maternity and women's health care*, ed 6, St Louis, 1997, Mosby.)

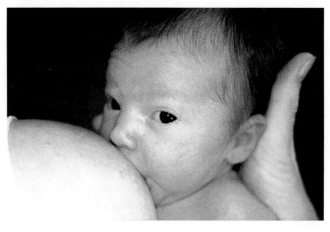

Fig. 21-4 Alert 1-week-old infant at breast. Note supporting head to maintain correct latch-on. (Courtesy Kim Molloy, San Jose, Calif.)

breast growth during pregnancy. In such cases, women may still be able to breastfeed and offer supplemental nutrition to support optimal infant growth. There are devices available to allow mothers to offer supplements while the baby is at the breast (Fig. 21-3).

I CARE MANAGEMENT: THE BREASTFEEDING MOTHER AND INFANT

Effective management of the breastfeeding mother and infant requires that the caregivers be knowledgeable about the benefits of breastfeeding, as well as about basic anatomy and the physiology of breastfeeding, how to assist the mother with feeding, and interventions for common problems. Ongoing support of the mother enhances her self-confidence and promotes a satisfying and successful breastfeeding experience. Planning care for the breastfeeding couple is based on thorough assessment of both the mother and infant.

Assessment and Nursing Diagnoses
Infant

Before the initiation of breastfeeding, the nurse needs to consider the following in preparing to effectively assist the breastfeeding infant:
- Maturity level: gestational age, term or preterm, birth weight (small for gestational age [SGA], large for gestational age [LGA])
- Labor and birth: length of labor, maternal medications (narcotics, magnesium sulfate [$MgSO_4$]); type of birth: vaginal with or without use of vacuum extraction or forceps; cesarean; type of anesthesia
- Birth trauma: fractured clavicle, bruising of face or head

- Maternal risk factors: diabetes, preeclampsia, infection, human immunodeficiency virus (HIV), herpes
- Congenital defects: cleft lip or palate, cardiac anomalies, Down syndrome
- Physical stability: vital signs within normal limits, unlabored respirations, bowel sounds present
- State of alertness: awake, sleepy, crying

Assessment during feeding: the infant is assessed for the following by direct observation while breastfeeding:
- Latch-on (Fig. 21-4)
- Position, alignment
- Sucking/swallowing

Ongoing assessment of the infant:
- Behavior after/between feedings: contented, sleepy
- Elimination patterns: six to eight wet diapers and two stools per day by day 4
- General assessment: presence of jaundice; weight loss <10%; regain birth weight by 10 to 14 days of age
- Normal versus pathologic jaundice

Mother

Before breastfeeding is begun, it is important that the nurse carefully assess the mother's knowledge of breastfeeding, as well as her physical and psychologic readiness to breastfeed. This assessment can be accomplished through interviews, discussion, and direct observation. Factors to consider include:
- Previous experience with breastfeeding: first baby; unsuccessful breastfeeding with previous infants
- Knowledge about breastfeeding: prenatal classes, support groups, books/pamphlets, videos, friends/relatives who breastfed; knowledge about positioning, latch-on, frequency/duration of feedings, etc.
- Cultural factors: belief that colostrum is bad, modesty issues, language barrier

- Feelings about breastfeeding: anxious, fear of failure; confident–expects to succeed
- Physical features: development of breast tissue, protractility of nipples (flat or inverted), previous breast surgery, chronic illness, carpal tunnel syndrome, visual or hearing impairment, physical limitations
- Physical/psychologic readiness: risk factors, time since giving birth, type of birth, complications, perineal discomfort, level of pain, medications, mood (eager, cheerful), energy level (tired, exhausted)
- Support: father of baby or family members/friends present and their level of knowledge about breastfeeding

As breastfeeding is becoming established, the nurse performs ongoing assessment of the mother and infant to determine appropriate interventions. During the time in the hospital, the nurse can help the mother to view each breastfeeding session as a "feeding lesson" or "practice session" that will foster maternal confidence and a satisfying breastfeeding experience for mother and baby. Items that need to be assessed are:

- Condition of nipples: during feeding, mother feels a "tugging" sensation, but no pain after the initial latch-on; presence of soreness, redness, cracking, bleeding
- Transition to mature milk: milk is "in" by day 4 or 5
- Breasts feel softer or lighter after feedings
- Mother states she feels relaxed or sleepy during feedings
- Mother reports uterine cramping and/or increased lochia flow during/after feeding
- Mother's comfort level with breastfeeding techniques including positioning and latch-on

Nursing diagnoses for the breastfeeding woman are listed in the nursing diagnoses box.

▌Nursing Diagnoses_____

The Breastfeeding Woman

Effective breastfeeding related to:
- Mother's knowledge of breastfeeding techniques
- Mother's appropriate response to infant's feeding-readiness cues
- Mother's ability to facilitate efficient breastfeeding

Risk for ineffective breastfeeding related to:
- Insufficient knowledge regarding newborn's reflexes and breastfeeding techniques
- Lack of support by father of baby
- Lack of maternal self-confidence; anxiety, fear of failure
- Poor infant sucking reflex
- Difficulty waking sleepy baby

Risk for altered nutrition: less than body requirements related to:
- Increased caloric and nutrient needs for breastfeeding (mother)
- Incorrect latch-on and inability to transfer milk (infant)

Expected Outcomes of Care

In planning care, the nurse discusses the desired outcomes with the parents. The expected outcomes include that the infant will:
- Latch on and feed effectively at least eight times per day
- Gain weight appropriately
- Remain well hydrated (have six to eight wet diapers and at least two to three bowel movements every 24 hours after day 4)
- Sleep or seem contented between feedings

Examples of expected outcomes for the mother include that she will:
- Verbalize/demonstrate understanding of breastfeeding techniques, including positioning and latch-on, signs of adequate feeding, self-care
- Report no nipple discomfort with breastfeeding
- Express satisfaction with the breastfeeding experience
- Consume a nutritionally balanced diet with appropriate caloric and fluid intake to support breastfeeding

Plan of Care and Interventions

Interventions are based on the expected outcomes and are influenced by the resources and time available to achieve the desired goals. In the early days after birth, interventions focus on helping the mother and the newborn to initiate breastfeeding and to achieve some degree of success/satisfaction before discharge from the hospital. Interventions to promote breastfeeding progress from basics such as latch-on and positioning to signs of adequate feeding and self-care measures such as prevention of engorgement. An important intervention is to provide the parents with a list of resources that they may contact after discharge from the hospital.

The ideal time to begin breastfeeding is within 1 hour after birth (AAP, 1997) when the infant is in the quiet, alert state. If this is not possible because of the effects of labor medications or anesthesia, it is advantageous to place the infant in skin-to-skin contact on the mother's chest for the first hour after birth. Each mother should receive instruction, assistance, and support in positioning and latching on until she is able to do so independently.

Positioning

There are four basic positions for breastfeeding: football hold, cradle, modified cradle or across-the-lap, and side-lying position (see Home Care box). Initially, it is advantageous to use the position that most easily facilitates latch-on while allowing maximum comfort for the mother. The football hold is often recommended for early feedings because the mother can easily visualize the baby's mouth as she guides the infant on to the nipple. The football hold is usually preferred by mothers who gave birth by cesarean. The modified cradle or across-the-lap hold also works well for early feedings. The side-lying position allows the mother to rest while breastfeeding and is often preferred by women experiencing perineal pain and swelling. Cradling is the most common

HOME CARE *Patient Instructions for Self-Care*
Breastfeeding
How to hold your baby for feeding.

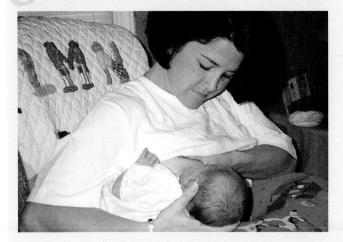

A, Football hold.

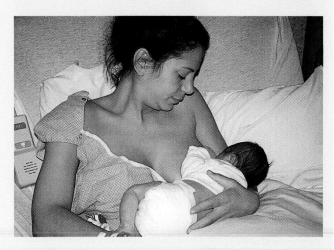

B, Cradling.

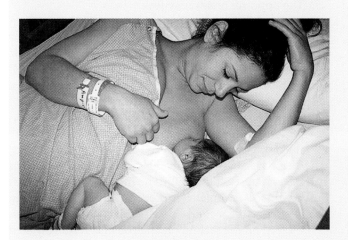

C, Lying down.

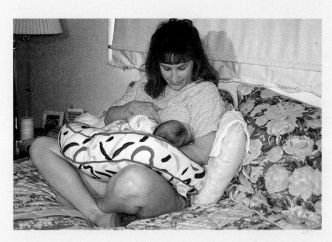

D, Across the lap. (*B, C, D,* Courtesy Marjorie Pyle, RNC, Lifecircle, Costa Mesa, Calif.)

breastfeeding position for infants who have learned to latch on easily and feed effectively. Before discharge from the hospital, the mother should be assisted in trying all of the positions so that she will feel confident in her ability to vary positions at home.

Whatever position is used, the mother should be comfortable, with pillows used as needed to provide support for her back and arms. The infant is placed at the level of the breast, supported by pillows or folded blankets, turned completely on his or her side, and facing the mother so that the infant is "belly to belly," with the arms "hugging" the breast. The baby's mouth is directly in front of the nipple (see Fig. 21-4). It is important that the mother support the baby's neck and shoulders with her hand and not push on the occiput. Pushing on the back of the head may result in bit-

ing, extension of the neck, or an aversion to being brought near the breast. The baby's body is held in correct alignment (ears, shoulders, and hips are in a straight line) during feeding.

Latching on
The mother supports the breast with a "**C-hold**": the four fingers are underneath the breast and the thumb is on top, all placed at the back edge of the areola. With the baby held close to the breast, the mother moves her breast slightly so that the tip of the nipple "tickles" the baby's lower lip, stimulating the mouth to open (**rooting reflex**). The tongue reflexively extrudes to pull the breast into the mouth. When the mouth is open wide and the tongue is down, the mother quickly pulls the baby onto the nipple. (She brings the baby

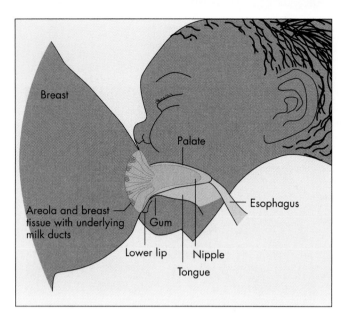

Fig. **21-5** Correct attachment (latch-on) of infant at breast.

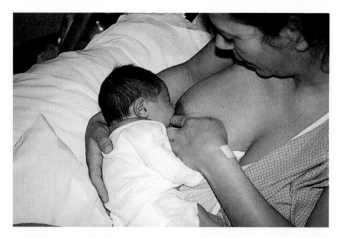

Fig. **21-6** Removing infant from the breast. (Courtesy Marjorie Pyle, RNC, Lifecircle, Costa Mesa, Calif.)

to the breast, not the breast to the baby.) The amount of areola in the baby's mouth depends on the size of the baby's mouth, the areola, and the nipple. During the early days it is helpful for the mother to continue to support the breast during feedings. This often helps prevent sore nipples.

With correct **latch-on** (1) the mother reports a firm, tugging sensation on her nipple but no pinching or pain; (2) as the baby sucks, the cheeks are rounded and not sucked in or dimpled; and (3) the infant's jaw glides smoothly with sucking (Fig. 21-5).

When the signs of adequate latch-on are not present, the infant is removed from the breast and latch-on is attempted again. To prevent nipple trauma as the baby is taken off the breast, the mother is instructed to break the suction by pushing a finger in between the baby's gums and leaving the finger there until the nipple is completely out of the infant's mouth (Fig. 21-6).

Milk ejection or let-down

As the baby begins sucking on the nipple, the let-down, or milk ejection, reflex is stimulated. The hormone oxytocin causes milk to be sent forward from the milk ducts to the nipple. Signs that let-down has occurred include:

1. The mother may feel a tingling sensation in the nipples, although many women never feel their milk let down.
2. The baby's suck changes from quick, shallow sucks to a slower, more drawing, sucking pattern.
3. Swallowing is heard as the baby sucks.
4. The mother experiences uterine cramping and may have increased lochia during and after feedings.
5. The mother feels relaxed, even sleepy, during feedings.

6. The breasts soften during feedings.
7. The opposite breast may leak.

Typical feedings

During a typical feeding, the baby begins with quick, shallow sucks that are followed by several bursts of 10 or more long, drawing sucks and swallows as let-down occurs. As the breast softens and the flow of milk slows, the baby has shorter bursts of sucks and swallows. If swallowing is not apparent, the baby's latch-on and positioning are reevaluated.

When the baby is feeding effectively, the breast softens as the baby nurses (Box 21-2). The infant stays on the first breast until it is completely softened. Burping is attempted before offering the second breast. The baby who is still hungry will feed on the second breast. The next feeding is then started on the breast that feels heavier. Some babies need to feed on only one breast at a feeding to feel satisfied and gain weight appropriately.

Frequency of feedings

Most newborns need 8 to 10 feedings every 24 hours for adequate weight gain. Parents are instructed that if babies do not awaken for feedings, they must wake them at least every 3 hours during the day and at least every 4 hours at night until feeding is well established. (Feeding frequency is determined by counting from the beginning of one feeding to the beginning of the next feeding.) **Demand feeding** means that the baby determines when feedings are needed; this is appropriate after feeding is well established and the baby is gaining weight well. As babies grow, they gradually space feedings wider apart.

Duration of feedings

The duration of breastfeeding sessions is highly variable, since the timing of milk transfer differs for each mother-baby

---

BOX 21-2 *Indicators of Effective Breastfeeding during the First Week*

INFANT

Physical assessment: alert; normal skin turgor; moist mucous membranes; fontanels soft and flat, strong and coordinated suck. Has periods of wakefulness and hunger alternating with periods of contentment/sleeping. Weight loss less than 8% before discharge; gains 15 to 30 gm per day after milk is "in."

Feeding frequency: 8 to 10 times per 24 hours

Feeding behavior: baby latches on easily, sucks with gliding jaw movements in bursts of 10 to 12 sucks/swallows at beginning of feeding, slows to bursts of 2 to 3 sucks/swallows at end of feeding. Swallowing is audible. Baby appears relaxed during feeding.

Output: six to eight wet diapers per 24 hours after milk is in; two to three bowel movements; stools transition to milk stools by 3 to 5 days.

MOTHER

Physical assessment: nipples intact (no redness, cracking, scabs, or bleeding), minimal nipple tenderness; breasts full, soft, without engorgement, no redness; minimal tenderness to palpation. No fever.

Milk is "in" by day 3 to 4. Breasts are full at beginning of feeding; soften as baby nurses. Baby softens at least one breast per feeding. No pinching or nipple pain with sucking.

Mother easily positions and latches baby on; experiences let-down with feeding; uterine cramping, increased lochia; leaking from opposite breast; feels relaxed during feeding.

---

pair. While some infants may complete a feeding in 5 to 10 minutes, others may require 45 minutes or longer. The average time for feeding is 30 minutes, or approximately 15 minutes per breast; this is a common recommendation. In reality, instructing mothers to feed for a set number of minutes is inappropriate. It is better to teach mothers how to determine when a baby has finished a feeding: the baby's suck/swallow pattern has slowed, the breast is softened, and the baby appears content and may fall asleep or release the nipple.

If a baby seems to be feeding effectively and the urine output is adequate but the weight gain is not, this may be due to the mother's switching to the second breast too soon. She may have been told to feed the baby for 10 minutes on each breast. Consequently, the baby is drinking only the foremilk (skim milk) and never reaches the rich, calorie-dense hindmilk. The foremilk is high in lactose and may cause the baby to have explosive stools, gas pains, and inconsolable crying. Feeding on the first breast until it softens ensures that the baby will receive the hindmilk and gain weight properly.

Engorgement

Primary **engorgement** is a common response of the breasts to the sudden change in hormones and the presence of an increased volume of milk. It usually occurs on the third to fifth postpartum day. The breasts are tender, swollen, hot, and hard, and may even be dry and red. The swelling can extend into the axilla. Some mothers may even run a fever and have a headache.

The nurse can teach the mother to treat engorgement aggressively by feeding the baby about every 2 hours, softening at least one breast at each feeding and pumping to soften the second breast. Because back pressure on full milk glands inhibits milk production, frequent emptying of the breasts in the first several days after birth is essential to establishing an adequate milk supply.

With treatment, engorgement usually lasts 12 to 24 hours. Use of an antiinflammatory pain reliever will decrease the swelling and also the pain and fever. The use of ice packs or raw cabbage leaves (Roberts, 1995) on the breasts can relieve both the pain and swelling and can soften the areola enough to allow the baby to latch on effectively. The decreased swelling also reduces the pressure on the ducts and promotes the flow of milk. Ice can be applied between feedings in a 15-minutes-on, 45-minutes-off rotation until the mother is comfortable. Fresh cabbage leaves can be placed on the breasts for up to 2 hours before a feeding and should be changed when they begin to wilt.

Although the exact mechanism of action of cabbage leaves in treatment of engorgement has not been identified, it is thought that continuous application might decrease the milk supply. The nonbreastfeeding mother may find it effective to keep cabbage leaves on her breasts continuously for several hours until the swelling has decreased.

Because heat increases blood flow, the application of heat to an already-congested area is usually counterproductive. Occasionally, however, standing in a warm shower will start the milk leaking and soften the breasts enough for the baby to latch on.

Special considerations

Sleepy baby. During the first few days of life, some babies need to be awakened for feedings. Parents are instructed to be alert for behavioral signs or feeding cues such as rapid eye movements under the eyelids, sucking movements, or hand-to-mouth motions. When these signs are present, it is a good time to attempt breastfeeding. If the infant is awakened from a sound sleep, attempts at feeding are more likely to be unsuccessful. Helpful hints to give parents as they are trying to bring the baby to an alert state for feeding include the following: unwrap the baby, change the diaper, sit the baby upright, talk to the baby with variable pitch, gently massage the baby's chest or back, and stroke the palms or soles.

Fussy baby. Babies sometimes awaken from sleep crying frantically. Although they may be hungry, they cannot focus on feeding until they are calmed. The nurse can encourage the parents to swaddle the baby, hold the baby close, talk soothingly, and allow the baby to suck on a clean finger until the baby is calmed enough to latch on to the breast. Dripping water on the infant's lower lip or tongue may facilitate latch-on.

Bottles and pacifiers. Because breastfeeding and bottle feeding require very different skills, it is best to avoid offering a bottle until the infant is proficient at breastfeeding. Although some infants can switch easily from breast to bottle and vice versa, many cannot. **Nipple confusion** (difficulty knowing how to latch on to the breast after having taken a bottle) can lead to frustration for infants and parents. It is safe to suggest that parents wait 4 to 6 weeks before offering a bottle to the breastfeeding infant. Breastfed infants do not necessarily need to ever have bottles. Even newborns and young infants can take expressed milk or formula from a cup.

If it becomes necessary to supplement breastfeeding with formula or expressed breast milk, a supplemental feeding system can be used (see Fig. 21-3). This eliminates the need for bottles and helps to prevent nipple confusion.

Pacifiers should be avoided during the first few weeks. They increase the risk of nipple confusion and may cause the infant to substitute nonnutritive sucking for actual breastfeeding, resulting in poor weight gain.

Jaundice. Jaundice (hyperbilirubinemia) in the newborn is discussed in detail in Chapter 19. **Physiologic jaundice** usually occurs after 24 hours of age and peaks by the third day. This has been referred to as early-onset jaundice, which in the breastfed infant may be associated with insufficient feeding and infrequent stooling. Colostrum has a natural laxative effect and promotes early passage of meconium. Bilirubin is excreted from the body primarily (98%) through the intestines. Infrequent stooling allows bilirubin in the stool to be reabsorbed into the infant's system, thus promoting hyperbilirubinemia. Infants who receive water or glucose water supplements are more likely to have hyperbilirubinemia, since only 2% of bilirubin is excreted through the kidneys. Decreased caloric intake (less milk) is associated with decreased stooling and increased jaundice.

To prevent early-onset breastfeeding jaundice from occurring, babies should be breastfed early and frequently during the first several days of life. More frequent feedings are associated with lower bilirubin levels.

To treat early-onset jaundice, breastfeeding is evaluated in terms of frequency and length of feedings, positioning and latch-on, and infant's ability to empty the breast. Factors such as a sleepy or lethargic baby or breast engorgement may interfere with effective breastfeeding and should be corrected. If the infant's intake of milk needs to be increased, a supplemental feeding device may be used to deliver additional breast milk or formula while the infant is nursing. Hyperbilirubinemia may reach levels that require treatment with phototherapy administered via light or blanket (see Chapter 20.)

Late-onset jaundice affects few breastfed infants and develops in the second week of life, peaking at about 10 days of age. These infants are typically thriving, gaining weight, and stooling normally, and all pathologic causes of jaundice have been ruled out. It was once postulated that an enzyme in the milk of some mothers caused the bilirubin level to increase. It now appears that a factor in human milk increases the intestinal absorption of bilirubin. In most cases no intervention is necessary, although some experts recommend temporary disruption of breastfeeding for 12 to 24 hours to allow bilirubin levels to decrease. During this time, the mother pumps her breasts and the baby is offered alternative nutrition, usually formula (Lawrence, 1994).

Preterm infants. Human milk is the ideal food for preterm infants, with benefits that are unique and in addition to those received by term, healthy infants. Benefits include protection against infection, necrotizing enterocolitis, and atopic disease. Breast milk enhances retinal maturation in the preterm infant and improves neurocognitive outcome. There is also greater physiologic stability with breastfeeding as compared with bottle feeding (Brown et al., 1996; Meier & Brown, 1996).

In addition, the mothers of preterm infants receive specific emotional benefits in breastfeeding or providing breast milk for their babies. They report rewards in knowing they can provide the healthiest nutrition for the infant and believe that breastfeeding enhances feelings of closeness to the infant (Kavanaugh et al., 1997).

Mothers of preterm infants should begin pumping their breasts as soon as possible after birth with a hospital-grade electric pump. To establish an optimal milk supply, the mother should use a dual collection kit and pump 8 to 10 times daily for 10 to 15 minutes and/or until the milk flow has ceased for a few minutes (Meier, 1997). These women are taught proper handling and storage of breast milk to minimize bacterial contamination and growth.

Nurses in neonatal intensive care units provide essential support to mothers of preterm infants as the babies progress from being held in skin-to-skin contact by their mothers to learning how to latch on and suck effectively. Clinical specialists and **lactation consultants** assigned to these units often prove invaluable in promoting effective breastfeeding by preterm infants.

Breastfeeding twins. Caring for twins takes some planning, but breastfeeding twins means that feedings are always ready instantly and no one has to wash bottles and fix formula. Some mothers are able to feed both babies at once. However, the mother of twins may need extra nourishment (200 to 500 kcal per day for each baby).

Each baby feeds from one breast per feeding, usually for about 20 to 30 minutes. Some mothers assign each baby a breast; others switch babies from one breast to the other, either on a schedule or randomly. The mother may find it easiest to use a modified demand feeding schedule. This involves feeding the first baby who wakes up and then waking the second baby for feeding.

During the early weeks, parents may find it helpful to keep a record of feeding times and which breast was used first by which baby. If one twin nurses more vigorously than the other, that twin should be alternated between breasts in order to equalize breast stimulation.

If the mother wants to feed the babies simultaneously, she may wish to experiment with positions. For example, one baby could be held in the football hold and the other in the cradle hold, or the babies could each be held in a cradling position. In another approach, each baby could be supported on firm pillows while in the football hold (Fig. 21-7), although, at first, some mothers who use this position may require help getting the babies off the breasts.

Diabetic mother. The diabetic mother is encouraged to breastfeed. In addition to benefits for the infant, and maternal satisfaction, breastfeeding has an antidiabetogenic effect. Blood glucose levels and insulin requirements are lower because of the carbohydrate used in milk production. During lactation, the diabetic woman may be able to eat more food and still take less insulin. However, insulin dosage must be adjusted as the baby is weaned. Some diabetic women are at increased risk for sore nipples caused by **monilial infections** and may have an increased risk for mastitis (Lawrence, 1994).

Expressing and storing breast milk

There are situations when expression of breast milk is necessary or desirable, such as when:
- Engorgement occurs.
- The mother and baby are separated (e.g., preterm or sick infant is in neonatal intensive care).
- The mother is employed outside the home and needs to maintain her milk supply.
- The nipples are severely sore or cracked.
- The mother is leaving the infant in the care of the father or other caregiver and will not be available to breastfeed.

Since pumping and hand expression are rarely as efficient as a baby in removing milk from the breast, the milk supply should never be judged based on the volume expressed.

Hand expression. After her hands are thoroughly washed, the mother places one hand on her breast at the edge of the areola. With her thumb above and fingers below, she presses in toward her chest wall and gently compresses the breast while rolling her thumb and fingers forward. These motions are repeated rhythmically until the milk begins to flow. The mother simply maintains steady, light pressure while the milk is flowing easily. The thumb and fingers should not pinch the breast or slip down to the nipple, and the mother should rotate her hand to reach all sections of the breast. After expressing milk from the second breast, she should return and express milk from the first

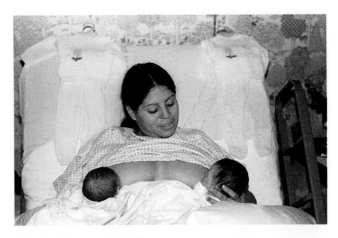

Fig. **21-7** Breastfeeding twins. (Courtesy Marjorie Pyle, RNC, Lifecircle, Costa Mesa, Calif.)

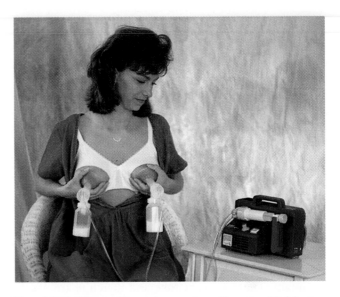

Fig. **21-8** Bilateral breast pumping. (Courtesy Medela, Inc., McHenry, Ill.)

breast, then repeat the second breast until all readily available milk is expressed.

Pumping. For most women, it is advisable to initiate pumping only after the milk supply is well established and the infant is latching on and breastfeeding well. When breastfeeding is delayed after birth, pumping is started as soon as possible and continued regularly until the infant is able to breastfeed effectively.

There are numerous ways to approach pumping. Some women pump on awakening in the morning, or when the baby has nursed but did not completely empty the breast. Others choose to pump after feedings or may pump one breast while the baby is nursing from the other. Double pumping (pumping both breasts at the same time) saves time and may stimulate the milk supply more effectively than single pumping (Fig. 21-8).

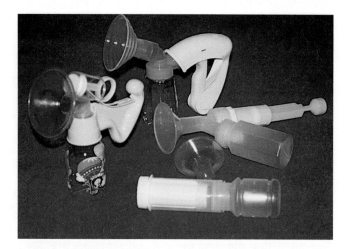

Fig. **21-9** Breast pumps. (Courtesy Marjorie Pyle, RNC, Life-circle, Costa Mesa, Calif.)

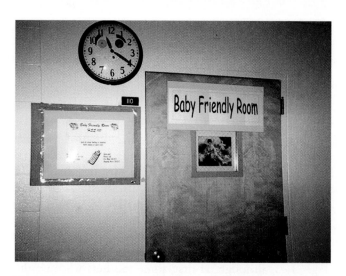

Fig. **21-10** Room on a university campus dedicated to parents and infants. The room contains comfortable furniture, a breast pump, a refrigerator, a baby changing table, and a television and VCR for instructional purposes. The room is available to students, faculty, and staff. (Courtesy Shannon Perry, Burlingame, Calif.)

The amount of milk obtained when pumping depends on the time of day, how long it has been since the baby breastfed, the mother's milk supply, how practiced she is at pumping, and her comfort level (pumping is uncomfortable for some women). Breast milk may vary in color and consistency, depending on the time of day, the age of the baby, and foods the mother has eaten (e.g., the milk may appear green after the mother eats a spinach salad).

Types of pumps. Numerous breast pumps are available, with wide variation in cost, effectiveness, and ease of operation. Before purchasing or renting a breast pump, the mother would benefit from counseling by a nurse or lactation consultant to determine which pump best suits her needs.

Full-service electric pumps, or hospital-grade pumps, are most similar to the sucking action and pressure of the nursing infant. These are expensive and therefore are usually rented. When breastfeeding is delayed after birth (e.g., the newborn is preterm or ill), or when mother and baby are separated for lengthy periods, these pumps are most appropriate.

Smaller electric or battery-operated pumps are also available (Fig. 21-9). Some have automatic suck/release cycling and others require use of a finger to regulate strength and speed of suction. These are typically used when pumping is done occasionally, but some models are satisfactory for working mothers or others who pump on a regular basis.

Manual or hand pumps are least expensive and most portable. These are most often used by mothers who are pumping for an occasional bottle.

Storage of breast milk. Breast milk can be safely stored in any clean glass or plastic container. Disposable bottle liners are easy and inexpensive to use when storing milk. When using bottle liners, doubling bagging is recommended to protect the milk most effectively.

Breast milk can be refrigerated safely for 48 hours after it is expressed. If it is not used within that time, it can be frozen (0° C) for up to 6 months; it should be kept in the middle or toward the back of the freezer to avoid variations in temperature. Milk can be stored for 2 years in a −20° C freezer. When storing breast milk, the container should be dated, and the oldest milk should be used first.

Frozen milk is thawed by placing the container in warm water or in the refrigerator. It cannot be refrozen, and it should be used within 24 hours. After thawing, the container should be shaken to mix the layers that have separated. It is never thawed or heated in a microwave oven. Microwaving does not heat evenly and can cause encapsulated boiling bubbles to form in the center of the liquid. This may not be detected when drops of milk are checked for temperature. Babies have sustained severe burns to the mouth, throat, and upper GI tract as a result of microwaved milk (Lawrence, 1994).

Being away from the baby

Many women are able to successfully combine breastfeeding with employment, attending school, or other commitments. If feedings are missed, the milk supply may be affected. Some women's bodies adjust the milk supply to the times she is with the baby for feedings, whereas others find they must pump or the supply diminishes quickly. Businesses are increasingly making available rooms where mothers can nurse their infants or use breast pumps (Fig. 21-10).

Breastfeeding mothers who work outside the home often feel a special connection to their babies even when they are separated. It is easy to continue breastfeeding while working. Planning ahead makes the transition back to work after birth much smoother and easier for both mother and baby.

Breastfed babies are healthier, and mothers are less likely to miss work; this is an added benefit for the family and the employer.

Weaning

Typically, weaning is initiated at a time chosen by the mother or the infant. Weaning can be accomplished with little effort and no discomfort when it is done gradually. Abrupt weaning is likely to be distressing for both mother and baby, as well as physically uncomfortable for the mother.

Infant-led weaning means that the infant moves at his or her own pace in omitting feedings. Drinking from a cup and increasing the amount of solid foods substitute for breastfeeding.

Mother-led weaning means that the mother decides which feedings to drop. This is most easily done by omitting the feeding of least interest to the baby or the one the infant is most likely to sleep through. It can also be the feeding most convenient for the mother to omit. After a week or more, another feeding is dropped, and so on, until the infant is weaned from the breast. Allowing time for the milk supply to adjust before omitting another feeding prevents discomfort for the mother as her supply gradually decreases.

Infants can be weaned directly from the breast to a cup. Bottles are usually offered to infants less than 6 months of age. If the infant is weaned before 1 year of age, formula should be offered instead of cow's milk.

If abrupt weaning is necessary, breast engorgement often occurs. The mother is instructed to take mild analgesics, wear a supportive bra, apply ice packs or cabbage leaves to the breasts, and pump if needed to increase comfort. The pump should not be used to empty the breasts, since they should remain full enough to promote a decrease in the milk supply.

Many women feel that weaning is the end to a special, satisfying relationship with the infant and benefit from time to adapt to the changes. Sudden weaning may evoke feelings of guilt and disappointment; some women go through a grieving period after weaning (Lorick, 1993). The nurse can assist the mother by discussing other ways to continue this nurturing relationship with the infant, such as skin-to-skin contact while bottle feeding, or holding and cuddling the baby. Support from the father of the baby and other family members is essential at this time.

Milk banking

For those infants who cannot be breastfed but who also cannot survive except on human milk, banked donor milk is critically important. Because of the antiinfective and growth-promoting properties of human milk, as well as its superior nutrition, donor milk is used in many neonatal intensive care units for preterm or sick infants when the mother's own milk is not available. Donor milk is also being used therapeutically for some medical purposes, such as in transplant recipients who are immunocompromised.

The Human Milk Banking Association of North America (HMBANA) has established annually reviewed guidelines for the operation of donor human milk banks (Arnold & Tully, 1996). Donor milk banks collect, screen, process, and distribute the milk donated by breastfeeding mothers who are feeding their own infants and pumping a few ounces extra each day for the milk bank. All donors are screened both by interview and serologically for communicable diseases. Donor milk is stored frozen until it is heat processed to kill potential pathogens; then it is refrozen for storage until it is dispensed for use. The heat processing adds a level of protection for the recipient that is not possible with any other donor tissue or organ. Banked milk is dispensed only by prescription. There is a per-ounce fee charged by the bank to pay for the processing costs, but the HMBANA guidelines prohibit payment to donors.

Care of the mother

Diet. The composition of human milk varies slightly among women, regardless of their diets. The mother's milk automatically contains everything the baby needs, except in rare cases of maternal nutrient deficiencies. For most women, only 200 to 500 extra calories per day need to be added to the diet to provide adequate nutrients for the infant while also protecting the mother's body stores (Riordan & Auerbach, 1993).

There are no specific foods or drinks that all breastfeeding mothers must either consume or avoid. Lactating mothers should ideally consume a balanced diet of nutrient-dense foods. Adequate amounts of calcium, minerals, and fat-soluble vitamins are important.

If the breastfeeding mother is drinking enough fluids to quench her thirst, she is likely drinking enough to support lactation. Typically, women find that they are drinking as much as 2 to 3 quarts of fluid each day, with the choice of fluid depending on the mother's preference. Because of her increased need for fluids, the breastfeeding mother may wish to keep a drink within reach during feedings. An indicator of adequate fluid intake is the color of the mother's urine. If she is drinking enough fluids, her urine should be clear to light yellow throughout the day.

Weight loss. Because it takes energy to produce milk, many mothers experience a gradual weight loss while breastfeeding as fat stores deposited during pregnancy are used. This fact can be an added incentive for breastfeeding in the mother who is overweight. However, the mother who wants to diet while lactating should avoid losing large amounts of weight quickly because fat-soluble environmental contaminants to which she has been exposed are stored in her body's fat reserves and these may be released into her milk. In addition, some mothers find that their milk supply decreases when their caloric intake is severely restricted.

Most mothers find that they can lose about 1 kg per week without affecting their milk supply.

Exercise. There is no reason for a breastfeeding woman to restrict her physical activity. Women can continue to engage in activities such as hiking, jogging, swimming, and aerobics with no detrimental effect on the milk supply or composition (Dewey et al., 1994). For comfort, mothers may find it beneficial to engage in exercise soon after breastfeeding, when their breasts are as empty as possible. Wearing a well-designed, supportive bra may also be helpful.

Rest. It is important for the breastfeeding mother to rest as much as possible, especially in the first 1 or 2 weeks after birth. Fatigue, stress, and worry can negatively affect milk production and let-down. The nurse can encourage the mother to sleep when the baby sleeps. Breastfeeding in a side-lying position promotes rest for the mother. Assistance with household chores and caring for other children can be done by the father, grandparents or other relatives, and friends.

Breast care. The breastfeeding mother's normal routine bathing is all that is necessary to keep her breasts clean. Although she should avoid soaping her breasts directly, the small amount of soap that runs down her breasts while she is washing her face and neck is of no concern.

Breast cream should not be used routinely because it may block the natural oil secreted from Montgomery's glands on the areola. In addition, some breast creams contain alcohol, which may irritate or dry the breasts. The use of vitamin E oil or cream is also not recommended because it is a fat-soluble vitamin and the infant could build up a toxic level of vitamin E by consuming it during feeding. In addition, some people are allergic to it.

Findings from research on moist wound healing indicate that purified lanolin may promote healing of a sore nipple (Huml, 1995). However, the oils in lanolin and other breast creams can foster the growth of yeast. Therefore it should first be determined that the soreness is not caused by a monilial infection before any breast cream is used (see Teaching Guidelines box on p. 570).

The mother with flat or inverted nipples will likely benefit by wearing breast shells in her bras. These hard, plastic devices put pressure around the base of the nipple to promote eversion (Fig. 21-11).

If a mother needs breast support, she will be uncomfortable unless she wears a bra, because the ligament that supports the breast (Cooper's ligament) will otherwise stretch and be painful. If she is comfortable without a bra, there is no reason for her to wear one. If a woman prefers to wear a bra, it needs to be comfortable and provide nonbinding support. A mother should breastfeed at least once each day without her bra on so that all milk ducts can be completely emptied.

Some breastfeeding mothers find that their breasts leak between feedings. The use of breast pads (available in either washable or disposable forms) inside a bra and the wearing

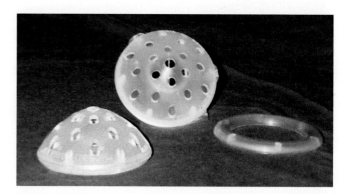

Fig. **21-11** Breast shells.

of layered or printed tops can help to camouflage the leaking. The nurse should warn the mother against using plastic-lined pads, however, because they trap moisture and this may cause nipples to become sore. To stop leaking, the mother can be alert to any sensation, such as a tingling, that might serve as a warning that her milk is letting down. If she experiences such a sensation, she can usually stop the let-down by pressing straight back on her nipples. In public, she can fold her arms across her chest to apply pressure unobtrusively.

Although only 1% to 2% of cases of breast cancer are diagnosed during pregnancy or lactation, a breastfeeding woman should perform monthly breast self-examination (BSE) (see Chapter 5). Prior to the resumption of menstrual periods, the woman needs to choose a convenient date on which to do her examination every month. She needs to become familiar with the normal lumpiness of her lactating breasts. Any lumps that match in location in both breasts are almost always breast tissue. Lumps that increase and decrease in size are milk glands or ducts. Because lactating breast tissue is very dense, mammography during lactation is of limited diagnostic value. Should a lump be discovered, a biopsy can usually be done without interrupting breastfeeding.

Effect of menstruation. The return of menstrual periods varies among lactating women. The majority will resume menstruation by 6 months postpartum. Menstruation has no effect on breastfeeding. There are no hormonal effects on the infant, although some babies may seem fussy for the first day. The quality of the milk is not affected (Lawrence, 1994).

Sexual sensations. Some women experience rhythmic uterine contractions during breastfeeding. Such sensations are not unusual because uterine contractions and milk ejection are both triggered by oxytocin, but they may be disturbing to some mothers who perceive them to be similar to orgasm.

Breastfeeding and contraception. Although breastfeeding confers a period of infertility, it is not considered an effective method of contraception. *Breastfeeding delays the* return of ovulation and menstruation; however, ovulation may occur even before the first menstrual period after childbirth. Thus the breastfeeding woman who is relying on the lactational amenorrhea (LAM) method of birth control needs to be knowledgeable about ways to determine when ovulation occurs (basal body temperature, cervical mucus, cervical position). Hormonal contraceptives, including pills, injectables, and implants, may cause a decrease in the milk supply and are best avoided during the first 6 weeks after birth. Oral contraceptives containing estrogen are not recommended for breastfeeding mothers. Progestin-only birth control pills are less likely to interfere with the milk supply. Some women find that the progestin-only injection (DepoProvera) or the implantable Norplant interfere with milk production, although others notice no alteration in the milk supply. Nonhormonal contraceptive methods (foam, condoms, nonhormonal intrauterine device [IUD], natural family planning, sterilization) are least likely to have a detrimental effect on breastfeeding (Kelsey, 1996).

Breastfeeding during pregnancy. It is possible for a breastfeeding woman to conceive and continue breastfeeding throughout the pregnancy if there are no medical contraindications (such as risk of preterm labor). Interestingly, when the baby is born, colostrum is produced. The practice of breastfeeding a newborn and an older child is called *tandem nursing.* The nurse should remind the mother to always feed the infant first to ensure that the newborn is receiving adequate nutrition. The supply-meets-demand principle works in this situation just as in the feeding of twins or triplets.

Drugs and breastfeeding. Although there is much concern about the compatibility of drugs and breastfeeding, there are in fact few drugs that are contraindicated during lactation. In evaluating the safety of a specific medication during breastfeeding, the health care provider considers the pharmacokinetics of the drug in the maternal system, as well as the absorption, metabolism, distribution, storage, and excretion in the infant. The gestational and chronologic age of the infant, body weight, and breastfeeding pattern are also considered (Lawrence, 1997).

The AAP (1994) has categorized commonly used medications according to their safety during breastfeeding (see Appendix C).

Drugs of abuse are contraindicated during lactation. These include amphetamine, cocaine, heroin, marijuana, nicotine, and phencyclidine hydrochloride ("angel dust," PCP) (AAP, 1994).

Nicotine can cause a decrease in the milk supply over time because of its effect on the milk ejection reflex. Mothers who continue to smoke tobacco when lactating should be advised not to smoke within 2 hours before breastfeeding and to never smoke in the same room with the infant (Lawrence, 1997).

Consumption of alcohol during lactation is approached with caution. Excessive amounts can have serious effects

on the infant and can adversely affect the mother's milk ejection reflex. The level of alcohol in breast milk decreases over time, unlike the levels of many drugs that remain in milk until it is removed from the breasts. If a mother chooses to consume alcohol, she should be advised to minimize its effects by having only one drink, and to consume the drink immediately after breastfeeding. The mother who is pumping for a sick or preterm infant should avoid alcohol until her infant is healthy.

Although only 1% of the caffeine ingested by the mother is passed into her breast milk, the infant's immature system limits the ability to excrete the caffeine. Caffeine accumulates in the infant's system and can cause irritability and poor sleeping patterns. Some infants are sensitive to even small amounts of caffeine. Mothers of such infants should limit caffeine intake. Caffeine is found in coffee, tea, chocolate, and many soft drinks (Lawrence, 1994).

Herbs and herbal teas are becoming more widely used during lactation. While some are considered safe, others contain pharmacologically active compounds that may have detrimental effects. A thorough history should include the consumption of any herbal remedies. Each remedy should then be evaluated for its compatibility with breastfeeding. The regional poison control center may provide information on the active properties of herbs (Lawrence, 1997).

Environmental contaminants. Chemicals that are lipophilic (dissolve in fat) are found in the lipid components of human milk. The amount depends on the mother's exposure to chemicals. Except under unusual circumstances, breastfeeding is not contraindicated because of exposure to environment contaminants such as DDT (an insecticide) and tetrachloroethylene (used in dry cleaning plants) (Lawrence, 1997).

Evaluation

Evaluation is based on the expected outcomes, and the plan of care is revised as needed based on the evaluation (see Plan of Care).

ROLE OF THE NURSE IN PROMOTING SUCCESSFUL LACTATION

Nurses who deal with women in prenatal settings are often the first to inquire about the mother's plans regarding infant feeding. It is the role of the nurse to educate the mother and her partner about the advantages of breastfeeding and to explore reasons why they may prefer formula feeding. Current reading materials and information about prenatal classes are made available to expectant parents. At each encounter the nurse offers to answer questions and provide additional information as needed.

Assessment of the mother's breasts and nipples during pregnancy are important. The nurse should inquire about breast changes during pregnancy, such as enlargement of

PLAN OF CARE   *Breastfeeding and Infant Nutrition*

> **NURSING DIAGNOSIS** Risk for ineffective breastfeeding related to limited maternal experience

Expected Outcomes *Infant is latched on correctly as evidenced by maternal comfort, signs of oxytocin and prolactin release, and sufficient milk transfer. Mother feels confident about signs of sufficient milk transfer, her own comfort, and a feeding plan after discharge.*

Nursing Interventions/*Rationales*

Explore the mother's knowledge about breastfeeding, her questions, and her assessment of feedings since birth and compare this information with the infant's feeding chart and appearance *to establish baseline to direct intervention.*

If the mother seems ambivalent about breastfeeding, explore her questions and the problems she is experiencing, assist her in solving the problems, and provide her with accurate information *to assist her in decision making and to decrease her anxiety, which could interfere with her ability to learn.*

If the woman is very anxious, spread teaching over several sessions, give her ongoing feedback during several feedings, coach her (possibly with a family member) to get her baby situated and latched on independent of your assistance, and provide her with written material she can review as needed *to ensure that she has a chance to express all of her needs and to feel competent after hospital discharge.*

Teach specific techniques that make feeding easier (i.e., how to wake a sleepy baby, how to position the baby at the breast, how to get the baby latched on without pain, how to recognize the milk transfer, how to keep the baby sucking, alternate breast massage during feeding, how to recognize when the baby is finished) *to increase her confidence in her ability to care for her baby and decrease the potential for inadequate feeding.*

Teach the mother to recognize release of oxytocin and prolactin (i.e., uterine contractions and increased lochia flow, drowsiness and thirst during feedings, baby's changing suck/swallow pattern) and why these hormones are important *to increase her confidence in her body's ability to produce milk.*

Teach the mother how to minimize and cope with engorgement if it should occur (i.e., regular 3-hour feeding schedule during the first week, thorough softening of one breast before switching to the second side, cabbage leaves or ice packs on swollen breasts before feeding, and pumping as necessary to soften breasts and provide comfort) *to minimize anxiety about engorgement and to ensure that the infant can continue to latch on successfully.*

Teach breast and nipple care (i.e., bras are necessary only if they provide comfort; dry the nipples before closing bra flaps; avoid soap on the areola and nipple; and how to heal sore or abraded nipples) *to ensure maternal comfort.*

Teach the mother what to expect in the first 2 weeks of breastfeeding (i.e., normal infant changes such as increased appetite and alertness, signs the baby is getting enough milk, why to avoid a pacifier until the baby is clearly showing signs of sufficient intake, and normal breast changes) *to establish milk supply and to increase her confidence that she can care for her baby.*

Supplement teaching with appropriate videos and other audiovisual aids, written material including how to get help after discharge, and demonstration/return demonstration as necessary *to increase maternal confidence and enhance learning.*

From Wong D & Perry S: *Maternal child nursing care,* St Louis, 1998, Mosby.

the breasts. Flat or inverted nipples are identified, and the mother is offered breast shells (see Fig. 21-11) to wear during the last trimester of pregnancy to encourage eversion of the nipples. These breast shells can also be worn postpartum between feedings.

In the immediate postpartum period, the nurse is instrumental in helping the mother to initiate breastfeeding as soon as possible after birth. Encouraging parents to keep the baby in the mother's room (rooming-in) allows the opportunity for the mother to learn to recognize feeding cues and to feed the baby when these cues are present. The nurse provides help with positioning and latch-on until the mother can do so independently. Explanations are given early on regarding frequency and duration of feedings, how to wake a sleepy baby, and how to determine if the baby is getting enough milk (Box 21-3). Before discharge, the nurse

verifies that the parents are knowledgeable about breastfeeding and are prepared for what to expect in the days ahead. For example, information about the transition to mature milk (milk coming in) and how to prevent engorgement is needed. The mother is also informed about prevention and treatment of sore nipples, and about signs of mastitis (including the importance of contacting the health care provider if these occur).

Parents often expect that because breastfeeding is "natural," it comes naturally for both mother and baby. This misconception needs to be clarified early on so that parents may view breastfeeding as a learning process. Then they are able to give themselves and their baby permission to learn, without unrealistic expectations. Nurses, physicians, and other health care providers who are knowledgeable about breastfeeding can offer needed support

Signs of Adequate Intake in the Breastfeeding Infant

- The mother's milk transitions from colostrum to mature milk. Milk "comes in" by 3 to 5 days after birth.
- The infant feeds at least eight times per day: approximately every 2 to 3 hours in the day and every 4 hours at night.
- After correctly latching on to the breast, the baby feeds for 15 to 20 minutes (per breast) with gliding jaw movements and audible swallowing. At least one breast is softened completely at each feeding.
- The infant appears relaxed and satisfied after feeding and is likely to fall asleep.
- By 24 hours after the milk has "come in," the infant urinates at least six to eight times (pale urine) and has at least two bowel movements per day. The stools transition from meconium to bright yellow, somewhat loose stools with a cottage cheese consistency by the fifth day.
- The infant gains 15 to 30 gm per day after the fourth or fifth day and surpasses the birth weight by 10 to 14 days of age.
- The mother reports a "tugging" sensation at the nipple with feeding and feels warm and relaxed during feeding.

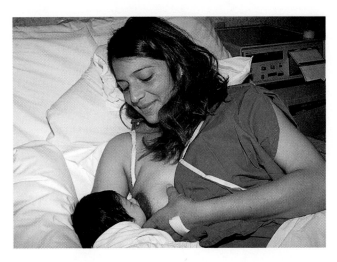

Fig. 21-12 Mother and infant enjoying breastfeeding. (Courtesy Marjorie Pyle, RNC, Lifecircle, Costa Mesa, Calif.)

and encouragement to parents, helping to instill a sense of confidence (Fig. 21-12).

Follow-Up after Hospital Discharge

The hospital nurse is instrumental in assisting mothers with positioning, latch-on, waking a sleepy baby, and establishing a feeding routine. Problems with sore nipples, engorgement, and jaundice are likely to occur after discharge. Thus it is the role of the hospital nurse to educate and prepare the mother for problems she may encounter once she is home (see Teaching Guidelines box). It is critical that the mother be given a list of resources for help with breastfeeding concerns and that she realizes when to call for assistance. Community resources for breastfeeding mothers include lactation consultants in hospitals, physicians' offices, or in private practice; nurses in pediatric or obstetric offices; support groups such as La Leche League; and peer counseling programs (such as those offered through WIC).

Telephone follow-up by hospital or office nurses within the first day or two after discharge can provide a means to identify any problems and offer needed advice and support. The AAP recommends that infants discharged before 48 hours of age be seen by a health care provider within 48 hours and have an office visit within 7 days after discharge. In some settings and circumstances, home care follow-up is available for mothers after hospital discharge.

FORMULA FEEDING

Reasons for Formula Feeding

The decision to feed a baby infant formula may be the result of the mother's or partner's personal preference, the influence of other significant family members, or simply a lack of familiarity with breastfeeding. Occasionally there is no other option: the mother may have extensive breast scarring or may have had a bilateral mastectomy; the mother may be on medications that preclude breastfeeding; or the baby may be adopted. Some mothers are able to induce lactation for an adopted baby. Rarely, an infant may have galactosemia and must be fed a lactose-free formula.

Infant formula may be used to supplement breastfeeding if the mother's milk supply is inadequate. It may also be fed to the baby if the mother will be away and wishes to leave a bottle of formula instead of expressed breast milk.

In the United States, formula feeding is also recommended for mothers who are infected with the human immunodeficiency virus (HIV). In Third World countries where the risks of the infant dying from diarrhea and dehydration are high because of unsafe water supplies, the mother who is HIV positive is advised to breastfeed her infant (Lawrence, 1997).

Parent Education

Inexperienced mothers and fathers who are formula feeding their infants usually need teaching, counseling, and support. They may need assistance with the feeding process and with any problems they may experience. Some parents who are formula feeding express concern that the baby will suffer as a result of their decision. Emphasis on the beneficial use of feeding times for close contact and socializing with the infant can help relieve some of this concern.

TEACHING GUIDELINES

Common Breastfeeding Problems

ENGORGED BREASTS

Engorgement usually occurs 3 to 5 days after birth and lasts 12 to 24 hours. It is the result of sudden hormonal changes and increased milk volume. Blood supply to the breasts increases and causes swelling of tissues surrounding the milk ducts. The ducts may be pinched shut, so that the milk does not flow. The breasts are firm, tender, hot, and may appear shiny and taut. The tenderness extends into the axilla. The unyielding areola makes it difficult for the infant to latch on. If milk is not removed from the breasts, milk production will decrease and the milk supply may suffer.

Prevention

1. Breastfeed frequently as milk is "coming in"—at least every 2 to 3 hours during the day, with only one longer interval at night of 4 to 5 hours.
2. Encourage baby to feed at least 15 to 20 minutes on each breast or until at least one breast softens per feeding.

Treatment

1. Feed every 2 hours, softening at least one breast per feeding, and pump as needed to soften second breast. Pumping during engorgement will not cause a problematic increase in milk supply.
2. Apply ice packs to breasts for 15 to 20 minutes in between feedings to reduce swelling.
3. Place raw cabbage leaves on breasts in between feedings; replace when wilting (Roberts, 1995). CAUTION: Continuous application may decrease milk supply.
4. It may be helpful to apply warm compresses or stand in warm shower just before feeding to foster relaxation and let-down. Use heat cautiously, since it may increase swelling.
5. Take an antiinflammatory analgesic (ibuprofen) to help decrease swelling and pain.
6. Gently massage breasts during nursing to help empty firmer areas.
7. To soften areola for easier latch-on, a manual or electric pump can be used if manual expression is not effective. If the baby is not effective in softening the breast, a pump can be used to remove residual milk. Milk can be fed to the baby or frozen for future use.

SORE NIPPLES

Mild nipple discomfort at the beginning of feedings or mild nipple tenderness during the first few days is not abnormal. Severe soreness and abraded, cracked, or bleeding nipples are not normal and most often result from poor positioning and/or incorrect latch-on. Monilial infection of the nipples causes severe soreness, stinging, or burning, and nipples appear shiny pink.

Prevention

1. Position baby at level of breast with baby's mouth directly in front of nipple.
2. Express milk to moisten nipple. Latch baby on only when mouth is open wide. Hold baby in close while nursing, with infant's nose, cheeks, and chin touching the breast. If sucking is painful after first 1 to 2 minutes, break suction and repeat latch-on.

Treatment

1. Assess positioning and latch-on. Position baby at level of breast with body in straight alignment and mouth directly in front of nipple. Support breast with C-hold: four fingers below areola and thumb on top. Express milk to lubricate nipple. Tickle baby's lower lip with nipple until mouth opens widely. Pull baby quickly onto breast so that mouth covers nipple and at least 2-cm diameter of areola. If nipple pain persists after first few sucks, break suction and latch on again; repeat until pain is eliminated and a "tugging" sensation is felt.
2. Evaluate baby's sucking during feeding, noting position of tongue.

TEACHING GUIDELINES—cont'd

SORE NIPPLES—cont'd

Treatment—cont'd

3. Begin feedings on least sore nipple. Apply ice to nipple 2 to 3 minutes before latch-on for numbing effect.
4. After feeding, wipe nipple with water to remove baby's saliva.
5. Express a few drops of milk and rub into nipples. Allow to air dry.
6. It may be helpful to blot a steeped, cooled caffeinated tea bag on nipples (tannic acid may help promote healing). Warm water compresses may also be comforting (Lavergne, 1997).
7. Modified lanolin can be applied to the nipples and areola. Do not use if allergic to wool or if a monilial infection on the nipples is suspected (Huml, 1995).
8. Breast shells may increase comfort by keeping clothing off nipples. Leave nipples open to air as much as possible.

PLUGGED MILK DUCT

A **milk duct** may become **plugged,** causing an area of the breast to be swollen and tender. There may be a small white pearl on the nipple; this is the curd of milk blocking the milk flow. Plugged ducts are caused by inadequate emptying of the breasts, poor positioning for feeding, always using the same position for feeding, or wearing a bra (underwire) or clothing that is too tight.

Treatment

1. Apply warm compresses to affected area of breast and to nipple before feeding.
2. Offer the sore breast first to foster more complete emptying.
3. Breastfeed more frequently and for longer periods. Massage swollen area while feeding.
4. Vary positions with every feeding

MASTITIS

Mastitis, or breast infection, is commonly caused by bacteria normally present in the baby's mouth *(Staphylococcus aureus).* Predisposing factors are cracked nipples, plugged ducts, breast trauma (poor latch-on, infant teething), and maternal exhaustion. Flulike symptoms, such as fever, chills, body aches, and headache, may occur, along with breast pain and redness.

Treatment

1. Notify the health care provider when symptoms occur. Antibiotic treatment for 10 days is often ordered.
2. Rest; increase fluid intake; take over-the-counter (OTC) analgesic/antipyretic.
3. Breastfeed more often. Apply warm compresses to breast before feedings.
4. If breastfeeding is too painful or ineffective in relieving fullness, use electric breast pump.

INSUFFICIENT MILK SUPPLY (OR SLOW WEIGHT GAIN IN INFANT)

Insufficient milk supply is often associated with slow weight gain or weight loss in the breastfed infant. Causes may include infrequent (fewer than eight feedings per day) or inadequate emptying of the breasts, poor positioning and/or latch-on, sleepy baby, abnormal sucking, unrelieved engorgement, sore nipples, maternal stress or exhaustion, pregnancy, use of oral contraceptives, or previous breast surgery. In addition to weight loss or poor weight gain, the infant may have fewer than six to eight wet diapers and fewer than two stools per day and may not seem satisfied after feedings.

Treatment

1. Increase number and length of feedings.
2. Awaken sleepy baby for feedings.
3. Examine positioning and latch-on techniques, and infant sucking.
4. Increase maternal fluid intake and nutrition, as well as rest.
5. Use imagery, relaxation, and breast massage to promote let-down reflex.
6. Use "alternate breast massage" during feedings (when baby stops sucking, massage breast from periphery toward nipple; continue throughout feeding).
7. If supplementation is needed, use nursing supplementer device to provide extra nutrition while nursing or offer supplement in cup, spoon, or bottle (use bottle only if no problems with latch-on and sucking).
8. Consult health care provider about maternal food supplements or medications that may help to increase milk supply.

Readiness for feeding

The first feeding of formula is ideally given after the initial transition to extrauterine life is made. Feeding readiness cues include such things as stability of vital signs, presence of bowel sounds, and an active sucking reflex.

Before the first formula feeding, some institutions have the policy of offering sips of water to the newborn to assess patency of the GI tract and absence of tracheoesophageal fistula. If the infant sucks and swallows the water without difficulty, formula is then offered.

Feeding patterns

Typically, a newborn will drink 7.5 to 15 ml of formula at a feeding at first, with the intake gradually increasing during the first week of life. Most babies are drinking 90 to 150 ml at a feeding by the end of the second week, or sooner. Generally, a baby who weighs less than 4.5 kg takes in about 840 ml of formula every 24 hours after the newborn period. A baby who weighs more than 4.5 kg ingests about 960 ml in 24 hours.

The newborn infant should be fed at least every 3 to 4 hours, even if that requires waking the baby for the feedings. The infant showing an adequate weight gain can be allowed to sleep at night and fed only on awakening. Most newborns need six to eight feedings in 24 hours, and the number of feedings decreases as the infant matures. Usually by 3 to 4 weeks after birth, a fairly predictable feeding pattern has developed. Scheduling feedings arbitrarily at predetermined intervals may not meet a baby's needs, but initiating feedings at convenient times often moves the baby's feedings to times that work for the family.

Mothers will usually notice increases in the infant's appetite between 10 days and 2 weeks, 6 and 9 weeks, and 3 and 6 months. These appetite spurts correspond to growth spurts. The amount of formula per feeding should be increased by about 30 ml to meet the baby's needs at these times.

Feeding technique

Parents who choose formula feeding often need education regarding feeding techniques. During feedings they should be encouraged to sit comfortably, holding the infant closely in a semiupright position. Feedings provide opportunities to bond with the baby through touching, talking, singing, or reading to the infant. Parents should consider feedings as a time of peaceful relaxation with the baby.

A bottle should never be propped with a pillow or other inanimate object and left with the infant. This practice may result in choking, and it deprives the infant of important interaction during feeding. Moreover, propping the bottle has been implicated in causing nursing bottle caries, or decay of the first teeth resulting from continuous bathing of the teeth with carbohydrate-containing fluid as the infant sporadically sucks the nipple.

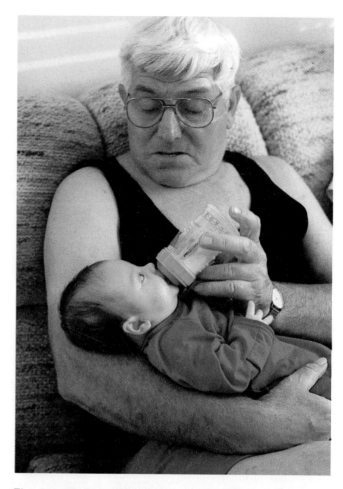

Fig. **21-13** Grandfather feeding infant granddaughter. Note angle of bottle that ensures milk covers nipple area. (Courtesy Kim Molloy, San Jose, Calif.)

The bottle should be held so that fluid fills the nipple and none of the air in the bottle is allowed to enter the nipple (Fig. 21-13). After the newborn period the infant who falls asleep, turns aside the head, or ceases to suck usually is signaling that enough formula has been taken. Parents should be taught to look for these cues and avoid overfeeding, which could contribute to obesity.

Most infants swallow air when fed from a bottle and should be given a chance to burp several times during a feeding (Fig. 21-14).

Bottles and nipples

There are various brands and styles of bottles and nipples available to parents. Most babies will feed well with any bottle and nipple. It is important that the bottles and nipples be washed in warm soapy water, using a bottle and nipple brush to facilitate thorough cleansing. Careful rinsing is necessary. Boiling of bottles and nipples is not needed unless there is some question about the safety of the water supply.

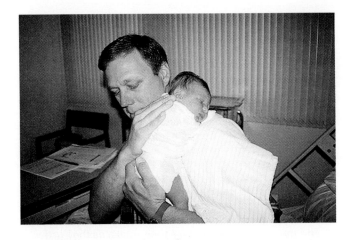

A

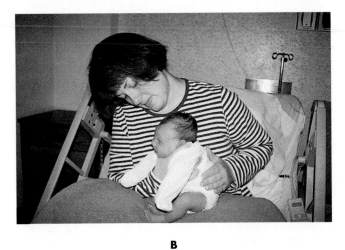

B

Fig. **21-14** Two positions for burping an infant. **A,** On the shoulder. **B,** Sitting. (Courtesy Marjorie Pyle, RNC, Lifecircle, Costa Mesa, Calif.)

Infant formulas

Commercial formulas. Because human milk is species specific to meet the needs of the human infant, it is used as the standard for all infant formulas. Commercial infant formulas are designed to resemble human milk as closely as possible, although none has ever duplicated it.

Infants who are not breastfed should be given commercial formulas. If this is too expensive, the family would likely be eligible for services through the WIC program, which provides iron-fortified infant formula. Cow's milk is the basis for most infant formulas, although soy-based and other specialized formulas are available for the infant who cannot tolerate cow's milk.

Commercial formulas are available in three forms: powder, concentrate, and ready-to-feed. All are equivalent in terms of nutritional content, but they vary considerably in cost:

- Powdered formula is the least expensive type. It is easily mixed by using one scoop for every 60 ml of water.

- Concentrated formula is more expensive than powder. It is diluted with equal parts of water and can be stored in the refrigerator for 24 hours after opening.
- Ready-to-feed formula is the most expensive and easiest to use. The desired amount is poured into the bottle. The opened can is safely refrigerated for 24 hours. This type of formula can be purchased in individual disposable bottles for the most convenient feeding.

Special formulas. Some infants have an allergic reaction to cow's milk formula. They may experience diarrhea, rash, colic, or vomiting, and, in extreme cases, fail to thrive. Some of these infants may better tolerate a soy milk formula; however, some then prove to be allergic to soy protein. If hypersensitivity to cow's milk protein is suspected, a hydrolyzed casein formula may be effective. Special formulas are very expensive. Some women may be able to begin breastfeeding or, in life-threatening cases, obtain human milk through a milk bank, at least temporarily.

Evaporated milk. Although evaporated milk is concentrated and less expensive than commercial formula, the mixing of evaporated milk and water to feed a baby is no longer recommended because evaporated milk does not provide adequate nutrition for an infant.

Unmodified cow's milk. Unmodified cow's milk is not suited to the nutritional needs of the human infant in the first year of life. Specific concerns include the excessive amounts of calcium, phosphorus, and other minerals it contains; an imbalance of calcium and phosphorus; its excessive protein content; the poor absorption of the fat it contains; and its low iron concentration. In addition, its use in infants is apt to cause microscopic hemorrhages that lead to GI blood loss. This blood loss, as well as the low levels of iron in the milk, increases the likelihood of iron deficiency anemia.

Formula preparation

Recent recommendations for the labeling of commercial infant formulas require that the directions for the preparation and use of the formula be communicated with pictures and symbols for the benefit of nonliterate people. In addition, manufacturers are translating the directions into various languages, such as Spanish, French, Vietnamese, Chinese, and Arabic, to prevent misunderstanding and errors in formula preparation. It is important to impress on families that the proportions must not be altered—neither diluted to expand the amount of formula nor concentrated to provide more calories.

Although manufacturers of commercial formula include directions for preparing their products, the nurse should review formula preparation with the mother. It is especially important that formula be mixed properly. The newborn's kidneys are immature, and giving the infant overly concentrated formula may provide protein and minerals in amounts that exceed the kidney's excretory ability. In contrast, if the formula is diluted too much (sometimes done in an effort to save money), the infant does not consume enough calories and does not grow well.

Sterilization of formula rarely is recommended for those families with access to a safe public water supply. Instead, the formula is prepared with attention to cleanliness. When water from a private well is used, parents should be advised to contact the health department to have a chemical and bacteriologic analysis of the water done before using the water in formula preparation. The presence of nitrates, excess fluoride, or bacteria may be harmful to the infant.

In addition, if the sanitary conditions in the home appear unsafe, it would be better to recommend the use of ready-to-feed formula or to teach the mother to sterilize the formula. The two traditional methods for sterilization are terminal heating and the aseptic method. In the terminal heating method, the prepared formula is placed in the bottles, which are topped with the nipples placed upside down and covered with the caps, and then sealed loosely with the rings. The bottles are then boiled together in a water bath for 25 minutes. In the aseptic method, the bottles, rings, caps, nipples, and any other necessary equipment, such as a funnel, are boiled separately, after which the formula is poured into the bottles. Any formula left in the bottle after the feeding should be discarded because the baby's saliva has mixed with it. (Instructions for formula preparation and feeding are provided in the Home Care box.)

Vitamin and mineral supplementation

Commercial iron-fortified formula has all of the nutrients the infant needs for the first 6 months of life. After 6 months, the only mineral supplementation required is 0.25 mg of fluoride daily if the local water supply is not fluoridated (AAP, 1997).

Weaning

The bottle-fed infant will gradually learn to use a cup, and the parents will find that they are preparing fewer bottles. Frequently the bottle feeding before bedtime is the last one to remain. Babies have a strong need to suck, and the baby who has the bottle taken away too early or abruptly will compensate with nonnutritive sucking on his or her fingers, thumb, a pacifier, or even his or her own tongue. Weaning from a bottle should therefore be done gradually because the baby has learned to rely on the comfort that sucking provides. This comfort helps a baby to cope with other events, such as toilet training or the birth of a sibling.

Introducing solid foods

The infant receives the right balance of nutrients from breast milk or formula during the first 4 to 6 months. It is not true that the feeding of solids will help the infant sleep through the night. Introduction of solid foods before the infant is 4 to 6 months of age may result in overfeeding

---

HOME CARE *Patient Instructions for Self-Care*
Formula Preparation and Feeding

Your newborn baby will be hungry about every 2 1/2 to 3 hours but sometimes may go 3 to 4 hours between feedings. The newborn should not go longer than 4 hours between feedings until a weight gain pattern is established—usually in about 2 weeks. Your baby needs to be awake before being fed. If your baby is sleepy, massage the baby's back and chest and talk to him or her.

Your baby's feedings will change a lot in the first week after birth. The first day, most babies only drink 7.5 to 15 ml of formula at a feeding. By the time they are a week old, most babies drink 30 to 60 ml at a feeding and then gradually increase their intake as they grow. If you do not use all of the formula at a feeding, throw away what is left, because it spoils once it has mixed with the baby's saliva.

You may want to write down how many milliliters your baby drinks each day. When you take the baby in for a checkup, the physician or nurse will ask you about how much formula the baby drinks. By 1 week of age, most babies who weigh 3 to 4.5 kg are drinking about 840 ml in 24 hours. Smaller babies drink a little less. Babies weighing more than 4.5 kg drink about 960 ml each day.

To feed your baby, place the nipple in the baby's mouth on the tongue. It should touch the roof of the mouth to stimulate the baby's sucking reflex. Hold the bottle like a pencil. Keep the bottle tipped so that the nipple stays filled with milk and the baby does not suck in air.

Hold your baby close for feedings. This should be a pleasant time for social interaction and cuddling. Some newborns take longer to feed than others. Be patient. It may be necessary to keep the baby awake and encourage continued sucking. Moving the nipple gently in the baby's mouth may stimulate more sucking.

Some newborns swallow air when sucking. Give your baby a chance to burp several times during early feedings. As your baby gets older and you get more experienced, you will know when to stop for burping.

If your baby fusses or cries in between feedings, check the diaper to see if he or she needs to be changed and see if the baby needs to be picked up and cuddled. If the baby continues to cry and acts hungry, then he or she needs to be fed. Babies do not get hungry on a schedule.

Place your baby on the right side after feedings so that air bubbles can come up easily. A rolled-up receiving blanket or small towel against the baby's back will keep him or her in the side-lying position. Some babies sleep better on their backs. To decrease the risk of SIDS, however, it is important not to put your baby to sleep stomach down.

The stools (bowel movements) of a formula-fed newborn are yellow and soft but formed. The baby will probably have a stool during or after each feeding in the first 2 weeks, but this will then gradually decrease to one to two stools each day.

HOME CARE *Patient Instructions for Self-Care*
Formula Preparation and Feeding—cont'd
SAFETY TIPS
- Babies should be held and never left alone while feeding. Do not prop the bottle. The baby could inhale formula or choke on any that was spit up.
- Know how to use the bulb syringe in case your baby should choke.
- Drinking bottles of formula or juice while falling asleep can cause tooth decay in young children (nursing bottle caries).

FORMULA PREPARATION
- Wash your hands and clean the bottle, nipple, and can opener carefully before preparing formula.
- If new nipples seem too hard, they can be softened by boiling them in water for 5 minutes before use.
- Read the label on the container of formula and mix it exactly according to the directions.
- Use tap water to mix concentrated or powdered formula unless directed otherwise by your baby's physician or nurse.
- Test the size of the nipple hole by holding a prepared bottle upside down. The formula should drip from the nipple. If it runs in a stream, the hole is too big and should not be used. If it has to be shaken for the formula to come out, the hole is too small. You can either buy a new nipple or enlarge the hole by boiling the nipple for 5 minutes with a sewing needle inserted in the hole.
- If a nipple collapses when your baby sucks, loosen the nipple ring a little to let in air.
- Opened cans of ready-to-feed or concentrated formula should be covered and refrigerated. Any unused portions must be discarded after 48 hours.
- Bottles or cans of unopened formula can be stored at room temperature.
- If the formula is refrigerated, warm it by placing the bottle in a pan of hot water. Never use a microwave to warm any food to be given to a baby. Test the temperature of the formula by letting a few drops fall on the inside of your wrist. If the formula feels comfortably warm to you, it is the correct temperature.

RESEARCH
Breastfeeding Incidence after Early Discharge
Although studies have demonstrated that early discharge is safe, health care providers have questioned the effect of early discharge on breastfeeding maintenance. The purpose of this study was to determine if the incidence of breastfeeding at 6 to 8 weeks postpartum differs for a mother who had a 48-hour length of hospital stay as compared with a mother with a 24-hour length of stay.

Factors that influenced the change from breastfeeding to bottle feeding were examined. A convenience sample of 101 primiparous breastfeeding women who had a vaginal birth of a healthy newborn were asked to complete a survey via the telephone between 6 and 8 weeks postpartum. There was no difference in the incidence of breastfeeding at 6 and 8 weeks postpartum for mothers who had a 48-hour length of stay and mothers who had a 24-hour length of stay with a home visit.

CLINICAL APPLICATION OF THE STUDY
Regardless of the length of hospital stay, mothers will decide on the method of feeding that best fits with herself, her baby, and the family situation. Nurses assisting patients with newborn nutrition and feeding need to give information to mothers about all feeding options so that they can make informed feeding choices, whether the choice is breastfeeding, bottle feeding, or a combination.

Source: Quinn A, Koepsell D & Haller S: Breastfeeding incidence after early discharge and factors influencing breastfeeding cessation, *J Obstet Gynecol Neonatal Nurs* 26(3):289, 1997.

*K*EY POINTS
- Human breast milk is species specific and is the recommended form of nutrition for infants, providing immunologic protection against many infections and diseases.
- Breast milk changes in composition with each stage of lactation, during each feeding, and as the infant grows.
- During the prenatal period, parents should be informed of the benefits of breastfeeding for infants, mothers, families, and society.
- Infants should be breastfed as soon as possible after birth and at least 8 to 10 times per day thereafter.
- There are specific, measurable indications that the infant is breastfeeding effectively.
- Breast milk production is based on a supply-meets-demand principle: the more the infant nurses, the greater the milk supply.

and decreased intake of breast milk or formula. The infant cannot communicate feeling full as can an older child, who is able to turn the head away. The proper balance of carbohydrate, protein, and fat for an infant to grow properly is in the breast milk or formula.

The infant's individual growth pattern should help determine the right time to start solids. The primary health care provider will advise when to introduce solid foods. The schedule for introducing solid foods and the type of foods to serve will be discussed during well-baby supervision visits with the pediatrician or pediatric nurse practitioner.

Continued

KEY POINTS—cont'd

- Commercial infant formulas provide satisfactory nutrition for most infants.
- All infants should be held for feedings.
- Parents should be instructed about the types of commercial infant formulas, proper preparation for feeding, and correct feeding technique.
- Unmodified cow's milk is inappropriate for infants during the first year of life.
- Solid foods should be started after 6 months of age.
- Nurses must be knowledgeable about feeding methods and provide education and support for families.

CRITICAL THINKING EXERCISES

1 *Develop a teaching plan for a prenatal breastfeeding class for first-time parents using culturally appropriate materials. List visual/teaching aids that might be useful. (Remember to include the fathers!) How would your plan differ for adolescents or older (over age 35 years) mothers and fathers?*

2 *Mrs. Alvarez, a multipara who gave birth 24 hours ago, is attempting to breastfeed her new daughter. With her first child, she "gave up" breastfeeding at 2 weeks because of cracked, bleeding nipples. Mrs. Alvarez states that she is determined to breastfeed this baby. What are factors that will affect her success or failure? What nursing interventions are appropriate to institute? How would you evaluate success or failure?*

3 *Mrs. Singer has a 1-week-old son who has been breastfeeding "well." She awoke this morning with headache, chills, fever of 38° C, and body aches. She noticed a reddened area on the inner aspect of her right breast after her shower. State the common breastfeeding complication she seems to be exhibiting. What is your plan of action, and what advice can you give her?*

References

American Academy of Pediatrics: The transfer of drugs and other chemicals into human breast milk, *Pediatrics* 93(1):137, 1994.

American Academy of Pediatrics, Work Group on Breastfeeding: Breastfeeding and the use of human milk, *Pediatrics* 100(6):1035, 1997.

Arnold L & Tully M: *Guidelines for the establishment and operation of a donor human milk bank,* ed 6, West Hartford, Conn, 1996, Human Milk Banking Association of North America.

Association of Women's Health, Obstetric, and Neonatal Nurses: *Standards and guidelines for professional nursing practice in the care of women and newborns,* ed 5, Washington, DC, 1998, The Association.

Barnard J: Gastrointestinal disorders due to cow's milk consumption, *Pediatr Ann* 26(4):244, 1997.

Bar-Yam N & Darby L: Fathers and breastfeeding: a review of the literature, *J Hum Lact* 13(1):45, 1997.

Brown L et al.: Use of human milk for low birthweight infants, *Online J Know Synth Nurs* 3(27):1, 1996.

Choudhry U: Traditional practices of women from India: pregnancy, childbirth, and newborn care, *J Obstet Gynecol Neonatal Nurs* 26(5):533, 1997.

Dewey K et al.: A randomized study of the effects of aerobic exercise by lactating women on breast-milk volume and composition, *N Engl J Med* 330(7):449, 1994.

Dewey K, Heinig M & Nommsen-Rivers L: *Differences in morbidity between breastfed and formula-fed infants,* J Pediatr 126(5 Part 1):696, 1995.

Florey C, Leech A & Blackhall A: Infant feeding and mental and motor development at 18 months of age in first born singletons, *Int J Epidemiol* (24 Suppl 1):S21, 1995.

Food and Nutrition Board: *Recommended dietary allowances,* Washington, DC, 1989, National Academy Press.

Ford R et al.: Breastfeeding and the risk of sudden infant death syndrome, *Int J Epidemiol* 22(5):885, 1993.

Fuchs S, Victoria C & Martines J: Case-control study of risk of dehydrating diarrhea in infant in the vulnerable period after full weaning, *BMJ* 313(7054):391, 1996.

Goldman A: The immune system of human milk: antimicrobial, antiinflammatory and immunomodulating properties, *Pediatr Infect Dis J* 12(8):664, 1993.

Grossman L et al.: The effect of postpartum lactation counseling on the duration of breast-feeding in low-income women, *Am J Dis Child* 144(4):471, 1990.

Hahn-Zoric M et al.: Antibody responses to parenteral and oral vaccines are impaired by conventional and low protein formulas as compared to breastfeeding, *Acta Paediatr Scand* 79(12):1137, 1990.

Halken S & Host A: Prevention of allergic disease: exposure to food allergens and dietetic intervention, *Pediatr Allergy Immunol* 7(9 suppl):102, 1996.

Hirose K et al.: A large-scale, hospital-based case-control study of risk factors of breast cancer according to menopausal status, *Jpn J Cancer Res* 86(2):146, 1995.

Howie P et al.: Protective effect of breastfeeding against infection, *Br Med J* 300(6716):11, 1990.

Huml S: Cracked nipples in the breastfeeding mother, *Adv Nurse Pract,* April:1, 1995.

Kavanaugh K et al.: The rewards outweigh the efforts: breastfeeding outcomes for mothers of preterm infants, *J Hum Lact* 13(1):15, 1997.

Kelsey J: Hormonal contraception and lactation, *J Hum Lact* 12(4):315, 1996.

Lavergne N: Does application of tea bags to sore nipples while breastfeeding provide effective relief? *J Obstet Gynecol Neonatal Nurs* 26(1):53, 1997.

Lawrence R: *Breastfeeding: a guide for the medical profession,* ed 4, St Louis, 1994, Mosby.

Lawrence R: *A review of the medical benefits and contraindications to breastfeeding in the United States,* Maternal and Child Health Technical Information Bulletin, US Department of Health and Human Services, 1997.

Lopez-Alarcon M, Villalpando S & Fajardo A: Breastfeeding lowers the frequency and duration of acute respiratory infections and diarrhea in infants under six months of age, *J Nutr* 127(3):436, 1997.

Lorick G: Untimely weaning: assisting the mother who may grieve, *Int J Childbirth Educ* 8(2):41, 1993.

Lucas A & Morley R: Breast milk and subsequent intelligence quotient in children born preterm, *Lancet* 339(8788):261, 1991.

Lucas A et al.: A randomised multicentre study of human milk versus formula and later development in preterm infants, *Arch Dis Child* 70(2):F141, 1994.

Meier P: *Professional guide to breastfeeding premature infants,* Columbus, Ohio, 1997, Ross Products Division, Abbott Laboratories.

Meier P & Brown L: State of the science: breastfeeding for mothers and low birthweight infants, *Nurs Clin North Am* 31(2):351, 1996.

Melton L et al.: Influence of breastfeeding and other reproductive factors on bone mass later in life, *Osteoporosis Int* 3(2):76, 1993.

Montgomery D & Splett P: Economic benefit of breastfeeding infants enrolled in WIC, *J Am Diet Assoc* 97(4):379, 1997.

Morse J, Jehle C & Gamble D: Initiating breastfeeding: a world survey of the timing of postpartum breastfeeding, *Int J Nurse Stud* 27(3):303, 1990.

Naylor A et al.: Oral water intoxication, *Am J Dis Child* 146(8):893, 1992.

Newman J: Water intoxication: a problem of bottle-feeding, *Am J Dis Child* 146(10):1131, 1992.

Rassin D et al.: Acculturation and the initiation of breastfeeding, *J Clin Epidemiol* 47(7):739, 1994.

Riordan J: The cost of not breastfeeding: a commentary, *J Hum Lact* 13(2):93, 1997.

Riordan J & Auerbach K: *Breastfeeding and human lactation,* Boston, 1993, Jones & Bartlett.

Roberts K: A comparison of chilled cabbage leaves and chilled gel-paks in reducing breast engorgement, *J Hum Lact* 11(1):17, 1995.

Rosenblatt K et al.: Prolonged lactation and endometrial cancer, *Int J Epidemiol* 24(3):499, 1995.

Ryan A: The resurgence of breastfeeding in the United States, *Pediatrics* 99(4):596, 1997.

Saarinen U & Kajosaari M: Breastfeeding as prophylaxis against atopic disease: prospective follow-up study until 17 years old, *Lancet* 346(8982):1065, 1995.

Sassen M, Brand R & Grote J: Breastfeeding and acute otitis media, *Am J Otolaryngol* 15(5):351, 1994.

Shu X et al.: Infant breastfeeding and the risk of childhood lymphoma and leukemia, *Int J Epidemiol* 24(1):27, 1995.

Tuttle C & Dewey K: Potential cost savings for Medi-Cal, AFDC, food stamps, and WIC programs associated with increasing breastfeeding among low-income Hmong women in California, *J Am Diet Assoc* 96(9):885, 1996.

Walker M: A fresh look at the risks of artificial infant feeding, *J Hum Lact* 9(2):97, 1993.

Widstrom A, Ransjo-Arvidsson A & Christensson K: *Breastfeeding is the baby's choice,* Richmond, Va, 1993, BGK Enterprises Production.

Worthington-Roberts B & Williams S: *Nutrition in pregnancy and lactation,* ed 5, St Louis, 1993, Mosby.

CHAPTER

Assessment for Risk Factors

CYNTHIA GARRETT

LEARNING OBJECTIVES

- *Define the key terms.*
- *Explore the scope of high-risk pregnancy.*
- *Discuss regionalization of health care services.*
- *Examine risk factors identified through history, physical examination, and diagnostic techniques.*
- *Describe diagnostic techniques and the implications of findings.*
- *Explain diagnostic techniques to patients and their families.*

KEY TERMS

acoustic stimulation test
alpha-fetoprotein (AFP)
amniocentesis
amniotic fluid index (AFI)
amniotic fluid volume (AFV)
biophysical profile (BPP)
biparietal diameter (BPD)
chorionic villus sampling (CVS)
contraction stress test (CST)
daily fetal movement count (DFMC)
Doppler ultrasound
fetal activity determination (FAD)
intrauterine growth restriction (IUGR)
magnetic resonance imaging (MRI)
meconium-stained amniotic fluid
nipple stimulation contraction test
nonstress test (NST)
percutaneous umbilical blood sampling (PUBS)
triple marker test
ultrasound
uteroplacental insufficiency (UPI)

Approximately 500,000 of the 4 million births that occur in the United States each year will be categorized as high risk because of maternal or fetal complications. Identification of the risks, together with appropriate and timely intervention during the perinatal period, can prevent morbidity and mortality among mothers and infants.

With the changing demographics in the United States, more women and families can be identified as at-risk because of factors other than biophysical criteria. The increasing numbers of homeless, single, or uninsured pregnant women who have no access to prenatal care during any stage of pregnancy and the behaviors and lifestyles that pose a risk to the health of the mother and fetus contribute to the problem (Fogel & Lewallen, 1995).

Care of these high-risk women requires the unified efforts of medical and nursing personnel. Factors associated with a diagnosis of high risk are identified in this chapter; diagnostic techniques used to monitor the maternal-fetal unit are emphasized.

▌ DEFINITION AND SCOPE OF THE PROBLEM

A high-risk pregnancy is one in which the life or health of the mother or fetus is jeopardized by a disorder coincidental with or unique to pregnancy. For the mother the high-risk status arbitrarily extends through the puerperium (30 days after childbirth). Maternal complications are usually resolved within 1 month of birth, but neonatal morbidity may continue for months or years.

Advances in the management of disorders that affect pregnant women have resulted in a significant decrease in maternal mortality and morbidity rates. In the United States, maternal mortality rates have declined from 376 deaths per 100,000 live births in 1940 to 8.3 per 100,000 in 1994 (March of Dimes StatBook, 1997).

However, the decline in perinatal mortality and morbidity is not as significant and needs to be examined when the scope of high-risk pregnancy is being considered. Infant mortality rates have shown improvement, dropping from 10 per 1,000 live births in 1970 to 7.2 per 1,000 live births in 1996, the lowest ever recorded in the United States (Guyer et al., 1997). Yet, compared with other developed countries, the United States ranks twentieth in infant mortality rate (Guyer et al., 1997).

High-risk pregnancy represents a critical problem in modern medical and nursing care. The new social emphasis on the quality of life and the wanted child has resulted in a reduction of family size and the number of unwanted pregnancies. At the same time, technologic advances have enabled pregnancies in previously infertile couples. As a consequence, emphasis is on the safe birth of normal infants who can develop to their fullest potential. Scientific and technologic advances have allowed perinatal health care to reach a level far beyond that previously available.

Although pregnancy is often referred to as a maturational crisis, the diagnosis of high risk imposes another crisis, a situational one (e.g., loss of pregnancy before the anticipated date, development of gestational diabetes mellitus with its potential complications, or birth of a neonate who does not meet cultural, societal, or familial norms and expectations).

Maternal Health Problems

The leading causes of maternal death attributable to pregnancy differ over the world. In general, three major causes have persisted for the last 35 years: hypertensive disorders, infection, and hemorrhage. The three leading causes of maternal mortality today are pregnancy-induced hypertension, hemorrhage, and pulmonary embolism (Grimes, 1994).

In 1994, 270 women in the United States died of complications of pregnancy, childbirth, and the puerperium (National Center for Health Statistics, 1995). Factors that are strongly related to maternal death include age (less than 20 years and greater than 40 years), low educational attainment, unmarried status, and nonwhite race (Grimes, 1994). Nonwhite women continue to have a maternal mortality rate higher than that of Caucasian women. African-American women were four times more likely to die than Caucasian women (Mortality Patterns—1993, 1996). The rates for anemia, chronic hypertension, and eclampsia were significantly higher for African-American mothers than for Caucasian mothers; the risk of a low-birth-weight (less than 2,500 gm) infant or a preterm birth was greater for African-American than for Caucasian mothers for each of the medical risk factors associated with these outcomes. Native-American mothers had the highest incidence of the four most frequently reported medical risk factors (anemia, diabetes, pregnancy-associated hypertension, and uterine bleeding) compared with all other racial or ethnic groups (National Center for Health Statistics, 1994). Effects of coagulation disorders, such as embolism, are also a significant cause of maternal morbidity and mortality. African-American women have a higher incidence of pregnancy complications associated with clotting problems.

Although the overall number of maternal deaths is small, maternal mortality remains a significant problem because a high proportion of deaths are preventable, primarily through improving the access to and use of prenatal care services. Educating the public about the importance of obtaining early and regular care during pregnancy is a function that nurses are well positioned to perform.

Fetal and Neonatal Health Problems

Fetal and neonatal health problems are described under certain categories: fetal death (demise), neonatal death, perinatal death, perinatal death rate, and infant mortality. (Definitions for these terms are found in Chapter 1.) The incidence of each disorder that results in infant mortality is expressed as the number of deaths per 1,000 live births. The infant mortality rate includes neonatal deaths.

The leading causes of death in the neonatal period are congenital anomalies, disorders relating to short gestation and low birth weight, respiratory distress syndrome, and the effects of maternal complications. African-American women are twice as likely as Caucasian women to have premature births, low-birth-weight infants, and infant and fetal deaths (National Center for Health Statistics, 1994).

Although a number of perinatal problems have benefited from improved treatment, congenital anomalies continue to be the leading cause of infant mortality. Some reduction in infant mortality rate might be achieved by a reduction in preterm birth (Wilcox et al., 1995), but progress has not yet been made in this area. Increased rates of survival during the neonatal period have resulted largely from high-quality prenatal care and the improvement in perinatal services, including technologic advances in neonatal intensive care and obstetrics. The four leading causes of death in the postneonatal period are sudden infant death syndrome, congenital anomalies, injuries, and infections.

Commitment at a national, state, and local level is required to reduce the infant mortality rate and eliminate racial and ethnic differences in pregnancy outcomes. Financial, educational, sociocultural, and logistic barriers to care must be removed so that pregnant women can seek and receive health services and infant mortality rates can be reduced.

Regionalization of Health Care Services

Mortality rate decreases when a woman's high-risk status is identified and intensive care is applied. Follow-up studies have shown that such identification and intervention can dramatically reduce serious residual handicaps (physical and mental) in surviving infants.

Each hospital cannot develop and maintain the full spectrum of medical, nursing, and health care specialists; laboratory capabilities; and equipment necessary to provide optimal care for all patients. As a consequence, regionalization of health care has emerged—facilities within a geographic region are organized to provide different levels of care. A regionalized system ideally includes primary care and three levels of facilities within the designated geographic area.

Centralized facilities with specialized personnel and equipment receive referrals from those facilities that provide care for low-risk conditions (level I facilities). Level I facilities have three primary functions: (1) management of normal pregnancy, labor, and childbirth; (2) early identification of high-risk pregnancy and high-risk neonates; and (3) provision of stabilization care in obstetric or neonatal emergencies.

Level II facilities provide care for specified types of maternal and neonatal complications and also offer a full range of maternity and neonatal care in uncomplicated cases. Staff members are educated and prepared for those particular complications, and appropriate equipment is available.

Level III facilities, the regional centers, have the capacity to manage complex disorders, both maternal and neonatal. Pregnant women are often transported to these centers before the birth of the baby to optimize maternal, fetal, and neonatal outcomes. The regional centers also provide outreach educational services for medical and nursing staff within the region.

Events occurring during the prenatal and intranatal periods can have adverse effects on the infant in later life. Serious biologic handicaps, health problems, obstetric disorders, and social deprivation may compromise the mother and infant in subtle or obvious ways. Identification of the high-risk patient is critical to minimize maternal and neonatal mortality or morbidity or both. By use of known risk factors that can identify high-risk patients prenatally or intrapartally, approximately 20% of pregnant women can be identified prenatally to be at risk; these women account for

55% of poor outcomes in pregnancy (American Academy of Pediatrics [AAP], American College of Obstetricians & Gynecologists [ACOG], 1997).

Assessment of Risk Factors

Pregnancies can be designated as high risk for any of several undesirable outcomes. Those considered to be at risk for uteroplacental insufficiency carry a serious threat for fetal growth restriction, intrauterine fetal death, intrapartum death, intrapartum fetal distress, and various types of neonatal morbidity.

In the past, risk factors were evaluated only from a medical viewpoint; thus only adverse medical, obstetric, or physiologic conditions were considered to place the patient at risk. Today, a more comprehensive approach to high-risk pregnancy is used. The factors associated with high-risk childbearing are grouped into broad categories based on threats to health and pregnancy outcome. Categories of risk include biophysical, psychosocial, sociodemographic, and environmental (Fogel & Lewallen, 1995) (Box 22-1).

- *Biophysical* risks include factors that originate within the mother or fetus and affect the development or functioning of either one or both.

BOX 22-1 *Categories of High-Risk Factors*

BIOPHYSICAL FACTORS

1. *Genetic considerations.* Genetic factors may interfere with normal fetal or neonatal development, result in congenital anomalies, or create difficulties for the mother. These factors include defective genes, transmissible inherited disorders and chromosome anomalies, multiple pregnancy, large fetal size, and ABO incompatibility.
2. *Nutritional status.* Adequate nutrition, without which fetal growth and development cannot proceed normally, is one of the most important determinants of pregnancy outcome. Conditions that influence nutritional status include young age; three pregnancies in the previous 2 years; tobacco, alcohol, or drug use; inadequate dietary intake because of chronic illness or food fads; inadequate or excessive weight gain; and hematocrit value less than 33%.
3. *Medical and obstetric disorders.* Complications of current and past pregnancies, obstetric-related illnesses, and pregnancy losses put the patient at risk (see Box 22-3).

PSYCHOSOCIAL FACTORS

1. *Smoking.* A strong, consistent, causal relationship has been established between maternal smoking and reduced birth weight. Risks include low-birth-weight infants, higher neonatal mortality rates, increased spontaneous abortions, and increased incidence of premature rupture of membranes. These risks are aggravated by low socioeconomic status, poor nutritional status, and concurrent use of alcohol.

2. *Caffeine.* Birth defects in humans have not been related to caffeine consumption. High intake (three or more cups of coffee per day) has been related to a slight decrease in birth weight.
3. *Alcohol.* Although its exact effects in pregnancy have not been quantified and its mode of action is largely unexplained, alcohol exerts adverse effects on the fetus, resulting in fetal alcohol syndrome, fetal alcohol effects, learning disabilities, and hyperactivity.
4. *Drugs.* The developing fetus may be adversely affected by drugs through several mechanisms. They can be teratogenic, cause metabolic disturbances, produce chemical effects, or cause depression or alteration of central nervous system function. This category includes medications prescribed by a health care provider or bought over the counter, as well as commonly abused drugs such as heroin, cocaine, and marijuana. (See Chapter 23 for more information about drug and alcohol abuse.)
5. *Psychologic status.* Childbearing triggers profound and complex physiologic, psychologic, and social changes, with evidence to suggest a relationship between emotional distress and birth complications. This risk factor includes conditions such as specific intrapsychic disturbances and addictive lifestyles; a history of child or spouse abuse; inadequate support systems; family disruption or dissolution; maternal role changes or conflicts; noncompliance with cultural norms; unsafe cultural, ethnic, or religious practices; and situational crises.

- *Psychosocial* risks are comprised of maternal behaviors and adverse lifestyles that have a negative effect on the health of the mother or fetus. These risks may include emotional distress and disturbed interpersonal relationships, as well as inadequate social support and unsafe cultural practices (Box 22-2).
- *Sociodemographic* risks arise from the mother and her family. These risks may place the mother and fetus at risk (Box 22-3).

- *Environmental* factors include hazards in the workplace and the woman's general environment.

Risk factors are interrelated and cumulative in their effects and are shown in Fig. 22-1. Risk factors of the postpartum woman and newborn are shown in Box 22-4. The development of a comprehensive database for pregnancy risk assessment will help generate appropriate nursing diagnoses. For example, use of functional health patterns can be the basis for an assessment tool (Box 22-5).

BOX 22-1 Categories of High-Risk Factors—cont'd

SOCIODEMOGRAPHIC FACTORS

1. *Low income.* Poverty underlies many other risk factors and leads to inadequate financial resources for food and prenatal care, poor general health, increased risk of medical complications of pregnancy, and greater prevalence of adverse environmental influences.
2. *Lack of prenatal care.* Failure to diagnose and treat complications early is a major risk factor arising from financial barriers or lack of access to care; depersonalization of the system, resulting in long waits, routine visits, variability in health care personnel, and unpleasant physical surroundings; lack of understanding of the need for early and continued care or cultural beliefs that do not support this need; and fear of the health care system and its providers.
3. *Age.* Women at both ends of the childbearing age spectrum have a higher incidence of poor outcomes; however, age may not be a risk factor in all cases. Both physiologic and psychologic risks should be evaluated.
   Adolescents—More complications are seen in young mothers (less than 15 years old), who have a 60% higher mortality rate than those over age 20, and in pregnancies occurring less than 3 years after menarche. Complications include anemia, pregnancy-induced hypertension (PIH), prolonged labor, and contracted pelvis and cephalopelvic disproportion. Long-term social implications of early motherhood are lower educational status, lower income, increased dependence on government support programs, higher divorce rates, and higher parity.
   Mature mothers—The risks to older mothers are not from age alone but from other considerations such as number and spacing of previous pregnancies; genetic disposition of the parents; and medical history, lifestyle, nutrition, and prenatal care. The increased likelihood of chronic diseases and complications that arise from more invasive medical management of a pregnancy and labor combined with demographic characteristics put an older woman at risk. Medical conditions more likely to be experienced by mature women include hypertension

and PIH, diabetes, extended labor, cesarean birth, placenta previa, abruptio placentae, and mortality. Her fetus is at greater risk for low birth weight and macrosomia, chromosomal abnormalities, congenital malformations, and neonatal mortality.

4. *Parity.* The number of previous pregnancies is a risk factor that is associated with age and includes all first pregnancies, especially a first pregnancy at either end of the childbearing-age continuum. The incidence of PIH and dystocia is higher with a first birth.
5. *Marital status.* The increased mortality and morbidity rates for nonmarried women, including a greater risk for PIH, are often related to inadequate prenatal care and a younger childbearing age.
6. *Residence.* The availability and quality of prenatal care varies widely with geographic residence. Women in metropolitan areas have more prenatal visits than those in rural areas, who have fewer opportunities for specialized care and consequently a higher incidence of maternal mortality. Health care in the inner city, where residents are usually poorer and begin childbearing earlier and continue longer, may be of lower quality than in a more affluent neighborhood.
7. *Ethnicity.* Although ethnicity itself is not a major risk factor, race is an indicator of other sociodemographic risk factors. Nonwhite women are more than three times as likely as Caucasian women to die of pregnancy-related causes. African-American babies have the highest rates of prematurity and low birth weight, with the infant mortality rate among African-Americans being more than double that for Caucasians.

ENVIRONMENTAL FACTORS

Various environmental substances can affect fertility and fetal development, the chance of a live birth, and the child's subsequent mental and physical development. Environmental influences include infections; radiation; chemicals such as pesticides, therapeutic drugs, illicit drugs, industrial pollutants, cigarette smoke; stress; and diet. Paternal exposure to mutagenic agents in the workplace has been associated with an increased risk of spontaneous abortion.

Antepartum Cultural Assessment

All cultures recognize pregnancy as a special transitional period and have particular customs and beliefs that dictate behavior during this time. In the antepartum period the nurse should assess the following:
- Beliefs of whether pregnancy is a state of illness or health
- Behavioral expectations of the mother and of the health care provider
- Dietary prescriptions or restrictions (e.g., hot/cold balance theory, pica)
- Activity restrictions or prescriptions (e.g., use of massage)
- Availability of advice (e.g., from whom and at what time advice will be sought and when prenatal care will begin [if at all])
- Considerations of modesty

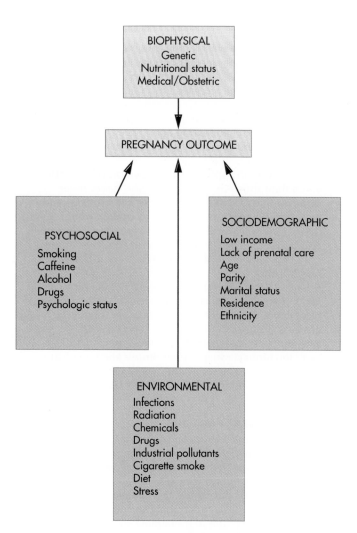

Fig. **22-1** Interrelationship of risk factors that may affect pregnancy outcome. (Modified from Fogel C & Woods N: *Health care of women,* Thousand Oaks, Calif, 1995, Sage).

Specific Pregnancy Problems and Related Risk Factors

PRETERM LABOR

Age less than 16 or more than 35 years
Low socioeconomic status
Maternal weight below 50 kg (110 lb)
Poor nutrition
Previous preterm birth
Incompetent cervix
Uterine anomalies
Smoking
Drug addiction and alcohol abuse
Pyelonephritis, pneumonia
Multiple gestation
Anemia
Abnormal fetal presentation
Premature rupture of membranes
Placental abnormalities
Infection

POLYHYDRAMNIOS

Diabetes mellitus
Multiple gestation
Fetal congenital anomalies
Isoimmunization (Rh or ABO)
Nonimmune hydrops
Abnormal fetal presentation

INTRAUTERINE GROWTH RESTRICTION (IUGR)

Multiple gestation
Poor nutrition
Maternal cyanotic heart disease
Chronic hypertension
Pregnancy-induced hypertension
Recurrent antepartum hemorrhage
Smoking
Maternal diabetes with vascular problems
Fetal infections
Fetal cardiovascular anomalies
Drug addiction and alcohol abuse
Fetal congenital anomalies
Hemoglobinopathies

OLIGOHYDRAMNIOS

Renal agenesis (Potter's syndrome)
Prolonged rupture of membranes
IUGR
Intrauterine fetal death

POSTTERM PREGNANCY

Anencephaly
Placental sulfatase deficiency
Perinatal hypoxia, acidosis
Placental insufficiency

CHROMOSOMAL ABNORMALITIES

Maternal age 35 years or more
Balanced translocation (maternal and paternal)

From DeCherney A & Pernol M, editors: *Current obstetric and gynecologic diagnosis and treatment,* ed 8, Norwalk, Conn, 1994, Appleton & Lange.

BOX 22-4   *Factors that Place the Postpartum Woman and Neonate at High Risk*

THE MOTHER
Hemorrhage
Infection
Abnormal vital signs
Traumatic labor or birth
Psychosocial factors

THE INFANT (FOR ADMISSION TO NICU)
High-Risk Category
Infants who continue with or develop signs of RDS or
  other respiratory distress
Asphyxiated infants (Apgar score <6 at 5 min),
  resuscitation required at birth
Preterm infants, dysmature infants
Infants with cyanosis or suspected cardiovascular
  disease, persistent cyanosis
Infants with major congenital malformations requiring
  surgery, chromosomal anomalies
Infants with convulsions, sepsis, hemorrhagic diathesis,
  or shock
Meconium aspiration syndrome

CNS depression for more than 24 hr
Hypoglycemia
Hypocalcemia
Hyperbilirubinemia

Moderate Risk
Dysmaturity
Prematurity (weight between 2,000 and 2,500 g)
Apgar score <5 at 1 min
Feeding problems
Multifetal birth
Transient tachypnea
Hypomagnesemia or hypermagnesemia
Hypoparathyroidism
Failure to gain weight
Jitteriness or hyperactivity
Cardiac anomalies not requiring immediate
  catheterization
Heart murmur
Anemia
CNS depression for less than 24 hr

NICU, Neonatal intensive care unit; *RDS,* respiratory distress syndrome; *CNS,* central nervous system.

BOX 22-5   *Assessment for High-Risk Pregnancy Using Functional Health Patterns*

For each of the following functional health patterns the
nurse includes questions that will provide data about
the individual woman, her family, her community, and
her cultural practices and beliefs:
• Health-perception/health management pattern
  Current health, past medical history, family medical
    history, environmental/chemical exposure, family
    decision making about health, community
    resources, beliefs about health care during
    pregnancy
• Nutritional-metabolic pattern
  Nutritional status, knowledge of pregnancy needs,
    pregnancy discomforts, community resources (WIC),
    cultural eating practices
• Elimination pattern
  Urinary and bowel patterns, family or cultural practices
    (laxatives), community waste/sanitation services
• Activity-exercise pattern
  Usual exercise, recreation, community resources,
    cultural practices or taboos for activities during
    pregnancy
• Sleep-rest pattern
  Usual sleep patterns, use of remedies, family sleep
    arrangements, cultural beliefs about sleep and rest in
    pregnancy

• Cognitive-perceptive pattern
  Communication problems, knowledge deficits about
    pregnancy and birth (individual and family),
    community resources for support for high-risk
    pregnant patients, cultural beliefs about pain and its
    management
• Self-perception/self-concept pattern
  Body image, responses of family to high-risk
    pregnancy, housing conditions, cultural practices
    about parenting
• Role-relationship pattern
  Feelings of security, occupation, hobbies, family living
    arrangements, community resources
• Sexuality-reproductive pattern
  Sexual activities, problems, restrictions, previous
    obstetric history, current obstetric status, cultural
    beliefs about sexual practices during pregnancy
• Coping-stress pattern
  Life stressors, losses experienced, coping mechanisms,
    support systems, community resources, spiritual or
    religious practices or beliefs that are important

Data from Gilbert E & Harmon J: *Manual of high risk pregnancy and delivery,* ed 2, St Louis, 1998, Mosby; Gordon M: *Nursing diagnosis: process and application,* ed 3, St Louis, 1994, Mosby.

ANTEPARTUM TESTING/ BIOPHYSICAL ASSESSMENT

The major expected outcome of antepartum testing is the detection of potential fetal compromise. Ideally, the technique used identifies fetal compromise before intrauterine asphyxia of the fetus so that the health care provider can take measures to prevent or minimize adverse perinatal outcomes. No single test can provide this information. The results of such tests must be interpreted in light of the complete clinical picture.

Daily Fetal Movement Count

Assessment of fetal activity by the mother is a simple yet valuable method for monitoring the condition of the fetus. The **daily fetal movement count (DFMC)** can be done at home, is noninvasive, is simple to understand, and usually does not interfere with a daily routine. The presence of movements is generally a reassuring sign of fetal health.

Several protocols are used for counting. Except for establishing a very low number of daily fetal movements or a trend toward decreased motion, the clinical value of the absolute number of fetal movements has not been established, except in the situation in which fetal movements cease entirely for 12 hours (the fetal alarm signal). Generally, a count of less than three fetal movements within 1 hour warrants further evaluation by nonstress or contraction stress testing, biophysical profile, or a combination of these. Patients should be taught the significance of fetal movements, the procedure for counting that is to be used, and how to record findings on a daily fetal movement record.

> **NURSE ALERT** *In assessing fetal movements it is important to remember that they are usually not present during the fetal sleep cycle; they may be temporarily reduced if the woman is taking depressant medications, drinking alcohol, or smoking a cigarette; and they do not decrease as the woman nears term.*

Ultrasonography

Sound is a form of wave energy that causes small particles in a medium to oscillate. The frequency of sound, which refers to the number of peaks or waves that traverse a given point per unit of time, is expressed in hertz (Hz). Sound with a frequency of one cycle, or one peak per second, has a frequency of 1 Hz. When directional beams of sound strike an object, an echo is returned. The time delay between the emission of the sound and the return of the echo and the direction of the echo are noted. From these data the distance and location of an object can be calculated.

Diagnostic ultrasonography is an important technique in antepartum fetal surveillance. **Ultrasound** is sound having a frequency higher than that detectable by humans, that is, greater than 20,000 Hz. Diagnostic ultrasound instruments operate within a frequency range of 2 million to 10 million Hz (or 2 to 10 MHz), which is below the range used by sonar and radar equipment.

Ultrasound can be done abdominally or transvaginally during pregnancy. Both produce a three-dimensional view from which a pictorial image is obtained. Abdominal ultrasonography is more useful after the first trimester when the pregnant uterus becomes an abdominal organ. For the procedure the woman usually needs to have a full bladder to get a better image of the fetus. Transmission gel or paste is applied to the abdomen before a transducer is moved over the skin to enhance transmission and reception of the sound waves.

Transvaginal ultrasonography, in which the probe is inserted into the vagina, allows pelvic anatomy to be evaluated in greater detail and intrauterine pregnancy to be diagnosed earlier (Cunningham et al., 1997). A transvaginal ultrasound examination is well tolerated by most patients because it alleviates the need for a full bladder. It is especially useful in obese patients whose thick abdominal layers cannot be penetrated adequately by an abdominal approach. Transvaginal ultrasonography is optimally used in the first trimester to detect ectopic pregnancies, monitor the developing embryo, help identify abnormalities, and help establish gestational age. In some instances, it may be used as an adjunct to abdominal scanning to evaluate second- and third-trimester pregnancies.

Levels of ultrasonography

Perinatal care providers and ultrasonographers have come to a tentative agreement on terminology describing two different levels of ultrasonography. The basic screening or limited examination is used most commonly and can be performed by ultrasonographers or other health care professionals, including nurses, who have had special training. Indications for limited ultrasonography are described in detail in the next section; its primary use is to detect fetal viability, determine the presentation of the fetus, assess gestational age, locate the placenta, and determine amniotic fluid volume. Targeted or comprehensive examinations are performed if a patient is suspected of carrying an anatomically or a physiologically abnormal fetus. Indications for a comprehensive examination include abnormal findings on clinical examination, especially with polyhydramnios or oligohydramnios, elevated alpha-fetoprotein (AFP) levels, and a history of offspring with anomalies that can be detected by ultrasound. Comprehensive ultrasonography is performed by highly trained and experienced personnel.

Indications for use

Major indications for obstetric sonography appear by trimester in Table 22-1. During the first trimester, ultrasound examination is performed to obtain information of (1) number, size, and location of gestational sacs; (2) presence or absence of fetal cardiac and body movements; (3) presence

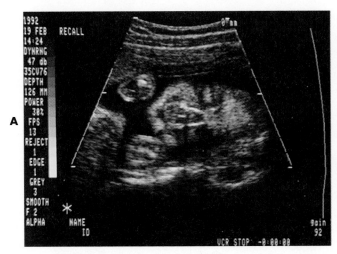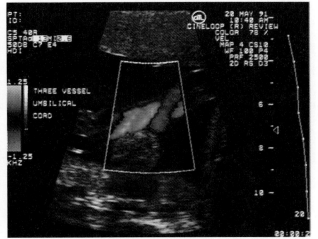

Fig. 22-2 Two views of the fetus during ultrasonography. **A,** Fetal face (20 weeks). **B,** Umbilical cord (26 weeks). (Courtesy Advanced Technology Laboratories, Bothell, Wash.)

TABLE 22-1	*Major Uses of Ultrasonography during Pregnancy*	
FIRST TRIMESTER	**SECOND TRIMESTER**	**THIRD TRIMESTER**
Confirm pregnancy	Establish or confirm dates	Confirm gestational age
Confirm viability	Confirm viability	Confirm viability
Determine gestational age	Detect polyhydramnios,	Detect macrosomia
Rule out ectopic pregnancy	oligohydramnios	Detect congenital anomalies
Detect multiple gestation	Detect congenital anomalies	Detect IUGR
Visualization during chorionic	Detect intrauterine growth	Determine fetal position
villus sampling	restriction (IUGR)	Detect placenta previa or abruptio
Detect maternal abnormalities	Confirm placenta placement	placentae
such as bicornuate uterus,	Visualization during amniocentesis	Visualization during amniocentesis,
ovarian cysts, fibroids		external version
		Biophysical profile
		Amniotic fluid volume assessment
		Doppler flow studies
		Detect placental maturity

or absence of uterine abnormalities (e.g., bicornuate uterus or fibroids) or adnexal masses (e.g., ovarian cysts or an ectopic pregnancy); (4) date of pregnancy (by measuring the crown-rump length); and (5) presence and location of an intrauterine contraceptive device.

During the second and third trimesters, information on the following conditions is sought: (1) fetal viability, number, position, gestational age, growth pattern, and anomalies (Fig. 22-2); (2) amniotic fluid volume; (3) placental location and maturity; (4) uterine fibroids and anomalies; and (5) adnexal masses.

Findings

Ultrasonography has led to earlier diagnoses, allowing therapy to be instituted early in the pregnancy and thereby decreasing the severity and duration of morbidity, both physical and emotional, for the family. For instance, early diagnosis of a fetal anomaly gives the family choices such as (1) intrauterine surgery or other therapy for the fetus, (2) termination of the pregnancy, or (3) preparation for the care of an infant with a disorder.

Fetal heart activity. Fetal heart activity can be demonstrated as early as 6 to 7 weeks by real-time echo scanners and at 10 to 12 weeks by Doppler mode. By 9 to 10 weeks, gestational trophoblastic disease can be diagnosed. Fetal death can be confirmed by lack of heart motion, the presence of fetal scalp edema, and maceration and overlap of the cranial bones.

Gestational age. Gestational dating by ultrasonography is indicated for conditions such as (1) uncertain dates for the last normal menstrual period, (2) recent discontinuation of oral contraceptives, (3) bleeding episode during the first trimester, (4) uterine size that does not agree with dates, and (5) other high-risk conditions.

During the first 18 weeks of gestation, ultrasonography provides an accurate assessment of gestational age because

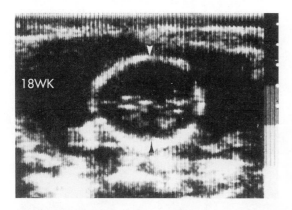

Fig. **22-3** Real-time image of fetal biparietal diameters at 18 weeks. (From Athay P & Haddock F: *Ultrasound in obstetrics and gynecology*, ed 2, St Louis, 1985, Mosby.)

TABLE 22-2	*Correlation of Fetal Weight and BPD*
BPD (CM)	**ESTIMATED FETAL WEIGHT**
8.2	2,290 gm
8.5	2,500 gm
8.8	2,730 gm
9.4	3,180 gm
10.0	3,630 gm
10.6	4,070 gm

most normal fetuses grow at the same rate. Accuracy is increased as the fetus ages because more than one variable is measured. The four methods of fetal age estimation used include: (1) determination of gestational sac dimensions (at about 8 weeks), (2) measurement of crown-rump length (between 7 and 14 weeks), (3) measurement of the **biparietal diameter (BPD)** (after 12 weeks), and (4) measurement of femur length (after 12 weeks). Fetal BPD at 36 weeks should be approximately 8.7 cm. Term pregnancy and fetal maturity can be diagnosed with some confidence if the biparietal measurement by ultrasound examination is greater than 9.8 cm (Fig. 22-3 and Table 22-2), especially when this is combined with appropriate femur length measurement.

In later gestational periods, serial measurements can provide a more accurate determination of fetal age. Two and preferably three composite measurements are recommended, at least 2 weeks apart, and these are plotted against standard fetal growth curves. This method, when applied between 24 and 32 weeks of gestation, yields an estimation error of 10 days more or less than the actual age (Manning, 1994).

Fetal growth. Fetal growth is determined by both intrinsic growth potential and environmental factors. Conditions that require ultrasound assessment of fetal growth include (1) poor maternal weight gain or pattern of weight gain, (2) previous **intrauterine growth restriction (IUGR)**, (3) chronic infections, (4) ingestion of drugs, (tobacco, alcohol, over-the-counter, and street drugs), (5) maternal diabetes mellitus, (6) hypertension, (6) multifetal pregnancy, and (7) other medical or surgical complications.

Serial evaluations of BPD and limb length can differentiate between size discrepancy resulting from inaccurate dates and true IUGR. IUGR may be symmetric (the fetus being small in all parameters) or asymmetric (head and body growth varying). Symmetric IUGR reflects a chronic or long-standing insult and may be caused by low genetic growth potential, intrauterine infection, undernutrition, heavy smoking, or chromosomal aberration. Asymmetric growth suggests an acute or late-occurring deprivation, such as

placental insufficiency resulting from hypertension, renal disease, or cardiovascular disease. Reduced fetal growth is still one of the most common conditions associated with stillbirth (Manning, 1994). Macrosomic infants (those weighing more than 4,000 g) are at increased risk for trauma during birth. In addition, fetal macrosomia associated with maternal glucose intolerance carries an increased risk of intrauterine fetal death (Manning, 1994).

Adjunct to amniocentesis, percutaneous umbilical blood sampling, and chorionic villus sampling. The safety of amniocentesis is increased when the positions of the fetus, placenta, and pockets of amniotic fluid can be identified accurately. Ultrasound scanning has reduced risks previously associated with amniocentesis, such as fetomaternal hemorrhage from a pierced placenta. Percutaneous umbilical blood sampling and chorionic villus sampling are also guided by ultrasonography to identify the cord and chorion frondosum accurately.

Fetal anatomy. Anatomic structures that may be identified by ultrasonography (depending on the gestational age) include the following: head (including ventricles and blood vessels), neck, spine, heart, stomach, small bowel, liver, kidneys, bladder, and limbs. Ultrasonography permits the confirmation of normal anatomy, as well as the detection of major fetal malformations. The presence of an anomaly may influence the location of birth (e.g., a delivery room versus a labor-delivery-recovery room or a level III center versus a level I institution) and the method of birth to optimize neonatal outcomes. More than 85% of all major anomalies can be detected by ultrasonography after 36 weeks of gestation. In general, the earlier in gestation a lesion is detected, the worse its prognostic significance (Manning, 1994).

The number of fetuses and their presentations may also be assessed by ultrasonography, allowing plans for therapy and mode of birth to be made in advance.

Placental position and function. The pattern of uterine and placental growth and the fullness of the maternal bladder influence the apparent location of the placenta by ultrasonography. During the first trimester, differentiation between the endometrium and small placenta is difficult. By 14 to 16 weeks the placenta is clearly defined, but if it is seen to be low lying, its relationship to the internal cervical os can sometimes be dramatically altered by varying the fullness of

BOX 22-6 *Placental Grading*

Third-trimester grading of placental maturation can be accomplished by ultrasound scanning. The placenta undergoes detectable maturational changes throughout gestation; a relationship has been noted between advancing placental grade and fetal pulmonary maturity. Placentas are graded as 0, I, II, and III (with grade III placentas being the most mature) on the basis of the identification and distribution of calcium deposits within the fetal portion (Manning, 1994). Ultrasound examination can identify changes in the chorionic plate, placental substance, and basal layer of the placenta that correspond to the various grades: (1) grade 0 placentas are seen in the first and second trimesters, (2) grade I placentas appear between 30 and 32 weeks and may even persist until term, (3) grade II placentas are observed at around 36 weeks and persist until term in 45% of pregnancies, and (4) grade III placentas are seen at 38 weeks and reflect the greatest maturation. However, only a small number of placentas are grade III.

the maternal bladder. In approximately 15% to 20% of all pregnancies in which ultrasound scanning is performed during the second trimester, the placenta seems to be overlying the os, but the incidence of placenta previa at term is only 0.5%. Thus the diagnosis of placenta previa can seldom be confirmed before 27 weeks, primarily because of the elongation of the lower uterine segment as pregnancy advances.

Another use for ultrasonography is grading of placental maturation (Box 22-6). Calcium deposits are of significance in postterm pregnancies because as they increase, the available surface area that can be adequately bathed by maternal blood decreases. The point at which this results in fetal wastage and hypoxia cannot be determined precisely; however, the effects are usually observable by 42 weeks and are progressive (Gilbert & Harmon, 1998).

Fetal well-being. Physiologic parameters of the fetus that can be assessed with ultrasound scanning include amniotic fluid volume, vascular waveforms from the fetal circulation, heart motion, fetal breathing movements, fetal urine production, and fetal limb and head movements. Assessment of these parameters, singly or in combination, yields a fairly reliable picture of fetal well-being. The significance of these findings is discussed in the following sections.

Amniotic fluid volume. Abnormalities of **amniotic fluid volume (AFV)** are frequently associated with fetal disorders. Subjective determinants of oligohydramnios (decreased fluid) include the absence of fluid pockets in the uterine cavity and the impression of crowding of small fetal parts. An objective criterion of decreased AFV is met if the largest pocket of fluid measured in two perpendicular planes is less than 1 cm. In the case of polyhydramnios (increased fluid), subjective criteria include multiple large pockets of fluid, the impression of a floating fetus, and free movement of

fetal limbs. The diagnosis may be made when the largest pocket of fluid exceeds 8 cm in two perpendicular planes (Fischer & Depp, 1995; Manning, 1994). The total AFV can be evaluated by a measurement in which the depths (in centimeters) of the amniotic fluid in all four quadrants surrounding the maternal umbilicus are totaled, providing an **amniotic fluid index (AFI)**. An AFI less than 5 cm indicates oligohydramnios, 5 to 19 cm is considered a normal measurement, and a measurement greater than 20 cm reflects polyhydramnios (Chervenak & Gabbe, 1996).

Oligohydramnios is associated with congenital anomalies (such as renal agenesis), growth restriction, and fetal distress during labor. Polyhydramnios is associated with neural tube defects, obstruction of the fetal gastrointestinal tract, multiple fetuses, and fetal hydrops (Brace, 1994; Fischer & Depp, 1995; Manning, 1994).

Doppler blood flow analysis. One of the major advances in perinatal medicine is the ability to study blood flow noninvasively in the fetus and placenta. **Doppler ultrasound** is a helpful adjunct in the management of pregnancies at risk because of hypertension, IUGR, diabetes mellitus, multiple fetuses, or preterm labor.

When a sound wave is reflected from a moving target, there is a change in frequency of the reflected wave relative to the transmitted wave. This is called the *Doppler effect.* An ultrasound beam scattered by a group of red blood cells (RBCs) is an example of this effect. The velocity of the RBCs can be determined by measuring the change in the frequency of the sound wave reflected off the cells (Trudinger, 1994).

The shifted frequencies can be displayed as a plot of velocity versus time, and the shape of these waveforms can by analyzed to give information about blood flow and resistance in a given circulation (Schulman, 1990). Velocity waveforms from umbilical and uterine arteries, reported as systolic/diastolic (S/D) ratios, can be first detected at 15 weeks of pregnancy. Because of the progressive decline in resistance in both the umbilical and uterine arteries, this ratio decreases as pregnancy advances. Most fetuses will achieve an S/D ratio of 3 or less by 30 weeks (Fig. 22-4). Persistent elevation of S/D ratios after 30 weeks is associated with IUGR, usually resulting from uteroplacental insufficiency (UPI). Abnormal results are also seen with certain chromosome abnormalities (trisomy 13 and 18) in the fetus and with lupus erythematosus in the mother (Schulman, 1990). Exposure to nicotine from maternal smoking has also been reported to increase the S/D ratio (Trudinger, 1994).

Biophysical profile. Real-time ultrasound permits detailed assessment of the physical and physiologic characteristics of the developing fetus and cataloging of normal and abnormal biophysical responses to stimuli. The **biophysical profile (BPP)** is a noninvasive dynamic assessment of a fetus and its environment by ultrasonography and external fetal monitoring.

BPP scoring is a method of fetal risk surveillance based on the assessment of both acute and chronic markers of

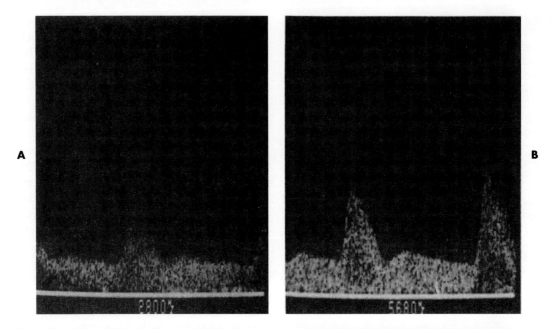

Fig. 22-4 Normal and abnormal uteroplacental vessels at 34 weeks. **A,** Normal S/D ratio of 2.2. **B,** S/D ratio of 3.4. (From Shulman H: Doppler ultrasound in Eden R & Boehm F, editors: *Assessment and care of the fetus: physiological, clinical and medical principles,* Norwalk, Conn, 1990, Appleton & Lange.)

fetal disease. The BPP includes fetal breathing movements, fetal movements, fetal tone, fetal heart rate (FHR) patterns by means of a nonstress test, and AFV. The procedure may be considered a physical examination of the fetus, including determination of vital signs. The fetal response to central hypoxia is alteration in movement, muscle tone, breathing, and heart rate patterns. The presence of normal fetal biophysical activities indicates that the central nervous system is functional and the fetus therefore is not hypoxemic (Manning & Harman, 1990). BPP variables and scoring are detailed in Table 22-3.

The BPP is an accurate indicator of impending fetal death. Fetal acidosis can be diagnosed early with a nonreactive nonstress test and absent fetal breathing movements (FBM). An abnormal BPP score and oligohydramnios are indications that labor should be induced (Manning & Harman, 1990). Fetal infection in women whose membranes rupture prematurely (at less than 37 weeks of gestation) can be diagnosed early by changes in biophysical activity that precede the clinical signs of infection and indicate the necessity for immediate birth (Gaffney, Salinger & Vintzileos, 1990). When the BPP score is normal and the risk of fetal death low, intervention is indicated only for obstetric or maternal factors.

Nursing role

Although a growing number of nurses with special training perform ultrasound scans and BPPs in certain centers, the main role of nurses is in counseling and educating women about the procedure.

Providing accurate information regarding the procedure is imperative to allay the mother's anxiety. Although ultrasound scanning has become a widely used diagnostic tool, recommendations for the procedure are based on expectations of a fetal problem and therefore may cause concern. Patients should be provided ample opportunity to ask questions and be reassured that the procedure is safe.

For an abdominal ultrasound the woman is usually directed to come for the examination with a full bladder because it supports the uterus in position for the imaging, particularly in the second trimester. She is then positioned comfortably with small pillows under her head and knees. The display panel is positioned so that the woman and/or her partner can observe the images on the screen if they desire.

A transvaginal ultrasound may be performed with the woman in a lithotomy position or with her pelvis elevated by towels, cushions, or a folded pillow. This pelvic tilt is optimal to image the pelvic structures. A protective cover such as a condom, the finger of a clean rubber surgical glove, or a special probe cover provided by the manufacturer is used to cover the transducer probe. The probe is lubricated with a water-soluble gel and placed in the vagina either by the examiner or by the woman herself. During the examination the position of the probe or the tilt of the examining table may be changed so that the complete pelvis is in view. The procedure is not physically painful, although the woman will feel pressure as the probe is moved (see the accompanying Teaching Guidelines box).

TABLE 22-3 *Biophysical Profile*

VARIABLES	NORMAL (SCORE = 2)	ABNORMAL (SCORE = 0)
Fetal breathing movements	One or more episodes in 30 min, each lasting ≥30 sec	Episodes absent or no episode ≥30 sec in 30 min
Gross body movements	Three or more discrete body or limb movements in 30 min (episodes of active continuous movement being considered as a single movement)	Less than three episodes of body or limb movements in 30 min
Fetal tone	One or more episodes of active extension with return to flexion of fetal limb(s) or trunk, opening and closing of hand being considered normal tone	Slow extension with return to flexion, movement of limb in full extension, or fetal movement absent
Reactive fetal heart rate	Two or more episodes of acceleration (≥15 beats/min) in 20 min, each lasting ≥15 sec and associated with fetal movement	Less than two episodes of acceleration or acceleration of <15 beats/min in 20 min
Qualitative amniotic fluid volume	One or more pockets of fluid measuring ≥1 cm in two perpendicular planes	Pockets absent or pocket < 1 cm in two perpendicular planes

SCORE

Normal	8-10 (if Amniotic Fluid Index is adequate)
Equivocal	6
Abnormal	<4

Data from Manning F: Dynamic ultrasound-based fetal assessment: the fetal biophysical profile score, *Clin Obstet Gynecol* 38(1):26, 1995.

TEACHING GUIDELINES

Preparing for an Ultrasound Examination

The woman should be informed of the necessity to have a full bladder during an abdominal ultrasound for better imaging of the fetus. She will be positioned comfortably, with pillows under her head and knees, ultrasonic gel will be applied to the abdomen, and the scanner will be passed over it while images are recorded. The woman (and her partner) will be able to watch if they wish to. She should not feel any discomfort.

For a transvaginal ultrasound, the woman should be informed that she may be placed in a lithotomy position or have her pelvis elevated because this position is optimal for imaging the pelvic structures. A transducer, with a protective sheath covering it, will be introduced into the vagina; if the woman wishes to, she may be permitted to insert it herself. The angle of the probe or the tilt of the table may be altered during the examination, but the procedure should not be painful.

Safety of diagnostic ultrasonography

In the 30 years that diagnostic ultrasonography has been used, no conclusive evidence of any harmful effects on humans has emerged. Although the possibility of unidentified biologic effects exists, the benefits to the patient of prudent use of diagnostic ultrasonography far outweigh any possible risk (Anthony, 1996).

LEGAL TIP **Performance of Limited Ultrasound Examinations**
Nurses who have the training and competence may perform limited ultrasound examinations if it is within the scope of practice in their state or area and consistent with regulations of the agencies in which they practice. Limited ultrasound examinations include identification of fetal number, fetal presentation, fetal cardiac activity, location of the placenta, and BPP including amniotic fluid volume assessment. Patients should be informed about the limited information provided by these examinations. They are not meant to evaluate or identify fetal anomalies, assess fetal age, or estimate fetal weight. The obstetric health care provider is responsible for obtaining a more comprehensive ultrasound examination when complete patient assessment is necessary (AWHONN, 1998).

Magnetic Resonance Imaging

Magnetic resonance imaging (MRI) is a noninvasive radiologic technique used for obstetric and gynecologic diagnosis. Like computed tomography (CT), MRI provides excellent pictures of soft tissue. Unlike CT, ionizing radiation is not used; thus vascular structures within the body can be visualized and evaluated without injection of an iodinated contrast medium, thus eliminating any known biologic risk. Like sonography, MRI is noninvasive and can provide

TABLE 22-4 *Summary of Biochemical Monitoring Techniques*

TEST	POSSIBLE FINDINGS	CLINICAL SIGNIFICANCE
MATERNAL BLOOD		
Coombs' test	Titer of 1:8 and rising	Significant Rh incompatibility
AFP	See below	
AMNIOTIC FLUID ANALYSIS		
Color	Meconium	Possible hypoxia or asphyxia
Lung profile		Fetal lung maturity
L/S ratio	>2	
Phosphatidylglycerol	Present	
Creatinine	>2 mg/dl	Gestational age >36 wk
Bilirubin (ΔOD 450/nm)	<0.015	Gestational age >36 wk, normal pregnancy
	High levels	Fetal hemolytic disease in Rh isoimmunized pregnancies
Lipid cells	>10%	Gestational age >35 wk
AFP	High levels after 15-wk gestation	Open neural tube or other defect
Osmolality	Decline after 20-wk gestation	Advancing gestational age
Genetic disorders	Dependent on cultured cells for	Counseling possibly required
Sex-linked	karyotype and enzymatic activity	
Chromosomal		
Metabolic		

images in multiple planes, but there is no interference from skeletal, fatty, or gas-filled structures, and imaging of deep pelvic structures does not require a full bladder.

MRI can be used in evaluation of (1) fetal structure (central nervous system, thorax, abdomen, genitourinary tract, musculoskeletal system) and overall growth; (2) placenta (position, density, and presence of gestational trophoblastic disease); (3) quantity of amniotic fluid; (4) maternal structures (uterus, cervix, adnexa, and pelvis); (5) biochemical status (pH, adenosine triphosphate content) of tissues and organs; and (6) soft tissue, metabolic, or functional anomalies.

The woman is placed on a table in the supine position and slid into the bore of the main magnet, which is similar in appearance to a CT scanner. Depending on the reason for the study, the procedure may take from 20 to 60 minutes, during which time the woman must be perfectly still except for short respites. Because of the long time needed to produce magnetic resonance images, the fetus will probably move, which will obscure anatomic details. The only way to ensure that this does not occur is to administer a sedative to the mother, but this approach should be reserved for selected cases in which visualization of fetal detail is critical.

BIOCHEMICAL ASSESSMENT

Biochemical assessment involves biologic examination (e.g., as chromosomes in exfoliated cells) and chemical determinations (e.g., L/S ratio and bilirubin level). Procedures used to obtain the needed specimens include amniocentesis, percutaneous umbilical blood sampling, chorionic villus sampling, and maternal sampling (Table 22-4).

Amniocentesis

Amniocentesis is performed to obtain amniotic fluid, which contains fetal cells. Under direct ultrasonographic visualization, a needle is inserted transabdominally into the uterus, amniotic fluid is withdrawn into a syringe, and the various assessments are performed. Amniocentesis is possible after week 14 of pregnancy, when the uterus becomes an abdominal organ and sufficient amniotic fluid is available for testing (Fig. 22-5). Indications for the procedure include prenatal diagnosis of genetic disorders or congenital anomalies (neural tube defects in particular), assessment of pulmonary maturity, and diagnosis of fetal hemolytic disease. Complications in the mother and fetus occur in fewer than 1% of the cases and include the following:

- Maternal–Hemorrhage, fetomaternal hemorrhage with possible maternal Rh isoimmunization, infection, labor, abruptio placentae, inadvertent damage to the intestines or bladder, and amniotic fluid embolism. Because of the possibility of fetomaternal hemorrhage, it is standard practice after an amniocentesis to administer Rh_0 D immune globulin (RhoGAM) to the woman who is Rh negative.
- Fetal–Death, hemorrhage, infection (amnionitis), direct injury from the needle, abortion or preterm labor, and leakage of amniotic fluid.

Many of the complications have been minimized or eliminated by using ultrasonography to direct the procedure.

Genetic problems

Prenatal assessment of genetic disorders is indicated in women more than 35 years old, with a previous child with a chromosomal abnormality, or with a family history of

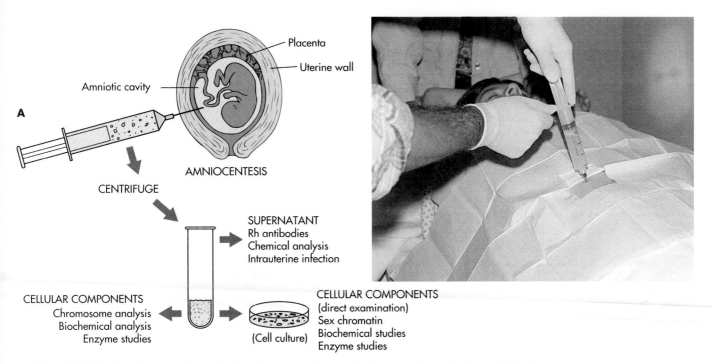

Fig. 22-5 **A,** Amniocentesis and laboratory use of amniotic fluid aspirant. **B,** Transabdominal amniocentesis. (Courtesy Marjorie Pyle, RNC, Lifecircle, Costa Mesa, Calif.)

chromosomal anomalies. Inherited errors of metabolism (such as Tay-Sachs disease, hemophilia, and thalassemia) and other disorders for which marker genes are known may also be detected.

Karyotyping of cultured fetal cells (see Chapter 8) reveals fetal chromosomal aberrations in 1% to 2% of women between 35 and 38 years old, 2% of women between 39 and 44 years old, and 10% of women more than 45 years old. Karyotyping also permits determination of fetal sex, which is important if an X-linked disorder (occurring almost always in a male fetus) is suspected.

Biochemical analysis of enzymes in amniotic fluid can detect inborn errors of metabolism. For example, **alpha-fetoprotein (AFP)** levels in amniotic fluid are assessed as a follow-up for elevated levels in maternal serum. High AFP levels in amniotic fluid help confirm the diagnosis of a neural tube defect such as spina bifida or anencephaly or an abdominal wall defect such as omphalocele. The elevation results from the increased leakage of cerebrospinal fluid into the amniotic fluid through the closure defect. In normal fetuses, circulatory levels of AFP are high, but amniotic fluid levels decrease to 18.5 μg/ml at 15 weeks and 0.26 μg/ml at term. AFP levels may also be elevated in a normal multifetal pregnancy and with intestinal atresia, presumably caused by lack of fetal swallowing.

A concurrent test for the presence of acetylcholinesterase almost always indicates a fetal defect (Simpson & Elias, 1994). In such instances, concurrent ultrasound examination is recommended.

Fetal maturity

Accurate assessment of fetal maturity is now possible through examination of amniotic fluid or its exfoliated cellular contents. The laboratory tests summarized in Table 22-4 are determinants of term pregnancy and fetal maturity.

Fetal hemolytic disease

Another indication for amniocentesis is the identification and follow-up of fetal hemolytic disease in cases of isoimmunization. The procedure is usually not done until the mother's antibody titer reaches 1:8 and is rising. However, percutaneous umbilical blood sampling (PUBS) is now the procedure of choice to evaluate and treat fetal hemolytic disease.

Meconium

The presence of meconium in the amniotic fluid is usually determined by visual inspection of the sample.

Antepartal period. Meconium in the amniotic fluid before the beginning of labor is not usually associated with an adverse fetal outcome. The finding may be the result of acute and subsequently corrected fetal stress, chronic continuing stress, or simply the physiologic passage of meconium. Because there has been some association between meconium in amniotic fluid in the third trimester and hypertensive disorders and postmaturity, the fetus should undergo further antepartum evaluation if the birth is not imminent (Woods & Glantz, 1994).

Intrapartal period. Intrapartal **meconium-stained amniotic fluid** is an indication for more careful evaluation by electronic fetal monitoring (EFM) and perhaps fetal scalp blood sampling. The presence of meconium, however, should not be the sole indicator for intervention (Scott et al., 1994).

Three possible reasons for the passage of meconium during the intrapartal period are as follows: (1) it is a normal physiologic function that occurs with maturity (meconium passage being uncommon before weeks 23 or 24, with an increased incidence after 38 weeks); (2) it is the result of hypoxia-induced peristalsis and sphincter relaxation; and (3) it may be a sequela to umbilical cord compression–induced vagal stimulation in mature fetuses.

The following criteria have been proposed for evaluating meconium-stained amniotic fluid during the intrapartal period (Scott et al., 1994):

1. *Consistency.* A thick, fresh consistency is more likely to be the result of fetal stress.
2. *Timing.* Thick, fresh meconium passed for the first time in late labor and in association with nonremediable severe variable or late FHR decelerations is an ominous sign. The presence of meconium alone, however, is not necessarily a sign of fetal distress.
3. *Presence of other indicators.* Meconium passage and nonremediable severe variable or late FHR decelerations (especially with poor baseline variability), with or without acidosis confirmed by scalp-blood sampling, are ominous signs of fetal distress.

The birth team should be ready to suction the nasopharynx of the neonate carefully at the time of birth, ideally before the first breath is taken. Suctioning at this time effectively reduces the incidence and severity of meconium aspiration in the neonate (Tepas & Cunningham, 1993).

Percutaneous Umbilical Blood Sampling

Direct access to the fetal circulation during the second and third trimesters is possible through **percutaneous umbilical blood sampling (PUBS),** or cordocentesis, which is the most widely used method for fetal blood sampling and transfusion (Baumann & McFarland, 1994). PUBS involves the insertion of a needle directly into a fetal umbilical vessel under ultrasound guidance. Ideally, the umbilical cord is punctured 1 to 2 cm from its insertion into the placenta (Fig. 22-6). At this point the cord is well anchored and will not move, and the risk of maternal blood contamination (from the placenta) is slight. Generally, 1 to 4 ml of blood is removed and tested immediately by the Kleihauer-Betke procedure to ensure that it is fetal in origin. Indications for use of PUBS include prenatal diagnosis of inherited blood disorders, karyotyping of malformed fetuses, detection of fetal infection, determination of the acid-base status of fetuses with IUGR, and

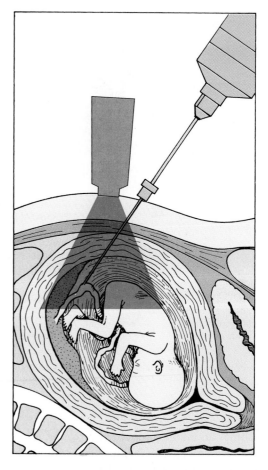

Fig. 22-6 Technique for PUBS guided by ultrasound.

assessment and treatment of isoimmunization and thrombocytopenia in the fetus. Complications that can occur include leaking of blood from the puncture site, cord laceration, thromboembolism, preterm labor, premature rupture of membranes, and infection.

PUBS may be the procedure of choice when time limitations do not permit amniotic fluid cultures to be used because a karyotype can be obtained from a fetal blood specimen in 2 to 3 days.

In fetuses at risk for isoimmune hemolytic anemia, PUBS permits precise identification of fetal blood type and RBC count and may prevent further intervention. If the fetus is positive for the presence of maternal antibodies, a direct blood test can confirm the degree of anemia resulting from hemolysis. Intrauterine transfusion of severely anemic fetuses can be done 4 to 5 weeks earlier using the umbilical route than through the intraperitoneal route.

Follow-up includes continuous FHR monitoring for several minutes to 1 hour and a repeat ultrasound examination 1 hour later to ensure that no further bleeding or hematoma formation has occurred.

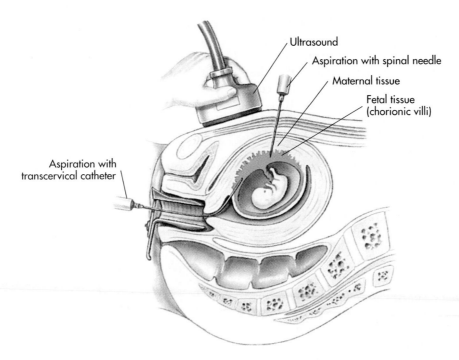

Fig. 22-7 Chorionic villus sampling. (Courtesy Medical and Scientific Illustration, Crozet, Va.)

Chorionic Villus Sampling

The combined advantages of earlier diagnosis and rapid results have made **chorionic villus sampling (CVS)** a popular technique for genetic studies, although some risks to the fetus exist.

The procedure is performed between 10 and 12 weeks of gestation and involves the removal of a small tissue specimen from the fetal portion of the placenta (Fig. 22-7). Because chorionic villi originate in the zygote, this tissue reflects the genetic makeup of the fetus (ACOG, 1995).

CVS procedures can be accomplished either transcervically or transabdominally. In transcervical sampling, a sterile catheter is introduced into the cervix under continuous ultrasonographic guidance and a small portion of the chorionic villi is aspirated with a syringe. The aspiration cannula and obturator must be placed at a suitable site, and rupture of the amniotic sac must be avoided.

If the abdominal approach is used, an 18-gauge spinal needle with stylet is inserted under sterile conditions through the abdominal wall into the chorion under ultrasound guidance. The stylet is then withdrawn and the chorionic tissue is aspirated into a syringe (Matthews & Smith, 1993) (see Fig. 22-7).

Complications of the procedure include vaginal spotting or bleeding immediately afterward, spontaneous abortion (in 0.3% of cases), rupture of membranes (in 0.1% of cases), and chorioamnionitis (in 0.5% of cases). Because of the possibility of fetomaternal hemorrhage, women who are Rh negative should receive immune globulin (RhoGAM) to avoid isoimmunization (National Institutes

| BOX 22-7 | *Fetal Rights* |

Amniocentesis, PUBS, and CVS are prenatal tests used for diagnosing fetal defects in pregnancy. They are invasive and carry risks to the mother and fetus. A consideration of abortion is linked to the performance of these tests because there is no treatment for genetically affected fetuses. Thus the issue of fetal rights is a key ethical concern in prenatal testing for fetal defects.

of Health CVS Study Group, 1989). An increased risk of limb anomalies (transverse digital anomalies) has been reported when CVS is done before 10 weeks of gestation (ACOG, 1995).

Indications for CVS are similar to those for amniocentesis. About 90% of the procedures are performed because of advanced maternal age (over age 35 years) (Simpson & Elias, 1994). Other indications include biochemical and molecular assays for infections or metabolic disorders (Box 22-7).

Maternal Assays

Maternal serum alpha-fetoprotein

Maternal serum AFP (MSAFP) levels are used to screen for neural tube defects (NTDs) in pregnancy. Through this technique, approximately 80% to 85% of all open NTDs and open abdominal wall defects can be detected early in pregnancy. Screening is recommended for all pregnant women (ACOG, 1996).

The cause of NTDs is not well understood; 95% of all affected infants are born to women with no previous family history of similar anomalies. The defect occurs in 1 to 2 per 1,000 births in most parts of the United States. The birth of one affected child increases the risk of NTD recurrence in future pregnancies to 2% to 3%, which is 10 to 15 times that for the general population. With two affected children, the risk rises to 6% to 8% (Simpson & Elias, 1994).

AFP is produced by the fetal liver and increasing levels are detectable in the serum of pregnant women from 14 to 34 weeks. Although amniotic fluid AFP is diagnostic for NTD, MSAFP is a screening tool only and identifies candidates for the more definitive procedures of amniocentesis and ultrasound examination. MSAFP screening can be done with reasonable reliability any time between 15 and 22 weeks of gestation (16 to 18 being ideal) (ACOG, 1996).

Once the maternal level of AFP is determined, it is compared with normal values for each week of gestation. Values should also be correlated with maternal age, weight, race, and whether the woman is an insulin-dependent diabetic (Covington et al., 1996). If findings are abnormal, follow-up procedures include genetic counseling for families with a history of NTD, repeat AFP, ultrasound examination, and possibly, amniocentesis.

Down syndrome and probably other autosomal trisomies are associated with lower-than-normal levels of MSAFP and amniotic fluid AFP. Another test, the **triple-marker test,** is also performed at 16 to 18 weeks of gestation and uses the levels of three markers, MSAFP, unconjugated estriol, and human chorionic gonadotropin (hCG), in combination with maternal age to calculate a new risk. In the presence of a fetus with Down syndrome, the MSAFP and unconjugated estriol levels are low, whereas the hCG level is elevated. With the two additional screening tests, approximately 60% of cases of Down syndrome can be identified (Ross & Elias, 1997).

As with MSAFP, these tests are screening procedures only and are not diagnostic. A definitive examination of amniotic fluid for AFP and chromosomal analysis combined with ultrasound visualization of the fetus is necessary for diagnosis.

Estriols

The steroid precursor produced by the fetal adrenal glands is synthesized into estriols in the placenta and is excreted by the mother's healthy kidneys. Estriol levels may also be assayed in maternal serum, which is the preferred method. At this time, unconjugated estriol levels are determined only as part of the triple-marker test described earlier.

Coomb's test

The Coomb's test for Rh incompatibility is discussed in Chapter 28. If the maternal titer for Rh antibodies is greater than 1:8, amniocentesis for determination of bilirubin in amniotic fluid is indicated to establish the severity of fetal hemolytic anemia. Coombs' test can also detect other antibodies that may place the fetus at risk for incompatibility with maternal antigens.

ELECTRONIC FETAL MONITORING

Indications

First- and second-trimester antepartal assessment is directed primarily at the diagnosis of fetal anomalies. The goal of third-trimester testing is to determine whether the intrauterine environment continues to be supportive to the fetus. The testing is often used to determine the timing of childbirth for patients at risk for **uteroplacental insufficiency (UPI)** (the gradual decline in delivery of needed substances by the placenta to the fetus). Gradual loss of placental function results first in inadequate nutrient delivery to the fetus, leading to IUGR. Subsequently, respiratory function is also compromised, resulting in fetal hypoxia. Indications for both the **nonstress test (NST)** (or **fetal activity determination [FAD]**) and the **contraction stress test (CST)** include the following:

- Maternal diabetes mellitus
- Chronic hypertension
- Pregnancy-induced hypertension
- Intrauterine growth restriction
- Sickle cell disease
- Maternal cyanotic heart disease
- Postmaturity
- History of previous stillbirth
- Decreased fetal movement
- Isoimmunization
- Meconium-stained amniotic fluid at third-trimester amniocentesis
- Hyperthyroidism
- Collagen disease
- Older pregnant woman
- Chronic renal disease

No clinical contraindications exist for the NST. Absolute contraindications for the CST are the following: rupture of membranes, previous classic incision for cesarean birth, preterm labor, placenta previa, and abruptio placentae. Other conditions in which CST may be contraindicated are multifetal pregnancy, previous preterm labor, hydramnios, and incompetent cervix. As a rule, reactive patterns with the NST or negative results with the CST are associated with favorable outcomes.

Fetal Responses to Hypoxia or Asphyxia

Hypoxia or asphyxia elicits a number of responses in the fetus. There is a redistribution of blood flow to certain vital organs. This series of responses (redistribution of blood flow favoring vital organs, decrease in total oxygen consumption, and switch to anaerobic glycolysis) is a temporary mechanism that enables the fetus to survive up to 30 minutes of limited oxygen supply without decompensation of vital organs. However, during more severe asphyxia or sustained hypoxemia, these compensatory responses are no longer maintained, and a decrease in the cardiac output, arterial blood pressure, and blood flow to the brain and heart occurs (Parer, 1994), with characteristic FHR patterns reflecting these changes.

Variability

Considerable evidence supports the clinical belief that FHR variability indicates an intact nervous pathway through the cerebral cortex, midbrain, vagus nerve, and cardiac conduction system. With a 98% accuracy in predicting fetal well-being, the presence of normal FHR variability is a reassuring indicator. Inputs from various areas of the brain decrease after cerebral asphyxia, leading to a decrease in variability after failure of the fetal hemodynamic compensatory mechanisms to maintain cerebral oxygenation (Parer, 1994).

Nonstress Test (Fetal Activity Determination)

The NST is the most widely applied technique for antepartum evaluation of the fetus. The basis for the NST, or FAD, is that the normal fetus will produce characteristic heart rate patterns in response to fetal movement. In the healthy fetus with an intact CNS, 90% of gross fetal body movements are associated with accelerations of the FHR. This response can be blunted by hypoxia, acidosis, drugs, (analgesics, barbiturates, and beta-blockers), fetal sleep, and some congenital anomalies.

Advantages

NST can be performed easily in an outpatient setting, including the home because it is noninvasive. It is also relatively inexpensive and has no known contraindications.

Disadvantages

Disadvantages center around the high rate of false-positive results for nonreactivity as a result of fetal sleep cycles, medications, and fetal immaturity. The test is also slightly less sensitive in detecting fetal compromise than are the CST or BPP.

Procedure

The woman is seated in a reclining chair (or in semi-Fowler's position) to avoid supine hypotension. The FHR is recorded by a Doppler transducer, and a tocotransducer is applied to detect uterine contractions or fetal movements. The strip chart is observed for signs of fetal activity and a concurrent acceleration of FHR. If evidence of fetal movement is not apparent on the strip, the woman may be asked to depress a button on a hand-held event marker connected to the monitor when she feels fetal movement. The movement is then noted on the strip. Because almost all accelerations are accompanied by fetal movement, the movements need not be recorded for the test to be considered reactive (Huddleston, Williams & Fabbri, 1993). The test is usually completed within 20 to 30 minutes, but it may take longer if the fetus needs to be awakened from a sleep state.

It has been suggested that the woman drink orange juice or be given glucose to raise her blood sugar and thereby stimulate fetal movements. In fact this practice is common; however, research has not proven this practice to be effective (McCarthy & Narrigan, 1995). Other methods that have been used to stimulate fetal activity such as manipulating the woman's abdomen or using a transvaginal light have not been very effective either. Only acoustic stimulation has had some impact (Marden et al., 1997).

Interpretation

Generally accepted criteria for a reactive tracing are as follows:
- Two or more accelerations of 15 beats/min lasting for 15 seconds over a 20-minute period
- Normal baseline rate
- Long-term variability amplitude of 10 or more beats per minute

If the test does not meet the criteria for 40 minutes, it is considered nonreactive (Fig. 22-8 and Table 22-5), in which case further assessments are needed with a CST or BPP. The current recommendation is that the NST be performed twice weekly (after 28 weeks' gestation) with patients who are diabetic or at risk for fetal death.

Fetal Acoustic Stimulation

The **acoustic stimulation test** is another method of testing antepartum FHR response, often used to change fetal state from quiet sleep to active sleep. The test takes approximately 15 minutes to complete, with the fetus monitored for 5 to 10 minutes before stimulation to obtain a baseline FHR. The sound source (usually a laryngeal stimulator) is then activated for 3 seconds on the maternal abdomen over the head. Monitoring continues for another 5 minutes, after which the monitor tracing is assessed. A test is considered reactive if there is an immediate and sustained increase in long-term variability and heart rate accelerations. The accelerations produced may have a significant increase in duration. The test may be repeated at 1-minute intervals up to three times when there is no response. Further evaluation is needed with BPP or CST if the pattern is still nonreactive.

Marden et al. (1997) found that fetuses who were exposed to vibracoustic stimulation exhibited significantly more movement than controls and therefore were more likely to have reactive NSTs.

Contraction Stress Test

The CST is one of the first electronic methods to be developed for assessment of fetal health. It was devised as a graded

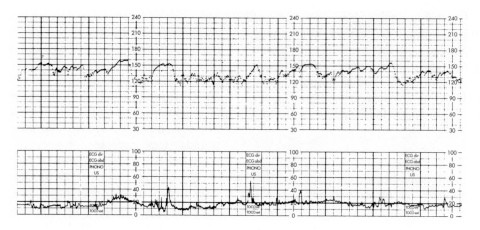

Fig. 22-8 Reactive NST (Fetal heart acceleration with movement). (From Tucker S: *Pocket guide to fetal monitoring and assessment*, ed 3, St Louis, 1996, Mosby.)

TABLE 22-5   *Interpretation of the Nonstress Test*

RESULT	INTERPRETATION	CLINICAL SIGNIFICANCE
Reactive	Two or more accelerations of FHR of 15 beats/min lasting 15 sec or more, associated with each fetal movement in a 20-min period (see Fig. 22-8)	As long as twice-weekly NSTs remain reactive, most high-risk pregnancies are allowed to continue
Nonreactive	Any tracing with either no FHR accelerations or accelerations <15 beats/min or lasting less than 15 sec throughout any fetal movement during testing period	Further indirect monitoring may be attempted with abdominal fetal electrocardiography in an effort to clarify FHR pattern and quantitate variability; external monitoring should continue, and CST or BPP should be done
Unsatisfactory	Quality of FHR recording not adequate for interpretation	Test is repeated in 24 hr or CST is done depending on clinical situation

stress test of the fetus, and its purpose was to identify the jeopardized fetus that was stable at rest but showed evidence of compromise after stress. Uterine contractions decrease uterine blood flow and placental perfusion. If this decrease is sufficient to produce hypoxia in the fetus, a deceleration in FHR will result, beginning at the peak of the contraction and persisting after its conclusion (late deceleration). In a healthy fetoplacental unit, uterine contractions usually do not produce late decelerations, whereas if there is underlying uteroplacental insufficiency, contractions will produce late decelerations.

Advantages

The CST provides an earlier warning of fetal compromise than the NST and with fewer false-positive results.

Disadvantages

In addition to the contraindications described earlier, the CST is more time consuming and expensive than the NST. It is also an invasive procedure if oxytocin stimulation is required.

Procedure

The woman is placed in semi-Fowler's position or sits in a reclining chair. She is placed on an external electronic monitor, and the strip is observed for 10 minutes for baseline rate, long-term variability, and the possible occurrence of spontaneous contractions. The two methods of CST are the **nipple stimulation contraction test** and the oxytocin-stimulated contraction test.

Nipple stimulation contraction test. After the procedure is explained to the woman, warm, moist washcloths are applied to both breasts for several minutes. The woman is then asked to massage one nipple for 10 minutes. Massaging the nipples causes a release of oxytocin from the posterior pituitary. An alternative approach is for her to massage the nipple for 2 minutes, rest for 2 minutes, and continue for four cycles of massage and rest. If unilateral stimulation does not achieve adequate contractions (three occurring within a 10-minute window), unilateral continuous stimulation should be tried (if the intermittent approach was used), followed by bilateral stimulation for 10 minutes. When adequate contractions or hyperstimulation occurs,

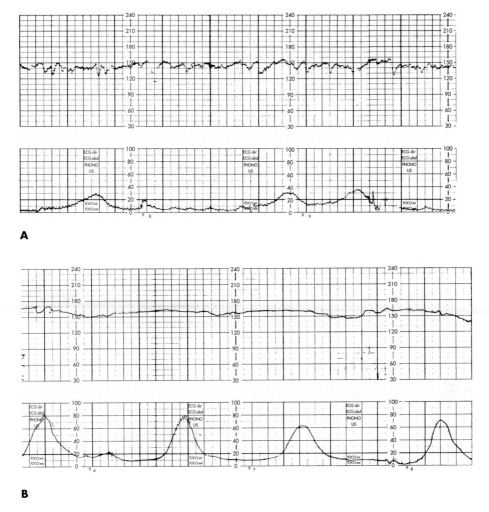

Fig. **22-9** CST. **A,** Negative CST. **B,** Positive CST. (From Tucker S: *Pocket guide to fetal monitoring and assessment,* ed 3, St Louis, 1996, Mosby.)

stimulation should be stopped. If the stimulation and rest cycle method is used, it can be performed indefinitely until considered unsuccessful (Devoe, 1995).

Oxytocin-stimulated contraction test. If nipple stimulation is not successful, an exogenous oxytocin-stimulated CST should be performed. An intravenous (IV) infusion is begun with a scalp needle. The oxytocin is diluted in an IV solution (usually 10 U to 1,000 ml fluid), infused into the tubing of the main IV device through a piggyback port, and delivered by an infusion pump to ensure accurate dosage. The oxytocin infusion is usually begun at 0.5 mU/min and increased by 0.5 mU/min at 15- to 30-minute intervals until three uterine contractions of good quality are observed within a 10-minute period. The typical rate of oxytocin infusion used to elicit uterine contractions is 4 to 5 mU/min, and rarely is more than 8 mU/min required.

The infusion rate should probably not be increased to more than 20 mU/min; however, each case should be assessed individually (Devoe, 1995).

Interpretation

If no late decelerations are observed with the contractions, the findings are considered negative. Repetitive late decelerations, occurring with most contractions, render the test results positive (Fig. 22-9 and Table 22-6).

After interpretation of the FHR pattern, the oxytocin infusion is halted and the maintenance IV solution infused until uterine activity has returned to the prestimulation level. If the CST is negative, the IV device is removed and the fetal monitor disconnected. If the CST is positive, continued monitoring and further evaluation of fetal well-being are indicated.

TABLE 22-6 *Guide for Interpretation of the CST*

INTERPRETATION	CLINICAL SIGNIFICANCE
NEGATIVE No late decelerations, with minimum of three uterine contractions lasting 40 to 60 sec within 10-min period (see Fig. 22-9)	Reassurance that the fetus is likely to survive labor should it occur within 1 wk; more frequent testing may be indicated by clinical situation
POSITIVE Persistent and consistent late decelerations occurring with more than half of contractions (see Fig. 22-9)	Management lies between use of other tools of fetal assessment such as BPP and termination of pregnancy; a positive test result indicates that fetus is at increased risk for perinatal morbidity and mortality; physician may perform expeditious vaginal birth after successful induction or may proceed directly to cesarean birth; decision to intervene is determined by fetal monitoring and presence of FHR reactivity
SUSPICIOUS Late decelerations occurring in less than half of uterine contractions once adequate contraction pattern established	NST and CST should be repeated within 24 hr; if interpretable data cannot be achieved, other methods of fetal assessment must be used*
HYPERSTIMULATION Late decelerations occurring with excessive uterine activity (contractions more often than every 2 min or lasting longer than 90 sec) or persistent increase in uterine tone	
UNSATISFACTORY Inadequate uterine contraction pattern or tracing too poor to interpret	

*Applies to results noted as suspicious, hyperstimulation, or unsatisfactory.

NURSING ROLE IN ANTEPARTAL ASSESSMENT FOR RISK

The nurse's role is that of educator and support person when the woman is undergoing such examinations as ultrasonography, MRI, CVS, PUBS, and amniocentesis. In some instances the nurse may assist the physician with the procedure. In many antepartal settings, nurses perform NSTs, CSTs, and BPPs; conduct an initial assessment; and begin necessary interventions for nonreassuring patterns. These nursing procedures are accomplished after additional education and training, under guidance of established protocols and in collaboration with physicians. Patient teaching, which is an integral component of this role, involves preparing the woman for the procedure, interpreting the findings, and providing psychosocial support when needed.

All women who undergo antepartal assessments are at risk for real and potential problems and may be in an anxious frame of mind. In most instances the tests are ordered because of suspected fetal compromise, deterioration of a maternal condition, or both. In the third trimester, pregnant women are most concerned about protecting themselves and their fetuses and consider themselves most vulnerable to outside influences. The label of high risk will increase this sense of vulnerability (Wright, 1994).

Most patients have incomplete knowledge of the assessment, whether it is regarding the procedure itself, the implications of findings, or the need for further evaluation or counseling. Perinatal nurses can provide the required education and, by keeping the patients well informed, can also promote a positive parental self-image in these high-risk individuals.

RESEARCH

Urinary Tract Infection in Pregnancy and Cerebral Palsy

Urinary tract infections (UTI) are a common occurrence during pregnancy. The purpose of this study was to assess a possible association of UTI during pregnancy and cerebral palsy in offspring. The study was a secondary analysis of a case-control study using structured telephone interviews and birth certificate reviews. The cases were from community-based agencies providing services to preschool children who were developmentally delayed. Participants in the study were 112 preschool children with cerebral palsy and 153 children without cerebral palsy. The results of the study showed a prevalence of UTI among case mothers of 17.9% compared with 5.2% among control mothers. The odds:risk ratio indicated that the risk of having a child with cerebral palsy for a mother with a UTI was 4 to 5 times greater than mothers who did not have a UTI during pregnancy. UTI during pregnancy was found to be a risk factor for development of cerebral palsy in offspring.

CLINICAL APPLICATION OF THE STUDY

Assessment for UTI should occur at the initial prenatal visit and more frequently for women with symptoms or who are at risk. Nurses should educate pregnant women about preventive measures for UTI.

Source: Polivka B, Nickel J & Wilkins J: Urinary tract infection during pregnancy: a risk factor for cerebral palsy?, *J Obstet Gynecol Neonatal Nurs* 26(4):405, 1997.

KEY POINTS

- A high-risk pregnancy is one in which the life or well-being of the mother or infant is jeopardized by a biophysical or psychosocial disorder coincidental with or unique to pregnancy.
- Factors that place the pregnancy and fetus or neonate at risk include biophysical, sociodemographic, psychosocial, and environmental ones.
- Psychosocial perinatal warning indicators include characteristics of the parents, the child, their support systems, and family circumstances.
- Maternal and perinatal mortality rates for Caucasians is considerably lower than for other ethnic groups in the United States.
- Mortality rate decreases when risk is identified early and intensive care is applied.

KEY POINTS—cont'd

- Biophysical assessment techniques include fetal movement counts, ultrasonography, and MRI.
- Biochemical monitoring techniques include amniocentesis, PUBS, CVS, and MSAFP.
- Reactive NSTs and negative CSTs suggest fetal well-being.
- Most assessment tests have some degree of risk for the mother and fetus, and usually cause some anxiety for the woman and her family.

CRITICAL THINKING EXERCISES

1 *Ms. Brown has been sent from the antepartum testing center for a CST to be performed after a nonreactive NST. She is frightened of this new test and its implications for the rest of her pregnancy and the health of her fetus. Explain the procedure and the rationale for doing the CST.*

2 *Formulate a teaching plan for a woman who has been advised to monitor fetal activity at home. Include the times monitoring is to take place and instruct her on the way to count movements and when to notify her health care provider.*

3 *Review several pregnant patients' charts. Identify risk factors (biophysical, psychosocial, sociodemographic, and environmental) and give your rationale for each choice.*

4 *Identify resources in your community for families who are experiencing a high-risk pregnancy, including support groups, home care agencies, and counseling facilities. Make a list for the antepartal clinic, including accessibility by public transportation and costs.*

References

American Academy of Pediatrics/American College of Obstetricians and Gynecologists: *Guidelines for perinatal care*, ed 4, Elk Grove Village, Ill, 1997, AAP and ACOG.

American College of Obstetricians and Gynecologists Committee on Genetics: Chorionic villi sampling, *Committee Opinion* 160, Washington, DC, 1995, ACOG.

American College of Obstetricians and Gynecologists: Management of isoimmunization in pregnancy, *Educational Bulletin* 227, Washington, DC, 1996, ACOG.

Anthony A: Biologic effects and safety. In Dubose T, editor: *Fetal sonography,* Philadelphia, 1996, WB Saunders.

Association of Women's Health, Obstetric and Neonatal Nurses (AWHONN): *Nursing practice competencies and educational guidelines for limited ultrasound examination in obstetric and gynecology/infertility settings,* ed 2, Washington, DC, 1998, AWHONN.

Athay P & Haddock F: *Ultrasound in obstetrics and gynecology,* ed 2, St Louis, 1985, Mosby.

Baumann P & McFarland B: Prenatal diagnosis, *J Nurse Midwifery,* 39(2):35, 1994.

Brace R: Amniotic fluid dynamics. In Creasy R & Resnik R, editors: *Maternal-fetal medicine: principles and practices,* ed 3, Philadelphia, 1994, WB Saunders.

Chervenak F & Gabbe S: Obstetric ultrasound: assessment of fetal growth and anatomy. In Gabbe S, Niebyl J & Simpson J, editors: *Obstetrics: normal and problem pregnancies,* ed 3, New York, 1996, Churchill Livingstone.

Covington C et al.: Family care related to alpha-fetoprotein screening, *J Obstet Gynecol Neonatal Nurs,* 25(2):125, 1996.

Cunningham F et al.: *Williams obstetrics,* ed 20, Stamford, Conn, 1997, Appleton & Lange.

DeCherney A & Pernoll M, editors: *Current obstetric and gynecologic diagnosis and treatment,* ed 8, Norwalk, Conn, 1994, Appleton & Lange.

Devoe L: Nonstress and contraction stress testing. In Sciarra J, editor: *Gynecology and obstetrics,* vol 3, Maternal and Fetal Medicine, Philadelphia, 1995, Lippincott.

Fischer R & Depp R: Amniotic fluid: physiology and assessment. In Sciarra J, editor: *Gynecology and obstetrics,* vol 3, Maternal and Fetal Medicine, Philadelphia, 1995, Lippincott.

Fogel C & Lewallen L: High-risk childbearing. In Fogel C & Woods N, editors: *Women's health care: a comprehensive handbook,* Thousand Oaks, Calif, 1995, Sage.

Gaffney S, Salinger L & Vintzileos A: The biophysical profile for fetal surveillance, *MCN Am J Matern Child Nurs* 15(6):356, 1990.

Gilbert E & Harmon J: *Manual of high risk pregnancy and delivery,* ed 2, St Louis, 1998, Mosby.

Grimes D: The morbidity and mortality of pregnancy: still risky business, *Am J Obstet Gynecol,* 170(5 Pt 2):1489, 1994.

Gordon M: *Nursing diagnosis: process and application,* ed 3, St Louis, 1994, Mosby.

Guyer B et al.: Annual summary of vital statistics, 1996, *Pediatrics* 100(6):905, 1997.

Huddleston J, Williams G & Fabri E: Antepartum assessment of the fetus. In Knuppel R & Drukker J, editors: *High risk pregnancy: a team approach,* ed 2, Philadelphia, 1993, WB Saunders.

Kochanek K & Hudson B: Advance report of final mortality statistics, 1992, *Monthly Vital Statistics Report* 43 (6) (suppl):1, 1995.

Manning F: General principles and application of ultrasound. In Creasy R & Resnik R, editors: *Maternal-fetal medicine: principles and practices,* Philadelphia, 1994, WB Saunders.

Manning F: Dynamic ultrasound-based fetal assessment: the fetal biophysical profile score, *Clin Obstet Gynecol* 38(1):26, 1995.

Manning F & Harman C: The fetal biophysical profile. In Eden R & Boehm F, editors: *Assessment and care of the fetus: physiological, clinical and medicolegal principles,* Norwalk, Conn, 1990, Appleton & Lange.

Marden D et al.: A randomized controlled trial of a new fetal acoustic stimulation test for fetal well-being, *Am J Obstet Gynecol* 176(6):1386, 1997.

Matthews A & Smith A: Genetic counseling. In Knuppel R & Drukker J, editors: *High risk pregnancy: a team approach,* Philadelphia, 1993, WB Saunders.

McCarthy K & Narrigan D: Is there scientific support for the use of juice to facilitate the nonstress test? *J Obstet Gynecol Neonatal Nurs* 24(4):303, 1995.

Mortality Patterns—1993: *MMWR* 45(87):1, 1996.

National Center for Health Statistics: Advance report of final natality statistics, 1992, *Monthly Vital Statistics Report* 43(5s):1, 1994.

National Center for Health Statistics: Births, marriages, divorces, and deaths for 1994, *Monthly Vital Statistics Report* 43(12):1, 1995.

National Institutes of Health CVS Study Group: The safety and efficacy of chorionic villus sampling for early prenatal diagnosis of cytogenic abnormalities, *N Eng J Med* 320(10):609, 1989.

Parer J: Fetal heart rate. In Creasy R & Resnik R, editors, *Maternal-fetal medicine: principles and practices,* ed 3, Philadelphia, 1994, WB Saunders.

Ross H & Elias S: Maternal serum screening for fetal genetic disorders, *Obstet Gynecol Clin NA* 24(1):33, 1997.

Schulman H: Doppler ultrasound. In Eden R & Boehm F, editors: *Assessment and care of the fetus: physiological, clinical and medicolegal principles,* Norwalk, Conn, 1990, Appleton & Lange.

Scott J et al., editors: *Danforth's obstetrics and gynecology,* ed 7, Philadelphia, 1994, Lippincott.

Simpson J & Elias S: Prenatal diagnosis of genetic disorders. In Creasy R & Resnik R, editors: *Maternal-fetal medicine: principles and practices,* Philadelphia, 1994, Saunders.

Tepas K & Cunningham M: Newborn care in the delivery room. In Knuppel R & Drukker J: *High risk pregnancy and delivery: a team approach,* ed 3, Philadelphia, 1993, WB Saunders.

Trudinger B: Doppler ultrasound assessment of blood flow. In Creasy R & Resnik R, editors: *Maternal-fetal medicine: principles and practices,* ed 2, Philadelphia, 1994, WB Saunders.

Tucker S: *Pocket guide to fetal monitoring and assessment,* ed 3, St Louis, 1996, Mosby.

Wilcox A et al.: Birth weight and perinatal mortality: a comparison of the United States and Norway, *JAMA* 273(9):709, 1995.

Woods J & Glantz J: Significance of amniotic fluid meconium. In Creasy R & Resnik R, editors: *Maternal-fetal medicine: principles and practices,* ed 3, Philadelphia, 1994, WB Saunders.

Wright L: Prenatal diagnosis in the 1990's, *J Obstet Gynecol Neonatal Nurs* 23(6):506, 1994.

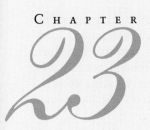

CHAPTER

23

Pregnancy at Risk: Preexisting Conditions

KITTY CASHION AND CAROL FOWLER DURHAM

LEARNING OBJECTIVES

- *Define the key terms.*
- *Differentiate the types of diabetes mellitus and their respective risk factors in pregnancy.*
- *Summarize the effects of pregnancy on insulin requirements.*
- *Discuss maternal and fetal risks or complications associated with diabetes in pregnancy.*
- *Discuss care management for the pregnant woman with pregestational or gestational diabetes.*
- *Explain the effects of thyroid disorders on pregnancy.*
- *Differentiate the management for pregnant women with class I to class IV cardiac disease.*
- *Describe the different types of anemia and their effects during pregnancy.*
- *Explain the care of pregnant women with pulmonary disorders.*
- *Discuss the effects of gastrointestinal disorders on pregnancy.*
- *Describe the effects of neurologic disorders on pregnancy.*
- *Outline the care of women whose pregnancies are complicated by autoimmune disorders.*
- *Explain effects on and management of pregnant women with human immunodeficiency virus (HIV).*
- *Discuss the care of pregnant women who use, abuse, or are dependent on alcohol or illicit or prescription drugs.*

KEY TERMS

adult respiratory distress syndrome (ARDS)
cardiac decompensation
diabetes mellitus
euglycemia
gestational diabetes mellitus (GDM)
glycosylated hemoglobin A1$_c$

KEY TERMS—cont'd

hyperglycemia
hyperthyroidism
hypertrophic cardiomyopathy (HCM)
hypoglycemia
hypothyroidism
idiopathic peripartum cardiomyopathy
ketoacidosis
macrosomia
Marfan syndrome
mitral valve prolapse (MVP)
mitral valve stenosis
oral glucose tolerance test (OGTT)
peripartum heart failure
pregestational diabetes mellitus
rheumatic heart disease (RHD)
sickle cell hemoglobinopathy
systemic lupus erythematosus (SLE)

For most women, pregnancy represents a normal part of life. This chapter, however, will discuss the care of women for whom pregnancy represents a significant risk because it is superimposed on a chronic illness. At one time, it was rare for women with a chronic illness such as diabetes or cardiac disease to achieve and maintain pregnancy and give birth to healthy infants. However, with the active participation of well-motivated women in the treatment plan and careful management from a multidisciplinary health care team, positive pregnancy outcomes are often possible today.

Providing safe and effective care for women experiencing high-risk pregnancy and their fetuses is quite a challenge. While unique needs related to the chronic illness exist in every individual situation, these women also experience many of the same pregnancy-related feelings, needs, and concerns as their "normal" counterparts. Nurses must guide and support the woman and her family in addressing both "normal pregnancy" and "chronic illness" issues. The primary objective of nursing care is to achieve optimal outcomes for both mother and fetus.

This chapter focuses on diabetes mellitus, cardiovascular disorders, and selected disorders of the respiratory,

601

gastrointestinal, integumentary, and central nervous systems. Substance abuse and HIV are also discussed.

DIABETES MELLITUS

Before the discovery of insulin in the early 1920s, it was uncommon for a diabetic woman to give birth to a healthy baby. Many diabetic women of childbearing age were infertile or sterile, and the majority of those who became pregnant were unable to carry to term. The perinatal mortality rate was approximately 65%, with stillbirth being the largest cause of fetal death (Gabbe, 1992; Landon, 1996).

Advances in medicine have greatly improved perinatal outcome. Today, the perinatal mortality rate for well-managed diabetic pregnancies, excluding major congenital malformations, is about the same as for any other pregnancy (Landon, 1996). The incidence of major congenital malformations in infants born to diabetic mothers has not changed significantly over time. Experts have concluded that the key to an optimal pregnancy outcome is strict maternal glucose control before conception, as well as throughout the gestational period. Consequently, much emphasis is currently being placed on preconceptional counseling for diabetic women.

Despite the advances in care, pregnancy complicated by diabetes is still considered high risk. It is most successfully managed by a multidisciplinary approach involving the obstetrician, internist or diabetologist, neonatologist, nurse, nutritionist, and social worker. A favorable outcome of diabetic pregnancy requires commitment and active participation by the woman and her family. The woman must comply with a schedule of frequent prenatal visits, strict adherence to the dietary regimen, regular self-monitoring of her blood glucose level, frequent laboratory evaluation, intensive fetal surveillance, and possible hospitalization.

Care of the pregnant woman with diabetes requires that the nurse fully understand the normal physiologic responses to pregnancy and the altered metabolism of diabetes. Furthermore, the nurse must understand the relationship between pregnancy and diabetes, including psychosocial implications, to assess the woman accurately, plan for her care, and intervene appropriately.

Pathogenesis

Diabetes mellitus is a group of metabolic diseases characterized by hyperglycemia resulting from defects in insulin secretion, insulin action, or both" (The Expert Committee on the Diagnosis and Classification of Diabetes Mellitus, 1997). Insulin, produced by the beta cells in the islets of Langerhans in the pancreas, regulates blood glucose levels by enabling glucose to enter adipose and muscle cells, where it is used for energy. Insulin also stimulates protein synthesis and storage of free fatty acids. When insulin is insufficient or ineffective in promoting glucose uptake by the muscle and adipose cells, glucose accumulates in the

bloodstream, and hyperglycemia results. Hyperglycemia causes hyperosmolarity of the blood, which attracts intracellular fluid into the vascular system, resulting in cellular dehydration and expanded blood volume. Consequently, the kidneys function to excrete large volumes of urine (polyuria) in an attempt to regulate excess vascular volume and to excrete the unusable glucose (glycosuria). Polyuria, along with cellular dehydration, causes excessive thirst (polydipsia).

The body compensates for its inability to convert carbohydrate (glucose) into energy by burning proteins (muscle) and fats. However, the end products of this metabolism are ketones and fatty acids, that, in excess quantities, produce ketoacidosis and acetonuria. Weight loss occurs as a result of the breakdown of fat and muscle tissue. This tissue breakdown causes a state of starvation that compels the individual to eat excessive amounts of food (polyphagia).

Over time, diabetes causes significant changes in both the microvascular and macrovascular circulations. These structural changes affect a variety of organ systems, particularly the heart, eyes, kidneys, and nerves. Complications resulting from diabetes include premature atherosclerosis, retinopathy, nephropathy, and neuropathy.

Diabetes may be caused by either impaired insulin secretion, when the beta cells of the pancreas are destroyed by an autoimmune process, or by inadequate insulin action in target tissues at one or more points along the metabolic pathway. Both of these conditions are frequently present in the same person, and it is unclear which, if either, abnormality is the primary cause of the disease (The Expert Committee on the Diagnosis and Classification of Diabetes Mellitus, 1997).

Classification

The classification and diagnosis of diabetes have been revised by an international Expert Committee working under the sponsorship of the American Diabetes Association (ADA). The Expert Committee report, published in July 1997, recommended that the old classification system developed by the National Diabetes Data Group in 1979 be revised to reflect current knowledge of the disease. The new classification system includes four groups: type 1 diabetes, type 2 diabetes, other specific types (e.g., diabetes caused by infection or drug induced), and gestational diabetes mellitus. A major change proposed by the Expert Committee is a move away from a system that classifies the disease by its pharmacologic management to one based on disease etiology. Therefore the terms *insulin-dependent diabetes mellitus* and *non-insulin-dependent diabetes mellitus* have been eliminated (The Expert Committee on the Diagnosis and Classification of Diabetes Mellitus, 1997).

Type 1 diabetes includes those cases that are primarily due to pancreatic islet beta cell destruction and that are prone to ketoacidosis. People with type 1 diabetes usually have an absolute insulin deficiency. Type 1 diabetes includes cases currently thought to be caused by an autoimmune process, as well as those for which the cause is unknown (The Expert Committee on the Diagnosis and Classification of Diabetes Mellitus, 1997).

Type 2 diabetes is the most prevalent form of the disease and includes individuals who have insulin resistance and usually relative (rather than absolute) insulin deficiency. Specific etiologies for type 2 diabetes are unknown at this time. Type 2 diabetes often goes undiagnosed for years because hyperglycemia develops gradually and often is not severe enough for the patient to recognize the classic signs of polyuria, polydipsia, and polyphagia. Many people who develop type 2 diabetes are obese or have an increased amount of body fat distributed primarily in the abdominal area. Other risk factors for the development of type 2 diabetes include aging, a sedentary lifestyle, hypertension, and prior gestational diabetes. Type 2 diabetes often has a strong genetic predisposition (The Expert Committee on the Diagnosis and Classification of Diabetes Mellitus, 1997).

Pregestational diabetes mellitus is the label sometimes given to type 1, or type 2 diabetes that existed before pregnancy.

Gestational diabetes mellitus (GDM) is any degree of glucose intolerance with the onset or first recognition occurring during pregnancy. This definition is appropriate whether or not insulin is used for treatment or the diabetes persists after pregnancy. It does not exclude the possibility that the glucose intolerance preceded the pregnancy. Women experiencing gestational diabetes should be reclassified 6 weeks or more after the pregnancy ends (The Expert Committee on the Diagnosis and Classification of Diabetes Mellitus, 1997).

Metabolic Changes Associated with Pregnancy

Normal pregnancy is characterized by complex alterations in maternal glucose metabolism, insulin production, and metabolic homeostasis. During normal pregnancy, adjustments in maternal metabolism allow for adequate nutrition for both the mother and the developing fetus. Glucose, the primary fuel used by the fetus, is transported across the placenta through the process of carrier-mediated facilitated diffusion. This means that the glucose levels in the fetus are directly proportional to maternal levels. Although glucose crosses the placenta, insulin does not. By the tenth week of gestation the embryo or fetus secretes its own insulin at levels adequate to use the glucose obtained from the mother. Thus as maternal glucose levels rise, fetal glucose levels are increased, resulting in increased fetal insulin secretion.

During the first trimester of pregnancy the pregnant woman's metabolic status is significantly influenced by the rising levels of estrogen and progesterone. These hormones stimulate the beta cells in the pancreas to increase insulin production, which promotes increased peripheral use of glucose and decreased blood glucose, with fasting levels being reduced by approximately 10% (Fig. 23-1, *A*). There is a concomitant increase in tissue glycogen stores and a decrease in hepatic glucose production, which further encourage lower fasting glucose levels. As a result of these normal metabolic changes of pregnancy, women who are diabetic and are insulin dependent are prone to hypoglycemia during the first trimester.

During the second and third trimesters, pregnancy exerts a "diabetogenic" effect on the maternal metabolic status. Because of the major hormonal changes, there is a decreased tolerance to glucose, an increased insulin resistance, decreased hepatic glycogen stores, and an increased hepatic production of glucose. Rising levels of human placental lactogen, estrogen, progesterone, prolactin, cortisol, and insulinase increase insulin resistance through their actions as insulin antagonists. Insulin resistance is a glucose-sparing mechanism that ensures an abundant supply of glucose for the fetus. Maternal insulin requirements may double or quadruple by the end of the pregnancy, usually leveling off or declining slightly after 36 weeks (Fig. 23-1, *B* and *C*).

At birth, expulsion of the placenta prompts an abrupt drop in levels of circulating placental hormones, cortisol, and insulinase (Fig. 23-1, *D*). Maternal tissues quickly regain their prepregnancy sensitivity to insulin. For the nonbreastfeeding mother the prepregnancy insulin-carbohydrate balance usually returns in about 7 to 10 days (Fig. 23-1, *E*). Lactation uses maternal glucose; thus the breastfeeding mother's insulin requirements will remain low for up to 6 to 9 months. On completion of weaning, the prepregnancy insulin requirement is reestablished (Fig. 23-1, *F*).

Pregestational Diabetes Mellitus

Women who have pregestational diabetes may have either type 1 or type 2 diabetes, which may or may not be complicated by vascular disease, retinopathy, nephropathy, or other diabetic sequelae. Almost all women with pregestational diabetes are insulin dependent during pregnancy.

The diabetogenic state of pregnancy imposed on the compromised metabolic system of the woman with pregestational diabetes has significant implications. The normal hormonal adaptations of pregnancy affect glycemic control, and pregnancy may accelerate the progress of vascular complications.

During the first trimester, when maternal blood glucose levels are normally reduced and the insulin response to glucose is enhanced, glycemic control is improved. The insulin dosage for the woman with well-controlled diabetes may need to be reduced to avoid **hypoglycemia** (low blood glucose levels). There is an increased incidence of hypoglycemic episodes in those with type 1 diabetes during early pregnancy. Nausea, vomiting, and cravings typical of early pregnancy result in dietary fluctuations, which influence maternal glucose levels and necessitate a reduction in insulin dosage.

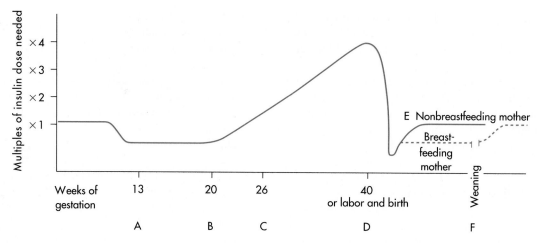

Fig. **23-1** Changing insulin needs during pregnancy. **A,** First trimester: insulin need is reduced because of increased insulin production by pancreas and increased peripheral sensitivity to insulin; nausea, vomiting, and decreased food intake by mother and glucose transfer to embryo or fetus contribute to hypoglycemia. **B,** Second trimester: insulin needs increase as placental hormones, cortisol, and insulinase act as insulin antagonists, decreasing insulin's effectiveness. **C,** Third trimester: insulin needs may double or even quadruple but usually level off after 36 weeks' gestation. **D,** Day of birth: maternal insulin requirements drop drastically to approach prepregnancy levels. **E,** Breastfeeding mother maintains lower insulin requirements, as much as 25% less than prepregnancy; insulin needs of nonbreastfeeding mother return to prepregnancy levels in 7 to 10 days. **F,** Weaning of breastfeeding infant causes mother's insulin needs to return to prepregnancy levels.

Because insulin requirements steadily increase after the first trimester, insulin dosage must be adjusted accordingly to prevent **hyperglycemia** (high blood glucose levels). Insulin resistance begins as early as 14 to 16 weeks and continues to rise until it stabilizes during the last few weeks of pregnancy.

In the past it was believed that pregnancy worsened microvascular complications. In fact, women who were diabetic and had vascular disease such as retinopathy or nephropathy were often encouraged to avoid or terminate pregnancy. With current management practices, however, women with vasculopathy other than coronary artery disease can achieve good pregnancy outcomes (Reece & Homko, 1994).

Diabetic nephropathy has more impact on perinatal outcome than any other vascular complication. Increased risks of preeclampsia, preterm labor, intrauterine growth restriction (IUGR), fetal distress, stillbirth, and neonatal death are associated with this condition (Kitzmiller & Coombs, 1993; Landon & Gabbe, 1992; Reece & Homko, 1993).

Although neuropathic complications are common in type 1 and type 2 diabetes, little information exists about the effect of pregnancy on diabetic neuropathy. An autonomic neuropathy such as gastroparesis (e.g., anorexia, vomiting of undigested food, belching, early satiety, and weight loss) may affect diabetic control because of its effects

on intake and absorption of adequate nutrition (Reece & Homko, 1993).

Preconceptional counseling

Preconceptional counseling, which is recommended for all diabetic women of reproductive age, is associated with an improved pregnancy outcome (Landon, 1996; Willhoite et al., 1993). Under ideal circumstances the pregestational diabetic woman is counseled before the time of conception to plan the optimal time for pregnancy, establish glycemic control before conception, and diagnose any vascular complications of diabetes. Unfortunately, it has been estimated that fewer than 20% of diabetic women in the United States participate in preconceptional counseling (Landon, 1996).

The partner of the diabetic woman should be included in the counseling to assess the couple's level of understanding related to the effects of pregnancy on the diabetic condition and of the potential complications of pregnancy as a result of diabetes. The couple should also be informed of the anticipated alterations in management of diabetes during pregnancy and the need for a multidisciplinary team approach to health care. Financial implications of diabetic pregnancy and other demands related to frequent maternal and fetal surveillance should be discussed. Contraception is another important aspect of preconceptional counseling to assist the couple in planning effectively for pregnancy.

Preconceptional counseling is particularly important because strict metabolic control before conception and in the early weeks of gestation is instrumental in decreasing the risk of congenital anomalies (Reece & Homko, 1993).

Some types of oral hypoglycemic agents (sulfonylureas such as tolbutamide) may have teratogenic effects on the fetus; they should be discontinued in the preconceptional period in type 2 diabetic women. These women are started on insulin before pregnancy when the pregnancy is planned, or as soon as the pregnancy is diagnosed when it is unplanned.

Maternal risks and complications

Although maternal morbidity and mortality rates have improved significantly, the pregnant diabetic woman remains at risk for the development of complications during pregnancy. Research has demonstrated repeatedly that the best predictor of pregnancy outcome for the diabetic woman and her neonate is the degree of maternal glycemic control during pregnancy.

Poor glycemic control around the time of conception and in the early weeks of pregnancy is associated with an increased incidence of spontaneous abortion in diabetic women. Those diabetic women with good glycemic control before conception and in the first trimester are no more likely than nondiabetic women to have a spontaneous abortion (Rosenn et al., 1994).

Poor glycemic control later in pregnancy, particularly in diabetic women without vascular disease, increases the rate of fetal macrosomia. Macrosomia occurs in 20% to 25% of diabetic pregnancies. These large infants of diabetic mothers tend to have a disproportionate increase in shoulder and trunk size. Because of this, the risk of shoulder dystocia is greater in these babies than in other macrosomic infants. Thus diabetic women face an increased likelihood of cesarean birth because of failure to progress or descend, or operative vaginal birth (delivery using episiotomy, forceps, or vacuum extractor) (Landon, 1996; Reece & Homko, 1993).

Pregnancy-induced hypertension (PIH), or preeclampsia, occurs more frequently during diabetic pregnancy. The highest incidence occurs in women with preexisting vascular changes related to diabetes (Cunningham et al., 1997).

Hydramnios (polyhydramnios) occurs about 10 times more often in diabetic than in nondiabetic pregnancies. Hydramnios—amniotic fluid more than 2,000 ml—increases the possibility of compression of maternal abdominal blood vessels (vena cava and aorta), causing supine hypotension. Maternal dyspnea may result from upward pressure on the diaphragm by the distended uterus. Premature rupture of membranes (PROM) and the onset of preterm labor are associated with hydramnios. Overdistention of the uterus caused by hydramnios may increase the incidence of postpartum hemorrhage.

Infections are more common and more serious in pregnant diabetic women. Disorders of carbohydrate metabolism alter the body's normal resistance to infection. The inflammatory response, leukocyte function, and vaginal pH are all affected. Vaginal infections, particularly monilial vaginitis, are more common in pregnant diabetic women. Urinary tract infections (UTIs) are also more prevalent. Infection is serious because it causes increased insulin resistance and may result in ketoacidosis. Postpartum infection is more common among diabetic women who are insulin dependent.

Ketoacidosis occurs most often during the second and third trimesters, when the diabetogenic effect of pregnancy is the greatest. When the maternal metabolism is stressed by illness or infection, the diabetic woman is at increased risk for diabetic ketoacidosis (DKA). Another factor that may contribute to the risk for hyperglycemia and subsequent DKA is the use of tocolytic drugs such as terbutaline to arrest preterm labor (magnesium sulfate is the preferred tocolytic agent for diabetic women) (Foley et al., 1993; Regenstein, Belluomini & Katz, 1993). DKA may also occur because of the woman's failure to take insulin appropriately. The onset of previously undiagnosed diabetes during pregnancy is another cause of DKA. DKA may occur with blood glucose levels barely exceeding 200 mg/dl, compared with 300 to 350 mg/dl in the nonpregnant state. In response to stress factors such as infection or illness, hyperglycemia occurs as a result of increased hepatic glucose production and decreased peripheral glucose use. Stress hormones, which act to impair insulin action and further contribute to insulin deficiency, are released. Fatty acids are mobilized from fat stores to enter into the circulation, and as they are oxidized, ketone bodies are released into the peripheral circulation. The woman's buffering system is unable to compensate, and metabolic acidosis develops. The excessive blood glucose and ketone bodies result in osmotic diuresis with subsequent loss of fluid and electrolytes, volume depletion, and cellular dehydration. Prompt treatment of DKA is necessary to avoid maternal coma or death. Ketoacidosis occurring at any time during pregnancy can lead to intrauterine fetal death and is also a cause of preterm labor. Perinatal mortality is about 20% with maternal ketoacidosis (Cunningham et al., 1997) (Table 23-1).

The risk of hypoglycemia is also increased. Early in pregnancy, when hepatic production of glucose is diminished and peripheral use of glucose is enhanced, hypoglycemia occurs frequently, often during sleep. Later in pregnancy, as insulin doses are adjusted to maintain normoglycemia, hypoglycemia may also result. Women with a prepregnancy history of severe hypoglycemia are at increased risk for severe hypoglycemia during gestation. Mild to moderate hypoglycemic episodes in pregnant diabetic women do not appear to have significant deleterious effects on fetal well-being. The long-term fetal effects of severe maternal hypoglycemia are as yet uncertain (Reece, Homko & Wiznitzer, 1994) (see Table 23-1).

TABLE 23-1 *Differentiation of Hypoglycemia (Insulin Shock) and Hyperglycemia (Diabetic Ketoacidosis)*

CAUSES	ONSET	SYMPTOMS	INTERVENTIONS
HYPOGLYCEMIA (INSULIN SHOCK)			

Excess insulin
Insufficient food (delayed or missed meals)
Excessive exercise or work
Indigestion, diarrhea, vomiting
	Rapid (regular insulin)
	Gradual (modified insulin or oral hypoglycemic agents)
		Irritability
		Hunger
		Sweating
		Nervousness
		Personality change
		Weakness
		Fatigue
		Blurred or double vision
		Dizziness
		Headache
		Pallor; clammy skin
		Shallow respirations
		Rapid pulse
		Laboratory values
		    Urine: negative for sugar and acetonze
		    Blood glucose: ≤60 mg/dl
			Check blood glucose level when symptoms first appear
			Eat or drink 10 to 15 gm simple carbohydrate immediately
			Recheck blood glucose level in 15 min and repeat if glucose remains low
			Notify primary health care provider if no change in glucose level
			If patient is unconscious, administer 50% dextrose IV push, 5% to 10% dextrose in water IV drip, or glucagon
			Obtain blood and urine specimens for laboratory testing

HYPERGLYCEMIA (DKA)			

Insufficient insulin
Excess or wrong kind of food
Infection, injuries, illness
Emotional stress
Insufficient exercise
	Slow (hours to days)	Thirst
		Nausea or vomiting
		Abdominal pain
		Constipation
		Drowsiness
		Dim vision
		Increased urination
		Headache
		Flushed, dry skin
		Rapid breathing
		Weak, rapid pulse
		Acetone (fruity) breath odor
		Laboratory value
		    Urine: positive for sugar and acetone
		    Blood glucose: ≥200 mg/dl
			Notify primary health care provider
			Administer insulin in accordance with blood glucose levels
			Give IV fluids such as normal saline solution or one-half normal saline solution; potassium when urinary output is adequate; bicarbonate for pH <7
			Monitor lab testing of blood and urine

Fetal and neonatal risks and complications

From the moment of conception, the infant of a diabetic woman faces an increased risk of complications that may occur during the antepartum, intrapartum, or neonatal periods. These complications may be mild and transient but are often life-threatening and may result in the infant's death. Infant morbidity and mortality rates associated with diabetic pregnancy are significantly reduced with strict control of maternal glucose levels before and during pregnancy.

Despite the improvements in care of diabetic pregnancy, sudden and unexplained stillbirth is still a major concern. Typically, this is observed in pregnancies after 36 weeks in women with vascular disease or poor glycemic control. It may also be associated with DKA, preeclampsia, hydramnios, or macrosomia. Although the exact cause of stillbirth is unknown, it may be related to chronic intrauterine hypoxia.

The most important cause of perinatal loss in diabetic pregnancy is congenital malformations. The incidence of congenital anomalies among infants of insulin-dependent diabetic women is from two to four times that of the general population. Up to 50% of all perinatal deaths among infants of diabetic mothers are the result of congenital malformations (Landon & Gabbe, 1995). The incidence of congenital malformations is related to the severity and duration of the diabetes. In addition to hyperglycemia, hyperketonemia and hypoglycemia may also play a role in the development of congenital anomalies (Landon, 1996). Anomalies commonly seen in infants of diabetic pregnancy primarily affect (1) the central nervous system,

(2) the cardiovascular system, (3) the urinary system, and (4) the gastrointestinal system. (see Chapter 28).

Macrosomia, excessive growth, is often defined as a weight ≥4,000 to 4,500 gm. Macrosomia may also be defined as large for gestational age (LGA), wherein the fetus or newborn is bigger than 90% of similar babies the same age (Landon, 1996). The fetal pancreas begins to secrete insulin at 10 to 14 weeks' gestation. The fetus responds to maternal hyperglycemia by secreting large amounts of insulin (hyperinsulinism). Insulin acts as a growth hormone, causing the fetus to produce excess stores of glycogen, protein, and adipose tissue, leading to increased fetal size. During birth, the macrosomic infant is at risk for a fractured clavicle, a liver or spleen laceration, a brachial plexus injury, facial palsy, phrenic nerve injury, or subdural hemorrhage (for further discussion, see Chapter 28) (Landon & Gabbe, 1995; Schwartz et al., 1994).

Intrauterine growth retardation (IUGR) is often seen in infants of diabetic mothers with vascular disease. It is related to compromised uteroplacental circulation and may be worsened in the presence of ketoacidosis and preeclampsia. The amount of oxygen available to the fetus is decreased as a result of maternal vascular changes (Bernstein & Gabbe, 1996).

Infants of diabetic mothers are at increased risk for respiratory distress syndrome (RDS). Hyperglycemia and hyperinsulinemia may be instrumental in delaying pulmonary maturation in the fetus of a diabetic mother (Landon & Gabbe, 1995; Piper & Langer, 1993).

For infants of a diabetic pregnancy the transition to extrauterine life is often beset with metabolic abnormalities. Within the first 30 to 60 minutes after birth, neonatal hypoglycemia often occurs. This is caused by the effects of fetal hyperinsulinism and the rapid use of glucose after birth. The incidence of neonatal hypoglycemia is related to the mother's glycemic control during pregnancy and to her glucose levels during labor and birth. Hypocalcemia, hypomagnesemia, hyperbilirubinemia, and polycythemia occur more frequently in infants of diabetic mothers, which places these neonates at increased risk (Landon, 1996).

▌CARE MANAGEMENT

Assessment and Nursing Diagnoses

Interview

When a pregnant woman with diabetes initiates prenatal care, a thorough evaluation of her health status is completed. In addition to the routine prenatal assessment, a detailed history regarding the onset and course of the diabetes and its management and the degree of glycemic control before pregnancy is obtained. Effective management of the diabetic pregnancy depends on the woman's adherence to a plan of care. For the woman to care for her diabetes on a daily basis, she must have an adequate understanding of her disease and the prescribed regimen. Thus with the initial prenatal visit the

woman's knowledge regarding diabetes and pregnancy, potential maternal and fetal complications, and the plan of care are thoroughly assessed. With subsequent visits follow-up assessments are completed. Data from these assessments are used to identify the woman's specific learning needs. The support person's knowledge of diabetes is also assessed, and teaching needs are identified.

The woman's emotional status is assessed to determine how she is coping with pregnancy superimposed on preexisting diabetes. Although normal pregnancy typically evokes some degree of stress and anxiety, pregnancy designated as "high risk" serves to compound anxiety and stress levels. Fear of maternal and fetal complications is a major concern. Strict adherence to the plan of care necessitates alterations in patterns of daily living and may be an additional source of stress.

The woman's support system is assessed to identify those people significant to the pregnant woman and their role in her life. It is important to assess reactions of the family or significant other to the pregnancy and to the strict management plan and their involvement in the treatment regimen. Socioeconomic factors are also reviewed. Any area of emotional stress is identified because such stress can precipitate complications.

Physical examination

At the initial visit a thorough physical examination is performed to assess the woman's current health status. In addition to the routine prenatal examination, specific efforts are made to assess the effects of the diabetes. A baseline electrocardiogram (ECG) may be done to assess cardiovascular status. Evaluation for retinopathy is done, with follow-up by an ophthalmologist each trimester and more frequently if retinopathy is diagnosed. Blood pressure is monitored carefully throughout pregnancy because of the increased risk for preeclampsia. The woman's weight gain is also monitored at each visit. Fundal height is measured, noting any abnormal increase in size for dates, which may indicate hydramnios or fetal macrosomia. Leopold's maneuvers may be performed to check for fetal size and possible hydramnios.

Laboratory tests

Routine prenatal laboratory examinations are performed. In addition, baseline renal function may be assessed with a 24-hour urine collection for total protein excretion and creatinine clearance. Urinalysis and culture are performed on the initial prenatal visit and throughout the pregnancy to assess for the presence of UTI, which is common in diabetic pregnancy. At each visit urine is also tested for the presence of glucose and ketones. Because of the risk of coexisting thyroid disease, thyroid function tests may also be performed (see later discussion of thyroid disorders).

For the woman with pregestational type 1 or type 2 diabetes, laboratory tests may be done to assess past glycemic

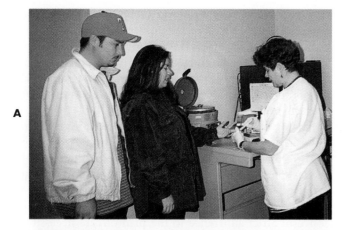

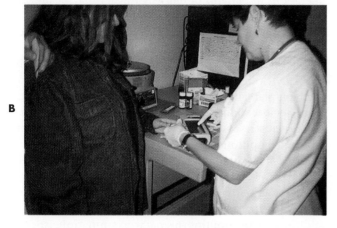

Fig. **23-2 A,** Clinic nurse collects blood to determine glucose level. **B,** Nurse interprets glucose value displayed by monitor. (Courtesy Dee Lowdermilk, UNC Ambulatory Care Clinics, Chapel Hill, NC.)

control. At the initial prenatal visit, **glycosylated hemoglobin A1$_c$** level may be measured. With prolonged hyperglycemia some of the hemoglobin remains saturated with glucose for the life of the red blood cell (RBC). Therefore a test for glycosylated hemoglobin provides a measurement of glycemic control over time, specifically over the previous 4 to 6 weeks. Regular measurements of glycosylated hemoglobin provide data for altering the treatment plan and lead to improvement of glycemic control. Values for the measurement of hemoglobin A1$_c$, the most commonly used index of glycosylated hemoglobin, are as follows (Pagana & Pagana, 1997):

Adult/elderly	4% to 8%
Good diabetic control	7%
Fair diabetic control	10%
Poor diabetic control	13% to 20%

Fasting blood glucose and/or random (1 to 2 hours after eating) glucose levels may be assessed during antepartum visits (Fig. 23-2). Self-blood glucose monitoring records may also be reviewed.

Nursing diagnoses for the woman with pregestational diabetes are listed in the Nursing Diagnoses box.

Nursing Diagnoses

The Woman with Pregestational Diabetes
Knowledge deficit related to:
- Diabetic pregnancy, management, and potential effects on pregnant woman and fetus
- Insulin administration and its effects
- Hypoglycemia and hyperglycemia
- Diabetic diet

Risk for ineffective individual coping related to:
- Woman's responsibility in managing her diabetes during her pregnancy

Anxiety, fear, dysfunctional grieving, powerlessness, body image disturbance, situational low self-esteem, spiritual distress, altered role performance, altered family processes related to:
- Stigma of being labeled "diabetic"
- Effects of diabetes and its potential sequelae on the pregnant woman and the fetus

Risk for noncompliance related to:
- Lack of understanding of diabetes and pregnancy and requirements of treatment plan
- Lack of financial resources to purchase blood glucose monitoring supplies or insulin and necessary supplies
- Insufficient funds or lack of transportation to grocery store to follow dietary regimen

Risk for injury to fetus related to:
- Uteroplacental insufficiency
- Birth trauma

Risk for injury to mother related to:
- Improper insulin administration
- Hypoglycemia and hyperglycemia
- Cesarean or operative vaginal birth
- Postpartum infection

Altered nutrition: less or more than body requirements related to:
- Noncompliance with dietary regimen
- Knowledge deficit regarding increased nutritional needs during pregnancy

Expected Outcomes of Care

Expected outcomes of management for the pregnant woman with pregestational diabetes include that she will:
- Demonstrate/verbalize understanding of diabetic pregnancy, the plan of care, and the importance of glycemic control
- Follow the plan of care
- Achieve and maintain glycemic control

- Demonstrate effective coping
- Experience no complications (maternal morbidity or mortality)
- Give birth to a healthy infant at term

Plan of Care and Interventions
Antepartum

Because of her high-risk status, a diabetic woman is monitored much more frequently and thoroughly than other pregnant women. During the first and second trimesters of pregnancy her routine prenatal care visits will be scheduled every 1 to 2 weeks. Throughout the last trimester she will likely be seen one to two times each week. In the past, routine hospitalization for management of the diabetes, such as insulin dose changes, was common. With the availability of better home glucose monitoring and the growing reluctance of third-party payers to reimburse for hospitalization, pregnant diabetic women are now generally managed as outpatients. Some patient and family education and maternal and fetal assessment may be done in the home, depending on the woman's insurance coverage and care provider preference.

Achieving and maintaining constant **euglycemia,** with blood glucose levels in the range of 60 to 120 mg/dl (Table 23-2), is the primary goal of medical therapy for the pregnant diabetic woman. Euglycemia is achieved through a combination of diet, insulin, exercise, and blood glucose determinations. Providing the patient with the knowledge, skill, and motivation she needs to achieve and maintain excellent blood glucose control is the primary nursing goal.

Achieving euglycemia requires commitment on the part of the patient and her family to make the necessary lifestyle changes, which can sometimes seem overwhelming. Maintaining tight blood glucose control necessitates that the patient follow a consistent daily schedule. She must get up and go to bed, eat, exercise, and take insulin at the same time each day. Blood glucose measurements are done frequently to determine how well the major components of therapy—diet, insulin, and exercise—are working together to control blood glucose levels.

In addition to the routine prenatal care provided to all pregnant women, the diabetic woman will receive additional counseling. She should wear an identification bracelet at all times and should carry insulin, syringes, and "glucose boosters" (see Home Care box) with her whenever she is away from home. She should also be given written instructions for reporting the development of problems such as nausea, vomiting, and infections, including directions for reaching her health care provider by phone at night and on weekends and holidays.

Because the diabetic woman is at risk for infections, eye problems, and neurologic changes, foot care and general skin care are important. A daily bath that includes good perineal care and foot care is important. For dry skin, lotions, creams,

TABLE 23-2	Target Blood Glucose Levels during Pregnancy
TIME OF DAY	TARGET GLUCOSE LEVEL (MG/DL)
Before breakfast (fasting)	60-90
Before lunch, dinner, bedtime	60-105
One to 2 hours after meals (postprandial)	100-120
2 AM to 4 AM	60-120

From American Diabetes Association: *Medical management of pregnancy complicated by diabetes,* ed 2, Alexandria, Va, 1994, The Association.

or oils can be applied. Tight clothing should be avoided. Shoes or slippers should be worn at all times, should fit properly, and are best worn with socks or stockings. Feet should be inspected regularly; toenails should be cut straight across, and professional help should be sought for any foot problems. Extremes of temperature should be avoided.

Diet. The woman with pregestational diabetes has likely been previously exposed to nutritional counseling regarding management of the diabetes. Because pregnancy precipitates special nutritional concerns and needs, the woman must be educated to incorporate these changes into dietary planning. Nutritional counseling is usually provided by a registered dietitian.

Dietary management during diabetic pregnancy must be based on blood (not urine) glucose levels. The diet is individualized to allow for increased fetal and metabolic requirements, with consideration of such factors as prepregnancy weight and dietary habits, overall health, ethnic background, lifestyle, stage of pregnancy, knowledge of nutrition, and insulin therapy. The dietary goal is to provide weight gain consistent with a normal pregnancy, to prevent ketoacidosis, and to minimize widely fluctuating blood glucose levels.

Energy needs are usually calculated on the basis of 30 to 35 calories per kilogram of ideal body weight, with the average diet including 2,200 (first trimester) to 2,500 calories (second and third trimesters). Total calories may be distributed among three meals and one evening snack, or more commonly, three meals and at least two snacks. Meals should be eaten on time and never skipped. Snacks must be carefully planned in accordance with insulin therapy to avoid fluctuations in blood glucose levels. A large bedtime snack of at least 25 gm of carbohydrate with some protein is recommended to help prevent hypoglycemia and starvation ketosis during the night.

The ratio of carbohydrate, protein, and fat is important to meet the metabolic needs of the woman and the fetus. Approximately 50% to 60% of the total calories should be carbohydrate, with a minimum of 250 gm per day. Simple carbohydrates are limited; complex carbohydrates that are high in fiber content are recommended because the starch

HOME CARE *Patient Instructions for Self-Care*

Dietary Management of Diabetic Pregnancy

- Follow the prescribed diet plan.
- Eat a well-balanced diet, including daily food requirements for a normal pregnancy.
- Divide daily food intake between three meals and two to four snacks, depending on individual needs.
- Eat a substantial bedtime snack to prevent a severe drop in blood glucose level during the night.
- Limit the intake of fats if weight gain occurs too rapidly.
- Take daily vitamins and iron as prescribed by the health care provider.
- Avoid foods high in refined sugar.
- Eat consistently each day; never skip meals or snacks.
- Reduce the intake of saturated fat and cholesterol.
- Eat foods high in dietary fiber.
- Avoid alcohol and caffeine.

and protein in such foods help to regulate the blood glucose level as a result of more sustained glucose release. Protein intake should constitute 12% to 20% of the total kilocalories. Twenty percent to 30% of the daily caloric intake should come from fat, with no more than 10% saturated fats (see Home Care box above). Weight gain for most women should be about 12 kg during the pregnancy (Gilbert & Harmon, 1998).

Exercise. Although it has been shown that exercise enhances the use of glucose and decreases insulin need in nonpregnant diabetic women, there are limited data regarding exercise in pregestational diabetes. Any prescription of exercise during diabetic pregnancy should be done by the primary health care provider and should be closely monitored to prevent complications. For those women with vasculopathy, only mild exercise is recommended because exercise causes a redistribution of blood flow, which increases the potential for ischemic injury to the placenta and already compromised organs. Also, women with vasculopathy typically depend completely on exogenous insulin and are at greater risk for wide fluctuations in blood glucose levels and ketoacidosis, which can be worsened by exercise.

When exercise is prescribed by the health care provider as part of the treatment plan, careful instructions are given to the woman. She should be told that exercise need not be vigorous to be beneficial: 15 to 30 minutes of walking four to six times a week is satisfactory for most pregnant women. Other exercises that may be recommended are non-weight-bearing activities such as arm ergometry or use of a recumbent bicycle. The best time for exercise is after meals, when the blood glucose level is rising. If the woman exercises at a time when the insulin is peaking or engages in prolonged exercise without carbohydrate intake, hypoglycemia may result. Hyperglycemia may occur when exercise is done at

a time when insulin action is waning. To monitor the effect of insulin on blood glucose levels, the woman can measure blood glucose before, during, and after exercise. The woman should be aware of the possibility of uterine contractions occurring during exercise and stop immediately if they are detected.

Insulin therapy. Adequate insulinization of the pregnant woman is the primary factor in the maintenance of normoglycemia during pregnancy, thus ensuring proper glucose metabolism of the mother and fetus. Insulin requirements during pregnancy change dramatically as the pregnancy progresses, necessitating frequent adjustments in insulin dosage. In the first trimester there is little or no change in prepregnancy insulin requirements; however, insulin dosage may need to be decreased because of hypoglycemia. During the second and third trimester, because of insulin resistance, dosage must be increased to maintain target glucose levels.

For the type 1 pregestational diabetic woman, who has typically been accustomed to one injection per day of intermediate-acting insulin, multiple daily injections of mixed insulin are a new experience. The type 2 diabetic woman, previously treated with oral hypoglycemics, is faced with the task of learning to administer self-injections of insulin. The nurse is instrumental in education and support of pregestational diabetic women with regard to insulin administration and adjustment of insulin dosage to maintain normoglycemia (see Home Care box at right).

More types of insulin are available today than ever before. Beef and pork insulin have largely been replaced by biosynthetic human insulin preparations (Humulin or Novolin), which are less likely to cause antibody formation. New-onset diabetic patients are almost always started on this type of insulin. Lispro (Humalog), a new rapid-acting insulin, is now available. It has a faster onset and shorter duration of action than regular insulin. Advantages of lispro include convenience, since it is injected immediately before mealtime; less hyperglycemia following meals; and fewer hypoglycemic episodes in some patients. Because its effects last ≤5 hours, most patients require a longer-acting insulin along with lispro to maintain optimal blood glucose levels (Eli Lilly & Co., 1996; Hoffmeister & Haines, 1996) (Table 23-3). Lispro can be used safely in pregnancy, but unlike other insulins, it is not available without a prescription.

Most insulin-dependent diabetic women are managed with two to three injections per day. Usually, two thirds of the daily insulin dose, with longer-acting (NPH) and short-acting (regular or lispro) insulin combined in a 2:1 ratio, is given before breakfast. Sometimes the remaining one third, again a combination of longer- and short-acting insulin, is administered in the evening before dinner. To reduce the risk of hypoglycemia during the night, often separate injections are administered, with short-acting insulin given before dinner, followed by longer-acting insulin at bedtime.

TABLE 23-3	*Insulin Administration during Pregnancy: Expected Time of Action*		
TYPE OF INSULIN	**ONSET**	**PEAK**	**DURATION**
Lispro (rapid acting)	Within 15 min	30-90 min	3 hr
Regular (rapid acting)	30 min-1 hr	2-4 hr	5-8 hr
Intermediate acting	2-4 hr	5-10 hr	12-24 hr
Long acting	3-4 hr	14-24 hr	24-36 hr

HOME CARE *Patient Instructions for Self-Care*

Self-Administration of Insulin

PROCEDURE FOR MIXING NPH (INTERMEDIATE-ACTING) AND REGULAR (SHORT-ACTING) INSULIN

- Wash hands thoroughly and gather supplies. Be sure the insulin syringe corresponds to the concentration of insulin you are using.
- Check insulin bottle to be certain it is the appropriate type and check the expiration date.
- Gently rotate (do not shake) the insulin vial to mix the insulin.
- Wipe off rubber stopper of each vial with alcohol.
- Draw into syringe the amount of air equal to total dose.
- Inject air equal to NPH (intermediate-acting) dose into NPH vial. Remove syringe from vial.
- Inject air equal to regular insulin dose into regular insulin vial.
- Invert regular insulin bottle and withdraw regular insulin dose.
- Without adding more air to NPH vial, carefully withdraw NPH dose.

PROCEDURE FOR SELF-INJECTION OF INSULIN

- Select proper injection site (remember to rotate sites).
- Cleanse injection site with alcohol.
- Pinch the skin up to form a subcutaneous pocket and, holding the syringe like a pencil, puncture the skin at a 45- to 90-degree angle. If there is a great deal of fatty tissue at the site, spread the skin taut and inject the syringe at a 90-degree angle.
- Slowly inject the insulin.
- As you withdraw the needle, cover the injection site with sterile gauze and apply gentle pressure to prevent bleeding.
- Record insulin dosage and time of injection.

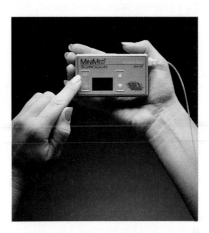

Fig. 23-3 Insulin pump shows basal rate for pregnant woman with diabetes. (Courtesy MiniMed, Inc, Sylmar, Calif.)

secreting insulin (Fig. 23-3). This portable, battery-powered device infuses regular insulin at a set basal rate and has the capacity to deliver up to four different basal rates in 24 hours. The pump also delivers bolus doses of insulin before meals to control postmeal blood glucose levels. The infusion tubing from the insulin pump can be left in place for several weeks without local complications. Insulin pumps are usually reserved for women whose diabetes cannot be controlled by multiple insulin injections and who are highly motivated, because meticulous blood glucose monitoring is required (Landon & Gabbe, 1995; Reece & Homko, 1993).

Monitoring blood glucose levels. Blood glucose testing at home is the commonly accepted method for monitoring blood glucose levels and the most important tool available to the woman to assess her degree of glycemic control. In addition, this monitoring provides motivation to continue the prescribed treatment plan, and the data obtained facilitates interaction with the health care team in maintaining glycemic control and minimizing fetal risk.

Pregestational diabetic women are often familiar with self-monitoring of blood glucose levels because it is typically included in the management plan for type 1 and some cases of type 2 diabetes. However, a thorough assessment of the woman's knowledge and skill related to blood glucose testing is essential to ensure accurate monitoring of glucose levels during pregnancy. The nurse observes the

Another alternative insulin regimen that works well for some women is to administer short-acting insulin before each meal and longer-acting insulin at bedtime (Jovanovic-Peterson & Peterson, 1992; Landon & Gabbe, 1995; Reece & Homko, 1993).

Although subcutaneous insulin injections are most commonly used, continuous insulin infusion systems may be used during pregnancy. The insulin "pump" is designed to mimic more closely the function of the pancreas in woman performing blood glucose monitoring to determine her accuracy and comfort with the system. The family is also included in the assessment and in subsequent instruction.

Pregnancy demands more frequent and judicious monitoring than many women have practiced previously. Willingness to comply with the monitoring schedule is essential to the management plan. Home glucose monitoring should be done using a glucose reflectance meter, which is battery powered and determines the blood glucose level by the amount of light reflected from a reacted test strip. Most insurance companies will cover the cost of a meter and necessary supplies. To perform blood glucose monitoring, a drop of blood is obtained by a finger stick and placed on a test strip. After a specified amount of time, the glucose level can be read by the meter (see Home Care box).

Meters that incorporate memory to store a large number of readings are available; however, the woman is still encouraged to keep written records of glucose levels. She should bring her written records and/or her meter containing stored test results with her to each appointment. It is important that the monitoring equipment be checked for accuracy at intervals by comparing the woman's results on her machine with the results of a laboratory test done at the same time on a capillary, whole blood sample.

Blood glucose levels are routinely measured at various times throughout the day, such as before breakfast, lunch, and dinner; 2 hours after each meal; at bedtime; and in the middle of the night. Because hyperglycemia is to be avoided, postprandial measurements are often performed. Hyperglycemia will most likely be identified in 2-hour postprandial values, because blood glucose levels peak about 2 hours after a meal. The health care provider will determine for each individual woman the number and timing of routine blood glucose determinations.

Special circumstances may necessitate more frequent testing. Women are instructed to check glucose levels at any sign of hypoglycemia or hyperglycemia. When there is any readjustment in insulin dosage or diet, more frequent measurement of blood glucose is warranted. If nausea, vomiting, or diarrhea occur, or if any infection is present, the woman will likely be asked to monitor her blood glucose levels more closely.

Target levels of blood glucose during pregnancy are lower than nonpregnant values. Acceptable fasting levels are generally between 60 and 90 mg/dl, and 2-hour postprandial levels should be between 90 and 120 mg/dl (see Table 23-2). The woman should be told to immediately report episodes of hypoglycemia (<60 mg/dl) and hyperglycemia (>200 mg/dl) to her health care provider so that adjustments in diet or insulin therapy can be made (ADA, 1994).

Pregnant diabetic women are much more likely to develop hypoglycemia than hyperglycemia, since the goal of therapy is to maintain the blood glucose in a narrow, low-normal range of 60 to 120 mg/dl. While a blood glucose level

---

HOME CARE *Patient Instructions for Self-Care*

Self-Testing of Blood Glucose Level

- Gather supplies, check expiration date, and read instructions on testing materials. Prepare glucose reflectance meter for use according to manufacturer's directions.
- Wash hands in warm water (warmth increases circulation).
- Select site on side of any finger (all fingers should be used in rotation).
- Pierce site with lancet (may use automatic, spring-loaded, puncturing device). Cleaning the site with alcohol is not necessary.
- Drop hand down to side; with other hand gently squeeze finger from hand to fingertip.
- Allow blood to drop onto testing strip. Be sure to cover entire reagent area.
- Determine blood glucose value using the glucose reflectance meter, following manufacturer's instructions.
- Record results.
- Repeat daily as instructed by health care provider and as needed for signs of hypoglycemia or hyperglycemia.

From American Diabetes Association: *Medical management of pregnancy complicated by diabetes,* ed 2, Alexandria, Va, 1995, The Association.

---

of >120 mg/dl is considered too high for a pregnant diabetic woman, it will not produce the classic signs and symptoms of hyperglycemia. On the other hand, many women will experience signs and symptoms of hypoglycemia with blood glucose levels <60 mg/dl (see Table 23-1).

Most episodes of mild or moderate hypoglycemia can be treated with oral intake of 10 to 15 gm of simple carbohydrate (see Home Care box at right). If severe hypoglycemia occurs, where the woman experiences a decrease or loss of consciousness or an inability to swallow, she will require a parenteral injection of glucagon or intravenous (IV) glucose (ADA, 1994; Becton Dickinson & Co., 1997). Because hypoglycemia can develop rapidly and because impaired judgment can be associated with even moderate episodes, it is vital that family members, friends, and work colleagues be able to quickly recognize signs and symptoms and initiate proper treatment if necessary (Becton Dickinson & Co., 1997).

While hyperglycemia is less likely to occur in compliant patients, it is still a dangerous complication. Hyperglycemia in the pregnant diabetic can rapidly progress to diabetic ketoacidosis. Women and family members should be particularly alert for signs and symptoms of hyperglycemia, especially when infections or other illnesses occur (see Table 23-1 and Home Care box at right).

Urine testing. Urine testing for ketones continues to have a place in diabetic management, since it may provide vital information for the pregnant woman, such as the onset of DKA. Women may be taught to perform urine testing daily with the first morning urine. Testing may also be done

HOME CARE *Patient Instructions for Self-Care*

Treatment for Hypoglycemia

- Be familiar with signs and symptoms of hypoglycemia (nervousness, headache, shaking, irritability, personality change, hunger, blurred vision, sweaty skin, tingling of mouth or extremities).
- Check blood glucose level immediately when hypoglycemic symptoms occur.
- If blood glucose is <60 mg/dl, immediately eat or drink something that contains 10 to 15 gm of simple carbohydrate. Examples are:
  —1/2 cup (4 ounces) unsweetened fruit juice
  —1/2 cup (4 ounces) regular (not diet) soda
  —5 to 6 LifeSavers candies
  —1 tablespoon honey or corn (Karo) syrup
  —1 cup (8 ounces) milk
  —2 to 3 glucose tablets
- Rest for 15 minutes, then recheck blood glucose.
- If glucose level is still <60 mg/dl, eat or drink another serving of one of the "glucose boosters" listed above.
- Wait 15 minutes, then recheck blood glucose. If it is still <60 mg/dl, notify health care provider immediately.

From American Diabetes Association: *Medical management of insulin-dependent (type 1) diabetes,* ed 2, Alexandria, Va, 1994, The Association; Becton Dickinson & Co: *Controlling low blood sugar reactions,* Franklin Lakes, NJ, 1997, Becton Dickinson.

HOME CARE *Patient Instructions for Self-Care*

What to Do When Illness Occurs

- Be sure to take insulin even though appetite and food intake may be less than normal. (Insulin needs are increased with illness or infection.)
- Call the health care provider and relay the following information:
  —Symptoms of illness (e.g., nausea, vomiting, diarrhea)
  —Fever
  —Most recent blood glucose level
  —Urine ketones
  —Time and amount of last insulin dose
- Increase oral intake of fluids to prevent dehydration.
- Rest as much as possible.
- If unable to reach health care provider and blood glucose exceeds 200 mg/dl with urine ketones present, seek emergency treatment at the nearest health care facility. Do not attempt to self-treat for this.

---

if a meal is missed or delayed, when illness occurs, or when the blood glucose level is greater than 200 mg/dl.

Spilling a trace or a small amount of ketones requires no treatment. However, if ketones appear repeatedly at the same time each day, some adjustment in diet may be needed. If testing shows a large amount of ketones, the health care provider should be contacted immediately (ADA, 1995).

Fetal surveillance. Diagnostic techniques for fetal surveillance are often performed to assess fetal growth and well-being. The goals of fetal surveillance are to detect fetal compromise as early as possible and to prevent intrauterine fetal death or unnecessary preterm birth. The majority of fetal surveillance measures are concentrated in the third trimester, when the risk of fetal compromise is greatest.

Early in pregnancy, efforts are made to determine the estimated date of birth. A baseline sonogram is done during the first trimester to assess gestational age. Follow-up ultrasound examinations are usually performed during the pregnancy, as often as every 4 to 6 weeks, to monitor fetal growth, estimate fetal weight, and detect hydramnios, macrosomia, and congenital anomalies.

Because diabetic pregnancies are at greater risk for neural tube defects (e.g., spina bifida, anencephaly, microcephaly), measurement of maternal serum alpha-fetoprotein is performed between 16 and 18 weeks' gestation. This is often done in conjunction with a detailed ultrasound study to examine the fetus for neural tube defects.

Fetal echocardiography may be performed between 18 and 22 weeks' gestation to detect cardiac anomalies. Some practitioners repeat this fetal surveillance test at 34 weeks. Doppler studies of the umbilical artery may be performed in women with vascular disease to detect placental compromise.

Maternal evaluation of fetal movements (kick counts) is used primarily as a screening technique in fetal surveillance. Few research studies have investigated the use of this method in diabetic pregnancies.

A commonly used measure of fetal well-being is the nonstress test, typically beginning around 28 to 30 weeks' gestation. After 32 weeks, testing may be done twice weekly. For the woman with vascular disease, testing may begin earlier and continue more frequently. In the presence of a nonreactive nonstress test, a contraction stress test or fetal biophysical profile may be used to evaluate fetal well-being (Landon, 1996; Landon & Gabbe, 1995; Reece & Homko, 1994).

Complications requiring hospitalization. Occasionally it becomes necessary to hospitalize a diabetic woman during pregnancy. A few days in the hospital early in pregnancy may be required to complete baseline cardiovascular, renal, and ophthalmologic evaluations and balance diet and insulin to achieve satisfactory glucose control. Infection, which can lead to hyperglycemia and diabetic ketoacidosis, is an indication for hospitalization, regardless of gestational age. At any time during the pregnancy, women who fail to maintain acceptable blood glucose levels may be hospitalized. A few days in a controlled environment often greatly increases patient compliance with diet and insulin therapy, resulting in marked improvement in blood glucose levels. Hospitalization during the third trimester for closer maternal and fetal observation may be indicated for women with vasculopathy, because of the increased risk for renal impairment, hypertensive disorders, and fetal compromise (ADA, 1994).

Determination of birth date and mode of birth. Today the majority of diabetic pregnancies are allowed to progress to term (38 to 40 weeks' gestation), as long as good metabolic control is maintained and all parameters of antepartum fetal surveillance remain within normal limits. Reasons to proceed with delivery before term include poor metabolic control, worsening hypertensive disorders, fetal macrosomia, or fetal growth restriction (Reece & Homko, 1994).

Many practitioners plan for elective labor induction between 38 and 40 weeks provided that maternal glucose levels are well controlled. To confirm fetal lung maturity before birth, an amniocentesis may be performed in pregnancies earlier than 39 weeks. For the pregnancy complicated by diabetes, fetal lung maturation is better predicted by the amniotic fluid phosphatidylglycerol than by the lecithin/sphingomyelin ratio. If the fetal lungs are still immature, birth should be postponed as long as the results of fetal assessment remain reassuring. Amniocentesis may be repeated to monitor lung maturity. Delivery despite poor fetal lung maturity may be essential when testing suggests fetal compromise or if preeclampsia (PIH), rapidly worsening retinopathy, or renal failure develops (Landon, 1996).

The mode of birth for pregestational diabetic women is a subject of controversy among practitioners. The cesarean rate for these women is exceedingly high, around 45%. Cesarean birth is often performed when antepartum testing suggests fetal distress or the estimated fetal weight is 4,000 to 4,500 gm. Also, when induction of labor is desired and the cervix fails to respond, cesarean birth is often necessary (Landon, 1996; Reece & Homko, 1994).

Intrapartum

During the intrapartum period the pregestational diabetic woman must be monitored closely to prevent complications related to dehydration, hypoglycemia, and hyperglycemia. Most women use large amounts of energy (calories) to accomplish the work and manage the stress of labor and birth; however, this calorie expenditure varies with the individual. Blood glucose levels and hydration must be carefully controlled during labor. An IV line is inserted for infusion of a maintenance fluid, such as lactated Ringer's or 5% dextrose in lactated Ringer's solution. Insulin may be administered by continuous infusion or intermittent subcutaneous injection. Determinations of blood glucose levels are made every hour, and fluids and insulin are adjusted to maintain blood glucose levels ≤100 mg/dl. It is essential that these target glucose levels be maintained because hyperglycemia during labor can precipitate metabolic problems, particularly hypoglycemia, in the neonate (Landon, 1996; Reece & Homko, 1993).

During labor, continuous fetal heart monitoring is necessary. The mother should assume a side-lying position during bed rest in labor to prevent supine hypotension because of a large fetus or polyhydramnios. Labor is allowed to progress provided normal rates of cervical dilatation, fetal descent, and fetal well-being are maintained. Failure to progress may indicate a macrosomic infant and cephalopelvic disproportion, which necessitates cesarean birth. The woman is observed and treated during labor for diabetic complications such as hyperglycemia, ketosis, ketoacidosis, and glycosuria. A neonatologist or pediatrician may be present at the birth to initiate assessment and neonatal care.

If a cesarean birth is planned, it should be scheduled in the early morning to facilitate glycemic control. The morning dose of insulin should be withheld and the woman given nothing by mouth. Epidural anesthesia is recommended because hypoglycemia can be detected earlier if the woman is awake. After surgery, glucose levels should be closely monitored, at least every 2 hours, and an IV solution containing 5% dextrose is infused (Landon & Gabbe, 1995).

Postpartum

In the immediate postpartum period, insulin requirements decrease substantially because the major source of insulin resistance, the placenta, has been removed. Women with type 1 diabetes may require only one half to two thirds the prenatal insulin dose on the first postpartum day, provided that they are eating a full diet. It takes several days after birth to reestablish carbohydrate homeostasis (see Fig. 23-1, *D, E*). Blood glucose levels are monitored in the postpartum period, and insulin dosage is adjusted accordingly. Blood glucose levels do not need to be as tightly controlled after birth. Usually insulin is not given until the blood glucose level is >200 mg/dl (American College of Obstetricians and Gynecologists [ACOG], 1994a; ADA, 1994). The insulin-dependent woman must realize the importance of eating on time even if the baby needs feeding or other pressing demands exist. Type 2 diabetic women often require no insulin in the postpartum period and are able to maintain normoglycemia through diet alone or with oral hypoglycemics.

Possible postpartum complications include preeclampsia-eclampsia, hemorrhage, and infection. Hemorrhage is a possibility if the mother's uterus was overdistended (hydramnios, macrosomic fetus) or overstimulated (oxytocin induction). Postpartum infections such as endometritis are more likely to occur in a woman with diabetes.

Postpartum thyroid dysfunction is more common among diabetic women (see later discussion of thyroid disorders). Routine thyroid screening may be performed during postpartum visits (Alvarez-Marfany et al., 1994; Gerstein, 1993).

Diabetic mothers are encouraged to breastfeed. In addition to the advantages of maternal satisfaction and pleasure, breastfeeding has an antidiabetogenic effect. Many mothers with diabetes find that their glucose levels are easier to control. Insulin requirements may be half the prepregnancy levels because of the carbohydrate used in human milk production. Because glucose levels are lower, breastfeeding women are at increased risk for hypoglycemia, especially in the early postpartum period and after breastfeeding sessions (Neubauer et al., 1993). It is important to remind the mother that continued dietary modification is needed to ensure adequate nutrition during lactation. Breastfeeding mothers with diabetes may be at increased risk for mastitis and yeast infections of the breast, particularly if glucose levels are not well controlled. Insulin dosage, which is decreased during lactation, must be recalculated at weaning (Landon, 1996; Lawrence, 1994) (see Fig. 23-1, *F*).

The diabetic mother may have early breastfeeding difficulties. Poor metabolic control may delay lactogenesis and contribute to decreased milk production (Neubauer et al., 1993). Many diabetic women give birth by cesarean, and the effects of anesthesia and postoperative discomfort may delay maternal attachment and make breastfeeding more difficult. In addition, initial contact and opportunity to breastfeed the infant are often delayed because many institutions place infants of diabetic mothers in neonatal intensive care units or special care nurseries for observation during the first few hours after birth. Support and assistance from nursing staff and lactation specialists can facilitate the mother's early experience with breastfeeding and encourage her to continue (Ferris et al., 1993).

The new mother needs information about family planning and contraception. Although family planning is important for all women, it is essential for the diabetic woman to safeguard her own health and to promote optimal outcomes in future pregnancies. The woman and her partner should be informed that the risks associated with pregnancy increase with the duration and severity of the diabetic condition and that pregnancy may contribute to vascular changes associated with diabetes.

The risks and benefits of contraceptive methods should be discussed with the mother and her partner before discharge from the hospital. The barrier method is the preferred method of contraception for the insulin-dependent diabetic woman. Barrier methods such as the diaphragm or condom and spermicide pose the least risk. The problem with these methods, however, is the inconsistency of use, which often leads to unplanned pregnancy (Landon, 1996; Mestman & Schmidt-Sarosi, 1993).

Use of oral contraceptives by diabetic women is controversial because of the risk of thromboembolic and vascular complications and the effect on carbohydrate metabolism. In women without vascular disease or other risk factors, low-dose oral contraceptives may be prescribed. Close monitoring of blood pressure and glucose levels is necessary to detect complications (Kjos, 1993; Landon & Gabbe, 1995).

Intrauterine contraceptive devices increase the risk of infection, especially during the first 4 months after insertion. However, they may be used for diabetic women who are older or who have hypertension or other vascular disease.

Such an individual should be parous, in a monogamous relationship, and at low risk for sexually transmitted diseases (STDs), with no history of pelvic infection. These women must be able to recognize the signs of pelvic infection and STDs and notify their health care providers promptly if these signs occur (Kjos, 1993).

There is no contraindication to use of the Norplant system in diabetic women who have no cardiovascular complications (Jovanovic-Peterson, 1993).

Sterilization should be discussed with the woman who has completed her family or who has significant vasculopathy (ADA, 1994).

Evaluation

Evaluation of the care of the pregnant woman with pregestational diabetes is based on the previously stated expected outcomes of care and are closely associated with the degree of maternal metabolic control during pregnancy (see Plan of Care).

Gestational Diabetes Mellitus

Gestational diabetes mellitus (GDM) complicates approximately 4% of all pregnancies in the United States and accounts for 90% of all cases of diabetic pregnancy. Prevalence varies by racial and ethnic groups. GDM is more likely to occur among Hispanic, Native American, Asian, and African-American populations than in Caucasians (The Expert Committee on the Diagnosis and Classification of Diabetes Mellitus, 1997). Persons with GDM are at significant risk of developing glucose intolerance later in life; about 50% will be diagnosed as diabetic within 22 to 28 years. This is especially true of women whose GDM is diagnosed early in pregnancy or who manifest fasting hyperglycemia (Landon, 1996). Classic risk factors for GDM include maternal age >30 years; obesity; family history of type 2 diabetes; and an obstetric history of a infant weighing >9 pounds, hydramnios, unexplained stillbirth, miscarriage, or an infant with congenital anomalies. Women at high risk for GDM are often screened at their initial prenatal visit and then rescreened later in pregnancy if the initial screen is negative.

The diagnosis of gestational diabetes is usually made during the second half of pregnancy. Because fetal nutrient demands rise during the late second and the third trimester, maternal nutrient ingestion induces greater and more sustained levels of blood glucose. At the same time, maternal insulin resistance is also increasing because of the insulin antagonistic effects of the placental hormones, cortisol, and insulinase. Consequently, maternal insulin demands rise as much as threefold. The majority of pregnant women are capable of increasing insulin production to compensate for insulin resistance and to maintain normoglycemia. When the pancreas is unable to produce sufficient insulin or the insulin is not used effectively, gestational diabetes can result.

≈≈≈ **PLAN OF CARE** *The Woman with Pregestational Diabetes*

NURSING DIAGNOSIS Knowledge deficit related to interaction of new health condition (pregnancy) with preexisting condition (diabetes mellitus)

Expected Outcomes *The patient will describe interaction of diabetes and pregnancy and potential effects on mother and fetus; follow plan of care for management of diabetes during pregnancy; and exhibit evidence of incorporation of care behaviors into daily routine.*

Nursing Interventions/Rationales

Review woman's general knowledge of diabetes and prepregnancy management routines *to assess baseline knowledge and evaluate effectiveness of treatment regimen.*

Explore woman's knowledge of effects of pregnancy on diabetes and what that means to her particular treatment regimen *to establish a teaching baseline.*

Discuss the potential sequelae of diabetes on mother and fetus, the management of a diabetic pregnancy, the need for careful adherence to the plan of care, and the importance of regular prenatal care *to ensure adequate understanding and promote adherence.*

Help woman plan any needed dietary changes *to promote adequate weight gain, maintain consistent blood glucose levels, and prevent ketoacidosis.*

Teach woman about likely insulin changes that will occur as body weight and gestational age increase and the importance of careful blood glucose monitoring *to ensure correct treatment and decrease chances of complications.*

Teach woman about importance of judicious exercise; the need for careful glucose monitoring before, during, and after exercise; and the need for close monitoring of any exercise program by a health care provider *to avoid ischemic injury to organs or placenta.*

Teach woman and significant other about potential complications and the need for prompt reporting of nausea, vomiting, infections, signs of dehydration, hypoglycemia or hyperglycemia, and any wide swings in blood glucose levels *to ensure early treatment of complications and prevent potential injury to mother and fetus.*

Use multiple teaching sessions, encourage questions, clarify misconceptions, use repetition of material, provide written supplements to teaching sessions, and include significant others *to optimize teaching effectiveness.*

Help woman individualize the knowledge and new treatment needs and integrate them into her existing management protocol *to ensure maximum treatment benefits.*

Have woman demonstrate use of new knowledge *to reinforce correct use of information and positive adaptations in behavior.*

NURSING DIAGNOSIS Fear/anxiety related to threat to maternal and fetal well-being

---

Expected Outcomes *The patient's feelings and symptoms of fear/anxiety will decrease or abate.*

Nursing Interventions/Rationales

Provide a calm, soothing atmosphere and teach family to provide emotional support *to facilitate coping.*

Encourage verbalization of fears *to decrease intensity of emotional response.*

Involve woman and family in the active management of her diabetes and pregnancy *to promote a greater sense of control.*

Encourage woman to differentiate between real and imagined threats to maternal and fetal well-being and detail what she can do to diminish the real threats *to promote a greater sense of control.*

Help woman identify and use appropriate coping strategies and support systems *to reduce fear/anxiety.*

Explore use of desensitization strategies such as progressive muscle relaxation, visual imagery, or thought stopping *to reduce fear-related emotions and related physical symptoms.*

From Wong D & Perry S: *Maternal child nursing care,* St Louis, 1998, Mosby.

Maternal-fetal risks

Women with gestational diabetes are at increased risk for preeclampsia, UTIs, and operative birth, including cesarean, forceps, or vacuum extraction (Mulford et al., 1993).

Hyperglycemia is associated with an increased risk for intrauterine fetal death and neonatal mortality. Perinatal morbidity and mortality are also higher among gestational diabetic women with a history of previous stillbirth, those who have preeclampsia, and those who were diagnosed with GDM late in pregnancy. Infants of gestational diabetic mothers are at risk for macrosomia with associated shoulder dystocia and birth trauma. Gestational diabetes places the neonate at increased risk for neonatal hypoglycemia, hypocalcemia, polycythemia, and hyperbilirubinemia. The infant of a gestational diabetic mother is more likely to be obese in childhood or later in life. There is also a greater chance that the infant will have glucose intolerance, specifically type 2 diabetes, in the future (Dorner & Plagmann, 1994; Silvermann et al., 1995).

The overall incidence of congenital anomalies among infants of gestational diabetic women approaches that of the nondiabetic population because gestational diabetes usually develops after the twentieth week of pregnancy—after the critical period of organogenesis (first trimester) has passed.

I CARE MANAGEMENT

Nurses involved in prenatal care delivery can be instrumental in the identification of women with GDM. Although protocols regarding which women will undergo screening and exactly how the screening will be done vary among care providers, nurses are often responsible for ensuring that the screen is performed on the identified group of women at the proper gestational age. Careful adherence to screening protocols is crucial in order to correctly identify women with GDM.

Screening for Gestational Diabetes Mellitus

Earlier recommendations from the ADA were that all pregnant women should be screened for the development of GDM. However, the Expert Committee on the Diagnosis and Classification of Diabetes Mellitus stated in its 1997 report that it is neither cost-effective nor necessary to screen certain women who are at low risk for GDM. This low-risk group includes normal-weight women <25 years of age who have no family history of diabetes and are not members of an ethnic or racial group known to have a high prevalence of the disease. The American College of Obstetricians and Gynecologists (ACOG) (1994a) has stated that selective screening may be appropriate in some low-risk settings (e.g., teen clinics), but that universal screening might be more appropriate for high-risk populations. ACOG also states that screening is unnecessary in certain populations with a high prevalence of GDM. Women in these groups may be considered to have an abnormal screen and proceed directly to diagnostic testing.

The screening test (glucola screening) most often used consists of a 50-gm oral glucose load, followed by a plasma glucose determination 1 hour later. Screening should be performed at 24 to 28 weeks' gestation. It is not necessary that the woman be fasting. A glucose value of ≥140 mg/dl is considered a positive screen.

A positive glucola screen requires follow-up with a 3-hour **oral glucose tolerance test (OGTT).** The 3-hour OGTT is administered after an overnight fast and at least 3 days of unrestricted diet (at least 150 gm of carbohydrate) and physical activity. The woman is instructed to avoid caffeine because it tends to increase glucose levels and to abstain from smoking for 12 hours before the test. A fasting blood glucose level is drawn before giving a 100-gm glucose load. Blood glucose levels are then drawn 1, 2, and 3 hours later. The woman is diagnosed a gestational diabetic if two or more values are met or exceeded (Fig. 23-4).

Controversy exists over the management of women with only one abnormal OGTT value. Many experts believe that these women are at increased risk for fetal macrosomia. Some experts immediately diagnose and treat these women as gestational diabetic patients. Other authorities prefer to retest them with another 3-hour OGTT 1 month later (Landon, 1996). Often women with one abnormal OGTT value will be placed on a modified diabetic diet that contains no concentrated sweets (candy, cookies, cake, pie, sugar-sweetened drinks) for the remainder of the pregnancy.

Nursing diagnoses are similar to those identified for women with pregestational diabetes (see Nursing Diagnoses box on p. 608).

Expected outcomes of care for the woman with GDM are basically the same as for pregestational diabetic patients except that the time frame for planning may be shortened with GDM because the diagnosis is usually made later in pregnancy.

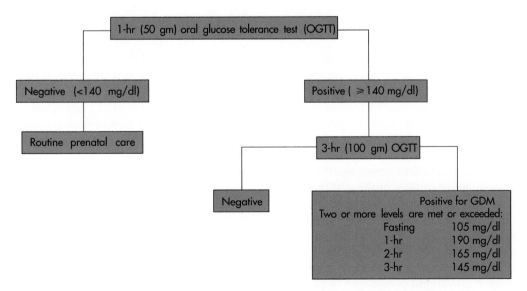

Fig. 23-4 Screening and diagnosis for gestational diabetes. (From American Diabetic Association: Position statement: gestational diabetes mellitus, *Diabetes care* 20 (suppl 1):S44, 1997.)

Antepartum

When the diagnosis of gestational diabetes is made, treatment begins immediately, allowing little or no time for the woman and her family to adjust to the diagnosis before they are expected to participate in the treatment plan. This is in contrast to the woman with pregestational diabetes, who may have had years to learn about the disease and to adapt to dietary modifications, self-monitoring glucose, and insulin administration. With each step of the treatment plan, the nurse and other health care providers should educate the woman and her family, providing detailed and comprehensive explanations to ensure understanding, participation, and adherence to the necessary interventions. Potential complications should be discussed, while the need for maintenance of normoglycemia throughout the remainder of the pregnancy is reinforced. It may be reassuring for the woman and her family to know that gestational diabetes typically disappears when the pregnancy is over.

As with pregestational diabetes, the aim of therapy in women with GDM is meticulous blood glucose control. Fasting blood glucose levels should be <105 mg/dl, and 2-hour postprandial blood levels should be <120 mg/dl (Landon, 1996).

Diet. Dietary modification is the mainstay of treatment for GDM. The woman with GDM is placed on a standard diabetic diet immediately on diagnosis. The usual prescription is for 30 to 35 kcal/kg of present pregnancy weight, which translates into 2,000 to 2,500 calories per day for most women. Some authorities recommend fewer calories for overweight or morbidly obese women, believing that such a diet will cause less hyperglycemia and reduce the need for insulin (Landon, 1996). Dietary counseling by a nutritionist is recommended. Most women with GDM do not require hospitalization for dietary instruction and management.

Exercise. Exercise in women with GDM appears to be safe. It helps to lower blood glucose levels and may be instrumental in eliminating the need for insulin. Women with GDM who already have an active lifestyle should be encouraged to continue an exercise program appropriate for pregnancy. Sedentary women may also be encouraged to increase their physical activity. The selected form of exercise should not stimulate uterine activity; arm exercises and walking are often recommended (ACOG, 1994a; Landon, 1996; Mulford et al., 1993). Of course, any exercise program should always be initiated or continued with the knowledge and consent of the primary health care provider.

Monitoring blood glucose levels. Continuous blood glucose monitoring is necessary to determine if euglycemia can be maintained by diet and exercise. Fasting and postprandial glucose levels should be monitored at least weekly (ACOG, 1994a). Some women with GDM are provided with reflectance meters and encouraged to perform frequent self-monitoring at home (see Home Care box), or monitoring may be done only at the clinic or office visit.

Insulin therapy. It is important to understand that many women with GDM will require insulin during the pregnancy to maintain adequate blood glucose levels, despite compliance with the prescribed diet. This is true because as pregnancy progresses, placental hormones increase blood glucose levels and cause insulin to work less effectively. Depending on the diet prescribed and the blood glucose thresholds used by the practitioner, as many as half of all women with GDM may require insulin at some point during pregnancy (Landon, 1996). Therefore the nurse should never assume that increased blood glucose levels in the woman with GDM have been caused by dietary indiscretion alone without first taking a thorough history.

ACOG (1994a) recommends that women who repetitively exceed the glucose thresholds of 105 mg/dl fasting and 120 mg/dl 2 hours postprandial be started on insulin therapy. In practice, however, many health care providers use either lower or higher thresholds for initiating insulin (Landon, 1996). The woman and her family should be taught the necessary skills to manage insulin administration (see previous discussion). Sometimes hospitalization may be required to regulate blood glucose levels and to educate the woman about glycemic control through insulin therapy in conjunction with dietary modification.

Fetal surveillance. There is no standard recommendation for fetal surveillance in pregnancies complicated by GDM. Women whose blood glucose levels are well controlled by diet are at low risk for fetal death. Many practitioners do not routinely perform antepartum fetal testing on them so long as their fasting and 2-hour postprandial blood glucose levels remain within normal limits and they have no other risk factors. More research must be done to determine if routine antepartum monitoring in this group of low-risk patients would be of benefit. Usually these women are allowed to progress to term and spontaneous labor without intervention. Once the woman reaches 40 weeks' gestation, fetal surveillance once or twice weekly is usually instituted (ACOG, 1994a; Landon, 1996).

Women with GDM whose blood glucose levels are not well controlled or who require insulin therapy, have hypertension, or have a history of previous stillbirth generally receive more intensive fetal biophysical monitoring. There is no standard recommendation regarding initiation of testing. Nonstress tests and biophysical profiles are often performed weekly, beginning anywhere from 32 to 36 weeks' gestation (ACOG, 1994a; Landon, 1996).

Intrapartum

During the labor and birth process, blood glucose levels are monitored at least every 2 hours to maintain levels at 100 mg/dl or less. Glucose levels within this range will decrease the severity of neonatal hypoglycemia. IV fluids containing glucose are not given as a bolus to the woman who is a gestational diabetic, although they may be necessary as maintenance fluids. Although gestational diabetes is not an indication for cesarean birth, it may be necessary in the presence of problems, such as preeclampsia or macrosomia.

Postpartum

More than 90% of women with GDM will return to normal glucose levels following childbirth (Reece & Homko, 1994). However, GDM is likely to recur in future pregnancies, and these women are at increased risk of developing overt diabetes later in life. Assessment for carbohydrate intolerance can be initiated 4 to 6 weeks' postpartum or after breastfeeding has stopped, and should be repeated at regular intervals throughout the woman's life (Dacus et al., 1994; Reece & Homko, 1994). Obesity is a major risk factor for the later development of diabetes. Thus women with a history of GDM, particularly those who are overweight, should be encouraged to make lifestyle changes that include weight loss and exercise to reduce this risk (Kaufmann et al., 1995; Reece & Homko, 1994; Ryan et al., 1995). Because infants born to mothers with GDM are at risk for obesity and future diabetes, regular health care for these children is also essential (Doshier, 1995; Jovanovic-Peterson, 1993).

Evaluation. Care of the woman with GDM is evaluated using the expected outcomes previously described.

THYROID DISORDERS

Hyperthyroidism

Hyperthyroidism occurs in approximately 1 or 2 of every 1,000 pregnancies (Landon, 1996). It is most often caused by Graves' disease, although other possible causes include acute thyroiditis, toxic solitary nodules, toxic multinodular goiter, and trophoblastic disease. Clinical manifestations of hyperthyroidism are associated with an increased basal metabolism rate (BMR) and increased sympathetic nervous system activity. Typical symptoms include nervousness, hyperactivity, weakness, fatigue, weight loss (or poor weight gain), diarrhea, tachycardia, shortness of breath, excessive perspiration, heat intolerance, and muscle tremors. Exophthalmos and enlargement of the thyroid gland (goiter) may also occur. Diagnosis may be difficult because many of the signs and symptoms of hyperthyroidism are typical of pregnancy. Laboratory findings include an elevated free thyroxine index and increased BMR (Landon, 1996; Lazarus, 1993; Molitch, 1995).

Hyperthyroidism in women may be responsible for anovulation and amenorrhea, but it is not a recognized cause of spontaneous abortion or fetal malformation. In women with uncontrolled hyperthyroidism there is an increased risk for congenital anomalies, preterm labor, and low-birth-weight infants. Hyperemesis gravidarum is often associated with elevated thyroid hormone levels (Landon, 1996; Lazarus, 1993).

The primary treatment of hyperthyroidism during pregnancy is drug therapy; the medication of choice is propylthiouracil (PTU). The usual starting dosage is 300 to 450 mg per day; the amount is gradually tapered to the smallest effective dosage to prevent unnecessary fetal hypothyroidism. PTU is usually well tolerated by the mother, with infrequent side effects of rash, nausea, pruritus, hepatitis, arthralgias, vasculitis, and cholestatic jaundice. The most severe side effect is agranulocytosis, which is more common with higher doses. Symptoms of agranulocytosis are fever and sore throat, which should be reported immediately to the health care provider, and at the same time the woman should cease taking PTU. Transient, benign leukopenia may occur as a result of thiouracil therapy. During therapy, thyroid activity is monitored every 2 weeks to prevent hypothyroidism and minimize the required dosage of medication. Thiouracil readily crosses the placenta and may induce fetal hypothyroidism and goiter, although these complications rarely occur (Landon, 1996; Lazarus, 1993; Molitch, 1995).

Beta-adrenergic blockers such as propranolol may be used in severe hyperthyroidism. Long-term use is not recommended because of the potential for IUGR, and altered response to anoxic stress, postnatal bradycardia, and hypoglycemia (Lazarus, 1993).

Radioactive iodine must not be used in diagnosis or treatment of hyperthyroidism because it may compromise the fetal thyroid. If a mother taking hyperthyroid medication chooses to breastfeed, she needs to be aware that physiologically significant doses of the drug are passed to the infant through the breast milk. The infant's thyroid status should be monitored periodically so that hypothyroidism can be prevented (Cunningham et al., 1997; Molitch, 1995).

In severe cases surgical treatment of hyperthyroidism, subtotal thyroidectomy, may be performed during the second or third trimester. Because of the increased risk of spontaneous abortion or preterm labor associated with major surgery, this treatment is usually reserved for women with severe disease, those for whom drug therapy proves toxic, and those who are unable to adhere to the prescribed medical regimen. Postoperative hypothyroidism is common, occurring in at least 20% of previously hyperthyroid women.

A serious but uncommon complication of undiagnosed or partially treated hyperthyroidism is *thyroid storm*, which may occur in response to stress such as infection, birth, or surgery. A woman with this emergency disorder may have fever, restlessness, tachycardia, vomiting, hypotension, or stupor. Prompt treatment is essential; IV fluids and oxygen are administered along with high doses of PTU. Potassium iodide, antipyretics, dexamethasone, and beta-blockers may also be given; sedation may be necessary for extreme restlessness (Landon, 1996; Molitch, 1995).

Hypothyroidism

Hypothyroidism during pregnancy is a rare phenomenon because women with this disorder are often infertile.

Hypothyroidism is usually caused by Hashimoto's disease, thyroid gland ablation by radiation, previous surgery, or antithyroid medications. Reduced thyroid function resulting from hypothalamic or pituitary failure is rare, with only a few reported cases. Iodine deficiency in the United States is also rare (Landon, 1996).

Characteristic symptoms of hypothyroidism include lethargy, weakness, anorexia, weight gain, cold intolerance, mental impairment, constipation, headache, and possibly goiter. Dry skin, thin brittle nails, alopecia, poor skin turgor, and delayed deep tendon reflexes are also common. Laboratory findings during pregnancy may reveal normal or reduced total thyroxine, free thyroxine, and triiodothyronine levels along with elevated thyroid-stimulating hormone levels (except in cases associated with hypopituitarism).

Pregnant women with hypothyroidism may be at increased risk for spontaneous abortion, preeclampsia, anemia, abruptio placentae, postpartum hemorrhage, and stillbirth. Infants born to hypothyroid mothers may be of low birth weight but for the most part are healthy, without evidence of thyroid dysfunction (Lazarus, 1993; Leung et al., 1993).

Thyroid hormone supplements are used to treat hypothyroidism. Levothyroxine (Synthroid) is most often prescribed during pregnancy, beginning with a dosage of 0.05 to 0.1 mg per day and increasing to a maximum of 0.2 mg per day over several weeks until normal levels of thyroid-stimulating hormone and thyroxine are reached. Women who were diagnosed as hypothyroid before pregnancy should continue their prepregnancy doses, although it is likely the dosage will need to be adjusted as pregnancy progresses (Lazarus, 1993; Molitch, 1995).

The fetus depends on maternal thyroid hormones until 12 weeks' gestation, when fetal production begins. Thus maternal hypothyroidism does not cause fetal hypothyroidism. However, maternal treatment of hypothyroidism may result in increased fetal levels of thyroid hormones. Careful monitoring of the neonate's thyroid status is important to detect any abnormalities.

CARDIOVASCULAR DISORDERS

During a normal pregnancy, the maternal cardiovascular system undergoes many changes that put a physiologic strain on the heart. The normal heart can compensate for the increased workload, so that pregnancy, labor, and birth are generally well tolerated, whereas the diseased heart is challenged hemodynamically. If the cardiovascular changes are not well tolerated, cardiac failure can develop during pregnancy, during labor, or during the postpartum period (Cunningham et al., 1997). In addition, if myocardial disease develops, if valvular disease exists, or if a congenital heart defect is present, cardiac decompensation (inability of the heart to maintain a sufficient cardiac output) is anticipated.

About 1% of pregnancies are complicated by heart disease (Cunningham et al., 1997). The degree of disability experienced by the woman with cardiac disease often is more important in the treatment and prognosis during pregnancy than is the diagnosis of the type of cardiovascular disease. The New York Heart Association's (NYHA) (1964) functional classification of organic heart disease, a widely accepted standard that is used to categorize disability, is as follows:

- Class I: asymptomatic at normal levels of activity
- Class II: symptomatic with increased activity
- Class III: symptomatic with ordinary activity
- Class IV: symptomatic at rest

No classification of heart disease can be considered rigid or absolute, but this one offers a basic practical guide for treatment, assuming that frequent prenatal visits, good patient cooperation, and appropriate obstetric care occur. Medical therapy is conducted as a team approach, including the cardiologist, obstetric physician, and nurses. The functional classification may change for the pregnant woman because of the hemodynamic changes that occur in the cardiovascular system. The functional classification of the disease is determined at 3 months and again at 7 or 8 months of gestation.

Spontaneous abortion is increased, and preterm labor and birth are more prevalent in the pregnant woman with cardiac problems. In addition, IUGR is common, probably because of low oxygen pressure in the mother. Maternal mortality rates for women with class IV cardiac disease approaches 50%; the perinatal mortality rate is even higher.

CARE MANAGEMENT

Assessment and Nursing Diagnoses

The presence of cardiac disease makes the decision to become pregnant more difficult. Planned pregnancy requires that the woman understand the peripartum risks. If the pregnancy is unplanned, the nurse needs to explore the woman's desire to continue the pregnancy after examining the risks in relation to the status of her cardiac condition. The woman's partner and family should be included in the discussion.

The pregnant woman with cardiac disease requires detailed assessment to determine the potential for optimal maternal health and a viable fetus throughout the peripartum period. If she chooses to continue the pregnancy, the high-risk pregnant woman's condition may be assessed as often as weekly.

The nurse assesses for factors that would increase stress on the heart, such as anemia, infection, and edema. In reviewing for symptoms, the nurse should assess how the woman is adapting to the physiologic changes of pregnancy. Special attention is given to the review of the cardiovascular and pulmonary systems. The nurse should determine whether the woman has experienced chest pain at rest or on exertion; edema of the face, hands, or feet; hypertension; heart murmurs; palpitations; paroxysmal nocturnal dyspnea; diaphoresis; pallor; or syncope. Pulmonary symptoms such as cough, hemoptysis, shortness of breath, and orthopnea can be signs of cardiac disease.

The nurse documents all medication taken by the woman—including over-the-counter (OTC) medications such as supplemental iron—and is alert to their potential side effects and interactions. The woman is also assessed for undue emotional stress that might further compromise her cardiac status. Examples are depression, anxiety/fear of morbidity or mortality for herself and her fetus, financial concerns related to extended hospitalization, anger because of impaired social interaction, and feelings of inadequacy regarding her inability to meet family and household demands.

The woman's cultural background may affect the amount of support that she is able to receive from significant others. Family size (number of children and extended family members in the home), as well as role expectations within the family, may be dictated by cultural norms. For the woman with cardiac impairment, family expectations may prove to be a cause of major stress if she is unable to bear the expected number of children or if it is unacceptable to receive help with domestic chores. The nurse should be aware of the cultural customs of the pregnant woman and her family.

Routine assessments continue during the prenatal period, including monitoring the amount and pattern of weight gain, edema, vital signs, and discomforts of pregnancy; urinalysis; and blood work. The woman with cardiac impairment requires a baseline ECG at the beginning of her pregnancy, if not before pregnancy, which permits vital diagnostic comparisons of subsequent ECGs. Echocardiograms and pulse oximetry studies may be performed as indicated.

The woman is observed for signs of **cardiac decompensation,** that is, progressive generalized edema, crackles at the base of the lungs, or pulse irregularity (see Signs of Potential Complications box). Symptoms of cardiac decompensation may appear abruptly or gradually. Medical intervention must be instituted immediately to maintain optimal cardiac status. Dyspnea, palpitations, syncope, and edema occur commonly in pregnant women and can mask the symptoms of a developing or worsening cardiovascular disorder. A woman's sudden inability to perform activities that she previously was comfortable doing may indicate cardiovascular decompensation.

During the intrapartum period, assessment includes the routine assessments for all laboring women, as well as assessments for cardiac decompensation, because labor and giving birth place an additional burden on an already-compromised cardiovascular system. In addition, arterial blood gases (ABGs) may be needed to assess for

signs of POTENTIAL COMPLICATIONS

CARDIAC DECOMPENSATION

Pregnant Woman: Subjective Symptoms

- Increasing fatigue or difficulty breathing, or both, with her usual activities
- Feeling of smothering
- Frequent cough
- Palpitations; feeling that her heart is "racing"
- Generalized edema: swelling of face, feet, legs, fingers (e.g., rings do not fit anymore)

Nurse: Objective Signs

- Irregular, weak, rapid pulse (≥ 100 beats/min)
- Progressive, generalized edema
- Crackles at base of lungs after two inspirations and exhalations that do not clear after coughing
- Orthopnea; increasing dyspnea
- Rapid respirations (≥ 25 breaths/min)
- Moist, frequent cough
- Cyanosis of lips and nail beds

adequate oxygenation. A Swan-Ganz catheter may be inserted to accurately monitor hemodynamic status during labor and birth.

> **NURSE ALERT** *The physician is alerted if the pulse rate is ≥ 100 beats/min or if respirations are ≥ 25 breaths/min. Respiratory status is checked frequently for developing dyspnea, coughing, or crackles at the base of the lungs. The color and temperature of the skin are noted. Pale, cool, clammy skin may indicate cardiac shock.*

The first 24 to 48 hours postpartum are the most hemodynamically difficult for the woman. Cardiac output increases rapidly as extravascular fluid is remobilized into the vascular compartment. At the moment of birth, intraabdominal pressure is reduced drastically, pressure on veins is removed, the splanchnic vessels engorge, and blood flow to the heart is increased. When blood flow to the heart increases, a reflex bradycardia (slowing of the heart in response to the increased blood flow) may result. In addition to routine postpartum assessments, hemodynamic monitoring may be continued. Monitoring for cardiac decompensation continues through the first week after birth because of hormonal shifts that affect hemodynamics. These shifts have been known to occur as late as the seventh postpartum day.

The woman's/family's response to the birth, and to the infant, needs to be observed. The woman's/couple's expectations for postpartum sexual activity and birth control need to be discussed in relation to her cardiovascular condition.

Nursing diagnoses for the pregnant woman with cardiovascular disease are listed in the Nursing Diagnoses box.

▌Nursing Diagnoses

The Pregnant Woman with Cardiac Disease

Fear related to:
- Increased peripartum risk

Risk for ineffective individual/family coping related to:
- The woman's cardiac condition
- Changes in relationships

Risk for altered tissue perfusion related to:
- Hypotensive syndrome

Activity intolerance related to:
- Cardiac condition

Knowledge deficit related to:
- Cardiac condition
- Pregnancy and how it affects cardiac condition
- Requirements to alter self-care activities

Impaired home maintenance management related to:
- Woman's confinement to bed and/or limited activity level

Anxiety related to:
- Fear for infant's safety

Fear of dying related to:
- Perceived physiologic inability to cope with stress of labor

Risk for impaired gas exchange related to:
- Cardiac condition

Risk for fluid volume excess related to:
- Extravascular fluid shifts

Self-care deficit (bathing, grooming, dressing) related to:
- Fatigue or activity intolerance
- Need for bed rest

Situational low self-esteem related to:
- Restriction placed on involvement in care of infant
- Ineffective (compromised) family coping

Ineffective breastfeeding (class I or II cardiac disease) related to:
- Fatigue from cardiac condition

Risk for altered mother/infant attachment related to:
- Separation due to prematurity
- Fatigue from cardiac condition

Expected Outcomes of Care

The pregnant woman with cardiovascular problems faces curtailment of her activities. These restrictions can have physical and emotional implications. The community health nurse, social worker, and physical or occupational therapist are some of the resource people whose services may need to be incorporated into the plan of care. Expected outcomes for the pregnant woman (and family, if appropriate) may include that she (they) will:
- Verbalize understanding of the disorder, management, and probable outcome

- Describe her role in management, including when and how to take medication, adjust diet, and prepare for and participate in treatment
- Cope with emotional reactions to the pregnancy and infant at risk
- Adapt to the physiologic stressors of pregnancy and labor and birth
- Identify and use support systems
- Carry her fetus to the point of viability or to term
- Develop no complications in the postpartum period

Plan of Care and Interventions
Antepartum

Therapy for the pregnant woman with heart disease is focused on minimizing stress on the heart, which is greatest between 28 and 32 weeks as the hemodynamic changes reach their maximum. Factors that increase the risk of cardiac decompensation are avoided. The workload of the cardiovascular system is reduced by appropriate treatment of any coexisting emotional stress, hypertension, anemia, hyperthyroidism, or obesity.

Signs and symptoms of cardiac decompensation are reviewed during the prenatal period. The woman with class I or II heart disease requires 8 to 10 hours of sleep every day and should take 30-minute naps after eating. Her activities are restricted, with housework, shopping, and exercise limited to the amount allowed for the functional classification of her heart disease.

The pregnant woman with class II cardiac disease should avoid heavy exertion and should stop any activity that causes even minor signs and symptoms of cardiac decompensation. She should also be admitted to the hospital near term (earlier if signs of cardiac overload or arrhythmia develop) for evaluation and treatment.

Bed rest for much of each day is necessary for pregnant women with class III cardiac disease. About 30% of these women experience cardiac decompensation during pregnancy. With this possibility the woman may require hospitalization for the remainder of the pregnancy.

Because decompensation occurs even at rest in persons with class IV cardiac disease, a major initial effort must be made to improve the cardiac status of the pregnant woman in this category who chooses to continue her pregnancy (see Teaching Guidelines box).

Infections are treated promptly because respiratory, urinary, or GI tract infections can complicate the condition by accelerating the heart rate and by direct spread of organisms (e.g., streptococci) to the heart structure. The woman should notify her physician at the first sign of infection or exposure to an infection. Hospitalization may be required until the infection is cured. Women who have valvular disorders should receive prophylactic antibiotics against bacterial endocarditis during gestation (Box 23-1).

Nutrition counseling is necessary, optimally with the woman's family present. The pregnant woman needs a well-

TEACHING GUIDELINES

The Pregnant Woman at Risk for Cardiac Decompensation

- Assess lifestyle patterns, emotional status, and environment of woman.
- Arrange for consultations as needed (i.e., dietitian, home care, child care, social work).
- Determine woman's and her family's understanding of her heart disease and how the disease affects her pregnancy.
- Determine stressors in the woman's life. Assist woman in identifying effective coping strategies.
- Instruct woman to report signs of cardiac decompensation or congestive heart failure: generalized edema, distention of neck veins, dyspnea, pulmonary crackles, cough, palpitations, weight gain of 4.4 kg in 1 day.
- Instruct woman to be watchful for signs of thromboembolism, such as redness, tenderness, pain or swelling of the legs. Instruct woman to seek medical help immediately if such symptoms occur.
- Instruct woman to avoid constipation and thus straining with bowel movements (Valsalva's maneuver) by taking in adequate fluids and fiber. A stool softener may be ordered.
- Explore with woman ways to obtain the needed rest throughout the day. Depending on the level of her cardiac disease, she may need to sleep 10 hours per night and rest 30 minutes after meals (class I or II) or rest for most of the day (class III or IV).
- Help woman make use of community resources, including support groups, as indicated.
- Emphasize the importance of keeping her prenatal visits.

From Gilbert & Harmon, 1998; Grohar, 1994; Health Care Resources, 1997. (See references for full citations.)

---

balanced diet high in iron and protein and adequate in calories to gain weight. The iron supplements tend to cause constipation. The pregnant woman should increase her intake of fluids and fiber. A stool softener may be prescribed. It is important for the cardiac woman to avoid straining during defecation, thus causing Valsalva's maneuver (forced expiration against a closed airway, which when released causes blood to rush to the heart and overload the cardiac system). Sodium intake may be restricted and accompanied by careful monitoring for hyponatremia. The woman's intake of potassium is monitored to prevent hypokalemia, which is associated with heart and other muscular weakness and dysfunction.

Cardiac medications are prescribed as needed for the pregnant woman, with attention to fetal well-being. The hemodynamic changes that occur during pregnancy, such as increased plasma volume and increased renal clearance of drugs, can alter the amount of medication needed to establish and maintain a therapeutic drug level (Jackson & Clark, 1993). The woman's size and ethnic background must also be taken into consideration. For example, women of short

---

> **BOX 23-1   Antibiotic Prophylaxis Against Infective Endocarditis**
>
> Antibiotic prophylaxis is given in active labor, with a follow-up dose 8 hours later and postpartum. The standard dose is ampicillin 2 gm IM or IV and gentamicin 1.5 mg/kg IV or IM up to 80 mg. For patients who are allergic to penicillin, vancomycin 1 gm IV may be substituted for the ampicillin.

From Landon M & Samuels P: Cardiac and pulmonary disease. In Gabbe S, Niebyl J & Simpson J, editors: *Obstetrics: normal and problem pregnancies*, ed 3, New York, 1996, Churchill Livingstone.

stature or of Asian descent require less medication for the desired physiologic response. Therefore the nurse must monitor the pregnant woman for adverse side effects, as well as the blood level of the medication.

If anticoagulant therapy is required during pregnancy, heparin should be used because this large-molecule drug does not cross the placenta (James et al., 1994). The nurse should closely monitor the woman's blood work, including clotting factors. The woman may need to learn to self-administer heparin. She also requires specific nutritional teaching to avoid foods high in vitamin K, such as raw, dark green, and leafy vegetables, which counteract the effects of the heparin. In addition, she will require a substitute source of folic acid in her diet.

Tests for fetal maturity and well-being, as well as placental sufficiency, may be necessary. Other therapy is directly related to the functional classification of heart disease. It may be important that the nurse reinforce the need for close medical supervision.

Intrapartum

Nursing care during labor and birth focuses on the promotion of cardiac function. Anxiety is minimized by maintaining a calm atmosphere in the labor and birth rooms. The nurse provides anticipatory guidance by keeping the woman and her family informed of labor progress and events that will probably occur, as well as answering any questions they have. The woman's childbirth preparation method should be supported to the degree it is feasible for her cardiac condition. Nursing techniques that promote comfort, such as back massage, are used.

Cardiac function is supported by keeping the woman's head and shoulders elevated and body parts resting on pillows. The side-lying position usually facilitates hemodynamics during labor. Discomfort is relieved with medication and supportive care. Epidural regional anesthesia provides better pain relief than narcotics and causes fewer alterations in hemodynamics (Cunningham et al., 1997). Hypotension must be avoided.

The woman may require other types of medication (e.g., anticoagulants, prophylactic antibiotics). If evidence of cardiac decompensation appears, the physician may order deslanoside (Cedilanid-D) for rapid digitalization, furosemide (Lasix) for rapid diuresis, and oxygen by intermittent positive pressure to decrease the development of pulmonary edema.

Beta-adrenergic agents (i.e., ritodrine and terbutaline) should not be used for tocolysis. These are associated with myocardial ischemia. Syntocinon, a synthetic oxytocin, can be used for induction of labor. This drug does not appear to cause significant coronary artery constriction in doses prescribed for labor induction or control of postpartum uterine atony.

Vaginal birth is recommended and may be accomplished with the woman in the side-lying position to facilitate uterine perfusion. If the supine position is used, a pad is positioned under the right hip to laterally displace the uterus and minimize the danger of supine hypotension. The knees are flexed, and the feet are flat on the bed. To prevent compression of popliteal veins and an increase in blood volume in the chest and trunk as a result of the effects of gravity, stirrups are not used. Valsalva's maneuver must be avoided when pushing during the second stage of labor because it reduces diastolic ventricular filling and obstructs left ventricular outflow (Cruikshank, 1994). Mask oxygen is important. Episiotomy and the use of outlet forceps may be used, since these procedures also decrease the work of the heart.

Penicillin prophylaxis may be ordered for nonallergic pregnant women with class II or higher cardiac disease to protect against bacterial endocarditis in labor and during the early puerperium. Dilute IV oxytocin immediately after birth may be employed to prevent postbirth hemorrhage. Ergot products should not be used because they increase blood pressure. If tubal sterilization is desired, surgery is delayed at least several days to ensure homeostasis.

Postpartum

Care in the postpartum period is tailored to the woman's functional capacity. Postpartum positioning of the woman with cardiac disease is the same as that for labor; that is, the head of the bed is elevated and the woman is encouraged to lie on her side. Bed rest may be ordered, with or without bathroom privileges. The nurse assesses the woman's affect, pulse rate, breath sounds, coughing, edema, and skin color, temperature, and dryness (e.g., pink, warm, and dry; or pale, cool, and clammy) before and after walking. The nurse may need to help the woman meet her grooming and hygiene needs and even help her with turning in bed, eating, and other activities. Respiratory and cardiovascular sequelae to immobility, as well as boredom, must be addressed. Progressive ambulation may be permitted as tolerated. Bowel movements without stress or strain are promoted with stool softeners, diet, and fluids, plus mild analgesia and local anesthetic spray.

The woman may direct a designated family member in the care of the infant. Women with class I or II heart disease may breastfeed; those whose functional capacity is classified as class III or IV are advised against breastfeeding because it requires considerable energy. If the woman is unable to breastfeed and her energies do not allow her to bottle feed the infant at this time, the fed baby can be brought regularly to the mother. The infant should be held at the mother's eye level and by her lips, and brought to her fingers so that she can establish an emotional bond with her baby with a low expenditure of energy. At the same time, involving the mother passively in her infant's care helps the mother feel vitally important—as she is—to the infant's well-being (e.g., "You can offer something no one else can: provide your baby with your sounds, touch, and rhythms, which are so comforting"). Perhaps the woman can be encouraged to make a tape recording of her talking, singing, or whispering, which can be played for the baby in the nursery to help the infant feel her presence and be in contact with her voice.

Preparation for discharge is carefully planned with the woman and family. Provision of help for the woman in the home by relatives, friends, and others must be addressed. If necessary, the nurse refers the family to community resources (e.g., for homemaking services). Rest and sleep periods, activity, and diet must be planned. The couple may need information about reestablishing sexual relations and contraception or sterilization (especially if the woman's condition is classified as class II, III, or IV).

Cardiopulmonary resuscitation of the pregnant woman

Trauma, pulmonary embolism, anesthesia complications, drug overdose, hypovolemia, or septic shock may result in cardiopulmonary arrest. Preexisting disorders, such as heart or pulmonary disease, hypertension, or autoimmune collagen vascular disease, increase this risk (Kulb, 1990). Some modifications of the procedure for cardiopulmonary resuscitation (CPR) (see Emergency box) and the Heimlich maneuver are needed during pregnancy (Fig. 23-5).

NURSE ALERT *In the event of cardiac arrest, standard resuscitative efforts with a few modifications are implemented. To prevent supine hypotension, the woman is placed on a firm surface with the uterus displaced to the left laterally either manually or with a wedge or rolled blanket or towel under the right hip (Association of Women's Health, Obstetric, and Neonatal Nurses [AWHONN], 1998; Bajo, 1997). If defibrillation is needed, the paddles need to be placed one rib interspace higher than usual because the heart is displaced slightly by the enlarged uterus. If possible, the fetus should be monitored during the cardiac arrest (Bajo, 1997).*

Complications may be associated with CPR of a pregnant woman. These complications may include laceration of the liver, rupture of the uterus, hemothorax, or hemoperitoneum. Fetal complications also may occur. These include cardiac arrhythmia or asystole related to maternal defibrillation and medications; CNS depression related to antiarrhythmic drugs and inadequate uteroplacental perfusion; and onset of preterm labor.

If there is successful resuscitation, the woman and her fetus must receive careful monitoring. The woman remains

EMERGENCY

CPR for the Pregnant Woman

CPR

Airway

Determine unresponsiveness.

Activate emergency medical system.

Position woman on flat, firm surface with uterus displaced laterally with a wedge (e.g., a rolled towel placed under her right hip) or manually.

Open airway with head-tilt–chin-lift maneuver.

Breathing

Determine breathlessness (look, listen, feel).

If the woman is not breathing, give two slow breaths.

Circulation

Determine pulselessness by feeling carotid pulse.

If there is no pulse, begin chest compressions at rate of 80 to 100/min.

After four cycles of 15 compressions and two breaths, check her pulse. If pulse is not present, continue CPR.

HEIMLICH MANEUVER

If the pregnant woman is unable to speak or cough, perform chest thrusts. Stand behind the woman and place your arms under her armpits to encircle her chest. Press backward with quick thrusts until the foreign body is expelled. (Fig. 23-5)

From American Heart Association: *Basic life support, heart saver guide,* Dallas, 1997, The Association.

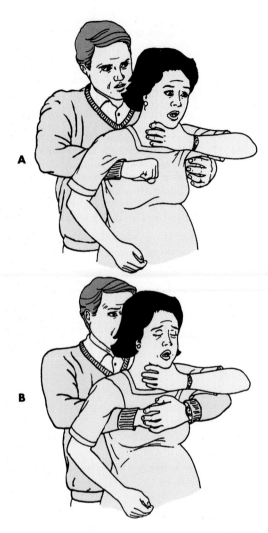

Fig. 23-5 Clearing airway obstruction in woman in late stages of pregnancy (can also be used in markedly obese victim). **A,** Standing behind victim, place your arms under woman's armpits and across chest. Place thumb side of your clenched fist against middle of sternum and place other hand over fist. **B,** Perform backward chest thrusts until foreign object is expelled or woman becomes unconscious. If pregnant women becomes unconscious because of foreign-body airway obstruction, place her on her back and kneel close to victim's side. (Be sure uterus is displaced laterally by using, for example, a rolled blanket under her right hip.) Open mouth with tongue-jaw lift, perform finger sweep, and attempt rescue breathing. If unable to ventilate, position hands as for chest compression. Deliver five chest thrusts firmly to remove obstruction. Repeat above sequence of Heimlich maneuver, finger sweep, and attempt to ventilate. Continue above sequence until pregnant woman's airway is clear of obstruction or help has arrived to relieve you (Chandra & Hazinski, 1997). If woman is unconscious, give chest compressions as for woman without pulse.

at increased risk for recurrent pulmonary arrest and arrhythmias (ventricular tachycardia, supraventricular tachycardia, bradycardia).

Evaluation

The nurse uses the previously stated expected outcomes as criteria to evaluate the care of the woman with cardiac disease (see Plan of Care).

ASSOCIATED CARDIOVASCULAR DISORDERS

Peripartum Heart Failure

Peripartum heart failure (failure of the heart to maintain an adequate cardiac output to maintain adequate circulation of blood) (Fig. 23-6) can result from an underlying chronic hypertension, previously unrecognized mitral valve stenosis, obesity, viral myocarditis, or idiopathic peripartum cardiomyopathy (Cunningham et al., 1997). It can develop from the last month of gestation to 5 months' postpartum. In addition, anemia and infection can predispose the woman to congestive heart failure (CHF).

Peripartum heart failure from an explainable cause such as an underlying heart disease usually responds well to

〰️ PLAN OF CARE *The Pregnant Woman with Cardiac Disease*

> **NURSING DIAGNOSIS** Activity intolerance related to effects of pregnant state on underlying cardiac condition

Expected Outcome *Patient will show no evidence of cardiac decompensation (i.e., no fatigue, shortness of breath, palpitations, edema, rapid irregular pulse, crackles, rapid respirations, cyanosis of nail beds and lips).*

Nursing Interventions/*Rationales*

Assist woman in identifying factors that decrease activity tolerance and explore extent of limitations *to establish a baseline for evaluation.*

Help woman to develop an individualized program of activity and rest *that maintains sufficient cardiac output.*

Teach woman to monitor physiologic response to activity (i.e., pulse rate, respiratory rate) and reduce activity that provokes fatigue and/or pain *to maintain sufficient cardiac output and prevent harm to fetus.*

Enlist significant others to assist woman in pacing activities and to provide support in performing role functions and self-care activities that are too strenuous *to increase chances of compliance with activity restrictions.*

Have woman maintain an activity log that records activities, time, duration, intensity, and physiologic response *to evaluate effectiveness of and adherence to activity program.*

> **NURSING DIAGNOSIS** Risk for altered tissue perfusion related to cardiac condition secondary to increased circulatory needs during pregnancy

Expected Outcomes *The mother will exhibit signs of hemodynamic stability (i.e., blood pressure, pulse, ABGs, and WBC counts are within normal limits). The fetus will exhibit signs of well-being (i.e., fetal activity and fetal heart rate [FHR] are within normal limits).*

Nursing Interventions/*Rationales*

Monitor heart rate and rhythm, blood pressure, skin color and temperature, WBCs, hemoglobin and hematocrit, ABGs *to detect early signs of cardiac failure/hypoxia.*

Monitor fetal activity and FHR, perform nonstress testing as indicated *to assess fetal status and detect uteroplacental insufficiency.*

Teach woman how to detect and report early signs of cardiac decompensation *to prevent maternal/fetal complications.*

> **NURSING DIAGNOSIS** Decreased cardiac output related to increased circulatory volume secondary to pregnancy and cardiac condition

Expected Outcome *The patient will exhibit signs of adequate cardiac output (i.e., normal pulse and blood pressure; normal heart and breath sounds; normal skin color, tone, and turgor; normal capillary refill; normal urine output; no evidence of edema).*

Nursing Interventions/*Rationales*

Reinforce importance of use of activity/rest cycles *to prevent cardiac complications.*

Teach woman to lie in left lateral position *to increase uterine blood flow* and to elevate legs while sitting *to promote venous return.*

Monitor intake and output and check for edema *to assess for renal complications or venous return problems.*

Monitor fetal activity and FHR, perform nonstress testing as indicated *to assess fetal status and detect uteroplacental insufficiency.*

From Wong D & Perry S: *Maternal child nursing care,* St Louis, 1998, Mosby.

therapy. The typical response is rapid reversal of heart failure with furosemide (Lasix) diuresis and correction of associated obstetric complications (Cunningham et al., 1997). Within days the heart size of these women returns to normal. Their long-term prognosis depends on the underlying heart disease (e.g., hypertrophic cardiomyopathy).

Hypertrophic cardiomyopathy (HCM) is a primary disease, classified on the basis of its structural abnormality and function. In this disorder the muscle tissue of the heart walls and the septum are hypertrophied, leaving relatively small chambers and causing impaired filling during diastole, resulting in decreased cardiac output. HCM usually is asymptomatic until late adolescence or early adulthood or, more rarely, middle age. Symptoms include angina, exertional dyspnea, dizziness, syncope, ventricular arrhythmias,

S_4 gallop, and mild cardiomegaly. HCM is associated with sudden death, unrelated to functional status. HCM may be precipitated by physical or emotional stress, and the myocardial ischemia resulting from stress may promote ventricular fibrillation. Propranolol is given if symptoms develop (Cunningham et al., 1997).

Idiopathic peripartum cardiomyopathy comprises a syndrome of heart failure (1) occurring during the peripartum period, (2) with no previous history of heart disease, and (3) with no specific etiologic factors.

The incidence of peripartum cardiomyopathies has been reported as 1/1,300 to 1/4,000 pregnancies (Mendelson & Lang, 1995). It occurs more often in the older, multiparous woman. Clinical findings are those of CHF (left ventricular failure). Signs include breathlessness, tachyarrhythmias,

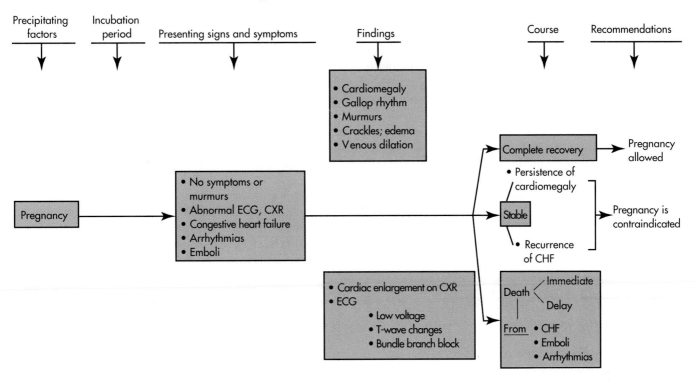

Fig. **23-6** Summary of course of peripartum cardiomyopathy.

and edema, with radiologic findings of cardiomegaly. The prognosis is good if cardiomegaly does not persist up to 6 months postpartum. The prognosis for women whose hearts remain enlarged after 6 months is poor (Mendelson & Lang, 1995). Recurrence of peripartum cardiomyopathy is likely; thus contraception is important until the ventricular function is restored (Mendelson & Lang, 1995).

Medical management of cardiomyopathy during pregnancy includes diuretics, potassium, anticoagulants, digitalis, and bed rest. Low sodium intake (1.5 to 2 gm per day) and fluid restriction are ordered for women with severe CHF (Brown & Bertolet, 1998). During labor the avoidance of IV fluid overload is important. Because all women experience some rise in blood pressure at the onset of lactation, suppression of lactation is recommended to minimize stress.

The nursing care of patients with peripartum cardiomyopathies is essentially the same as for those with other types of cardiac problems. Because sudden death can occur with this condition, the family needs to be trained in CPR (see Emergency box).

Rheumatic Heart Disease

Rheumatic fever usually develops suddenly, several symptom-free weeks after an inadequately treated group A beta-hemolytic streptococcal infection of the throat. Episodes of rheumatic fever create an autoimmune reaction in the heart tissue, leading to permanent damage of heart valves (usually the mitral valve) and the chordae tendineae cordis.

This damage is referred to as **rheumatic heart disease (RHD)**. Rheumatic heart disease may be evident during acute rheumatic fever or discovered years later. Recurrences of rheumatic fever are common, each with the potential to increase the severity of heart damage. If a woman has had rheumatic fever in the past, a recurrence can occur during pregnancy; most likely, early in the pregnancy. The American Heart Association recommends lifelong prophylaxis with benzathine penicillin, even during pregnancy. For penicillin allergies, erythromycin is an acceptable alternative during pregnancy. Heart murmurs, resulting from stenosis, valvular insufficiency, or thickening of the walls of the heart, characterize rheumatic heart disease. Abnormal pulse rate and rhythm, as well as CHF, are common.

Mitral Valve Stenosis

Mitral valve stenosis (narrowing of the opening of the mitral valve due to stiffening of valve leaflets, obstructing blood flow from the atrium to the ventricles) is caused almost entirely by rheumatic fever (McAnulty, Metcalfe & Ueland, 1995). Even though a history of rheumatic fever may be absent, it remains the most likely cause of mitral stenosis. As the mitral valve narrows, dyspnea worsens, occurring first on exertion and eventually at rest. A tight stenosis, plus the increase in blood volume and thus cardiac output of normal pregnancy, may cause ventricular failure and pulmonary edema; hemoptysis may occur.

The occurrence of atrial fibrillation can precipitate a drop in the cardiac output. IV verapamil, cardioversion, and digitalis therapy may be used to treat atrial fibrillation (McAnulty, Metcalfe & Ueland, 1995). Cardiac failure occurs for the first time during pregnancy in 25% of women with mitral valve stenosis. The care of the woman with mitral stenosis typically is managed by reducing her activity, by restricting dietary sodium, and by increasing bed rest. The pregnant woman with mitral stenosis should be followed clinically for symptoms and by echocardiograms to monitor the atrial and ventricular size, as well as heart valve function. Prophylaxis for intrapartum endocarditis and pulmonary infections is provided (see Box 23-1).

Beta-blockers may be used to blunt heart rate response to exercise and anxiety. Adverse fetal and neonatal effects include IUGR, delayed neonatal breathing, and bradycardia. Epidural anesthesia for labor and avoidance of IV fluid overload are appropriate (Cunningham et al., 1997). Even with close monitoring, the woman with moderate to severe mitral stenosis will commonly have pulmonary edema for the first 1 or 2 days after giving birth because of volume shifts after birth (Mendelson & Lang, 1995).

Mitral Valve Prolapse

Mitral valve prolapse (MVP) is a common, usually benign, condition occurring in nearly 10% of women of reproductive age (Cunningham et al., 1997). The mitral valve leaflets prolapse into the left atrium during ventricular systole, allowing some backflow of blood. Midsystolic click and late systolic murmur are hallmarks of this syndrome. Most cases are asymptomatic. A few women have atypical chest pain (sharp and located in the left side of the chest) that occurs at rest and does not respond to nitrates. They may also have anxiety, palpitations, dyspnea on exertion, and syncope. Patients usually are treated with beta-blockers such as propranolol (Inderal). Pregnancy and its associated hemodynamic changes may change or alleviate the murmur and click of MVP, as well as symptoms. Pregnancy usually is well tolerated unless bacterial endocarditis occurs. As with RHD, antibiotic prophylaxis is given before invasive procedures for at-risk patients and for complicated vaginal births in patients with MVP (see Box 23-1).

Marfan Syndrome

Marfan syndrome is an autosomal dominant disorder characterized by generalized weakness of the connective tissue, resulting in joint deformities, ocular lens dislocation, and weakness of the aortic wall and root (McAnulty, Metcalfe & Ueland, 1995). About 90% of individuals with this syndrome have MVP, and 25% have aortic insufficiency. There is an increased risk of aortic dissection and rupture during pregnancy (McAnulty, Metcalfe & Ueland, 1995). Excruciating chest pain is the most common symptom of aortic dissection. Preconceptional genetic counseling is recommended to make patients aware of the risks of pregnancy with this condition. The woman should have baseline data gathered about the aortic root before pregnancy or at the first prenatal visit by noninvasive imaging with transesophageal echocardiography, computed tomography, or magnetic resonance imaging (MRI). Management during pregnancy includes restricted activity and beta-blockers; surgery may be indicated in some women. Antibiotic prophylaxis is suggested for labor; regional anesthesia is well tolerated. Mortality rates may be as high as 50% in women who have significant cardiac disease.

❙ ANEMIA

Anemia is the most common medical disorder of pregnancy, affecting at least 20% of pregnant women. Women with anemia have a higher incidence of puerperal complications, such as infection, than do pregnant women with normal hematologic values.

Anemia results in reduction of the oxygen-carrying capacity of the blood. Because the oxygen-carrying capacity of the blood is decreased, the heart tries to compensate by increasing the cardiac output. This effort increases the workload of the heart and stresses ventricular function. Therefore anemia that occurs with any other complication (e.g., preeclampsia) may result in CHF.

An indirect index of the oxygen-carrying capacity is the packed RBC volume, or hematocrit level. The normal hematocrit range in nonpregnant women is 38% to 45%. However, normal values for pregnant women with adequate iron stores may be as low as 34%. This has been explained by hydremia (dilution of blood), or the physiologic anemia of pregnancy.

At or near sea level, the pregnant woman is anemic when her hemoglobin level is less than 11 gm/dl or hematocrit is less than 33%. In areas of high altitude, much higher values indicate anemia; for example, at 1,500 m (5,000 feet) above sea level, a hemoglobin level less than 14 gm/dl indicates anemia (Pagana & Pagana, 1997).

When a woman has anemia during pregnancy, the loss of blood at birth, even if minimal, is not well tolerated. She is at an increased risk for requiring blood transfusions. About 90% of cases of anemia in pregnancy are of the iron deficiency type. The remaining 10% of cases embrace a considerable variety of acquired and hereditary anemias, including folic acid deficiency, sickle cell anemia, and thalassemia.

Nursing care of the anemic pregnant woman requires that the nurse be able to distinguish between the normal physiologic anemia of pregnancy and the disease states. During prenatal visits the nurse should take a diet history and provide dietary teaching as appropriate. Pregnancy may cause increased fatigue, stress, and financial difficulties for a woman with anemia as she copes with her activities of daily living. The nurse should assess the woman's needs and provide her with appropriate resources and/or referral.

Iron Deficiency Anemia

Pathologic anemia of pregnancy is mainly due to iron deficiency (James et al., 1994). Without iron therapy even pregnant women who enjoy excellent nutrition will end pregnancy with an iron deficit because iron for the fetus comes from the maternal serum (Duffy, 1995). Diet alone cannot replace gestational iron losses. Inadequate nutrition without therapy will certainly mean iron deficiency anemia during late pregnancy and the puerperium.

Successful iron therapy during pregnancy can be carried out in most cases with oral iron supplements (e.g., ferrous sulfate, 30 to 60 mg per day). It is important to teach the woman the significance of the iron therapy (see Home Care box, p. 278). In addition, it is necessary to instruct the woman in dietary ways to decrease GI side effects of iron. Some pregnant women cannot tolerate the prescribed oral iron because of nausea and vomiting. In such cases the woman should receive parenteral iron such as an iron-dextran complex (Imferon) (Duffy, 1995).

Folate Deficiency

Even in well-nourished women, it is common to have a folate deficiency. Poor diet, cooking with large volumes of water, or home canning of food (especially vegetables) may lead to folate deficiency. Malabsorption may play a part in the development of anemia caused by a lack of folic acid. Folic acid deficiency anemia is common in multiple gestations. Periconception folate deficiency has been associated with increases in the incidence of neural tube defects, cleft lip, and cleft palate (Letsky, 1995). During pregnancy the recommended daily intake is 400 to 800 μg of folic acid per day.

Sickle Cell Hemoglobinopathy

Sickle cell hemoglobinopathy is a disease caused by the presence of abnormal hemoglobin in the blood. Sickle cell trait (SA hemoglobin pattern) is sickling of the RBCs but with a normal RBC life span, and it usually causes only mild clinical symptoms. Sickle cell anemia (sickle cell disease) is a recessive, hereditary, familial hemolytic anemia that affects those of African-American or Mediterranean ancestry. These individuals usually have abnormal hemoglobin types (SS or SC). Persons with sickle cell anemia have recurrent attacks (crises), beginning in childhood, of fever and pain in the abdomen or extremities. These attacks are attributed to vascular occlusion (from abnormal cells), tissue hypoxia, edema, and RBC destruction. Crises are associated with normochromic anemia, jaundice, reticulocytosis, a positive sickle cell test, and the demonstration of abnormal hemoglobin (usually SS or SC).

Almost 10% of African-Americans in North America have the sickle cell trait, but fewer than 1% have sickle cell anemia. The anemia often is complicated by iron and folic acid deficiency.

Nurses working in women's health clinics should encourage patients with sickle cell trait to undergo genetic counseling before pregnancy is undertaken because pregnancy

usually results in a worsening of most aspects of the disease (Cruikshank, 1994). The anemia that occurs in normal pregnancies may aggravate sickle cell anemia and bring on more crises. Fetal loss is high, because of impaired oxygen supply and sickling, as well as infarcts in the placental circulation (James et al., 1994). Pregnant women with sickle cell anemia are prone to pyelonephritis, leg ulcers, bone abnormalities, strokes, cardiopathy, CHF, and preeclampsia. UTIs and hematuria are common. An aplastic crisis may follow serious infection. Prophylactic transfusions of the mother to decrease the sickle cells and to increase the hemoglobin are not used as readily as in the past and require close monitoring of the woman for complications (Duffy, 1995).

Table 23-4 identifies some potential problems faced by the woman with sickle cell disease and some preventive and maintenance interventions.

Thalassemia

Thalassemia (Mediterranean or Cooley's anemia) is a relatively common anemia in which an insufficient amount of hemoglobin is produced to fill the RBCs. The condition eventually manifests itself in severe bone deformities caused by massive marrow tissue expansion (Letsky, 1995). For the infant born with severe thalassemia, death from cardiac failure is common (Letsky, 1995). Thalassemia is a hereditary disorder that involves the abnormal synthesis of the alpha or beta chains of hemoglobin. Beta-thalassemia is the more common variety in the United States and often is diagnosed in persons of Italian, Greek, or southern Chinese, Mediterranean, North African, African-American, Middle Eastern, southern Asian, or Indo-Pakistani descent. The unbalanced synthesis of hemoglobin leads to premature RBC death, resulting in severe anemia. Thalassemia major is the homozygous form of this disorder; thalassemia minor is the heterozygous form. Couples with the thalassemia trait should seek genetic counseling.

Thalassemia major complicates pregnancy. Preeclampsia is more common in women with thalassemia major. Thalassemia major may be associated with low-birth-weight infants and increased fetal death. Placental weight often is increased, perhaps secondary to maternal anemia. The frequency of fetal distress from hypoxia is greater than in women without thalassemia major.

Pregnant patients are managed similarly to those who have sickle cell disease. Folic acid should be given to avoid folate deficiency. The anemia will not respond to iron therapy. Prolonged parenteral iron can lead to harmful, excessive iron storage. Regular transfusion may be necessary.

▌PULMONARY DISORDERS

As pregnancy advances and the uterus impinges on the thoracic cavity, any pregnant woman may experience increased respiratory difficulty. This difficulty will be compounded by pulmonary disease.

TABLE 23-4 *Sickle Cell Anemia: Potential Problems, Prevention, and Maintenance*

POTENTIAL PROBLEM	PREVENTION AND MAINTENANCE
1. Inadequate oxygen to meet needs of labor and prevent sickling	1. a. Monitor Hb level and HCT to maintain Hb at ≥8 gm and HCT at ≥20% b. Have typed and crossmatched blood available c. Assist with transfusions d. Administer oxygen continuously during labor e. Coach for relaxation and to lessen anxiety
2. Infection: UTI, pyelonephritis, pneumonia	2. a. Continue actions as under No. 1 b. Maintain adequate hydration c. Administer antibiotics as ordered d. Maintain strict asepsis e. Encourage frequent voiding to keep bladder empty
3. Sequestration crisis caused by need for and destruction of RBCs	3. Administer folic acid supplement (15-30 mg) to decrease erythropoietic demands and reduce probability of capillary stasis
4. Crisis caused by hypoxia, hypotension, acidosis, dehydration, exertion, sudden cooling, low-grade fever	4. a. Continue actions as under No. 1 b. Avoid supine hypotension c. Maintain adequate hydration d. Maintain comfortable room temperature: use warm blankets or cool cloths as needed e. Assist with analgesia and anesthesia
5. Pseudotoxemia (hypertension, proteinuria, *no* large weight gain); often accompanying bone pain crisis	5. a. If true PIH occurs, care is the same as for PIH b. Monitor blood pressure and urine
6. Thromboembolism (from increased blood viscosity)	6. a. Monitor for positive Homans' sign b. Initiate bed rest if Homans' sign is positive or if reddened, warm areas, or lump appears in the calf c. Maintain adequate hydration d. Administer heparin, as ordered e. Apply warm compresses f. Apply antiembolism stockings
7. Congestive heart failure	7. a. Assess pulse, respiratory rate b. Place in semirecumbent position; lateral position for labor c. Auscultate the lungs frequently for crackles d. Administer oxygen and medications (e.g., digitalis, antibiotics, diuretics, analgesics) e. Regional anesthesia for pain relief in labor
8. Pulmonary infarction (hemoptysis, cough, temperature to 38.9° C, friction rub)	8. Assess for this possible complication to facilitate early diagnosis
9. Postpartum hemorrhage (resulting from heparin therapy)	9. Administer ordered oxytocic medication

UTI, Urinary tract infection; *Hb,* hemoglobin; *HCT,* hematocrit; *PIH,* pregnancy-induced hypertension; *RBCs,* red blood cells.

Asthma

Bronchial asthma is an acute respiratory illness caused by allergens, marked change in ambient temperature, or emotional tension. In many cases the actual cause may be unknown. A family history of allergy is likely in about 50% of all persons with asthma. In response to stimuli, there is widespread but reversible narrowing of the hyperreactive airways, making it difficult to breathe. The clinical manifestations are expiratory wheezing, productive cough, thick sputum, and/or dyspnea.

Fewer than 0.4% to 1.3% of pregnant women have asthma (Gilbert & Harmon, 1998). However, it is a major problem for adolescents who become pregnant. Physiologic alterations induced by pregnancy do not make the pregnant women more prone to asthmatic attacks. With good care, the morbidity and mortality rate of the woman with asthma is equivalent to that of the general population of pregnant women (ACOG, 1996; Niswander & Evans, 1995).

Therapy for asthma has three objectives: (1) relief of the acute attack, (2) prevention or limitation of later attacks, and (3) adequate maternal and fetal oxygenation. In all persons with asthma, known allergens should be eliminated and a comfortable home temperature maintained.

Respiratory infections should be treated and mist or steam inhalation employed to aid expectoration of mucus. Acute episodes may require albuterol, steroids, aminophylline, oxygen, beta-adrenergic agents, and correction of fluid-electrolyte imbalance. Precautions specific for obstetrics include the following:

- Morphine should not be used in labor because it may cause bronchospasm; meperidine (Demerol) usually will relieve bronchospasm.
- The use of ephedrine and corticotropin (pressor drugs) in preeclampsia and eclampsia should be avoided or limited.
- Vaginal birth with use of local or regional anesthesia is recommended.

Adult Respiratory Distress Syndrome

Adult respiratory distress syndrome (ARDS), or shock lung, occurs when the lungs are unable to maintain levels of oxygen and carbon dioxide within normal limits. Marked tachycardia, dyspnea, and cyanosis that do not respond to nasal oxygen or intermittent positive pressure breathing are the most noted signs. ARDS is not a condition specific to pregnancy; it can also result from chest trauma, drug ingestion, or pneumonia. When ARDS is associated with pregnancy, pulmonary embolism, disseminated intravascular coagulation (DIC), and aspiration pneumonia are the precipitators.

The postpartum incidence of ARDS is not affected by the means of birth but by the amount of trauma experienced during pregnancy and birth. It may also occur after spontaneous or medically induced abortion.

Laboratory reports are important in identifying the origin of acute pulmonary problems. The important observations for the nurse to note are vital signs, signs of thrombophlebitis, and hemorrhage. During the postpartum period, symptoms such as apprehension, distended neck veins, cyanosis, diaphoresis, and pallor provide clues. Mental confusion or disorientation also may be noted.

The pulse rate increases to compensate for respiratory insufficiency of any origin. The severity of the pulmonary problem increases as the pulse rate rises. An initial rise in blood pressure occurs as cardiac output increases in an attempt to supply the tissue with oxygen. When lung damage is severe, the blood pressure drops.

Respiratory changes are the most important indicators of ARDS. The rate, depth, respiratory pattern, symmetry of chest movement, and use of accessory muscles should be noted; therefore observation of respiratory characteristics after activity is important. If there is any indication of abnormality, respirations are counted for a full minute; an error in rate of plus or minus 4 respirations per minute may be highly significant. On auscultation, crackles, rhonchi, wheezes, or a pleural friction rub should be reported, especially when they have occurred after an earlier normal assessment. The pregnant woman should be positioned for breathing comfort. Oxygen and emergency equipment should be available. The woman should be reassured and coached in relaxation techniques so that her anxiety is lessened.

The lower extremities need to be checked for swelling, pain, inflammation, venous distention, and Homans' sign. Temperature elevation may indicate the development of thrombophlebitis. If thrombophlebitis is suspected, the woman should be maintained on bed rest. Sudden movement or straining can dislodge a clot and lead to pulmonary embolism.

Alterations in vein distensibility have been noted, possibly because of softening of collagen induced by hormonal influences. The combination of vein distensibility and obstruction of venous blood return from the lower extremities (caused by fetal pressure on veins, especially in the last trimester) predisposes a woman to pooling of blood. In addition, hypercoagulation and pooling may lead to thrombophlebitis. Thrombophlebitis can result in ARDS (emboli cause obstruction in the pulmonary circulation).

It has been noted that during pregnancy there is an increase in some of the coagulation factors. This increase in coagulation results in shortening of the partial thromboplastin time (PTT). This state predisposes the woman to an increase in rapidity of blood clotting and an increased tendency to form blood clots (hypercoagulability). Petechiae, ecchymosis, hematuria, and epistaxis are important indications of DIC. Replacement of clotting factors and heparin therapy may be required for DIC. Sources of trauma should be identified and eliminated so that outside causes of hemorrhage are avoided.

Aspiration pneumonia can be caused by changes in the GI system during pregnancy. Progesterone relaxes smooth muscles of the GI tract. When the resting tone is lowered, the cardiac sphincter becomes weak and reflux of the stomach contents can easily occur. Increased intraabdominal pressure (because of fetal growth) further predisposes the mother to gastric reflux.

Food eaten as long as 24 to 48 hours before labor can be vomited and then aspirated. Aspiration of solid foods and liquids may cause bronchial obstruction leading to bronchoconstriction, which in turn can result in ARDS. Large particles can be removed by coughing, suctioning, or bronchoscopy, but liquids are harder to remove. The hydrochloric acid in the aspirated stomach contents may cause an asthmatic-like syndrome with necrotizing bronchitis. For this reason, an antacid is given preoperatively as a prophylactic measure.

ARDS carries a high rate of mortality. The prognosis is good if the woman is otherwise healthy and if ventilator support can be maintained until the underlying disease can be treated (Cunningham et al., 1997).

Cystic Fibrosis

Cystic fibrosis is a common autosomal recessive genetic disorder in which the exocrine glands produce excessive viscous secretions. There are problems with both respiratory and digestive functions within the individual. Respiratory failure and early death (early 20s) are outcomes.

Improvements in diagnosis and treatment of cystic fibrosis have allowed an increasing number of females to survive to adulthood. Most are infertile; however, pregnancy can occur. The pregnancy is often complicated by chronic hypoxia and frequent pulmonary infections. Women with cystic fibrosis show a decrease in their residual volume during pregnancy, as do normal pregnant women. However, persons with cystic fibrosis are unable to maintain vital capacity. Presumably, the pulmonary vasculature cannot accommodate the increased cardiac output of pregnancy. The results are decreased oxygen to the myocardium, decreasing cardiac output, and an increase in hypoxemia. Severe pulmonary infection is related to increased maternal and perinatal mortality rates.

During labor, monitoring for fluid and electrolyte balance is required. The amount of sodium lost through sweat can be significant, and hypovolemia can occur. Conversely, if the woman has any degree of cor pulmonale, she must be guarded against fluid overload. Oxygen is administered by face mask during labor. Epidural or local anesthesia is the preferred analgesic for birth.

Newborns with cystic fibrosis may be born with meconium ileus. The neonate may also "taste salty" when kissed and have a positive sweat test. Genetic counseling is encouraged to identify carriers of the disease.

Breastfeeding appears to be safe as long as the sodium content of the milk is not abnormal (Lawrence, 1994). Pumping and discarding the milk is done until the sodium content has been determined.

INTEGUMENTARY DISORDERS

The skin surface may exhibit many physiologic and pathologic conditions during pregnancy. Dermatologic disorders induced by pregnancy include melasma (chloasma), herpes gestationis, noninflammatory pruritus of pregnancy, vascular "spiders," palmar erythema, and pregnancy granuloma (including epulides). Skin problems generally aggravated by pregnancy are acne vulgaris (acne) (in the first trimester), erythema multiforme, herpetiform dermatitis (fever blisters and genital herpes), granuloma inguinale (Donovan bodies), condylomata acuminata (genital warts), neurofibromatosis (von Recklinghausen's disease), and pemphigus. Dermatologic disorders usually improved by pregnancy include acne vulgaris (in the third trimester), seborrheic dermatitis (dandruff), and psoriasis. An unpredictable course during pregnancy may be expected in atopic dermatitis, lupus erythematosus, and herpes simplex.

NURSE ALERT *Isotretinoin (Accutane), commonly prescribed for cystic acne, is highly teratogenic. There is a risk for craniofacial, cardiac, and CNS malformations in exposed fetuses. This drug should not be taken during pregnancy.*

Explanation, reassurance, and commonsense measures should suffice for normal skin changes. In contrast, disease processes during and soon after pregnancy may be extremely difficult to diagnose and treat.

NEUROLOGIC DISORDERS

The pregnant woman with a neurologic disorder needs to deal with potential teratologic effects of prescribed medications, changes of mobility during pregnancy, and ability to care for the baby. The nurse should be aware of all drugs the patient is taking and the associated potential for producing congenital anomalies. As the pregnancy progresses, the woman's center of gravity shifts and causes balance and gait changes. The nurse needs to advise the woman of these expected changes and to suggest safety measures as appropriate. Familial and community resources should be assessed to provide child care for the neurologically impaired woman.

Epilepsy

Epilepsy is a disorder of the brain causing recurrent seizures and is the most common neurologic disorder accompanying pregnancy (Cartlidge, 1995). Epilepsy may result from developmental abnormalities or injury, as well as having no known cause. Convulsive seizures may be more frequent or severe during complications of pregnancy, such as edema, alkalosis, fluid-electrolyte imbalance, cerebral hypoxia, hypoglycemia, and hypocalcemia. On the other hand, the effects of pregnancy on epilepsy are unpredictable.

The differential diagnosis between epilepsy and eclampsia may pose a problem. Epilepsy and eclampsia can coexist. However, a history of seizures and a normal plasma uric acid level, as well as the absence of hypertension, generalized edema, or proteinuria, point to epilepsy. Electroencephalography rarely is diagnostic.

During pregnancy, the risk of vaginal bleeding is doubled, and there is a threefold risk of abruptio placentae. Abnormal presentations are more common in labor and birth, and there is an increased possibility that the fetus will experience seizures in utero (Mishell & Brenner, 1994).

Metabolic changes in pregnancy usually alter pharmacokinetics. In addition, nausea and vomiting may interfere with ingestion and absorption of medication. All anticonvulsants have a significant teratogenic risk and thus are not considered safe. Research is unclear about the teratogenic effects, but the major malformations are cleft lip and cleft palate, facial abnormalities, deformities of the extremities, and some neural tube defects (Donaldson, 1995). On the other hand, tonic-clonic convulsions may be injurious to the fetus or mother and may lead to miscarriage. Antiepileptic drugs should be monotherapeutic and should be used in the smallest therapeutic dose with the least side effects. Daily folic acid supplementation is important because of the depletion that occurs when taking anticonvulsants (Cartlidge, 1995).

Multiple Sclerosis

Multiple sclerosis (MS), a patchy demyelinization of the spinal cord and CNS, may be a viral disorder. MS has a greater prevalence in females and is more common during the childbearing years, between the ages of 20 and 40 years (Cartlidge, 1995). Infertility, abortion, stillbirth, and fetal anomalies do not appear to be increased in women with MS; however, most women with MS choose not to become pregnant (James et al., 1994).

MS may occasionally complicate pregnancy, but exacerbations and remissions are unrelated to the pregnant state. Steroids are commonly used to treat acute exacerbations. Nursing care of the pregnant woman with MS is similar to the care of the normal pregnant woman. Women with MS occasionally may have an almost painless labor. The character of uterine contractions is unaffected by the disease, however.

Bell's Palsy

An association between Bell's palsy (idiopathic facial paralysis) and pregnancy was first cited by Bell in 1830. The incidence of Bell's palsy in pregnancy is about 57 per 100,000 per year. The incidence usually peaks during the third trimester and the puerperium (Cartlidge, 1995).

No effects of maternal Bell's palsy have been observed in infants. Maternal outcome is generally good unless there is a complete block in nerve conduction. Steroids sometimes are prescribed for the condition, but they do not hasten recovery. In most affected women, 90% or more of facial function can be expected to return (Cunningham et al., 1997). Supportive care includes prevention of injury to the exposed cornea, facial muscle massage, careful chewing and manual removal of food from inside the affected cheek, and reassurance that return of total neurologic function is likely.

I AUTOIMMUNE DISORDERS

Autoimmune disorders make up a large group of diseases that disrupt the function of the immune system of the body. In these types of disorders the body develops antibodies that attack its normally present antigens, causing tissue damage. Autoimmune disorders have a predilection for women in their reproductive years; therefore associations with pregnancy are not uncommon (James et al., 1994; Varner, 1994). Pregnancy may affect the disease process. Some disorders adversely affect the course of pregnancy or are detrimental to the fetus. Autoimmune disorders include rheumatoid arthritis, systemic lupus erythematosus, hyperthyroidism, myasthenia gravis, and immunologic thrombocytopenic purpura.

Rheumatoid Arthritis

The peak age of onset of rheumatoid arthritis (RA) is between 35 and 40 years. RA affects women more often than men (Gilbert & Harmon, 1998). During pregnancy, women with RA experience an increase in alpha$_2$-glycoprotein. In addition, total plasma and free cortisol (especially estrogens and progesterone) show an increase. Two thirds of women with RA find that the severity of symptoms decreases during pregnancy, but in many women exacerbation often follows childbirth (Lockshin & Druzin, 1995).

Management of RA during pregnancy includes an appropriate balance of rest and exercise, heat and physical therapy, salicylates and low-dose steroids (Scott & Branch, 1994). Low-dose aspirin probably remains the safest and most useful antiinflammatory drug for these women.

Systemic Lupus Erythematosus

One of the most common serious disorders of childbearing age, **systemic lupus erythematosus (SLE)** is a chronic, multisystem inflammatory disease characterized by autoimmune antibody production that affects the skin, joints, kidneys, lungs, CNS, liver, and other body organs (James et al., 1994). More than 250,000 persons are known to have SLE, with an estimated 50,000 new cases per year. The exact cause is unknown, but viral infection and hormonal and genetic factors may be related.

Early symptoms, such as fatigue, weight loss, skin rashes, and arthralgias may be overlooked. Pericarditis is often the presenting symptom. Eventually all organs become involved. The condition is characterized by a series of exacerbations and remissions.

If the diagnosis has been established and the woman desires a child, she is advised to wait until she has been in remission for at least 6 months before attempting to get pregnant (Gilbert & Harmon, 1998). An exacerbation of SLE during pregnancy or postpartum occurs in 15% to 60% of women (James et al., 1994). Complications such as spontaneous abortion, preeclampsia, HELLP syndrome, and preterm labor are common.

Medical therapy is kept to a minimum in women who are in remission or who have a mild form of SLE. Antiinflammatory drugs such as prednisone and aspirin may be used. Immunosuppressive drugs are not recommended during pregnancy but may be used in some situations. Nursing care focuses on early recognition of signs of SLE exacerbation and pregnancy complications, education and support of the woman and her family, and assessment of fetal well-being.

Myasthenia Gravis

Myasthenia gravis (MG), an autoimmune motor (muscle) end-plate disorder that involves acetylcholine use, affects the motor function at the myoneural junction. Muscle weakness, particularly of the eyes, face, tongue, neck, limbs, and respiratory muscles, results. MG occurs in 40 persons per 1 million and in women twice as often as in men (Cartlidge, 1995). The peak age of onset of MG is about the third decade. Pregnancy may complicate the disorder, although some women experience a remission during gestation. The experience in one pregnancy does not predict the course of the pregnancy in relation to the disease in subsequent pregnancies (Donaldson, 1995).

The nurse and physician should be alert to symptoms, which include easy fatigability, intermittent double vision, upper eyelid drooping, and facial muscle weakness. Patients present with easy fatigability, diplopia, difficulty speaking, and difficulty swallowing and clearing secretions (James et al., 1994). In more serious cases, upper arm weakness and breathing difficulty occur. Infections may precipitate onset or relapse and must be treated aggressively during pregnancy.

Women with MG usually tolerate labor well because they already have some degree of muscle relaxation. Meperidine is the obstetric analgesic of choice. Local anesthesia is preferred. Oxytocin may be given, but magnesium sulfate is contraindicated because it worsens the neuromuscular blockade. After birth, women must be carefully supervised because relapses often occur during the puerperium.

The effects of MG on pregnancy are usually minor, and there is no effect on fertility (Cartlidge, 1995). Occasionally an infant born to a mother with severe MG also shows myasthenic signs sufficient to require neostigmine treatment for 1 to 2 months. The nurse should observe the baby for a feeble cry, respiratory difficulties, and poor sucking. Neonatal MG is transient, and complete recovery of the infant is expected.

▌GASTROINTESTINAL DISORDERS

Compromise of gastrointestinal (GI) function during pregnancy is a concern. Obvious physiologic alterations, such as the greatly enlarged uterus, and less apparent changes, such as hormonal differences and hypochlorhydria (deficiency of hydrochloric acid in the stomach's gastric juice), require understanding for proper diagnosis and treatment. Gallbladder disease and inflammatory bowel disease are two GI disorders that may occur during pregnancy.

Cholelithiasis and Cholecystitis

Women are twice as likely to have cholelithiasis (presence of gallstones in the gallbladder) as men (Baker, 1995), and pregnancy seems to make the woman more vulnerable to gallstone formation (see Home Care box). Decreased muscle tone allows gallbladder distention, thickening of the bile, and prolonged emptying time. Increased progesterone levels result in a slight hypercholesterolemia. Cholecystitis (inflammation of the gallbladder) does not commonly occur during pregnancy. Pregnancy, however, poses a risk of worsening gallbladder disease that is preexisting.

Generally, gallbladder surgery should be postponed until the puerperium. The woman presenting with cholelithiasis

> ### ⊙ HOME CARE *Patient Instructions for Self-Care*
>
> **Nutritional Counseling for the Pregnant Woman with Cholecystitis or Cholelithiasis**
> - Assess your diet for foods that cause discomfort and flatulence and omit foods that trigger episodes.
> - Reduce dietary fat to 40- to 50-gm intake per day.
> - Limit protein to 10% to 12% of total calories.
> - Choose foods so that most of the calories come from carbohydrates.
> - Prepare food without adding fats or oils as much as possible.
> - Avoid fried foods.

or cholecystitis in the first trimester should be treated conservatively with IV fluids, bowel rest, nasogastric (NG) suctioning, and antibiotics. Meperidine or atropine alleviates ductal spasm and pain.

Inflammatory Bowel Disease

Inflammatory bowel disease can be acute or chronic. Infection or antibiotic therapy can induce acute inflammation of the bowel. Chronic inflammatory bowel disease can be classified as regional enteritis (Crohn's disease) or ulcerative colitis.

Chronic inflammatory bowel diseases are prone to periods of exacerbation and remission. The cause is unknown. The clinical manifestations for this chronic disorder are liquid diarrhea, urgency of defecation, and crampy lower abdominal pain. Blood, mucus, and/or pus may be seen in the stool.

Treatment and therapy are the same for the pregnant woman as for the nonpregnant woman. Medications include sulfasalazine and prednisone. Folic acid and vitamin supplementation is especially important because of the problems with malabsorption and malnutrition associated with chronic inflammatory bowel disease.

The effect of inflammatory bowel disease on pregnancy is minimal unless there is marked debilitation, whereupon spontaneous abortion, fetal death, or preterm birth may occur. In general, when pregnancy coincides with active ulcerative colitis, most women will experience a severe exacerbation of the disease. When pregnancy occurs during a period of inactivity of the disorder, a flare-up is unlikely.

▌HUMAN IMMUNODEFICIENCY VIRUS AND ACQUIRED IMMUNODEFICIENCY SYNDROME

Infection with the human immunodeficiency virus (HIV) and the resultant acquired immunodeficiency syndrome (AIDS) are increasingly occurring in women. Although HIV and AIDS have been traditionally associated with homosexual populations, about 12% of all current cases of HIV infection in the United States have been diagnosed in women. Women are most likely to have acquired the infection through IV drug use or heterosexual contact with a high-risk man. Women of color are disproportionately affected; about 75% of HIV-infected women are black or Hispanic. In the United States, AIDS is found 13 times more frequently in African-American women than in Caucasian women; the occurrence rate in Hispanic women is 6 times greater than in Caucasian women (Duff, 1996; Flagler et al., 1997). This chapter addresses management of the pregnant woman who is HIV positive or has developed full-blown AIDS. See Chapter 6 for more information about the diagnosis and management of nonpregnant women with HIV and Chapter 28 for a discussion of HIV/AIDS in infants.

Preconceptional Counseling

Pregnancy is not encouraged in HIV-positive women; preconceptional counseling is recommended. Exposure to the virus has a significant impact on the pregnancy, neonatal feeding method, and neonatal health status. HIV-positive women should be counseled extensively about the risk of perinatal transmission and possible obstetric complications. Pregnancy itself does not appear to significantly accelerate the progression of HIV infection (Duff, 1996). HIV-positive women should be encouraged to seek prenatal care immediately if they suspect pregnancy in order to maximize chances for a positive outcome.

Incidence

In the general obstetric population in the United States, about 1 in 1,000 women are HIV positive. In some inner-city populations, however, 1% to 1.5% of all pregnant women are infected with the virus (Duff, 1996).

Pregnancy Risks

Perinatal transmission

About 90% of all pediatric AIDS cases are due to transmission of the virus from mother to child during the perinatal period. Exposure may occur to the fetus through the maternal circulation as early as the first trimester of pregnancy, to the infant during labor and birth by inoculation or ingestion of maternal blood and other infected fluids, or to the infant through breast milk. The frequency of perinatal transmission has been reported from a low of 5% to 10% to a high of 50% to 60%. Most researchers report transmission rates of 20% to 30% (Duff, 1996; Lamphear, 1994). Factors that increase the likelihood of perinatal viral transmission are listed in Box 23-2.

Further information regarding perinatal transmission of the HIV virus was provided in a landmark study published in 1994. In this study, known as the AIDS Clinical Trials Group Protocol 076, treatment of HIV-infected women with the antiviral drug zidovudine (AZT) during pregnancy and intrapartum and treatment of their infants for the first 6 weeks of life with zidovudine remarkably decreased the rate

---

BOX 23-2	*Factors That Increase the Risk of Perinatal HIV Transmission*

- Previous history of a child with HIV infection
- AIDS
- Preterm birth
- Decreased maternal CD_4 count
- Firstborn twin
- Chorioamnionitis
- Intrapartum blood exposure
- Failure to treat mother and fetus with zidovudine during the perinatal period

From Duff P: Maternal and perinatal infection. In Gabbe S, Niebyl J & Simpson J, editors: *Obstetrics: normal and problem pregnancies,* ed 3, New York, 1996, Churchill Livingstone.

of viral transmission from 25.5% in study subjects who received a placebo to 8.3% in those who were given zidovudine. This represented a 67% reduction in the risk of perinatal HIV transmission (Connor et al., 1994).

Obstetric complications

It is difficult to determine obstetric risk in persons with HIV infection because so many confounding variables are often present. Many HIV-positive women also suffer from drug and alcohol addiction, poor nutrition, limited access to prenatal care, and/or concurrent STDs. HIV-positive women are probably at risk for preterm labor and birth, premature rupture of membranes (PROM), IUGR, perinatal mortality, and postpartum endometritis (Duff, 1996).

I CARE MANAGEMENT

HIV counseling and testing should be offered to all women at their initial entry into prenatal care (Centers for Disease Control and Prevention [CDC] 1998). Most states in the United States have enacted legislation to ensure this is offered. If only those presumed to be at high risk are screened, about half of all HIV-positive women will not be detected (Duff, 1996). Identification of HIV-positive pregnant women is especially important, since antepartum and intrapartum antiviral drug therapy has been shown to greatly decrease the risk of viral transmission to the fetus.

HIV-infected women should also be tested for other STDs, such as gonorrhea; syphilis; chlamydial infection; hepatitis B, C, and D; and herpes. Cytomegalovirus (CMV) and toxoplasmosis antibody testing should be done because both infections can cause significant maternal and fetal complications and can be successfully treated with antimicrobial agents. Any history of vaccination and immune status should be documented, and chickenpox (varicella) and rubella titers should be determined. A tuberculin skin test should be performed; a positive test necessitates a chest x-ray film to identify active pulmonary disease. Also, a Papanicolaou (Pap) smear should be done (Duff, 1996).

All HIV-infected women should be treated with zidovudine during pregnancy, regardless of their CD_4 counts (Boyer et al., 1994; CDC, 1994). The major side effect of this drug is bone marrow suppression; periodic hematocrit, white blood cell (WBC) count, and platelet count assessments should be performed (Duff, 1996). Women with CD_4 counts <200 cells/mm³ should receive prophylactic treatment for *Pneumocystis carinii* pneumonia with daily trimethoprim-sulfamethoxazole (Duff, 1996). Any other opportunistic infections should be treated with medications specific for the infection; often dosages must be higher for women with HIV infection or AIDS.

Women who are HIV positive should also be vaccinated against hepatitis B, pneumococcal infection, hemophilus B influenza, and viral influenza. To support any pregnant woman's immune system, appropriate counseling is provided about optimal nutrition, sleep, rest, exercise, and stress reduction. The HIV-infected woman needs a greater amount of nutritional support and counseling about diet choices, food preparation, and food handling. Weight gain or maintenance in pregnancy is a challenge with the HIV-infected patient. The infected patient is counseled regarding "safer sex" techniques. Use of condoms and nonoxynol-9 spermicide is encouraged to minimize further exposure to HIV if her partner is the source. Orogenital sex is discouraged.

The woman is referred for drug rehabilitation as necessary to discontinue substance abuse. Abuse of alcohol, methamphetamines (speed, ice), marijuana, cocaine, nitrites (poppers, snappers), or other drugs compromises the body's immune system and increases the risks of AIDS and associated conditions. It also interferes with many medical and alternative therapies for AIDS. In addition, alcohol and other drugs affect the judgment of abusers, who may be more likely to engage in activities that place them at high risk for AIDS or increased exposure to HIV.

IV zidovudine will be administered to the HIV-positive woman during the intrapartum period. A loading dose is initiated on her admission in labor, followed by a continuous maintenance dose throughout labor (Duff, 1996).

Every effort should be made during the birthing process to decrease the neonate's exposure to infected maternal blood and secretions. If feasible, the membranes should be left intact until the birth. Women who give birth within 4 hours after membrane rupture are less likely to transmit the virus to their neonates than women who experience a longer interval between rupture and birth (Gilbert & Harmon, 1998). Fetal scalp electrode and scalp pH sampling should be avoided, since these procedures may result in inoculation of the virus into the fetus. Likewise, the use of forceps and a vacuum extractor should be avoided when possible. Episiotomy and cesarean birth do not seem to greatly influence the infection rate (Gilbert & Harmon, 1998).

Immediately after birth, infants should be wiped free of all body fluids and then bathed as soon as they are in stable condition. All staff members working with the mother or infant must strictly adhere to infection control techniques and observe Standard Precautions for blood and body fluid (Craven et al., 1994; Duff, 1996).

The postpartum period for the woman infected with HIV may be notable for infection, hemorrhage, or both (Bastin et al., 1992). Women without symptoms may have an unremarkable postpartum course; on the other hand, immunosuppressed women with symptoms may be at increased risk for postpartum UTIs, vaginitis, postpartum endometritis, and poor wound healing. HIV-related thrombocytopenias may also increase hemorrhage risk (Mandelbrot et al., 1994).

The cleansed neonate can be with the mother after birth, but breastfeeding is discouraged because of possible HIV transmission in breast milk. (The World Health Organization has not discouraged breastfeeding in nonindustrialized nations because of the decreased availability of infant formula and hygiene risks in its preparation but may be changing their recommendation.) After discharge, the woman and her infant are referred to physicians who are experienced in the treatment of AIDS and associated conditions.

▌ SUBSTANCE ABUSE

Substance abuse among women of childbearing age is increasing throughout all segments of society. ACOG (1994b) estimates that substance abuse is a problem in 10% of all pregnancies. Care of the pregnant substance abuser offers a tremendous nursing challenge. Many substance abusers are deeply depressed, sometimes because of previous negative life experiences. Often, substance abuse has provided a way for the woman to relieve psychologic distress and blunt the feelings of loneliness and emptiness that are part of depression. Sometimes, substance abusers have grown up in an environment where such behavior was considered "normal"; consequently, they may have had little opportunity to learn sober living skills. Inadequate role models, particularly coupled with continued substance abuse, greatly impact on a woman's ability to parent. She may require much assistance to care for, nurture, and form a warm, close, intimate relationship with her child. Chapter 28 discusses neonatal effects of maternal substance abuse. The care needed by each woman varies according to her particular circumstances and the substance(s) abused. However, the nursing process is similar for all. Chapter 4 discusses several commonly abused illicit and prescription drugs.

▌ CARE MANAGEMENT

Every pregnant woman should be screened, at least verbally, for substance abuse. Ideally, drug and alcohol use should be identified at the first prenatal visit so that intervention can begin early in pregnancy. Unfortunately, this ideal situation frequently does not occur. Women who are heavily involved in substance abuse often receive no prenatal care or make only a limited number of visits beginning late in pregnancy.

During the initial prenatal visit, questions about alcohol and drug use should be incorporated into the overall prenatal history. Because women frequently deny or greatly underreport usage when asked directly about drug or alcohol consumption, it is crucial that the nurse display a nonjudgmental and matter-of-fact attitude while taking the history in order to gain the woman's trust and hopefully elicit a reasonably accurate estimate (Cefalo & Moos, 1995). Information about drug use should be obtained by asking first about the woman's intake of OTC and prescribed medications. Next, her usage of "legal" drugs, such as caffeine, nicotine, and alcohol, should be ascertained. Finally, the woman should be questioned about her use of illicit drugs, such as cocaine, heroin, and marijuana. The approximate frequency and amount should be documented for each drug used (Redding & Selleck, 1993).

Screening for alcohol use is best done by the use of self-reporting questionnaires because there is currently no reliable biochemical marker for alcohol use. Urine screening is unreliable because alcohol is undetectable within a few hours following ingestion (Redding & Selleck, 1993; Russell et al., 1996). Screening questionnaires generally ask about consequences of heavy drinking, alcohol intake, or both. The Michigan Alcoholism Screening Test (MAST) and the CAGE test are two well-known screens that are often used. Two screening tests, the T-ACE (Box 23-3) and the TWEAK (Box 23-4), have been developed to screen specifically for alcohol use during pregnancy (Russell, 1994).

Urine toxicology testing is often performed to screen for illicit drug use. Drugs may be found in urine days to weeks after ingestion, depending on how quickly they are metabolized and excreted from the body. Meconium (from the neonate) and hair can also be analyzed to determine past drug use over a longer period of time (Gilbert & Harmon, 1998).

There is no state requirement for a health care provider to test either the mother or the newborn for the presence of drugs. It is most important that nurses be aware of laws regarding prenatal drug use in the states in which they practice. In some states a woman with a positive urine drug screen who is pregnant or has just given birth must be referred to child protective services. If the mother is not in a drug treatment program or is judged unable to provide newborn care, her infant may be placed in foster care.

While the ideal long-term outcome is total abstinence, it is not likely that the woman will either desire or be able to stop alcohol and drug use suddenly. Indeed, it may be harmful to the fetus for her to do so. In some situations, the goal may be to decrease substance use, and short-term outcomes will be necessary.

Intervention with the pregnant substance abuser begins with education about specific effects on pregnancy, the fetus, and the newborn for each drug used. Consequences of perinatal drug use should be clearly communicated and abstinence recommended as the safest course of action. Women are frequently more receptive to making lifestyle

---

BOX 23-3 T-ACE Test

- How many drinks can you hold before getting sleepy or passing out? (TOLERANCE)
- Have people ANNOYED you by criticizing your drinking?
- Have you ever felt you ought to CUT DOWN on your drinking?
- Have you ever had a drink first thing in the morning to steady your nerves or get rid of a hangover? (EYE-OPENER)

Scoring: Two points are given for the TOLERANCE question for the ability to hold at least a six pack of beer or a bottle of wine. A "yes" answer to any of the other questions receives one point. An overall score of ≥2 indicates a high probability that the woman is a risk drinker.

From Hankin J & Sokol R: Identification and care of problems associated with alcohol ingestion in pregnancy, *Semin Perinatol* 19(4):286, 1995.

BOX 23-4 TWEAK Test

- How many drinks can you hold before getting sleepy or passing out? (TOLERANCE)
- Have close friends or relatives WORRIED or complained about your drinking during the past year?
- Do you sometimes take a drink in the morning when you first get up? (EYE-OPENER)
- Has a friend or family member ever told you about things you said or did while you were drinking that you could not remember? (AMNESIA)
- Do you sometimes feel the need to KUT/CUT down on your drinking?

Scoring: Two points are given for the TOLERANCE question for the ability to hold more than five drinks. A "yes" answer to the WORRY question receives two points. A "yes" answer to any of the other questions receives one point. An overall score of ≥2 indicates the woman is likely to be a risk drinker.

From Russell M: New assessment tools for risk drinking during pregnancy: T-ACE, TWEAK, and others, *Alcohol Health Res World* 18(1):55, 1994.

---

changes during pregnancy than at any other time in their lives. The casual, experimental, or recreational drug user is frequently able to achieve and maintain sobriety when she receives education, support, and continued monitoring throughout the remainder of the pregnancy. Periodic screening throughout pregnancy of women who have admitted to drug use may help them to continue abstinence (Gilbert & Harmon, 1998; Redding & Selleck, 1993).

Women who are unlikely to abstain from the use of alcohol and/or other drugs despite education and support should be confronted about the danger of this behavior during pregnancy and offered referral for substance abuse treatment. The goal of confrontation is to have the woman admit that she has an alcohol and/or drug problem and become willing to do something about it. Treatment will be individualized for each woman depending on the type of drug used and the frequency and amount of use. Detoxification, short-term inpatient or outpatient treatment, long-term residential treatment, aftercare services, and 12-step, self-help support groups such as Alcoholics Anonymous are all possible options. In general, long-term treatment of any sort is becoming increasingly more difficult to obtain, particularly for women who lack insurance coverage. Although some programs allow a woman to keep her children with her at the treatment facility, there are far too few available to meet the demand (Gilbert & Harmon, 1998; Redding & Selleck, 1993).

Alcohol withdrawal treatment consists of the administration of benzodiazepines, an improvement in the woman's nutritional intake (folic acid and other vitamins), and psychotherapy. Detoxification with disulfiram (Antabuse) is not used in pregnant women because of its teratogenic effects (Lewis & Woods, 1994).

Methadone treatment for pregnant women dependent on heroin or other narcotics is controversial. If women withdraw from heroin during pregnancy, blood flow to the placenta is impaired. The substitution of methadone for the heroin not only promotes withdrawal from heroin but also does not cause impaired blood flow to the placenta. Methadone, however, can cause detrimental fetal effects, and withdrawal from it after birth can be worse for the newborn than heroin withdrawal (Gilbert & Harmon, 1998; Glantz & Woods, 1993; Stuart & Sundeen, 1998).

While cocaine is powerfully psychologically addictive, use of the drug does not result in physical dependence. Therefore women who abuse cocaine can stop its use abruptly without developing symptoms of withdrawal. Most cocaine abusers will need a great deal of assistance, such as an alcohol and drug treatment program, individual or group counseling, and participation in self-help support groups, in order to successfully accomplish this major lifestyle change.

Because of the lifestyle often associated with drug use, substance-abusing women are at risk for STDs, including HIV. Laboratory assessments will likely include screening for STDs such as gonorrhea and chlamydial infection and antibody determinations for hepatitis B and HIV. A chest x-ray film may be taken to assess for pulmonary problems such as hilar lymphadenopathy, pulmonary edema, bacterial pneumonia, and foreign-body emboli. A skin test to screen for tuberculosis may also be ordered.

Initial and serial ultrasound studies are usually performed to determine gestational age, because the woman may have had amenorrhea as a result of her drug use or may not know when her last menstrual period occurred. Because of concerns about stillbirth, an increased frequency of the birth of small-for-gestational-age (SGA) infants, and the potential for hypoxia, some experts recommend that nonstress testing be done in women who are known substance abusers (Glantz & Woods, 1993).

While substance abusers may be difficult to care for at any time, they are often particularly challenging during the

---

| BOX 23-5 | *Dealing with Pregnant Substance Abusers* |

- Realize that the decision to become and remain sober can *only* be made by the substance abuser.
- Understand that nurses do not have the power to cure anyone. We are only cheerleaders and supporters!
- Educate yourself about the effects of drug use in general and its effect on pregnancy and the newborn specifically.
- Confront substance abusers openly and honestly with the facts regarding their drug use. Do not make threats or pile on guilt.
- Treat substance abusers with the same respect and consideration you show other people.
- Become familiar with your local treatment centers. Learn which of them will accept pregnant women. Keep an up-to-date list of 12-step groups meeting in your community.
- Remember that there are no "hopeless cases." It is *never* too late to quit!
- Practice patience and persistence. It may take months or years to see the effects of your work.

---

intrapartum and postpartum periods because of manipulative and demanding behavior. Typically, these women display poor control over their behavior and a low threshold for pain. Increased dependency needs and poor parenting skills may also be apparent.

Nurses must understand that substance abuse is an illness and that these women deserve to be treated with patience, kindness, consistency, and firmness when necessary (Box 23-5). Even women who are actively abusing drugs will experience pain during labor and after giving birth. Withholding analgesia and/or anesthesia in an attempt to "punish" them for prenatal substance abuse is not helpful and should be avoided. It is helpful to develop a standardized plan of care so that patients have limited opportunities to play staff members against each other. Mother-infant attachment should be promoted by identifying the woman's strengths and reinforcing positive maternal feelings and behaviors. Staffing should be sufficient to ensure strict surveillance of visitors and prevent unsupervised drug use.

Advice regarding breastfeeding must be individualized. Although all abused substances appear in breast milk, some in greater amounts than others (Brody, Larner & Minneman, 1998), breastfeeding is definitely contraindicated in women who use amphetamines, alcohol, cocaine, heroin, or marijuana. The baby's nutrition and safety needs are of primary importance in this consideration. For some women, a desire to breastfeed may provide strong motivation to achieve and maintain sobriety.

Before a known substance abuser is discharged with her baby, the home situation must be assessed to determine that the environment is safe and that someone will be available to meet the infant's needs if the mother proves unable to do so. Usually the hospital's social services department will be involved in interviewing the mother before discharge to ensure that the infant's needs will be met. Sometimes family members or friends will be asked to become actively involved with the mother and infant after discharge. A home care or public health nurse may be asked to make home visits to assess the mother's ability to care for the baby and provide guidance and support. If serious questions about the infant's well-being exist, the case will probably be referred to the state's child protective services agency for further action.

KEY POINTS

- Lack of maternal glycemic control before conception and in the first trimester of pregnancy may be responsible for fetal congenital malformations.

- Maternal insulin requirements increase as the pregnancy progresses and may quadruple by term as a result of insulin resistance created by placental hormones, insulinase, and cortisol.

- Poor glycemic control before and during pregnancy can lead to maternal complications such as spontaneous abortion, infection, and dystocia (difficult labor) caused by fetal macrosomia.

- Careful glucose monitoring, insulin administration when necessary, and dietary counseling are used to create a normal intrauterine environment for fetal growth and development in the pregnancy complicated by diabetes mellitus.

- Because gestational diabetes mellitus is asymptomatic in most cases, many women undergo routine screening during pregnancy.

- Thyroid dysfunction during pregnancy requires close monitoring of thyroid hormone levels to regulate therapy and prevent fetal insult.

- The stress of the normal maternal adaptations to pregnancy on a heart whose function is already taxed may cause cardiac decompensation.

- In the case of cardiac arrest in a pregnant woman, the standard advanced cardiac life support (ACLS) guidelines should be implemented with the modification of positioning the woman so that the uterus is displaced laterally.

- Maternal morbidity or mortality is a significant risk in a pregnancy complicated by mitral stenosis.

- The chance of developing adult respiratory distress syndrome increases with the amount of trauma experienced during pregnancy or birth.

KEY POINTS—cont'd

- The normal hemodynamic values are significantly altered as a result of pregnancy.

- Anemia, the most common medical disorder of pregnancy, affects at least 20% of pregnant women.

- Autoimmune disorders (e.g., systemic lupus erythematosus, myasthenia gravis) show a predilection for women in their reproductive years; therefore associations with pregnancy are not uncommon.

- Acquired immunodeficiency syndrome (AIDS) is becoming increasingly prevalent among heterosexuals and women, particularly women of color.

- Human immunodeficiency virus (HIV) may be transmitted through blood, semen, and perinatal events.

- Perinatal administration of zidovudine (AZT) is recommended to decrease transmission of the HIV virus from mother to fetus.

- Because medical history and examination cannot reliably identify all persons with HIV or other blood-borne pathogens, blood and body fluid precautions should be consistently used for everyone.

- Much support from a variety of sources, including family and friends, health care providers, and the recovery community, is needed to help perinatal substance abusers achieve and maintain sobriety.

- It is crucial that health care providers provide compassionate, nonjudgmental care to substance abusers.

CRITICAL THINKING EXERCISES

1 Carmelita Hershey is admitted to the antepartum unit. She is a type 1 diabetic who is 30 weeks pregnant. She receives insulin twice a day. Her blood glucose level on admission is 220 mg/dl. This admission is to control her blood glucose and assess both her status and that of her fetus.

 a What assessment would you need to do in order to determine why Carmelita's blood glucose levels are out of control?

 b How would Carmelita's fetus respond to increased maternal glucose levels? What complications might this cause in the fetus?

 c Carmelita is from Mexico, and she likes to eat tortillas and beans and spicy foods. Prepare a diet exchange list for a 2,200-calorie ADA diet that would incorporate foods that she prefers.

CRITICAL THINKING EXERCISES—cont'd

2 Attend a high-risk prenatal clinic on a day when diabetic women are scheduled. Interview several women with gestational diabetes and talk with their significant others. Ask them the following questions, and then analyze your interview data and present a clinical conference on the impact of gestational diabetes.

a How did you feel when you were first told that you had gestational diabetes?

b What changes in your lifestyle have you made as a result of being a gestational diabetic? Which change has been the hardest to make?

c What was the best thing that your health care provider did to help you adjust to being a gestational diabetic?

d What could your health care provider(s) have done differently that might have helped you adjust more quickly or easily to having gestational diabetes?

3 You are assigned to a woman who has a history of class III cardiac disease (New York Heart Association classification). She has come to the clinic, where she is diagnosed to be 8 weeks pregnant. She has a 2-year-old at home and a husband (who is not present today) who thinks that she is healthy and that she does not need any help with household or child care activities during her pregnancy.

a Identify inconsistencies in the above scenario.

b Explain how you can help the husband understand the status of his wife's condition.

c Identify three community resources for the woman and her family. Describe the services available, costs, and accessibility.

d Discuss ways the woman can cope with activity limitations without giving up all household and child care activities.

4 Michelle Mann is admitted to the labor and delivery unit at 37 weeks' gestation in active labor. Michelle is HIV positive and has a past history of IV cocaine and heroin use. She has been sober now for the past 18 months. She tells you that she has been taking "some AIDS drug" during this pregnancy, but she doesn't seem to know much about it.

a Which drug has Michelle probably been taking during pregnancy, and why? Will this drug therapy continue during the intrapartum and postpartum periods? What about the baby?

CRITICAL THINKING EXERCISES—cont'd

b Describe the precautions you would be certain to observe in order to protect yourself as you provide care for Michelle.

c What changes will occur in Michelle's health if she progresses from "being HIV positive" to actually "having AIDS"?

d What risk factors for acquiring HIV infection are present in Michelle's background? What advice would you give her in terms of lifestyle and future planning?

References

Alvarez-Marfany M et al: Long-term prospective study of postpartum thyroid dysfunction in women with insulin dependent diabetes mellitus, *J Clin Endocrinol Metab* 79(1):10, 1994.

American College of Obstetricians and Gynecologists: Diabetes and pregnancy, *ACOG Tech Bull* 200:1, 1994a.

American College of Obstetricians and Gynecologists: Substance abuse in pregnancy, *ACOG Tech Bull* 195:1, 1994b.

American College of Obstetricians and Gynecologists: Pulmonary disease in pregnancy, *ACOG Tech Bull* 224, Part 1, 1996.

American Diabetes Association: *Medical management of insulin-dependent (type 1) diabetes*, ed 2, Alexandria, Va, 1994, The Association.

American Diabetes Association: *Medical management of pregnancy complicated by diabetes*, ed 2, Alexandria, Va, 1995, The Association.

American Diabetes Association: Position statement: gestational diabetes mellitus, *Diabetes Care* 20(suppl 1):S44, 1997.

American Heart Association: *Basic life support, heart saver guide*, Dallas, 1997, The Association.

Association of Women's Health, Obstetric, and Neonatal Nurses: *Standards and guidelines for professional nursing practice in the care of women and newborns*, ed 5, Washington, DC, 1998, The Association.

Bajo T: Cardiopulmonary resuscitation of the pregnant patient. In Foley M & Strong T, editors: *Obstetric intensive care*, Philadelphia, 1997, WB Saunders.

Baker A: Liver and bilary tract disease. In Barron W & Lindheimer M, editors: *Medical disorders during pregnancy*, ed 2, St Louis, 1995, Mosby.

Bastin N et al.: HIV disease and pregnancy. III. Postpartum care of the HIV-positive woman and her newborn, *J Obstet Gynecol Neonatal Nurs* 21(2):105, 1992.

Becton Dickinson & Co: *Controlling low blood sugar reactions*, Franklin Lakes, NJ, 1997, Becton Dickinson & Co.

Bernstein I & Gabbe S: Intrauterine growth restriction. In Gabbe S, Niebyl J & Simpson J, editors: *Obstetrics: normal and problem pregnancies*, ed 3, New York, 1996, Churchill Livingstone.

Boyer P et al.: Factors predictive of maternal-fetal transmission of HIV-1: preliminary analysis of zidovudine given during pregnancy and/or delivery, *JAMA* 271(24):1925, 1994.

Brody T, Larner J & Minneman K: *Human pharmacology: molecular to clinical*, ed 3, St Louis, 1998, Mosby.

Brown C & Bertolet B: Peripartum cardiomyopathy: a comprehensive review, *Am J Obstet Gynecol* 178(2):409, 1998.

Cartlidge N: Neurologic disorders. In Barron W & Lindheimer M, editors: *Medical disorders during pregnancy,* ed 2, St Louis, 1995, Mosby.

Cefalo R & Moos M: *Preconceptional health care, a practical guide,* ed 2, St Louis, 1995, Mosby.

Centers for Disease Control and Prevention: Recommendations of the U.S. Public Health Service Task Force on the use of zidovudine to reduce perinatal transmission of human immunodeficiency virus, *MMWR* 43(RR-11):1, 1994.

Centers for Disease Control and Prevention: 1998 guidelines for treatment of sexually transmitted diseases, *MMWR* 47(RR-1):1, 1998.

Chandra N & Hazinski M, editors: *American Heart Association textbook of basic life support for healthcare providers,* Dallas, 1997, The Association.

Connor E et al: Reduction of maternal-infant transmission of human immunodeficiency virus type 1 with zidovudine treatment, *N Engl J Med* 331(8):1173, 1994.

Craven D et al.: Human immunodeficiency virus infection in pregnancy: epidemiology and prevention of vertical transmission, *Infect Control Hosp Epidemiol* 15(1):36, 1994.

Cruikshank D: Cardiovascular, pulmonary, renal and hematologic disease in pregnancy. In Scott J et al., editors: *Danforth's obstetrics and gynecology,* ed 7, Philadelphia, 1994, JB Lippincott.

Cunningham F et al.: *Williams obstetrics,* ed 20, Stamford, Conn, 1997, Appleton & Lange.

Dacus J et al.: Gestational diabetes: postpartum glucose tolerance testing, *Am J Obstet Gynecol* 171(4):927, 1994.

Donaldson J: Neurologic complications. In Burrow G & Ferris T, editors: *Medical complications during pregnancy,* Philadelphia, PA, 1995, WB Saunders.

Dorner G & Plagemann A: Perinatal hyperinsulinism as a possible predisposing factor for diabetes mellitus, obesity, and enhanced cardiovascular risk in later life, *Horm Metab Res* 26(5):213, 1994.

Doshier S: What happens to the offspring of diabetic pregnancies? *MCN Am J Matern Child Nurs* 20(1):25, 1995.

Duff P: Maternal and perinatal infection. In Gabbe S, Niebyl J & Simpson J, editors: *Obstetrics: normal and problem pregnancies,* ed 3, New York, 1996, Churchill Livingstone.

Duffy T: Hematologic aspects of pregnancy. In Burrow G & Ferris T, editors: *Medical complications during pregnancy,* Philadelphia, 1995, WB Saunders.

Eli Lilly & Co: *Humalog,* Indianapolis, 1996, Eli Lilly & Co.

The Expert Committee on the Diagnosis and Classification of Diabetes Mellitus: Report of the expert committee on the diagnosis and classification of diabetes mellitus, *Diabetes Care* 20(7):1183, 1997.

Ferris A et al.: Perinatal lactation protocol and outcome in mothers with and without insulin-dependent diabetes mellitus, *Am J Clin Nutr* 58(1):43, 1993.

Flagler S et al.: Toward an understanding of addiction, *J Obstet Gynecol Neonatal Nurs* 26(4):441, 1997.

Foley M et al.: Effect of prolonged oral terbutaline therapy on glucose tolerance in pregnancy, *Am J Obstet Gynecol* 168(1 Part 1):100, 1993.

Gabbe S: A story of two miracles: the impact of the discovery of insulin on pregnancy in women with diabetes mellitus, *Obstet Gynecol* 79(2):295, 1992.

Gerstein H: Incidence of postpartum thyroid dysfunction in patients with type 1 diabetes mellitus, *Ann Intern Med* 118(6):419, 1993.

Gilbert E & Harmon J: *Manual of high risk pregnancy and delivery,* ed 2, St Louis, 1998, Mosby.

Glantz C & Woods J: Cocaine, heroin, and phencyclidine: obstetric perspectives, *Clin Obstet Gynecol* 36(2):279, 1993.

Grohar J: Nursing protocols for antepartum home care, *J Obstet Gynecol Neonatal Nurs* 23(8):687, 1994.

Hankin J & Sokol R: Identification and care of problems associated with alcohol ingestion in pregnancy, *Semin Perinatol* 19(4):286, 1995.

Health Care Resources: *Handbook of high-risk perinatal home care,* St Louis, 1997, Mosby.

Hoffmeister A & Haines S: The newest insulin: Lispro, *Diabetes Wellness Lett* 2(12):1, 1996.

Jackson G & Clark S: Cardiac and pulmonary disorders and pregnancy. In Moore T et al, editors: *Gynecology and obstetrics: a longitudinal approach,* New York, 1993, Churchill Livingstone.

James D et al., editors: *High risk pregnancy: management options,* Philadelphia, 1994, WB Saunders.

Jovanovic-Peterson L, editor: *Medical management of pregnancy complicated by diabetes,* Alexandria, Va, 1993, American Diabetes Association.

Jovanovic-Peterson L & Peterson C: Pregnancy in the diabetic woman, *Endocrinol Metab Clin North Am* 21(2):433, 1992.

Kaufmann R et al.: Gestational diabetes diagnostic criteria: long-term maternal follow-up, *Am J Obstet Gynecol* 172(2):621, 1995.

Kitzmiller J & Coombs C: Maternal and perinatal implications of diabetic nephropathy, *Clin Perinatol* 20(3):561, 1993.

Kjos S: Contraception in the diabetic woman, *Clin Perinatol* 20(3):649, 1993.

Kulb N: Cardiac disorders. In Buckley K & Kulb N, editors: *High risk maternity nursing manual,* Baltimore, 1990, Williams & Wilkins.

Lamphear B: Trends and patterns in the transmission of blood-borne pathogens to health care providers, *Epidemiol Rev* 16(2):437, 1994.

Landon M: Diabetes mellitus and other endocrine diseases. In Gabbe S, Niebyl J & Simpson J, editors: *Obstetrics: normal and problem pregnancies,* ed 3, New York, 1996, Churchill Livingstone.

Landon M & Gabbe S: Diabetes mellitus and pregnancy, *Obstet Gynecol Clin North Am* 19(4):633, 1992.

Landon M & Gabbe S: Diabetes mellitus. In Barron W & Lindheimer M, editors: *Medical disorders during pregnancy,* ed 2, St Louis, 1995, Mosby.

Landon M & Samuels P: Cardiac and pulmonary disease. In Gabbe S, Niebyl J & Simpson J, editors: *Obstetrics: normal and problem pregnancies,* ed 3, New York, 1996, Churchill Livingstone.

Lawrence R: *Breastfeeding: a guide for the medical profession,* ed 4, St Louis, 1994, Mosby.

Lazarus J: Treatment of hyper- and hypothyroidism in pregnancy, *J Endocrinol Invest* 16(5):391, 1993.

Letsky E: Hematologic disorders. In Barron W & Lindheimer M, editors: *Medical disorders during pregnancy,* ed 2, St Louis, 1995, Mosby.

Leung A et al.: Perinatal outcome in hypothyroid pregnancies, *Obstet Gynecol* 81(3):349, 1993.

Lewis D & Woods S: Fetal alcohol syndrome, *Am Fam Physician* 50(5):1025, 1994.

Lockshin M & Druzin M: Rheumatic disease. In Barron W & Lindheimer M, editors: *Medical disorders during pregnancy,* ed 2, St Louis, 1995, Mosby.

Mandelbrot L et al.: Thrombocytopenia in pregnant women infected with human immunodeficiency virus: maternal and neonatal outcome, *Am J Obstet Gynecol* 171(1):252, 1994.

McAnulty J, Metcalfe J & Ueland K: Cardiovascular disease. In Burrow G & Ferris T, editors: *Medical complications during pregnancy,* Philadelphia, 1995, WB Saunders.

Mendelson M & Lang R: Pregnancy and heart disease. In Barron W & Lindheimer M, editors: *Medical disorders during pregnancy,* ed 2, St Louis, 1995, Mosby.

Mestman J & Schmidt-Sarosi C: Diabetes mellitus and fertility control: contraception management issues, *Am J Obstet Gynecol* 168(6 Part 2):2012, 1993.

Mishell D & Brenner P, editors: *Management of common problems in obstetrics and gynecology,* ed 3, Boston, 1994, Blackwell Scientific Publications.

Molitch M: Pituitary, thyroid, adrenal, and parathyroid disorders. In Barron W & Lindheimer M, editors: *Medical disorders during pregnancy,* ed 2, St Louis, 1995, Mosby.

Mulford M et al.: Alternative therapies for the management of gestational diabetes, *Clin Perinatol* 20(3):619, 1993.

Neubauer S et al.: Delayed lactogenesis in women with insulin-dependent diabetes mellitus, *Am J Clin Nutr* 58:(1)54, 1993.

New York Heart Association: *Diseases of the heart and blood vessels: nomenclature and criteria for diagnosis,* ed 6, Boston, 1964, Little, Brown.

Niswander K & Evans S: *Manual of obstetrics,* Boston, 1995, Little, Brown.

Pagana K & Pagana T: *Mosby's diagnostic and laboratory test reference,* ed 3, St Louis, 1997, Mosby.

Piper J & Langer O: Does maternal diabetes delay fetal pulmonary maturity? *Am J Obstet Gynecol* 168(3 Part 1):783, 1993.

Redding B & Selleck C: Perinatal substance abuse: assessment and management of the pregnant woman and her children, *Nurs Pract Forum* 4(4):216, 1993.

Reece E & Homko C: Diabetes-related complications of pregnancy, *J Natl Med Assoc* 85(7):537, 1993.

Reece E & Homko C: Assessment and management of pregnancies complicated by pregestational and gestational diabetes mellitus, *J Assoc Acad Minority Phys* 5(3):87, 1994.

Reece E, Homko C & Wiznitzer A: Hypoglycemia in pregnancies complicated by diabetes mellitus: maternal and fetal considerations, *Clin Obstet Gynecol* 37(1):50, 1994.

Regenstein A, Belluomini J & Katz M: Terbutaline tocolysis and glucose intolerance, *Obstet Gynecol* 81(5 Part 1):739, 1993.

Rosenn B et al.: Glycemic thresholds for spontaneous abortion and congenital malformations in insulin dependent diabetes, *Obstet Gynecol* 84(4):515, 1994.

Russell M: New assessment tools for risk drinking during pregnancy: T-ACE, TWEAK, and others, *Alcohol Health Res World* 18(1):55, 1994.

Russell M et al.: Detecting risk drinking during pregnancy: a comparison of four screening questionnaires, *Am J Public Health* 86(10):1435, 1996.

Ryan A et al.: Defects in insulin secretion and action in women with a history of gestational diabetes, *Diabetes* 44(5):506, 1995.

Schwartz R et al.: Hyperinsulinemia and macrosomia in the fetus of the diabetic mother, *Diabetes Care* 17(7):640, 1994.

Scott J & Branch D: Immunologic disorders. In Scott J et al., editors: *Danforth's obstetrics and gynecology,* ed 7, Philadelphia, 1994, JB Lippincott.

Silvermann B et al.: Impaired glucose tolerance in adolescent offspring of diabetic mothers, *Diabetes Care* 18(5):611, 1995.

Stuart G & Sundeen S: *Principles and practice of psychiatric nursing,* ed 6, St Louis, 1998, Mosby.

Varner M: General medical and surgical diseases in pregnancy. In Scott J et al., editors: *Danforth's obstetrics and gynecology,* ed 7, Philadelphia, 1994, JB Lippincott.

Willhoite M et al.: The impact of preconception counseling on pregnancy outcomes: the experience of the Maine Diabetes in Pregnancy Program, *Diabetes Care* 16(2):450, 1993.

Wong D & Perry S: *Maternal child nursing care,* St Louis, 1998, Mosby.

CHAPTER

24

Pregnancy at Risk: Gestational Conditions

KITTY CASHION

LEARNING OBJECTIVES

- Define the key terms.
- Describe the pathophysiology of preeclampsia and eclampsia.
- Differentiate the management of the woman with mild preeclampsia and the woman with severe preeclampsia.
- Identify the priorities for management of eclamptic seizures.
- Describe HELLP syndrome, including appropriate nursing actions.
- Explain the effects of hyperemesis gravidarum on maternal and fetal well-being.
- Discuss the management of the woman with hyperemesis gravidarum in the hospital and at home.
- Differentiate among causes, signs and symptoms, possible complications, and management of spontaneous abortion, ectopic pregnancy, incompetent cervix, and hydatidiform mole.
- Compare and contrast placenta previa and abruptio placentae in relation to signs and symptoms, complications, and management.
- Discuss the diagnosis and management of disseminated intravascular coagulation (DIC).
- Explain the basic principles of care for a pregnant woman undergoing abdominal surgery.
- Discuss implications of trauma on mother and fetus during pregnancy.
- Identify priorities in assessment and stabilization measures for the pregnant trauma victim.
- Differentiate signs and symptoms, effects on pregnancy and the fetus, and management during pregnancy of common STDs.
- Describe signs, symptoms, and management of pregnant woman with TORCH infections.

KEY TERMS

abortion
abruptio placentae
arteriolar vasospasm
cerclage
cervical funneling
chronic hypertension
clonus
Couvelaire uterus
deep tendon reflexes (DTRs)
disseminated intravascular coagulation (DIC)
eclampsia
ectopic pregnancy
edema
HELLP syndrome
hydatidiform mole (molar pregnancy)
hyperemesis gravidarum
hypertension
incompetent cervix
placenta previa
preeclampsia
pregnancy-induced hypertension (PIH)
proteinuria
succenturiate placenta
TORCH infections
transient hypertension
velamentous insertion of the cord

For most women pregnancy represents a normal part of life rather than an illness. There are, however, women who experience significant problems during the months of gestation that can greatly affect pregnancy outcome. Some of these conditions develop as a result of the pregnant state, while others are problems that could happen to anyone, at any time of life, but occur in this woman during pregnancy.

This chapter discusses a wide variety of disorders that did not exist before pregnancy, all of which have at least one thing in common: their occurrence in pregnancy puts the woman and fetus at risk. Hypertension in pregnancy, hyperemesis gravidarum, hemorrhagic complications of early and late pregnancy, surgery during pregnancy, trauma, and sexually transmitted diseases (STDs) are discussed.

HYPERTENSION IN PREGNANCY

Significance and Incidence

Hypertensive disorders are the most commonly occurring medical complications of pregnancy. They occur in 5% to 10% of all pregnancies, and the incidence varies among different hospitals, regions, and countries (Sibai, 1996). Hypertensive disease accounts for 15% of all maternal deaths in the United States (ACOG, 1996).

The term "hypertension in pregnancy" covers a wide range of disorders that can be generally divided into two groups: chronic hypertensive disorders and gestational hypertension or **pregnancy-induced hypertension (PIH).** Although all affected women may experience hypertension and proteinuria, these symptoms are caused by very different disease processes. Hypertension and proteinuria usually develop after 20 weeks of gestation in women with PIH, whereas these symptoms preexist pregnancy in women who have chronic hypertension, renal disease, or autoimmune diseases such as lupus erythematosus (Sibai, 1996).

Preeclampsia contributes to intrauterine fetal death and perinatal mortality. The main causes of neonatal death from preeclampsia are placental insufficiency and abruptio placentae. Iatrogenic preterm delivery, performed because of worsening maternal condition, is another important cause of perinatal morbidity and mortality (ACOG, 1996). Intrauterine growth restriction (IUGR) is also common among infants of preeclamptic women (Roberts, 1994).

Eclampsia (characterized by seizures) from profound cerebral effects of preeclampsia is the major maternal hazard. As a rule, maternal and perinatal morbidity and mortality are highest among cases in which eclampsia is seen early in gestation (before 28 weeks), maternal age is greater than 25 years, the woman is a multigravida, and chronic hypertension or renal disease is present. The fetus of the eclamptic woman is at increased risk from abruptio placentae, preterm birth, IUGR, and acute hypoxia (Gilbert & Harmon, 1998).

Classification

The hypertensive disorders of pregnancy encompass a variety of conditions featuring an elevation of maternal blood pressure with a corresponding risk to maternal and fetal well-being. Originally, hypertensive disorders of pregnancy were referred to as "toxemia"; this term is inappropriate, however, because no toxic agents or toxins have been identified. Confusion regarding classification continues today, causing difficulties in establishing a clinical diagnosis of the specific hypertensive disorder (ACOG, 1996; Scott, 1994a; Sibai, 1996). The two classification systems most commonly

TABLE 24-1	*Classification of Hypertensive States of Pregnancy*
TYPE	**DESCRIPTION**
GESTATIONAL HYPERTENSIVE DISORDERS: PREGNANCY-INDUCED HYPERTENSION (PIH)	
Transient hypertension	Development of mild hypertension during pregnancy in previously normotensive patient without proteinuria or pathologic edema
Gestational proteinuria	Development of proteinuria after 20 wks of gestation in previously nonproteinuric patient without hypertension
Preeclampsia	Development of hypertension and proteinuria in previously normotensive patient after 20 wks of gestation or in early postpartum period; in presence of trophoblastic disease it can develop before 20 wks of gestation
Eclampsia	Development of convulsions or coma in preeclamptic patient
CHRONIC HYPERTENSIVE DISORDERS	
Chronic hypertension	Hypertension and/or proteinuria in pregnant patient with chronic hypertension
Superimposed preeclampsia/eclampsia	Development of preeclampsia or eclampsia in patient with chronic hypertension

From: Gilbert E & Harmon J: *Manual of high risk pregnancy and delivery,* ed 2, St Louis, 1998, Mosby.

used in the United States today are based on reports from the American College of Obstetricians and Gynecologists (ACOG, 1996) and the Working Group on High Blood Pressure in Pregnancy (1990). These classification systems are summarized in Table 24-1.

Preeclampsia

Preeclampsia, a pregnancy-specific condition in which hypertension develops after 20 weeks of gestation in a previously normotensive woman, is a multisystem, vasospastic disease process characterized by hemoconcentration, hypertension, and proteinuria. The diagnosis of preeclampsia has traditionally been based on the presence of hypertension with proteinuria, pathologic edema, or both. Preeclampsia is usually categorized as mild or severe in terms of management (Table 24-2.)

TABLE 24-2 *Differentiation between Mild and Severe Preeclampsia*

	MILD PREECLAMPSIA	SEVERE PREECLAMPSIA
MATERNAL EFFECTS		
Blood pressure	Rise in systolic blood pressure ≥30 mm Hg; rise in diastolic blood pressure ≥15 mm Hg or reading of 140/90 mm Hg × 2, 6 hr apart	Rise to ≥160/110 mm Hg on two separate occasions 6 hr apart with pregnant woman on bed rest
Mean arterial pressure (MAP)	>105 mm/Hg or >20 mm Hg above baseline	>105 mm/Hg or >20 mm Hg above baseline
Weight gain	Weight gain of more than 0.5 kg/wk during the second and third trimesters or sudden weight gain of 2 kg/wk at any time.	Same as mild preeclampsia
Proteinuria —Qualitative dipstick —Quantitative 24-hr analysis	Proteinuria of 0.3 gm/L in a 24-hr specimen or >0.1 gm/L in a random daytime specimen of two or more occasions 6 hr apart (because protein loss is variable); with dipstick, values varying from 2+ to 3+	Proteinuria of >5 gm/L in 24 hr or >4+ protein on dipstick
Edema	Dependent edema, some puffiness of eyes, face, fingers; pulmonary edema absent	Generalized edema, noticeable puffiness; eyes, face, fingers; pulmonary edema possibly present
Reflexes	May be normal	Hyperreflexia ≥3+, possible ankle clonus
Urine output	Output matching intake, ≥30 ml/hr or <650 ml/24 hr	<20 ml/hr or <500 ml/24 hr
Headache	Absent/transient	Severe
Visual problems	Absent	Blurred, photophobia, blind spots on fundoscopy
Irritability/changes in affect	Transient	Severe
Epigastric pain	Absent	Present
Serum creatinine	Normal	Elevated
Thrombocytopenia	Absent	Present
AST elevation	Minimal	Marked
Hematocrit	Normal	Increased
FETAL EFFECTS		
Placental perfusion	Reduced	Decreased perfusion expressing as IUGR in fetus, FHR: late decelerations
Premature placental aging	Not apparent	At birth placenta appearing smaller than normal for duration of pregnancy, premature aging apparent with numerous areas of broken syncytia, ischemic necroses (white infarcts) numerous, intervillous fibrin deposition (red infarcts)

AST, Aspartate aminotransferase; *FHR,* fetal heart rate.

An elevated blood pressure is often the first sign of preeclampsia to develop. **Hypertension** is defined as a blood pressure greater than or equal to 140/90 mm Hg. When first trimester blood pressures are known, they serve as the woman's baseline values. With this information, an alternative definition for hypertension is a rise in systolic blood pressure of greater than or equal to 30 mm Hg or a greater than or equal to 15 mm Hg diastolic increase above the woman's baseline values (Working Group on High Blood Pressure in Pregnancy, 1990). ACOG's Committee on Terminology has also defined hypertension as an increase in mean arterial pressure (MAP) of 20 mm Hg; if previous blood pressures are unknown, a MAP of 105 mm Hg is considered definitive of

hypertension (see Box 9-2). The blood pressure elevation must be present on two occasions at least 4 to 6 hours apart (Fairlie & Sibai, 1992). One of the difficulties in diagnosing hypertension has been a lack of standardization in blood pressure measurement. The accompanying Protocol box presents recommendations for standardizing this procedure.

Proteinuria is defined as a concentration of 0.1 gm/L (1+ to 2+ on dipstick measurement) or more in at least two random urine specimens collected at least 6 hours apart. In a 24-hour specimen, proteinuria is defined as a concentration of 0.3 gm/L per 24 hours.

Pathologic **edema** is clinically evident, generalized accumulation of fluid of the face, hands, and/or abdomen that

PROTOCOL *Blood Pressure Measurement*

1. Measure blood pressure with the woman seated (ambulatory) or in a 30-degree tilt on her left side.
2. After positioning, allow the woman at least 5 minutes of quiet rest before blood pressure measurement, to encourage relaxation.
3. Use the right arm for blood pressure measurement.
4. Hold the arm in a roughly horizontal position at heart level.
5. Use the proper-sized cuff (cuff should cover approximately 80% of the upper arm).
6. Maintain a slow, steady deflation rate.
7. Take the average of two readings at least 6 hours apart to minimize recorded blood pressure variations across time.
8. Use Korotkoff phase V (disappearance of sound) for recording the diastolic value (some sources recommend recording both phase IV [the muffled sound] and phase V).
9. Use accurate equipment.
10. If interchanging manual and electronic devices, use caution in interpreting different blood pressure values.

is not responsive to 12 hours of bed rest. It may also be manifested as a rapid weight gain of more than 2 kg in 1 week.

Eclampsia

Eclampsia is the occurrence of seizures or coma in a patient with preeclampsia that cannot be attributed to other causes. Approximately half of all cases of eclampsia occur before labor begins, with the other half equally divided between the intrapartum and postpartum periods.

Chronic hypertension

Chronic hypertension is defined as hypertension present before the pregnancy or diagnosed before the twentieth week of gestation. Hypertension that persists longer than 6 weeks postpartum is also classified as chronic hypertension.

Chronic hypertension with superimposed preeclampsia

Women with chronic hypertension may acquire preeclampsia or eclampsia. Superimposed preeclampsia is defined as an increase in blood pressure (30 mm Hg systolic or 15 mm Hg diastolic or 20 mm Hg MAP) along with proteinuria or generalized edema in women with chronic hypertension (Sibai, 1996).

Transient hypertension

Transient hypertension is the development of hypertension during pregnancy or the first 24 hours postpartum without other signs of preeclampsia or preexisting hypertension. Blood pressure must return to normal levels by the tenth postpartum day (Sibai, 1996). The presence of transient hypertension may be predictive of the eventual development of essential hypertension.

Etiology

Causes of hypertension in pregnancy are multiple and have been the subject of extensive research and much speculation. The ultimate cause remains unknown. Preeclampsia is a condition unique to human pregnancy; signs and symptoms usually develop only during pregnancy and disappear

---

BOX 24-1　　**Risk Factors Associated with the Development of Pregnancy-Induced Hypertension**

Chronic renal disease
Chronic hypertension
Family history of PIH
Twin gestation
Primigravidity
Maternal age <19 years; >40 years
Diabetes
Rh incompatibility

Data from American College of Obstetricians and Gynecologists: Hypertension in pregnancy, *Technical Bulletin* 219, Washington DC, 1996, ACOG; Gilbert E & Harmon J: *Manual of high risk pregnancy and delivery*, ed 2, St Louis, 1998, Mosby; and Roberts J: Current perspectives on preeclampsia, *J Nurse Midwifery* 39(2):70, 1994.

---

quickly after birth of the fetus and passage of placenta. No single patient profile identifies the woman who will have preeclampsia. Box 24-1 lists factors associated with increased incidence of PIH.

Several major concepts that contribute to current theories regarding the etiology of PIH are increased vasoconstrictor tone (Gilstrap & Gant, 1990; Scott 1994a), abnormal prostaglandin action (Friedman, 1988), and endothelial cell activation (Creasy & Resnik, 1994; Tsukimori et al., 1992). Immunologic factors may play an important role (Sibai, 1991a).

In part, vasospasms are the underlying mechanism for the signs and symptoms present with preeclampsia. Vasospasms result from an increased sensitivity to circulating pressors, such as angiotensin II, and possibly an imbalance between the prostaglandins, prostacyclin and thromboxane A$_2$ (Cunningham & Lindheimer, 1992; Magness & Gant, 1994; Working Group on High Blood Pressure in Pregnancy, 1990).

Endothelial cell dysfunction, believed to result from decreased placental perfusion, may account for many preeclampsia changes, as depicted in Fig. 24-1. In addition

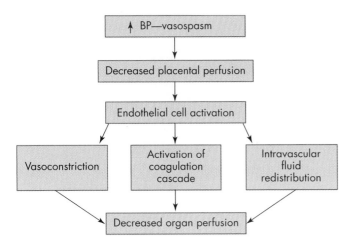

Fig. 24-1 Etiology of PIH. Endothelial cell dysfunction and preeclampsia.

to endothelial damage, arteriolar vasospasm may contribute to an increased capillary permeability. This increases edema and further decreases intravascular volume, predisposing the woman with preeclampsia to pulmonary edema (Dildy et al., 1991).

Immunologic factors may play an important role in the development of preeclampsia. The presence of foreign protein, the placenta, or the fetus may trigger an adverse immunologic response. This theory is supported by the increased incidence of preeclampsia or eclampsia in first-time mothers (first exposure to fetal tissue) and women pregnant by a new partner (different genetic material) and increased incidence among daughters and granddaughters of women with a history of eclampsia (Sibai, 1991a).

Pathophysiology

The pathophysiology of preeclampsia or eclampsia is somehow related to the physiologic changes of pregnancy. Normal physiologic adaptations to pregnancy include increased blood plasma volume, vasodilation, decreased systemic vascular resistance, elevated cardiac output, and decreased colloid osmotic pressure (Box 24-2).

Preeclampsia is quite different from chronic hypertension. Pathologic changes in the endothelial cells of the glomeruli (glomeruloendotheliosis) are uniquely characteristic of preeclampsia, particularly in nulliparous women (85%). The main pathogenic factor is not an increase in blood pressure but poor perfusion as a result of vasospasm. **Arteriolar vasospasm** diminishes the diameter of blood vessels, which impedes blood flow to all organs and raises blood pressure (Working Group on High Blood Pressure in Pregnancy, 1990). Function in organs such as the placenta, kidneys, liver, and brain is depressed by as much as 40% to 60%. The pathophysiologic sequelae are shown in Fig. 24-2.

Impaired placental perfusion leads to early degenerative aging of the placenta and possible IUGR of the fetus. Reduced kidney perfusion decreases the glomerular filtration rate and leads to degenerative glomerular changes and oliguria. Protein, primarily albumin, is lost in the urine. Uric acid clearance is decreased; however, blood urea nitrogen, serum creatinine, and serum uric acid levels increase (Dildy et al., 1991). Sodium and water are retained. Plasma colloid osmotic pressure decreases as serum albumin levels decrease. Intravascular volume is reduced as fluid moves out of the intravascular compartment, resulting in hemoconcentration, increased blood viscosity, and tissue edema. The hematocrit value increases as fluid leaves the intravascular space (Cunningham et al., 1997). The hematocrit value therefore rises as the condition worsens; a drop in hematocrit value (to normal levels) accompanies improvement of the condition. In severe preeclampsia, blood volume may fall to or below nonpregnancy levels; severe edema develops and rapid weight gain is seen (Scott, 1994a).

Decreased liver perfusion causes impaired function. Hepatic edema and subcapsular hemorrhage, felt by the pregnant woman as epigastric or right upper quadrant pain, is one sign of impending eclampsia (convulsion). Liver enzyme levels (e.g., aspartate aminotransferase [AST]) rise in the wake of liver damage.

Arteriolar vasospasms and decreased blood flow to the retina lead to visual symptoms such as scotoma (blind spots)

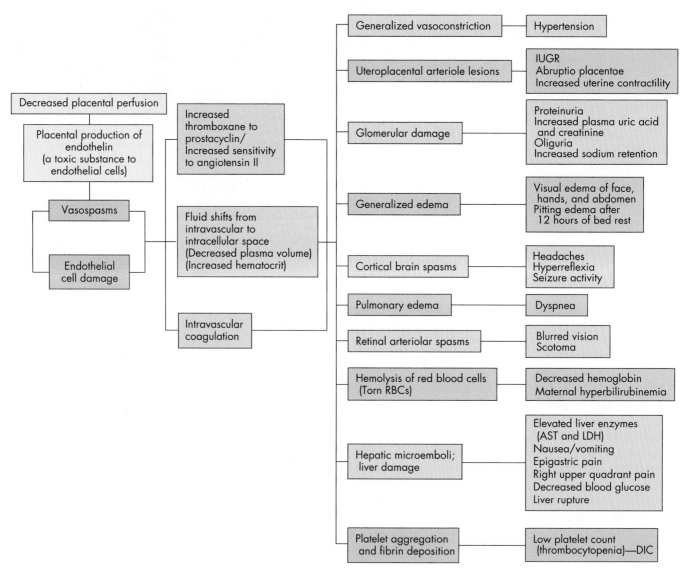

Fig. 24-2 Pathophysiology of PIH. Modified from Gilbert E & Harmon J: *Manual of high risk pregnancy and delivery,* ed 2, St Louis, 1998, Mosby.)

and blurring. The same pathologic condition leads to cerebral edema and hemorrhages, as well as to increased central nervous system (CNS) irritability (Dildy et al., 1991). CNS irritability manifests as headache, hyperreflexia, positive ankle clonus, and occasionally the development of eclampsia. Changes in affect (changes in emotion, mood, and consciousness) are typical symptoms of cerebral edema (Scott, 1994a).

If the hypertension is difficult to bring under control, cardiac and pulmonary complications can occur. Heart failure, a common cause of maternal death attributed to preeclampsia, is rare among young, otherwise healthy women (Scott, 1994a). Sudden circulatory collapse and shock may occur in women with a history of repeated hypertensive pregnancies.

HELLP Syndrome

HELLP syndrome (*H*, hemolysis; *EL*, elevated liver enzymes; *LP*, low platelet count) is a variant of severe preeclampsia that has been reported in 2% to 12% of pregnancies complicated by preeclampsia (Sibai, 1996). Arteriolar vasospasm, endothelial damage, and platelet aggregation with resultant tissue hypoxia are the underlying mechanisms for the pathophysiology of HELLP syndrome (Poole, 1993).

Most commonly, HELLP syndrome is seen in white, multigravid women. About 90% of patients report a history of malaise for several days. Many women (65%) experience epigastric or right upper quadrant abdominal pain (possibly related to hepatic ischemia), and approximately half develop nausea and vomiting. It is extremely important to understand

TABLE 24-3 *Common Laboratory Changes in Preeclampsia*

	NORMAL	PIH	HELLP
Hemoglobin/hematocrit	12 to 16 gm/dl 37% to 47%	May ↑	↓
Platelets	150,000 to 400,000/mm³	Unchanged	<100,000/mm³
PT/PTT	12 to 14 sec/60 to 70 sec	Unchanged	Unchanged
Fibrinogen	150 to 400 mg/dl	300 to 600 mg/dl	↓
Fibrin split products (FSP)	Absent	Absent	Present
Blood urea nitrogen (BUN)	10 to 20 mg/dl	<10 mg/dl	↑
Creatinine	0.5 to 1.1 mg/dl	<1 mg/dl	↑
Lactate dehydrogenase (LDH)	45 to 90 U/L	Unchanged	↑
Aspartate aminotransferase (AST) (formerly SGOT)	4 to 20 U/L	Unchanged	↑
Alanine aminotransferase (ALT) (formerly SGPT)	3 to 21 U/L	Unchanged	↑
Creatinine clearance	80 to 125 ml/min	130 to 180 ml/min	↓
Burr cells/schistocytes	Absent	Absent	Present
Uric acid	2 to 6.6 mg/dl	4.5 to 6 mg/dl	>10 mg/dl
Bilirubin (Total)	0.1 to 1 mg/dl	Unchanged or ↑	↑

that many patients with HELLP syndrome may present without signs or symptoms of severe preeclampsia. For example, many of these women are normotensive or have only slight elevations in blood pressure. Proteinuria also may be absent. As a result, women with HELLP syndrome are often misdiagnosed with a variety of other medical or surgical disorders (Sibai, 1996).

HELLP syndrome is a laboratory, not a clinical, diagnosis. In order to make a diagnosis of HELLP syndrome, a woman's platelet count must be less than 100,000/mm³, her liver enzyme levels (aspartate aminotransferase [AST] and alanine aminotransferase [ALT]) must be elevated, and there must be some evidence of intravascular hemolysis (burr cells on peripheral smear or elevated bilirubin level). A unique form of coagulopathy (not DIC) occurs with HELLP syndrome. While the platelet count is low, coagulation factor assays, prothrombin time (PT), partial thromboplastin time (PTT), and bleeding time, remain normal (Leduc et al., 1992; Perry & Martin, 1992).

Recognition of the clinical and laboratory findings associated with HELLP syndrome is important if early, aggressive therapy is to be initiated to prevent maternal and neonatal mortality (Sibai, 1992). Maternal mortality as high as 24% has been reported, while perinatal mortality has ranged from about 8% to 60%. Complications reported with HELLP syndrome include renal failure, pulmonary edema, ruptured liver hematoma, DIC, and placental abruption (Sibai, 1996). Common laboratory findings in preeclampsia are listed in Table 24-3.

CARE MANAGEMENT

Assessment and Nursing Diagnoses

Hypertensive disorders of pregnancy can occur without warning or with the gradual development of symptoms. Because currently the cause is unknown and proven methods to prevent the illness are nonexistent, a key goal is early detection of the disease to prevent the catastrophic maternal and fetal sequelae that can occur. One strategy to meet this goal is the identification of high-risk individuals at the initial prenatal visit (see Box 24-1). During each subsequent visit the woman is assessed for signs or symptoms that suggest the onset or presence of preeclampsia.

Interview

In both inpatient and outpatient settings, the nurse begins the assessment process by completing and/or reviewing the woman's medical record. Personal medical history is reviewed, especially the presence of diabetes mellitus, renal disease, and hypertension. Family history is explored for occurrence of preeclamptic or hypertensive conditions, diabetes mellitus, and other chronic conditions. The social and experiential history provides information about the woman's marital status, nutritional status, cultural beliefs, activity level, and health habits such as smoking, alcohol, and illicit drug consumption.

A review of systems adds to the database for detecting blood pressure changes from baseline, abnormal weight gain and pattern of weight gain, increased signs of edema, and presence of proteinuria. Noting whether the woman is having unusual, frequent, or severe headaches; visual disturbances; or epigastric pain is also important.

Physical examination

Accurate and consistent blood pressure assessment is important for establishing a baseline and monitoring subtle changes throughout pregnancy. Many variables can influence blood pressure measurements, such as position, cuff size, arm used, and emotional state of the patient. Personnel caring for pregnant women need to be consistent in taking and recording blood pressure measurements in the standardized manner (see Protocol box, p. 646).

Observation of edema in addition to hypertension warrants additional investigation. Edema is assessed for distribution, degree, and pitting. If periorbital or facial edema is not obvious, the pregnant woman is asked whether it was present when she awoke. Edema may be described as dependent or pitting.

Dependent edema is edema of the lowest or most dependent parts of the body, where hydrostatic pressure is greatest. If a pregnant woman is ambulatory, this edema may first be evident in the feet and ankles. If the pregnant woman is confined to bed, the edema is more likely to occur in the sacral region.

Pitting edema is edema that leaves a small depression or pit after finger pressure is applied to the swollen area. The pit, which is caused by movement of fluid to adjacent tissue away from the point of pressure, normally disappears within 10 to 30 seconds. Although the amount of edema is difficult to quantitate, the method described in Fig. 24-3 may be used to record relative degrees of edema formation in the lower extremities.

Symptoms reflecting CNS and visual system involvement usually accompany facial edema. Although it is not a routine assessment during the prenatal period, evaluation of the fundus of the eye yields valuable data. An initial baseline finding of normal eye grounds assists in differentiating preexisting disease from a new disease process.

Deep tendon reflexes (DTRs) are evaluated if preeclampsia is suspected. The biceps and patellar reflexes and ankle clonus are assessed and the findings recorded (Fig. 24-4). The evaluation of DTRs is especially important if the woman is being treated with magnesium sulfate; absence of DTRs is an early indication of impending magnesium toxicity. To elicit the biceps reflex, the examiner strikes a downward blow over the thumb, which is situated over the biceps tendon. Normal response is flexion of the arm at the elbow, described as a 2+ response (Table 24-4). The patellar reflex is elicited with the woman's legs hanging freely over the end of the examining table or with the woman lying on her left side with the knee slightly flexed. A blow with a percussion hammer is dealt directly to the patellar

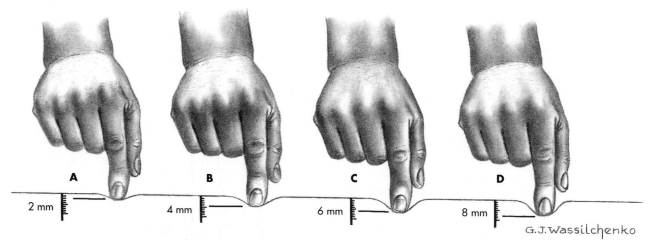

Fig. **24-3** Assessment of pitting edema of lower extremities: **A,** +1; **B,** +2; **C,** +3; **D,** +4.

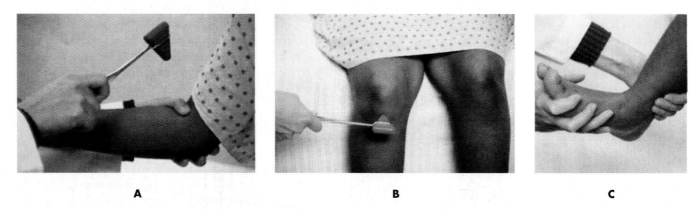

Fig. **24-4 A,** Biceps reflex; **B,** patellar reflex with patient's legs hanging freely over end of examining table; **C,** test for ankle clonus. (Seidel H et al.: *Mosby's guide to physical examination,* ed 4, St Louis, 1999, Mosby.)

tendon, inferior to the patella. Normal response is the extension or kicking out of the leg. To assess for hyperactive reflexes **(clonus)** at the ankle joint, the examiner supports the leg with the knee flexed. With one hand, the examiner sharply dorsiflexes the foot, maintains the position for a moment, and then releases the foot. Normal (*negative clonus*) response is elicited when no rhythmic oscillations (jerks) are felt while the foot is held in dorsiflexion. When the foot is released, no oscillations are seen as foot drops to the plantar flexed position. Abnormal (positive clonus) response is recognized by rhythmic oscillations of one or more "beats" felt when the foot is in dorsiflexion and seen as the foot drops to the plantar flexed position.

An important assessment is determination of fetal status. Uteroplacental perfusion is decreased in women with preeclampsia, placing the fetus in jeopardy. The fetal heart rate (FHR) is assessed for baseline rate and variability and accelerations, which indicate an intact, oxygenated fetal CNS. Abnormal baseline rate, decreased or absent variability, and late decelerations are indications of fetal intolerance to the intrauterine environment. Biophysical or biochemical monitoring such as nonstress testing, contraction stress testing, biophysical profile, and serial ultrasonography are all used to assess fetal status.

Doppler flow velocimetry studies also may be used to evaluate maternal and fetal well-being (see Chapter 22). Uteroplacental perfusion is assessed by measuring the velocity of blood flow through the uterine artery, umbilical artery, or both. A systolic/diastolic ratio greater than 3 after 26 weeks of gestation is considered abnormal, and ratios of 3.8

TABLE 24-4	*Assessing Deep Tendon Reflexes*
GRADE	**DEEP TENDON REFLEX RESPONSE**
0	No response
1+	Sluggish or diminished
2+	Active or expected response
3+	More brisk than expected, slightly hyperactive
4+	Brisk, hyperactive, with intermittent or transient clonus

From Seidel H et al.: *Mosby's guide to physical examination,* ed 4, St Louis, 1999, Mosby.

have been associated with preeclampsia (Fairlie, 1991; Farmakides et al., 1992).

Uterine tonicity is evaluated for signs of labor and abruptio placentae. If labor is suspected, a vaginal examination for cervical changes is indicated.

During the physical examination, the pregnant woman is examined for signs of progression of mild preeclampsia to severe preeclampsia or eclampsia. Signs of worsening liver involvement, renal failure, worsening hypertension, cerebral involvement, and developing coagulopathies must be assessed and documented. Respirations are assessed for crackles or diminished breath sounds, which may indicate pulmonary edema. (Warning signs of preeclampsia and the differentiation of mild from severe preeclampsia are summarized in Table 24-2.) Eclampsia is usually preceded by various premonitory symptoms and signs, including headache, severe epigastric pain, hyperreflexia, and hemoconcentration. However, convulsions can appear suddenly and without warning in a woman in seemingly stable condition who has only minimum blood pressure elevation (Sibai, 1996).

The convulsions that occur in eclampsia are frightening to observe. Increased hypertension and tonic contraction of all body muscles (seen as arms flexed, hands clenched, legs inverted) precede the tonic-clonic convulsions (Fig. 24-5). During this stage, muscles alternatively relax and contract. Respirations are halted and then begin again with long, deep, stertorous inhalation. Hypotension follows, and coma ensues. Nystagmus and muscular twitching persist for a time. Disorientation and amnesia cloud the immediate recovery. Oliguria and anuria are notable. Seizures may recur within minutes of the first convulsion, or the woman may never have another. Eclamptic seizures can result in tissue damage to the mother during the convulsion, especially if she is in a bed with unpadded side rails. During the convulsion the mother and fetus are not receiving oxygen, so eclamptic seizures produce a marked metabolic insult to both mother and fetus.

Laboratory tests

The nurse assists in obtaining a number of blood and urine specimens to aid in the diagnosis and treatment of preeclampsia, HELLP syndrome, and chronic hypertension. Baseline laboratory test information is useful in cases of

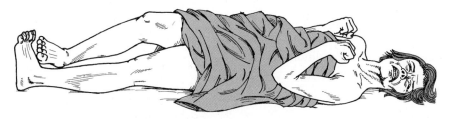

Fig. **24-5** Eclampsia (convulsions or seizures).

early diagnosis of preeclampsia because it can be compared with later results to evaluate progression and severity of disease (see Table 24-3). An initial blood specimen is obtained for the following tests to assess the disease process and its effect on renal and hepatic functioning:

- Complete blood cell count (including a platelet count)
- Clotting studies (including bleeding time, PT, PTT, and fibrinogen)
- Liver enzymes (lactate dehydrogenase [LDH], AST, ALT)
- Chemistry panel (blood urea nitrogen, creatinine, glucose, uric acid)
- Type and screen, possible crossmatch

The hematocrit, hemoglobin, and platelet levels are monitored closely for changes indicating a worsening of patient status.

Proteinuria is determined from dipstick testing of a clean-catch or catheterized urine specimen. A reading of 2+ on two or more occasions at least 6 hours apart should be followed by a 24-hour urine collection (Gilbert & Harmon, 1998). A 24-hour collection for protein and creatinine clearance is more reflective of true renal status. Proteinuria is usually a late sign in the course of preeclampsia (Working Group on High Blood Pressure in Pregnancy, 1990). Protein readings are designated as follows:

0	Negative
Trace	Trace
+1	30 mg/dl (equivalent to 300 mg/L)
+2	100 mg/dl
+3	300 mg/dl
+4	>1,000 mg (1 gm)/dl

Urine output is assessed for volume of at least 30 ml/hr or 120 ml/4 hr.

Nursing Diagnoses for the woman with hypertensive disorders in pregnancy are listed in the accompanying box.

❙ Nursing Diagnoses

Woman Experiencing a Hypertensive Disorder in Pregnancy

Anxiety related to:
- Preeclampsia and its effect on woman and infant

Knowledge deficit related to:
- Management (diet, medications, activity restrictions)

Ineffective individual/family coping related to:
- Woman's restricted activity and concern over a complicated pregnancy
- Woman's inability to work outside the home

Powerlessness related to:
- Inability to prevent or control condition and outcomes

Altered tissue perfusion related to:
- Hypertension
- Cyclic vasospasms

- Cerebral edema
- Hemorrhage

Risk for impaired gas exchange related to:
- Magnesium sulfate therapy
- Pulmonary edema

Risk for injury to fetus related to:
- Uteroplacental insufficiency
- Preterm birth
- Abruptio placentae
- Adverse effects of maternal medications

Risk for injury to mother related to:
- CNS irritability secondary to cerebral edema, vasospasm, decreased renal perfusion
- Magnesium sulfate and antihypertensive therapies
- Abruptio placentae

Expected Outcomes of Care

Expected outcomes for care of women with hypertensive disorders of pregnancy include that the woman will do the following:
- Recognize and immediately report signs and symptoms indicative of worsening condition
- Adhere to the medical regimen to minimize risk to herself and her fetus
- Identify and use available support systems
- Verbalize her fears and concerns to cope with the condition and situation
- Develop no signs of eclampsia and its complications
- Give birth to healthy infant.
- Develop no sequelae to her condition or its management

Plan of Care and Interventions

Preeclampsia

The only definitive cure for preeclampsia is delivery. The goals of therapy are first, to assure maternal safety, and next, to deliver a healthy newborn as close to term as possible, who will not require prolonged intensive care (Sibai, 1996). At or near term, the plan of care for a woman with preeclampsia is most likely to be induction of labor, preceded, if necessary, by cervical ripening.

When preeclampsia is diagnosed in a woman who is less than 37 weeks of gestation, however, immediate delivery may not be in the best interest of the fetus. In this situation, the initial intervention is usually a thorough evaluation of both the maternal and fetal condition. Women may be hospitalized during this initial evaluation or the evaluation may be done in a high-risk clinic or the physician's office. A multidisciplinary plan of care is then developed, based on the assessment findings. Whenever possible, the plan should take into account the wishes of the woman and her family.

HOME CARE *Patient Instructions for Self-Care*

Assessing and Reporting Clinical Signs of Preeclampsia

Report immediately any increase in your blood pressure, protein in urine, weight gain greater than 1 lb/wk, or edema.

Take your blood pressure on the same arm in a sitting position each time for consistent and accurate readings. Support arm on a table in a horizontal position at heart level.

Use the same scale, wearing the same clothes, at the same time each day, after voiding, before breakfast, for reliable daily weights.

Dipstick test your clean-catch urine sample to assess proteinuria; report frequency or burning on urination.

Report to your health care provider if proteinuria is +2 or more or if you have a decrease in urine output.

Assess your baby's activity daily. Decreased activity (three or fewer movements per hour) may indicate fetal distress.

It is important to keep your scheduled prenatal appointments so that any changes in your or your baby's condition can be detected immediately.

Keep a daily log or diary of your assessments for your home health care nurse, or bring it with you to your next prenatal visit.

Emotional and psychologic support are essential in assisting the woman and her family to cope. Their perception of the disease process, the reasons for it, and the care received will affect their compliance with and participation in therapy. The family needs to use coping mechanisms and support systems to help them through this crisis. It is also important to remember that, although this woman has a high-risk condition, she is first of all having a baby. A plan of care specifically designed for the woman with preeclampsia must be superimposed on the nursing care all women need during labor and the birth process.

Mild preeclampsia and home care

If the woman has mild preeclampsia (blood pressure is stable, urine protein is <500 mg in a 24-hour collection, and no subjective complaints), she may be managed expectantly, usually at home. The maternal-fetal condition needs to be assessed two to three times per week. Many agencies are available to provide this assessment in the home. Arrangements for this service may be made, depending upon the woman's insurance coverage. If home nursing care is not possible, the woman may be asked to perform self-assessment daily, including weight, urine dipstick protein determinations, blood pressure measurement, and fetal movement counting. In addition, she will be asked to immediately report the development of any

subjective symptoms (see Home Care box at left). In this case, she will likely return to the physician's office or high-risk clinic at least twice each week for continued fetal assessment.

The fetal condition is also closely monitored because the only reason for expectant management of preeclampsia is to allow additional time for fetal growth and maturation. An ultrasound for evaluation of fetal growth should be obtained every 3 weeks. Fetal movement is counted daily. Other fetal assessment tests include a nonstress test once or twice a week and a biophysical profile as needed. Fetal jeopardy as evidenced by inappropriate growth or abnormal testing necessitates immediate delivery (Sibai, 1996).

Activity restriction. Bed rest in the lateral recumbent position is a standard therapy for preeclampsia and maximizes uteroplacental blood flow during pregnancy. However, bed rest recommendations for all high-risk pregnant women are becoming more controversial. Maloni (1994) documented adverse physiologic outcomes related to complete bed rest, including cardiovascular deconditioning; diuresis with accompanying fluid, electrolyte, and weight loss; muscle atrophy; and psychologic stress. These changes begin on the first day of bed rest and continue for the duration of therapy. Sibai (1996) recommends rest at home, rather than strict bed rest, and allows patients hospitalized with mild preeclampsia to be out of bed.

Bed rest has been shown to be beneficial in decreasing blood pressure and promoting diuresis. Women with mild preeclampsia feel reasonably well; boredom from the restriction is therefore common. Diversionary activities, visits from friends, telephone conversations, and creation of a comfortable and convenient environment are just a few ways of coping with this boredom (see the Home Care box on next page). Gentle exercise (e.g., range of motion, stretching, Kegel, pelvic tilts) is important in maintaining muscle tone, blood flow, regularity of bowel function, and a sense of well-being (Grohar, 1994; Maloni, 1998).

Relaxation techniques can help reduce the stress associated with the high-risk condition and prepare the woman for labor and birth.

Diet. Diet and fluid recommendations are much the same as for healthy pregnant women. The efficacy of a high-protein diet, avoidance of foods high in sodium, and forgoing additional salt at the table have not been proven (Fairlie & Sibai, 1992). Therefore, Sibai (1996) now recommends a regular diet with no salt restriction. Because pregnant women with hypertension have a lower plasma volume than do normotensive women, sodium restriction is not necessary. Women need salt for maintenance of blood volume and placental perfusion. The exception may be the woman with chronic hypertension that was successfully controlled with a low-salt diet before the pregnancy. Adequate fluid intake helps maintain optimum fluid volume and aids in

HOME CARE *Patient Instructions for Self-Care*

Coping with Bed Rest

In bed, lie on your side. This allows more blood to get to your uterus (womb) and baby. The bed or sofa should be near a window and a bathroom.

Increase your fluid intake to 8 glasses/day and add roughage (bran, fruits, leafy vegetables) to your diet to decrease constipation. Keep a bowl of fruit and a large container full of water close by.

Include diversionary activities, such as puzzles, reading, and crafts, to reduce boredom. Place a box or table within reach to store magazines, books, telephone, etc.

Do gentle exercises, such as circling your hands and feet or gently tensing and relaxing arm and leg muscles. This improves muscle tone, circulation, and sense of well-being.

Encourage family participation in your care.

Have significant others assist you with care of the house, children, etc.

Use relaxation to help cope with stress. Relax your body one muscle at a time, or imagine some pleasant scene, word, or image. Soothing music can also help you relax.

HOME CARE *Patient Instructions for Self-Care*

Nutrition

Eat a nutritious, balanced diet (60 to 70 gm protein, 1,200 mg calcium, and adequate zinc, magnesium, and vitamins). Consult with registered dietitian on the diet best suited for you as an individual.

There is no sodium restriction; however, consider limiting excessively salty foods (luncheon meats, pretzels, potato chips, pickles, sauerkraut).

Eat foods with roughage (whole grains, raw fruits, and vegetables).

Drink 6 to 8 8-oz glasses of water per day.

Avoid alcohol.

renal perfusion and filtration. The nurse uses assessment data regarding the woman's diet to counsel her as needed in areas of deficiency (Home Care box at right).

Successful home care requires the woman to be well educated about preeclampsia and motivated to follow the plan of care. She must also be reliable about keeping appointments. For home care to be effective, the home environment must be assessed and the woman's ability to assume responsibility determined. In addition, the effects of illness, language, age, culture, beliefs, and support systems must be considered. The woman's support systems must be mobilized and involved in planning and implementing her care (see Plan of Care).

Severe Preeclampsia and HELLP Syndrome

If the woman's condition worsens or she already has severe preeclampsia or HELLP syndrome and is critically ill, she should receive appropriate management (usually in a tertiary care center), ranging from immediate birth to conservative management of the pregnancy (Harvey & Burke, 1992; Sibai, 1991b). Recognition of the clinical and laboratory findings of severe preeclampsia or HELLP syndrome is important if early, aggressive therapy is to be initiated to prevent maternal and perinatal mortality. An unfavorable (uneffaced and undilated) cervix, resulting from the gestational age and the aggressive nature of this disorder, support cesarean birth. Prolonged induction of labor could increase maternal morbidity.

Important components of management include the administration of magnesium sulfate as prophylaxis against seizures and an antihypertensive agent if diastolic blood pressure is higher than 100 to 110 mm Hg.

Hospital care. The woman with severe preeclampsia or HELLP syndrome has multiple problems and provides a complex challenge for the health care team. Nursing care must focus on both mother and fetus.

Antepartum care focuses on stabilization and preparation for birth. The woman may be admitted to an antepartum or a labor and delivery unit, depending on the hospital. If the woman's condition is severe, she may be placed in an obstetric critical care unit or medical intensive care unit (if an obstetric critical care unit is not available) for any necessary hemodynamic monitoring. Maternal and fetal surveillance, patient education regarding the disease process, and supportive measures directed toward the woman and her family are initiated. Assessments include review of the cardiovascular system, pulmonary system, renal system, hematologic system, and CNS. Fetal assessments for well-being (e.g., nonstress test, biophysical profile, Doppler velocimetry) are important because of the potential for hypoxia related to uteroplacental insufficiency. Baseline laboratory assessments include metabolic studies for liver enzyme (AST, ALT, LDH) determination, complete blood count with platelets, coagulation profile to assess for DIC, and electrolyte studies to establish renal functioning (Farmakides et al., 1990).

Weight is measured on admission and every day thereafter. An indwelling urinary catheter facilitates monitoring of renal function and effectiveness of therapy. If appropriate, vaginal examination may be done to check for cervical changes. Abdominal palpation establishes uterine tonicity and fetal size, activity, and position. Electronic monitoring to determine fetal status is initiated at least once a day. The nurse's skill in implementing the techniques described here can be reassuring to the woman and her family. The woman's room must be close to staff and emergency drugs, supplies, and equipment. Noise and external stimuli must be minimized. Seizure precautions are taken (Box 24-3).

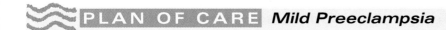

PLAN OF CARE *Mild Preeclampsia*

Home Care

> **NURSING DIAGNOSIS** Risk for injury related to signs of preeclampsia

Expected Outcomes *Patient will demonstrate ability to assess self and fetus for signs of worsening preeclampsia; no adverse sequelae will occur as result of preeclamptic condition.*

Nursing Interventions/*Rationales*

Review warning signs/symptoms of preeclampsia *to ensure adequate knowledge base exists for decision making.*

Assess home environment, including woman's ability to assume self-care responsibilities, support systems, language, age, culture, beliefs, and effects of illness, *to determine if home care is viable option.*

Teach woman how to do a self-assessment for clinical signs of preeclampsia (take and record blood pressure, measure urine protein, maintain daily weight log, assess edema formation, assess fetal activity) *to provide immediate evidence of a worsening condition.*

Teach woman to report any increases in blood pressure, +2 proteinuria, weight gain greater than 1 lb per week, presence of edema, and decreased fetal activity to her health care provider immediately *to prevent worsening of preeclamptic condition.*

Teach woman about use of bed rest, relaxation, and diet as palliative treatment options *to decrease blood pressure and promote diuresis.*

> **NURSING DIAGNOSIS** Fear/anxiety related to preeclampsia and its effect on the fetus

Expected Outcome *Patient's feelings and symptoms of fear/anxiety will decrease/ease.*

Nursing Interventions/*Rationales*

Provide a calm, soothing atmosphere and teach family to provide emotional support *to facilitate coping.*

Encourage verbalization of fears *to decrease intensity of emotional response.*

Involve woman and family in the management of her preeclamptic condition *to promote a greater sense of control.*

Help woman identify and use appropriate coping strategies and support systems *to reduce fear/anxiety.*

Explore use of desensitization strategies such as progressive muscle relaxation, visual imagery, or thought stopping *to reduce fear-related emotions and related physical symptoms.*

> **NURSING DIAGNOSIS** Diversional activity deficit related to imposed bed rest.

Expected Outcome *Patient will verbalize diminished feelings of boredom.*

Nursing Interventions/*Rationales*

Assist woman to explore creatively personally meaningful activities that can be pursued from the bed *to ensure activities that have meaning, purpose, and value to the individual.*

Maintain emphasis on personal choices of woman *to promote control and minimize imposition of routines by others.*

Evaluate what support and system resources are available in the environment *to assist in providing diversional activities.*

Explore ways for woman to remain an active participant in home management and decision making *to promote control.*

Engage support of family and friends in carrying out chosen activities and making necessary environmental alterations *to ensure success.*

Teach woman about stress management and relaxation techniques *to help manage tension of confinement.*

From Wong D & Perry S: *Maternal child nursing care,* St Louis, 1998, Mosby.

Bed rest is commonly ordered. The nurse's ingenuity may be called on to help the woman cope physically and psychologically with the side effects of immobility and an environment limited in stimuli and support. Thromboembolic events, a risk factor during normal pregnancy, pose an even greater risk with preeclampsia (see Plan of Care on next page).

Intrapartum nursing care of the woman with severe preeclampsia or HELLP syndrome involves continuous monitoring of maternal and fetal status as labor progresses. The assessment and prevention of tissue hypoxia and hemorrhage, both of which can lead to permanent compromise of vital organs, continue throughout the intrapartum and postpartum periods (Harvey & Burke, 1992).

Magnesium sulfate. One of the important goals of care for the woman with severe preeclampsia is prevention or

BOX 24-3	*Hospital Precautionary Measures*

Environment
—Quiet
—Nonstimulating
—Lighting subdued
Seizure precautions
—Padded side rails
—Suction equipment tested and ready to use
—Oxygen administration equipment tested and ready to use
Call button within easy reach
Emergency medication tray immediately accessible
—Hydralazine and magnesium sulfate in or adjacent to woman's room
—Calcium gluconate immediately available
Emergency birth pack accessible

PLAN OF CARE   *Severe Preeclampsia: Hospital Care*

NURSING DIAGNOSIS Risk for injury to mother and fetus related to CNS irritability

Expected Outcome *Patient will show diminished signs of CNS irritability (e.g., DTRs 2+, absence of clonus) and have no convulsions.*

Nursing Interventions/*Rationales*

Establish baseline data (e.g., DTRs, clonus) *to use as basis for evaluating effectiveness of treatment.*

Administer IV MgSO₄ per physician's orders *to decrease hyperreflexia and minimize risk of convulsions.*

Monitor maternal vital signs, FHR, urine output, DTRs, IV flow rate, and serum levels of MgSO₄ *to assess for and prevent MgSO₄ toxicity* (e.g., depressed respirations, oliguria, sudden drop in blood pressure, hyporeflexia, fetal distress).

Have calcium gluconate at bedside if needed *as antidote for MgSO₄ toxicity.*

Maintain a quiet, darkened environment *to avoid stimuli that may precipitate seizure activity.*

NURSING DIAGNOSIS Altered tissue perfusion related to preeclampsia secondary to arteriolar vasospasm

Expected Outcome *Patient will exhibit signs of increased vasodilation (i.e., diuresis, decreased edema, weight loss).*

Nursing Interventions/*Rationales*

Establish baseline data (i.e., weight, degree of edema) *to use as basis for evaluating effectiveness of treatment.*

Administer intravenous magnesium sulfate per physician order, *which serves to relax vasospasms and increase renal perfusion.*

Place woman on bed rest in a side-lying position *to maximize uteroplacental blood flow, reduce blood pressure, and promote diuresis.*

Monitor intake and output, edema, and weight *to assess for evidence of vasodilation and increased tissue perfusion.*

NURSING DIAGNOSIS Risk for
- fluid volume excess related to increased sodium retention secondary to administration of MgSO₄
- impaired gas exchange related to pulmonary edema secondary to increased vascular resistance
- decreased cardiac output related to use of antihypertensive drugs
- injury to fetus related to uteroplacental insufficiency secondary to use of antihypertensive medications

Expected Outcomes *Patient will exhibit signs of normal fluid volume (i.e., balanced intake and output, normal serum creatinine levels, normal breath sounds); adequate oxygenation (i.e., normal respirations, fully oriented to person, time, and place); normal range of cardiac output (i.e., normal pulse rate and rhythm); and fetal well-being (i.e., adequate fetal movement, normal FHR).*

Nursing Interventions/*Rationales*

Monitor woman for signs of fluid volume excess (increased edema, decreased urine output, elevated serum creatinine level, weight gain, dyspnea, crackles) *to prevent complications.*

Monitor woman for signs of impaired gas exchange (i.e., increased respirations, dyspnea, altered blood gases, hypoxemia) *to prevent complications.*

Monitor woman for signs of decreased cardiac output (i.e., altered pulse rate and rhythm) *to prevent complications.*

Monitor fetus for signs of difficulty (i.e., decreased fetal activity, decreased FHR) *to prevent complications.*

Record findings and report signs of increasing problems to physician *to enable timely interventions.*

From Wong D & Perry S: *Maternal child nursing care,* St Louis, 1998, Mosby.

---

control of convulsions. Magnesium sulfate (MgSO₄) is the drug of choice in the prevention and treatment of convulsions caused by preeclampsia or eclampsia (ACOG, 1996). Benefits of magnesium sulfate therapy include an increase in uterine blood flow to protect the fetus and an increase in prostacyclins to prevent uterine vasoconstriction (Gilbert & Harmon, 1998).

Magnesium sulfate is administered as a secondary infusion to the main IV line by volumetric infusion pump. An initial loading dose of 4 to 6 gm magnesium sulfate in 100 ml of 5% dextrose in water or other IV fluid per protocol or physician's order is infused over 20 to 30 minutes. This dose is followed by a maintenance dose of magnesium sulfate that is diluted in an IV solution per physician's order (e.g., 40 gm magnesium sulfate in 1,000 ml lactated Ringer's solution) and administered by infusion pump at 2 gm/hr (Fairlie & Sibai, 1992; Gilbert & Harmon, 1998). This dose should maintain a therapeutic serum magnesium level of 4 to 8 gm/dl. Serum magnesium levels are obtained after the patient has received magnesium sulfate for 4 to 6 hours. The infusion rate is adjusted to maintain the therapeutic level (Sisson & Sauer, 1996) (see the accompanying Protocol box).

After the loading dose, there may be a transient lowering of the arterial blood pressure as a result of relaxation of smooth muscle. Within an hour of initiation of therapy,

PROTOCOL *Care of Preeclamptic Patient Receiving Magnesium Sulfate*

MAGNESIUM SULFATE ADMINISTRATION

Patient and Family Teaching

Explain technique, rationale, and reactions to expect

- Route and rate
- Purpose of "piggyback"

Reasons for use

- Tailor information to patient's readiness to learn
- Explain it is to prevent disease progression
- Explain it is to prevent seizures

Reactions to expect from medication

- Initially patient will feel flushed, hot, sedated, nauseated, especially during the bolus
- Sedation will continue

Monitoring to anticipate

- Maternal: blood pressure, pulse, DTRs, level of consciousness, urine output (indwelling catheter), presence of headache, visual disturbances, epigastric pain
- Fetal: FHR and activity

Administration

- Position woman in side-lying position
- Prepare solution and administer with an infusion control device (pump)
- Piggyback initial bolus of magnesium sulfate, 4 to 6 gm in 100 ml 5% dextrose in water over 20 to 30 min
- Piggyback a solution of 40 gm magnesium sulfate in 1,000 ml 5% dextrose in water or lactated Ringer's solution with an infusion control device at the ordered rate, usually 2 gm/hr

Maternal and Fetal Assessments

- Monitor blood pressure, pulse, respiratory rate, FHR, and contractions every 15 to 30 min, depending on patient condition
- Monitor intake and output, proteinuria, DTRs, presence of headache, visual disturbances, level of consciousness and epigastric pain at least hourly
- Restrict hourly fluid intake to a total of 100 to 125 ml/hr; urinary output should be at least 30 ml/hr

Reportable Conditions

- Blood pressure: systolic >160 mm Hg, diastolic >110 mm Hg, or both
- Respiratory rate: ≤12 breaths/min
- Urinary output <30 ml/hr
- Presence of headache, visual disturbances, or epigastric pain
- Increasing severity or loss of DTRs; increasing edema, proteinuria
- Any abnormal laboratory values (magnesium levels, platelet count, creatinine clearance, levels of uric acid, AST, ALT, prothrombin time, partial thromboplastin time, fibrinogen, fibrin split products)
- Any other significant change in maternal or fetal status

Emergency Measures

- Keep emergency drug tray at bedside with calcium gluconate and intubation equipment
- Keep side rails up and padded
- Keep lights dimmed and maintain a quiet environment

Documentation

- All of the above

---

however, arterial blood pressure will return to pretherapy levels. Magnesium sulfate is not an antihypertensive drug; it is an anticonvulsant drug.

Intramuscular (IM) magnesium sulfate is rarely used because absorption rate cannot be controlled, injections are painful, and tissue necrosis may occur. The IM route may be used with some women who are being transported to a tertiary care center. The IM dose is 4 to 5 gm given in each buttock, a total of 10 gm (with 1% procaine possibly being added to the solution to reduce injection pain), and can be repeated at 4-hour intervals. Z-track technique should be used for the deep IM injection, followed by gentle massage at the site.

Magnesium sulfate interferes with the release of acetylcholine at the synapses, decreasing neuromuscular irritability, depressing cardiac conduction, and decreasing CNS irritability (Dildy et al., 1991). Because magnesium circulates free and unbound to protein and is excreted in the urine, accurate recordings of maternal urine output must be obtained. Because magnesium sulfate is a CNS depressant, the nurse assesses for signs and symptoms of magnesium toxicity (see Protocol box).

NURSE ALERT *Loss of patellar reflexes, respiratory depression, oliguria, and decreased level of consciousness are signs of magnesium toxicity. Actions are needed to prevent respiratory or cardiac arrest. If magnesium toxicity is suspected, the infusion should be discontinued immediately. Calcium gluconate, the antidote for magnesium sulfate, may also be ordered and given by slow IV push over at least 3 minutes (Sibai, 1996).*

Because magnesium sulfate is also a tocolytic agent, its use may increase the duration of labor.

NURSE ALERT *A preeclamptic woman receiving magnesium sulfate may need augmentation with oxytocin during labor. The amount of oxytocin needed to stimulate labor may be more than that needed for a woman who is not on magnesium sulfate.*

If eclampsia develops after the initiation of magnesium sulfate therapy, the treatment of choice is to administer an additional 2 gm of magnesium sulfate IV push over 3 to 5 minutes (see Emergency box). Occasionally, it is necessary

EMERGENCY

Eclampsia

TONIC-CLONIC CONVULSION SIGNS

Stage of invasion: 2 to 3 sec, eyes are fixed, twitching of facial muscles occurs

Stage of contraction: 15 to 20 sec, eyes protrude and are bloodshot, all body muscles are in tonic contraction

Stage of convulsion: muscles relax and contract alternately (clonic), respirations are halted and then begin again with long, deep, stertorous inhalation, coma ensues

INTERVENTION

Keep airway patent: turn head to one side, place pillow under one shoulder or back if possible

Call for assistance

Protect with side rails up and padded

Observe and record convulsion activity

AFTER CONVULSION OR SEIZURE

Observe for postconvulsion coma, incontinence

Use suction as needed

Administer oxygen via face mask at 10 L/min

Start IV fluids and monitor for potential fluid overload

Give magnesium sulfate or other anticonvulsant drug as ordered

Insert indwelling urinary catheter

Monitor blood pressure

Monitor fetal and uterine status

Expedite laboratory work as ordered to monitor kidney function, liver function, coagulation system, and drug levels

Provide hygiene and a quiet environment

Support and keep woman and family informed

Be prepared for delivery when woman is in stable condition

---

to repeat the dose because the woman will experience additional seizures. Rarely, the woman will continue to experience seizures despite adequate blood magnesium levels. In that case, sodium amobarbital 250 mg may be administered by slow IV push over 3 to 5 minutes (Sibai, 1996). Diazepam is sometimes used to treat eclamptic seizures. However, this drug can cause phlebitis and venous thrombosis. If administered too rapidly, it can also lead to apnea and/or cardiac arrest (Sibai, 1996).

Both sodium amobarbital and diazepam have fetal and neonatal effects as well. FHR demonstrates a loss of variability, a reflection of fetal oxygenation. High levels of these drugs in the neonate depress sucking ability, cause hypotonia, and may result in temperature instability. The neonate's respiratory rate may be decreased. Careful surveillance of both maternal and fetal or neonatal status is warranted.

Control of blood pressure. For the severely hypertensive preeclamptic woman, antihypertensive medications may be ordered to lower the diastolic blood pressure. Initiation of antihypertensive therapy reduces maternal morbidity and mortality associated with left ventricular failure and cerebral hemorrhage (Harvey & Burke, 1992). Because a degree of maternal hypertension is necessary to maintain uteroplacental perfusion, antihypertensive therapy must not decrease the arterial pressure too much or too rapidly. The target range for the diastolic pressure is therefore 90 to 100 mm Hg (Harvey & Burke, 1992).

Intravenous hydralazine remains the antihypertensive agent of choice for the treatment of hypertension in severe preeclampsia. Intravenous labetalol hydrochloride and oral methyldopa and nifedipine are also used (Cunningham et al., 1997; Sibai, 1996; Sisson & Sauer, 1996). The choice of agent used depends on patient response and physician preference. Table 24-5 compares antihypertensive agents used to treat hypertension in pregnancy.

Eclampsia

Immediate care. The immediate care during a convulsion is to ensure a patent airway (see the accompanying Emergency box). When convulsions occur, the woman is turned onto her side to prevent aspiration of vomitus and supine hypotension syndrome. After the convulsion ceases, food and fluid are suctioned from the glottis or trachea, and oxygen is administered by face mask. Magnesium sulfate and/or other anticonvulsant is given as ordered (Sibai, 1996). If an IV infusion is not in place, one is begun with a large-bore needle. Time, duration, and description of convulsions are recorded, and any urinary or fecal incontinence is noted. The fetus is monitored for adverse effects. Transient fetal bradycardia and decreased FHR variability are common.

Aspiration is a leading cause of maternal morbidity and mortality after eclamptic seizure. After initial stabilization and airway management, the nurse should anticipate orders for a chest radiograph and possibly arterial blood gases to rule out the possibility of aspiration.

A rapid assessment of uterine activity, cervical status, and fetal status is performed after a convulsion. During the convulsion, membranes may have ruptured; the cervix may have dilated because the uterus becomes hypercontractile and hypertonic; birth may be imminent. If not, once a woman's seizure activity and blood pressure are controlled, a decision should be made regarding whether birth should take place. The more serious the condition of the woman, the greater the need to proceed to birth. The route of birth—induction of labor versus cesarean birth—depends on maternal and fetal condition. If fetal lungs are not mature and the birth can be delayed for 48 hours, steroids such as betamethasone may be given.

The woman may have been incontinent of urine and stool during the convulsion; she will need assistance with hygiene and a change of gown. Oral care with a soft toothbrush may be of comfort.

Immediately following a seizure, the woman may be very confused and can be combative, necessitating the temporary

TABLE 24-5	*Pharmacologic Control of Hypertension in Pregnancy*

ACTION	TARGET TISSUE	EFFECTS		NURSING ACTIONS
		MATERNAL	FETAL	
HYDRALAZINE (APRESOLINE, NEOPRESOL)				
Arteriolar vasodilator	Peripheral arterioles: to decrease muscle tone, decrease peripheral resistance; hypothalamus and medullary vasomotor center for minor decrease in sympathetic tone	Headache, flushing, palpitation, tachycardia, some decrease in uteroplacental blood flow, increase in heart rate and cardiac output, increase in oxygen consumption, nausea and vomiting	Tachycardia; late decelerations and bradycardia if maternal diastolic pressure <90 mm Hg	Assess for effects of medications, alert mother (family) to expected effects of medications, assess blood pressure frequently because precipitous drop can lead to shock and perhaps abruptio placentae; assess urinary output; maintain bed rest in a lateral position with side rails up
LABETALOL HYDROCHLORIDE (NORMODYNE)				
β-blocking agent causing vasodilation without significant change in cardiac output	Peripheral arterioles (see hydralazine)	Minimal: flushing, tremulousness	Minimal, if any	See hydralazine; less likely to cause excessive hypotension and tachycardia
METHYLDOPA (ALDOMET)				
Maintenance therapy if needed: 250 to 500 mg orally every 8 hr (α₂-receptor agonist)	Postganglionic nerve endings: interferes with chemical neurotransmission to reduce peripheral vascular resistance, causes CNS sedation	Sleepiness, postural hypotension, constipation; rare: drug-induced fever in 1% of women and positive Coombs' test result in 20%	After 4 mo maternal therapy, positive Coombs' test result in infant	See hydralazine
NIFEDIPINE (PROCARDIA)				
Calcium-channel blocker	Arterioles: to reduce systemic vascular resistance by relaxation of arterial smooth muscle	Headache, flushing; possible potentiation of effects on CNS if administered concurrently with magnesium sulfate, may interfere with labor	Minimal	See hydralazine; use caution if patient also getting magnesium sulfate

use of restraints. It may take several hours for the woman to regain her usual level of mental functioning. The health care provider explains procedures briefly and quietly. The woman is never left alone. The family is also kept informed of management, rationale for treatment, and the woman's progress.

Determination of central venous pressure or pulmonary arterial wedge pressure (Swan-Ganz catheter) may occasionally be required for accurate fluid monitoring in the presence of pulmonary edema or acute renal failure (ACOG, 1996). No oral intake is permitted if the woman is convulsing or has symptoms of severe preeclampsia. An indwelling catheter is required for accurate measurement of urinary output. For correction of hypovolemia, crystalloids (0.9% saline solution or lactated Ringer's solution) are infused IV at a rate that maintains a urine output of at least 30 ml/hr, and the maternal response is recorded.

Medications (such as magnesium sulfate) are given as directed. The woman's response is monitored and recorded, and all drugs, dosages, and times are noted. Laboratory tests are ordered to assess for HELLP syndrome and to have blood typed and cross-matched for administration of packed red blood cells as needed. Blood is kept available for emergency transfusion; abruptio placentae, with accompanying hemorrhage and shock, often occurs in women with eclampsia. Other tests include determination of electrolyte levels, liver function battery, and complete hemogram and clotting profile, including platelet count and fibrin split product levels (to assess for DIC).

Postpartum nursing care

After birth the symptoms of preeclampsia or eclampsia resolve quickly, usually within 48 hours. The hematopoietic and hepatic complications of HELLP syndrome may persist longer. These patients often show an abrupt decrease in platelet count, with a concomitant increase in LDH and AST levels, after a trend toward normalization of values has begun. Generally the laboratory abnormalities seen with HELLP syndrome resolve in 72 to 96 hours.

The nursing care of the woman with hypertensive disease differs from that required in the usual postpartum period in a number of respects. The following variations in the nursing process are described.

Careful assessment of the woman with a hypertensive disorder continues throughout the postpartum period. Blood pressure is measured at least every 4 hours for 48 hours or more frequently as the woman's condition warrants. Even if no convulsions occurred before the birth, they may occur within this period. Magnesium sulfate infusion may be continued 12 to 24 hours after the birth. The same assessments continue until the medication is discontinued. The woman is at risk for a boggy uterus and a large lochia flow as a result of the magnesium sulfate therapy. Assessments of uterine tone and lochia flow must be monitored closely. The preeclamptic woman is hemoconcentrated and unable to tolerate excessive postpartum blood loss. Oxytocin or prostaglandin products are used to control bleeding. Ergot products (e.g., Ergotrate and Methergine) are contraindicated because they can increase blood pressure. The woman is asked to report symptoms such as headaches and blurred vision. The nurse assesses affect, level of consciousness, blood pressure, pulse, and respiratory status before an analgesic is given for headache. Magnesium sulfate potentiates the action of narcotics, CNS depressants, and calcium-channel blockers; these drugs must be administered with caution. The woman may need to continue an antihypertensive medication regimen if her diastolic blood pressure exceeds 100 mm Hg at discharge.

The woman's and family's responses to labor, birth, and the neonate are monitored. Interactions and involvement in the care of the neonate are encouraged to the extent that the woman and her family desire. In addition, the woman and her family need opportunities to discuss their emotional response to complications. The nurse provides information concerning the prognosis. Preeclampsia and eclampsia do not necessarily recur in subsequent pregnancies (recurrence rate is approximately 30%), but careful prenatal care is essential.

Prevention

Although there is no known etiology for preeclampsia, research offers some suggestions for preventing the disease. These include:

- Adequate nutrition in pregnancy, including daily intake of 60 to 70 gm protein, 1,200 mg calcium, and adequate intake of magnesium, sodium, and other vitamins and minerals and drinking 6 to 8 glasses of fluid a day
- Adequate rest including 8 hours of sleep a night and a rest period during the day
- Water therapy (shoulder-deep immersion), to mobilize extravascular fluid; initiate diuresis; and increase renin, angiotensin, aldosterone, and vasopressin levels in women with severe edema to prevent or slow progression of preeclampsia
- Early prenatal care for identification of women at risk and early detection of development of preeclampsia
- Low-dose aspirin (60 to 80 mg/day) to reduce incidence of preeclampsia in women at risk. This is still a controversial suggestion and is not recommended for women at low risk (CLASP Collaborative Group, 1995; Cunningham et al., 1997; Katz et al., 1990; Sanchez-Ramos et al., 1994; Sibai et al., 1993; Zuspan & Samuels, 1993).

Further research is needed to determine what effects, if any, these suggestions have on prevention of preeclampsia.

Evaluation

Evaluation of the effectiveness of care of the woman with preeclampsia is based on the expected outcomes.

❘ HYPEREMESIS GRAVIDARUM

Nausea and vomiting complicate about 70% of all pregnancies and are usually confined to the first trimester (Cruikshank et al., 1996). Although these manifestations are distressing, they are typically benign, with no significant metabolic alterations or risks to the mother or fetus.

When vomiting during pregnancy becomes excessive enough to cause weight loss and fluid, electrolyte, and acid-base imbalances, the disorder is termed **hyperemesis gravidarum.** The estimated incidence varies from 0.5 to 10 per 1,000 births. Although most cases are mild and resolve with time, approximately 1 in every 1,000 pregnant women requires hospitalization as a result of severe, intractable vomiting. Hyperemesis gravidarum is generally self-limiting, but recovery is slow and frequent relapses are common. It occurs most frequently among primigravidas and tends to recur in subsequent pregnancies. Other predisposing factors include maternal age less than 20 years, obesity, multifetal gestation, and trophoblastic disease (hydatidiform mole) (Abell & Riely, 1992; Hod et al., 1994).

The effects of hyperemesis gravidarum on perinatal outcome vary with the severity of the disorder. Women who lose weight are more likely to have low-birth-weight infants. There may be some relationship between hyperemesis gravidarum and the development of CNS and skeletal anomalies in the fetus (Hod et al., 1994).

Etiology

The etiology of hyperemesis gravidarum remains obscure. Several theories have been proposed as to the cause, although none of them adequately explains the disorder. Hyperemesis gravidarum may be related to high levels of estrogen or human chorionic gonadotropin (hCG) and may be associated with transient hyperthyroidism during pregnancy. It may be accompanied by liver dysfunction with elevation in transaminase and bilirubin levels. Esophageal reflux, reduced gastric motility, and decreased secretion of free hydrochloric acid may contribute to the disorder. Other possible causes may be vitamin B deficiencies or disturbances of carbohydrate metabolism (Hod et al., 1994; Modigliani & Bernades, 1995).

Psychologic factors may be instrumental in the development of hyperemesis gravidarum. Ambivalence toward the pregnancy and conflicting feelings regarding prospective motherhood, body changes, and lifestyle alterations, all normal reactions to pregnancy, may contribute to episodes of vomiting, particularly if these feelings are excessive or unresolved. Women with psychologic problems whose normal reaction patterns to stress involve gastrointestinal disturbances are often affected. However, in some women psychologic causes cannot be identified (Deuchar, 1995; Hod et al., 1994).

I CARE MANAGEMENT

Whenever a pregnant woman presents for care with a complaint of nausea and vomiting, the first priority is a thorough assessment to determine the severity of the problem. In most cases, the woman should be told to come immediately to the health care provider's office or to the emergency department, because the severity of the illness is often difficult to determine by phone conversation.

The history includes information about the frequency, severity, and duration of episodes of nausea and vomiting. Other symptoms such as diarrhea, indigestion, and abdominal pain or distention are also identified. The woman is asked to report any precipitating factors relating to the onset of her symptoms. Any pharmacologic or nonpharmacologic treatment measures should be recorded. Prepregnancy weight and documented weight gain or loss during pregnancy are important to note.

The woman's weight and vital signs are measured and a complete physical examination is performed, with attention to signs of fluid and electrolyte imbalance and nutritional status. The most important initial laboratory test to be obtained is a dipstick determination of ketonuria. Other laboratory tests that may be ordered are a urinalysis, a complete blood cell count, electrolytes, liver enzymes, and bilirubin levels. These tests help rule out the presence of underlying diseases such as pyelonephritis, pancreatitis, cholecystitis, and hepatitis (Cruikshank et al., 1996). Because of the recognized association between hyperemesis gravidarum and hyperthyroidism, thyroid levels may also be measured.

Psychosocial assessment includes asking the woman about anxiety, fears, and concerns related to her own health and the effects on pregnancy outcome. Family members should be assessed both for anxiety and in regard to their role in providing support for the woman.

Hospital care

The woman with hyperemesis who is unable to keep down clear fluids by mouth is usually admitted to the hospital for intravenous therapy. The woman should be kept NPO until dehydration has been resolved and for at least 48 hours after vomiting has stopped to prevent rapid recurrence of the problem (Cruikshank et al., 1996). Feedings are started in small amounts at frequent intervals, and the diet is slowly advanced as tolerated. Antiemetic medications may be used if nausea and vomiting are uncontrolled; recommended medications are promethazine or metoclopramide. Some women may benefit from psychotherapy such as hypnotherapy or behavior modification (Modigliani & Bernades, 1995; Torem, 1994).

Nursing care of the hospitalized hyperemetic woman involves implementing the medical plan of care: initiating and monitoring IV therapy, administering drugs and nutritional supplements, and monitoring the woman's response to interventions. The nurse observes the woman for any signs of complications such as metabolic acidosis, jaundice, or hemorrhage and alerts the physician should these occur.

Accurate measurement of intake and output, including the amount of emesis, is an important aspect of nursing care. Oral hygiene while the woman is receiving nothing by mouth, and after episodes of vomiting, helps allay associated discomforts. Assistance with positioning and providing a quiet, restful environment, free from odors, may increase the woman's comfort. When the woman begins responding to therapy, limited amounts of oral fluids and bland foods such as crackers or toast are begun. The diet is progressed slowly as tolerated by the woman until she is able to consume a nutritionally sound diet. Because sleep disturbances may accompany hyperemesis gravidarum, promoting adequate rest is important. The nurse can assist in coordinating treatment measures and periods of visitation to provide opportunity for rest periods.

In severe cases of hyperemesis gravidarum, enteral or parenteral nutrition may be necessary to correct maternal nutritional deprivation. Central or peripheral infusions of total parenteral nutrition may be administered for a rapid therapeutic effect (Charlin et al., 1993).

Home care

After several days of treatment in the hospital, most women are able to return home, taking nourishment by mouth. Education before hospital discharge is very important to prevent rapid readmission because of recurrent nausea and vomiting. Women should be encouraged to eat small, frequent meals and low-fat protein foods, to avoid greasy and highly seasoned foods, and to increase their dietary intake of potassium and magnesium. Herbal teas such as chamomile or raspberry leaf may decrease nausea. Taking fluids between meals, rather than with them sometimes helps decrease nausea. Many pregnant women find exposure to cooking odors nauseating. If other family members can take over cooking chores, even temporarily, the woman's nausea and vomiting may decrease. Finally, the woman should be told to contact her health care provider immediately if the nausea and vomiting recurs, especially if accompanied by abdominal pain, dehydration, and/or significant weight loss.

A few women will continue to experience intractable nausea and vomiting throughout pregnancy. Rarely, it may be necessary to maintain a woman on enteral, parenteral, or total parenteral nutrition (TPN) in order to provide adequate nutrition for the mother and fetus. Many home health agencies are able to provide these services, and arrangements for service may be made depending upon the woman's insurance coverage.

Regardless of the site of care, the nurse must remain calm, compassionate, and sympathetic, recognizing that the manifestations of hyperemesis can be physically and emotionally debilitating. Irritability, tearfulness, and mood changes are often consistent with this disorder. Fetal well-being is a primary concern of the woman. The nurse can provide an environment conducive to discussion of those concerns and assist the woman in identifying and mobilizing sources of support. The family should be included in the plan of care whenever possible. Encouraging their participation may help alleviate some of the emotional stress associated with this disorder. Psychologic counseling may be needed, as well as referral to a social worker. Education of the woman and her family about hyperemesis, its causes, potential complications, and management plan is necessary at the onset because understanding enhances adherence to the treatment plan and influence maternal and fetal outcomes.

▌HEMORRHAGIC COMPLICATIONS

Maternal adaptations in the hematologic and cardiovascular systems during pregnancy result in a hypervolemic state. The increased blood volume serves (1) to meet the metabolic demands of the mother and fetus, (2) to protect against the potentially deleterious impairment in venous return caused by the pressure of an enlarging uterus, and (3) to

safeguard the mother against the effects of blood loss at birth (Knuppel & Hatangadi, 1995). Any bleeding in pregnancy may therefore jeopardize both maternal and fetal well-being. Maternal blood loss decreases oxygen-carrying capacity, which predisposes the woman to increased risk for hypovolemia, anemia, infection, preterm labor, and preterm birth and adversely affects oxygen delivery to the fetus. Fetal risks from maternal hemorrhage include blood loss or anemia, hypoxemia, hypoxia, anoxia, and preterm birth. If the bleeding involves fetal blood loss, the effects are exponential because of the smaller fetal blood volume. It is estimated that one in every five pregnancies is complicated by bleeding; the incidence and type of bleeding vary by trimester (Thorp, 1993). Hemorrhagic disorders in pregnancy are medical emergencies. Prompt, expert teamwork by the health care team is required to save the life of mother and/or fetus. For a discussion of postpartum hemorrhage, see Chapter 26.

Early Pregnancy Bleeding

Bleeding during early pregnancy is alarming to the woman and of concern to the health care provider and nurse. The common bleeding disorders of early pregnancy include spontaneous abortion, incompetent cervix, ectopic pregnancy, and hydatidiform mole (molar pregnancy).

Spontaneous abortion

Spontaneous **abortion** is defined as termination of a pregnancy that occurs before the fetus is able to survive outside the uterus. In the United States, this period is before 20 weeks of gestation. A fetal weight less than 500 gm may also be used to define spontaneous abortion (Cunningham et al., 1997). A spontaneous abortion results from natural causes; it is generally referred to by the lay public as a miscarriage. Induced abortion (intentional interruption of pregnancy) is discussed in Chapter 7.

Incidence and etiology. About 10% to 15% of all clinically recognized pregnancies end in spontaneous abortion (Simpson, 1996). An early spontaneous abortion is one that occurs before 12 weeks of gestation.

At least 50% of all clinically recognized pregnancy losses result from chromosomal abnormalities (Simpson, 1996). The majority (over 90%) of spontaneous abortions occur early, before 8 weeks of gestation (Simpson, 1996). Possible causes of early abortion include endocrine imbalance (as in women who have luteal phase defects or insulin-dependent diabetes mellitus with high blood glucose levels in the first trimester), immunologic factors (such as antiphospholipid antibodies), infections (such as bacteriuria and *Chlamydia trachomatis*), systemic disorders (such as lupus erythematosus), and genetic factors (ACOG, 1995; Gilbert & Harmon, 1998).

A late spontaneous abortion is one that occurs between 12 and 20 weeks of gestation. Late spontaneous abortions

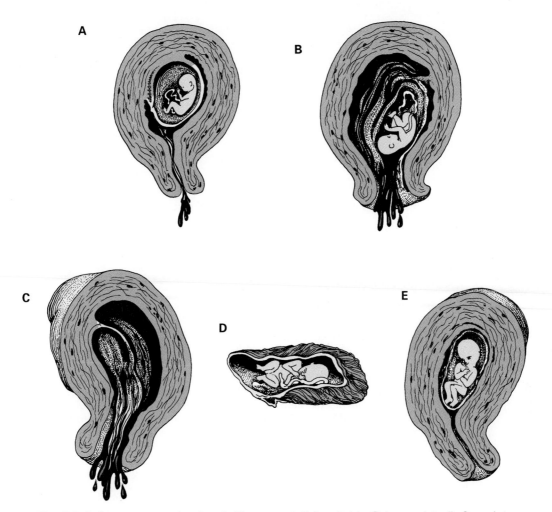

Fig. **24-6** Spontaneous abortion. **A,** Threatened. **B,** Inevitable. **C,** Incomplete. **D,** Complete. **E,** Missed.

usually result from maternal causes, such as advancing maternal age and parity, chronic infections, incompetent cervix and other anomalies of the reproductive tract, chronic debilitating diseases, nutrition, and recreational drug use (Cunningham et al., 1997). Little can be done to avoid genetically caused pregnancy loss, but correction of maternal disorders, immunization against infectious diseases, adequate early prenatal care, and treatment of pregnancy complications can do much to prevent spontaneous abortion.

Types. The types of spontaneous abortion include threatened, inevitable, incomplete, complete, and missed. Abortions (both early and late) can recur; all but the threatened abortion can lead to infection (Fig. 24-6).

Signs and symptoms. Signs and symptoms of spontaneous abortion depend on the duration of pregnancy. Once pregnancy has been diagnosed, the presence of uterine bleeding, uterine contractions, and uterine pain are ominous signs that must be considered a threatened abortion until proved otherwise.

If abortion occurs before the sixth week of pregnancy, the woman may report a heavy menstrual flow. Abortion that occurs between the sixth and twelfth weeks of pregnancy causes moderate discomfort and blood loss. After the twelfth week, abortion is typified by more severe pain, similar to that of labor, because the fetus must be expelled. Diagnosis of the type of abortion is based on the signs and symptoms present (Table 24-6).

Symptoms of a threatened abortion (see Fig. 24-6, *A*) include spotting of blood but with the cervical os closed. Mild uterine cramping may be present.

Inevitable (see Fig. 24-6, *B*) and incomplete (see Fig. 24-6, *C*) abortions involve a moderate to heavy amount of bleeding with an open cervical os. Tissue may be present with the bleeding. Mild to severe uterine cramping may be present. An inevitable abortion is often accompanied by rupture of membranes (ROM) and cervical dilatation; passage of the products of conception is a certainty. An incomplete abortion involves the expulsion

TABLE 24-6 *Assessing Abortion*

TYPE OF ABORTION	AMOUNT OF BLEEDING	UTERINE CRAMPING	PASSAGE OF TISSUE	CERVICAL DILATATION
Threatened	Slight, spotting	Mild	No	No
Inevitable	Moderate	Mild to severe	No	Yes
Incomplete	Heavy, profuse	Severe	Yes	Yes, with tissue in cervix
Complete	Slight	Mild	Yes	No
Missed	None, spotting	No	No	No
Septic	Varies, usually malodorous	Varies	Varies	Yes, usually
Recurrent	Varies	Varies	Yes	Yes, usually

From: Gilbert E & Harmon J: *Manual of high risk pregnancy and delivery,* ed 2 St Louis, 1998, Mosby.

TABLE 24-7 *Types of Spontaneous Abortion and Usual Management*

TYPE OF ABORTION	MANAGEMENT
Threatened	Bed rest, sedation, and avoidance of stress and orgasm usually recommended. Further treatment depends on woman's response to treatment.
Inevitable and incomplete	Prompt termination of pregnancy is accomplished, usually by dilatation and curettage (D&C).
Complete	No further intervention may be needed if uterine contractions are adequate to prevent hemorrhage and there is no infection.
Missed	If spontaneous evacuation of the uterus does not occur within 1 month, pregnancy is terminated by method appropriate to duration of pregnancy. Blood clotting factors are monitored until uterus is empty. Disseminated intravascular coagulation (DIC) and incoagulability of blood with uncontrolled hemorrhage may develop in cases of fetal death after the twelfth week, if products of conception are retained for longer than 5 weeks.
Septic	Immediate termination of pregnancy by method appropriate to duration of pregnancy. Cervical culture and sensitivity studies are done and broad-spectrum antibiotic therapy (such as ampicillin) is started. Treatment for septic shock is initiated if necessary.

of the fetus with retention of the placenta (Cunningham et al., 1997).

In a complete abortion (see Fig. 24-6, *D*), all fetal tissue is passed, the cervix is closed, and there may be slight bleeding. Mild uterine cramping may be present.

The term *missed abortion* (see Fig. 24-6, *E*) refers to a pregnancy in which the fetus has died but spontaneous abortion does not occur. It may be diagnosed by ultrasonic examination after the uterus stops increasing in size or even decreases in size. There may be no bleeding or cramping, and the cervical os remains closed.

Recurrent early (habitual) spontaneous abortion is the loss of three or more previable pregnancies.

Spontaneous abortions can become septic, although this is not a common occurrence. Symptoms of a septic abortion include fever and abdominal tenderness. Vaginal bleeding, which may be slight to heavy, is usually malodorous.

Medical management. Medical management (Table 24-7) depends on the classification of spontaneous abortion and on signs and symptoms. Traditionally, threatened abortions have been managed with bed rest and supportive care, although this treatment has not been scientifically shown to improve pregnancy outcome. Follow-up treatment depends on whether the threatened abortion progresses to actual abortion or symptoms subside and the pregnancy remains intact. Dilatation and curettage (D&C) is commonly used to treat inevitable and incomplete abortions. Complete abortions usually require no treatment unless the woman hemorrhages or becomes infected. A missed abortion usually terminates spontaneously, but if this does not occur, the primary health care provider evacuates the uterus to prevent disseminated intravascular coagulation (DIC) or sepsis. If infection occurs, antibiotic therapy and treatment for septic shock are initiated.

CARE MANAGEMENT

Assessment and Nursing Diagnoses

Whenever a woman with vaginal bleeding early in pregnancy presents for care, a thorough assessment should be performed (Box 24-4). Information to be obtained includes chief complaint, type and location of pain, quantity and

| BOX 24-4 | *Assessment of Bleeding in Pregnancy* |

INITIAL DATABASE
Chief complaint
Vital signs
Gravidity, parity
LMP/estimated date of birth
Pregnancy history (previous and current)
Allergies
Nausea and vomiting
Pain (onset, quality, precipitating event)
Bleeding or coagulation problems
Level of consciousness
Emotional status

EARLY PREGNANCY
Confirmation of pregnancy
Bleeding (bright or dark, intermittent or continuous)
Pain (type, intensity, persistence)
Vaginal discharge

LATE PREGNANCY
Estimated date of birth
Bleeding (quantity, associated pain)
Vaginal discharge
Amniotic membrane status
Uterine activity
Abdominal pain
Fetal status/viability

Nursing Diagnoses for the woman experiencing spontaneous abortion are listed in the accompanying box.

Nursing Diagnoses

Woman Experiencing Spontaneous Abortion
Anxiety/fear related to:
* Unknown outcome and unfamiliarity with medical procedures
Fluid volume deficit related to:
* Excessive bleeding secondary to spontaneous abortion
Acute pain related to:
* Uterine contractions
Anticipatory grieving related to:
* Unexpected pregnancy outcome
Situational low self-esteem related to:
* Inability to successfully carry a pregnancy to term gestation
Risk for altered health maintenance related to:
* Lack of knowledge of risk factors and preventive measures for spontaneous early abortion

Expected Outcomes of Care

Expected outcomes of care for the woman experiencing spontaneous abortion may include the following. The woman will:
* Discuss the impact of the loss on her and her family
* Identify and use available support systems
* Have no signs and symptoms of complications (such as hemorrhage or infection)
* Identify health promotion measures that decrease her risk of spontaneous abortion and state understanding of reasons for diagnostic and genetic follow-up if needed
* Report relief from pain

Plan of Care and Interventions

Hospital care

Immediate nursing care focuses on physiologic stabilization. The nurse reinforces explanations given by the primary health care provider and carries out appropriate orders. An intravenous line is started and blood is drawn for laboratory testing. At a minimum, hematocrit and/or hemoglobin values, blood type and Rh status, and an atypical antibody screen are obtained. An ultrasound scan is performed to confirm the diagnosis.

If D&C or dilatation and evacuation is scheduled, the nurse reinforces explanations, answers any questions or concerns, and prepares the woman for surgery. D&C is a surgical procedure in which the cervix is dilated and a curette is inserted to scrape the uterine walls and remove uterine contents. Dilatation and evacuation, performed after 16 weeks

nature of bleeding, and date of last menstrual period (LMP) to determine approximate gestational age. The initial database should also include vital signs, previous pregnancies, previous pregnancy losses, allergies, and emotional status. Frequently the woman is anxious and fearful of what may happen to her and to her pregnancy.

Various laboratory findings are characteristic of abortion. Evaluation of hCG, a placental hormone, is used in the diagnosis of pregnancy and pregnancy loss. Human chorionic gonadotropin is produced by the syncytiotrophoblast, and the β subunit of hCG (β-hcg) can be detected in maternal plasma and urine 8 to 9 days after ovulation if the woman is pregnant. In early pregnancy, the concentration of β-hcg should double every 1.4 to 2 days until about 60 or 70 days of gestation (Cunningham et al., 1997). Before 8 weeks of gestation, if spontaneous abortion is suspected, two serum quantitative β-hcg levels are drawn 48 hours apart. If a normal pregnancy is present, the β-hcg level doubles in this time frame. Ultrasonography can then be used to determine the presence of a viable gestational sac. With considerable or persistent blood loss, anemia is likely (hemoglobin level less than 10.5 gm/dl). If infection is present, the white blood cell (WBC) count is greater than 12,000 cells/mm^3.

of gestation, consists of wide cervical dilatation followed by instrumental removal of the uterine contents.

Before either surgical procedure is performed, a full history should be obtained and general and pelvic examinations should be performed. General preoperative and postoperative care are appropriate for the woman requiring surgical intervention for spontaneous abortion. Analgesics or anesthesia appropriate to the procedure are used.

For late incomplete or inevitable abortions (16 to 20 weeks) and missed abortions, prostaglandins may be administered into the amniotic sac or by vaginal suppository to induce or augment labor and cause the products of conception to be expelled. Intravenous oxytocin may also be used.

Nursing care is similar to care for any woman whose labor is being induced. Special care may be needed for management of side effects of prostaglandin such as nausea and vomiting and diarrhea. If the products of conception are not passed in entirety, the woman may be prepared for manual or surgical evacuation of the uterus.

After evacuation of the uterus, 10 to 20 U of oxytocin in 1,000 ml of intravenous fluids may be given to prevent hemorrhage. For excessive bleeding after the abortion, ergot products such as ergonovine or a prostaglandin derivative such as carboprost tromethamine may be given to contract the uterus. Three or four doses of ergonovine, 0.2 mg orally or intramuscularly every 4 hours, may be given if the woman is normotensive. A 25-mg dose of carboprost may be given intramuscularly every 15 to 90 minutes for as many as eight doses (Cunningham et al., 1997). Antibiotics are given as necessary. Analgesics, such as antiprostaglandin agents, may decrease discomfort from cramping. Transfusion therapy may be required for shock or anemia. The woman who is Rh negative and does not have isoimmunization is given an intramuscular injection of Rh_o (D) immune globulin within 72 hours of the abortion.

Psychosocial aspects of care focus on what the pregnancy loss means to the woman and her family. Explanations are provided regarding the nature of the abortion, expected procedures, and possible future implications for childbearing.

As with the other fetal or neonatal losses, the woman should be offered the option of seeing the products of conception. She may also want to know what the hospital does with the products of conception or whether she needs to make a decision about final disposition.

Home care

The woman will likely be discharged home within a few hours of undergoing D&C or as soon as her vital signs are stable, vaginal bleeding is minimal, and she has recovered from anesthesia. Discharge teaching should emphasize the need for rest. If significant blood loss has occurred, iron supplementation may be ordered. Teaching includes information about normal physical findings, such as cramping, type and amount of bleeding, resumption of sexual activity,

---

TEACHING GUIDELINES

Discharge Teaching for the Woman after Spontaneous Abortion

- Advise woman to report any heavy, profuse, or bright red bleeding to health care provider.
- Reassure woman that a scant, dark discharge may persist for 1 to 2 weeks.
- To reduce the risk of infection, remind the woman not to put anything into the vagina until bleeding has stopped. She should take antibiotics as prescribed.
- Acknowledge that the woman has experienced a loss and that time is required for recovery. She may have mood swings and depression.
- Refer the woman to support groups, clergy, or professional counseling as needed.
- Advise woman that attempts at pregnancy should be postponed for at least 2 months to allow body to recover.

From Gilbert E & Harmon J: *Manual of high risk pregnancy & delivery,* ed 2, St Louis, 1998, Mosby.

---

and family planning. Follow-up care should assess the woman's physical and emotional recovery. Referrals to local support groups should be provided as needed (see the Teaching Guidelines box).

Follow-up phone calls after a loss are important. The woman may appreciate a phone call on what would have been her due date. These calls provide opportunities for the woman to ask questions, seek advice, and receive information to help process her grief.

Incompetent cervix

Another cause of late abortion is **incompetent cervix,** which has traditionally been defined as passive and painless dilatation of the cervix during the second trimester. This definition assumes an "all or nothing" role for the cervix; it is either "competent" or "incompetent." Newer thinking contends that cervical competence is variable and exists as a continuum that is determined in part by cervical length. Other related factors include composition of the cervical tissue and the individual circumstances associated with the pregnancy in terms of maternal stress and lifestyle. Iams (1996) refers to this condition as abnormal or reduced cervical competence. Freda (1995) suggests the term recurrent premature dilatation of the cervix.

Etiology. Etiologic factors include a history of previous cervical lacerations during childbirth, excessive cervical dilatation for curettage or biopsy, or the patients' mother's ingestion of diethylstilbestrol during pregnancy with the patient. Other instances may result from a congenitally short cervix or cervical or uterine anomalies. Reduced cervical competence is a clinical diagnosis, based on history. Short labors and recurring loss of the pregnancy at progressively earlier gestational ages are characteristics of

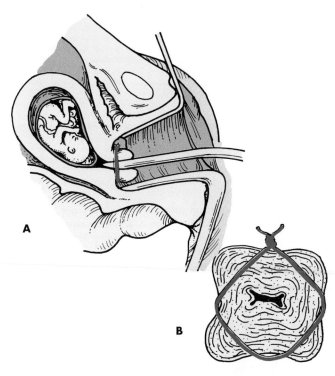

Fig. **24-7 A,** Cerclage correction of premature dilatation of the cervical os. **B,** Cross-sectional view of closed internal os.

reduced cervical competence. Ultrasound is being used to diagnose this condition objectively. A short cervix (less than 20 mm in length) is indicative of reduced cervical competence. Often, but not always, the short cervix is accompanied by **cervical funneling,** or effacement of the internal cervical os (Iams, 1996).

Medical management. Women with a history of painless cervical dilatation and effacement in a previous pregnancy or with a previous second trimester loss in which short cervix and funneling were documented by ultrasound are candidates for prophylactic **cerclage,** a technique that uses suture material to constrict the internal os of the cervix (Fig. 24-7). Prophylactic cerclage is placed at 10 to 14 weeks of gestation, after which the woman is told to refrain from intercourse, prolonged (more than 90 minutes) standing, and heavy lifting. She is followed during the course of her pregnancy with ultrasound scans to assess for cervical shortening and funneling. The cerclage is electively removed (usually an office/clinic procedure) when the woman reaches 37 weeks of gestation or it may be left in place and a cesarean birth will be performed. Eighty to 90% of pregnancies treated with cerclage result in live, viable births (Iams, 1996). If removed, cerclage placement will need to be repeated with each successive pregnancy.

A woman whose reduced cervical competence is diagnosed during the current pregnancy may undergo emergency cerclage placement. Risks of the procedure include premature rupture of membranes, preterm labor, and

chorioamnionitis. Because of these risks, and because bed rest and tocolytic therapy can be used to prolong the pregnancy, cerclage is rarely performed after 26 weeks of gestation (Iams, 1996).

I CARE MANAGEMENT

The nurse assesses the woman's feelings about her pregnancy and her understanding of reduced cervical competence. It is also important to evaluate the woman's support systems. Because the diagnosis of reduced cervical competence is usually not made until the woman has lost one or two previous pregnancies, she may feel guilty or to blame for this impending loss. It is therefore important to assess for previous reactions to stresses and appropriateness of coping responses. The woman needs the support of her health care providers, as well as that of her family.

Hospital care

Care of the woman with reduced cervical competence focuses on the patient's self-concept, her ability to cope with possible pregnancy loss, and her ability to understand treatment regimens.

If a cervical cerclage is performed, the woman is monitored after operation for contractions, signs of ROM, and infection. Referrals are made as appropriate for assistance once she is discharged to her home. It is important that the woman understand the rationale for the treatment and the needed follow-up care.

Discharge teaching focuses on signs and symptoms of preterm labor, ROM, and infection. If home uterine monitoring is used, the woman should receive initial instructions from the home health agency before discharge.

Home care. The woman must understand the importance of activity restriction at home and the need for close observation and supervision. Instruction includes the rationale for bed rest, activity restriction, and warning signs of preterm labor, ROM, and infection to report (Grohar, 1994; Simpson, 1992). The woman must be instructed on the importance of taking oral tocolytic medication if prescribed, the expected response, and possible side effects. Tocolytics may be given prophylactically to prevent uterine contractions and further dilatation of the cervix. If home uterine monitoring is implemented, the woman is taught how to apply a uterine contraction monitor and transmit the monitor tracing by telephone to the monitoring center. Nurses at the monitoring center assess the tracing for contractions, answer questions, provide emotional support and education, and report information to the woman's physician or midwife. The woman should know the signs that would warrant immediate transfer to the hospital, including strong contractions less than 5 minutes apart, rupture of membranes, severe perineal pressure, and an urge to push (Health Care Resources, 1997). If management is unsuccessful and the fetus is born before viability, appropriate grief support should be provided. If the fetus is born prematurely, appropriate anticipatory guidance and support will be necessary.

Ectopic pregnancy

Incidence and etiology. **Ectopic pregnancy** is one in which the fertilized ovum is implanted outside the uterine cavity (Fig. 24-8). About 95% of ectopic pregnancies occur in the uterine (fallopian) tube, with most located on the ampullar or largest portion of the tube. Other sites include the abdominal cavity (3% to 4%), ovary (1%), and cervix (1%).

Ectopic pregnancy is responsible for 10% of all maternal mortality, and it is the leading pregnancy-related cause of first trimester maternal mortality (Simpson, 1996; Powell & Spellman, 1996). Moreover, ectopic pregnancy is a leading cause of infertility. Only about 60% of women who have been treated for ectopic pregnancy are able to conceive afterwards, and approximately 40% of those pregnancies are ectopic (Powell & Spellman, 1996).

The incidence of ectopic pregnancy has increased during the past 15 to 20 years. In 1992, 1 of every 50 (2%) of reported pregnancies was ectopic (Powell & Spellman, 1996). In part, this increase is due to improved diagnostic techniques, such as more sensitive β-hCG assays and the availability of transvaginal ultrasound. Other reasons include an increased incidence of STDs, better treatment of pelvic inflammatory disease (PID) (which formerly would have caused sterility), increased numbers of tubal sterilizations, and surgical reversal of tubal sterilizations (Simpson, 1996).

Ectopic pregnancy is classified according to site of implantation (e.g., tubal or ovarian). The uterus is the only organ capable of containing and sustaining a term pregnancy. However, abdominal pregnancy with birth by laparotomy may result occasionally in a living infant (Fig. 24-9) in 5% to 25% of such pregnancies; however, the risk of deformity is as high as 40% (Gilbert & Harmon, 1998).

Signs and symptoms. A missed period, adnexal fullness, and tenderness may suggest an unruptured tubal pregnancy. The tenderness can progress from a dull pain to a colicky pain when the tube stretches. Pain may be unilateral, bilateral, or diffuse over the abdomen. Abnormal vaginal bleeding that is dark red or brown occurs in 50% to 80% of women. If the ectopic pregnancy ruptures, pain increases. This pain may be generalized, unilateral, or acute deep lower quadrant pain caused by blood irritating the peritoneum. Referred shoulder pain can occur as a result of diaphragmatic irritation caused by blood in the peritoneal cavity. The woman may exhibit signs of shock related to the amount of bleeding in the abdominal cavity and not necessarily related to obvious vaginal bleeding. An ecchymotic blueness around the umbilicus, indicating hematoperitoneum, may develop in a neglected ruptured intraabdominal ectopic pregnancy.

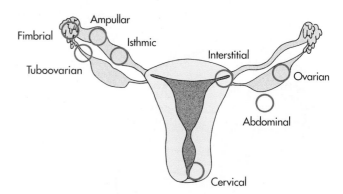

Fig. 24-8 Sites of implantation of ectopic pregnancies. Order of frequency of occurrence is ampulla, isthmus, interstitium, fimbria, tuboovarian ligament, ovary, abdominal cavity, and cervix (external os).

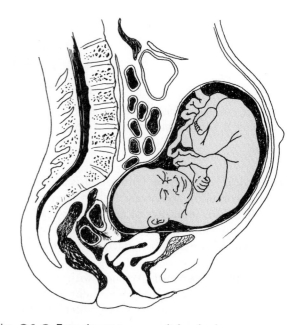

Fig. 24-9 Ectopic pregnancy, abdominal.

Medical diagnosis and management. The differential diagnosis of ectopic pregnancy involves consideration of numerous disorders that share many signs and symptoms. The physician, nurse midwife, or nurse practitioner must consider abortion, ruptured corpus luteum cyst, appendicitis, salpingitis, ovarian cysts, torsion of the ovary, and urinary tract infection (Table 24-8). Diagnostic evaluation for an ectopic pregnancy includes laboratory testing and vaginal sonography.

Most ectopic pregnancies occur in the uterine tube. In the past, these tubal pregnancies were usually diagnosed at the time of rupture, when the major management problem was hemorrhage. Often, laparotomy, followed by removal of the entire uterine tube, was the treatment necessary to control bleeding and save the woman's life.

TABLE 24-8 *Differential Diagnosis of Ectopic Pregnancy*

	ECTOPIC PREGNANCY	APPENDICITIS	SALPINGITIS	RUPTURED OVARIAN CYST	SPONTANEOUS ABORTION
Pain	Unilateral cramps and tenderness before rupture May be colicky after rupture Sudden sharp abdominal pelvic pain Abdominal tenderness	Epigastric, periumbilical, then right lower quadrant pain, tenderness localizing at McBurney's point, rebound tenderness	Usually in both lower quadrants with or without rebound Mild to severe pelvic pressure	Unilateral, becoming general with progressive bleeding, dull cramping	Mild uterine cramps to severe uterine pain
Nausea and vomiting	Occasionally before, frequently after rupture	Usual, precedes shift of pain to right lower quadrant	Infrequent	Rare	Almost never
Menstruation	Some aberration, missed period, spotting	Unrelated to menses	Hypermenorrhea, metrorrhagia, or both	Period delayed, then bleeding, often with pain	Amenorrhea then spotting, then brisk bleeding
Temperature, pulse, and blood pressure	37.2°-37.8° C, pulse variable, normal before and rapid after rupture, ↓ BP after rupture	37.2°-37.8° C, pulse rapid, 99-100 beats/min	37.2°-40° C: pulse elevated in proportion to fever	Not over 37.2° C, pulse normal unless blood loss marked, then rapid	To 37.2° C Signs of shock related to obvious bleeding
Pelvic examination	Unilateral tenderness, especially on movement of cervix, crepitant mass on one side or in cul-de-sac; dark red or brown vaginal discharge	No masses, rectal tenderness high on right side No vaginal discharge	Bilateral tenderness on movement of cervix Purulent discharge	Tenderness over affected ovary, no masses	Cervix open or closed, uterus slightly enlarged, irregularly softened, tender with infection, vaginal bleeding
Laboratory findings	WBC to 15,000/mm³ Pregnancy test positive Ultrasound to rule out pregnancy after 6 weeks	WBC 10,000-18,000/mm³ (rarely normal) Pregnancy test negative	WBC 15,000-30,000/mm³ Pregnancy test negative	WBC normal to 10,000/mm³ Pregnancy test negative unless also pregnant Ultrasound will show ovarian cyst	WBC normal Pregnancy test positive

Modified from Gilbert E & Harmon J: *Manual of high risk pregnancy and delivery*, ed 2, St Louis, 1998, Mosby.

With the development of laparoscopy, removal of the ectopic pregnancy by salpingostomy is possible before rupture. Residual tissue that remains after surgery is treated with methotrexate, a drug that causes the tissue to dissolve. Medical therapy, in the form of a single or multiple doses of methotrexate, has also been used to treat unruptured ectopic pregnancies (Minnick-Smith & Cook, 1997). It is usually injected intramuscularly but may be injected directly into the ectopic tissue. Methotrexate, a folic acid antagonist that has been used for years to treat actively proliferating

trophoblastic disease, destroys the rapidly dividing cells. It has been shown to produce similar results to surgical therapy, in terms of high success rate, low complication rate, and good reproductive potential (Simpson, 1996).

Advanced ectopic abdominal pregnancy requires laparotomy as soon as the woman has been stabilized for operation. If the placenta of a second- or third-trimester abdominal pregnancy is attached to a vital organ, such as the liver, separation is usually not attempted because of the risk of hemorrhage. The cord is cut flush with the placenta and the abdomen is closed, with the placenta left in place. Degeneration and absorption of the placenta usually occur without complication, although infection and intestinal obstruction may occur. Methotrexate may be given to dissolve the residual tissue (Cunningham et al., 1997).

I CARE MANAGEMENT

The key to early detection of ectopic pregnancy is having a high index of suspicion for this condition. Any woman presenting for care with complaints of abdominal pain, vaginal spotting or bleeding, and a positive pregnancy test should undergo screening for ectopic pregnancy, especially if she has any of the risk factors previously mentioned. Laboratory screening includes determination of serum progesterone and β-hCG levels. If either of these values is lower than would be expected for a normal pregnancy, the woman is asked to return within 48 hours for serial measurements. At this time, the woman will also undergo transvaginal ultrasound to confirm intrauterine or tubal pregnancy (Powell & Spellman, 1996).

The woman should also be assessed for the presence of active bleeding, associated with tubal rupture. If internal bleeding is present, assessment may reveal vertigo, shoulder pain, hypotension, and tachycardia. A vaginal examination should be performed only once, and then with great caution. Approximately half of patients with a tubal pregnancy have a palpable mass on exam. It is possible to rupture the mass during a bimanual exam, so gentleness is critical (Simpson, 1996).

Hospital care

Once an ectopic pregnancy is suspected, the physician is notified of assessment findings. Vital signs (pulse, respirations, and blood pressure) are assessed every 15 minutes or as needed, according to severity of the bleeding and the woman's condition. Laboratory tests include determination of blood type and Rh factor, complete blood cell count, and serum quantitative β-hCG assay. Ultrasonography is used to confirm an extrauterine pregnancy. General preoperative and postoperative care is appropriate for the woman requiring surgical intervention for an ectopic pregnancy. Blood replacement may be necessary. The nurse needs to verify the woman's Rh and antibody status and administer Rh$_o$ (D) immune globulin if appropriate. The woman should be encouraged to verbalize her feelings related to the loss. Referral to community resources may be appropriate.

Home care

Hemodynamically stable women with ectopic pregnancies are eligible for methotrexate therapy if the mass is unruptured and measures less than 4 cm in diameter by ultrasound (Simpson, 1996). Methotrexate therapy avoids surgery and is a safe, effective, and cost-conscious way of managing many cases of tubal pregnancy. Management is almost always accomplished on an outpatient basis.

The woman is informed how the medication works, what adverse effects are possible, who to call if she has concerns or problems develop, and the importance of follow-up care. After receiving the methotrexate injection, the woman will need to return at least weekly for follow-up laboratory studies for an average of 2 to 8 weeks. During that time, she is instructed to put nothing in the vagina (no tampons, douches, or intercourse) and to avoid sun exposure because the drug will make her more photosensitive (Powell & Spellman, 1996).

NURSE ALERT *The woman on methotrexate therapy who drinks alcohol and takes vitamins containing folic acid (such as prenatal vitamins) increases her risk of experiencing side effects of the drug or exacerbating the ectopic rupture.*

The issue of future fertility should be discussed. Any woman who has been diagnosed with an ectopic pregnancy should be told to contact her health care provider as soon as she suspects that she might be pregnant, because of the increased risk for recurrent ectopic pregnancy. These women may need referral to grief or infertility support groups. In addition to the loss of the current pregnancy, they are faced with the possibility of future pregnancy losses or infertility.

Hydatidiform mole (molar pregnancy)

Hydatidiform mole (molar pregnancy) is a gestational trophoblastic disease. There are two distinct types of hydatidiform moles: complete (or classic) mole and partial mole.

Incidence and etiology. Hydatidiform mole occurs in 0.6 to 1.1 of every 1,000 pregnancies in the United States and Europe, but a higher incidence has been reported in Asian countries (Cunningham et al., 1997). The etiology is unknown, although there may be an ovular defect or nutritional deficiency (such as carotene or protein) (Hammond & Bachus, 1994). Women at higher risk for hydatidiform mole formation are those who have undergone ovulation stimulation with clomiphene (Clomid) and those who are in their early teens or older than 40 years of age. The risk of a second mole is 1% to 2%.

Types. The complete mole results from fertilization of an egg whose nucleus has been lost or inactivated (Fig. 24-10, *A*). The nucleus of a sperm (23X) duplicates itself (resulting in the diploid number, 46XX) because the ovum has no genetic material or the material is inactive. The mole resembles a bunch of white grapes (Fig. 24-10, *B*). The fluid-filled vesicles grow rapidly, causing the uterus to be larger than expected for the duration of the pregnancy. Usually the complete mole contains no fetus, placenta, amniotic membranes, or

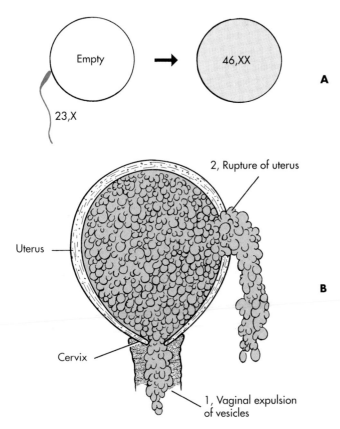

Fig. **24-10** **A,** Chromosomal origin of complete mole. Single sperm (color) fertilizes an "empty" ovum. Reduplication of sperm's 23,X set gives completely homozygous diploid 46,XX. Similar process follows fertilization of empty ovum by two sperm with two independently drawn sets of 23,X or 23,Y; both karyotypes of 46,XX and 46,XY can therefore result. **B,** Uterine rupture with hydatidiform mole. 1, Evacuation of mole through cervix. 2, Rupture of uterus and spillage of mole into peritoneal cavity (rare).

fluid. Maternal blood has no placenta to receive it; hemorrhage into the uterine cavity and vaginal bleeding therefore occur. In about 20% of cases of complete mole, progression toward choriocarcinoma occurs.

Partial moles often have embryonic or fetal parts and an amniotic sac present. Congenital anomalies are usually present. The potential for malignant transformation is much less (less than 5%) than that associated with the complete hydatidiform mole (Hammond & Bachus, 1994).

Signs and symptoms. The signs and symptoms of a complete hydatidiform mole in the early stages cannot be distinguished from those of normal pregnancy. Later, vaginal bleeding occurs in almost 95% of cases. The vaginal discharge may be dark brown (resembling prune juice) or bright red and either scant or profuse. It may continue for only a few days or intermittently for weeks. Early in pregnancy the uterus in approximately half of affected women is

significantly larger than expected from menstrual dates. The percentage of women with an excessively enlarged uterus increases as length of time since LMP increases. Approximately 25% of affected women have a uterus smaller than would be expected from menstrual dates.

Anemia from blood loss, excessive nausea and vomiting (hyperemesis gravidarum), and abdominal cramps caused by uterine distention are relatively common findings. Preeclampsia occurs in about 15% of cases, usually between 9 and 12 weeks of gestation, but any symptoms of PIH before 20 weeks of gestation may suggest hydatidiform mole. Hyperthyroidism and pulmonary embolization of trophoblastic elements occur infrequently but are serious complications of hydatidiform mole. Partial moles cause few of these symptoms and may be mistaken for an incomplete or missed abortion.

Passage of vesicles may occur around 16 weeks of gestation. There is no fetal movement, fetal heart rate, or palpable fetal parts. Some women have signs and symptoms of hyperthyroidism. A trophoblastic pulmonary embolus may develop in about 20% of women with hydatidiform mole (Berkowitz, Goldstein & Bernstein, 1991).

I CARE MANAGEMENT

Nursing assessments during prenatal visits should include observation for signs of molar pregnancy during the first 24 weeks. If hydatidiform mole is suspected, ultrasonography and serial β-hCG immunoassays will be used to confirm the diagnosis. The sonographic pattern of a molar pregnancy is characterized by a diffuse "snow storm" pattern. A β-hCG titer will remain high or rise above normal peak after the time at which it normally drops (70 to 100 days) (Cunningham et al., 1997).

Hospital care

Although most moles abort spontaneously, suction curettage offers a safe, rapid, and effective method of evacuation of hydatidiform mole if necessary (Hammond & Bachus, 1994). Induction of labor with oxytocic agents or prostaglandins is not recommended because of the increased risk of embolization of trophoblastic tissue (Copeland & Landon, 1996). Administration of Rh$_o$ (D) immune globulin to women who are Rh negative is necessary to prevent isoimmunization.

The nurse provides the woman and her family with information about the disease process, the necessity for a long course of follow-up, and the possible consequences of the disease. The nurse helps the woman understand and cope with pregnancy loss and recognize that the pregnancy was abnormal. The woman and her family are encouraged to express their feelings, and information is provided about support groups or counseling resources if needed. Explanations about the importance of the need to postpone a

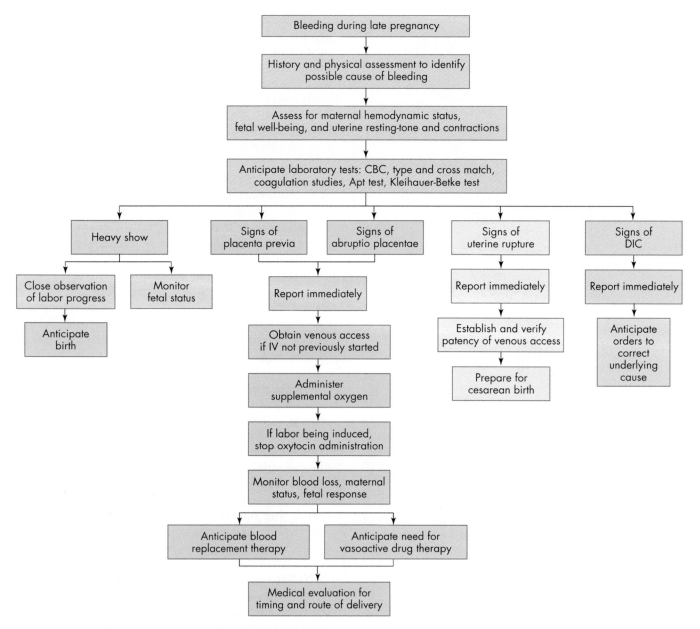

Fig. **24-11** Bleeding during late pregnancy. *CBC,* Complete blood count; *IV,* intravenous.

subsequent pregnancy and contraceptive counseling are provided to emphasize the importance of consistent and reliable use of the method chosen.

Home care

Follow-up management includes frequent physical and pelvic examinations along with biweekly measurements of β-hCG level until the level drops to normal and remains normal for 3 weeks. Monthly measurements are taken for 6 months, then every 2 months for a total of 1 year. A rising titer and an enlarging uterus may indicate choriocarcinoma.

To avoid confusion with signs of pregnancy, pregnancy should be avoided for 1 year. Any contraceptive method except an intrauterine device is acceptable. Oral contraceptives are highly effective. Referral to community support resources may be needed.

Late Pregnancy Bleeding

Late pregnancy bleeding disorders include placenta previa, premature separation of placenta (abruptio placentae), and cord insertion and placental variations. Expedient assessment for and diagnosis of the cause of bleeding are

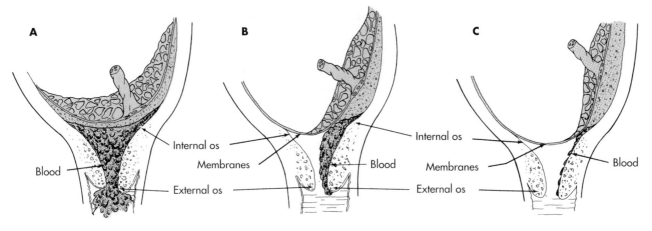

Fig. **24-12** Types of placenta previa after onset of labor. **A,** Complete, or total. **B,** Incomplete, or partial. **C,** Marginal, or low lying.

essential to reduce maternal and perinatal morbidity and mortality (Fig. 24-11).

Placenta previa

In **placenta previa,** the placenta is implanted in the lower uterine segment near or over the internal cervical os. The degree to which the internal cervical os is covered by the placenta has traditionally been used to classify three types of placenta previa (Fig. 24-12). Placenta previa often is described as *total* or complete if the internal os is entirely covered by the placenta when the cervix is fully dilated. *Partial* placenta previa implies incomplete coverage of the internal os. *Marginal* placenta previa indicates that only an edge of the placenta extends to the internal os but may extend onto the os during dilatation of the cervix during labor. The term *low-lying placenta* is used when the placenta is implanted in the lower uterine segment but does not reach the os.

Incidence and etiology. The incidence of placenta previa is 1 in 200 pregnancies (Scott, 1994b). The most important risk factor is previous cesarean birth possibly related to endometrial scarring. The risk increases with the number of previous cesarean births; in women with four or more, the risk of previa is nearly 10% (Benedetti, 1996). Other risk factors include multiple gestation, because of the larger placental area, closely spaced pregnancies, previous placenta previa, and advanced maternal age (older than 35 years) (Scott, 1994b).

Clinical manifestations. About 70% of women with placenta previa will have painless vaginal bleeding; 20% will have vaginal bleeding associated with uterine activity. Previa should be suspected whenever vaginal bleeding occurs after 24 weeks of gestation. This bleeding is associated with the stretching and thinning of the lower uterine segment that occurs during the third trimester. Placental attachment is gradually disrupted and bleeding occurs when the uterus is not able to adequately contract and stop blood flow from open vessels (Benedetti, 1996). The initial bleeding is usually a small amount and stops as clots form; however, it can recur at any time (Table 24-9). It is bright red in color.

Vital signs may be normal, even with heavy blood loss, because a pregnant woman can lose up to 40% of blood volume without showing signs of shock. Clinical presentation and decreasing urinary output may be better indicators of acute blood loss than vital signs alone (Veronikis & O'Grady, 1994). The fetal heart rate is reassuring unless there is a major detachment of the placenta.

Abdominal examination usually reveals a soft, relaxed, nontender uterus with normal tone. If the fetus is lying longitudinally, the fundal height is usually greater than expected for gestational age because the low placenta hinders descent of the presenting fetal part. Leopold's maneuvers may reveal a fetus in an oblique or breech position or lying transverse because of the abnormal site of placental implantation.

Maternal and fetal outcome. Maternal morbidity is about 5% and mortality is less than 1% with placenta previa (Scott, 1994b). Complications associated with placenta previa include preterm ROM, preterm birth, surgery-related trauma to structures adjacent to the uterus, anesthesia complications, blood transfusion reactions, overinfusion of fluids, other placental problems (such as placenta accreta, placenta percreta, and placenta increta), postpartum hemorrhage, anemia, and infection.

The greatest risk of fetal mortality is caused by preterm birth. Other fetal risks include hypoxia in utero and congenital anomalies. Infants who are small for gestational age or have IUGR have been associated with placenta previa; this association may be related to poor placental exchange or hypovolemia resulting from maternal blood loss and maternal anemia (Scott, 1994b).

TABLE 24-9 *Summary of Findings: Abruptio Placentae and Placenta Previa*

	ABRUPTIO PLACENTAE			
	GRADE 1 **MILD SEPARATION** **(10% TO 20%)**	**GRADE 2** **MODERATE SEPARATION** **(20% TO 50%)**	**GRADE 3** **SEVERE SEPARATION** **(>50%)**	**PLACENTA PREVIA**
Bleeding, external, vaginal	Minimal	Absent or moderate	Absent to moderate	Minimal to severe and life-threatening
Total amount of blood loss	<500 ml	1,000 to 1,500 ml	>1,500 ml	Varies
Color of blood	Dark red	Dark red	Dark red	Bright red
Shock	Rare; none	Mild shock	Common, often sudden, profound	Uncommon
Coagulopathy	Rare, none	Occasional DIC	Frequent DIC	None
Uterine tonicity	Normal	Increased, may be localized to one region or diffuse over uterus, uterus fails to relax between contractions	Tetanic, persistent uterine contraction, boardlike uterus	Normal
Tenderness (pain)	Usually absent	Present	Agonizing, unremitting uterine pain	Absent
Ultrasonographic findings				
Location of placenta	Normal, upper uterine segment	Normal, upper uterine segment	Normal, upper uterine segment	Abnormal, lower uterine segment
Station of presenting part	Variable to engaged	Variable to engaged	Variable to engaged	High, not engaged
Fetal position	Usual distribution*	Usual distribution*	Usual distribution*	Commonly transverse, breech, or oblique
PIH or chronic hypertension	Usual distribution*	Commonly present	Commonly present	Usual distribution*
Fetal effects	Normal FHR pattern	Nonreassuring FHR pattern	Nonreassuring FHR pattern, death can occur	Normal FHR pattern

Usual distribution refers to the usual variations of incidence seen when there is no concurrent problem.

I CARE MANAGEMENT

Assessment and Nursing Diagnoses

A woman who presents for care with third trimester vaginal bleeding requires immediate evaluation. Necessary history data include gravidity, parity, and a description of the bleeding (how long, precipitating event, estimation of amount). Other assessment data to be collected are the woman's general status, estimated gestational age, current amount of bleeding, vital signs, and fetal status (see Box 24-4). Laboratory studies include a complete blood count, determination of blood type and Rh status, a coagulation profile, and a possible type and crossmatch.

Placenta previa can be diagnosed using transabdominal ultrasound, which is accurate 93% to 97% of the time. False-negative and false-positive results usually occur as a result of factors such as an engaged cephalic presentation,

a posteriorly implanted placenta, maternal obesity, and compression of the lower uterine segment by an over-distended bladder. If the ultrasound reveals a normally implanted placenta, a speculum examination may be performed to rule out local causes of bleeding (such as cervicitis, polyps, or carcinoma of the cervix). Nursing Diagnoses for the woman experiencing placenta previa are listed in the accompanying box.

I Nursing Diagnoses

Woman Experiencing Placenta Previa
Decreased cardiac output related to:
• Excessive blood loss secondary to placenta previa
Fluid volume deficit related to:
• Excessive blood loss secondary to placenta previa

Continued

Risk for fluid volume excess related to:
- Fluid resuscitation

Altered peripheral tissue perfusion related to:
- Hypovolemia and shunting of blood to central circulation

Risk for injury (fetal) related to:
- Decreased placental perfusion secondary to placenta previa

Anxiety/fear related to:
- Maternal condition and pregnancy outcome

Knowledge deficit related to:
- Hospitalization and treatment regimens

Altered family processes related to:
- Mother's condition and hospitalization

Anticipatory grieving related to:
- Actual/perceived threat to self, pregnancy, or infant

Expected Outcomes of Care

Expected outcomes for the woman experiencing placenta previa may include the following. The woman will:
- Verbalize understanding of her condition and its management
- Identify and use available support systems
- Demonstrate compliance with prescribed activity limitations
- Develop no complications related to bleeding
- Carry the pregnancy to term or near term
- Give birth to a healthy infant

Plan of Care and Interventions

Hospital care

Active management. Once placenta previa has been diagnosed a management plan is developed based on gestational age, amount of bleeding, and fetal condition. If the woman is at term (greater than or equal to 37 weeks of gestation) and in labor or bleeding persistently, immediate delivery by cesarean is almost always indicated. In women with partial or marginal previas who have minimal bleeding, vaginal birth may be attempted. Vaginal birth may also be indicated for previable gestations or births involving intrauterine fetal demise (Benedetti, 1996).

If cesarean birth is undertaken, the nurse continuously assesses maternal and fetal status while preparing the woman for surgery. Maternal vital signs are assessed frequently for decreasing blood pressure, rising pulse rate, changes in level of consciousness (LOC), and oliguria. Fetal assessment is maintained by continuous electronic fetal monitoring to assess for signs of hypoxia.

Blood loss may not cease with the birth of the infant. The large vascular channels in the lower uterine segment may continue to bleed because of that segment's diminished muscle content. The natural mechanism to control bleeding so characteristic of the upper part of the uterus—the interlacing muscle bundles, the "living ligature" contracting around open vessels—is absent in the lower part of the uterus. Postpartum hemorrhage may therefore occur even if the fundus is contracted firmly.

Emotional support for the woman and her family is extremely important. The actively bleeding patient is concerned not only for her own well-being but for the well-being of her fetus. All procedures should be explained, and a support person should be present. The woman should be encouraged to express her concerns and feelings. If the woman and her support person or family desire pastoral support, the nurse can notify the hospital chaplain service or provide information about other supportive resources.

Expectant management. If the woman is less than 36 weeks of gestation, not in labor, and the bleeding is mild or has stopped, expectant management is generally the treatment of choice to give the fetus time to mature in utero.

Expectant management consists of rest and close observation. The woman is usually placed on bed rest, although she may be allowed bathroom privileges and limited activity (up in a wheelchair for an hour or so daily). Bleeding is assessed by checking the amount of bleeding on perineal pads, bed pads, and linens. Weighing pads, although not frequently used, is one way to more accurately assess blood loss: 1 gm represents 1 ml blood.

Ultrasonographic examinations may be done every 2 to 3 weeks. Fetal surveillance may include nonstress testing or biophysical profiles once or twice weekly. Serial laboratory values are evaluated for falling hemoglobin and hematocrit levels and changes in coagulation studies. Venous access with an IV infusion or heparin lock may be placed in case blood or blood component therapy is needed. Antepartum steroids (betamethasone) may be ordered to promote fetal lung maturity if the woman is less than 34 weeks of gestation.

No vaginal or rectal exams are performed, and the woman is placed on pelvic rest (nothing in the vagina). Once she reaches 37 weeks of gestation and fetal lung maturity is documented, cesarean birth can be scheduled. During her hospitalization, the woman with placenta previa should always be considered a potential emergency because massive blood loss with resulting hypovolemic shock can occur quickly if bleeding resumes. The possibility that she may require an emergency cesarean for delivery always exists. Placenta previa in a preterm gestation may be an indication for transfer to a tertiary perinatal center because many community hospitals are not equipped to perform emergency cesarean births 24 hours per day, 7 days per week.

Home care

Criteria for home care management vary with primary perinatal provider and home care agency. To be considered

PLAN OF CARE *Placenta Previa*

> **NURSING DIAGNOSIS** Decreased cardiac output related to bleeding secondary to placenta previa

Expected Outcomes *Patient will exhibit signs of increased blood volume and restoration of cardiac output (i.e., normal pulse and blood pressure, normal heart and breath sounds, normal skin color, tone and turgor, normal capillary refill).*

Nursing Interventions/*Rationales*

Palpate uterus for tenderness and tone; assess bleeding rate, amount, color, degree of bleeding, CBC values, and coagulation profile, to *determine severity of situation.* (Do not perform vaginal examination, because it may stimulate further bleeding)

Establish baseline data for cardiac output (vital signs; heart and breath sounds; skin color, tone, turgor; capillary refill; level of consciousness; urinary output; pulse oximetry) *to use as basis for evaluating effectiveness of treatment.*

Initiate intravenous therapy and/or blood transfusions and medications per physician order *to restore blood volume and prevent organ compromise to mother and fetus.*

Place woman on bed rest *to decrease oxygen demands.*

Monitor vital signs, intake and output, hemodynamic status and laboratory values *to evaluate treatment response.*

Provide emotional support to woman and her family (i.e., explain procedures and their rationale; explain what is happening and what to expect; keep support person present) *to allay fears and provide the family with some sense of control.*

After stabilization, teach woman home management, including bed rest, watching for spotting/bleeding, close follow-up with her health care provider and preparation for immediate return to hospital if needed *to prevent or stem further complications.*

> **NURSING DIAGNOSIS** Risk for injury to the fetus related to decreased uterine/placental perfusion secondary to bleeding

Expected Outcome *Patient will exhibit ongoing signs of fetal well-being (i.e., adequate fetal movement, normal FHR, reactive NST, normal BPP).*

Nursing Interventions/*Rationales*

Monitor fetus daily for signs of tachycardia, decreased movement, loss of reactivity on NST *to identify and treat changes in fetal status early.*

Obtain BPP per physician order *to assess for signs of chronic asphyxia.*

Maintain maternal side-lying position *to prevent compression of aorta and vena cava.*

> **NURSING DIAGNOSIS** Risk for infection related to anemia and bleeding secondary to placenta previa

Expected Outcome *Patient will show no signs of intrauterine infection.*

Nursing Interventions/*Rationales*

Monitor vital signs for elevated temperature, pulse, and blood pressure; monitor laboratory results for elevated WBC count, differential shift; check for uterine tenderness and malodorous vaginal discharge *to detect early signs of infection resulting from exposure of placental tissue.*

Provide/teach perineal hygiene *to decrease the risk of ascending infection.*

From Wong D & Perry S: *Maternal child nursing care,* St Louis, 1998, Mosby.

---

for home care referral, the woman must be in stable condition with no evidence of active bleeding and must have resources to be able to return to the hospital immediately if active bleeding resumes (Grohar, 1994; Simpson, 1992).

She must have close supervision by family or friends in the home. The woman should be taught how to assess fetal and uterine activity and bleeding and told to avoid intercourse, douching, and enemas. She should limit her activities according to the advice of her physician and be informed to keep all appointments for fetal testing, laboratory assessments, and prenatal care. Visits by a perinatal home care nurse may be arranged.

If hospitalization or home care with activity restriction is prolonged, the woman may have concerns about her work- or family-related responsibilities or may become bored with inactivity. She should be encouraged to participate in her own care and decisions about care as much as possible. Provision of diversionary activities or encouragement to participate in activities she enjoys and can do during bed rest is needed (see suggestions for activities in the box on p. 654).

Evaluation

The expected outcomes of care are used to evaluate the care for the woman with placenta previa (see Plan of Care).

Premature separation of placenta

Premature separation of the placenta, also termed **abruptio placentae** is the detachment of part or all of the placenta from its implantation site (Fig. 24-13). Separation

Abruptio placentae (premature separation)

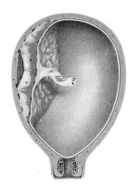
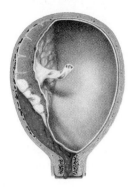
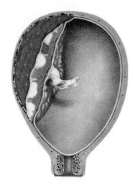

Partial separation
(concealed hemorrhage)

Partial separation
(apparent hemorrhage)

Complete separation
(concealed hemorrhage)

Fig. 24-13 Abruptio placentae. Premature separation of normally implanted placenta.

occurs in the area of the decidua basalis after the twentieth week of pregnancy and before the birth of the baby.

Incidence and etiology. Premature separation of the placenta is a serious event that accounts for significant maternal and fetal morbidity and mortality. Current literature reports that 1% of all pregnancies are complicated by abruption. Approximately 10% of cases of abruption are severe enough to threaten fetal viability (Hunter & Weiner, 1996), and premature separation of the placenta accounts for about 15% of all perinatal deaths. Approximately one third of infants born to women with premature separation of the placenta die. More than 50% of these deaths are the result of preterm birth; many others are the result of intrauterine hypoxia.

Maternal hypertension is probably the most consistently identified risk factor for abruption (Benedetti, 1996). Cocaine is also a risk factor, which is likely in part because cocaine use is associated with the development of hypertension. Blunt external abdominal trauma, most often the result of motor vehicle accidents or maternal battering, is an increasingly significant cause of placental abruption (Benedetti, 1996). Maternal smoking and poor nutrition may be associated with an increased risk. In the past, advanced maternal age and parity, short umbilical cord, and folic acid deficiency were all thought to cause increased risk; however, more recent research has failed to confirm this (Benedetti, 1996). There is a significantly high (10% to 30%) recurrence risk for placental abruption, which yields a relative risk of 30 to 40 times that in the general population (Thorp, 1993). A woman who has had two previous premature separations has a recurrence risk of 25% in the next pregnancy (Benedetti, 1996).

Classification systems. The most common classification of placental abruption is according to type and severity. This classification system grades an abruption as follows (Green, 1994; Hunter & Weiner, 1996).

Grade 1. The woman has vaginal bleeding perhaps with uterine tenderness and mild tetany, but neither mother nor baby is in distress. Approximately 10% to 20% of the total placental surface area is detached.

Grade 2. The woman has uterine tenderness and tetany, with or without external evidence of bleeding. The mother is not in shock, but there is fetal distress. Approximately 20% to 50% of the total surface area is detached.

Grade 3. Uterine tetany is severe, the woman is in shock (although the bleeding may not be obvious), and the fetus is dead. Often the woman has coagulopathy. Greater than 50% of the placental surface area detaches (Gilbert & Harmon, 1998).

These grades are often classified as mild (grade 1), moderate (grade 2), and severe (grade 3) (Hunter & Weiner, 1996).

Clinical manifestations. The separation may be partial or complete, or only the margin of the placenta may be involved. Bleeding from the placental site may dissect (separate) the membranes from the decidua basalis and flow out through the vagina, it may remain concealed (retroplacental hemorrhage), or it may do both (see Fig. 24-13). Clinical symptoms vary with degree of separation (see Table 24-9).

Classic symptoms of abruptio placentae include vaginal bleeding, abdominal pain, and uterine tenderness and contractions. Vaginal bleeding is present in as many as 70% to 80% of women with abruption (Green, 1994). It should be remembered that although abdominal pain and uterine tenderness are characteristic for this complication, either finding may be absent in the presence of a silent abruption (Konje & Walley, 1995). Bleeding may result in maternal hypovolemia (shock, oliguria, anuria) and coagulopathy. Mild to severe uterine hypertonicity is present. Pain is mild to severe and localized over one region of the uterus or diffuse over the uterus with a boardlike abdomen.

Extensive myometrial bleeding damages the uterine muscle. If blood accumulates between the separated placenta and the uterine wall, it may produce a **Couvelaire uterus.** The uterus appears reddish or purplish, it is ecchymotic, and contractility is lost. Shock may occur and is out of proportion to blood loss. Laboratory findings include a positive result of Apt test (blood in amniotic fluid); a drop in hemoglobin and hematocrit levels (which may appear later); and a drop in coagulation factor levels. Clotting defects (such as DIC) develop in 10% or 30% of patients. A Kleihauer-Betke stain may be ordered to determine the presence of fetal-to-maternal bleeding (transplacental hemorrhage).

Maternal, fetal, and neonatal outcomes. Maternal mortality approaches 1% for abruptio placentae; this condition remains a leading cause of maternal death. The mother's prognosis depends on the extent of placental detachment, overall blood loss, degree of DIC, and time between placental detachment and birth.

Maternal complications are associated with the abruption or its treatment. Hemorrhage, hypovolemic shock, hypofibrinogenemia, and thrombocytopenia are associated with severe abruption. Couvelaire uterus, DIC, and infection may occur. Renal failure and pituitary necrosis may result from ischemia. In rare cases, women who are Rh negative can become sensitized if fetal to maternal hemorrhage occurs and the fetal blood type is Rh positive.

Perinatal mortality ranges from 15% to 30% and occurs as a result of fetal hypoxia, preterm birth, and status as small for gestational age. Risks of neurologic defects are increased (Cunningham et al., 1997).

❙ CARE MANAGEMENT

Abruptio placentae should be highly suspected in the woman who presents with a sudden onset of intense, usually localized, uterine pain, with or without vaginal bleeding. Initial assessment is much the same as for placenta previa. Physical examination usually reveals abdominal pain, uterine tenderness, and contractions. The fundal height may be measured over time, since increasing fundal height indicates concealed bleeding. Vaginal bleeding is present in about 80% of cases (Benedetti, 1996). About 60% of live fetuses exhibit nonreassuring signs on the electronic fetal heart monitor, such as loss of variability and late decelerations; uterine hyperstimulation and increased resting tone may also be noted on the monitor tracing (Benedetti, 1996). Many women demonstrate coagulopathy, as evidenced by abnormal clotting studies (fibrinogen, platelet count, PT, PTT, fibrin split products). Sonographic examination is used to rule out placenta previa; however, it is not always diagnostic for abruption. A retroplacental mass may be detected by ultrasonographic examination, but negative findings do not rule out a life-threatening abruption (Cunningham et al., 1997; Scott, 1994b). Better imaging technology has made it possible to demonstrate ultrasonographic evidence of hemorrhage in more than 50% of cases of confirmed placental abruption (Benedetti, 1996).

Nursing diagnoses and expected outcomes of care are similar to those described for placenta previa.

Hospital care

Once abruption has been diagnosed, a management plan is developed. Treatment depends on the severity of blood loss and fetal maturity and status. If the abruption is mild and the fetus is less than 36 weeks of gestation and not in distress, expectant management may be implemented. The woman is hospitalized and observed closely for signs of bleeding and labor. The fetal status is also monitored with intermittent fetal heart rate monitoring and NST or biophysical profiles until fetal maturity is determined or until the woman's condition deteriorates and immediate birth is indicated. Use of corticosteroids to accelerate fetal lung maturity is appropriately included in the plan of care for expectant management (ACOG, 1994; Hunter & Weiner, 1996). Women who are Rh negative may be given Rh_o (D) immune globulin if fetal-to-maternal hemorrhage occurs and the fetal blood is Rh positive.

Delivery is the treatment of choice if the fetus is at term gestation or if the bleeding is moderate to severe and mother or fetus is in jeopardy. At least one large bore (16-gauge) intravenous line should be started. Maternal vital signs are monitored frequently to observe for signs of declining hemodynamic status, such as increasing pulse rate and decreasing blood pressure. Serial laboratory studies include hematocrit or hemoglobin determinations and clotting studies. Continuous electronic fetal monitoring is mandatory. An indwelling Foley catheter is inserted for continuous assessment of urine output, an excellent indirect measure of maternal organ perfusion (Benedetti, 1996).

Blood and fluid volume replacement will most likely be ordered, with a goal of maintaining the urine output at greater than or equal to 30 ml/hr and the hematocrit at greater than or equal to 30%. If this goal is not reached despite vigorous attempts at replacement, hemodynamic monitoring may be necessary (Benedetti, 1996). Fresh frozen plasma or cryoprecipitate may be given to maintain the fibrinogen level at a minimum of 100 to 150 mg/dl.

Vaginal birth is usually feasible and is especially desirable in cases of fetal demise. Cesarean birth should be reserved for cases of fetal distress or other obstetric indications. Cesarean birth should not be attempted when the woman has severe and uncorrected coagulopathy because it may well result in surgically uncontrollable bleeding (Benedetti, 1996).

Nursing care of patients experiencing moderate-to-severe abruption is demanding because it requires meticulous assessment of maternal and fetal condition, as described above. Information about abruptio placentae, including cause, treatment, and expected outcome, is given to the woman and her family. Emotional support is also extremely important because the woman and her family may be experiencing fetal loss in addition to the mother's critical illness.

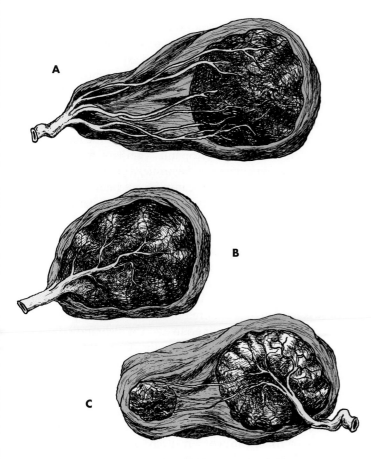

Fig. 24-14 Cord insertion and placental variations. **A,** Velamentous insertion of cord. **B,** Battledore placenta. **C,** Placenta succenturiate.

Home care

Women with abruptio placentae are not managed out of the hospital because the placenta can separate further at any time and immediate intervention or delivery may be necessary.

Cord insertion and placental variations

Velamentous insertion of the cord is a rare placental anomaly associated with placenta previa and multiple gestation. The cord vessels begin to branch at the membranes and then course onto the placenta (Fig. 24-14, *A*). ROM or traction on the cord may tear one or more of the fetal vessels. As a result the fetus may quickly bleed to death. Battledore (marginal) (Fig. 24-14, *B*) insertion of the cord increases the risk of fetal hemorrhage, especially after marginal separation of the placenta.

Rarely, the placenta may be divided into two or more separate lobes, resulting in **succenturiate placenta** (Fig. 24-14, *C*). Each lobe has a distinct circulation; the vessels collect at the periphery, and the main trunks unite eventually to form the vessels of the cord. Blood vessels joining the lobes may be supported only by the fetal membranes and

are therefore in danger of tearing during labor, birth, or expulsion of the placenta. During recovery of the placenta, one or more of the separate lobes may remain attached to the decidua basalis, preventing uterine contraction and increasing the risk of postpartum hemorrhage.

Clotting Disorders in Pregnancy
Normal clotting

Normally, there is a delicate balance (homeostasis) between the opposing hemostatic and fibrinolytic systems. The hemostatic system is involved in the lifesaving process. This system stops the flow of blood from injured vessels, in part through the formation of insoluble fibrin, which acts as a hemostatic platelet plug. The phases of the coagulation process involve an interaction of the coagulation factors in which each factor sequentially activates the factor next in line, the "cascade effect" sequence. The fibrinolytic system is the process through which the fibrin is split into fibrinolytic degradation products and circulation is restored.

Clotting problems

A history of abnormal bleeding, inheritance of unusual bleeding tendencies, and a report of significant aberrations of laboratory findings indicate a bleeding or clotting problem. For the obstetric patient, bleeding disorders are suspected if the woman has PIH, HELLP syndrome, retained dead fetus syndrome, amniotic fluid embolism, sepsis, or hemorrhage. Determination of hemostasis is made by testing the usual mechanisms for the control of bleeding, the function of platelets and the necessary clotting factors.

Disseminated intravascular coagulation. Disseminated intravascular coagulation (DIC) is a pathologic form of clotting that is diffuse and consumes large amounts of clotting factors, causing widespread external bleeding, internal bleeding, or both. DIC is an overactivation of the clotting cascade and the fibrinolytic system that results in depletion of platelets and clotting factors. This results in the formation of multiple fibrin clots throughout the body's vasculature, even in the microcirculation. Blood cells are destroyed as they pass through these fibrin-choked vessels. Thus, DIC results in a clinical picture of hemorrhage, anemia, and ischemia.

It is important to understand that DIC is always a secondary diagnosis. In the obstetric population, DIC is most often triggered by the release of large amounts of tissue thromboplastin, which occurs, for example, in abruptio placentae, retained dead fetus, and amniotic fluid embolus. Severe preeclampsia, HELLP syndrome, and gram-negative sepsis are examples of conditions that can also trigger DIC because of widespread damage to vascular integrity.

Medical management. The diagnosis of DIC is made according to clinical findings and laboratory markers. Physical examination reveals unusual bleeding; spontaneous bleeding from the woman's gums or nose may be noted. Petechiae may appear around a blood pressure cuff placed on the patient's arm. Excessive bleeding may occur from the site of a slight trauma (such as venipuncture sites, intramuscular or subcutaneous injection sites, nicks from shaving of perineum or abdomen, and injury from insertion of urinary catheter). Maternal symptoms may include tachycardia and diaphoresis.

Laboratory assessment includes a battery of tests often referred to as "clotting studies." These tests evaluate both the clotting and lysing systems and include PT, PTT, platelet count, fibrinogen level, and presence of fibrin split (or degradation) products. The clot retraction test, which is often performed when blood is drawn for clotting studies, provides a quick assessment of the body's ability to clot. Blood placed in a plain (red top) vacutainer tube should form a solid clot within 10 minutes. A positive clot retraction test indicates a fibrinogen level of at least 100 mg/dl. The clot retraction test can assist in clinical decision making while awaiting the results of laboratory tests.

In DIC, usually all of the clotting studies are abnormal. Both the PT and PTT are prolonged. The platelet count and the fibrinogen level are decreased. Fibrin split products are present.

Primary management in all cases of DIC involves correction of the underlying cause, which may be removal of the dead fetus, treatment of existing infection or of preeclampsia or eclampsia, or removal of a placental abruption. Other treatment is aimed at supporting physiologic functioning and replacing essential factors faster than the body can consume them. Intravenous fluids are given to replace volume lost through severe bleeding. Packed cells are administered to maintain enough circulating red blood cells to assure tissue oxygenation. Fresh frozen plasma or cryoprecipitate is given to replace fibrinogen and coagulation factors. Platelets may also be administered.

Clotting studies are repeated every couple of hours to determine the effects of therapy on the coagulation process. The aim of replacement therapy is to maintain a urine output of greater than or equal to 30 ml/hr, a hematocrit of greater than or equal to 30%, a fibrinogen level of greater than or equal to 150 mg/dl, and a platelet count of greater than or equal to 100,000 cells/mm^3 (Benedetti, 1996).

Nursing care. The nurse caring for the woman at risk for DIC must be aware of risk factors. Careful and thorough assessment is required, with particular attention to signs of bleeding (petechiae, oozing from injection sites, and hematuria). Because renal failure is one consequence of DIC, urinary output is carefully monitored, using an indwelling Foley catheter. Vital signs are assessed frequently.

If the woman is still pregnant, she will be maintained in a side-lying tilt to maximize blood flow to the uterus. Oxygen may be administered through a tight-fitting, rebreathing mask at 10 to 12 L/min, or per hospital protocol or physician order. Blood and blood products must be administered safely.

The educational and emotional needs of the woman and her family must be recognized and supported. They need information about her condition and explanations of unfamiliar equipment and procedures and will most likely be very anxious about the health of mother and baby.

Autoimmune thrombocytopenic purpura. Autoimmune thrombocytopenic purpura is an autoimmune disorder in which antiplatelet antibodies decrease the life span of the platelets. Thrombocytopenia, capillary fragility, and increased bleeding time are diagnostic. Autoimmune thrombocytopenic purpura may cause severe hemorrhage after cesarean birth or from cervical or vaginal lacerations. Incidences of postpartum uterine bleeding and vaginal hematomas are also increased.

Medical management focuses on control of platelet stability. Platelet transfusions are given to maintain the platelet count at 100,000 cells/mm^3. Corticosteroids are given if the diagnosis is made before or during pregnancy. If splenectomy is needed, it is deferred until after the puerperium.

von Willebrand's disease. von Willebrand's disease, a type of hemophilia, is probably the most common of all hereditary bleeding disorders (Cunningham et al., 1997). It results from a factor VIII deficiency and platelet dysfunction that is transmitted as an incomplete autosomal dominant trait to both sexes. Although von Willebrand's disease is rare, it is among the most common congenital clotting defects in American women of childbearing age. Symptoms include a familial bleeding tendency, previous bleeding episodes, prolonged bleeding time (the most important test), factor VIII deficiency (mild to moderate), and bleeding from mucous membranes. Factor VIII increases during pregnancy, and this increase may be sufficient to offset danger from hemorrhage during childbirth. von Willebrand's disease is variable in its clinical course, severity, and laboratory values, so it is possible for this condition to go undetected throughout pregnancy until bleeding problems develop following birth. If the woman is known to have von Willebrand's disease before labor, factor VIII levels should be monitored and cryoprecipitate given as needed to maintain activity at 40% of normal near term (Benedetti, 1996).

SURGERY DURING PREGNANCY

The incidence of surgery requiring anesthesia during pregnancy ranges from 0.2% to 2.2%, affecting an estimated 50,000 pregnant women each year. It is difficult to determine the true incidence because many surgeries may occur very early in gestation, before women recognize the pregnancy (Kendrick, 1994). The need for abdominal surgery occurs as frequently among pregnant women as among nonpregnant women of comparable age. However, pregnancy may make diagnosis more difficult. An enlarged uterus and displaced internal organs may make abdominal palpation more difficult, alter the position of an affected organ and/or change the usual signs and symptoms associated with a particular disorder. Three common conditions necessitating abdominal surgery during pregnancy are discussed: appendicitis, acute cholecystitis, and gynecologic problems.

Appendicitis

Appendicitis is the most common acute surgical condition seen in pregnancy, occurring approximately once in 2,000 pregnancies. This condition occurs in approximately the same frequency during each trimester of pregnancy and the postpartum period (Depp, 1996). The diagnosis of appendicitis is often delayed because the usual signs and symptoms mimic some normal changes of pregnancy such as nausea and vomiting and increased WBC count. As pregnancy progresses, the appendix is pushed upward and to the right from its usual anatomic location (see Fig. 9-14). Because of these changes, appendiceal rupture and peritonitis occur two to three times more often in pregnant women than in nonpregnant women.

The woman with appendicitis most commonly presents with abdominal pain, nausea and vomiting, and loss of appetite. Approximately half of these affected women have muscle guarding. Moving the uterus tends to increase the pain. Temperature may be normal or mildly increased (to 38.3° C). Because of the physiologic increase in WBCs that occurs in pregnancy, significant increases associated with appendicitis must be documented either by rising levels on serial samples or by an increasing left shift.

The diagnosis of appendicitis requires a high level of suspicion because the typical signs and symptoms are similar to those found in many other conditions, including pyelonephritis, round ligament pain, placental abruption, torsion of an ovarian cyst, cholecystitis, and preterm labor (Depp, 1996) (see Table 24-8).

Appendectomy before rupture usually does not require either antibiotic or tocolytic therapy. If surgery is delayed until after rupture, multiple antibiotics are ordered. Rupture is likely to result in preterm labor, perhaps necessitating the use of tocolytic agents. However, the value of prophylactic tocolytic therapy in cases of rupture has not been proven (Depp, 1996).

Acute Cholecystitis

Women are twice as likely to have cholelithiasis (presence of gallstones in the gallbladder) as men (Baker, 1995). Maternal adaptation significantly alters gallbladder function and the pregnant woman may be more vulnerable to gallstone formation (Varner, 1994). Decreased muscle tone allows gallbladder distention, thickening of bile, and prolonged emptying time. Increased progesterone levels result in a slight hypercholesterolemia.

Cholecystitis (inflammation of the gallbladder) is also more common in pregnancy, probably because pressure of the enlarged uterus interferes with the normal circulation and drainage of the gallbladder. Acute cholecystitis occurs in about 1 in 4,000 pregnancies, most often in older women who have been pregnant several times and who have a history of previous attacks (Depp, 1996).

Women with acute cholecystitis usually present with colicky abdominal pain, nausea, and vomiting. Fever and an increased leukocyte count may also be present. Ultrasound is often used to detect the presence of stones or dilatation of the common bile duct (Depp, 1996).

Usually the woman can be treated with medical therapy, consisting of antibiotics, antispasmodics, intravenous fluids, bowel rest, and nasogastric suctioning (Depp, 1996; Gleicher, 1992). Morphine should not be used as an analgesic because it may cause ductal spasm (Gleicher, 1992). The woman's condition should improve significantly within 48 hours of beginning treatment. Impaction of a stone in the cystic or common bile duct or development of pancreatitis may necessitate immediate cholecystectomy or cholecystotomy. If surgery is necessary, there is significant risk of subsequent preterm labor (Depp, 1996).

Gynecologic Problems

Ovarian cysts and twisting of ovarian cysts or adnexal tissues may occur. Pregnancy predisposes a woman to ovarian problems, especially during the first trimester. Problems include retained or enlarged cystic corpus luteum of pregnancy, ovarian cyst, and bacterial invasion of reproductive or other intraperitoneal organs.

Laparotomy or laparoscopy may be required to discriminate between ovarian problems and early ectopic pregnancy, appendicitis, or other infectious processes.

▌CARE MANAGEMENT

Initial assessment of the pregnant woman requiring surgery focuses on her presenting signs and symptoms. A thorough history and physical examination are performed as described above. Laboratory testing includes, at a minimum, a complete blood count with differential and a urinalysis. Additional laboratory and other diagnostic tests may well be necessary to reach a diagnosis. In addition, fetal heart rate and activity, along with uterine activity should be monitored and constant vigilance for symptoms of impending obstetric complications maintained. The extent of presurgery assessment is determined by the immediacy of surgical intervention and the specific disorder that requires surgery.

Hospital care

When surgery becomes necessary during pregnancy, the woman and her family are concerned about the effects of the procedure and medication on fetal well-being and the course of pregnancy. Kendrick (1994) reported that every participant in her study of women undergoing surgery during pregnancy described her greatest fear related to surgery as the fear of losing her baby. An important part of preoperative nursing care is encouraging the woman to express her fears, concerns, and questions.

Preoperative care for a pregnant woman differs from that for a nonpregnant woman in one significant aspect: the presence of at least one other person, the fetus. Continuous FHR and uterine contraction monitoring should be performed if the fetus is considered viable. Procedures such as preparation of the operative site and time of insertion of IV lines and urinary retention catheters vary with the physician and the facility. However, in every instance there is a total restriction of solid foods and liquids or a clear specification of the type, amount, and time at which clear liquids may be taken before surgery. Food by mouth is restricted for several hours before a scheduled procedure. Even if she has had nothing by mouth–but more important, if surgery is unexpected–the woman is in danger of vomiting and aspirating, and special precautions are taken before anesthetic is administered (e.g., administering an antacid).

Intraoperatively, perinatal nurses may collaborate with the surgical staff to increase their knowledge about the special needs of pregnant women undergoing surgery. One intervention to improve fetal oxygenation is positioning the woman on the operating table with a lateral tilt to avoid maternal venacaval compression (Kendrick, 1994). Perinatal nurses may also recommend continuous fetal and uterine monitoring during the procedure because the risk of preterm labor, especially following abdominal surgery, is great. Monitoring may be accomplished using sterile aquasonic gel and a sterile sleeve for the transducer. During abdominal surgery, uterine contractions may be manually palpated (Kendrick, 1994).

In the immediate recovery period, general observations and care pertinent to postoperative recovery are initiated. Frequent assessments are carried out for several hours following surgery. Whether the woman is cared for in the surgical postanesthesia recovery area or in labor and delivery, continuous fetal and uterine monitoring will likely be initiated or resumed because of the increased risk of preterm labor. Tocolysis may be necessary if preterm labor occurs (see Chapter 25).

Home care

Plans for the woman's return home and for convalescent care should be completed as early as possible before discharge. Depending on her insurance coverage, nursing care may be provided through a home health agency. If not, the woman and other support persons need to be taught necessary skills and procedures, such as care of the incision and/or dressing changes. Ideally, the woman and other caregivers should have opportunities for supervised practice before discharge, so they can feel comfortable with their knowledge and ability before being totally

---

BOX 24-5 *Discharge Teaching for Home Care*

- Care of incision site
- Diet and elimination related to gastrointestinal function
- Signs and symptoms of developing complications: wound infection, thrombophlebitis, pneumonia
- Equipment needed and technique for assessing temperature
- Recommended schedule for resumption of activities of daily living
- Treatments and medications ordered
- List of resource persons and their telephone numbers
- Schedule of follow-up visits
If birth has not occurred:
- Assessment of fetal activity (kick counts)
- Signs of preterm labor

---

responsible for providing care. Box 24-5 lists information that should be included in discharge teaching for the postoperative patient. The woman may also need referrals to various community agencies for evaluation of the home situation, child care, home health care, and financial or other assistance.

TRAUMA DURING PREGNANCY

Trauma continues to be a common complication during pregnancy because of the continuation of usual activities by the majority of pregnant women in the United States. Pregnant women are at the same risk as other citizens for vehicular crashes, falls, industrial mishaps, violence, and other injuries in the home and community.

Significance

Approximately 7% of pregnancies have been reported to be complicated by physical trauma (Esposito, 1994). As pregnancy progresses, the risk of trauma seems to increase because more cases of trauma are reported in the third trimester than earlier in gestation. Approximately 10% of injuries are reported in the first trimester, 40% during the second, and 50% during the third (Troiano, 1991).

Acts of violence are increasing in record numbers throughout the United States. Violence is now viewed as a major public health problem (Huzel & Remsburg-Bell, 1996). About 17% (1 in 6) adult pregnant women are physically or sexually abused during pregnancy. Abuse that is already occurring frequently escalates during pregnancy (Greenberg et al., 1997; McFarlane, 1993).

The majority of maternal injuries are a result of motor vehicle crashes, followed by falls and direct assaults to the abdomen (Coleman, Trianfo & Rund, 1997). Statistics show that trauma is the leading nonobstetric cause of maternal death (Depp, 1996). Maternal death caused by trauma is usually the result of head injury or hemorrhagic shock (Lavery & Staten-McCormick, 1995).

Trauma increases the incidence of spontaneous abortion, preterm labor, abruptio placentae, and stillbirth (Greenberg et al., 1997; Pearlman & Tintinalli, 1991). The effect of trauma on pregnancy is influenced by the length of gestation, type and severity of the trauma, and degree of disruption of uterine and fetal physiologic features. Fetal death as a result of trauma is more common than the occurrence of both maternal and fetal death. Less serious trauma is associated with numerous complications for pregnancy, including fetomaternal hemorrhage, abruptio placentae, intrauterine fetal death, and preterm labor and delivery (Pearlman & Tintinalli, 1991). Careful evaluation of mother and fetus after all types of trauma is imperative.

Etiology

Motor vehicle accidents and battering most often result in blunt abdominal trauma. Maternal and fetal mortality and morbidity associated with motor vehicle accidents are directly correlated with whether the mother remains inside the vehicle or is ejected. Death is usually the result of a head injury or exsanguination from a major vessel rupture. Maternal death usually results in fetal death. The most common fetal injury in severe trauma is skull fracture with subsequent intracranial hemorrhage (Pearlman & Tintinalli, 1991). Serious retroperitoneal hemorrhage after lower abdominal and pelvic trauma is reported more frequently during pregnancy. Serious maternal abdominal injuries are usually the result of splenic rupture or liver or renal injury.

When maternal survival of trauma occurs, fetal death is usually the result of abruptio placentae occurring within 48 hours of the accident (Pearlman & Tintinalli, 1991). Placental separation is thought to be a result of deformation of the elastic myometrium around the relatively inelastic placenta (ACOG, 1991). Shearing of the placental edge from the underlying decidua basalis results and is worsened by the increased intrauterine pressure resulting from the impact. It is imperative that all pregnant victims be carefully evaluated for signs and symptoms of abruptio placentae after even minor blunt abdominal trauma. Signs and symptoms of abruptio placentae include uterine tenderness or pain, uterine irritability, uterine contractions, vaginal bleeding, leaking of amniotic fluid, or a change in fetal heart rate characteristics. A second-generation fetal monitor with autocorrelation for continuous EFM may show early signs of abruptio placentae, including characteristics such as a change in baseline rate, loss of accelerations or the presence of late decelerations.

Pelvic fracture may result from severe injury and may produce bladder trauma or retroperitoneal bleeding with the two-point displacement of pelvic bones that usually occurs. One point of displacement is commonly at the symphysis pubis and the second point is posterior because of the structure of the pelvis. Careful evaluation for clinical signs of internal hemorrhage is indicated.

Uterine rupture as a result of trauma is rare, occurring in only 0.6% of all reported cases of trauma during pregnancy. Uterine rupture depends on numerous factors, including gestational age and the intensity of the impact and the presence of a predisposing factor such as a distended uterus caused by polyhydramnios or multiple gestation or the presence of a uterine scar resulting from previous uterine surgery (Pearlman, Tintinalli & Lorenz, 1990). When uterine rupture occurs, the force responsible is usually a direct, high-energy blow. Fetal death is common with traumatic uterine rupture. However, maternal death occurs less than 10% of the time, and when it occurs it is usually the result of massive injuries sustained from an impact severe enough to rupture the uterus.

▌ CARE MANAGEMENT

Immediate stabilization

Immediate priorities for stabilization of the pregnant woman after trauma should be identical to those of the nonpregnant trauma patient. Pregnancy should not result in any restriction of the usual diagnostic, pharmacologic, or resuscitative procedures or maneuvers (ACOG, 1991). Priorities of care for the pregnant woman after trauma must be to resuscitate the woman and stabilize her condition **FIRST** and then consider fetal needs. The trauma team should follow a methodic evaluation of maternal status to ensure complete assessment and stabilization of the mother. Fetal survival depends on maternal survival, and stabilization of the mother improves fetal chance of survival.

In cases of minor trauma, the woman is evaluated for vaginal bleeding, uterine irritability, abdominal tenderness, abdominal pain or cramps, and evidence of hypovolemia. A change in the absence of FHR or fetal activity, leakage of amniotic fluid, and presence of fetal cells in the maternal circulation are also included in the assessment.

In cases of major trauma, the systematic evaluation begins with a primary survey and the initial "ABCs" of resuscitation: establishment of and maintaining an *airway*, ensuring adequate *breathing*, and maintenance of an adequate *circulatory volume*.

After immediate resuscitation and successful stabilization measures, a more detailed secondary survey of the mother and fetus should be accomplished. A complete physical assessment including all body systems is performed. The evaluation and care is usually performed by two teams of care providers. The first team focuses on the mother and the second focuses on the fetus and any pregnancy-related problems. Table 24-10 summarizes posttrauma care for the pregnant woman and fetus.

TABLE 24-10 *Priorities for Perinatal TRAUMA Management*

ACTIVITY	TEAM A (MOTHER)	TEAM B (FETUS)
T = Triage*	Assess ABCs —Airway —Breathing —Circulation	Assess fetus —Cardiac activity —Gestational age Assess placenta for abruption

R = Resuscitation	Perform CPR
	Infuse crystalloid fluids
	Administer oxygen at 8-10 L/m in by mask
	Administer blood as indicated
	  (in emergency situation, O-negative
	  blood can be used)
		Position mother in left lateral tilt

A = Assessment	Assess for maternal injuries
	  (similar to that in nonpregnant patient)
	Assess vital signs; level of consciousness;
	  respiratory status as to depth,
	  irregularity, and breath sounds
		Assess FHR and uterine contractions
		  with EFM
		Assess for vaginal bleeding and rupture
		  of membranes
		Kleihauer-Betke test may be done to rule
		  out fetal hemorrhage

U = Ultrasound/uterine evaluation	Evaluate uterine cavity for hemorrhage	Evaluate fundal height
		Palpate for uterine tenderness,
		  contractions, or irritability
		Ultrasound may be done to determine
		  placental or fetal injury and placental
		  location
		Amniocentesis may be done to assess
		  fetal lung maturity or intrauterine
		  bleeding

M = Management/monitor	Decide initial management and needed
	  continual monitoring
		Decide to monitor or deliver depending
		  on status of mother and fetus and risk
		  of prematurity

A = Activate transport/transfer	After stabilization, transport/transfer
	  to critical care, operating suite, or
	  level III perinatal unit
		Activate neonatal team for consultation,
		  transfer, or transport as necessary

From Gilbert E & Harmon J: *Manual of high risk pregnancy and delivery*, ed 2, St Louis, 1998, Mosby.
CPR, Cardiopulmonary resuscitation; *FHR*, fetal heart rate; *EFM*, electronic fetal monitor.
*Mother is first priority, then fetus.

The perinatal nurse is often called on to function collaboratively with emergency department or trauma unit staff members in providing care for the pregnant trauma victim.

In addition to assisting with stabilization of the woman, the nurse will likely be providing emotional support for the injured woman and her family. If the trauma is the result of a motor vehicle accident, other family members may also have been critically injured or killed. The nurse collaborates with staff members in other units of the same hospital, as well as at other hospitals, to make sure that questions are answered and consistent information given. Grief support may also be necessary.

The woman may be discharged home after several hours of evaluation following minor trauma. Her vital signs should be stable, with no evidence of bleeding at the time of discharge. The fetal tracing should be reassuring before monitoring is discontinued and the woman discharged.

Education for the woman and her family is very important. She should be instructed to contact her health care provider immediately if changes in fetal movement or signs and symptoms indicative of preterm labor, premature rupture of membranes or placental abruption develop. If the trauma occurred as a result of a motor vehicle accident, the woman should be instructed about the importance of wearing a seat belt and given directions for using it correctly during pregnancy (position the lap belt over hips and thighs, rather than across the abdomen) (see Fig. 10-17). If the trauma occurred as a result of domestic violence, the woman may need information about the abuse cycle (Chapter 4); referral to a crisis center, law enforcement agency, or counseling center; and help in forming a safety plan (Greenberg et al., 1997; Huzel & Remsburg-Bell, 1996). It is important that the woman be allowed to make her own decisions in regard to seeking help and filing

TABLE 24-11 *Pregnancy and Fetal Effects of Common STDs*

INFECTION	PREGNANCY EFFECTS	FETAL EFFECTS
Chlamydia	Premature rupture of membranes* Preterm labor*	Preterm birth* Conjunctivitis Pneumonia
Gonorrhea	Intraamniotic infection Preterm labor Premature rupture of membranes Postpartum endometritis Spontaneous abortion	Preterm birth Sepsis Conjunctivitis
Group B streptococcus	Preterm labor Premature rupture of membranes Chorioamnionitis Postpartum sepsis Urinary tract infections	Preterm birth* Early-onset sepsis
Herpes simplex	Rare—infection	Systemic infection
Human papillomavirus (HPV)	Dystocia from large lesions Excessive bleeding from lesions following birth trauma	Respiratory papillomatosis (rare)
Syphilis	Preterm labor Spontaneous abortion	Preterm birth Stillbirth Congenital infection

Data from Cunningham F et al.: *Williams obstetrics,* ed 20, Stamford, Conn, 1997, Appleton & Lange; Gilbert E & Harmon J: *Manual of high risk pregnancy and delivery,* ed 2, St Louis, 1998, Mosby; and Walker C & Sweet R: HIV and other sexually transmitted diseases in pregnancy. In Reece E et al., editors: *Medicine of the fetus and mother,* Philadelphia, 1992, JB Lippincott.
*Controversial.

criminal charges. At the same time, she should be reassured that no one deserves abuse, whether physical, sexual, or emotional (ACOG, 1993).

SEXUALLY TRANSMITTED INFECTIONS IN PREGNANCY

Sexually transmitted infections in pregnancy are responsible for significant morbidity and mortality. Some consequences of maternal infection, such as infertility and sterility, last a lifetime. Psychosocial sequelae may include altered interpersonal relationships and lowered self-esteem. Congenitally acquired infection may affect a child's length and quality of life.

Chapter 6 discusses the diagnosis and management of STDs. Chapter 28 discusses neonatal effects and management. This discussion focuses only on the effects of several common STDs on pregnancy and the fetus (Table 24-11). It is sometimes difficult to predict these effects with certainty. Published studies vary in their findings, perhaps because many confounding variables are often involved. Maternal age, coinfection with other STDs, coexisting alcohol and illicit drug use, single marital status, minority status, urban residence, and low socioeconomic status are examples of often quoted risk factors that may confound research results (Adimora et al., 1994). Effects on preg-

nancy and the fetus also vary according to whether the infection has been treated at the time of labor and birth. The effects of STDs on pregnancy and the fetus definitely need further investigation.

CARE MANAGEMENT

Factors that influence the development and management of STDs during pregnancy include previous history of STD or PID, number of current sexual partners, frequency of intercourse, and anticipated sexual activity during pregnancy. Lifestyle choices also may affect STDs in the perinatal period. Women who use intravenous drugs or have partners who use intravenous drugs are at risk. Other lifestyle factors that increase susceptibility to STDs (through suppressive effects on the immune system) include smoking, alcohol use, inadequate or poor nutrition, and high levels of fatigue or personal stress.

Physical examination and laboratory studies to determine the presence of STDs in the pregnant woman are the same as those done in nonpregnant women (see Chapter 6).

Treatment of specific STDs may be different for the pregnant woman and may even be different at different stages of pregnancy. Table 24-12 describes the treatment of common STDs during pregnancy. Infected women need instruction on how to take prescribed medications, information on

| TABLE 24-12 | *Treatment of Common STDs in Pregnancy* |

STD	TREATMENT	NURSING CONSIDERATIONS
Chlamydia	Erythromycin 500 mg PO qid × 7 days; or amoxicillin 500 mg PO tid × 14 days	Instruct patient to take after meals and with 8 oz water; instruct partner to be tested and treated if needed.
Herpes	Acyclovir is not approved for use in pregnancy unless patient is in research studies; treat symptoms	Instruct patient in comfort measures: keep lesions clean and dry; use compresses to lesions (cold milk, colloidal oatmeal) every 2 to 4 hr, sitz baths; patient should abstain from intercourse while lesions are present; if woman has active lesions at time of labor, a cesarean birth will usually be performed to prevent perinatal transmission.
Gonorrhea	Ceftriaxone 125 mg IM × 1 dose, followed by erythromycin 500 mg PO qid × 7 days or amoxicillin 500 mg PO tid × 14 days	Screening is done at first prenatal visit; repeated in third trimester if high risk. Instruct partner to be tested and treated if needed. Infants are treated within 1 hour of birth with ophthalmic erythromycin or tetracycline ointment.
Group B streptococcus	Penicillin G 5 million U IV initial dose followed by 2.5 million U IV q4h during labor or ampicillin 2 gm IV initial dose followed by 1 gm IV q4h	Pregnant women should be screened at 36-37 weeks' gestation; if positive or status unknown at time of labor, the woman is treated.
Hepatitis B	For exposure, hepatitis B immune globulin 0.06 mg/kg IM; repeat in 1 month, followed by hepatitis B vaccine series	Screening should be at first prenatal visit and prescreening in third trimester for high-risk patients; treatment is supportive—bed rest, high-protein, low-fat diet, increased fluid intake; the woman should avoid medications that are metabolized in the liver.
Human papillomavirus	Trichoacetic acid (TCA) 80% to 90% applied topically to warts 1 to 3 times a week; xylocaine jelly applied for burning sensations; cryotherapy with liquid nitrogen in second and third trimesters; CO_2 laser therapy	Podophyllum and 5-fluorouracil are possibly teratogenic and should not be used in pregnancy; inform partners to be tested and treated if needed; couples should use condoms for intercourse; inform patients that smoking can decrease effects of therapy.
Syphilis	Benzathine penicillin G 2.4 million U IM × 1 No proven alternatives to penicillin in pregnancy; women who have a history of allergy to penicillin should be desensitized and treated with penicillin	Treatment cures maternal infection and prevents congenital syphilis 98% of the time; routine screening during pregnancy should be at the first prenatal visit and in the third trimester in women at high risk; partners should be tested and treated if needed.
Trichomonas	Metronidazole 2 gm PO × 1	Inform partners to be treated; patients should avoid alcohol and vinegar products to avoid nausea and vomiting, intestinal cramping, and headaches; not recommended during lactation; stop breastfeeding, treat; resume in 48 hours after last dose. Women may use breast pump and discard milk to prevent interruption of milk supply.
Candidiasis	Over-the-counter topical agents; butoconazole, clotriamazole, miconazole, or terconazole; use for 7 days	May be used during lactation.
Bacterial vaginosis	Metronidazole 250 mg PO tid × 7 days	See Trichomonas; infection may increase risk of preterm labor; women are usually asymptomatic.

whether their partner(s) also need to be evaluated and treated, and a review of preventive measures to avoid reinfection.

Effects on Pregnancy and the Fetus
TORCH infections

*T*oxoplasmosis, *o*ther infections (such as hepatitis), *r*ubella virus, *c*ytomegalovirus (CMV), and *h*erpes simplex virus, known collectively as **TORCH infections,** comprise a group of organisms capable of crossing the placenta and adversely affecting the development of the fetus. Generally, all TORCH infections produce influenza-like symptoms in the mother, but fetal and neonatal effects are more serious. TORCH infections and their maternal, fetal, and neonatal effects are discussed in Table 24-13.

Toxoplasmosis

Toxoplasmosis is a protozoan infection associated with the consumption of infested raw or undercooked meat and with poor handwashing after handling infected cat litter. Pregnant women with HIV antibodies are at higher risk because toxoplasmosis is a common accompanying opportunistic infection. The presence of toxoplasmosis can be determined through blood studies, although laboratory diagnosis is difficult. Women at risk for infection should have toxoplasmosis titers evaluated. Acute infection in pregnancy produces influenza-like symptoms and lymphadenopathy in some women but no symptoms in others. Spontaneous abortion may occur.

The pharmaceutic treatment of choice for toxoplasmosis is a combination of pyrimethamine and sulfadiazine. Although pyrimethamine may be potentially harmful to the fetus, treatment of the parasitemia is essential (Fanaroff & Martin, 1997).

Other infections

The primary infection included in the category of other infections is hepatitis. Hepatitis A, or infectious hepatitis, a virus spread by droplets or hands, is associated with poor handwashing after defecation. Hepatitis A is an uncommon complication of pregnancy, and perinatal transmission is rare but can occur. Pregnancy effects include spontaneous abortion and influenza-like symptoms of fever, malaise, nausea. Possible effects of untreated exposure to the fetus in the first trimester include fetal anomalies, preterm birth, fetal or neonatal hepatitis, and intrauterine fetal death. Gamma-globulin is given to infected mothers and exposed neonates for prophylaxis (Fanaroff & Martin, 1997).

Hepatitis B virus (HBV) was discussed in Chapter 6. It is a major concern in pregnancy. Acute HBV infection occurs in 1 to 2 per 10,000 pregnancies, while chronic infections occur in 5 to 15 per 1,000 pregnancies. The rate of transmission to the fetus varies. The infection is rarely trans-

mitted to the fetus in the second trimester. Women in the third trimester have up to a 60% chance of transmitting the infection to the fetus (Fanaroff & Martin, 1997). Most infections are transmitted during vaginal birth when the newborn infant is exposed to contaminated blood and genital secretions.

During pregnancy, common symptoms include fever, rash, anorexia, malaise, myalgias, and, if the liver is acutely affected, jaundice, right upper quadrant pain, and nausea and vomiting. Fetal and neonatal effects include maternal-fetal transmission (approximately 90% transmission rate), sequelae of prematurity, and fetal or neonatal hepatitis.

The CDC (1998) recommends that *all* women be screened for HBV (serum HBsAg) early in pregnancy and those at high risk rescreened in the third trimester. Approximately 10% of women are chronic HBV carriers. Populations at risk who are seronegative should be given the three-dose series of HBV recombinant vaccine. Plasma-derived vaccines are no longer produced in the United States; use of such vaccines are now limited to immunocompromised and yeast-allergic patients. Vaccination during pregnancy is not thought to pose risks to the fetus. Hepatitis B immune globulin may be combined with HBV vaccination within 14 days of HBV exposure to prevent infection (see Table 24-12).

Hepatitis C is another type of viral hepatitis prevalent chiefly among users of intravenous drugs and recipients of multiple blood transfusions. This infection is of growing concern because perinatal transmission has been implicated in a few cases but no immunoprophylaxis is yet available. Hepatitis D is similarly found among users of intravenous drugs and recipients of multiple transfusions; however, immunization against HBV is also protective against vertical perinatal transmission of hepatitis D.

Infections other than hepatitis may also be identified as "other" TORCH infections. These include group B streptococci, varicella, and HIV.

Rubella

Rubella, also called German measles or 3-day measles, is a viral infection transmitted by droplets (such as from an infected person's sneeze). Fever, rash, and mild lymphedema are usually seen in the infected mother. Consequences for the fetus are much more serious and include spontaneous abortion, congenital anomalies (referred to as congenital rubella syndrome), and death. Vaccination of pregnant women is contraindicated because a rubella infection may develop after the vaccine is administered. Rubella vaccine is given to women who are not immune as part of preconceptional counseling, with instructions to use contraception for at least 3 months after vaccination.

TABLE 24-13 *Maternal Infection: TORCH*

INFECTION	MATERNAL EFFECTS	FETAL EFFECTS	COUNSELING:PREVENTION, IDENTIFICATION, AND MANAGEMENT
Toxoplasmosis (protozoa)	Acute infection similar to influenza, lymphadenopathy Woman immune after first episode (except in immunocompromised patients)	With maternal acute infection, parasitemia Less likely to occur with maternal chronic infection Abortion likely with acute infection early in pregnancy	Use good handwashing technique Avoid eating raw meat and exposure to litter used by infected cats; if cats in house, have toxoplasma titer checked If titer is rising during early pregnancy, abortion may be considered an option
Other Hepatitis A (infectious hepatitis) (virus)	Abortion, cause of liver failure during pregnancy Fever, malaise, nausea, and abdominal discomfort	Exposure during first trimester, fetal anomalies, fetal or neonatal hepatitis, preterm birth, intrauterine fetal death	Usually spread by droplet or hand contact especially by culinary workers; gamma-globulin can be given as prophylaxis for hepatitis A
Hepatitis B (serum hepatitis) (virus)	May be transmitted sexually, symptoms variable—fever, rash, arthralgia, depressed appetite, dyspepsia, abdominal pain, generalized aching, malaise, weakness, jaundice, tender and enlarged liver	Infection occurs during birth Maternal vaccination during pregnancy should present no risk for fetus (however, data are not available)	Generally passed by contaminated needles, syringes, or blood transfusions; also can be transmitted orally or by coitus (but incubation period is longer); hepatitis B immune globulin can be given prophylactically after exposure Hepatitis B vaccine recommended for populations at risk Populations at risk are women from Asia, Pacific islands, Indochina, Haiti, South Africa, Alaska (women of Eskimo descent); other women at risk include health care providers, users of intravenous drugs, those sexually active with multiple partners or single partner with multiple risks
Rubella (3-day German measles) (virus)	Rash, fever, mild symptoms; suboccipital lymph nodes may be swollen; some photophobia Occasionally arthritis or encephalitis Spontaneous abortion	Incidence of congenital anomalies—first month 50%, second month 25%, third month 10%, fourth month 4% Exposure during first 2 months—malformations of heart, eyes, ears, or brain, abnormal dermatoglyphics Exposure after fourth month—systemic infection, hepatosplenomegaly, intrauterine growth restriction, rash	Vaccination of pregnant women contraindicated; pregnancy should be prevented for 3 months after vaccination; pregnant women nonreactive to hemagglutinin-inhibition antigen can be safely vaccinated after birth

TABLE 24-13 *Maternal Infection: TORCH—cont'd*

INFECTION	MATERNAL EFFECTS	FETAL EFFECTS	COUNSELING:PREVENTION, IDENTIFICATION, AND MANAGEMENT
Cytomegalovirus (CMV) (a herpes virus)	Respiratory or sexually transmitted asymptomatic illness or mononucleosis-like syndrome, may have cervical discharge No immunity develops	Fetal death or severe, generalized disease—hemolytic anemia and jaundice, hydrocephaly or microcephaly, pneumonitis, hepatosplenomegaly, deafness	Virus may be reactivated and cause disease in utero or during birth in subsequent pregnancies; fetal infection may occur during passage through infected birth canal; disease is commonly progressive through infancy and childhood
Herpes genitalis (herpes simplex virus, type 2 [HSV-2])	Primary infection with painful blisters, rash, fever, malaise, nausea, headache; pregnancy risks include spontaneous abortion, preterm labor, stillbirths	Transplacental infection is rare; congenital effects include skin lesions and scarring, IUGR, mental retardation, microcephaly	Risk of transmission is greatest during vaginal birth if woman has active lesions Acyclovir not recommended in pregnancy; treat symptomatically (see Table 24-12)

Cytomegalovirus

Maternal infection with cytomegalovirus (CMV) may begin as a mononucleosis-like syndrome. In most adults the onset of CMV infection is uncertain and asymptomatic; however, the disease may remain subclinical for years. This virus is primarily transmitted by respiratory droplets but has also been isolated from semen, cervical and vaginal secretions, breast milk, placental tissue, urine, feces, and banked blood. Maternal CMV infection may be diagnosed serologically because many women have evidence of CMV infection. Women who show CMV infection in pregnancy (by positive viral titers) usually have chronic or recurrent infections (Fanaroff & Martin, 1997).

Women at risk for infection include those who work in or have children in day care centers, institutions for the mentally retarded, or certain health settings (such as nursery, dialysis, laboratories, and oncology).

In the United States 1% to 2% of infants have congenital CMV infection. Fetal infection can cause microcephaly; eye, ear, and dental defects; and mental retardation.

There is no treatment available during pregnancy.

Herpes simplex virus

Herpes simplex virus (HSV) was discussed in Chapter 6. The potential pregnancy effects of primary genital herpes infection include spontaneous abortion, preterm labor, and IUGR. The main route of HSV transmission from mother to neonate is through an infected birth canal. The risk of maternal-infant transmission is greater during a primary HSV-2 infection than during a recurrent episode (Fanaroff &

Martin, 1997). Cesarean birth is not recommended for all mothers with HSV. Only mothers with clinical evidence of active lesions during labor should have cesarean birth. Prenatal HSV cultures do not predict the presence of a live virus at time of birth. Cultures in women with HSV lesions at or near term may be done to assure the absence of the virus at time of birth and increase the likelihood of a vaginal birth.

Acyclovir has been used since 1977 to treat life-threatening HSV infections in adults and neonates; however, data are not clear regarding its safety or efficacy in pregnancy. Treatment of symptoms includes acetaminophen for fever and malaise and 5% lidocaine gel, local heat, or warm boric acid soaks for lesion discomfort (see Table 24-12).

RESEARCH

Fathers' Experience of Their Partners' Antepartum Bed Rest

In an effort to reduce the incidence of preterm birth, over 700,000 pregnant women in the United States are placed on bed rest. Studying the effects of bed rest on mothers is a recent development, and even less information exists about how fathers respond to having a partner on bed rest during pregnancy. Paternal worries, concerns, stresses or problems, and the type of support received by men whose partners were prescribed antepartum bed rest at home, in the hospital, or both were surveyed. A national subsample of 59 men whose mates were on

Continued

RESEARCH—cont'd

pregnancy bed rest were randomly selected from a nonrandom select sample of individuals who had contacted a bed rest support group for information. The Paternal Bed Rest Questionnaire of nine open-ended questions and one problem checklist detailing paternal concerns, stresses, and supports was mailed to fathers. Data from the study were analyzed using content analysis of the open-ended questions. The researchers found that the major problems for fathers were assuming multiple roles, managing emotional responses, and caring for their partner. The major paternal worry was for the health of the mate and the fetus. The fathers reported receiving little help from health care providers.

CLINICAL APPLICATION OF THE STUDY

Nurses must remember that while caring for mothers on bed rest that the fathers experience extreme stress when pregnancy bed rest is prescribed for a partner. Nurses need to use a family-centered care approach to include the father; interventions that reduce worry for the couple should be provided.

Source: Maloni J & Ponder M: Fathers' experience of their partners' antepartum bed rest, *Image J Nurs Scholar* 29(2):183, 1997.

KEY POINTS

- Hypertensive disorders during pregnancy are a leading cause of infant and maternal morbidity and mortality worldwide.
- The cause of PIH is unknown, and there are no known reliable tests for predicting which women are at risk for preeclampsia.
- Preeclampsia is a multisystem disease rather than only an increase in blood pressure.
- HELLP syndrome, which usually becomes apparent during the third trimester, is a variant of severe preeclampsia and is considered life threatening.
- Magnesium sulfate, the anticonvulsive agent of choice for preventing eclampsia, requires careful monitoring of reflexes, respirations, and urinary output; its antidote, calcium gluconate, should be available at the bedside.
- Intent of emergency interventions for eclampsia is to prevent self-injury, ensure adequate oxygenation, reduce aspiration risk, establish seizure control with magnesium sulfate, and correct maternal acidemia.
- The woman hospitalized with hyperemesis gravidarum is discharged home when fluid and electrolyte balance is restored and weight gain begins.

KEY POINTS—cont'd

- Some spontaneous abortions occur for unknown reasons, but fetal or placental maldevelopment and maternal factors account for many others.
- The type of spontaneous abortion directs care management.
- Ectopic pregnancy is a significant cause of maternal morbidity and mortality, even in developed countries.
- There are two distinctive types of hydatidiform mole, complete and partial.
- Premature separation of the placenta and placenta previa are differentiated by type of bleeding, uterine tonicity, and presence or absence of pain.
- Clotting disorders are associated with many obstetric complications.
- In the pregnant woman an enlarged uterus, displaced internal organs, and altered laboratory values may confound differential diagnosis when the need for immediate abdominal surgery occurs.
- Preoperative care for a pregnant woman differs from that for a nonpregnant woman in one significant aspect; the presence of at least one other person, the fetus.
- Domestic violence and battering increase during pregnancy.
- Pregnancy does not limit or restrict resuscitative, diagnostic, or pharmacologic treatment after trauma.
- Fetal survival depends on maternal survival; after trauma the first priority is resuscitation and stabilization of the mother before consideration of fetal concerns.
- Minor trauma is associated with major complications for the pregnancy, including abruptio placentae, fetomaternal hemorrhage, preterm labor and birth, and fetal death.
- Pregnancy confers no immunity against infection, and both mother and fetus must be considered when the pregnant woman contracts an infection.

CRITICAL THINKING EXERCISES

1 *Angie T., a 16-year-old G2 P0 A1, comes into clinic for a routine prenatal visit at 32 weeks' gestation. You find that her blood pressure is 150/96, she has 1+ proteinuria on a urine dipstick, and she has gained 6 pounds since her last clinic visit 10 days ago.*

   a *During your initial assessment, what other signs and symptoms of preeclampsia might you find?*

CRITICAL THINKING EXERCISES—cont'd

b *Develop a plan for Angie's care at home. What would you teach her about diet, rest, self-assessment, and fetal assessment?*

c *What danger signs should Angie be told to report immediately?*

2 *Angie talks daily on the phone with the clinic nurse and is seen twice-weekly at the clinic for evaluation. At her visit 2 weeks later, she reports a "blinding headache," "terrible heartburn," and blurred vision. Her blood pressure is 190/115. She is immediately admitted to the labor and delivery unit.*

a *What other assessment tests will most likely be performed on Angie and her fetus upon admission to the hospital?*

b *Discuss MgSO₄ administration: dosage, route, aim of therapy, side effects, indications for discontinuing.*

c *What other medications might this patient receive?*

3 *Susie P. is a 27-year-old G6 P3 A2 at 28 weeks' gestation admitted to labor and delivery with bright red vaginal bleeding.*

a *What possible diagnoses does Susie have?*

b *What physical assessment, laboratory tests, and diagnostic procedures would you expect to see done in order to reach a final diagnosis?*

c *Under what circumstances could Susie be transferred to the antepartum unit or be discharged home?*

4 *Denise S. is a 19-year-old G1 P0 at 34 weeks' gestation who was involved in a minor motor vehicle accident earlier today while taking her husband to work. (Someone rear-ended her car while she was stopped at a light.) Denise is brought to the hospital by ambulance and initially evaluated and cleared by the trauma service. She is then transferred to the labor and delivery unit for prolonged fetal monitoring (at least 4 hours). At this point, Denise threatens to sign herself out of the hospital against medical advice, stating, "I feel fine and I want to go home." Pretend that you are the nurse assigned to care for Denise and role play how you might handle this situation. Ask the group to suggest different strategies.*

5 *The nurse on the antepartal unit is called to the desk to admit a new patient. The nurse recognizes the patient right away because it is her third admission this month for excessive vomiting (hyperemesis gravidarum). Suzanne M. smiles weakly as the nurse approaches. She is pale, her eyes appear sunken, skin turgor is poor, and she*

CRITICAL THINKING EXERCISES—cont'd

is clutching an emesis basin. The nurse recalls that this is Suzanne's first pregnancy; it was unplanned and happened just as her husband found out he was being "laid off" from his job.

a *Develop a plan of care for Suzanne while she is in the hospital.*

b *What teaching do Suzanne and her husband need before discharge?*

c *What lifestyle changes would you recommend to help Suzanne stay out of the hospital?*

6 *The nurse is assigned to admit a woman with abdominal pain in the second trimester of pregnancy. She has two children at home, ages 2 and 5 years. Her chief complaint is fatigue, right-sided pain, and nausea.*

a *What would be focused assessment questions?*
   What physical assessments would the nurse make?
   What laboratory values would be expected to be ordered and why?

b *Given a diagnosis of appendicitis, what would be the top priority nursing diagnosis? Formulate a plan of care.*

c *List home care concerns as the woman is prepared to be discharged.*

References

Abell T & Riely C: Hyperemesis gravidarum, *Gastroenterol Clin North Am* 21(4):835, 1992.

Adimora A et al.: *Sexually transmitted diseases* (companion handbook), ed 2, New York, 1994, McGraw-Hill.

American College of Obstetricians and Gynecologists: Trauma during pregnancy, *Technical Bulletin 161*, Washington, DC, 1991, ACOG.

American College of Obstetricians and Gynecologists. *Clinical aspects of domestic violence for the obstetrician/gynecologist* (continuing education program), Washington DC, 1993, ACOG.

American College of Obstetricians and Gynecologists: Antenatal corticosteroid therapy for fetal maturation, *Technical Bulletin 147*, Washington, DC, 1994, ACOG.

American College of Obstetricians and Gynecologists: Early pregnancy loss, *Technical Bulletin 212*, Washington, DC, 1995, ACOG.

American College of Obstetricians and Gynecologists: Hypertension in pregnancy, Technical Bulletin 219, Washington DC, 1996, ACOG.

Baker A: Liver and biliary tract disease. In Barron W & Lindheimer M, editors: *Medical disorders during pregnancy*, St Louis, 1995, Mosby.

Benedetti T: Obstetric hemorrhage. In Gabbe S, Niebyl J & Simpson J, editors: O*bstetrics: normal and problem pregnancies*, ed 3, New York, 1996, Churchill Livingstone.

Berkowitz R, Goldstein D & Bernstein M: Advances in management of partial molar pregnancy, *Contemp OB/GYN* 38(5):33, 1991.

Caritis S et al.: Low dose aspirins to prevent preeclampsia in women at high risk, *New Eng J Med* 338(11):701, 1998.

Centers for Disease Control and Prevention (CDC): 1998 Guidelines for treatment of sexually transmitted diseases, *MMWR* 47(R-R 1):1, 1998.

Charlin V et al.: Parenteral nutrition in hyperemesis gravidarum, *Nutrition* 9(1):29, 1993.

Coleman M, Trianfo V & Rund D: Nonobstetric emergencies in pregnancy: trauma and surgical conditions, *Am J Obstet Gynecol* 177(3):497, 1997.

Copeland L & Landon M: Malignant diseases and pregnancy. In Gabbe S, Niebyl J & Simpson J, editors: *Obstetrics: normal and problem pregnancies,* ed 3, New York, 1996, Churchill Livingstone.

Creasy R & Resnik R: *Maternal-fetal medicine: principles and practice,* ed 3, Philadelphia, 1994, WB Saunders.

Cruikshank D et al.: Maternal physiology in pregnancy. In Gabbe S, Niebyl J & Simpson J, editors: *Obstetrics: normal and problem pregnancies,* ed 3, New York, 1996, Churchill Livingstone.

Cunningham F et al.: *Williams obstetrics,* ed 20, Stamford, Conn, 1997, Appleton & Lange.

Cunningham F & Lindheimer M: Hypertension in pregnancy, *N Engl J Med* 326(14):927, 1992.

Depp R: Cesarean delivery. In Gabbe S, Niebyl J & Simpson J, editors: *Obstetrics: normal and problem pregnancies,* ed 3, New York, 1996, Churchill Livingstone.

Deuchar N: Nausea and vomiting in pregnancy: a review of the problem with particular regard to psychological and social aspects, *Br J Obstet Gynaecol* 102(1):6, 1995.

Dildy N et al.: Complications in pregnancy-induced hypertension. In Clark S et al., editors: *Critical care obstetrics* ed 2, Boston, 1991, Blackwell Scientific.

Esposito T: Trauma during pregnancy, *Emerg Med Clin North Am* 12(1):167, 1994.

Fairlie F: Doppler flow velocimetry in hypertension in pregnancy, *Clin Perinatol* 18(4):749, 1991.

Fairlie F & Sibai B: Hypertensive diseases in pregnancy. In Reece E et al., editors: *Medicine of the fetus and mother,* Philadelphia, 1992, JB Lippincott.

Fanaroff A & Martin R: *Neonatal-perinatal medicine: diseases of the fetus and infant,* ed 6, St Louis, 1997, Mosby.

Farmakides G et al.: Pregnancy surveillance with Doppler velocimetry, *Female Patient* 15(5):49, 1990.

Farmakides G, Schulman H & Schneider E: Surveillance of the pregnant hypertensive patient with Doppler flow velocimetry, *Clin Obstet Gynecol* 35(2):387, 1992.

Freda M: Arrest, trial, and failure, *J Obstet Gynecol Neonatal Nurs* 24(5); 383, 1995.

Friedman S: Preeclampsia: a review of the role of prostaglandins, *Obstet Gynecol* 71(1):122, 1988.

Gilbert E & Harmon J: *Manual of high risk pregnancy and delivery,* ed 2, St Louis, 1998, Mosby.

Gilstrap L & Gant N: Pathophysiology of preeclampsia, *Semin Perinatol* 14(2):147, 1990.

Gleicher N, editor: *Principles and practice of medical therapy in pregnancy,* ed 2, Norwalk, Conn, 1992, Appleton & Lange.

Green J: Placenta previa and abruptio placenta. In Creasy R & Resnik R, editors: *Maternal-fetal medicine: principles and practice,* Philadelphia, 1994, WB Saunders.

Greenberg E et al.: Vaginal bleeding and abuse: assessing pregnant women in the emergency department, *MCN Am J Matern Child Nurs* 22(4):182, 1997.

Grohar J: Nursing protocols for antepartum home care, *J Obstet Gynecol Neonatal Nurs* 23(8):687, 1994.

Hammond C & Bachus K: Ectopic pregnancy. In Scott J et al., editors: *Danforth's obstetrics and gynecology,* Philadelphia, 1994, JB Lippincott.

Harvey C & Burke M: Hypertensive disorders in pregnancy. In Mandeville L & Troiano N, editors: *High-risk intrapartum nursing,* Philadelphia, 1992, JB Lippincott.

Health Care Resources: *Handbook of high risk prenatal home care,* St Louis, 1997, Mosby.

Hod M et al.: Hyperemesis gravidarum, *J Reprod Med* 39(8):605, 1994.

Hunter S & Weiner C: Obstetric hemorrhage. In Repke J, editor: *Intrapartum obstetrics,* New York, 1996, Churchill Livingstone.

Huzel P & Remsburg-Bell E: Fetal complications related to minor maternal trauma, *J Obstet Gynecol Neonatal Nurs* 25(2):121, 1996.

Iams J: Preterm birth. In Gabbe S, Niebyl J & Simpson J, editors: *Obstetrics: normal and problem pregnancies,* ed 3, New York, 1996, Churchill Livingstone.

Katz V et al.: A comparison of bed rest and immersion for treating edema of pregnancy, *Obstet Gynecol* 75(2):147, 1990.

Kendrick J: Fetal and uterine response during maternal surgery, *MCN Am J Matern Child Nurs* 19(3):165, 1994.

Knuppel R & Hatangadi S: Acute hypotension related to hemorrhage in the obstetric patient, *Obstet Gyncol Clin North Am* 22(1):111, 1995.

Konje J & Walley R: Bleeding in late pregnancy. In James D et al., editors: *High risk pregnancy: management options,* Philadelphia, 1995, WB Saunders.

Lavery J & Staten-McCormick M: Management of moderate to severe trauma in pregnancy. *Obstet Gynecol Clin North Am* 22(1):69, 1995.

Leduc L et al.: Coagulation profile in severe preeclampsia, *Obstet Gynecol* 79(1):14, 1992.

Magness R & Gant N: Control of vascular reactivity in pregnancy: the basis for therapeutic approaches to prevent pregnancy-induced hypertension, *Semin Perinatol* 18(2):45, 1994.

Maloni J: Antepartum bed rest: case studies, research & nursing care, Washington, DC, 1998, AWHONN.

Maloni J: Home care of the high-risk pregnant woman requiring bed rest, *J Obstet Gynecol Neonatal Nurs* 23(8):696, 1994.

McFarlane J: Abuse during pregnancy: the horror and the hope, *NAACOG's Clin Issu Perinat Women's Health Nurs* 4(3):350, 1993.

Minnick-Smith K & Cook F: Current treatment options for ectopic pregnancy, *MCN Am J Matern Child Nurs* 22(1):21, 1997.

Modigliani R & Bernades P: Gastrointestinal and pancreatic diseases. In Barron W & Lindheimer M, editors: *Medical disorders during pregnancy,* ed 2, St Louis, 1995, Mosby.

Pearlman M & Tintinalli J: Evaluation and treatment of the gravida and fetus following trauma during pregnancy, *Obstet Gynecol Clin North Am* 18(2):371, 1991.

Pearlman M, Tintinalli J & Lorenz R: Blunt trauma during pregnancy, *N Engl J Med* 323(23):1609, 1990.

Pickles C, Broughton P & Symonds E: A randomized placebo controlled trial of labetalol in the treatment of mild to moderate pregnancy induced hypertension, *Br J Obstet Gynaecol* 99(12):964, 1992.

Poole J: HELLP syndrome and coagulopathies of pregnancy, *Crit Care Nurs Clin North Am* 5(3):457, 1993.

Powell M & Spellman J: Medical management of the patient with an ectopic pregnancy, *J Perinat Neonatal Nurs* 9(4):31, 1996.

Roberts J: Current perspectives on preeclampsia, *J Nurse Midwifery* 39(2):70, 1994.

Sanchez-Ramos L et al.: Prevention of pregnancy-induced hypertension by calcium supplementation in angiotensin II-sensitive patients, *Obstet Gynecol* 84(3):349, 1994.

Scott J: Hypertensive disorders of pregnancy. In Scott J et al., editors: *Danforth's obstetrics and gynecology,* ed 7, Philadelphia, 1994a, JB Lippincott.

Scott J: Placenta previa and placental abruption. In Scott J et al., editors: *Danforth's obstetrics and gynecology,* Philadelphia, 1994b, JB Lippincott.

Seidel H et al.: *Mosby's guide to physical examination,* ed 4, St Louis, 1999, Mosby.

Sibai B: The HELLP syndrome (hemolysis, elevated liver enzymes, and low platelets): much ado about nothing? *Am J Obstet Gynecol* 162(2):311, 1990.

Sibai B: Immunologic aspects of preeclampsia, *Clin Obstet Gynecol* 34(1):27, 1991a.

Sibai B: Management of preeclampsia, *Clin Perinatol* 18(4):793, 1991b.

Sibai B: Hypertension in pregnancy, *Obstet Gynecol Clin North Am* 19(2):615, 1992.

Sibai B: Hypertension in pregnancy. In Gabbe S, Niebyl J & Simpson J, editors: *Obstetrics: normal and problem pregnancies,* ed 3, New York, 1996, Churchill Livingstone.

Sibai B et al.: Prevention of preeclampsia with low-dose aspirin in healthy, nulliparous pregnant women, *N Engl J Med* 329(17):1213, 1993.

Simpson J: Fetal wastage. In Gabbe S, Niebyl J & Simpson J, editors: *Obstetrics: normal and problem pregnancies,* ed 3, New York, 1996, Churchill Livingstone.

Simpson K: *Protocols for homecare management of high-risk pregnancies,* St Louis, 1992, Healthy Homecomings.

Sisson M & Sauer P: Pharmacologic therapy for pregnancy-induced hypertension, *J Perinat Neonatal Nurs* 9(4):1, 1996.

Thorp J: Third-trimester bleeding. In Moore T et al., editors: *Gynecology and obstetrics: a longitudinal approach,* New York, 1993, Churchill Livingstone.

Torem M: Hypnotherapeutic techniques in the treatment of hyperemesis gravidarum, *Am J Clin Hypn* 37(1):1, 1994.

Troiano N: Trauma during pregnancy. In Harvey C, editor: *Critical care obstetrical nursing,* Gaithersburg, Md, 1991, Aspen.

Tsukimori K et al.: The possible role of endothelial cells in hypertensive disorders during pregnancy, *Obstet Gynecol* 80(2):229, 1992.

Varner M: General medical and surgical diseases in pregnancy. In Scott J et al.: *Danforth's obstetrics and gynecology,* Philadelphia, 1994, Lippincott.

Veronikis D & O'Grady J: What to do—or not to do—for postpartum hemorrhage, *Contemp OB/GYN* 39:11, 1994.

Walker C & Sweet R: HIV and other sexually transmitted diseases in pregnancy. In Reece E et al., editors: *Medicine of the fetus and mother,* Philadelphia, 1992, JB Lippincott.

Wong D & Perry S: *Maternal child nursing care,* St Louis, 1998, Mosby.

Working Group on High Blood Pressure in Pregnancy: Consensus Report: National high blood pressure education program working group report on high blood pressure in pregnancy, *Am J Obstet Gynecol* 163(5 Part 1):1691, 1990.

Zuspan F & Samuels P: Preventing preeclampsia, *N Engl J Med* 329(17):1265, 1993.

CHAPTER

25

Labor and Birth at Risk

KAREN A. PIOTROWSKI

LEARNING OBJECTIVES

- Define the key terms.
- Compare the assessment and care management of women with preterm labor carried out at home and in the hospital setting.
- Identify the assessments for women experiencing different types of abnormal labor.
- Formulate nursing diagnoses based on the assessment of abnormal labor.
- Describe the nursing interventions for a trial of labor, the induction of labor, forceps-assisted birth, vacuum-assisted birth, cesarean birth, and vaginal birth after a cesarean birth.
- Discuss the criteria for evaluating the nursing care of women experiencing at-risk labor and birth.
- Describe the assessment and care management of women experiencing a postterm pregnancy.
- Discuss possible obstetric emergencies and their appropriate management.
- Identify measures a nurse can use to facilitate family coping following fetal, newborn, or maternal death during childbirth.

KEY TERMS

amniotic fluid embolism (AFE)
amniotomy
artificial rupture of membranes (AROM)
augmentation of labor
Bishop score
cephalopelvic disproportion (CPD)
cesarean birth
dysfunctional labor
dystocia
external cephalic version (ECV)
forceps-assisted birth
hypertonic uterine dysfunction
hypotonic uterine dysfunction
induction of labor
multifetal pregnancy

KEY TERMS—cont'd

oxytocin
postterm pregnancy
precipitous labor
premature rupture of membranes (PROM)
preterm labor
preterm pregnancy
prolapse of the umbilical cord
prolonged labor
prostaglandins
rupture of the uterus
shoulder dystocia
therapeutic rest
tocolytic agents
trial of labor (TOL)
vacuum-assisted birth
vaginal birth after cesarean (VBAC)

The development of complications during labor and birth is associated with an increase in perinatal morbidity and mortality. Some complications are anticipated, especially if the mother is identified as being at risk for a particular complication during the antepartum period; others are unexpected or unforeseen. The woman, her family, and the health care team can feel devastated when things go wrong. Nurses must recognize these feelings if they are to provide effective support. It is crucial for nurses to understand the normal birth process in order to be able to prevent and detect deviations from normal labor and birth and to implement nursing measures if complications arise. Optimal care of the laboring woman experiencing complications, as well as of her fetus and family, is possible only when the nurse and other members of the obstetric team use their knowledge and skills in a concerted effort to provide care.

PRETERM LABOR AND BIRTH

Preterm labor is defined as the onset of regular uterine contractions that cause cervical changes between 20 and 37 weeks' gestation. **Preterm birth** is a birth that occurs before the end of 37 weeks' gestation. Although the overall incidence of preterm birth in the United States is approximately

---

BOX 25-1 *Risk Factors for Preterm Labor*

DEMOGRAPHIC RISKS
- Nonwhite race
- Age ($<17, >35$)
- Low socioeconomic status
- Unmarried
- Less than high school education

BIOPHYSICAL RISKS
- Previous preterm labor or birth
- Second-trimester abortion (more than two spontaneous or therapeutic); still births
- Grand multiparity; short interval between pregnancies (≤ 1 year since last birth); family history of preterm labor and birth
- Progesterone deficiency
- Uterine anomalies or fibroids; uterine irritability
- Cervical incompetence, trauma, shortened length
- Exposure to DES or other toxic substances
- Medical diseases (e.g., diabetes, hypertension, anemia)
- Small stature (< 119 cm in height; <45.5 kg or underweight for height)
- Current pregnancy risks:
  - Multifetal pregnancy

- Hydramnios
- Bleeding
- Placental problems (e.g., placenta previa, abruptio placentae)
- Infections (e.g., pyelonephritis, recurrent urinary tract infections, asymptomatic bacteriuria, bacterial vaginosis, chorioamnionitis)
- Pregnancy-induced hypertension
- Premature rupture of the membranes
- Fetal anomalies
- Inadequate plasma volume expansion; anemia

BEHAVIORAL-PSYCHOSOCIAL RISKS
- Poor nutrition; weight loss or low weight gain
- Smoking (>10 cigarettes a day)
- Substance abuse (e.g., alcohol; illicit drugs, especially cocaine)
- Inadequate prenatal care
- Commutes of more than $1\frac{1}{2}$ hours each way
- Excessive physical activity (heavy physical work, prolonged standing, heavy lifting, young child care)
- Excessive lifestyle stressors

From Heffner L et al.: Clinical and environmental predictors of preterm labor, *Obstet Gynecol* 81:750, 1993; Jones D & Collins B: The nursing management of women experiencing preterm labor: clinical guidelines and why they are needed, *J Obstet Gynecol Neonatal Nurs* 25(7):569, 1996; Lang J, Lieberman E & Cohen A: A comparison of risk factors for preterm labor and term small-for-gestational-age birth, *Epidemiology* 7(4):369, 1996; Simpson K: Preterm birth in the United States: current issues and future perspectives, *J Perinat Neonat Nurs* 10(4):11, 1997; Varney H: *Varney's textbook for midwives*, ed 3, Sudberry, Mass, 1997, Jones and Bartlett Publishers; and Wheeler D: Preterm birth prevention, *J Nurse Midwifery* 38(suppl 2):66S, 1994.

10%, preterm birth is responsible for 83% of infant deaths, not counting those associated with congenital anomalies (Creasy, 1993; Ventura et al., 1997). Preterm infants born weighing less than 1,500 gm are much more likely to die or, if they survive, to experience neurologic impairment than infants born weighing more than 2,500 gm (ACOG 1995a).

The infant born before term has not yet achieved the growth and development necessary for uncomplicated adjustment to extrauterine life. As a result, his or her prospects for survival or good health may be severely compromised. For those who do survive, the emotional and financial costs to families and health care systems are phenomenal. The average neonatal intensive care cost for one preterm infant is estimated to be $40,000 to $50,000. Total annual costs of neonatal intensive care is estimated to be $5 billion a year, with most costs attributed to care of preterm infants (Gilbert & Harmon, 1998).

Etiologic Factors

No definite precipitating cause can be identified in approximately 50% of preterm births. However, a history of preterm birth has been identified as the single most important predisposing risk factor for preterm labor and birth. Additional risk factors closely associated with preterm labor and birth include bacterial vaginosis, intraamniotic infection, premature rupture of the membranes (PROM), multiple gestation, bleeding, and uterine/cervical abnormalities (Simpson, 1997).

Research findings indicate that genital tract infections are strongly associated with PROM and preterm labor and birth, especially in pregnancies less than 30 weeks' gestation. Early identification and prompt treatment of these infections has the potential for reducing the occurrence of preterm birth (Andrews, Goldenburg & Hauth, 1995, McGregor et al., 1995).

Risk factors commonly related to preterm labor may be classified in several ways. For this discussion, the categories of demographic risks, biophysical risks, and behavioral-psychosocial risks are used. Box 25-1 lists the possible risk factors for preterm labor.

I CARE MANAGEMENT

Assessment and Nursing Diagnoses

The obstetric management of preterm birth involves detecting preterm labor early, suppressing uterine activity, and improving the intrapartum care of the fetus destined to be born early.

All pregnant women are screened at their initial prenatal visit for the presence of risk factors associated with preterm labor. Women then need to be reassessed at each subsequent visit. Many risk-scoring systems have been developed to help identify women who might be at risk for preterm labor. Based on their risk status, women at risk for preterm labor are then enrolled into a program of ongoing, more frequent

---

BOX 25-2   *Signs and Symptoms of Preterm Labor*

UTERINE ACTIVITY
- Uterine contractions more frequent than every 10 minutes persisting for 1 hour or more
- Uterine contractions may be painful or painless

DISCOMFORT
- Lower abdominal cramping similar to gas pains; may be accompanied by diarrhea
- Dull, intermittent low back pain (below the waist)
- Painful, menstrual-like cramps
- Suprapubic pain or pressure
- Pelvic pressure or heaviness
- Urinary frequency

VAGINAL DISCHARGE
- Change in character and amount of usual discharge: thicker (mucoid) or thinner (watery), bloody, brown or colorless, increased amount, odor
- Rupture of amniotic membranes

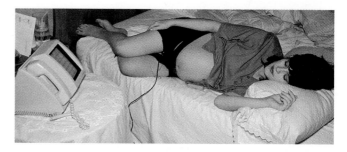

Fig. 25-1 Home uterine activity monitoring. Tocodynamometer is in place at center of abdomen below umbilicus. Recording unit and transmitter are on the bedside table. (Courtesy Michael S. Clement, MD, Mesa, Ariz.)

---

assessment of health status, education, prematurity prevention, home visits, and hotlines (Edenfeld et al., 1995). These risk-scoring systems have been used with limited success; therefore, all women should be educated about the signs and symptoms of preterm labor (Box 25-2), what to do if they occur, and shown the way to palpate and time uterine contractions.

The signs and symptoms of preterm labor are vague, and it is not unusual for both high-risk and low-risk women to interpret them as typical experiences associated with pregnancy unless they are educated about their significance and the correct action to take if they occur. In addition, all pregnant women should be taught to use measures found to be effective in preventing the onset of preterm labor. These prevention measures include adequate nutrition and fluid intake; appropriate weight gain; avoidance of smoking, nontherapeutic drugs, alcohol, and strenuous activity; use of techniques to reduce stress; and use of infection control measures, especially with regard to genital tract infections (Freston et al., 1997; Iams, Johnson & Parker, 1994; Jones & Collins, 1996; Varney, 1997).

Home uterine activity monitoring (HUAM) using an ambulatory tocodynamometer (Fig. 25-1) may be implemented to detect any excessive uterine contractions before they can be perceived by the woman herself. Women using these devices record their uterine activity twice a day, or more often if necessary; the data are then transmitted by telephone to the hospital or to a monitoring service for analysis. Appropriate therapy is instituted if labor is suspected (Hill et al., 1990). Before initiating a HUAM program, the health care provider must ensure that the woman has a telephone or that arrangements have been made to install one. The woman and her family should be instructed

in the correct use of the monitor, including how to transmit uterine activity data (Jones & Collins, 1996). Although some studies have shown that the use of home uterine activity monitoring is associated with a lower incidence of preterm birth, others speculate that the decrease is the result of more frequent contact with health care providers (ACOG, 1995a, Creasy & Merkatz, 1990, Freston et al., 1997). The cost of home uterine monitoring using the tocodynamometer is estimated to be $450 per day, thus also calling into question whether this type of monitoring is actually cost effective in detecting preterm labor (Wheeler, 1994). Based on the lack of data indicating the beneficial effects of HUAM, ACOG (1995a) does not recommend its use, but rather considers it to be an investigational device. Continued study of the effectiveness of this technology is needed.

The common nursing diagnoses for the woman in preterm labor are listed in the box.

| Nursing Diagnoses_____

Preterm Labor
Knowledge deficit related to:
- Recognition of preterm labor and/or management of preterm labor

Risk for maternal or fetal injury related to:
- Preterm labor and birth
- Prescribed maternal bed rest
- Administration of tocolytic drugs to suppress preterm labor

Anxiety related to:
- Possible preterm birth

Impaired physical mobility related to:
- Prescribed bed rest

Anticipatory grieving related to:
- Potential loss of fetus

Situational low self-esteem related to:
- Inability to carry pregnancy to term

Altered family processes related to:
- Demands of preterm labor treatment regimen

PROTOCOL Home Management of Preterm Labor

ASSESSMENTS—TO BE DONE DAILY UNLESS OTHERWISE SPECIFIED

- Monitor uterine contractions two to three times a day for 30 minutes to 1 hour, as instructed (using self-palpation or home uterine activity monitoring [HUAM] device). If HUAM device is used, transmit data as instructed.
- Assess for fetal activity daily by counting fetal movements, as instructed. If nurse is visiting, FHR and nonstress testing may be done as prescribed.
- Review signs and symptoms of preterm labor. Report their occurrence to your primary health care provider.
- Weigh yourself; take your blood pressure and/or pulse as instructed.
- Blood tests, urine checks, and/or cervical assessments may be done by the visiting nurse, as prescribed.

INTERVENTIONS

- Follow instructions about limiting your activities as prescribed; for example, remain on bed rest on your side, except to go to the bathroom.
- Practice relaxation techniques.
- Eat well-balanced meals and nutritious snacks; be sure to include roughage in your diet.
- Drink 8 to 10 (8-oz) cups of fluids a day.
- Empty bladder when fullness is first noted.
- Limit caffeine intake.
- Eliminate smoking, alcohol, nontherapeutic drugs.
- Delegate tasks to others.
- Use measures to prevent infection.
- Avoid or limit activities that could stimulate labor, as instructed (e.g., sexual activity that causes orgasm, nipple stimulation).
- Take medications as prescribed. Report side effects to your health care provider.
- Keep appointments with your health care provider.

Data from Grohar J: Nursing protocols for antepartum home care, *J Obstet Gynecol Neonatal Nurs* 23(8):687, 1994; Jones D & Collins B: The nursing management of women experiencing preterm labor: clinical guidelines and why they are needed, *J Obstet Gynecol Neonatal Nurs* 25(7):569, 1996.

Expected Outcomes of Care

The nurse develops a plan of care based on whether the woman's care is to be managed at home or in the hospital. Common expected outcomes are that the woman will:

- Follow instructions for activity limitations, uterine monitoring (self-palpation or home monitoring equipment), and/or medication schedules
- Communicate concerns, fears, questions, and perceptions to her health care providers and to members of her support system
- Experience no complications as the result of the medication management prescribed or the activity restrictions
- Carry the fetus to term or near term
- Give birth to a healthy, mature infant

Plan of Care and Interventions

Identifying preterm labor

Pregnant women should be instructed to notify their health care provider if they experience signs and symptoms of preterm labor, particularly uterine contractions occurring more frequently than every 10 minutes (Protocol box). If signs and symptoms of preterm labor are experienced, the woman should be instructed to empty her bladder; drink three glasses of fluid; and lie down on her side to increase blood flow to the uterus, eliminate myometrial hypoxia, and decrease uterine activity. If the woman continues to have more than four to six uterine contractions after 1 hour of these interventions, she should contact her primary health care provider at which time she usually is instructed to come to the health care provider's office or hospital for further evaluation (Jones & Collins, 1996; Freston et al.,

1997). There the woman is positioned on her side and an external fetal and uterine monitor is applied to assess uterine activity and the fetal heart rate (FHR). Her vital signs are also monitored. An intravenous infusion may be started to provide additional hydration in order to expand fluid volume and thereby suppress uterine activity, although the effectiveness of this measure has not been proven.

NURSE ALERT *Caution must be used when administering intravenous fluids to women in preterm labor because this practice can increase the risk for tocolytic-induced pulmonary edema. It is recommended that the total oral and intravenous fluid intake in 24 hours should be restricted to 2,400 to 3,000 ml. Strict intake and output measurement, daily weight determination, and assessment of pulmonary function should be instituted (ACOG, 1995a; Freda & DeVore; 1996; Hill, 1995).*

A clean-catch or catheterized urine specimen is obtained and examined for evidence of a urinary tract infection. If substance abuse is suspected, a urine toxicology screen may be performed. A sterile speculum examination usually is performed to obtain cervical or vaginal specimens for culture to detect an infection such as those caused by group B streptococcus, *Chlamydia*, or gonococcus. A cervical examination is performed to determine whether dilatation, effacement, or both are occurring.

The diagnosis of preterm labor is based on the presence of uterine contractions resulting in the effacement and/or dilatation of the cervix (Jones & Collins, 1996). If uterine activity subsides and the status of dilatation and effacement does not change from that noted at the initial examination, the woman may be discharged home. She may be given instructions to limit her activities (see Protocol box) and medications to prevent preterm labor. If labor continues, her care is continued in the hospital until her condition is stable and she can go home or until the infant is born.

Home care

If the preterm labor subsides and the woman is discharged home, her care will be continued in the outpatient setting and consist of frequent visits and cervical examinations. The nurse reviews the signs and symptoms of preterm labor with her at each visit. Inclusion of the woman's family in this process is essential because of the effect preterm labor has on the entire family. For example, the woman may have small children at home who need care and supervision, or she may work outside the home and be forced to take a leave of absence or even give up her job. The restriction on her activities can also disrupt the daily lives of all family members, necessitating that they assume different roles and responsibilities.

The home care of the woman with preterm labor may or may not be supervised by a home health caregiver. The plan of care prescribed for the woman is shared with all caregivers and family members so that all have the information needed to help the woman stay motivated to comply with the plan. The woman's condition is assessed daily, unless otherwise specified (see Protocol).

Activity restriction in terms of varying degrees of bed rest has long been prescribed as a means to prevent preterm birth by relieving cervical pressure and enhancing uterine blood flow. Goldenberg and associates (1994) estimated that more than 700,000 high-risk pregnant women are placed on bed rest each year by their health care providers. Research findings, however, fail to demonstrate the effectiveness of this treatment measure and at the same time indicate that bed rest can have adverse effects on the woman and her support system, including her partner. These adverse effects are added to the stressors already associated with the experience of high-risk pregnancy. Bed rest often requires an abrupt change in maternal and family routines. Box 25-3 summarizes the adverse effects encountered by the woman on bed rest and her family (Goldenberg, 1994; Maloni, 1994).

When a woman is placed on bed rest, the primary health care provider must clearly define the extent of activity restriction, including the number of hours to be spent in bed and the woman's ability to go to the bathroom, shower, go outdoors, engage in limited exercise, and have meals with her family. Women who have strong support systems and who are placed on partial rather than complete bed rest are more likely to comply with the required activity restrictions (Josten et al., 1995; Schroeder, 1996).

The woman placed on bed rest needs emotional support and help with household management, time management, and child care. Nurses need to help the woman deal with these problems by keeping the woman informed about the status of her pregnancy; assisting her to mobilize her support system; making referrals to home care agencies; and

---

| BOX 25-3 | *Adverse Effects of Bed Rest* |

MATERNAL EFFECTS (PHYSICAL)
- Weight loss
- Muscle wasting, weakness
- Bone demineralization and calcium loss
- Decreased plasma volume and cardiac output
- Increased clotting tendency; risk for thrombophlebitis
- Alteration in bowel function
- Sleep disturbance, fatigue
- Prolonged postpartum recovery

MATERNAL EFFECTS (PSYCHOSOCIAL)
- Loss of control associated with role reversals
- Dysphoria—anxiety, depression, hostility, and anger
- Guilt associated with difficulty complying with activity restriction and inability to meet role responsibilities
- Boredom, loneliness
- Emotional lability (mood swings)

EFFECTS ON SUPPORT SYSTEM
- Stress associated with role reversals, increased responsibilities, and disruption of family routines
- Financial strain associated with loss of maternal income and cost of treatment
- Fear and anxiety regarding the well-being of the mother and fetus

---

providing the woman with opportunities to voice her concerns, questions, frustrations, and anger. The woman should be encouraged to actively participate in decision making regarding her care and the care of her family as a means of preserving her sense of control over her life (Gupton, Heaman & Ashcroft, 1997) (Home Care box, p. 699, left).

If there are children at home to be cared for, the nurse can suggest activities to keep the children entertained without causing the woman to exert herself (Home Care box, p. 699, right). The woman on prolonged bed rest may also have to deal with boredom. The nurse can help her relieve this boredom by assessing her interests in activities that are acceptable within her limitations. The Home Care box provides ideas for activities that can be performed while the woman is on bed rest. Women who have preterm labor may also benefit from a referral to a high-risk support group.

Partners of women placed on bed rest report that this activity restriction represents a major stressor in their lives, resulting in constant worry about the well-being of their partner and baby and feeling overwhelmed with the need to take on additional responsibilities, including the care of their partner and children and the performance of household maintenance tasks. Nurses need to recognize the concerns and feelings of partners and provide them with needed support by keeping them informed about the well-being of the woman and fetus, making referrals to assist them to meet their new responsibilities, and encouraging them to voice their feelings and concerns (Maloni & Ponder, 1997).

HOME CARE *Patient Instructions for Self-Care*

Suggested Activities for Women on Bed Rest

- Set a routine for daily activities (e.g., getting dressed, moving from the bedroom to a "day bed rest place," having social time, eating meals, self-monitoring fetal and uterine activity).
- Do passive exercises as allowed.
- Review childbirth education information or have a childbirth class at home, if this can be arranged.
- Plan menus and make up grocery shopping lists.
- Shop by phone.
- Read books about high-risk pregnancy or other topics.
- Keep a journal of the pregnancy.
- Keep a calendar of your progress.
- Reorganize files, recipes, household budget.
- Update address book.
- Do mending, sewing.
- Listen to audiotapes, watch videos or TV.
- Do crossword puzzles, jigsaw puzzles, etc.
- Do craft projects; make something for the baby.
- Put pictures in photo albums.
- Call a friend, family member, or support person each day.
- Treat yourself to a facial, manicure, neck massage, or other special treat when you need a lift.

From Gilbert E & Harmon J: *Manual of high risk pregnancy and delivery,* ed 2, St Louis, 1998, Mosby; Isennock P: *Bed rest before baby: what's a mother to do?* Perry Hall, Md, 1992, Mustard Seed Publications; and Maloni J: Home care of the high-risk pregnant woman requiring bed rest, *J Obstet Gynecol Neonatal Nurs* 23(8):696, 1994.

HOME CARE *Patient Instructions for Self-Care*

Activities for Children of Women on Bed Rest

- Schedule brief play periods throughout the day.
- Keep a few favorite toys in a box or basket close to the bed or couch.
- Read to the child(ren).
- Put puzzles together.
- Watch videos, play video games (remote control for TV is ideal).
- Play cards or board games.
- Color in coloring books.
- Cut out pictures from magazines and paste on cardboard.
- Play bed basketball with a soft (sponge) ball or rolled up sock and a trash can or empty laundry basket.

Adapted from Isennock P: *Bed rest before baby: what's a mother to do?* Perry Hall, Md, 1992, Mustard Seed Publications; Bolane J & Furlong J: *Coping with bedrest in pregnancy,* Waco, Texas, 1994, Childbirth Graphics.

Hospital care

The nursing assessments for the woman hospitalized for the management of preterm labor are similar to those carried out in the home setting. The nurse assesses the woman's vital signs, lung function (signs of pulmonary edema), fundal height, fluid balance (weight, intake and output, presence of edema) gastrointestinal function, deep tendon reflexes, and psychosocial adaptation. The nurse also assesses fetal health status by evaluating FHR pattern and fetal movement. A speculum examination is performed to detect effacement and dilatation, and uterine activity monitoring is initiated. The urine is checked for the presence and concentration of glucose, protein, and ketones. Prolonged hospitalization can have the same negative physiologic and psychologic effects as home care with the woman on bed rest. It is important to remember that involving the woman in as many decisions regarding her care as possible usually is beneficial to her self-esteem and preserves her sense of control (see Plan of Care).

Suppression of uterine activity

If uterine contractions persist, or if significant cervical changes occur, tocolytic treatment may be initiated to stop labor. **Tocolytic agents** are medications that inhibit uterine contractions. *Toko-* and *toco-* are combining forms derived from the Greek word for 'childbirth' or 'labor'; *-lytic* is a word termination that also comes from the Greek and means 'to break down' or 'stop.' The agents most commonly used include β-sympathomimetics such as ritodrine, terbutaline, and magnesium sulfate.

Despite their widespread use, tocolytic agents are fairly ineffective as a means of suppressing labor and preventing preterm birth. Their use is associated with significant maternal, fetal, and neonatal risks and complications. Research findings, however, do justify the use of tocolytic agents as a means of suppressing labor long enough (24 to 48 hours) to facilitate the transfer of the woman in preterm labor to an appropriate facility with the capability of caring for a preterm newborn, to treat a contributing medical disorder such as an infection, and to administer corticosteroids to stimulate fetal lung maturation (de Veciana et al., 1995; Hill, 1995; Iams, 1996; Sandmire, 1996).

β-Sympathomimetics. β-Sympathomimetics work by acting on type II β-adrenergic receptors of the sympathetic nervous system, which has the effect of inhibiting uterine muscle activity and causing vasodilation, bronchodilation, and muscle glycogenolysis. However, because of the presence of β-receptor sites in other organs, they also cause certain side effects. The cardiovascular system is the system most affected.

Cardiopulmonary complications are potential consequences of β-sympathomimetic therapy. In fact, some deaths in pregnant women with unrecognized preexisting cardiovascular disease have been attributed to the use of these medications. Careful assessment and monitoring are essential in all women receiving these agents, especially when given intravenously. Because of these possible cardiopulmonary effects, the primary health care provider may

PLAN OF CARE *Preterm Labor*

NURSING DIAGNOSIS Knowledge deficit related to recognition of preterm labor

Expected Outcome *Woman and significant other delineate the signs and symptoms of preterm labor.*

Nursing Interventions/*Rationales*

Assess what the partners know about abnormal signs and symptoms during pregnancy *to identify areas of deficit.*

Discuss signs and symptoms that serve as warning signs of preterm labor *so that the woman or her partner has adequate information to identify problems early.*

Provide written supplemental materials that include a list of warning signs and instructions regarding what to do if any of the listed signs occur *so that the couple can reinforce and review learning and act swiftly and appropriately should a sign occur.*

Discuss and demonstrate how to assess and time the contractions *to provide needed skills to assess the signs of labor.*

NURSING DIAGNOSIS Risk for maternal/fetal injury related to recurrence of preterm labor

Expected Outcomes *Woman demonstrates ability to assess self and fetus for signs of recurring labor; maternal-fetal well-being is maintained.*

Nursing Interventions/*Rationales*

Teach woman/partner how to monitor fetal and uterine contraction activity daily *to provide immediate evidence of a worsening condition.*

Have woman/partner report rupture of membranes, vaginal bleeding, cramping, pelvic pressure, or low backache to appropriate health care resource immediately *because such symptoms are signs of labor.*

If home uterine activity monitoring is to be used, teach woman/partner how to use the monitoring device and how to transmit the data to the health care provider via telephone *to enhance correct use of monitoring device and increase the accuracy of detection of early labor.*

Have woman monitor her weight, diet, fluid intake, and vital signs on a daily basis to *evaluate for potential problems.*

Limit activities to bed rest with bathroom privileges *to decrease the likelihood of onset of labor.*

Use a side-lying position *to enhance placental perfusion.*

Abstain from sexual intercourse and nipple stimulation *because such activities may stimulate uterine contractions.*

Practice relaxation techniques *to decrease uterine tone and decrease anxiety and stress.*

Take tocolytic or other medications per physician's orders *to inhibit uterine contractions.*

Teach woman/partner about and have them report any medication side effects immediately *to prevent medication-induced complications.*

Have family arrange for alternative strategies in carrying out the woman's usual roles and functions *to decrease stress and limit temptations to increase activity.*

If small children are part of the household, encourage family to make alternative arrangements for child care *to enhance woman's adherence to bedrest protocol.*

NURSING DIAGNOSIS Fear/anxiety related to preterm labor and potentially premature neonate

Expected Outcomes *Feelings and symptoms of fear/anxiety abate.*

Nursing Interventions/*Rationales*

Provide a calm, soothing atmosphere and teach family to provide emotional support *to facilitate coping.*

Encourage verbalization of fears *to decrease intensity of emotional response.*

Involve woman and family in the home management of her condition *to promote a greater sense of control.*

Help the woman identify and use appropriate coping strategies and support systems *to reduce fear/anxiety.*

Explore the use of desensitization strategies such as progressive muscle relaxation, visual imagery, or thought stopping *to reduce fear-related emotions and related physical symptoms.*

NURSING DIAGNOSIS Diversional activity deficit related to imposed bed rest

Expected Outcomes *Verbalization of diminished feelings of boredom.*

Nursing Interventions/*Rationales*

Assist woman to creatively explore personally meaningful activities that can be pursued from the bed *to ensure activities that have meaning, purpose, and value to the individual.*

Maintain emphasis on personal choices of the woman *because doing so promotes control and minimizes imposition of routines by others.*

Evaluate what support and system resources are available in the environment *to assist in providing diversional activities.*

Explore ways for the woman to remain an active participant in home management and decision making *to promote control.*

Engage support of family and friends in carrying out chosen activities and making necessary environmental alterations *to ensure success.*

Teach woman about stress management and relaxation techniques *to help manage tension of confinement.*

From Wong D & Perry S: *Maternal child nursing care*, St Louis, 1998, Mosby.

EMERGENCY

Tocolytic-Induced Pulmonary Edema

SIGNS

Tightness in chest
Dyspnea, orthopnea
Crackles
Cough, frothy sputum

INTERVENTIONS

Discontinue medication immediately
Administer oxygen by face mask
Give intravenous diuretics as ordered
Restrict fluid intake
Position to facilitate breathing

BOX 25-4 *Risks and Complications of β-Sympathomimetic Therapy*

MATERNAL SIDE EFFECTS

Cardiovascular System

Widening pulse pressure (increase in systolic, decrease in diastolic)
Continuous palpitations, chest pain, tachycardia of 120 beats/min or more

Respiratory System

Shortness of breath, coughing, respirations exceeding 24/min, pulmonary edema (life-threatening)

Central Nervous System

Severe dizziness, drowsiness, headache, nervousness, restlessness

Metabolic Effects

Hyperglycemia, hypokalemia

Musculoskeletal System

Severe muscle cramps and weakness

Gastrointestinal System

Continuous nausea and vomiting

FETAL SIDE EFFECTS

Tachycardia of more than 180 beats/min
Hypoglycemia
Hyperinsulinemia

From Lowdermilk D, Perry S & Bobak I: *Maternity and women's health care*, ed 6, St Louis, 1997, Mosby.

---

order that an electrocardiogram be obtained before the first dose is given. A cardiac monitor for the mother may also be called for during intravenous administration to continuously assess her for the development of tachycardia, arrhythmia, or pulmonary edema (Emergency box).

Metabolic effects can occur because there are also receptor sites in the liver and pancreas. In addition, β-sympathomimetics can cause a decrease in the serum potassium levels, resulting in arrythmias. Other risks and complications are listed in Box 25-4 (Hill, 1995).

Maternal contraindications to the use of β-sympathomimetics include cardiovascular disease, severe preeclampsia, severe antepartum hemorrhage, chorioamnionitis, and hyperthyroidism. Fetal death and gestational age of less than 20 weeks confirmed by ultrasound scan are two fetal contraindications.

Ritodrine (Yutopar) was the first and remains the only β-sympathomimetic drug approved by the U.S. Food and Drug Administration (FDA) for use in the United States for the purpose of inhibiting preterm labor (Cunningham et al., 1997; Hill, 1995). When used, ritodrine is most often administered intravenously at an initial dose of 50 μg/min, which is increased every 10 to 20 minutes until contractions stop or a maximum dose of 350 μg/min is reached). Then it is administered intramuscularly, orally, or both, once the woman's condition has stabilized (Mongra & Creasy, 1995). The maintenance dose is determined by the primary health care provider and by the woman's response to the medication. The oral dosage is 10 to 20 mg given every 4 to 6 hours. The woman should be instructed to count her pulse before every dose and not to take the dose, but rather call her primary health care provider for further instructions, if her pulse rate is greater than 120 beats/min (Jones & Collins, 1996).

Terbutaline (Brethine) is another β-adrenergic agent that is used for the management of preterm labor. Although it has not been approved by the FDA for this purpose, most health care providers prefer it to ritodrine because its long-term clinical use has been observed to be associated with fewer serious side effects than ritodrine therapy. As a result, terbutaline is now the more commonly used of the two agents for this purpose and is usually given subcutaneously.

Because prolonged and continuous high-dose ritodrine and terbutaline treatment causes desensitization of the β-adrenergic receptors, preterm labor usually recurs as a result of tocolytic breakthrough. However, the continuous subcutaneous administration of low-dose terbutaline by pump infusion for long-term tocolysis has been reported to be effective in preventing recurrence and reducing the occurrence and severity of side effects, including tachycardia (Gilbert & Harmon; 1998; Hill, 1995). Pump infusion decreases desensitization by delivering a continuous low dose, with intermittent bolus doses administered at those times when uterine activity is known to occur in that particular woman. The average daily dose of terbutaline delivered by the pump is 3 to 4 mg (not including bolus doses); a daily oral dose of 30 to 60 mg is given in divided doses (Romero & Jones, 1994).

Women using the terbutaline pump (Fig. 25-2) need to be instructed in its use, self-injection techniques, and site care. Such techniques require that women have the fine motor skills and hand strength to handle and use the equipment

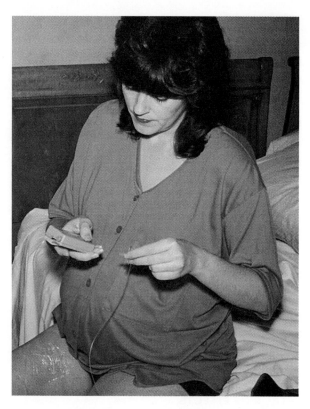

Fig. **25-2** Subcutaneous terbutaline pump attached to patient. (Courtesy Michael S. Clement, MD, Mesa, Ariz.)

required for this form of tocolytic therapy. In addition, they need to know the signs of preterm labor and the way to palpate uterine contractions and to recognize the warning signs and symptoms of β-sympathomimetic risks and complications (see Box 25-4). They also need to know that they must observe activity restrictions (Jones & Collins, 1996).

Nursing considerations. Nursing interventions for women receiving ritodrine or terbutaline depend on whether the drug is administered intravenously, subcutaneously, or orally. Before intravenous therapy, the woman may undergo hydration with intravenous fluid. The type and amount of solution depends on agency policy and practice of the primary health care provider. As stated previously, hydration can increase the woman's risk for pulmonary edema. Therefore, appropriate assessment measures should be instituted. When administered intravenously, the medication is mixed in an intravenous solution and piggybacked to the primary infusion at the part closest to the IV insertion site. The amount of medication given is controlled by an infusion pump. The dose is increased in increments, as ordered, with the minimum amount of the drug administered that will stop uterine contractions. After 12 to 24 hours of successful therapy, oral therapy usually is instituted as the intravenous therapy is tapered off (ACOG, 1995a; Gilbert & Harmon, 1998; Jones & Collins, 1996).

During intravenous therapy, the nurse continuously monitors uterine activity and FHR, which should not exceed 180 beats/min. Maternal vital signs, including blood pressure, are assessed per the hospital protocol; pulse should not exceed 120 beats/min. The woman's breath sounds are assessed and her lungs auscultated every 8 to 12 hours. The nurse assesses the woman for other signs of drug side effects, such as fluid overload, dyspnea, pulmonary edema, cardiac arrhythmias, and chest pain or pressure. If any signs of these are noted, the medication is stopped and the primary health care provider notified. An antidote, a β-blocking agent such as propranolol (Inderal), may be prescribed. The maximum intravenous rate of infusion is 125 ml/hr. Blood samples may be drawn for laboratory analysis of glucose and potassium levels to detect hypokalemia or hyperglycemia, two common side effects of the drug. Diabetic women who are being treated with ritodrine or terbutaline require careful monitoring and may require intravenous insulin administration. The woman is maintained on bed rest in a side-lying position to optimize placental perfusion and to decrease pressure on the cervix. Intake and output and daily weights are monitored to detect overhydration. The woman should be told about the potential side effects of the medication to avert undue anxiety if they occur.

If the women is taking either oral or subcutaneous therapy, maternal vital signs and FHR, fetal activity, and uterine activity are assessed per the hospital routine, or as ordered. If the woman's pulse is persistently above 120 beats/min, the primary health care provider is usually consulted before another dose is administered. The tocolytic medications need to be given on time every 4 to 6 hours to prevent the recurrence of uterine activity.

Magnesium sulfate. Magnesium sulfate also can decrease uterine activity, and it is a safer tocolytic agent than ritodrine or terbutaline. It is the most commonly used intravenous tocolytic in the United States today, almost replacing ritodrine and terbutaline as the first-line medication used to suppress preterm labor. Although maternal risks and complications can occur (Box 25-5), fetal-newborn side effects are rare. Magnesium oxide or gluconate is used whenever the drug is administered orally; the main side effect is diarrhea. This form of treatment, however, has had very limited success (Creasy, 1993, Hill, 1995).

For intravenous therapy, magnesium sulfate is mixed with normal saline and an initial dose of 4 to 6 gm is infused over a 20-minute period. The drug is then infused by a pump at a rate of 1 to 2 gm/hr and the dose increased per the hospital protocol (usually 0.5 gm/hr every 15 to 30 minutes) until contractions stop. Serum magnesium levels should be checked every 4 to 6 hours to ensure that the therapeutic level of 5 to 8 mEq/L has been reached but not exceeded. Intravenous tocolysis with magnesium sulfate is usually continued for at least 48 hours but should not exceed 7 days (de Veciana et al., 1995).

BOX 25-5

BOX 25-5 *Maternal Risks and Complications of Magnesium Sulfate Therapy*

CARDIOVASCULAR SYSTEM
- Vasodilation—flushing, hypothermia
- Chest pain, palpitations
- Hypotension
- Cardiac arrest

RESPIRATORY SYSTEM
- Respiratory depression
- Pulmonary edema

CENTRAL NERVOUS SYSTEM
- Decreased deep tendon reflexes
- Headaches

METABOLIC EFFECTS
- Electrolyte imbalances: hypermagnesemia, hypocalcemia

MUSCULOSKELETAL SYSTEM
- Drowsiness, lethargy

GASTROINTESTINAL SYSTEM
- Dry mouth
- Nausea and vomiting
- Paralytic ileus

BOX 25-6 *Risks and Complications of Nifedipine Therapy*

Headache
Fatigue
Hypotension, tachycardia
Dizziness
Peripheral edema
Vasodilation, flushing
Nausea

Nursing considerations. Nursing assessments during the intravenous administration of magnesium sulfate therapy include monitoring blood pressure, pulse, respiratory rates, heart and breath sounds; checking deep tendon reflexes; evaluating fluid balance (measuring intake and output, and weight); assessing level of consciousness; and checking laboratory results to see whether therapeutic levels of the magnesium have been reached and whether hypocalcemia has occurred. Hourly urine outputs may be determined because magnesium sulfate is excreted through the renal system. Poor renal function can lead to magnesium toxicity (Jones & Collins, 1996). Calcium gluconate should be available to reverse serious side effects. Uterine activity and FHR also are monitored. Neonatal side effects are rare but include slight muscle flaccidity and hypocalcemia.

Calcium channel blockers. Calcium channel blockers prevent preterm labor by blocking the movement of calcium into the smooth muscles of the uterus, thereby preventing contractions of the uterus. Nifedipine (Procardia) is the calcium channel blocker usually given for this purpose, although its use for preterm labor is still considered investigational (Mongra & Creasy, 1995). It is administered either orally or sublingually at a dosage of 10 to 20 mg every 3 to 8 hours (Gilbert & Harmon, 1998). Fewer risks and complications are reported for nifedipine than for β-agonists (Box 25-6). However, more research is needed

to determine the potential benefits and risks of nifedipine treatment to the woman and fetus (Hill, 1995; Jones & Collins, 1996).

Prostaglandin inhibitors. Prostaglandin antagonists (indomethacin, nonsteroidal antiinflammatory agents [naproxen], and salicylates) are being investigated for the treatment of preterm labor because these drugs are known to be as effective in relaxing the uterus as β-agonists. The maternal side effects that have been observed are minimal but may include gastrointestinal upset, prolonged bleeding time, headache, tinnitus, vertigo and rash. However, concern about their potential effects on the fetus (especially premature closing of the ductus arteriosus and renal compromises that can lead to oligohydramnios) and their potential to cause bleeding and to mask infection as a result of their antipyretic effect continue to be responsible for limiting their use (Hill, 1995; Jones & Collins, 1996; Mongra & Creasy, 1995). Studies investigating their use have shown that their administration for short periods ≤ 48 hours) may limit the fetal effects (Keirse, 1995).

Oxytocin antagonists. Oxytocin antagonists are tocolytic agents whose efficacy is still being investigated. Atosiban is a synthetic form of this new class of tocolytic drugs. The effect of oxytocin antagonists is to block oxytocin receptors thereby decreasing the contractility of the uterus. The route of administration at present is by intravenous infusion. These agents have demonstrated fewer serious maternal, fetal, and neonatal side effects. Maternal side effects documented have included nausea and vomiting, headache, uterine atony, and urinary tract infection (Hill, 1995; Simpson, 1997).

Promotion of fetal lung maturity

Respiratory distress syndrome (RDS) is common in small preterm infants whose lungs are immature. However, it has been found that the incidence and severity of RDS are reduced if glucocorticoids (e.g., betamethasone) are administered to the mother at least 24 to 48 hours, but no more than 7 days, before the birth. The fetus must be at less than 34 weeks' gestation.

Neither tocolytic nor steroidal therapy is universally recommended for the management of preterm labor after premature rupture of membranes (PROM) (Hannah, 1996;

Hill, 1995; Jones & Collins, 1996; Simpson, 1997). The woman who has received both tocolytics and glucocorticoids is at risk for cardiac decompensation because of the side effects of the drugs. Therefore, the nurse should be vigilant in monitoring the woman for signs of cardiac decompensation (see p. 621) and pulmonary edema.

Care during preterm labor and birth

If labor cannot be stopped, the primary health care provider makes every attempt to help the woman give birth to the preterm infant safely and without trauma. If needed, and if time permits, the woman is usually transferred to a center with adequate neonatal services to provide care for her preterm infant. During labor, drugs such as narcotics or barbiturates that can depress the fetus's state are avoided. Epidural analgesia is commonly used during labor, but pudendal block or local anesthetic may be administered for the birth. An episiotomy may be performed to shorten the second stage of labor and to reduce excessive pressure on the fragile fetal head. The route of birth is a subject of controversy, but cesarean birth may be performed in the event of malpresentation or fetal distress.

Parental concern for the well-being of the infant is apparent during labor. Such parents need to be aware of the interest and support of staff members to help them through this difficult time. However, false assurance of fetal health must be avoided. For some parents the reality of the situation is not fully appreciated until they see their daughter or son in the intensive care unit. For those who experience fetal or neonatal death, the loss intensifies once the stress of labor and childbirth is over (see later discussion).

During the postpartum period, the physical care of the mother is similar to that required after any vaginal or cesarean birth. However, if the woman gives birth while still receiving tocolytics or shortly after they have been discontinued, she is at increased risk for postpartum hemorrhage. Frequent palpation of the fundus for uterine atony is critical (Hill, 1995). The family will be very anxious about the health of and prognosis for their infant. Care of the preterm infant involves not only medical and nursing personnel but also the participation of the parents. The nurse must be aware of the effect that preterm birth may have on family dynamics. Parents must be helped to accept that the infant has special needs, and they must learn to meet these needs before discharge so that they will have more realistic expectations when they are at home (Weingarten et al., 1990). Additionally, prolonged treatment of the woman with activity restriction increases the time it will take her to reach her prepregnant level of functioning.

Evaluation

Evaluation of the effectiveness of nursing care for women with preterm labor is based on the previously stated expected outcomes.

I PREMATURE RUPTURE OF MEMBRANES

Premature rupture of membranes (PROM) is the rupture of the amniotic sac before labor begins. It occurs in approximately 2% to 18% of all pregnancies and is the most common cause of preterm labor (Gaute & Spellacy, 1994; Varney, 1997). At term, uterine contractions begin in most women within 24 hours after the rupture of membranes; however, labor may not start for up to 1 week after the rupture of membranes in women who are between 28 and 34 weeks of gestation. The earlier in pregnancy that rupture of the membranes occurs, the longer the time before the onset of labor. Rupture of the membranes before term is called preterm PROM (PPROM). If the membranes are ruptured for more than 24 hours before birth, it is called prolonged rupture of the membranes (Gaute & Spellacy, 1994; Varney, 1997).

Etiologic Factors

The cause of PROM is unknown in most instances. However, factors that are associated with its occurrence include amnionitis, placenta previa, multifetal gestation, malpresentation, polyhydramnios, bacterial vaginal/cervical infections, and maternal smoking (Andrews et al., 1995; Gilbert & Harmon, 1998; King, 1994; McGregor et al., 1995). PROM may also occur after cervical cerclage or amniocentesis (Gaute & Spellacy, 1994). PROM can result in preterm labor and birth and in intrauterine infection and compression of the umbilical cord as a result of prolapse or oligohydramnios (Varney, 1997).

I CARE MANAGEMENT

If PROM is suspected, a sterile speculum examination is done. Visualization of amniotic fluid from the cervix, a positive nitrazine test result (litmus paper turns blue), or the presence of ferning (a fernlike pattern assumed by dried amniotic fluid on a slide and seen under a microscope) (Gilbert & Harmon, 1998) are all signs of ruptured membranes.

The treatment of PROM continues to be a controversial matter. The woman may be hospitalized until the birth of the infant, or she may return home (Home Care box). Expectant management is often instituted if there are no signs of infection, or fetal distress. This approach includes daily assessments of maternal temperature, pulse, respirations, and blood pressure, as well as the FHR (tachycardia may be a sign of infection) and fetal movements; palpation to evaluate for uterine tenderness; assessment of vaginal discharge for color, odor, and amount; and assessment for signs of preterm labor (Grohar, 1994). Biophysical profiles every 2 days to weekly may be done to assess fetal well-being and to monitor the amniotic fluid index.

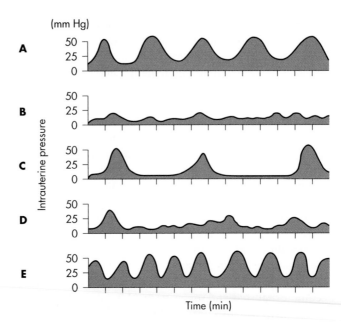

Fig. 25-3 Uterine contractility patterns in labor. **A,** Typical normal labor. **B,** Subnormal intensity, with frequency greater than needed for optimum performance. **C,** Normal contractions but too infrequent for efficient labor. **D,** Incoordinate activity. **E,** Hypercontractility.

If infection is identified, treatment with broad-spectrum antibiotics is usually initiated. Induction of labor with birth accomplished vaginally or cesarean birth may be necessary to improve the chances of a good fetal outcome, even if the fetus is premature (Varney, 1997).

DYSTOCIA

Dystocia is defined as long, difficult, or abnormal labor and is caused by various conditions associated with the five factors affecting labor. It is estimated that dystocia occurs in approximately 8% to 11% of women during the first stage of labor when the fetus is in a vertex presentation. Second-stage dystocia is equally as common (Wiznitzer, 1995). Dystocia can be caused by any of the following:

1. *Dysfunctional labor,* resulting in ineffective uterine contractions or maternal bearing-down efforts (the powers).
2. *Alterations in the pelvic structure* (the passage).
3. *Fetal causes,* including abnormal presentation or position, anomalies, excessive size, and number of fetuses (the passenger).
4. *Maternal position* during labor and birth.
5. *Psychologic responses* of the mother to labor related to past experiences, preparation, culture and heritage, and support system.

These five factors are interdependent. In assessing the woman for an abnormal labor pattern, the nurse must consider the way in which these factors interact and influence labor progress. Dystocia is suspected when there is a lack of progress in the rate of cervical dilatation, a lack of progress in fetal descent and expulsion, or an alteration in the characteristics of uterine contractions.

Dysfunctional Labor

Dysfunctional labor is described as abnormal uterine contractions that prevent the normal progress of cervical dilatation, effacement (primary powers), or descent (secondary powers), or a combination of these. Dysfunction of uterine contractions can be further described as being hypertonic or hypotonic.

Hypertonic uterine dysfunction

The woman who is experiencing **hypertonic uterine dysfunction,** or primary dysfunctional labor, often is an anxious first-time mother who is having painful contractions that are out of proportion to their intensity and that are not causing cervical dilatation or effacement. These contractions usually occur in the latent stage (cervical dilatation of <4 cm) and usually are uncoordinated and frequent (Fig. 25-3). The force of the contraction may be in the midsection of the uterus rather than in the fundus, and the uterus may not relax completely between contractions (Varney, 1997).

Women experiencing hypertonic uterine dysfunction may be exhausted and express concern about loss of control because of the intense pain they are experiencing and the lack of progress. **Therapeutic rest,** which is achieved through the administration of effective analgesics such as morphine or meperidine to reduce the pain and encourage sleep, is usually prescribed for the management of hypertonic uterine dysfunction. Often uterine activity will be normal when these women awaken.

Hypotonic uterine dysfunction

The second and more common type of uterine dysfunction is **hypotonic uterine dysfunction,** or secondary uterine inertia. In this form of uterine dysfunction, the woman initially makes normal progress into the active stage of labor, then the contractions become weak and inefficient or stop altogether (see Fig. 25-3). The uterus is easily indented, even at the peak of contractions. Cephalopelvic disproportion and malpositions are common causes of this type of uterine dysfunction.

Women experiencing hypotonic uterine dysfunction may become exhausted and are at particular risk for infection. Management usually consists of performing an ultrasound or x-ray examination to rule out cephalopelvic disproportion and assessing the FHR pattern, characteristics of amniotic fluid if membranes are ruptured, and maternal well-being. If findings are normal, then measures can be used to augment the progress of labor, including ambulation, hydrotherapy, enema, stripping or rupture of membranes, nipple stimulation, and oxytocin infusion (Varney, 1997).

Secondary powers

Secondary powers, or bearing-down efforts, are compromised when large amounts of analgesic are given. Anesthesia may also block the bearing-down reflex and, as a result, alter the effectiveness of voluntary efforts. Exhaustion resulting from lack of sleep or long labor and fatigue resulting from inadequate hydration and food intake also affect the woman's voluntary efforts. In addition, maternal position can work against the forces of gravity, as well as decrease the strength and efficiency of contractions. The characteristics of dysfunctional labor are summarized in Table 25-1.

Alterations in Pelvic Structure

Pelvic dystocia

Pelvic dystocia can occur whenever there are contractures of the pelvic diameters that reduce the capacity of the bony pelvis, including the inlet, midpelvis, outlet, or any combination of these planes. Pelvic contractures may be caused by congenital abnormalities, maternal malnutrition, neoplasms, or lower spinal disorders. An immature pelvic size predisposes some adolescent mothers to pelvic dystocia. Pelvic deformities may also be the result of automobile or other accidents.

An inlet contracture occurs in 1% to 2% of term births and is diagnosed whenever the diagonal conjugate is less than 11.5 cm. The incidence of face and shoulder presentation is increased. Because these presentations prevent engagement and fetal descent, the risk of prolapse of the umbilical cord is increased during such births. Inlet contracture is associated with maternal rickets and a flat pelvis. Weak uterine contractions may be noted during the first stage of labor in affected women.

Midplane contracture, the most common cause of pelvic dystocia, is diagnosed whenever the sum of the interischial spinous and posterior sagittal diameters of the midpelvis is 13.5 cm or less. Fetal descent is arrested (transverse arrest of the fetal head) in such births because the head cannot rotate internally. These infants are usually born by cesarean, but vacuum-assisted birth has been used safely if the cervix is fully dilated. Midforceps-assisted birth usually is not done because of the increased perinatal morbidity associated with this intervention.

Outlet contracture occurs when the interischial diameter is 8 cm or less. It rarely occurs in the absence of midplane contracture, however. Women with outlet contracture have a long, narrow pubic arch and an android pelvis, and this causes fetal descent to be arrested. Maternal complications include extensive perineal lacerations during vaginal birth because the fetal head is pushed posteriorly.

Soft-tissue dystocia

Soft-tissue dystocia results from obstruction of the birth passage by an anatomic abnormality other than that involving the bony pelvis. The obstruction may result from placenta previa (low-lying placenta) that partially or completely obstructs the internal os of the cervix. Other causes, such as leiomyomas (uterine fibroids) in the lower uterine segment, ovarian tumors, and a full bladder or rectum, may prevent the fetus from entering the pelvis. Occasionally, cervical edema occurs during labor when the cervix is caught between the presenting part and the symphysis or when the woman engages in bearing-down efforts prematurely, thereby preventing complete dilatation.

Bandl's ring, a pathologic retraction ring, is associated with prolonged rupture of membranes and protracted labor (Cunningham et al., 1997).

Fetal Causes

Dystocia of fetal origin may be caused by anomalies, excessive fetal size and malpresentation, malposition, or multifetal pregnancy. Complications associated with dystocia of fetal origin include neonatal asphyxia, fetal injuries or fractures, and maternal vaginal lacerations. Although spontaneous vaginal birth is possible in these instances, a low-forceps or vacuum-assisted birth or cesarean birth often is necessary.

Anomalies

Gross ascites, abnormal tumors, myelomeningocele, and hydrocephalus are fetal anomalies that can also cause dystocia. The anomalies affect the relationship of the fetal anatomy to the maternal pelvic capacity, with the result that the fetus is unable to descend through the birth canal.

TABLE 25-1 *Dysfunctional Labor: Primary and Secondary Powers*

HYPERTONIC UTERINE DYSFUNCTION	HYPOTONIC UTERINE DYSFUNCTION	INADEQUATE VOLUNTARY EXPULSIVE FORCES
DESCRIPTION		
Usually occurs before 4 cm dilatation; cause not known, may be related to fear and tension (primary powers)	Cause may be contracture and fetal malposition, overdistention of uterus (e.g., twins), or unknown (primary powers)	Involves abdominal and levator ani muscles Occurs in second stage of labor; cause may be related to conduction anesthetic, heavy analgesic, exhaustion
CHANGE IN PATTERN OF PROGRESS		
Pain out of proportion to intensity of contraction Pain out of proportion to effectiveness of contraction in effacing and dilatating the cervix Contractions increase in frequency Contractions uncoordinated Uterus is contracted between contractions, cannot be indented	Contractions decrease in frequency and intensity Uterus easily indentable even at peak of contraction Uterus relaxed between contractions (normal)	No voluntary urge to push or bear down or else inadequate/ineffective pushing
POTENTIAL MATERNAL EFFECTS		
Loss of control related to intensity of pain and lack of progress Exhaustion	Infection Exhaustion Psychologic trauma	Spontaneous vaginal birth prevented
POTENTIAL FETAL EFFECTS		
Fetal asphyxia with meconium aspiration	Fetal infection Fetal and neonatal death	Fetal asphyxia
MEDICAL MANAGEMENT		
Analgesic (e.g., morphine, meperidine) if membranes not ruptured or cephalopelvic disproportion not present Relief of pain permits mother to rest; when she awakens, normal uterine activity may begin	Rule out cephalopelvic disproportion Oxytocic stimulation of labor (p. 716)	Coach mother in bearing down with contractions Position mother in favorable position for pushing Low forceps or vacuum-assisted birth if assistance is needed Cesarean birth only if nonreassuring fetal status occurs

Cephalopelvic disproportion

Cephalopelvic disproportion (CPD), also called *fetopelvic disproportion (FPD),* is related to excessive fetal size (4,000 gm or more) and occurs in about 5% of term births. When CPD is present, the fetus cannot fit through the maternal pelvis to be born vaginally. Excessive fetal size, or macrosomia, is associated with maternal diabetes mellitus, obesity, multiparity, or the large size of one or both parents. If the maternal pelvis is too small, abnormally shaped, or deformed, CPD may be of maternal origin.

Malposition

The most common fetal malposition is the persistent occipitoposterior position (right occipitoposterior [ROP] or left occipitoposterior [LOP]; see Fig. 12-2), occurring in about 25% of all labors. Labor in these women, especially the second stage, is prolonged; the mother typically complains of severe back pain resulting from the fetal head pressing against her sacrum. Counterpressure to the sacral area and frequent position changes may decrease the pain. The hands-and-knees or lateral position has been used to facilitate rotation of the fetus from a posterior to an anterior position (Simpkin, 1995).

Malpresentation

Breech presentation is the most common form of malpresentation, occurring in 3% to 4% of all births and in up to 25% of preterm births. There are four main types of breech presentation: frank breech (thighs flexed, knees extended), complete breech (thighs and knees flexed), and two types of incomplete breech, one in which the knee extends below the buttocks and the other in which the foot extends below the buttocks (Fig. 25-4). Breech presentations are associated with multifetal gestation, preterm birth, fetal

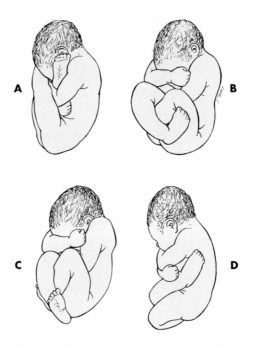

Fig. **25-4** Types of breech presentation. **A,** Frank breech: thighs are flexed on hips; knees are extended. **B,** Complete breech: thighs and knees are flexed. **C,** Incomplete breech: foot extends below buttocks. **D,** Incomplete breech: knee extends below buttocks.

and maternal anomalies, hydramnios, and oligohydramnios. Diagnosis is made on the basis of the findings yielded by abdominal palpation and vaginal examination and usually is confirmed by ultrasound scan (Laros, Flanagan & Kilpatrick, 1995; Lydon et al., 1993).

During labor, the descent of the fetus in a breech presentation may be slow because the breech is not as good a dilating wedge as the fetal head, but the labor itself usually is not prolonged. There is risk of the cord prolapsing if the membranes rupture in early labor. The presence of meconium in amniotic fluid is not necessarily a sign of fetal distress, however, because it results from the pressure being exerted on the fetal abdominal wall as it traverses the birth canal. The fetal heart tones of such infants are best heard at or above the umbilicus. Vaginal birth is accomplished by mechanisms of labor that manipulate the buttocks and lower extremities as they emerge from the birth canal (Varney, 1997) (Fig. 25-5). Piper forceps sometimes are used to deliver the head (see Fig. 25-11).

Besides the vaginal birth of the fetus in breech presentation, external cephalic version (ECV) may be tried to turn the fetus to a vertex presentation. Cesarean birth may also prove necessary (Laros et al., 1995).

Although opinions vary regarding the conditions calling for cesarean birth, it is commonly performed for nulliparas, women with fetuses estimated to be larger than 3,800 gm or smaller than 1,500 gm if labor is ineffective or complications occur (Scott, 1994). Although cesarean birth reduces the risks to the fetus, the maternal risks are increased. ECV also poses risks and is not always successful.

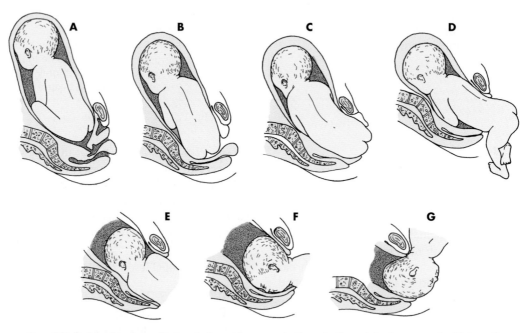

Fig. **25-5** Mechanism of labor in breech presentation. **A,** Breech before onset of labor. **B,** Engagement and internal rotation. **C,** Lateral flexion. **D,** External rotation or restitution. **E,** Internal rotation of shoulders and head. **F,** Face rotates to sacrum when occiput is anterior. **G,** Head is born by gradual flexion during elevation of fetal body.

Women whose breech presentation occurs late in pregnancy need to be informed of the options for birth, as well as the risks associated with each.

Face and brow presentations (Fig. 25-6) are uncommon and are associated with fetal anomalies, pelvic contractures, and CPD. Vaginal birth is possible if the fetus flexes to a vertex presentation, although forceps often are used. Cesarean birth is indicated if the presentation persists, there is fetal distress, or labor stops progressing.

Cesarean birth is usually necessary for fetuses in shoulder presentations (the fetus is in a transverse lie), although ECV may be attempted after 38 weeks' gestation (Cunningham et al., 1997; Varney, 1997).

Multifetal pregnancy

Multifetal pregnancy is the gestation of twins, triplets, quadruplets, or more infants. In 1995, the number of multiple births rose to 26.1 per 1,000 live births. This represents a slight decrease in twin births but an increase in the number of triplets, quadruplets, and more. It is speculated that this trend is related to use of fertility-enhancing drugs and procedures (Ventura et al., 1997). Their births are associated with more complications, including dysfunctional labor, than are single births. This high incidence of complications and risk of perinatal mortality primarily stems from the birth of low-birth-weight infants resulting from preterm birth or intrauterine growth restriction (IUGR). In addition, fetal complications such as congenital anomalies and abnormal presentations can result in dystocia and cause the incidence of cesarean birth to be increased. For example, in only half of all twin pregnancies do both fetuses present in the vertex position, the most favorable for vaginal birth; in one third of the pregnancies, one twin may present in the vertex position and one in the breech. To accomplish the vaginal birth of both twins, an intrapartum version (internal or external) may be attempted for the twin in a nonvertex position if the presenting twin's position is vertex. If the presenting twin is not in a vertex position, a cesarean birth often is performed (Cunningham et al., 1997; Varney, 1997).

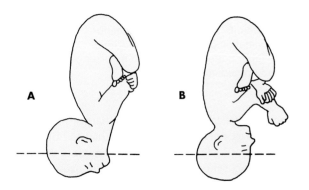

Fig. **25-6** Extension of normally flexed head. Face **(A)** and brow **(B)** presentations.

Position of the Mother

The functional relationships between the uterine contractions, the fetus, and the mother's pelvis are altered by the maternal position. In addition, the position can have either a mechanically advantageous or disadvantageous effect on the mechanisms of labor by altering the effects of gravity and the relationships among body parts that are important to the progress of labor. For example, the hands-and-knees position more effectively facilitates rotation of the fetus from a posterior occiput position than does the lateral position. Sitting and squatting facilitate fetal descent during pushing and shorten the second stage of labor (Biancuzzo, 1993). In addition, discouraging maternal movement or restricting the woman's position during labor to the recumbent or lithotomy position may only compromise labor. The incidence of dystocia is also increased in women confined to these positions, resulting in an increased need for augmentation of labor, the use of forceps or vacuum-assisted or cesarean birth (Andrews & Chrzanowski, 1990).

Psychologic Response

Hormones released in response to stress can also bring about dystocia. Sources of stress vary for each woman, but pain and the absence of a support person are two accepted factors. Confinement to bed and the restriction of maternal movement can also be a source of psychologic stress that only compounds the physiologic stress caused by immobility in the unmedicated laboring woman. If the woman's anxiety is excessive, it can cause normal cervical dilatation to be inhibited, resulting in **prolonged labor** and increased pain perception. Anxiety also causes an increase in the levels of stress-related hormones (β-endorphin, adrenocorticotropic hormone, cortisol, and epinephrine). These hormones act on the smooth muscles of the uterus; when the levels are increased, this can lead to dystocia by reducing uterine contractility (Biancuzzo, 1993).

Abnormal Labor Patterns

Abnormal labor patterns occur in 8% of pregnancies, with the highest incidence among nulliparous women (Friedman, 1989). These patterns may result from the following previously described causes: ineffective uterine contractions, pelvic contractures, CPD, abnormal fetal presentations or position, early use of analgesics, conduction anesthesia, and anxiety and stress. In these women, progress in either the first or second stage of labor can be either protracted (prolonged) or arrested (stopped). Abnormal progress can be identified by plotting cervical dilatation on a labor graph at various intervals after the onset of labor and comparing the resulting curve with a normal labor curve. Figure 25-7, *A* is a labor graph showing a normal labor progress in a first-time mother. Fig. 25-7, *B* shows major types of deviation from the normal progress of labor. If a woman exhibits an abnormal labor

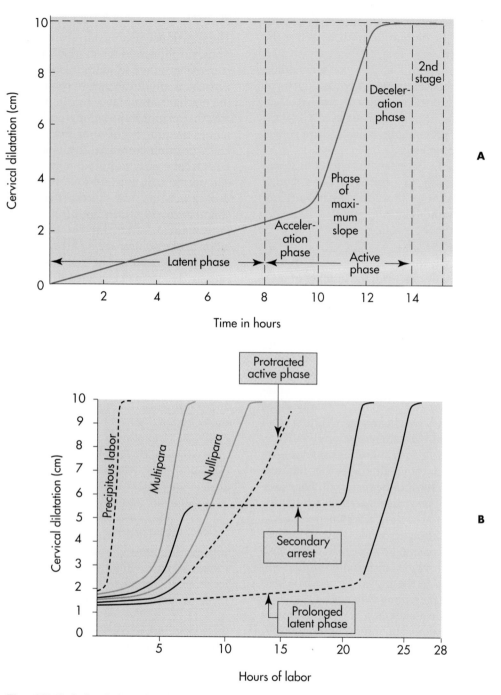

Fig. **25-7 A,** Depiction of a normal labor for a primigravida. **B,** Major types of deviation from normal progress of labor may be detected by noting dilatation of cervix at various intervals after labor begins. If a woman exhibits an abnormal labor pattern, as depicted by broken lines, primary health care provider should be notified immediately.

pattern, as depicted by the broken lines, the primary health care provider is notified.

Six abnormal labor patterns have been identified and classified by Friedman (1989) according to the nature of the cervical dilatation and fetal descent. The labor patterns seen in normal and abnormal labor are described in Table 25-2.

The risk of fetal death increases sharply whenever the active first stage of labor lasts for more than 15 hours. Maternal morbidity and death may occur as a result of uterine rupture, infection, serious dehydration, and postpartum hemorrhage. A long and difficult labor also can have an adverse psychologic effect on the mother, father, and family.

TABLE 25-2 *Labor Patterns in Normal and Abnormal Labor*

NORMAL LABOR

1. Dilatation: continues
   a. Latent phase: <4 cm and low slope
   b. Active phase: >5 cm or high slope
   c. Deceleration phase: ≥9 cm
2. Descent: active at ≥9 cm dilatation

ABNORMAL LABOR

PATTERN	NULLIPARAS	MULTIPARAS
Prolonged latent phase	>20 hr	>14 hr
Protracted active phase dilatation	<1.2 cm/hr	<1.5 cm/hr
Secondary arrest: no change	≥2 hr	≥2 hr
Protracted descent	<1 cm/hr	<2 cm/hr
Arrest of descent	≥1 hr	≥½ hr
Failure of descent	No change during deceleration phase and second stage	
Precipitous labor	>5 cm/hr	10 cm/hr

Precipitous labor

Precipitous labor is defined as labor that lasts less than 3 hours from the onset of contractions to the time of birth. Precipitous labor may result from hypertonic uterine contractions that are tetanic-like in intensity. Maternal and fetal complications can occur as a result. Maternal complications include uterine rupture, lacerations of the birth canal, amniotic fluid embolism, and postpartum hemorrhage. Fetal complications include hypoxia resulting from decreased periods of uterine relaxation between contractions and intracranial hemorrhage related to rapid birth (Cunningham et al., 1997).

Women who experience precipitous labor often describe feelings of disbelief that their labor began so quickly, alarm that their labor progressed so rapidly, panic about the possibility they would not make it to the hospital on time to give birth, and finally, relief when they arrived at the hospital. In addition, women expressed frustration when nurses would not believe them when they reported their readiness to push. Some women have difficulty remembering the details of their labor and birth and require others, including caregivers, to help them to fill in the gaps in their memory (Rippin-Sisler, 1996).

I CARE MANAGEMENT

The care management of the woman at risk for problems related to abnormal labor or birth, or both, involves all members of the health care team. The rendering of nursing care is facilitated through the use of the nursing process.

Assessment and Nursing Diagnoses

Risk assessment is a continuous process in the laboring woman. Review of the findings gleaned during the initial interview conducted at the woman's admission to the labor unit and ongoing observations of her psychologic response to labor may reveal factors that can be a source of dysfunctional labor, for example, anxiety or fear, a complication of pregnancy, or previous labor complications. The initial physical assessment and ongoing assessments provide information about the frequency, duration, and intensity of uterine contractions; the cervical status; the FHR; the presentation and station of the fetus; and the status of membranes.

The health care provider can use laboratory data such as the scalp pH to identify fetal distress and ultrasound scanning to identify potential dysfunctional labor problems related to the fetus or maternal pelvis. All these assessments help in the accurate identification of potential and actual nursing diagnoses related to dystocia and maternal-fetal compromise.

Nursing diagnoses vary with the type of dystocia, as well as with the individual needs of the woman and her family. Potential or actual nursing diagnoses that might be identified in women experiencing dystocia are listed in the box.

I Nursing Diagnoses

Dystocia

Anxiety related to:
• Slowed labor progress
• Perceived threat to well-being of self or fetus
Pain related to:
• Dystocia
• Obstetric procedures
Risk for fetal injury related to:
• Obstetric procedures
Risk for maternal injury related to:
• Interventions implemented for dystocia
Risk for infection related to:
• Premature rupture of membranes
• Operative procedures
Fatigue related to:
• Prolonged labor
Risk for altered parent-infant attachment related to:
• Unplanned cesarean birth
Ineffective individual coping related to:
• Lack of knowledge regarding measures to enhance labor and facilitate birth
• Pain
• Fatigue
• Lack of support system
Situational low self-esteem related to:
• Inability to labor and give birth as expected

Expected Outcomes of Care

Nursing diagnoses provide the direction for care. After they have been identified, expected outcomes are formulated. They are phrased in patient-centered terms and prioritized. Nursing actions are selected with the woman, as appropriate, to meet the expected outcomes.

Expected outcomes for the woman who is experiencing dystocia include that she will:

- Verbalize understanding of the causes and treatment of dysfunctional labor
- Use measures recommended by the health care team to enhance the progress of labor and birth
- Use positive patterns of coping to maintain a positive self-concept
- Demonstrate diminished or minimal anxiety
- Verbalize relief of pain
- Experience labor and birth with minimal or no complications, such as infection, injury, or hemorrhage
- Give birth to a healthy infant who has not experienced fetal distress

Plan of Care and Interventions

Nurses assume many caregiving roles when labor is complicated. Knowledge of the medical management required for each condition is essential to implementing the nursing process. This knowledge enables the nurse to work collaboratively with the other health care providers and to meet the woman's knowledge and emotional needs. Interventions that the nurse may implement or assist with implementing include external cephalic version; trial of labor; induction or augmentation with oxytocin; amniotomy; and operative procedures such as forceps-assisted birth, vacuum-assisted birth, and cesarean birth. The nursing role is identified with each of the procedures described.

LEGAL TIP **Standard of Care—Labor and Birth at Risk**

- *Document all assessment findings, interventions, and patient responses on patient record, and monitor strips according to unit protocols, procedures, and/or policies.*
- *Assess whether the woman is fully informed about procedures to which she is consenting.*
- *Maintain safety in administering medications and treatments correctly.*
- *Get verbal orders signed as soon as possible.*
- *Provide care at the acceptable standard (e.g., according to hospital protocols, professional standards).*
- *If short staffing occurs in the unit and the nurse is assigned additional patients, the nurse should document that rejecting these assignments would have placed the patient in danger as a result of abandonment.*
- *Maternal and fetal monitoring continues until birth according to the policies, procedures, and/or protocols of the birthing facility, even when a decision to carry out cesarean birth is made.*

Version

Version is the turning of the fetus artificially from one presentation to another and may be done either externally or internally.

External cephalic version. External cephalic version (ECV) is used to attempt to turn the fetus from a breech or shoulder presentation to a vertex presentation for birth. It may be attempted in a labor and birth setting after 37 weeks' gestation. Before it is attempted, however, ultrasound scanning is done to determine the fetal position, to locate the umbilical cord, to rule out placenta previa, and to assess the amount of amniotic fluid, the fetal age, and the presence of any anomalies. A nonstress test is also performed to confirm fetal well-being or the FHR pattern is monitored for a period of time, usually 10 to 20 minutes. Informed consent must be obtained for the maneuver to be done. Contraindications to its use include uterine anomalies, previous cesarean birth, CPD, placenta previa, multifetal gestation, and oligohydramnios (Cunningham et al., 1997; Laros et al., 1995).

ECV is accomplished by the exertion of gentle, constant pressure on the abdomen while the FHR is continuously monitored (Fig. 25-8). A tocolytic agent, such as magnesium sulfate or terbutaline usually is given to relax the uterus and facilitate the maneuver. Ultrasound scanning usually is done to identify potential problems, such as cord entanglement and placental separation (Cunningham et al., 1997; Laros et al., 1995).

During an attempted ECV, the nurse continuously monitors the FHR, especially for bradycardia; frequently checks the maternal vital signs; and assesses the woman's level of comfort because the procedure may cause discomfort. After the procedure is completed, the nurse continues to monitor maternal vital signs, uterine activity, and FHR and watches for vaginal bleeding until the woman's condition is stable. Women who are Rh negative should receive Rh immune globulin because the manipulation can cause fetomaternal bleeding (Cunningham et al., 1997; Laros et al., 1995).

Internal version. With internal version, the fetus is turned by the physician who inserts a hand into the uterus and changes the presentation to a cephalic (head) or podalic (foot) one. Internal version may be used in multifetal pregnancies to deliver the second fetus. The safety of this procedure has not been documented; maternal and fetal injury are possible. Cesarean birth is the usual method for managing malpresentation in multifetal pregnancies. The nurse's role is to monitor the status of the fetus and to provide support to the woman.

Trial of labor

A **trial of labor (TOL)** is the allowance of a reasonable period (4 to 6 hours) of spontaneous active labor so that the safety of a vaginal birth for the mother and infant can be

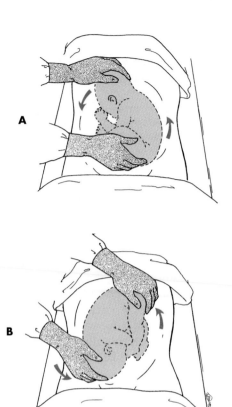

Fig. **25-8** External version of fetus from breech to vertex presentation. This must be achieved without force. **A,** Breech is pushed up out of pelvic inlet while head is pulled toward inlet. **B,** Head is pushed toward inlet while breech is pulled upward.

assessed. TOL may be initiated if the mother's pelvis is of questionable size or shape, if she wishes to give birth vaginally after a previous cesarean birth, or if the fetus is in an abnormal presentation. Fetal sonography or maternal pelvimetry, or both, may be done before a TOL to rule out CPD. The cervix must be soft and dilatable. During TOL, the woman is evaluated for the occurrence of active labor, including adequate contractions, engagement and descent of the presenting part, and effacement and dilatation of the cervix. Augmentation of labor seldom is implemented.

During a TOL the nurse assesses uterine activity, cervical changes, maternal vital signs, and fetal status. If maternal or fetal complications are identified, the nurse is responsible for initiating appropriate actions, including notifying the primary health care provider, and for evaluating and documenting the maternal or fetal response to the interventions. Nurses must recognize that the woman and her partner are often anxious about her health and well-being and that of their baby. Supporting and encouraging the woman and her partner and providing information regarding progress can reduce stress and enhance the labor process and facilitate a successful outcome.

TABLE 25-3	**Bishop Score**			
	SCORE			
	0	1	2	3
Dilatation (cm)	0	1 to 2	3 to 4	5 to 6
Effacement (%)	0 to 30	40 to 50	60 to 70	80
Station (cm)	−3	−2	−1	−1
Cervical consistency	Firm	Medium	Soft	
Cervix position	Posterior	Midline	Anterior	

Induction of labor

Induction of labor is the initiation of uterine contractions before their spontaneous onset for the purpose of bringing about the birth. In 1993, the rate of labor induction was estimated to be 134 per 1,000 live births (Ventura et al., 1995).

Labor can be induced by both chemical and mechanical methods. Intravenous oxytocin and amniotomy are the most common methods used in the United States. Less commonly used methods include nipple stimulation (manual or with a breastpump), the ingestion of castor oil or herbal preparations, a soap-suds enema, stripping of the membranes, and acupuncture (Summers, 1997). Prostaglandins are also used for inducing labor, but their use for this purpose continues to be investigated (Day & Snell, 1993; Mastrogiannis & Knuppel, 1995; Summers, 1997).

The success of the induction of labor is greater if the condition of the cervix is favorable, or inducible. A rating system such as the **Bishop score** (Table 25-3) can be used to evaluate inducibility. For example, a score of 9 or more on this 13-point scale indicates that the cervix is soft, anterior, 50% effaced, and dilated 2 cm or more, and that the presenting part is engaged. Induction of labor is likely to be more successful if the score for nulliparas is 9 or more and the score for multiparas is 5 or more.

Cervical ripening methods

Chemical agents. Different **prostaglandins** (hormones) have been applied to the cervix before induction to induce or "ripen" (soften and thin) the cervix. Since 1993, a prostaglandin gel has been approved by the FDA for use as a cervical ripening agent (ACOG, 1995b) The gel is available in a 2.5-ml syringe that contains 0.5 mg of dinoprostone (Prepidil), which is a form of prostaglandin E_2. After being brought to room temperature, the gel is inserted into the cervical canal just below the internal os using a catheter. The woman should be instructed to remain in the supine position for at least 15 to 30 minutes after administration. The dose may be repeated in 6 hours if there is no cervical response. A maximum of 1.5 mg of dinoprostone can be given in a 24-hour period. Induction of labor using an intravenous infusion of oxytocin can begin in 6 to 12 hours after the instillation if cervical ripening has occurred (ACOG, 1995b; Summers, 1997).

Prostaglandin E_2 may also be administered in the form of a vaginal insert (Cervidil), which contains 10 mg of dinoprostone. The insert is placed in the posterior fornix of the vagina where it absorbs moisture, swells, and slowly releases the dinoprostone. It can be easily removed by pulling its string after 12 hours, when active labor begins, or if hyperstimulation of the uterus occurs. The manufacturer recommends that the woman remain in a supine position for 2 hours after insertion. Labor induction can begin 30 minutes after the insert is removed.

Systemic maternal side effects related to prostaglandin use, which include vomiting, fever, and diarrhea, are negligible. Hyperstimulation of the uterus with or without fetal distress can occur, usually within 1 hour of administration. Terbutaline 0.25 mg can be given subcutaneously or intravenously to reduce uterine activity if hyperstimulation occurs. Prostaglandin E_2 should be used with caution in women who have a history of asthma, glaucoma, renal disease, hepatic disease, and cardiovascular disease (ACOG, 1995b).

After the gel or insert has been administered, the nurse should monitor uterine activity and the FHR pattern continuously for 30 minutes to 2 hours and periodically thereafter. Maternal vital signs are taken every hour for 2 hours or for 4 hours if uterine contractions occur and continue. The woman should remain in the supine position with her hips elevated for the recommended length of time. Then the woman may be ambulatory and allowed to go home if no signs of labor or fetal distress are exhibited. She is instructed to return the next day for oxytocin induction of her labor (Home Care box). If contractions are still occurring, the oxytocin infusion should be postponed or used with great caution in a very low dose (ACOG, 1995b).

Misoprostol (Cytotec) is a synthetic prostaglandin analog that can be administered intravaginally. It is not approved by the FDA for cervical ripening, but it is effective, especially when membranes are ruptured (Mundle & Young, 1996).

Mechanical methods. Hygroscopic dilators (substances that absorb fluid from surrounding tissues and then enlarge) also can be used for cervical ripening. These consist of laminaria tents (natural cervical dilators made from seaweed) and synthetic dilators (Dilakan), which are inserted into the endocervix without rupturing the membranes. As they absorb fluid, they expand and cause the cervix to dilate. These dilators are left in place for 6 to 12 hours before being removed to assess cervical dilatation. Fresh dilators are inserted if further cervical dilatation is necessary (ACOG, 1995b, AWHONN, 1993, Summers, 1997). Hydroscopic dilators compare favorably with prostaglandins in terms of

their effectiveness in ripening the cervix but are associated with a higher incidence of postpartum maternal and newborn infections (Reichler, Romem & Divon, 1995).

Nursing responsibilities for women who have dilators inserted include documenting the number of dilators and sponges (used to hold the dilators in place) inserted during the procedure.

Amniotomy

Amniotomy (artificial rupture of membranes [AROM]) can be used to stimulate labor when the condition of the cervix is favorable. Labor usually begins within 12 hours of the rupture; however, if amniotomy does not stimulate labor, the resulting prolonged rupture may lead to infection. Once an amniotomy is performed, the woman is committed to giving birth. For this reason, amniotomy often is used in combination with oxytocin induction. Before the procedure, the woman should be told what to expect; she should also be assured that the procedure is painless for her and the fetus (Procedure box). The presenting part of the fetus should be well applied to the cervix to reduce the risk of cord prolapse (ACOG, 1995b; Summers, 1997). The membranes are ruptured with an amnihook or other sharp instrument, and the amniotic fluid allowed to drain slowly. The color, odor, and consistency of the fluid is assessed (i.e., for the presence or absence of meconium or blood). The time of rupture is recorded. The FHR is assessed before and immediately after the procedure to detect any changes (such as variable decelerations) that may indicate the occurrence of cord compression or prolapse. The woman's temperature should be checked at least every 2 hours to rule out possible infection. The primary health care provider is notified if her temperature is found to be 38° C or higher. The nurse also assesses for other signs and symptoms of infection, such as maternal chills, fetal tachycardia, uterine tenderness on palpation, and foul-smelling vaginal drainage (AWHONN, 1993). Comfort measures, such as frequently changing the woman's underpads, and perineal cleansing

---

HOME CARE *Patient Instructions for Self-Care*

Instructions for after Intravaginal Insertion of Prostaglandin Gel for Cervical Ripening

Return to the hospital if true labor begins spontaneously.

Return to the hospital immediately if your membranes rupture or if you have vaginal bleeding, decreased fetal movement, or severe abdominal pain.

If you do not experience labor, return for your scheduled induction.

From Lowdermilk D, Perry S & Bobak I: *Maternity and women's health care,* ed 6, St Louis, 1997, Mosby.

PROCEDURE

Assisting with an Amniotomy

PROCEDURE

Explain to the woman what will be done.

Assess FHR before procedure begins to obtain a baseline reading.

Place several underpads under the woman's buttocks to absorb the fluid.

Position the woman on a padded bed pan, fracture pan, or rolled up towel to elevate her hips.

Assist the health care provider who is performing the procedure by providing sterile gloves and lubricant for the vaginal examination.

Unwrap sterile package containing Amnihook or Allis clamp and pass instrument to the primary health care provider, who inserts it alongside the fingers and then hooks and tears the membranes.

Reassess the FHR.

Assess the color, consistency, and odor of the fluid.

Assess the woman's temperature every 2 hours or per protocol.

Assess the woman for signs and symptoms of infection.

DOCUMENTATION

Chart the following:

Time of rupture

Color, odor, and consistency of the fluid

FHR before and after the procedure

Maternal status (how well procedure was tolerated)

From Lowdermilk D, Perry S & Bobak I: *Maternity and women's health care,* ed 6, St Louis, 1997, Mosby

---

should be implemented, because the amniotic fluid will continue to leak from the vagina until the birth.

Oxytocin

Oxytocin is a hormone normally produced by the posterior pituitary gland that stimulates uterine contractions. It may be used either to induce the labor process or to augment a labor that is progressing slowly because of inadequate uterine contractions.

The indications for oxytocin induction or augmentation of labor may include, but are not limited to, the following:

- Suspected fetal jeopardy
- Inadequate uterine contractions; dystocia
- PROM
- Postterm pregnancy
- Chorioamnionitis
- Maternal medical problems (e.g., woman with severe Rh isoimmunization, diabetes, renal disease, or chronic pulmonary disease)

- Pregnancy-induced hypertension
- Fetal demise
- Multiparous women with a history of precipitous labor who live far from the hospital

The management of stimulation of labor is the same regardless of the indication. Because of the potential dangers associated with the injection of oxytocin in the prenatal and intrapartal periods, however, the FDA has issued certain restrictions to its use.

Contraindications to oxytocin stimulation of labor include, but are not limited to, the following:

- CPD, prolapsed cord, transverse lie
- Nonreassuring FHR
- Placenta previa or vasa previa
- Prior classic uterine incision or uterine surgery
- Active genital herpes infection
- Invasive cancer of the cervix

Certain maternal and fetal conditions, although not contraindications to the use of oxytocin to stimulate labor, do require special caution during its administration. These conditions include the following:

- Multifetal presentation
- Breech presentation
- Presenting part above the pelvic inlet
- Abnormal FHR pattern not requiring emergency delivery
- Polyhydramnios
- Grand multiparity
- Maternal cardiac disease; hypertension

Oxytocin use can pose hazards to the mother and fetus. These hazards are primarily dose related, with high doses given rapidly creating the most problems. Maternal hazards include water intoxication and tumultuous labor with tetanic contractions, which may cause premature separation of the placenta, rupture of the uterus, lacerations of the cervix, or postbirth hemorrhage. These complications can lead to infection, disseminated intravascular coagulation, or amniotic fluid embolism. Women also may become anxious or fearful if the induction is not successful because of concerns they may then have about the method of birth.

Uterine hyperstimulation reduces the blood flow through the placenta and results in fetal heart rate decelerations (bradycardia, diminished variability, late decelerations), fetal asphyxia, and neonatal hypoxia. If the estimated date of birth is inaccurate, physical injury, neonatal hyperbilirubinemia, and prematurity are other hazards.

It is the primary health care provider who is responsible for initiating the induction or augmentation of labor with oxytocin, although the nurse often administers the medication. The aim of induction in the past has been to achieve a contraction pattern that simulates the active phase of labor as quickly as possible. However, research

PATIENT/FAMILY TEACHING

Explain technique, rationale, and reactions to expect:
- Route and rate
- What "piggyback" is for
- Reasons for use:
  Induce labor, improve labor
- Reactions to expect concerning the nature of contractions: the intensity of contraction increases more rapidly, holds the peak longer, and ends more quickly; contractions will come regularly and more often
- Monitoring to anticipate:
  Maternal: blood pressure, pulse, uterine contractions, uterine tone
  Fetal: heart rate, activity
- Success to expect: a favorable outcome will depend on inducibility of the cervix (Bishop score of 9 for nulliparas and 5 for multiparas)
- Keep woman and support person informed of progress

ADMINISTRATION (FIG. 25-9)

Position woman in side-lying position
Prepare solutions and administer with pump delivery system according to prescribed orders:
- Infusion pump and solution are set up (e.g., 10 U/1,000 ml isotonic solution)
- Piggyback solution is connected to IV line at proximal port
- Solution with oxytocin is flagged with a medication label
- Begin induction at 0.5 to 1 mU/min
- Increase dose 1 to 2 mU/min at intervals of 30 to 60 minutes until either a dose of up to 20 mU/min or 300 montevideo units (MVUs) is reached (see Box 25-7)

MAINTAIN DOSE IF

- Intensity of contractions results in intrauterine pressures of 40 to 90 mm Hg (shown by internal monitor)
- Duration of contractions is 40 to 90 seconds
- Frequency of contractions is 2- to 3-minute intervals
- Cervical dilatation of 1 cm/hr in the active phase

MATERNAL/FETAL ASSESSMENTS

- Monitor blood pressure and pulse every 30 to 60 minutes
- Monitor contraction pattern and uterine resting tone every 15 minutes
- Assess intake and output; limit IV intake to 1,000 ml/8 hr; output should be 120 ml or more every 4 hours
- Monitor for nausea, vomiting, headache, hypotension
- Assess fetal status according to hospital protocol; electronic fetal monitoring is recommended

REPORTABLE CONDITIONS

- Uterine hyperstimulation
- Nonreassuring FHR pattern
- Suspected uterine rupture

EMERGENCY MEASURES

Discontinue use of oxytocin per hospital protocol:
- Turn woman on her side
- Increase primary IV rate up to 200 ml/hr, unless patient has water intoxication, in which case, the rate is decreased to one that keeps the vein open
- Give woman oxygen by face mask at 8 to 10 L/min or per protocol or physician's order

DOCUMENTATION

- Medication: kind, amount, time of beginning, increasing dose, maintaining dose, and discontinuing medication in patient record and on monitoring strip
- Reactions of mother and fetus
  Pattern of labor
  Progress of labor
  FHR
  Maternal vital signs
  Nursing interventions and woman's response
- Notification of primary health care provider

From American College of Obstetricians and Gynecologists: Induction of labor, *Technical Bulletin* 217, Washington, DC, 1995b, ACOG; Association of Women's Health, Obstetric, and Neonatal Nurses: *Cervical ripening and induction and augmentation of labor,* Practice Resource, Washington, DC, Dec 1993, AWHONN; Davis L: Protocol for the nursing management of the patient requiring oxytocin for induction and augmentation of labor. In Mandeville L & Troiano N, editors: *High-risk intrapartum nursing,* Philadelphia, 1992, Lippincott; and Summers L: Methods of cervical ripening and labor induction, *J Nurse Midwifery* 42(2):71, 1997.

on uterine tolerance to oxytocin has now shown that lower doses given over a longer time are as effective as previous protocols and are less likely to cause uterine hyperstimulation and dysfunctional labor (ACOG, 1995b; Summers, 1997).

Nursing considerations. A written protocol for the preparation and administration of oxytocin should be established by the obstetric department (physicians, nurses) at each institution. Procedures that are recommended for a woman who is eligible for induction of labor are discussed in Box 25-7 and the Protocol box. Policies, protocols, and procedures of individual institutions will also dictate set-up and administration, the frequency of administration, and documentation.

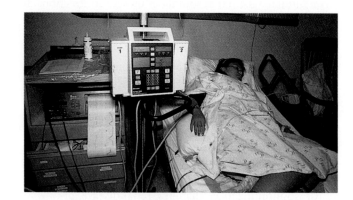

Fig. 25-9 Woman in side-lying position receiving oxytocin. (Courtesy Michael S. Clement, MD, Mesa, Ariz.)

| BOX 25-7 | *Calculation of Montevideo Units* |

Montevideo units (MVUs) can be used to describe uterine intensity when an intrauterine pressure gauge is being used. To calculate them, the baseline uterine pressure (resting tone) is first subtracted from the peak contraction pressure for each contraction recorded on a 10-minute monitor tracing. These adjusted pressures are then added, and the sum is the number of Montevideo units (average, 180 to 240 MVUs).

For example, if the resting tone is 5 mm Hg and three contractions occur in 10 minutes with peaks of 80, 85, and 90 mm Hg, the resulting numbers are $80 - 5 + 85 - 5 + 90 - 5$, which total 240 MVUs.

From Lowdermilk D, Perry S & Bobak I: *Maternity and women's health care,* ed 6, St Louis, 1997, Mosby.

EMERGENCY

Uterine Hyperstimulation with Oxytocin

SIGNS

Uterine contractions lasting more than 90 seconds and occurring more frequently than every 2 minutes
Uterine resting tone greater than 20 mm Hg
Nonreassuring FHR:
  Abnormal baseline
  Absent variability
  Repeated late decelerations or prolonged decelerations

INTERVENTIONS

Maintain woman in side-lying position
Turn off oxytocin infusion; keep maintenance IV line open; increase rate
Start administering oxygen by face mask, per protocol or physician's order
Notify primary health care provider
Continue monitoring FHR and uterine activity
Document responses to actions

| NURSE ALERT | *Oxytocin is discontinued immediately and the primary health care provider notified if uterine hyperstimulation or a nonreassuring FHR occurs.* |

Other nursing interventions, such as administering oxygen by face mask, positioning the woman on her side and infusing more intravenous fluids are implemented immediately (Emergency box). Based on the status of the maternal-fetal unit, the primary health care provider may restart the infusion once the FHR and uterine activity return to acceptable levels (ACOG, 1995b).

Augmentation

Augmentation of labor is the stimulation of uterine contractions after labor has started spontaneously yet progress proves unsatisfactory. It usually is implemented for the management of hypotonic dysfunctional labor. The procedures and nursing assessments called for are the same as those called for during oxytocin induction of labor (Plan of Care box).

Some physicians advocate the active management of labor, that is, the augmentation of labor to establish efficient labor so that the woman gives birth within 12 hours of admission (ACOG, 1995c). Advocates of active management believe that intervening early (as soon as a nulliparous labor is not progressing at least 1 cm/hr) with the aggressive use of oxytocin (e.g., a starting dose of 6 mU/min with increases of 6 mU/min, every 15 minutes to a maximum dose of 40 mU/min shortens labor and is associated with a lower incidence of cesarean birth (ACOG, 1995c). Additional components of the active management of labor include strict criteria to diagnose that the woman is in labor, that abnormal progress is occurring and fetal compromise is present, amniotomy within 1 hour of admission of a woman in labor, and the continuous presence of a personal nurse who cares for the woman in labor. Active management continues to be under study in the United States to determine effectiveness and impact on perinatal morbidity and mortality.

Forceps-assisted birth

A **forceps-assisted birth** is one in which an instrument with two curved blades is used to assist in the birth of the fetal head. The cephalic-like curve of the forceps commonly used is similar to the shape of the fetal head, with a pelvic curve to the blades conforming to the curve of the pelvic axis. The blades are joined by a pin, screw, or groove arrangement. These locks prevent the forceps from compressing the fetal skull. Maternal indications for forceps-assisted birth include the need to shorten the second stage of labor in the event of dystocia (difficult labor) or to compensate for the woman's deficient expulsive efforts (e.g., if she is tired or has been given spinal or epidural anesthesia), as well as to reverse a dangerous condition (e.g., cardiac decompensation).

Fetal indications include birth of a fetus in distress, in certain abnormal presentations, or in arrest of rotation, as well as to deliver an aftercoming head in a breech presentation.

Certain conditions are required for a forceps-assisted birth to be successful. The woman's cervix must be fully dilated to avert lacerations and hemorrhage. This also requires that her bladder be empty. The presenting part must be engaged, and a vertex presentation is desired. Membranes must be ruptured so that the position of the fetal head can be determined and the forceps can firmly grasp the head during birth. In addition, CPD should not be present.

There are different definitions of forceps applications. According to ACOG (1991), it is appropriate to use *outlet* forceps if the fetal scalp is visible on the perineum without

PLAN OF CARE *Dysfunctional Labor: Secondary Inertia*

> **NURSING DIAGNOSIS**   Risk for injury to mother and/or fetus related to oxytocin stimulation secondary to dysfunctional labor

Expected Outcomes   *Maternal-fetal well-being is maintained; labor progresses and birth occurs.*

Nursing Interventions/*Rationales*

Explain oxytocin protocol to woman and her labor partner *to allay apprehension and enhance participation.*

Encourage woman to void before beginning protocol *to prevent discomfort and remove a barrier to labor progress.*

Apply the electronic fetal monitor per hospital protocol and obtain a 15- to 20-minute baseline strip *to ensure adequate assessment of FHR and contractions.*

Position woman in a side-lying position and administer the oxytocin per physician order using an IV infusion pump *to stimulate uterine activity and provide adequate control of the flow rate.*

Regulate the oxytocin per protocol and advancing the dose in increments of 1 to 2 mU/min every 30 to 60 minutes *to allow adequate evaluation of the woman's response to stimulation and to prevent hyperstimulation and fetal hypoxia.*

Maintain oxytocin dose and rate when contractions occur every 2 to 3 minutes with a duration of 40 to 90 seconds and intrauterine pressures of 40 to 90 mm Hg *to produce effective uterine stimulation without risk of hyperstimulation.*

If infusion rate is advanced to 20 mU/min without achieving the desired contractility pattern, notify physician *because woman is at risk for hyperstimulation and water intoxication.*

Monitor maternal vital signs every 30 to 60 minutes *to assess for oxytocin-induced hypertension.*

Monitor contractility pattern and FHR pattern every 15 minutes *to assess uterine activity for possible hypertonicity or ineffective uterine response to oxytocin and to detect evidence of fetal distress.*

Monitor intake, output, and specific gravity (limit intake to 1,000 ml/8 hr; output should be at least 120 ml/4 hr) *to assess for urinary retention and prevent water intoxication.*

Monitor cervical dilatation, effacement, and station *to assess progress of labor.*

If hypertonicity or signs of fetal distress are detected, discontinue oxytocin immediately *to arrest the progress of hypertonicity;* turn woman on her side *to increase placental blood flow;* increase primary IV rate to 200 ml/hr (unless signs of water toxicity are present); administer oxygen per face mask *to enhance placental perfusion;* notify physician; and continuously monitor maternal vital signs and FHR *to provide ongoing assessment of maternal/fetal status.*

> **NURSING DIAGNOSIS**   Pain related to increasing frequency, regularity, intensity, and prolonged peak of contractions

Expected Outcomes   *The woman exhibits signs of decreased discomfort.*

Nursing Interventions/*Rationales*

Prepare woman and labor partner for the change in the nature of the contractions once the oxytocin drip is initiated *to prepare them and allow for more effective coping.*

Remind woman and labor partner that analgesics are available for use during labor *to provide knowledge to help them make decisions about pain control.*

Review the use of specific techniques such as conscious relaxation, focused breathing, effleurage, massage, and application of sacral pressure *to increase relaxation, decrease intensity of pain of contractions, and promote use of controlled thought and direction of energy.*

Provide comfort measures such as frequent mouth care *to prevent dry mouth,* application of damp cloth to forehead and changing of damp gown or bed covers *to relieve diaphoresis,* and positioning *to reduce stiffness.*

Encourage conscious relaxation between contractions *to prevent fatigue, which contributes to increased pain perceptions.*

> **NURSING DIAGNOSIS**   Anxiety/ineffective coping related to prolonged labor, increased pain, and fatigue

Expected Outcomes   *Woman's anxiety is reduced; woman actively participates in the labor process.*

Nursing Interventions/*Rationales*

Provide ongoing feedback to woman and partner *to allay anxiety and enhance participation.*

Present care options when possible *to increase feelings of control.*

Continue to provide comfort measures *to maintain a posture of support and caring and to aid woman in focusing on the labor process.*

Encourage woman and partner to continue to use those mechanisms that promote effective labor (e.g., breathing, positioning) *to keep woman and partner actively involved in process.*

> **NURSING DIAGNOSIS**   Risk for maternal/fetal infection related to prolonged rupture of membranes or possible invasive procedures (e.g., use of fetal scalp electrodes, use of forceps, episiotomy, cesarean birth)

Expected Outcomes   *There is no evidence of infection.*

Nursing Interventions/*Rationales*

Monitor temperature *because elevation is early indicator of infection.*

Monitor FHR/variability *because rates greater than 160 beats/minute and minimal variability may be indicative of maternal fever and infection.*

Monitor intake and output for dehydration *because signs of infection closely resemble those of dehydration, and differentiation is needed.*

≋ PLAN OF CARE *Dysfunctional Labor: Secondary Inertia—cont'd*

Maintain Standard Precautions and use scrupulous handwashing techniques when providing care *to prevent spread of infection.*

Use strict aseptic technique when performing invasive procedures such as urinary catheterization, insertion of intravenous lines, or application of scalp electrodes *to reduce risk of nosocomial infection.*

Monitor IV sites, electrode sites, and incision sites for signs such as pain, redness, edema, heat, and drainage, *which are indicative of infection.*

Monitor urine for color, concentration, odor, clouding, casts, and sediment, *which may indicate a urinary tract infection.*

When membranes rupture, assess fluid for color, amount and odor, and for the presence of meconium stain *because alterations may be indicative of intrauterine infection.*

After membrane rupture, keep vaginal examinations to a minimum and use sterile gloves *to decrease risk of uterine infection.*

Assist woman to maintain good personal hygiene habits (e.g., wiping perineal region from front to back, keeping area dry *to reduce introduction of bacteria.*

Monitor laboratory values (e.g., white blood cell count, culture) *for indicators of infection.*

From Wong D & Perry S: *Maternal child nursing care,* St Louis, 1998, Mosby.

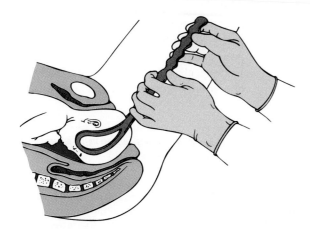

Fig. **25-10** Outlet forceps–assisted extraction of the head.

manually separating the labia (Fig. 25-10). Outlet forceps are used to shorten the second stage of labor. *Low forceps* refers to the application of forceps to the fetal head that is at least at the +2 cm station. *Midforceps* refers to the application of forceps to the fetal head that is engaged (no higher than station 0) but above the +2 cm station. There are no instances in which forceps should be applied to an unengaged presenting part.

Nursing considerations. When a forceps-assisted birth is deemed necessary, the nurse obtains the type of forceps requested by the physician (Fig. 25-11). The FHR is checked, reported, and recorded *before* the forceps are applied. The nurse may explain to the mother that the forceps blades fit like two tablespoons around an egg, with the blades coming over the baby's ears. Because compression of the cord between the fetal head and the forceps would cause a drop in FHR, the FHR is rechecked, reported, and recorded *before* and *after* application of the forceps. If a drop in FHR occurs, the physician would then remove and reapply the forceps. Ordinarily traction is applied during contractions.

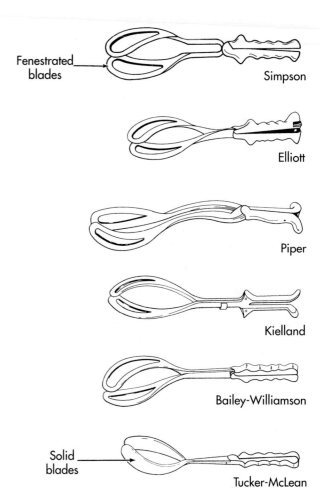

Fig. **25-11** Types of forceps. Piper forceps are used to assist delivery of the head in a breech birth.

After birth, the mother is assessed for vaginal and cervical lacerations (bleeding that occurs even with a contracted uterus) and urine retention, which may result from bladder injuries. The infant should be assessed for bruising or abrasions at the site of the blade applications, facial palsy resulting from pressure of the blades on the facial nerve (cranial nerve VII), and subdural hematoma. Newborn and postpartum caregivers should be told that forceps-assisted birth has been performed.

Vacuum-assisted birth

Vacuum-assisted birth, or vacuum extraction, is a birth method involving the attachment of a vacuum cup to the fetal head, using negative pressure. Indications for its use are similar to those for the use of outlet forceps. Prerequisites for use include a vertex presentation, ruptured membranes, and absence of CPD (Cunningham et al., 1997).

When vacuum extraction is to be done, the woman is prepared for a vaginal birth in the lithotomy position to allow for sufficient traction. The cup is applied to the fetal head, and a caput develops inside the cup as the pressure is initiated (Fig. 25-12). Traction is then applied to facilitate descent of the fetal head, and the woman is encouraged to push as suction is applied. As the head crowns, an episiotomy is performed if necessary. The vacuum cup is released and removed after birth of the head. If vacuum extraction is not successful, a forceps-assisted or cesarean birth is then performed.

Risks to the newborn include cephalhematoma, scalp lacerations, and subdural hematoma. Maternal complications are uncommon but can include perineal, vaginal, or cervical lacerations.

Nursing considerations. The nurse's role in the care of the woman who has given birth with the assistance of vacuum extraction is one of support person and educator. The nurse can prepare the woman for birth and encourage her to remain active in the birth process by pushing during contractions. In addition, the nurse assesses the FHR frequently during the procedure. After birth, the newborn should be observed for signs of infection at the application site and for cerebral irritation (e.g., poor sucking, listlessness). The newborn may be at risk for cephalohematoma and neonatal jaundice as bruising resolves. The parents may need to be reassured that the caput succedaneum will begin to disap-

pear in a few hours. Neonatal caregivers should be alerted that the birth was achieved by vacuum extraction.

Cesarean birth

Cesarean birth is the birth of a fetus through a transabdominal incision of the uterus. Although the myth persists that Julius Caesar was born in this manner, the name is more likely derived from the Latin word *caedo*, meaning 'to cut.' Whether cesarean birth is planned (scheduled) or unplanned (emergency), the loss of the experience of giving birth to a child in the traditional manner may have a negative effect on a woman's self-concept. An effort is therefore made to maintain the focus on the birth of a child rather than on the operative procedure.

The basic aim of cesarean birth is to preserve the life or health of the mother and her fetus (Box 25-8) and may be the best choice for birth when there is evidence of maternal or fetal complications. Since the advent of modern surgical methods and care, there has been a decrease in the maternal and fetal morbidity and mortality associated with cesarean birth. In addition, today incisions are made into the lower uterine segment rather than into the muscular body of the uterus to promote more effective healing. However, despite

---

| BOX 25-8 | *Forced Cesarean Birth: Ethical Consideration* |

A woman's refusal to undergo cesarean birth for fetal reasons is often described as a maternal-fetal conflict. Health care providers are ethically obliged to protect the well-being of both the mother and the fetus; it is difficult to make a decision for one without affecting the other. If a woman refuses a cesarean birth that is needed, health care providers need to make every effort to find out why she is refusing and provide information that may persuade her to change her mind. If the woman continues to refuse surgery, then health care providers must decide if it is ethical to get a court order for the surgery. Every effort should be made to avoid this legal step, however.

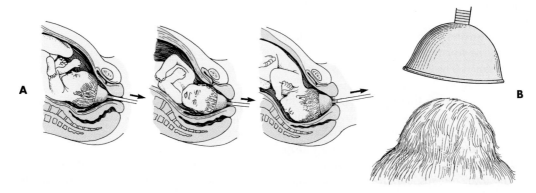

Fig. **25-12** Use of vacuum extraction to rotate fetal head and assist with descent. **A,** Arrow indicates direction of traction on the vacuum cup. **B,** Caput succedaneum formed by the vacuum cup.

these advances, cesarean birth still poses threats to the health of the mother and infant.

The incidence of cesarean births has increased dramatically from less than 5% in 1965 to more than 24% in 1990 (Taffel et al., 1992). Factors cited as sources of this increase include use of electronic fetal monitoring and epidural anesthesia; an increase in the number of first-time pregnancies, as well as pregnancy at an older age; and the high incidence of repeat cesarean births. In addition, women who have private insurance, are of a higher socioeconomic status, or deliver in a private hospital are more likely to experience cesarean birth than are women who are poor, have no insurance, are on public assistance (e.g., Medicaid), or deliver in public hospitals. (DiMatteo et al., 1996; Porreco & Thorp, 1996; Scott, 1994). In 1995 the rate dropped to 20.8% (Ventura, 1997), although it is still the most common major surgery performed in the United States. This decline may be attributed, in part, to more attempts at vaginal births in mothers who have previously given birth by cesarean. From 1989 to 1995, the rate of vaginal births after cesarean increased 46% (Ventura, 1997).

The type of nursing care may also influence the rate of cesarean births. A study by Radin, Harmon, and Hanson (1993) revealed that cesarean rates were lower for women whose nurses provided supportive care during labor. A labor management approach that uses female labor coaches (doulas) and emphasizes ambulation, maternal position changes, relaxation measures, and nonpharmacologic pain relief, facilitates the progress of labor and reduces the incidence of dystocia, a major cause for cesarean birth, especially in first-time labors (Albers, Lydon-Rochelle & Krulewitch 1995; Porreco & Thorp, 1996).

Indications. There are few absolute indications for cesarean birth. Today most are performed primarily for the benefit of the fetus. The most common indications for cesarean birth are dystocia, repeat cesarean, breech presentation, and fetal distress. Other indications for the procedure include active herpes viral infection, prolapsed umbilical cord, medical complications such as PIH, placental abnormalities such as placenta previa and premature separation (abruption), malpresentations such as shoulder presentation, fetal anomalies such as hydrocephaly, and multiple gestation (Porreco & Thorp, 1996).

Surgical techniques. There are two main types of cesarean operation—classic and lower-segment cesarean births. Classic cesarean birth is rarely performed today, although it may be used when rapid birth is necessary and in some cases of shoulder presentation and placenta previa. The incision is made vertically into the upper body of the uterus (Fig. 25-13, *A*). Because the procedure is associated with a higher incidence of blood loss, infection, and uterine rupture in subsequent pregnancies than is lower-segment cesarean birth, vaginal birth after a classic cesarean birth is contraindicated.

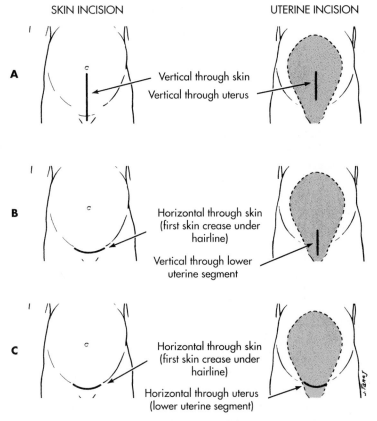

Fig. **25-13** Cesarean birth: skin and uterine incisions. **A,** Classic: vertical incisions of skin and uterus. **B,** Low cervical: horizontal incision of skin; vertical incision of uterus. **C,** Low cervical: horizontal incisions of skin and uterus.

Lower-segment cesarean birth can be achieved through a vertical or transverse incision (Fig. 25-13, *B* and *C*) into the uterus. The transverse incision is more popular, however, because it is easier to perform, is associated with less blood loss and fewer postoperative infections, and is less likely to rupture in subsequent pregnancies (Cunningham et al., 1997, Scott, 1994).

Complications and risks. Cesarean births are not without complications, either for the mother or the fetus. Maternal complications occur in 25% to 50% of births and include aspiration, pulmonary embolism, wound infection, wound dehiscence, thrombophlebitis, hemorrhage, urinary tract infection, injuries to the bladder or bowel, and complications related to anesthesia. There also is a risk that the fetus will be born prematurely if the gestational age has not been accurately determined; in addition, fetal injuries can occur during the surgery (Scott, 1994). Besides these risks, the woman is at economic risk because the cost of cesarean birth is higher than that of vaginal birth and a longer recovery period may necessitate additional expenditures.

Many women who experience a cesarean birth speak of having feelings that interfere with their maintaining an adequate self-concept. These feelings include fear, disappointment, frustration at losing control, anger (the "why me" syndrome), and loss of self-esteem related to a change in body image and perceived inability to give birth as they had expected and hoped. Often the ability to interact with their newborns after birth is delayed. Women who experience cesarean birth are less likely to breastfeed and may even have some difficulty expressing positive feeling about their newborns for some time after birth. They are often less satisfied with their childbirth experience and report more fatigue and poor physical functioning during the first few weeks after discharge. These reactions are more pronounced among women who had unplanned or emergency cesarean birth (DiMatteo et al., 1996). Success at mothering and in the recovery process can do much to restore the self-esteem of these women. Some women see the scar as mutilating, and worries concerning sexual attractiveness may surface. Some men are fearful of resuming intercourse because of the fear of hurting their mates. Parents may wonder if a cesarean birth was absolutely necessary, and such feelings may surface even years later. They should therefore be given opportunities to discuss the experience to try to understand and resolve concerns after the birth.

Anesthesia. Spinal, epidural, and general anesthetics are used for cesarean births. Epidural blocks are popular because women want to be awake for and aware of the birth experience. However, the choice of anesthetic depends on several factors. The mother's medical history or present condition, such as a spinal injury or hemorrhage, may rule out the use of regional anesthesia. Time is another factor, especially if there is an emergency and the life of the mother or infant is at stake. In this event, general anesthesia will most likely be used, unless the woman already has an epidural block in effect. The woman herself is a factor. Either she may not know all the options or she may have fears about having "a needle in her back" or about being awake and feeling pain. The woman needs to be fully informed about the risks and benefits of the different types of anesthesia so that she can participate in the decision whenever there is a choice.

Scheduled cesarean birth. Cesarean birth is scheduled or planned if labor is contraindicated (e.g., complete placenta previa), if birth is necessary but labor is not inducible (e.g., hypertensive states, which cause a poor intrauterine environment that threatens the fetus), or if this has been decided upon by the primary health care provider and the woman (e.g., a repeat cesarean birth).

Women who are scheduled to have a cesarean birth have time to prepare for it psychologically. However, the psychologic responses of these women may differ. Those having a repeat cesarean birth may have disturbing memories of the conditions preceding the initial surgical birth and of their experiences in the postoperative recovery period. They may be very concerned about the added burden of caring for an infant while recovering from a surgical operation. Others may feel glad that they have been relieved of the uncertainty about the date and time of the birth and of the pain of labor.

Unplanned cesarean birth. The psychosocial outcomes of unplanned or emergency cesarean birth are usually more pronounced and negative in nature when compared with the outcomes associated with a scheduled or planned cesarean birth (DiMatteo et al., 1996). Women and their families both experience abrupt changes in their expectations for birth, postbirth care, and the care of the new baby at home. This may be an extremely traumatic experience for all. The woman usually approaches the procedure tired and discouraged after a fruitless labor. She is worried about her own and the infant's condition. She may be dehydrated, with low glycogen reserves. Because all preoperative procedures must be done quickly and competently, however, the time for an explanation of the procedures and the operation is short. In addition, because maternal and family anxiety levels are high at this time, much of what is said is forgotten or perhaps misconstrued. After surgery, therefore, time must be spent reviewing the events preceding the operation and the operation itself to ensure that the woman understands what has happened and that gaps in her recollections are filled. Fatigue is often noticeable in these women. They need much supportive care.

Prenatal preparation. Concerned professional and lay groups in the community have established councils for cesarean birth to meet the needs of these women and their families. Such groups advocate that a discussion of cesarean birth be included in all parenthood preparation classes. No woman can be guaranteed a vaginal birth, even if she is in good health and there is no indication of danger to the fetus before the onset of labor. For this reason, every woman needs to be aware of and prepared for this eventuality. The unknown and unexpected are only ego weakening.

Childbirth educators stress the importance of emphasizing the similarities as well as the differences between cesarean and vaginal birth. In support of the philosophy of family-centered birth, many hospitals have instituted policies that permit fathers and other partners to share in these births as they do in vaginal ones. Women who have undergone cesarean birth agree that the continued presence and support of their partners helped them respond positively to the entire experience. In addition to preparing women for the possibility of cesarean birth, childbirth educators should empower women to believe in their ability to give birth vaginally and to seek care measures during labor that will enhance the progress of their labors and reduce their risk for cesarean birth.

Preoperative care. Family-centered care is the goal for the woman who is to undergo cesarean birth and for her family. The preparation of the woman for cesarean birth is the same as that done for either elective or emergency surgery. The primary health care provider discusses the need for the cesarean birth and the prognosis for the mother and infant with the woman and her family. The anesthesiologist assesses the woman's cardiopulmonary system and describes the options for anesthesia. Informed consent is obtained for the procedure.

Maternal vital signs and blood pressure and FHR continue to be assessed per the hospital routine until the operation begins. Physical preoperative preparation usually includes the insertion of a retention catheter to keep the bladder empty and the administration of prescribed preoperative medications. Additionally, the abdominal-mons area may be shaved or pubic hair clipped. An antacid is administered as a precautionary measure if general anesthesia is anticipated to neutralize gastric secretions in case of aspiration. Intravenous fluids are started to maintain hydration and to provide an open line for the administration of blood or medications, if this proves necessary. Blood and urine samples are collected and sent to the laboratory for analysis. Laboratory tests, which are usually ordered to establish baseline data, include a complete blood cell count and chemistry, blood typing and cross-matching, and urinalysis.

Removal of dentures, nail polish, and jewelry may be optional, depending on hospital policies. If the woman wears glasses and is going to be awake, the nurse should make sure her glasses accompany her to the operating room so she can see her infant. If the woman wears contact lenses, the nurse can find out whether they can be worn for the birth.

During the preoperative preparation the support person is encouraged to remain with the woman as much as possible to provide continuing emotional support. The nurse also provides essential information about the preoperative procedures during this time. Although the nursing actions may be carried out quickly if a cesarean birth is unplanned, verbal communication, particularly explanations, is important. Silence can be frightening to the woman and her support person. The nurse's use of touch can communicate feelings of care and concern for the woman.

The nurse can assess the woman's and her partner's perceptions about cesarean birth. For example, the woman may feel that she is a failure because she did not have a vaginal birth. As the woman expresses her feelings, the nurse may identify a potential for a disturbance in self-concept during the postpartum period that may need to be addressed.

If there is time before the birth, the nurse can teach the woman about postoperative expectations as well as pain relief, turning, coughing, and deep breathing measures.

Intraoperative care. Cesarean births occur in operating rooms in the surgical unit or in the labor and birth units. Once the woman has been taken to the operating room, her care becomes the responsibility of the obstetric team, surgeon, anesthesiologist, pediatrician, and surgical nursing staff (Fig. 25-14). If possible, the partner, who is gowned appropriately, accompanies the mother to the surgical unit and remains close to her so that he or she can provide continued support and comfort.

The nurse who is circulating may assist with positioning the woman on the birth (surgical) table. It is important to position her so that the uterus is displaced laterally to prevent compression of the inferior vena cava, which causes placental perfusion to decrease. This is usually accomplished by placing a wedge under the hip. A Foley catheter is inserted into the bladder at this time if one is not already in place.

If the partner is not allowed or chooses not to be present, the nurse can stay in communication with him or her and give progress reports whenever possible. If the mother is awake during the birth, the nurse can tell her what is happening and provide support. The mother may be anxious about the sensations she is experiencing, such as the coldness of solutions used to prepare the abdomen and pressure or pulling during the actual birth of the infant. She also may be apprehensive because of the bright lights and the presence of unfamiliar equipment and masked and gowned personnel in the room.

Care of the infant usually is delegated to a pediatrician or a nurse team skilled at neonatal resuscitation, because these infants are considered to be at risk until there is evidence of physiologic stability after the birth.

A crib with resuscitation equipment is readied before the birth. Those responsible for care are expert not only in resuscitative techniques but also in their ability to detect normal and abnormal infant responses. After birth, if the infant's

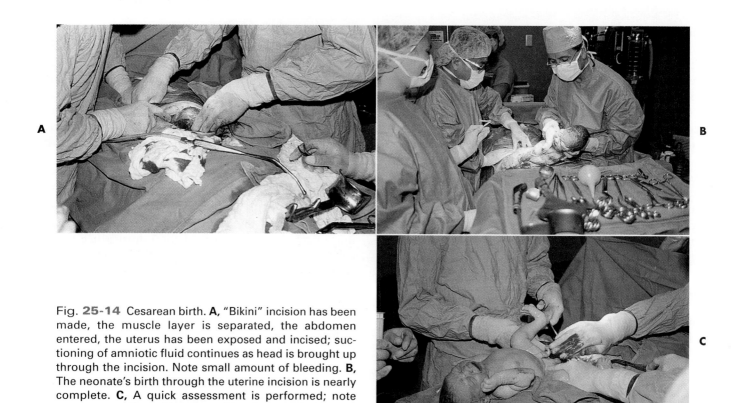

Fig. **25-14** Cesarean birth. **A,** "Bikini" incision has been made, the muscle layer is separated, the abdomen entered, the uterus has been exposed and incised; suctioning of amniotic fluid continues as head is brought up through the incision. Note small amount of bleeding. **B,** The neonate's birth through the uterine incision is nearly complete. **C,** A quick assessment is performed; note extreme molding of head resulting from cephalopelvic disproportion. (Courtesy Marjorie Pyle, RNC, Lifecircle, Costa Mesa, Calif.)

condition permits, the baby can be given to the woman's partner to hold. If the mother is awake, she can see and touch the baby (Fig. 25-15). The infant whose condition is compromised is transported after initial stabilization to the nursery for observation and the implementation of appropriate interventions. In some institutions the partner may accompany the infant; if not, personnel keep the family informed of the infant's progress and parent-infant contacts are initiated as soon as possible.

If the family cannot accompany the woman during surgery, the family is directed to the surgical or obstetric waiting room. The physician then reports on the condition of the mother and child to the family members after the birth is completed. Family members may accompany the infant as she or he is transferred to the nursery, giving the family an opportunity to see and admire the new baby.

Immediate postoperative care. Once surgery is completed, the mother is transferred to a recovery room or back to her labor room. The care of the woman after cesarean birth combines surgical and obstetric nursing. Nursing assessments in this immediate postbirth period include the degree of recovery from the effects of anesthesia, the postoperative and postbirth status, and the degree of pain. A patent airway is maintained, and the woman is positioned to prevent possible aspiration. Vital signs are taken every 15 minutes for 1 to 2 hours, or until stable. The condition of the incisional

dressing, the fundus, and the amount of lochia are assessed, as well as the intravenous intake and the urine output via the Foley catheter. The woman is helped to turn and do coughing and deep-breathing and leg exercises. Medications to relieve pain may be administered.

If the baby is present, the mother and her partner are given some time alone with him or her to facilitate bonding and attachment. Breastfeeding can be initiated if the mother feels like trying. The woman usually is transferred to the postpartum unit after 1 to 2 hours, or once her condition is stable and the effects of anesthesia have worn off (e.g., alert, oriented, moving all extremities) (see Care Path).

Postpartum care. The attitude of the nurse and other health team members can influence the perception the woman has of herself after a cesarean birth. The caregivers should stress that the woman is a new mother first and a surgical patient second. This will help the woman perceive herself as having the same problems and needs as other new mothers.

The women's physiologic concerns for the first few days may be dominated by pain at the incision site and pain resulting from intestinal gas, and hence the need for pain relief. If epidural anesthesia was used for the surgery, epidural narcotics can be given in the recovery period to provide pain relief for approximately 24 hours. Otherwise, pain medications usually are given every 3 to 4 hours, or patient-controlled

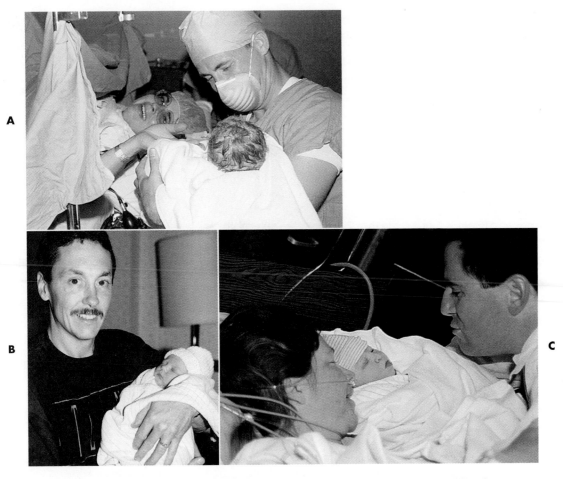

Fig. **25-15 A,** Parents and their newborn. The physician manually removes the placenta, suctions the remaining amniotic fluid and blood from uterine cavity, and closes the uterine incision, peritoneum, muscle layer, fatty tissue, and finally the skin, while new family shares some private time. **B,** Father-infant bonding is important. **C,** Parents become better acquainted with their newborn while mother rests after surgery. (**A** and **C** courtesy Marjorie Pyle, RNC, Lifecircle, Costa Mesa, Calif.; **B** courtesy J. Zipfel.)

analgesia may be ordered instead. Other comfort measures such as position changes, splinting of the incision with pillows, and relaxation techniques may be implemented. Women are often the best judges of what their bodies need and can tolerate, including the ingestion of foods and fluids postoperatively. If desired by the woman, the early introduction of solid food is safe. Women who eat early have been found to require less analgesia. Gastrointestinal problems do not occur (Burrows et al., 1995). Ambulation and rocking in a rocking chair may relieve gas pains, and avoiding the consumption of gas-forming foods and carbonated beverages may help minimize them (Thomas et al., 1990) (Home Care box, p. 728). Other physiologic concerns of women after cesarean birth may include fatigue, activity intolerance, and incisional problems (Miovech et al., 1994).

Daily care includes perineal care, breast care, and routine hygienic care, including showering after the dressing has been removed (if showering is acceptable according to the women's cultural prescriptions). The nurse assesses the woman's vital signs, incision, fundus, and lochia in accordance with hospital policies, procedures, or protocols. Breath sounds, bowel sounds, circulatory status of lower extremities, and urinary and bowel elimination also are assessed.

During the postpartum period the nurse can also provide care that meets the psychologic and teaching needs of mothers who have had cesarean births. For instance, the nurse can explain postpartum procedures to the woman to help elicit her cooperation in her recovery from surgery. The nurse can help the woman plan care and visits from family and friends that will allow for adequate rest periods. In addition, the nurse can give her information on infant care and assist her with infant care to facilitate her adjustment to the mothering role. The woman should be encouraged to breastfeed her baby by receiving one-on-one assistance to comfortably hold and position the baby at her breast. The partner can be included in infant care teaching

CARE PATH   *Cesarean Birth without Complications: Expected Length of Stay—48 to 72 Hours*

	IMMEDIATE POST-OP CESAREAN	BY 4TH HOUR AFTER ADMISSION TO PP UNIT	5 TO 24 HOURS	25 TO 48 HOURS	BY DISCHARGE
ASSESSMENTS	Recovery room/ PACU admission assessment completed	PP admission assessment and care plan completed			
Vital Signs	q15min × 1 hr; q30min × 4 hr, WNL	q1h × 3, WNL	q4 to 8h, WNL	q8h, WNL	q8h, WNL
Postpartum Assessment	q15min × 1 hr, WNL	q1h × 3, WNL	q8h, WNL	q8 to 12 h, WNL	q8 to 12 h, WNL
Abdominal Incision	Dressing dry and intact	Dressing dry and intact	Dressing dry and intact	Dressing off or changed, incision intact	Incision intact; staples may be removed and steri-strips in place, incision WNL
Genitourinary	Retention catheter output >30 ml/hr	Retention catheter output >30 ml/hr	Retention catheter output >30 ml/hr	Catheter discontinued, output >100 ml/ void or 240 ml/8 hr	Urine output >240 ml/8 hr
Gastrointestinal		Absent or hypoactive BS	Hypoactive to active BS	Active BS + flatus	Active BS + flatus; may or may not have BM
Musculoskeletal	Alert or easily aroused, can move legs	Alert and oriented, moving all extremities	Ambulating with help	Ambulating unassisted	Ambulating ad lib
Bonding	Evidence of parent-infant bonding; first breastfeeding if desired		Parent-infant bonding continues	Parent-infant bonding progressing	
Laboratory Tests			Intrapartal CBC results on chart/computer; determine Rh status and need for anti-Rh globulin; check for rubella immunity	PP HCT WNL, all lab results on chart, give anti-Rh globulin if indicated	Give rubella vaccine if indicated
INTERVENTIONS					
IV	IV continues	IV continues	IV continues	IV may be discontinued	
Diet	NPO	Ice chips, sips of clear liquids	Clear liquids	Regular diet or as tolerated	Regular diet
Perineal		Peri-care by nurse	Peri-care with help	Self-peri-care	
Activity	Bed rest	Bed rest	OOB × 3 with help, ADLs assisted, assisted to comfortable position to hold and feed baby	Holds baby comfortably, ambulates without assistance, ADLs unassisted	Activity ad lib

CARE PATH	Cesarean Birth without Complications: Expected Length of Stay—48 to 72 Hours—cont'd

	IMMEDIATE POST-OP CESAREAN	BY 4TH HOUR AFTER ADMISSION TO PP UNIT	5 TO 24 HOURS	25 TO 48 HOURS	BY DISCHARGE
INTERVENTIONS—cont'd					
Pulmonary Care	Patent airway; O$_2$ discontinued	TCDB q2h with splinting, incentive spirometry q1h if ordered, lungs clear	TCDB q2h while awake; lungs clear	TCDB as needed; lungs clear	
Medications	Oxytocin added to IV Pain control: analgesics, IV, or epidural narcotic	Oxytocin continued Pain control: analgesics— PCA, IM, PO, or epidural narcotic	Oxytocin may be discontinued Pain control: IM, PO, PCA narcotics or analgesics	Oxytocin discontinued Pain control: PO analgesics, NSAIDs; PCA discontinued; stool softener, PNV	Rx filled or given to take home
Teaching, Discharge Plan	Breastfeeding, positioning, leg exercises	Verbalize understanding/ unit routines, how to achieve rest, TCDB, involution, pain control	*Self:* comfort measures and care; reinforce TCDB and positioning; introduce teaching videos, lactation promotion or suppression *Infant:* Hand-washing, infant safety, positioning for feeding and burping; if breastfeeding, then positioning baby, latching on, timing, removing from breast	*Self:* diet; activity/ rest; bowel/ bladder function *Infant:* bonding; parent concerns; feeding; infant bath, cord care; need for car seat; newborn characteristics; circumcision, if requested; answer questions	*Self:* home care, signs of complications (infections, bleeding), normal psychologic adjustments, normal ADLs; resumption of sexual activities; contraception; identification of support system at home; self-concept issues related to cesarean birth. Inform whom to call if problems; review need to keep follow-up appointment; provide information about community resources; provide copy of home care *Infant:* parents to demonstrate infant care; reinforce use of booklets for infant care, whom to call if problems; discuss immu-nization needs; review need to keep follow-up appointments

ADLs, Activities of daily living; *BM,* bowel movement; *BS,* bowel sounds; *CBC,* complete blood count; *HCT,* hematocrit; *IV,* intravenous; *NPO,* nothing by mouth; *NSAIDs,* nonsteroidal antiinflammatory agents; *OOB,* out of bed; *PCA,* patient-controlled analgesia; *PNV,* prenatal vitamins; *PP,* postpartum; *TCDB,* turn, cough, deep breathe; *WNL,* within normal limits.

HOME CARE *Patient Instructions for Self-Care*

Postpartum Pain Relief after Cesarean Birth

INCISIONAL

Splint incision with a pillow when moving or coughing.
Use relaxation techniques such as music, breathing, and dim lights.
Apply a heating pad to the abdomen.

GAS

Walk as often as you can.
Do not eat or drink gas-forming foods, carbonated beverages, or whole milk.
Do not use straws for drinking fluids.
Take antiflatulence medication if prescribed.
Lie on your left side to expel gas.
Use a rocking chair.

HOME CARE *Patient Instructions for Self-Care*

Signs of Postoperative Complications after Discharge

Report the following signs to your health care provider:
Fever exceeding 38° C
Painful urination
Lochia heavier than a normal period
Wound separation
Redness or oozing at the incision site
Severe abdominal pain

---

sessions, as well as explanations about the woman's recovery. The couple should also be encouraged to express their feelings about the birth experience. Some parents are angry, frustrated, or disappointed that a vaginal birth was not possible. Some women express feelings of low self-esteem or a negative self-image. Others express relief and gratitude that the baby is healthy and was born safely. It may be helpful for them to have the nurse who was present during the birth visit and help fill in "gaps" about the experience. Other psychologic and lifestyle concerns that have been reported include depression, feeling limited in activities, and changes in family interactions (Miovech et al., 1994).

Discharge after cesarean birth is usually by the third postoperative day. The time is often determined by criteria established by the woman's insurance carrier or the federal government (e.g., diagnosis-related groups). These criteria may not coincide with the woman's physical or psychosocial readiness for discharge. The nurse must provide discharge teaching to prepare women for self-care and newborn care in a limited time, while trying to ensure that the woman is comfortable and able to rest. The nurse needs to assess the woman's information needs and coordinate the health care team's efforts to meet them. Discharge teaching includes information about diet, exercise and activity restrictions, breast care, sexual activity and contraception, medications, signs of complications (Home Care box, above right), and infant care. The nurse also assesses the woman's need for continued support or counseling to facilitate her emotional recovery from the birth. Referral to support groups or to community agencies may be indicated to further promote this process. A postdischarge program of telephone follow-up and home visits can facilitate the woman's physical and psychosocial recovery following cesarean birth.

Vaginal birth after cesarean

Indications for primary cesarean birth, such as dystocia, breech presentation, or fetal distress, often are nonrecurring.

Therefore a woman who has had a cesarean birth may not have any contraindications to labor and vaginal birth at a subsequent pregnancy.

Most obstetricians no longer adhere to the belief that "once a cesarean, always a cesarean." ACOG (1994) recommends that a trial of labor and **vaginal birth after cesarean (VBAC)** be routinely attempted in women who have had one previous cesarean birth by low transverse incision. As proof of the merits of this approach vaginal births after previous cesarean birth increased 46% from 1989 to 1995. In 1995, 27.2% of women who had one previous cesarean birth were able to give birth vaginally at their second pregnancy (Ventura, 1995). Studies have shown that such vaginal birth is relatively safe, with only a 0.5% risk of uterine rupture through a lower uterine segment scar (Knuppel & Drukker, 1993). Labor and vaginal birth are not recommended if there are contraindications, such as a previous fundal classic cesarean scar or evidence of CPD.

According to Scott (1994), 60% to 88% of women can give birth vaginally after a trial of labor. Women are most often the primary decision makers with regard to choice of birth method. During the antepartal period, the women should be given information about VBAC and encouraged to choose it as an alternative to repeat cesarean birth, as long as no contraindications occur. VBAC support groups and prenatal classes can help prepare the woman psychologically for labor and vaginal birth.

Women not only need to believe that their efforts during a TOL will be successful but also that they are fully capable of doing what is necessary to give birth vaginally (self-efficacy). They need to be given the opportunity to discuss their previous labor experience, including feelings of failure and loss of control and to express any uncertainty and concern they may have about how they will manage during their upcoming labor and birth (Dilks & Beal, 1996).

This labor should occur in a hospital facility that has the equipment and personnel available to begin cesarean birth within 30 minutes from the time a decision is made to perform cesarean birth. Ideally the woman is admitted to the labor and birth unit at the onset of spontaneous labor. In the latent phase of labor, the nurse encourages her to engage in normal activities such as ambulation. In the active phase of labor, FHR and uterine activity usually are monitored electronically and intravenous access such as a heparin lock may be established. Collaboration among the woman in labor, the nurse, and other health care providers often results in a successful VBAC.

There is no evidence that administering oxytocin to induce or augment labor or the use of epidural anesthesia is contraindicated, although some physicians may elect not to use these measures (Cunningham et al., 1997).

Attention should be paid to the woman's psychologic, as well as physical, needs during the TOL. Anxiety can inhibit the release of oxytocin, thus delaying the progress of labor and possibly leading to a repeat cesarean birth. To alleviate such anxiety, the nurse can encourage the woman to use breathing and relaxation techniques and to change positions to promote labor progress. The woman's partner can be encouraged to provide comfort measures and emotional support (Fawcett, Tulman & Spedden, 1994). If a TOL is unsuccessful, the woman will need support and encouragement to express her feelings about once again not achieving her desired outcome.

Evaluation

To evaluate the effectiveness of nursing care for a woman experiencing dystocia, the nurse reviews the expected outcomes that were met and assesses the woman's and the family's level of satisfaction with the care received.

I POSTTERM PREGNANCY, LABOR, AND BIRTH

A **postterm** or postdate **pregnancy** is one that extends beyond the end of week 42 of gestation, or 294 days from the first day of the last menstrual period. The incidence of postterm pregnancy is estimated to be between 4% and 14% with an average of 10% (Cunningham et al., 1997). The most common cause is inaccurate dating of the pregnancy because the woman had an irregular ovulatory pattern (Spellacy, 1994). Deficiency of placental estrogen may also be a cause.

Maternal and Fetal Risks

Maternal risks are related to the birth of an excessively large infant. The woman is at increased risk for dysfunctional labor or lacerations related to vaginal birth; induction of labor, forceps- or vacuum-assisted birth, and cesarean birth are also more likely to be necessary (Spellacy, 1994, Wood, 1994). The woman also may experience psychologic risks because she may become anxious about going past her estimated date of birth (EDB).

The fetal risks appear to be twofold. The first is the possibility of birth trauma and asphyxia stemming from macrosomia. The second risk is the compromising effects an "aging" placenta is believed to have on the fetus. Spellacy (1994) notes that placental function gradually decreases after 37 weeks of gestation. Amniotic fluid volume (AFV) declines to approximately 800 ml by 40 weeks of gestation and to

about 400 ml by 42 weeks of gestation (Resnik, 1994). The resulting oligohydramnios can lead to fetal hypoxia related to cord compression. If placental insufficiency is present, there is a high likelihood of fetal distress occurring during labor. Neonatal problems may include asphyxia, meconium aspiration syndrome, dysmaturity syndrome, and respiratory distress (Gilbert & Harmon, 1998). Whether an infant born after a postterm pregnancy has neurologic, behavioral, or intellectual development problems needs to be further investigated. There are no conclusions in the literature about the long-term effects (Wood, 1994).

I CARE MANAGEMENT

The management of postterm pregnancy is still a controversial matter. The induction of labor at 41 to 42 weeks is suggested by some authorities as a means of reducing the rate of cesarean birth as well as still birth or neonatal death (Hannah et al., 1996). Others allow pregnancy to proceed to 43 weeks as long as tests of fetal well-being are performed and the results are normal.

LEGAL TIP Informed Consent Regarding Care during Postterm Pregnancy

The woman with a postterm pregnancy should be informed of the risks and benefits of both treatment and nontreatment. In the usual standard of practice, antepartal surveillance (maternal assessments and tests of fetal well-being) must begin by 14 days after the EDB, no matter how the date has been derived. A plan of care should be mutually agreed upon by the woman and her primary health care provider (Wood, 1994).

Antepartum assessments for postterm pregnancy may include daily fetal movement counts. Nonstress testing followed by stress testing, when indicated, is usually performed twice weekly. Assessment of amniotic fluid volume is usually done weekly. The AFV (see p. 587) should be greater than 8 with at least one pocket of amniotic fluid greater than 2 cm and amniotic fluid should be present throughout the uterine cavity (Gilbert & Harmon, 1998). The biophysical profile may be the best way of gauging fetal well-being because it combines nonstress testing with real-time ultrasound scanning to assess fetal movements, fetal breathing movements, and the AFV. Determining the AFV is critical in women with postterm pregnancies because, as just mentioned, a decreased AFV has been associated with fetal stress (Spellacy, 1994).

Cervical checks usually are performed weekly after 40 weeks' gestation to determine whether the condition of the cervix is favorable for induction (>5 on the Bishop score for multiparas and 9 for nulliparas) (see Table 25-3). Amniocentesis or amnioscopy may be performed to detect meconium in the amniotic fluid (Spellacy, 1994).

During the postterm period the woman is encouraged to assess fetal activity daily, assess for signs of labor, and keep appointments with her primary health care provider (Home Care box). The woman and her family should be encouraged to express their feelings about the prolonged pregnancy. Referral to a support group or other supportive resource may be needed.

If the woman's cervix is ripe, labor is usually induced with oxytocin. If her cervix is not ripe, a cervical ripening agent (e.g., prostaglandin gel) may be applied before the oxytocin induction (Gilbert & Harmon, 1998; Hannah et al., 1996).

During the labor of a woman with a postterm pregnancy, the fetus should be monitored electronically for a more accurate assessment of the FHR pattern. Fetal scalp pH sampling may be done to determine whether there is acidosis. If oligohydramnios is present, amnioinfusion may be implemented to restore amniotic fluid volume thereby preventing or treating cord compression or a variable deceleration pattern. This procedure can prevent meconium aspiration as a result of meconium passage by a hypoxic fetus. (Gilbert & Harmon, 1998; Wenstrom, Andrews & Maher, 1995). Accurate assessment of the woman's labor pattern also is important because dysfunctional labor is common (Spellacy, 1994).

Emotional support is essential for the woman with a postterm pregnancy and her family. Although a vaginal birth is anticipated, the couple should be prepared for the possibility of a forceps- or vacuum-assisted birth or a cesarean birth if complications arise.

Expected outcomes include that the woman uses appropriate coping mechanisms to deal with the emotional aspects of her postterm pregnancy and that the woman and her newborn experience no injury during the birth.

OBSTETRIC EMERGENCIES

Shoulder Dystocia

Etiologic factors and clinical manifestations

Shoulder dystocia is a rare emergency that can result in injury to the fetus or the woman, or both, during the attempt to deliver the fetus vaginally. It is estimated that 0.23% to 2.09% of all vaginal births are complicated by shoulder dystocia (Naef & Martin, 1995). In this condition, the head is born, but the anterior shoulder cannot pass under the pubic arch. Fetopelvic disproportion related to excessive fetal size or maternal pelvic abnormalities may be a cause (Hall, 1997; Wiznitzer, 1995), although shoulder dystocia can occur in the absence of any known risk factors. The nurse should be observant for signs that could indicate the presence of shoulder dystocia, including slowing of the progress of labor and formation of a caput succedaneum that increases in size. When the head emerges it retracts against the perineum (turtle sign) and external rotation does not occur (Hall, 1997; Wiznitzer, 1995).

CARE MANAGEMENT

Many maneuvers such as maternal position changes have been suggested and tried to free the anterior shoulder, although no one maneuver has been found to be most effective (Naef & Morrison, 1994). Having the woman move to a hands-and-knees position, a squatting position, or lateral recumbent position has resolved shoulder dystocia (Hall, 1997; Piper & McDonald, 1994). The two most frequently described maneuvers are the application of suprapubic pressure and the McRoberts maneuver. In the former, suprapubic pressure is applied to the anterior shoulder (Fig. 25-16) in an attempt to push it under the symphysis pubis (Naef & Morrison, 1994). In the McRoberts maneuver (Fig. 25-17), the woman's legs are flexed apart, with her knees on her abdomen (Piper & McDonald, 1994). This causes the sacrum to straighten and the symphysis pubis to rotate toward the mother's head; the angle of pelvic inclination is thereby decreased, freeing the shoulder. In other alternatives, the primary health care provider implements rotation procedures to move the shoulder and deliver the posterior arm. Fundal pressure usually is not advised (Naef & Morrison, 1994; Piper & McDonald, 1994). The nurse helps the woman to assume the position(s) that may facilitate birth of the shoulders and assists the primary health care provider with these maneuvers during the birth. In addition the nurse documents the maneuvers performed as well as other birth information according to the hospital policy. Newborn assessment should include examination for fracture of the clavicle or humerus as well as brachial plexus injuries, and asphyxia (Hall, 1997).

Prolapsed Umbilical Cord

Etiologic factors and clinical manifestations

Prolapse of the umbilical cord occurs when the cord lies below the presenting part of the fetus. Umbilical cord prolapse may be occult (hidden, not visible) at any time during labor whether or not the membranes are ruptured (Fig. 25-18, *A* and *B*). It is most common to see frank (visible) prolapse directly after ROM, when gravity washes the cord in front of the presenting part (Fig. 25-18, *C* and *D*). This occurs in 1 of 400 births. Contributing factors are a long cord (>100 cm), malpresentation (breech), transverse lie, or unengaged presenting part.

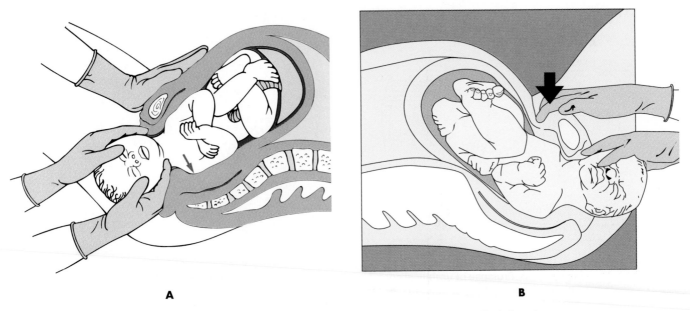

A

B

Fig. **25-16** Application of suprapubic pressure. **A,** Mazzanti technique. Pressure is applied directly posteriorly and laterally above the symphysis pubis. **B,** Rubin technique. Pressure is applied obliquely posteriorly against the anterior shoulder.

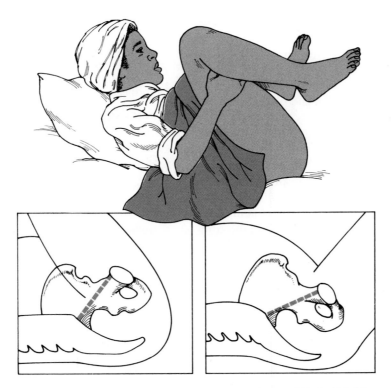

Fig. **25-17** McRoberts maneuver. (Modified from Gabbe S, Niebyl J & Simpson J: *Obstetrics, normal and problem pregnancies,* ed 3, New York, 1996, Churchill Livingstone.)

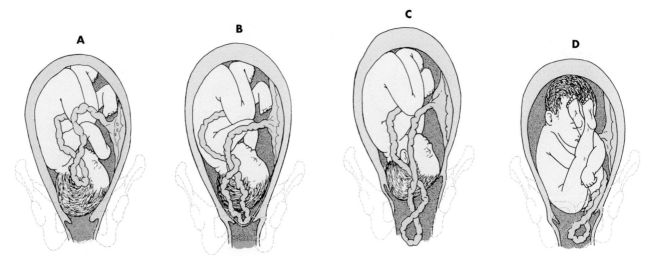

Fig. 25-18 Prolapse of umbilical cord. Note pressure of presenting part on umbilical cord, which endangers fetal circulation. **A**, Occult (hidden) prolapse of cord. **B**, Complete prolapse of cord. Note membranes are intact. **C**, Cord presenting in front of fetal head may be seen in vagina. **D**, Frank breech presentation with prolapsed cord.

When the presenting part does not fit snugly into the lower uterine segment, as can occur in hydramnios or ROM, a sudden gush of amniotic fluid may cause the cord to be displaced downward. Similarly the cord may prolapse during amniotomy if the presenting part is high. A small fetus may not fit snugly into the lower uterine segment; as a result, cord prolapse is more likely to occur. Other factors predisposing to cord prolapse that are associated with a high presenting part are multiparity, CPD, and placenta previa.

▌CARE MANAGEMENT

Prompt recognition of a prolapsed umbilical cord is important because fetal hypoxia resulting from prolonged cord compression (occlusion of blood flow to and from the fetus for more than 5 minutes) usually results in central nervous system damage or death of the fetus. Pressure on the cord may be relieved by the examiner putting a sterile gloved hand into the vagina and holding the presenting part off of the umbilical cord (Fig. 25-19, *A* and *B*). The woman is assisted into a position such as a modified Sims' (Fig. 25-19, *C*), Trendelenburg, or knee-chest (Fig. 25-19, *D*) position, in which gravity keeps the pressure of the presenting part off of the cord. If the cervix is fully dilated, forceps- or vacuum-assisted birth can be performed for the fetus in a cephalic presentation; otherwise a cesarean birth is likely to be performed. Nonreassuring fetal status, inadequate uterine relaxation, and bleeding can also occur as a result of a prolapsed umbilical cord. Indications for immediate interventions are presented in the Emergency box.

▌EMERGENCY

Prolapsed Cord

SIGNS
Fetal bradycardia with variable deceleration during uterine contraction.
Woman reports feeling the cord after membranes rupture.
Cord is seen or felt in or protruding from the vagina.

INTERVENTIONS
Call for assistance.
Notify health care provider immediately.
Glove the examining hand quickly and insert two fingers into the vagina to the cervix. With one finger on either side of the cord or both fingers to one side, exert upward pressure against the presenting part to relieve compression of the cord (Fig. 25-19, *A* and *B*). Place a rolled towel under the woman's right hip.
Place woman into the extreme Trendelenburg's or a modified Sims' position (Fig. 25-19, *C*), or a knee-chest position (Fig. 25-19, *D*).
If cord is protruding from vagina, wrap loosely in a sterile towel saturated with warm sterile normal saline solution.
Administer oxygen to the woman by mask at 10 to 12 L/min until birth is accomplished.
Start IV fluids or increase existing drip rate.
Continue to monitor FHR by internal fetal scalp electrode, if possible.
Explain to woman and support person what is happening and the way it is being managed.

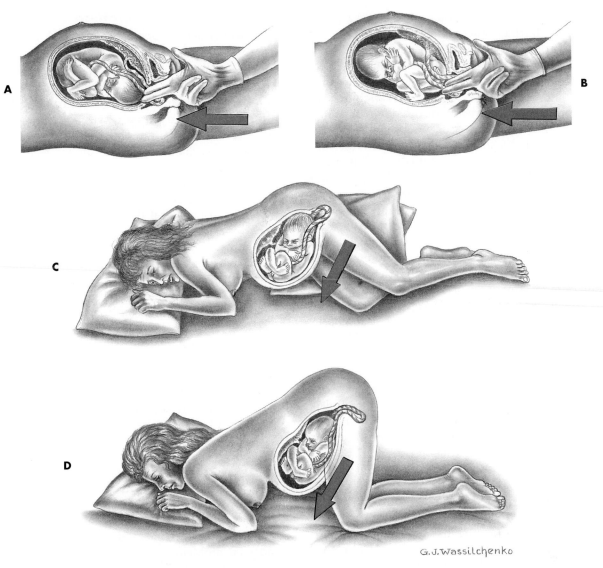

G.J.Wassilchenko

Fig. 25-19 Arrows indicate direction of pressure against presenting part to relieve compression of prolapsed umbilical cord. Pressure exerted by examiner's fingers in **A,** vertex presentation, and **B,** breech presentation. **C,** Gravity relieves pressure when woman is in modified Sims' position with hips elevated as high as possible with pillows. **D,** Knee-chest position.

Rupture of the Uterus

Etiologic factors and clinical manifestations

Rupture of the uterus is a rare but very serious obstetric injury that occurs in 1 to 1,500 to 2,000 births. The most frequent causes of uterine rupture during pregnancy are separation of the scar of a previous classic cesarean birth, uterine trauma (e.g., accidents, surgery), and a congenital uterine anomaly. During labor and birth, uterine rupture may be caused by intense spontaneous uterine contractions, labor stimulation (e.g., oxytocin), an overdistended uterus

(e.g., multifetal gestation), malpresentation, external or internal version, or a difficult forceps-assisted birth. It occurs more frequently in multigravidas than primigravidas (Varney, 1997).

A uterine rupture is classified as either complete or incomplete. A complete rupture extends through the entire uterine wall into the peritoneal cavity or broad ligament. An incomplete rupture extends into the peritoneum but not into the peritoneal cavity or broad ligament. Bleeding is usually internal. An incomplete rupture may also be a partial separation at an old cesarean scar and may go unnoticed unless the woman undergoes a subsequent cesarean birth or other uterine surgery.

Signs and symptoms vary with the extent of the rupture and may therefore be silent or dramatic. In an incomplete rupture, pain may not be present. The fetus may or may not show late decelerations, decreased variability, an increased or decreased heart rate, or other nonreassuring signs. The woman may experience vomiting, faintness, increased abdominal tenderness, hypotonic uterine contractions, and lack of progress. Eventually, bleeding and the effects of blood loss will be noted. Fetal heart tones may be lost. In a complete rupture the woman may complain of sudden, sharp shooting pain in her lower abdomen and may state that "something tore" or "gave way." If she is in labor, her contractions will cease and pain is relieved. She may exhibit signs of hypovolemic shock caused by hemorrhage (hypotension, tachypnea, pallor, cool, clammy skin). If the placenta separates, the FHR will be absent. Fetal parts may be palpable through the abdomen. The nurse should suspect pulmonary embolism if the woman complains of chest pain (Varney, 1997).

I CARE MANAGEMENT

Prevention is the best treatment. Women who have undergone a classic cesarean birth are advised not to attempt vaginal birth in subsequent pregnancies. Women at risk for uterine rupture are assessed closely during labor. In addition, women whose labor is induced with oxytocin are monitored for signs of uterine hyperstimulation, because this also can precipitate uterine rupture. If hyperstimulation occurs, the oxytocin infusion is discontinued or decreased and a tocolytic drug may be given to decrease the intensity of the uterine contractions. After giving birth, women are assessed for excessive bleeding, especially if the fundus is firm and there are signs of hemorrhagic shock.

If rupture occurs, the type of medical management implemented depends on the severity. A small rupture may be managed with a laparotomy and birth of the infant, repair of the laceration, and blood transfusions, if needed. In the event of complete rupture, hysterectomy and blood replacement is the usual treatment.

The nurse's role may include starting intravenous fluids, transfusing blood products, administering oxygen and assisting with the preparation for immediate surgery. Supporting the woman's family and giving them information about the treatment are also important during this emergency (Varney, 1997). The associated fetal mortality rates are high (>80%), and the maternal mortality rate may be as high as 50% to 75% (Cunningham et al., 1997). Providing information about spiritual support services or suggesting that the family contact their own support system may therefore be warranted.

Amniotic Fluid Embolism
Etiologic factors and clinical manifestations

An **amniotic fluid embolism (AFE)** occurs when amniotic fluid containing particles of debris (e.g., vernix, hair, skin cells, meconium) enters the maternal circulation and obstructs pulmonary vessels, causing respiratory distress and circulatory collapse. This can happen because fluid can enter the maternal circulation any time there is an opening in the amniotic sac or an opening in the maternal uterine veins, accompanied by enough intrauterine pressure to force the amniotic fluid into the veins (e.g., if the placenta separates of if there are rapid or strong contractions that cause the uterus to rupture or lacerate). This complication is estimated to be associated with a maternal mortality rate as high as 86% and a fetal mortality rate of 50% (Sisson, 1992).

Amniotic fluid is more damaging if it contains meconium and other particulate matter such as mucus, fat globules, lanugo, bacterial products, or debris from a dead fetus because emboli can then form more readily. Maternal death occurs most often, however, if thick meconium is present in the amniotic fluid because it clogs the pulmonary veins more completely than other debris. Even if death does not occur immediately, serious coagulation problems such as disseminated intravascular coagulopathy usually occur. The substances in the amniotic fluid can also adversely affect pulmonary blood vessels, by causing venospasm or pulmonary hypertension, and cardiac function, by causing left ventricular failure. Hemorrhage is an additional problem that often accompanies AFE.

Maternal factors, including multiparity, tumultuous labor, abruptio placentae, and oxytocin induction of labor, and fetal problems, including macrosomia, death, and meconium passage, have been associated with an increased risk for the development of AFE (Clark, 1990; Cunningham et al., 1997; Sisson, 1992).

I CARE MANAGEMENT

The immediate interventions for AFE are summarized in the Emergency box. Such medical management must be instituted immediately. Cardiopulmonary resuscitation is often necessary. The woman is usually placed on mechanical ventilation, and blood replacement is initiated and coagulation defects treated. Although the incidence of possible complications is small, the alert nurse can be important in their immediate recognition and the prompt initiation of treatment.

The nurse's immediate responsibility is to assist with the resuscitation efforts. If the woman survives, she is usually moved to a critical care unit, where hemodynamic monitoring and blood replacement and coagulopathy treatment are implemented.

EMERGENCY

Amniotic Fluid Embolism

SIGNS

Respiratory Distress
- Restlessness
- Dyspnea
- Cyanosis
- Pulmonary edema
- Respiratory arrest

Circulatory Collapse
- Hypotension
- Tachycardia
- Shock
- Cardiac arrest

Hemorrhage
- Coagulation failure: bleeding from incisions, venipuncture sites, trauma (lacerations); petechiae, ecchymoses, purpura
- Uterine atony

INTERVENTIONS

Oxygenate
- Administer oxygen by face mask (8-10 L/min) or resuscitation bag delivering 100% oxygen
- Prepare for intubation and mechanical ventilation
- Initiate or assist with cardiopulmonary resuscitation. Tilt pregnant woman 30 degrees to side to displace uterus

Maintain Cardiac Output and Replace Fluid Losses
- Position woman on her side
- Administer IV fluids
- Administer blood: packed cells, fresh frozen plasma
- Insert indwelling catheter, and measure hourly urine output

Correct coagulation failure

Monitor fetal and maternal status

Prepare for emergency birth once woman's condition is stabilized

Provide emotional support to woman, her partner, and family

From Lowdermilk D, Perry S & Bobak I: *Maternity and women's health care,* ed 6, St Louis, 1997, Mosby.

Support of the woman's partner and family is needed because they will be anxious and distressed. Brief explanations of what is happening are important during the emergency, with reexplanation and further explanation given after the immediate crisis. If the woman dies, emotional support and involvement of the perinatal loss support team or other resource is needed.

LOSS AND GRIEF IN THE INTRAPARTAL PERIOD

The risk of maternal and fetal and newborn death is increased in high-risk labor and birth. Death is a crisis that is then superimposed on the experience of childbearing.

Neonatal Death

From the perspective of the parents, their perceived loss may be the most terrible thing that has ever happened. They never thought such a thing could happen to them. Instead of celebrating, they are mourning at a birth. They have experienced a loss and are bereaved. The feelings and emotions that are associated with bereavement are called grief responses.

The critical intervention time is during the immediate crisis period after the loss. The goal of the nurse is to provide care, support, information, and anticipatory guidance to help with decision making. Families usually do not expect a loss to happen to them. The sudden and unexpected nature of their loss leaves them unprepared, both in life experiences and knowledge about grief responses and the mourning process. More important, they are unaware of what they might need for positive memories of this tragic time in their lives.

Assessment of the feelings, the perception of the loss, and the events surrounding the loss are important. Listening to the words that are used to describe the experience can help the nurse formulate appropriate nursing diagnoses and a plan of care. Mothers, fathers, and extended families look to the medical and nursing staff for support and understanding during the time of loss. It is rare for a mother or family to know exactly what is needed and to be willing to verbalize those needs. However, all families can make a choice once it has been offered and they have some time to consider what their needs might be. The nurse should do everything in his or her power to see that the needs are met. Unmet needs can form the basis of "if only" that may plague a mother or family for a lifetime or be the foundation for the development of complicated bereavement.

The nurse should listen patiently during the story of loss or grief. Questions helping the person talk specifically about grief and the experiences surrounding the loss may be needed. Bereaved persons should be encouraged to talk about their loved one and about what the loss means to them. The nurse should resist the temptation to give advice or to use clichés in offering support to the bereaved (Box 25-9).

Nurses need to be comfortable with their own feelings of grief and loss to effectively support and care for bereaved persons. It is appropriate to express such feelings with bereaved families and to share in the moment with them.

BOX 25-9	*What to Say and What Not to Say*

WHAT TO SAY

"I'm sad for you."
"How are you doing with all of this?"
"This must be hard for you."
"What can I do for you?"
"I'm sorry."
"I'm here, and I want to listen."

WHAT NOT TO SAY

"You're young, you can have others."
"You have an angel in heaven."
"This happened for the best."
"Better for this to happen now, before you knew the baby."
"There was something wrong with the baby anyway."
Calling the baby a "fetus" or "it."

Copyright 1998 Lutheran Hospital-LaCrosse, Inc. Used with permission of RTS Bereavement Services, LaCrosse, Wis.

Counseling techniques.

A number of counseling techniques have been identified that are effective in helping families share and express their grief. Box 25-10 lists some of these interventions.

Caring interventions

Physical comfort. Coping with loss and grief after childbirth can be an overwhelming experience for the woman and her family. Many times, these families request that the mother be moved off the maternity unit or discharged to her home. Their baby has died, and the thought of being on the same unit with other mothers and babies is more than they want to handle. Other mothers, however, may want to remain on the maternity unit, where the staff nurses are better prepared to meet their physical and emotional needs. The mother should be offered the option to choose where she wants to spend her postpartum stay.

Options for memories

Families need to be involved in the decision-making process. The decisions made during the time of their loss will provide their memories for a lifetime. Sensitivity to cultural and religious beliefs needs to be incorporated into the decision-making process.

It is sometimes difficult for the nurse to offer bereaved persons information about their rights regarding options without making them feel guilty if they do not choose to exercise those rights. Communicating with parents that options are their right, not their obligation, is vitally important.

Seeing and holding. One of the first options to discuss is whether the family wants to see their baby. A statement such as, "Some parents have found it helpful to see their baby," may be all the encouragement needed. Parents

BOX 25-10	*Counseling and Caring Interventions to use with Grieving Families*

- Ask the bereaved questions that help them express the experience of the loss. The nurse should use the name of the baby. In the case of a death, the nurse should make sure to see the baby first, before speaking with family members.
- When a bereaved person expresses feelings of anger, it can be helpful to identify the feeling by simply saying, "You sound angry," or "You look angry" or, "Where is this anger coming from?" The nurse's willingness to sit down and talk about these feelings of anger can help the bereaved move past those surface feelings into the underlying feelings of powerlessness and helplessness in not being able to control many aspects of the situation.
- Provide time to see and hold their baby in private, make arrangements for their baby to be returned to them for further viewing, and delay the processing of consent forms for autopsy or removal from the hospital. These actions by the nurse gives the family the opportunity for further acceptance of the reality of the loss and a last good-bye.
- Provide reading material on the grief process, responses of family and friends, talking with children, planning a special good-bye, and the differences between men's and women's grief.

appreciate explanations as to how their baby will look, for example, red, peeling skin like a bad sunburn; dark discoloration similar to bruises; or any defects. This helps them know what to expect. The nurse should make the baby look as normal as possible.

When bringing the baby to the parents, it is important to treat the baby as one would a live baby. Holding the baby close, touching a hand or cheek, using the baby's name, and talking with the parents about the special features of their child conveys that it is all right for them to do likewise.

Parents need to be offered time alone with their baby. Parents need to know when the nurse will return and how to call if they should need anything. The nurse should watch for cues that the parents have had enough time with their baby, such as when parents are no longer holding their child close to them or have placed the baby back in the crib. Asking parents whether they have had enough time usually makes the parents feel that the nurse thinks they have had enough time, which may not be the case. Sensitivity to their needs in actualizing the loss and coping with the reality of the death is essential for their healing.

Naming the baby. Naming the baby is an important decision parents can make. Choosing a name helps to make the baby a member of their family, the loss becomes more real, and the baby can more easily be remembered in a special way.

Autopsy and organ donation. An autopsy can be instrumental in determining the cause of death. For some families this information is helpful in understanding why their loss occurred, processing their grief, and perhaps preventing another loss. Other parents may feel that their baby has been through enough. They prefer not to have further information about the cause of death. Some religions prohibit autopsy. Options for the type of autopsy, such as excluding the head, are available to parents. Parents may need time to make this decision. There is no need to rush them, unless there was evidence of contagious disease or maternal infection at the time of death.

Organ donation can be an aid to grieving and an opportunity for the family to see something positive associated with this experience. The physician is usually the first to offer this opportunity to the family. Organ donation of eyes from a baby can occur if the baby was born alive at 36 weeks or more of gestation.

Privacy. If at all possible, the family should be placed in a private room, and when possible the room should have a rocking chair for the parents to sit in when holding their baby. This offers the mother and father special time together with their baby and with other family members. Marking the door to the room with a special card can be helpful in reminding the staff that this family has experienced a loss.

Rituals of remembrance. The spiritual aspect in meeting many families' needs at the time of a loss can be an important part of their care. Support from the clergy is an option that should be offered to all parents. Parents may wish to have their own pastor, priest, rabbi, or spiritual leader contacted, or they may wish to see the hospital's chaplain. They may also choose to do none of these.

Members from the clergy may offer the parents the opportunity for baptism when appropriate. Other rituals that may be offered include blessing, naming ceremony, anointing, ritual of the sick, memorial service, prayer, or just physical presence as a representative of a higher being.

Funeral arrangements. Parents should be given information about the choices for the final disposition of their baby's body. The choices are cremation or burial. Depending on the cemetery's policies, casketed babies or the ashes from cremated babies can be buried in a special place designated for babies, at the foot of an already deceased relative, in a separate plot, or in a mausoleum. Ashes may also be scattered in a designated area; many states have regulations regarding where ashes can be scattered. A local funeral director or a state's Vital Statistics Bureau should have information about the state's rules, codes, and regulations regarding live births, burial requirements, transportation of the deceased by parents, and cremation.

In making final arrangements for their baby, parents may want a special service. They may choose to have a service in the hospital chapel, visitation at a funeral home or their own home, a funeral service, or a graveside service. Parents can make any of these services as special, personal, and

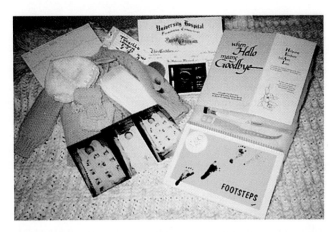

Fig. **25-20** A memory kit assembled at the University of Connecticut Health Center, Farmington, Conn. It includes pictures of the infant, clothing, death certificate, footprints, ID bands, fetal monitor printout, and ultrasound picture. (From Dickason E., Silverman B & Kaplan J: *Maternal-infant nursing care,* ed 3, St Louis, 1998, Mosby.)

memorable as they like. They can choose special music, poetry, or prose written by others or themselves.

Special memories. Parents need tangible mementos of their baby to allow them to actualize the loss. Parents may want to bring in a previously purchased baby book. Special memory books, cards, and information on grief and mourning are available for purchase by parents or hospitals or clinics through national perinatal bereavement organizations.

The nurse provides information about the baby's weight, length, and head circumference to the family. Footprints and handprints are taken and placed with the other information on a special card or in a memory or baby book (Fig. 25-20).

Any article that comes in contact with or is used in caring for the baby should be saved, placed in a sealable bag, and given to the parents. Articles should not be washed or cleaned beforehand, so the parents will be able to keep the smell of their baby. Articles parents have appreciated receiving include the tape measure used to measure the baby, lotions, combs, clothing, hats, blankets, pacifier, crib cards, and identification bands. A lock of hair may be an important keepsake for the parents' memories. Parents need to be asked for permission before cutting a lock of hair, which can be removed from the nape of the baby's neck, where it is not noticeable.

Pictures are the most important memento a parent can have. Photographs should be taken whenever there is an identifiable baby, and when it is culturally acceptable to the family. It does not matter how tiny the baby is, what the baby looks like, or how long the baby has been dead.

Pictures should be taken by an instant-print camera as well as a 35 mm camera. To provide as many different memories of the baby as possible, pictures should include close-ups of the baby's face, hands, and feet. The baby should be clothed in some of the pictures, and wrapped in a blanket with a hat or gown. Pictures should also be taken of the unclothed baby. If there are any congenital anomalies, close-ups of the anomalies should also be taken. Flowers, blocks, stuffed animals, or toys can be placed in the background to make the picture more special (Primeau & Recht, 1994).

Follow-up after discharge

Follow-up phone calls after a loss are important. The grief of the mother and her family does not end with discharge; rather it really begins once they return home, attend the funeral, and start to live their lives without their baby. Follow-up calls are made to let the parents know they are still thought of and cared about. The calls are made at predictably difficult times such as the first week at home, 1 month to 6 weeks later (parents should be invited to attend a support group at this time), 4 to 6 months after the loss, and at the anniversary of the death.

Maternal Death

It is extremely rare for a woman to die in childbirth, but it does happen. The occurrence of maternal deaths is 7 per 100,000 each year (National Center for Health Statistics, 1997). Families may be faced with not only mourning the death of a wife and mother but also the death of the baby. Or they may be faced with parenting a baby without a surviving mother. The family structure is completely disrupted; the father is left to care for the baby when his emotional reserves are the lowest. The same bereavement process and tasks need to be accomplished for the surviving partner, children, grandparents, other family members, and friends for them to heal after such a devastating loss.

The nursing care of families at this time is similar to that already described. Options need to be offered, memories made, and mementos obtained and held for the family until they are ready for them. These families are at risk for complicated bereavement and altered parenting of the surviving baby and other children in the family. Referral to social services to help the family mobilize support systems and for counseling can help combat potential problems before they develop. Such a referral may be beneficial not only at the time of the loss but also in the future.

The emotional toll that a maternal death can take on the nursing and medical staff must also be addressed. Guilt, anger, fear, sadness, and depression are all common responses to a maternal death. The staff may want to review the situation surrounding the events, the chart, and their responses in the forum of a mortality-morbidity review and a critical incident debriefing to help in coping with the feelings and emotions that result after a maternal death. Attending memorial or funeral services may benefit staff and family.

KEY POINTS

- The pregnant woman and her family can be taught to manage preterm labor at home with bed rest and the avoidance of activities that stimulate the uterus. Tocolytic therapy may also be implemented along with HUAM.
- In-hospital treatment for preterm labor involves bed rest, the administration of tocolytics, and pharmacologic stimulation of fetal lung maturity.
- Dystocia occurs if there are differences in the normal relationships among any of the five factors affecting labor.
- Dystocia and normal labor are characterized by differences in the pattern of progress in labor.
- Uterine dysfunction can be either hypertonic or hypotonic in nature.
- The functional relationships among the uterine contractions, the fetus, and the mother's pelvis are altered by maternal positioning.
- Uterine contractility is augmented by the effects of oxytocin and prostaglandin and is decreased by the effects of tocolytic agents (magnesium sulfate, β-sympathomimetic agents, calcium channel blockers, and prostaglandin inhibitors).
- The risk of infection is increased when PROM is prolonged without the onset of labor.
- All expectant parents benefit from learning about operative obstetrics (e.g., forceps-assisted and cesarean birth) and preterm labor during the prenatal period.
- The basic purpose of cesarean birth is to preserve the life or health of the mother and her fetus.
- Unless contraindicated, vaginal birth is possible after a cesarean birth. Women must be empowered to recognize their ability to give birth vaginally and to choose a TOL when appropriate.
- A postterm pregnancy poses a risk to both the mother and the fetus.
- Obstetric emergencies (e.g., shoulder dystocia, prolapsed cord, rupture of the uterus, and amniotic fluid embolism) occur rarely but require immediate intervention to preserve the health or life of the mother and newborn.
- Death of a woman in childbirth is rare. When a baby or a mother dies, each family member is affected, but no two family members grieve in the same way.

KEY POINTS—cont'd

- Therapeutic communication and counseling techniques can help families to identify their feelings, feel comfortable in expressing their grief, and understand their bereavement process.
- Follow-up after discharge is an essential component in providing care to families who have experienced a loss.

CRITICAL THINKING EXERCISES

1 You have been invited to present a class to a group of pregnant women and their partners who are beginning their second trimester. The topic of the class is the Identification and Prevention of Preterm Labor and Birth.
   a What risk factors would you emphasize in your class?
   b Describe three measures you would recommend to the couples to prevent the occurrence of preterm labor and birth.
   c Identify signs and symptoms that strongly suggest the onset of preterm labor. Describe the actions these couples should take should these signs and symptoms begin to occur.
   d Discuss the role of the partner in terms of assisting the pregnant woman to use appropriate measures to prevent preterm labor.

2 Describe the measures the nurse manager of a labor and birth unit could teach the nursing staff of the unit in an effort to reduce the incidence of prolonged labor and the rate of cesarean births.

3 A woman, G 2 P 1-0-0-1, had an unplanned cesarean birth as an outcome of her first pregnancy. She asks the nurse midwife about the possibility of a vaginal birth with this pregnancy because there are no factors in her health history that would contraindicate a TOL and a VBAC. She also expresses concern about how successful she would be in giving birth to her baby the "right way," since she failed to give birth vaginally the last time.
   a What factors influence a woman's decision to choose a TOL with the expected outcome of a vaginal birth or to schedule a cesarean birth.
   b What measures could the nurse use to empower this woman to attempt a vaginal birth?

CRITICAL THINKING EXERCISES—cont'd

4 You are preparing a woman and her partner for an unplanned cesarean birth necessitated by fetal distress.
   a Describe the possible reaction of the woman and her partner to this situation and how these reactions should influence the nursing care provided.
   b Describe the feelings you might have regarding this situation and how these feelings could influence the care you administer.
   c How would your preparation of this couple differ from the way in which you would prepare a couple for a planned cesarean birth?
   d Discuss how this woman's postpartum care would differ from a woman who experienced a vaginal birth.
   e How would you involve the woman's partner in assisting with her care?

5 A pregnant woman, G 4 P 0-2-1-2, at 30 weeks' gestation is being treated at home for preterm labor. She is married and has two children, aged 3 years and 9 years. The treatment regimen includes bed rest with bathroom privileges, terbutaline subcutaneous pump, and home uterine activity monitoring. Develop a plan of care that includes each of the following:
   a Safe and effective administration of terbutaline
   b Adherence to activity restrictions
   c Accurate monitoring of uterine activity
   d Avoidance of behaviors that could stimulate uterine activity and interfere with the effort to suppress labor
   e Home maintenance; care of young children
   f Supportive measures to help the family deal with the adverse outcomes of high-risk pregnancy and bed rest

6 Investigate community and support groups that exist to assist parents who have experienced the death of a baby through stillbirth, newborn death, or maternal death. Identify information that will be useful in providing care to families experiencing loss.

References

Albers L, Lydon-Rochelle M & Krulewitch C: Maternal age and labor complications in healthy primigravidas at term, *J Nurse Midwifery* 40(1):4, 1995.

American College of Obstetricians and Gynecologists: Operative vaginal delivery, *Technical Bulletin* 152, Washington, DC, Feb 1991, ACOG.

American College of Obstetricians and Gynecologists: Committee Opinion: Vaginal delivery after a previous cesarean birth, *Committee on Obstetrics Practice* 143, Washington, DC, Oct 1994, ACOG.

American College of Obstetricians and Gynecologists: Preterm labor, *Technical Bulletin* 206, Washington, DC, 1995a, ACOG.

American College of Obstetricians and Gynecologists: Induction of labor, *Technical Bulletin* 217, Washington, DC, 1995b, ACOG.

American College of Obstetricians and Gynecologists: Dystocia and the augmentation of labor, *Technical Bulletin* 218, Washington, DC, 1995c, ACOG.

Andrews C & Chrzanowski M: Maternal position, labor, and comfort, *Appl Nurs Res* 3(1):7, 1990.

Andrews W, Goldenburg R & Hauth J: Preterm labor: emerging role of genital tract infections, *Infect Agents Dis* 4(4):196, 1995.

Association of Women's Health, Obstetric, and Neonatal Nurses: *Cervical ripening and induction and augmentation of labor,* Practice Resource, Washington, DC, Dec 1993, AWHONN.

Biancuzzo M: Six myths of maternal position during labor, *MCN Am J Matern Child Nurs* 18(5):264, 1993.

Bolane J & Furlong J: *Coping with bedrest in pregnancy,* Waco, Texas, 1994, Childbirth Graphics.

Burrows W et al.: Safety and efficacy of early postoperative solid food consumption after cesarean section, *J Reprod Med* 40(6):463, 1995.

Clark S: New concepts of amniotic fluid embolism: a review, *Obstet Gynecol* 45(6):360, 1990.

Creasy R: Preterm birth prevention: where are we? *Am J Obstet Gynecol* 168(4):1223, 1993.

Creasy R & Merkatz I: Prevention of preterm labor: clinical opinion, *Obstet Gynecol* 76(suppl 1):25, 1990.

Cunningham F et al.: *Williams obstetrics,* ed 20 Stamford, Conn, 1997, Appleton & Lange.

Davis L: Protocol for the nursing management of the patient requiring oxytocin for induction and augmentation of labor. In Mandeville L & Troiano N, editors: *High-risk intrapartum nursing,* Philadelphia, 1992, Lippincott.

Day M & Snell B: Use of prostaglandin for induction of labor, *J Nurse Midwifery* 38(2) (suppl):42S, 1993.

de Veciana M et al.: Tocolysis in advanced pretern labor: impact on neonatal outcome, *Am J Perinatol* 12(4):294, 1995.

Dilks F & Beal J: Role of self-efficacy in birth choice, *J Perinat Neonat Nurs* 11(1):1, 1997.

DiMatteo M et al.: Cesarean childbirth and psychosocial outcomes: a meta-analysis, *Health Psychol* 15(4):303, 1996.

Edenfield S et al.: Validity of the Creasy Risk Appraisal Instrument for prediction of preterm labor, *Nurs Res* 44(2):76, 1995.

Fawcett J, Tulman L & Spedden J: Responses to vaginal birth after cesarean section, *J Obstet Gynecol Neonatal Nurs* 23(3):253, 1994.

Freda M & De Vore N: Should intravenous hydration be the first line of defense with threatened preterm labor? A critical review of the literature, *J Perinatol* 16(5):385, 1996.

Freston M et al.: Responses of pregnant women to potential preterm labor symptoms, *J Obstet Gynecol Neonatal Nurs* 26(1):35, 1997.

Friedman E: Normal and dysfunctional labor. In Cohen W et al., editors: *Management of labor,* ed 2, Rockville, Md, 1989, Aspen.

Gabbe S, Niebyl J & Simpson G: *Obstetrics, normal and problem pregnancies,* ed 3, New York, 1996, Churchill Livingstone.

Gaute T & Spellacy W: Premature rupture of membranes. In Scott J et al., editors: *Danforth's obstetrics and gynecology,* ed 7, Philadelphia, 1994, Lippincott.

Gilbert E & Harmon J, *Manual of high risk pregnancy and delivery,* ed 2, St Louis, 1998, Mosby.

Goldenberg R et al.: Bed rest in pregnancy, *Obstet Gynecol* 84(1):131, 1994.

Grohar J: Nursing protocols for antepartum home care, *J Obstet Gynecol Neonatal Nurs* 23(8):687, 1994.

Gupton A, Heaman M & Ashcroft T: Bed rest from the perspective of the high-risk pregnant woman, *J Obstet Gynecol Neonatal Nurs* 26(4):423, 1997.

Hall S: The nurse's role in the identification of risks and treatment of shoulder dystocia, *J Obstet Gynecol Neonatal Nurs* 26(1):25, 1997.

Hannah M: Tocolytics—more good than harm or is it the reverse? *Birth* 23(1):41, 1996.

Hannah M et al.: Postterm pregnancy: putting the merits of a policy of induction of labor into perspective, *Birth* 23(1):13, 1996.

Heffner L et al.: Clinical and environmental predictors of preterm labor, *Obstet Gynecol* 81(5 part 1): 750, 1993.

Hill W: Risks and complications of tocolysis, *Clin Obstet Gynecol* 38(4):725, 1995.

Hill W et al.: Home uterine activity monitoring is associated with a reduction in preterm birth, *Obstet Gynecol* 76(suppl 1):13S, 1990.

Iams J: The role of tocolysis in the prevention of preterm birth, *Birth* 23(1):40, 1996.

Iams J, Johnson F & Parker M: A prospective evaluation of the signs and symptoms of preterm labor, *Obstet Gynecol* 84(2):227, 1994.

Isennock P: *Bed rest before baby: what's a mother to do?* Perry Hall, Md, 1992, Mustard Seed Publications.

Jones D & Collins B: The nursing management of women experiencing preterm labor: clinical guidelines and why they are needed, *J Obstet Gynecol Neonatal Nurs* 25(7):569, 1996.

Josten L et al.: Bed rest compliance for women with pregnancy problems, *Birth* 22(1):1, 1995.

Keirse M: New perspectives for the effective treatment of preterm labor, *Am J Obstet Gynecol* 173(2):618, 1995.

King T: Clinical management of premature rupture of membranes, *J Nurse Midwifery* 39(suppl 2):81S, 1994.

Knuppel R & Drukker J: *High-risk pregnancy: a team approach,* ed 2, Philadelphia, 1993, WB Saunders.

Lang J, Lieberman E & Cohen A: A comparison of risk factors for preterm labor and term small-for-gestational-age birth, *Epidemiology* 7(4):369, 1996.

Laros R, Flanagan T & Kilpatrick J: Management of term breech presentation: a protocol of external cephalic version and selective trial of labor, *Am J Obstet Gynecol* 172(6):1916, 1995.

Lydon M et al.: Accuracy of Leopold maneuvers in screening for malpresentation: a prospective study, *Birth* 20(3):132, 1993.

Maloni J: Home care of the high-risk pregnant woman requiring bed rest, *J Obstet Gynecol Neonatal Nurs* 23(8):696, 1994.

Maloni J & Ponder B: Fathers' experience of their partners' antepartum bed rest, *Image: J Nurs Sch* 29(2):183, 1997.

Mastrogiannis D & Knuppel R: Labor induced using methods that do not involve oxytocin, *Clin Obstet Gynecol* 38(2):259, 1995.

McGregor J et al.: Prevention of premature birth by screening and treatment for common genital tract infections: results of a prospective controlled evaluation, *Am J Obstet Gynecol* 173(1):157, 1995.

Miovech S et al.: Major concerns of women after cesarean delivery, *J Obstet Gynecol Neonatal Nurs* 23(1):53, 1994.

Mongra M & Creasy R: Pharmacologic management of preterm labor, *Semin Perinatol* 19(1):84, 1995.

Mundle W & Young D: Vaginal misoprostol for induction of labor: a randomized, controlled trial, *Obstet Gynecol* 88(4 part 1):521, 1996.

Naef R & Martin J: Emergent management of shoulder dystocia, *Obstet Gynecol Clin North Am* 22(2):247, 1995.

Naef R & Morrison J: Guidelines for the management of shoulder dystocia, *J Perinatol* 14(6):435, 1994.

National Center for Health Statistics: *Health, United States, 1995-1996,* Hyattsville, Md, 1997, Public Health Service.

Piper D & McDonald P: Management of anticipated and actual shoulder dystocia: interpreting the literature, *J Nurse Midwifery* 39(suppl 2):91S, 1994.

Porreco R & Thorp J: The cesarean birth epidemic: trends, causes, and solutions, *Am J Obstet Gynecol* 175(2):369, 1996.

Primeau M & Recht K: Professional bereavement photographs: one aspect of a perinatal bereavement program, *J Obstet Gynecol Neonatal Nurs* 23(1):22, 1994.

Radin T, Harmon J & Hanson D: Nurses' care during labor: its effects on the cesarean birth rate of healthy nulliparous women, *Birth* 20(1):14, 1993.

Reichler A, Romem Y & Divon M: Induction of labor, *Curr Opin Obstet Gynecol* 7(6):432, 1995.

Resnik R: Posterm pregnancy. In Creasy R & Resnik R, editors: *Maternal fetal medicine: principle and practice,* ed 3, Philadelphia, 1994, WB Saunders.

Rippin-Sisler C: The experience of precipitate labor, *Birth* 23(4):224, 1996.

Romero C & Jones P: Home infusion therapies for obstetric patients, *J Obstet Gynecol Neonatal Nurs* 23(8):675, 1994.

Sandmire H: Whither tocolysis, *Birth* 23(1):38, 1996.

Schroeder C: Women's experience of bed rest in high-risk pregnancy, *Image: J Nurs Sch* 28(3):253, 1996.

Scott J: Cesarean delivery. In Scott J et al., editors: *Danforth's obstetrics and gynecology,* ed 7, Philadelphia, 1994, Lippincott.

Simpkin P: Reducing pain and enhancing progress in labor: a guide to nonpharmacologic methods for maternity caregivers, *Birth* 22(3):161, 1995.

Simpson K: Preterm birth in the United States: current issues and future perspectives, *J Perinat Neonat Nurs* 10(4):11, 1997.

Sisson M: Amniotic fluid embolism, *NAACOG's Clin Issues Perinat Women's Health Nurs* 3(3):469, 1992.

Spellacy W: Postdate pregnancy. In Scott J et al., editors: *Danforth's obstetrics and gynecology,* ed 7, Philadelphia, 1994, Lippincott.

Summers L: Methods of cervical ripening and labor induction, *J Nurse Midwifery* 42(2):71, 1997.

Taffel S, Placek P & Kosary C: US cesarean section rates 1990: an update, *Birth* 19(1):21, 1992.

Thomas L et al.: The effects of rocking, diet modifications, and antiflatulent medication on postcesarean section gas pain, *J Perinat Neonatal Nurs* 4(3):12, 1990.

Varney H: *Varney's textbook for midwives,* ed 3, Sudberry, Mass, 1997, Jones and Bartlett Publishers.

Ventura J et al.: Report of final natality statistics, 1995, *Monthly Vital Statistics Report,* 45(11s):97, 1997, Public Health Service.

Ventura J et al.: Advance report of final natality statistics, 1993, *Monthly Vital Statistics Report,* 44(35):1, 1995, Public Health Service.

Weingarten C et al.: Married mothers perceptions of their premature or term infants and the quality of their relationships with their husbands, *J Obstet Gynecol Neonatal Nurs* 19(1):64, 1990.

Wenstrom K, Andrews W & Maher J: Amnioinfusion survey: prevalence, protocols, and complications, *Obstet Gynecol* 86(4, part 1):572, 1995.

Wheeler D: Preterm birth prevention, *J Nurse Midwifery* 38(suppl 2):66S, 1994.

Wiznitzer A: Obstructed labor and shoulder dystocia, *Curr Opin Obstet Gynecol* 7(6):486, 1995.

Wood C: Postdate pregnancy update, *J Nurse Midwifery* 39(suppl 2):110S, 1994.

CHAPTER

26

Postpartum Complications

DEITRA LEONARD LOWDERMILK AND ANNE HOPKINS FISHEL

Collaborative efforts of the health care team are needed to provide safe and effective care to the woman and family experiencing postpartum complications. This chapter focuses on hemorrhage, infection, sequelae of childbirth trauma, and psychologic complications.

POSTPARTUM HEMORRHAGE

Postpartum hemorrhage (PPH) continues to be a leading cause of maternal morbidity and mortality in the United States today (Berg et al., 1996). It is a life-threatening event that can occur with little warning and is often unrecognized until the mother has profound symptoms (Grimes, 1994; Norris, 1997). PPH is traditionally defined as the loss of greater than 500 ml of blood in the first 24 hours after vaginal birth. However, defining PPH is not a clear-cut issue; even the American College of Obstetricians and Gynecologists (ACOG) states that there is "no universally accepted definition" of PPH (ACOG, 1990). In defining PPH, the cliniciaon must recognize that blood loss (which is traditionally underestimated by as much as 50%) is as important as clinical signs and symptoms. Reports cited in Roberts (1995) indicate that a postpartum blood loss as great as 1,000 ml is generally well tolerated by the woman without significant changes in blood pressure and cardiac output because of the increased blood volume in pregnancy. A more realistic definition suggested for PPH is a postpartum blood loss exceeding 1,000 ml, independent of the mode of birth (Roberts, 1995). Clinically, a more objective criterion for determining PPH is bleeding that is in excess of the health care provider's definition of normal bleeding that cannot be controlled by uterine massage or oxytocic use (Zahn & Yeomans, 1990). Another clinical definition of PPH is a decrease in hematocrit of 10 or more percentage points or the need for transfusion therapy (Roberts, 1995).

PPH may be sudden and even exsanguinating. With blood flow of approximately 650 ml/min to the uterine vasculature and placenta, disruption of vascular integrity has the potential for maternal exsanguination within a matter of minutes (Knuppel & Hatangadi, 1995). The nurse must therefore be alert to the symptoms of hemorrhage and hypovolemic shock and be prepared to act quickly to minimize blood loss.

Traditionally, PPH has been classified as early or late with respect to the birth. Early, acute, or primary PPH occurs within 24 hours of the birth. Late or secondary PPH occurs more than 24 hours but less than 6 weeks postpartum (Hunter & Weiner, 1996). Today's health care environment encourages shortened stays after birth, thereby increasing the potential for acute episodes of PPH to occur outside the traditional hospital or birth center setting.

The most common cause of PPH is uterine atony, which complicates approximately 1 in 20 births (Hunter & Weiner, 1996). Less common causes include retained placenta, abnormal placentation, uterine lacerations and rupture, lower genital tract lacerations and hematomas, infection, and coagulopathies. Predisposing factors for PPH are listed in Box 26-1.

It is helpful to consider the problem of excessive bleeding with reference to the stages of labor. From birth of the infant until separation of the placenta, the character and quantity of blood passed may suggest excessive bleeding. For example, dark blood is probably of venous origin, perhaps from varices or superficial lacerations of the birth canal. Bright blood is arterial and may indicate deep lacerations of the cervix. Spurts of blood with clots may indicate partial placental separation. Failure of blood to clot or remain clotted indicates a pathologic condition or coagulopathy such as disseminated intravascular coagulation.

Excessive bleeding may occur during the period from the separation of the placenta to its expulsion or removal. Commonly, such excessive bleeding is the result of incomplete placental separation, undue manipulation of the fundus, or excessive traction on the cord. After the placenta has been expelled or removed, persistent or excessive blood loss usually is the result of atony of the uterus (its failure to contract well or maintain contraction) or prolapse of the uterus into the pelvis. Late PPH may be a result of incomplete involution of the uterus and unrecognized lacerations of the birth canal, but it is most often due to retained placental fragments.

Uterine Atony

Uterine atony is marked hypotonia of the uterus. Normally, placental separation and expulsion are facilitated by contraction of the uterus, which also prevents hemorrhage from the placental site. The corpus is in essence a basket weave of strong, interdigitating smooth muscle bundles through which many large maternal blood vessels pass. If the uterus is flaccid after detachment of all or part of the placenta, brisk venous bleeding occurs and normal coagulation of the open vasculature is impaired and continues until the uterine muscle is contracted.

Uterine atony is the leading cause of PPH, accounting for greater than 90% of all cases of PPH (Norris, 1997). It is associated with grand multiparity, hydramnios, a macrosomic fetus, and multifetal gestation. In such conditions the uterus is "overstretched" and contracts poorly after the birth. Other

---

| BOX 26-1 | *Risk Factors for Postpartum Hemorrhage* |

Uterine atony
- Overdistended uterus
  - —Large fetus
  - —Multiple fetuses
  - —Hydramnios
  - —Distention with clots
- Anesthesia and analgesia
  - —Conduction anesthesia
- Previous history of uterine atony
- High parity
- Prolonged labor, oxytocin-induced labor
- Trauma during labor and birth
  - —Forceps birth
  - —Vacuum-assisted birth
  - —Cesarean birth

Chorioamnionitis
Retained placental fragments
Abnormal adherent placenta
Lacerations of the birth canal
Ruptured uterus
Inversion of the uterus
Placental abruption
Placenta previa
Coagulation disorders
Manual removal of a retained placenta
Uterine subinvolution
Magnesium sulfate administration during labor or postpartum

---

causes of atony include traumatic birth, use of halogenated anesthesia (e.g., halothane) or magnesium sulfate, rapid or prolonged labor, chorioamnionitis, and use of oxytocin for labor induction or augmentation.

Lacerations of the Genital Tract

Lacerations of the cervix, vagina, and perineum are also causes of PPH. Hemorrhage related to lacerations should be suspected if bleeding continues despite a firm, contracted uterine fundus. This bleeding can be a slow trickle, an oozing, or frank hemorrhage.

Factors that influence the causes and incidence of obstetric lacerations of the lower genital tract include operative birth; precipitous birth; congenital abnormalities of the maternal soft parts; contracted pelvis; size, abnormal presentation, and position of the fetus; relative size of the presenting part and the birth canal; previous scarring from infection, injury, or operation; and vulvar, perineal, and vaginal varicosities.

Extreme vascularity in the labial and periclitoral areas often results in profuse bleeding if laceration occurs. Hematomas may also be present.

Lacerations of the perineum are the most common of all injuries in the lower portion of the genital tract. These are classified as first, second, third, and fourth degree (see

Chapter 15). An episiotomy may extend to become either a third- or fourth-degree laceration.

Prolonged pressure of the fetal head on the vaginal mucosa ultimately interferes with the circulation and may produce ischemic or pressure necrosis. The state of the tissues in combination with the type of birth may result in deep vaginal lacerations and sulci tears (see p. 395), with consequent predisposition toward vaginal hematomas.

Vaginal **hematomas** (collections of blood in the connective tissue) occur more commonly in association with a forceps-assisted birth, an episiotomy, or primigravidity (Ridgeway, 1995). During the postpartum period, if the woman reports a persistent perineal or rectal pain or a feeling of pressure in the vagina, a careful examination is made. However, a subperitoneal hematoma may cause minimal pain, and the initial symptoms may be signs of shock (Ridgeway, 1995).

Cervical lacerations usually occur at the lateral angles of the external os. Most are shallow, and bleeding is minimal. More extensive lacerations may extend into the vaginal vault or into the lower uterine segment.

Retained Placenta

Nonadherent retained placenta

The normally implanted placenta separates with the first or second strong uterine contraction after birth of the infant. Placental separation occurs within 15 minutes in about 90% of women; within 30 minutes after birth, about 95% of women will have a separated placenta, and within 45 minutes, about 98% will have achieved placental separation. If the placenta has not been recovered within 30 minutes of birth, most health care providers attempt to remove it manually.

Retained placenta may result from partial separation of a normal placenta, entrapment of the partially or completely separated placenta by an hourglass constriction ring of the uterus, mismanagement of the third stage of labor, or abnormal adherence of the entire placenta or a portion of the placenta to the uterine wall. Placental retention because of poor separation is common in very preterm births (20 to 24 weeks' gestation).

Management of nonadherent retained placenta is by manual separation and removal by the primary health care provider. Supplementary anesthesia is not usually needed for women who have had regional anesthesia for birth. For other women, administration of light nitrous oxide and oxygen inhalation anesthesia or intravenous (IV) thiopental facilitates uterine exploration and placental removal. After this removal the woman is at continued risk for PPH or for infection.

Adherent retained placenta

Abnormal adherence of the placenta occurs for reasons unknown, but it is thought to result from zygotic implantation in an area of defective endometrium so that there is no zone of separation between the placenta and the decidua. Attempts to remove the placenta in the usual manner are unsuccessful, and laceration or perforation of the uterine wall may result, putting the woman at great risk for severe PPH and infection (Cunningham et al., 1997).

Predisposing factors for abnormal placental attachment include scarring of the uterus, such as occurs after cesarean birth, myomectomy, or vigorous curettage; endometritis associated with tuberculosis; abnormal site of implantation, such as the cervix or lower uterine segment (placenta previa); and malformation of the placenta.

Unusual placental adherence may be partial or complete. The following degrees of attachment are recognized:
* *Placenta accreta*—slight penetration of myometrium by placental trophoblast.
* *Placenta increta*—deep penetration of myometrium by placenta.
* *Placenta percreta*—perforation of uterus by placenta.

Bleeding with complete or total placenta accreta may not occur unless separation of the placenta is attempted. With more extensive involvement, bleeding will become profuse when delivery of the placenta is attempted. Treatment includes blood component replacement therapy, and hysterectomy may be indicated (Cunningham et al., 1997).

Inversion of the Uterus

Inversion of the uterus (turning inside out) after birth is a potentially life-threatening complication. The incidence of uterine inversion is approximately 1 in 2,000 to 2,500 births (Wendel & Cox, 1995), and inversion may recur with a subsequent birth.

Uterine inversion may be partial or complete. Complete inversion of the uterus is obvious; a large, red, rounded mass (perhaps with the placenta attached) protrudes 20 to 30 cm outside the introitus. Incomplete inversion cannot be seen but must be felt; a smooth mass will be palpated through the dilated cervix.

Contributing factors to uterine inversion include fundal pressure, traction applied to the cord, uterine atony, leiomyomas, and abnormally adherent placental tissue (Cunningham et al., 1997). Uterine inversion occurs most often in multiparous women and with placenta accreta or increta. Although proper management of the third stage of labor prevents most cases of uterine inversion, some are unavoidable.

The primary presenting signs of uterine inversion are hemorrhage, shock, and pain. Hemorrhage is the primary presenting sign in as many as 94% of women with uterine inversion, with blood loss estimated to range from 800 to 1,800 ml. As many as 40% of these women may also have shock (Wendel & Cox, 1995; Zahn & Yeomans, 1990).

Prevention—always the easiest, least expensive, and most effective therapy—is especially appropriate for uterine inversion. *The umbilical cord should not be pulled on strongly unless the placenta has definitely separated.*

Subinvolution of the Uterus

Late postpartum bleeding may occur as a result of subinvolution of the uterus. **Subinvolution** is defined as the delayed return of the enlarged uterus to normal size and function. Recognized causes of subinvolution include retained placental fragments and pelvic infection.

Signs and symptoms include prolonged lochial discharge, irregular or excessive bleeding, and sometimes hemorrhage. A pelvic examination usually reveals a uterus that is larger than normal and one that may be boggy.

CARE MANAGEMENT

Assessment and Nursing Diagnoses

PPH can progress rapidly to shock; therefore the nurse must assess the patient carefully and thoroughly (Fig. 26-1 and Box 26-2). The woman's history should be reviewed for factors that cause predisposition to PPH (see Box 26-1).

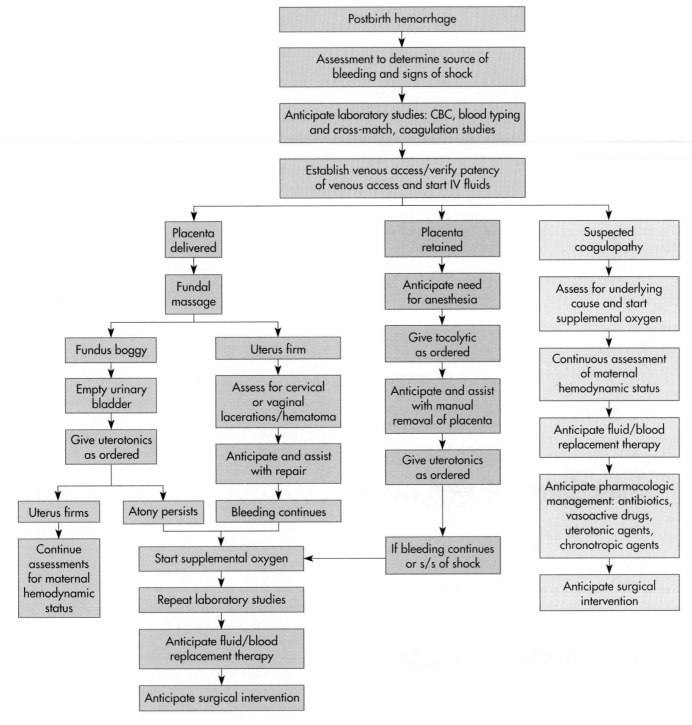

Fig. **26-1** Nursing assessments for postpartum bleeding. *CBC,* Complete blood count; *IV,* intravenous; *s/s,* signs and symptoms.

BOX 26-2   Noninvasive Assessments of Cardiac Output in Postpartum Patients Who Are Bleeding

Palpation of pulses (rate, quality, equality)
• Arterial
• Blood pressure
Auscultation
• Heart sounds/murmurs
• Breath sounds
Inspection
• Skin color, temperature, turgor
• Level of consciousness (LOC)
• Capillary refill
• Urinary output
• Neck veins
• Pulse oximetry
• Mucous membranes
Presence or absence of anxiety, apprehension, restlessness, disorientation

---

The fundus is assessed to determine whether it is firmly contracted at or near the level of the umbilicus. Bleeding should be assessed for color and amount. The perineum is inspected for signs of lacerations or hematomas to determine the possible source of bleeding.

Vital signs may not be reliable indicators of shock immediately postpartum because of the physiologic adaptations of this period. However, frequent vital sign measurements during the first 2 hours after birth may identify trends related to blood loss (e.g., tachycardia, tachypnea, falling blood pressure).

Assessment for bladder distention is important because a distended bladder can displace the uterus and prevent contraction. The skin is examined for warmth and dryness; nail beds are checked for color and promptness of capillary refill. Laboratory studies include determination of hemoglobin and hematocrit levels.

Late PPH may develop within 24 hours of birth or later in the postpartum period. The woman may be at home when the symptoms occur. Discharge teaching should emphasize the signs of normal involution, as well as potential complications. Suggested nursing diagnoses for women experiencing PPH are listed in the Nursing Diagnoses box.

Nursing Diagnoses

Women Experiencing Postpartum Hemorrhage
Fluid volume deficit (immediate) related to:
• Excessive blood loss secondary to uterine atony, lacerations, or uterine inversion
Risk for fluid volume excess related to:
• Blood and fluid volume replacement therapy
• Excessive blood loss or exposed placental attachment site

Risk for injury (maternal) related to:
• Attempted manual removal of retained placenta
• Administration of blood products
• Operative procedures
Fear/anxiety related to:
• Threat to self
• Lack of knowledge regarding procedures and operative management
Risk for altered parenting related to:
• Separation from infant secondary to treatment regimen
Altered peripheral tissue perfusion related to:
• Excessive blood loss and shunting of blood to central circulation

Expected Outcomes of Care
Expected outcomes for the woman experiencing PPH may include that the woman will:
• Identify and use available support systems
• Maintain normal vital signs and laboratory values
• Develop no complications related to excessive bleeding
• Express understanding of her condition, its management, and discharge instructions

Plan of Care and Interventions
Medical management
Early recognition and acknowledgment of the diagnosis of PPH are critical to care management. The first step is to evaluate the contractility of the uterus. If the uterus is hypotonic, management is directed toward increasing contractility and minimizing blood loss.

Hypotonic uterus. The initial management of excessive postpartum bleeding is firm massage of the uterine fundus, expression of any clots in the uterus, elimination of any bladder distention, and rapid IV infusion of 20 units of oxytocin in 1,000 ml of lactated Ringer's or normal saline solution. If the uterus fails to respond to oxytocin, a 0.2-mg dose of ergonovine (Ergotrate) or methylergonovine (Methergine) may be given intramuscularly or intravenously to produce sustained uterine contractions. If first-line drugs are not effective, a derivative of prostaglandin $F_2\alpha$ (carboprost tromethamine) may be given intramuscularly. Most hemorrhages can be controlled after one or two injections of 0.25 mg intramuscularly or intramyometrially (Doan-Wiggins, 1994). (See Table 26-1 for a comparison of drugs used to manage PPH.) In addition to the medications used to contract the uterus, rapid administration of crystalloid solutions and/or blood will be needed to restore the woman's intravascular volume.

TABLE 26-1 *Drugs Used to Manage Postpartum Hemorrhage*

	OXYTOCIN (PITOCIN)	METHYLERGONOVINE (METHERGINE)	PROSTAGLANDIN $F_{2\alpha}$ (PROSTIN/15M; HEMABATE)
ACTION	Contraction of uterus; decreases bleeding	Contraction of uterus	Contraction of uterus
SIDE EFFECT	Infrequent; water intoxication; nausea and vomiting	Hypertension, nausea, vomiting, headache	Headache, nausea, vomiting, fever
CONTRAINDICATIONS	None for PPH	Hypertension, cardiac disease	Asthma, hypersensitivity
DOSAGE; ROUTE	20-40 U/L diluted in lactated Ringer's solution or normal saline at 125-200 mU/min IV or 10-20 U IM	0.2 mg IM every 2-4 hr up to 5 doses; 0.2 mg IV only for emergency	0.25 mg IM or intramyometrially every 15 min up to 5 doses
NURSING CONSIDERATIONS	Continue to monitor vaginal bleeding and uterine tone	Check blood pressure before giving and do not give if >140/90; continue monitoring vaginal bleeding and uterine tone	Continue to monitor vaginal bleeding and uterine tone

NURSE ALERT *Use of ergonovine or methylergonovine is contraindicated in the presence of hypertension or cardiovascular disease. Prostaglandin $F_2\alpha$, should be used cautiously in women with cardiovascular disease or asthma (Bowes, 1994).*

If bleeding persists, bimanual compression may be considered by the obstetrician or nurse-midwife. This procedure involves inserting a fist into the vagina and pressing the knuckles against the anterior side of the uterus, and then placing the other hand on the abdomen and massaging the posterior side of the uterus with it. If the uterus still does not become firm, manual exploration of the uterine cavity for retained placental fragments is implemented. If the preceding procedures are ineffective, surgical management may be the only alternative. Surgical management options include vessel ligation (uteroovarian, uterine, hypogastric), angiographic embolization (placement of autologous blood clots in vessel), and hysterectomy (Roberts, 1995).

Bleeding with a contracted uterus. If the uterus is firmly contracted and bleeding continues, the source of bleeding still needs to be identified and treated. Assessment may include visual or manual inspection of the perineum, vagina, uterus, cervix, or rectum and laboratory studies (e.g., hemoglobin, hematocrit, coagulation studies, platelet count) (Roberts, 1995). Treatment depends on the source of the bleeding. Lacerations are usually sutured. Hematomas may be managed with observation, application of cold therapy, or ligation of the bleeding vessel. Fluids and/or blood replacements may be needed (Akins, 1994; Druelinger, 1994; Roberts, 1995).

Uterine inversion. Uterine inversion is an emergency situation requiring immediate recognition, replacement of the uterus within the pelvic cavity, and correction of associated clinical conditions. Medical management of this condition involves all of the following interventions (Wendel & Cox, 1995; Zahn & Yeomans, 1990):

- Shock is treated. Usually lactated Ringer's solution is infused intravenously; blood component products may also be transfused.
- The fundus of the uterus is repositioned. This is often accomplished manually after the placenta has already separated. However, tocolytic agents such as terbutaline or magnesium sulfate or general anesthesia may be needed to relax the uterus for repositioning. As soon as the uterus is repositioned, these relaxing agents are discontinued.
- Oxytocic agents are given only after the uterus is repositioned. These may include oxytocin, prostaglandin $F_{2\alpha}$, or Prostin/15M (0.25 mg intramuscularly or intramyometrially). Bimanual compression may be effective in controlling bleeding until these oxytocic drugs take effect.
- Vaginal manual replacement is usually successful in about 75% of women who experience uterine inversion. If it is not successful, abdominal or vaginal surgery may be necessary to reposition or even remove the uterus.
- Broad-spectrum antibiotic therapy may be initiated to prevent infection, and a nasogastric tube may be inserted to minimize the risk of paralytic ileus that may occur as a result of repositioning the uterus.

BOX 26-3	*Herbal Remedies for Postpartum Hemorrhage*

HERBS	ACTION
Witch hazel	Hemostatic
Lady's mantel	Hemostatic
Blue cohosh	Oxytocic
Cotton root bark	Oxytocic
Motherwart	Promotes uterine contraction; vasoconstrictive
Shepherd's purse	Promotes uterine contraction
Alfalfa leaf	Increases availability of vitamin K; increases hemoglobin
Nettle	Increases availability of vitamin K; increases hemoglobin

Suggested reading: Weed S: *Wise woman herbal for the childbearing year,* Woodstock, NY, 1986, Ash Tree Publishing.

Subinvolution. Treatment of subinvolution depends on the cause. Ergonovine 0.2 mg every 4 hours for 2 or 3 days and antibiotic therapy are the most common medications used (Cunningham et al., 1997). Dilatation and curettage (D&C) may be needed to remove retained placental fragments or to debride the placental site.

Herbal remedies

Herbal remedies have been used with some success to control PPH in some settings. Some herbs have hemostatic actions, whereas others work as oxytocic agents to contract the uterus (Akins, 1994, Weed, 1986). Box 26-3 lists herbs that have been used and their actions.

Nursing interventions

Immediate nursing care of the woman with PPH includes assessment of vital signs and uterine consistency and administration of oxytocin or other drugs to stimulate uterine contraction. The primary health care provider is notified if not present. Labor and birth units have standing orders or protocols for the nurse to implement interventions, such as starting IV infusions and administering medications. If bleeding is not controlled, the nurse may be responsible for preparing the woman for operative intervention.

The woman and her family will be anxious about her condition. The nurse can intervene by calmly providing explanations about interventions being performed and the need to act quickly.

After the bleeding has been controlled, the care of the woman with lacerations of the perineum is similar to that for women with episiotomies (analgesia as needed for pain and hot or cold applications as necessary). The need for increased roughage in the diet and increased intake of fluids is emphasized. Stool softeners may be used to assist the woman in reestablishing bowel habits without straining and putting stress on the suture lines.

NURSE ALERT *To avoid injury to the suture line, a woman with third- or fourth-degree lacerations is not given rectal suppositories or enemas.*

The care of the woman who has experienced an inversion of the uterus focuses on immediate stabilization of hemodynamic status. This requires close observation of her response to treatment to prevent shock or fluid overload. If the uterus has been repositioned manually, care must be taken after the birth to avoid aggressive fundal massage.

Discharge instructions for the woman who has had PPH are similar to those for any postpartum woman. In addition, she should be told that she will probably feel fatigue, even exhaustion, and will need to limit her physical activities to conserve her strength. She may need instructions in increasing her dietary iron and protein intake, as well as iron supplementation to rebuild lost red blood cell (RBC) volume. She may need assistance with infant care and household activities until she has regained strength. Some women have problems with delayed or insufficient lactation and postpartum depression (Akins, 1994). Referrals for home care follow-up or to community resources may be needed.

Evaluation

The nurse can be reasonably assured that care was effective to the extent that the expected outcomes were achieved.

HEMORRHAGIC (HYPOVOLEMIC) SHOCK

Hemorrhage may result in **hemorrhagic (hypovolemic) shock.** Shock is an emergency situation in which the perfusion of body organs may become severely compromised and death may occur. Physiologic compensatory mechanisms are activated in response to hemorrhage. The adrenal glands release catecholamines, causing arterioles and venules in the skin, lungs, gastrointestinal (GI) tract, liver, and kidneys to constrict. The available blood flow is diverted to the brain and heart and away from other organs, including the uterus. If shock is prolonged, the continued reduction in cellular oxygenation results in an accumulation of lactic acid and acidosis (from anaerobic glucose metabolism). Acidosis (lowered serum pH) causes arteriolar vasodilation; venule vasoconstriction persists. A circular pattern is established; that is, decreased perfusion, increased tissue anoxia and acidosis, edema formation, and pooling of blood further decrease the perfusion. Cellular death occurs. (See Emergency box for signs of hemorrhagic shock.)

Medical Management

Vigorous treatment is necessary to prevent adverse sequelae. Medical management of hypovolemic shock involves restoring circulating blood volume and treating the cause of the hemorrhage (such as lacerations, uterine atony, or inversion). To restore circulating blood volume, a rapid IV infusion of

Hemorrhagic Shock

ASSESSMENTS	CHARACTERISTICS	INTERVENTION
Respirations	Rapid and shallow	Summon assistance and equipment.
Pulse	Rapid, weak, irregular	Start IV infusion per standing orders.
Blood pressure	Decreasing (late sign)	Ensure patent airway; administer oxygen.
Skin	Cool, pale, clammy	Continue to monitor status.
Urinary output	Decreasing	
Level of consciousness	Lethargy → coma	
Mental status	Anxiety → coma	
Central venous pressure	Decreased	

From Wong D & Perry S: *Maternal child nursing care,* St Louis, 1998, Mosby.

crystalloid solution is given at a rate of 3 ml infused for every 1 ml of estimated blood loss (e.g., 3,000 ml infused for 1,000 ml of blood loss). Packed RBCs are usually infused if the woman is still actively bleeding and no improvement in her condition is noted after the initial crystalloid infusion (Roberts, 1995). Infusion of fresh-frozen plasma may be needed if clotting factors and platelet counts are below normal values (Cunningham et al., 1997).

Nursing Interventions

Hemorrhagic shock can occur rapidly, but the classic signs of shock may not appear until the postpartum woman has lost 30% to 40% of blood volume. The nurse needs to continue to reassess the woman's condition, as evidenced by the degree of measurable and anticipated blood loss, and mobilize appropriate resources.

Most interventions are instituted to improve or monitor tissue perfusion. The nurse continues to monitor the woman's pulse and blood pressure. If invasive hemodynamic monitoring is ordered, the nurse may assist with the placement of the central venous pressure (CVP) or pulmonary artery (Swan-Ganz) catheter and monitor CVP, pulmonary artery pressure, or pulmonary artery wedge pressure as ordered (Clark et al., 1994; White & Poole, 1996).

Additional assessments to be made include evaluation of skin temperature, color, and turgor, as well as assessment of the woman's mucous membranes. Breath sounds should be auscultated before fluid volume replacement, if possible, to provide a baseline for future assessment. Inspection for oozing at the sites of incisions or injections and assessment of the presence of petechiae or ecchymosis in areas not associated with surgery or trauma are critical in the evaluation for disseminated intravascular coagulopathy.

Oxygen is administered, preferably by nonrebreathing face mask, at 10 to 12 L/min to maintain oxygen saturation. Oxygen saturation should be monitored with a pulse oximeter, although measurements may not always be accurate in a patient with hypovolemia or decreased perfusion. Level of consciousness is assessed frequently and provides additional indications of blood volume and oxygen saturation. In early stages of decreased blood flow, the woman may report "seeing stars" or feeling dizzy or nauseated. She may become restless and orthopneic. As cerebral hypoxia increases, she may become confused and react slowly or not at all to stimuli. Some women complain of headaches. An improved sensorium is an indicator of improved perfusion.

Continuous electrocardiographic monitoring may be indicated for the woman who is hypotensive or tachycardic, continues to bleed profusely, or is in shock. A Foley catheter with a urometer is inserted to allow hourly assessment of urinary output. The most objective and least invasive assessment of adequate organ perfusion and oxygenation is urinary output of at least 30 ml/hr (White & Poole, 1996). Blood may need to be drawn and sent to the laboratory for studies that include hemoglobin and hematocrit levels, platelet count, and coagulation profile.

Fluid or Blood Replacement Therapy

Critical to successful management of the woman with a hemorrhagic complication is establishment of venous access, preferably with a large-bore IV catheter. The establishment of two IV lines facilitates fluid resuscitation. Vigorous fluid resuscitation includes the administration of crystalloids (lactated Ringer's, normal saline solutions), colloids (albumin), blood, and blood components. Fluid resuscitation must be carefully monitored because fluid overload may occur. Intravascular fluid overload occurs more frequently with colloid therapy.

Transfusion therapy is used to restore oxygen-carrying capacity and intravascular volume. Packed RBCs (250 to 300 ml/unit) may be administered to increase vascular volume and improve oxygen-carrying capacity. Each unit of packed RBCs increases the hematocrit level by 3%. Fresh-frozen plasma contains clotting factors and fibrinogen and is the only source of factors V, XI, and XII. Each unit (250 ml/unit) of fresh-frozen plasma increases intravascular volume and fibrinogen (10 mg/dl per unit). Platelets increase the platelet count by 5,000 to 10,000 cells/unit and provide limited volume expansion. Cryoprecipitate is used to correct specific clotting disorders; it contains factor VIII, von Willebrand's factor, and fibrinogen. Administration of cryoprecipitate increases fibrinogen 10 mg/dl per unit.

Administration of blood and blood components is not without risk. Banked blood is cold (4° C) and has an acid pH (6.6 to 6.8), which can result in hypothermia, arrhythmias, and acidosis. In addition, banked blood can result in electrolyte imbalances because of the electrolyte composition of the blood (sodium 150 to 160 mEq/L, potassium 10 to 15 mEq/L, no ionized calcium, and low levels of 2,3-diphosphoglyceric acid). Coagulopathies may result from massive transfusion therapies because banked blood is deficient in platelets and clotting factors.

Transfusion reactions may follow administration of blood or blood components, including cryoprecipitates. Even in an emergency, each unit should be checked per hospital protocol. Complications include hemolytic reactions, febrile reactions, allergic reactions, circulatory overloading, and air embolism.

LEGAL TIP Standard of Care for Bleeding Emergencies

The standard of care for obstetric emergency situations, such as PPH or hypovolemic shock, is that provision should be made for the nurse to implement actions independently. Policies, procedures, standing orders or protocols, and clinical guides should be established by each health care facility in which births occur and should be agreed on by health care providers involved in the care of obstetric patients.

COAGULOPATHIES

When bleeding is continuous and there is no identifiable source, a coagulopathy may be the cause. The woman's coagulation status needs to be assessed quickly and continuously. The nurse may draw and send blood to the laboratory for studies. Abnormal results depend on the cause and may include increased prothrombin time, increased partial prothrombin time, decreased platelets, decreased fibrinogen level, increased fibrin degradation products, and prolonged bleeding time (Druelinger, 1994). Causes of coagulopathies may be pregnancy complications such as idiopathic thrombocytopenic purpura or von Willibrand's disease.

Idiopathic Thrombocytopenic Purpura

Idiopathic thrombocytopenic purpura (ITP) is an autoimmune disorder in which antiplatelet antibodies decrease the life span of the platelets. Thrombocytopenia, capillary fragility, and increased bleeding time are diagnostic findings. ITP may cause severe hemorrhage after cesarean birth or from cervical or vaginal lacerations. Incidences of postpartum uterine bleeding and vaginal hematomas are also increased.

Medical management focuses on control of platelet stability. Platelet transfusions are given to maintain the platelet count at 100,000 cells/mm^3. Corticosteroids are given if the diagnosis has been made before or during pregnancy. If splenectomy is needed, it is deferred until after the puerperium. Neonatal thrombocytopenia, a result of the maternal disease process, occurs in about 50% of cases and is associated with a high mortality rate.

von Willebrand's Disease

von Willibrand's disease, a type of hemophilia, is probably the most common of all hereditary bleeding disorders (Kleinert et al., 1997). It results from a factor VIII deficiency and platelet dysfunction that is transmitted as an incomplete autosomal dominant trait to both sexes. Although von Willebrand's disease is rare, it is among the most common congenital clotting defects in American women of childbearing age. Symptoms include familial bleeding tendency, previous bleeding episodes, prolonged bleeding time (the most important test), factor VIII deficiency (mild to moderate), and bleeding from mucous membranes. Factor VIII increases during pregnancy, and this increase may be sufficient to offset danger from hemorrhage during childbirth. However, the woman's condition should be observed for at least 1 week after childbirth. Treatment of von Willebrand's disease may include replacement of factor VIII if it is at less than 30% of normal levels and administration of cryoprecipitate or fresh-frozen plasma.

Disseminated Intravascular Coagulation

Disseminated intravascular coagulation (DIC) is a pathologic form of clotting that is diffuse and consumes large amounts of clotting factors, causing widespread external bleeding, internal bleeding, or both. DIC is an overactivation of the clotting cascade and the fibrinolytic system that results in depletion of platelets and clotting factors. In the obstetric population DIC may occur as a result of abruptio placentae, amniotic fluid embolism, dead fetus syndrome, severe preeclampsia, septicemia, cardiopulmonary arrest, and hemorrhage.

The diagnosis of DIC is made according to clinical findings and laboratory markers. Physical examination reveals unusual bleeding; spontaneous bleeding from the woman's gums or nose may be noted. Petechiae may appear around a blood pressure cuff placed on the woman's arm. Excessive bleeding may occur from the site of a slight trauma (such as venipuncture sites, intramuscular or subcutaneous injection sites, nicks from shaving of the perineum or abdomen, and injury from insertion of a urinary catheter). Symptoms may also include tachycardia and diaphoresis.

Laboratory tests reveal decreased levels of platelets, fibrinogen, proaccelerin, antihemophilic factor, and prothrombin (the factors consumed during coagulation). Levels of other factors should be normal. Fibrinolysis is increased at first but is later severely depressed. Degradation of fibrin leads to the accumulation of fibrin-split products in the blood. Fibrin-split products have anticoagulant properties and prolong the prothrombin time. Bleeding time is normal, coagulation time shows no clot, clot retraction time shows no clot, and partial thromboplastin time is increased. DIC must be distinguished from other clotting disorders before therapy is initiated.

Primary medical management in all cases of DIC involves correction of the underlying cause (e.g., removal of the dead fetus, treatment of existing infection or of preeclampsia or eclampsia, or removal of a placental abruption). Volume replacement, blood component therapy, optimization of oxygenation and perfusion status, and continued reassessment of laboratory parameters are the usual forms of treatment (Clark et al., 1994; Richey, Gilstrap & Ramin, 1995).

Nursing interventions include assessment for signs of bleeding and signs of complications from the administration of blood and blood products. Because renal failure is one consequence of DIC, urinary output is monitored, usually by insertion of an indwelling urinary catheter. Urinary output must be maintained at more than 30 ml/hr. Oxygen is administered through a tight-fitting nonrebreathing mask at 10 to 12 L/min, or per hospital protocol or physician order.

The woman and her family will be anxious or concerned about her condition and prognosis. The nurse offers explanations about care and provides emotional support to the woman and her family through this critical time.

THROMBOEMBOLIC DISEASE

A thrombosis is the formation of a blood clot or clots inside a blood vessel and is caused by inflammation (**thrombophlebitis**) or partial obstruction of the vessel. Three thromboembolic conditions are of concern in the postpartum period:

- *Superficial venous thrombosis*—involvement of the superficial saphenous venous system.
- *Deep venous thrombosis*—involvement varies but can extend from the foot to the iliofemoral region.
- *Pulmonary embolism*—complication of deep venous thrombosis occurring when part of a blood clot dislodges and is carried to the pulmonary artery, where it occludes the vessel and obstructs blood flow to the lungs.

Incidence and Etiology

The incidence of thromboembolic disease in the postpartum period varies from about 1 in 1,000 to 1 in 2,000 women (Cunningham et al., 1997). The incidence has declined in the last 20 years as early ambulation after childbirth has become the standard practice. The major causes of thromboembolic disease are venous stasis and hypercoagulation, both of which are present in pregnancy and continue into the postpartum period. Other risk factors include cesarean birth, history of venous thrombosis or varicosities, obesity, maternal age over 35, multiparity, and smoking.

Clinical Manifestations

Superficial venous thrombosis is characterized by pain and tenderness in the lower extremity. Physical examination may reveal warmth, redness, and an enlarged, hardened vein over the site of the thrombosis. Deep venous thrombosis is characterized by unilateral leg pain, calf tenderness, and swelling (Fig. 26-2). Physical examination may reveal redness and warmth, but women may also have a large amount of clot and have few symptoms (Mishell et al., 1997). A positive Homan's sign may be present, but further evaluation is needed because the calf pain may be attributed to other causes, such as a strained muscle resulting from the birthing position.

Physical examination is not a sensitive diagnostic indicator for thrombosis. Venography is the most accurate

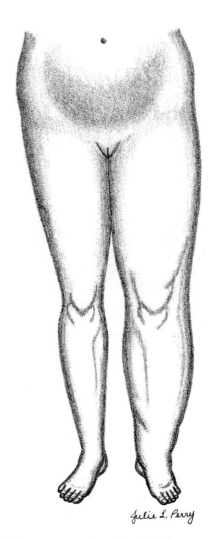

Fig. 26-2 Deep venous thrombophlebitis.

method for diagnosing deep venous thrombosis, but it is associated with serious complications. Noninvasive diagnostic methods are more commonly used; these include real-time and color Doppler ultrasound (Cunningham et al., 1997).

Medical Management

Superficial venous thrombosis is treated with analgesia (nonsteroidal antiinflammatory agents), rest with elevation of the affected leg, and elastic stockings. Local application of heat may also be used. Deep venous thrombosis is initially treated with anticoagulant (usually continuous IV heparin) therapy, bed rest with the affected leg elevated, and analgesia. After the symptoms have decreased, the woman may be fitted with elastic stockings to use when she is allowed to ambulate. IV heparin therapy continues for 5 to 7 days. Oral anticoagulant therapy (warfarin) is started during this time and continued for about 3 months.

Nursing Interventions

Nursing care in the hospital setting of the woman with a thrombosis consists of continued assessments: inspection and palpation of the affected area; palpation of peripheral pulses; checking for Homan's sign; measurement and comparison of leg circumferences; inspection for signs of bleeding; monitoring for signs of pulmonary embolism, including chest pain, coughing, dyspnea, and tachypnea; and assessment of respiratory status for presence of crackles. Laboratory reports are monitored for prothrombin or partial prothrombin times. The woman and her family are assessed for their level of understanding about the diagnosis and their ability to cope during the unexpected extended period of recovery.

Interventions include explanations and education about the diagnosis and the treatment. The woman will need assistance with personal care as long as she is on bed rest; the family should be encouraged to participate in the care if that is what they wish. While the woman is on bed rest, she should be encouraged to change positions frequently, but not to place the knees in a sharply flexed position that could cause pooling of blood in the lower extremities. She should also be cautioned not to rub the affected area, since this action could cause the clot to dislodge. Once the woman is allowed to ambulate, she is taught how to prevent venous congestion by putting on the elastic stockings before getting out of bed.

The nurse administers heparin as ordered and notifies the physician if clotting times are outside the therapeutic level. If the woman is breastfeeding, she is assured that heparin is not excreted in breast milk. (If the infant has been discharged, the family is encouraged to bring the infant for feedings as permitted by hospital policy; the mother can also express milk to be sent home.)

Pain can be managed with a variety of measures. Position changes, elevating the leg, and application of moist warm heat may decrease discomfort. Administration of analgesics and antiinflammatory medications may be needed.

> **NURSE ALERT** *Drugs containing aspirin are not given to women receiving anticoagulant therapy because aspirin inhibits synthesis of clotting factors and can lead to prolonged clotting time and increased risk of bleeding.*

The woman is usually discharged home while taking oral anticoagulants and will need explanations about the treatment schedule and possible side effects. She and her family should also be given information about safe care practices to prevent bleeding and injury while she is receiving anticoagulant therapy, such as using a soft toothbrush and an electric razor. She will also need information about the need for follow-up with her health care provider to monitor clotting times and to make sure the correct dose of anticoagulant therapy is maintained.

POSTPARTUM INFECTIONS

Postpartum or **puerperal infection** (puerperal sepsis or childbed fever) is any clinical infection of the genital canal that occurs within 28 days after abortion or childbirth. The first symptom of postpartum infection is usually a fever of 38° C or more on 2 successive days of the first 10 postpartum days (not counting the first 24 hours after birth) (Hamadeh, Dedmon & Mozley, 1995). Puerperal infection is probably the major cause of maternal morbidity and mortality throughout the world; however, it occurs after only 6% of births in the United States. Common postpartum infections include endometritis, wound infections, mastitis, urinary tract infections, and respiratory tract infections.

The most common infecting organisms are the numerous streptococcal and anaerobic organisms. *Staphylococcus aureus*, gonococci, coliform bacteria, and clostridia are less common but serious pathogenic organisms that also cause puerperal infection (Clark, 1995). Factors that predispose the woman to postpartum infection are listed in Box 26-4.

Endometritis

Endometritis (uterine infection) is the most common postpartum infection. It usually begins as a localized infection at the placental site (Fig. 26-3), but it can spread to involve the entire endometrium. Incidence is higher after cesarean birth. Assessment for signs of endometritis may reveal a fever (usually greater than 38° C), increased pulse, chills, anorexia, nausea, fatigue and lethargy, pelvic pain, uterine tenderness, or foul-smelling, profuse lochia (Calhoun & Brost, 1995). Leukocytosis and a markedly increased RBC sedimentation rate are typical laboratory findings of postpartum infections. Anemia may also be present. Blood cultures or intracervical or intrauterine bacterial cultures

BOX 26-4 *Predisposing Factors for Postpartum Infection*

PRECONCEPTION OR ANTEPARTUM FACTORS
History of previous venous thrombosis, urinary tract infection, mastitis, pneumonia
Diabetes mellitus
Alcoholism
Drug abuse
Immunosuppression
Anemia
Malnutrition

INTRAPARTUM FACTORS
Cesarean birth
Prolonged rupture of membranes
Chorioamnionitis
Prolonged labor
Bladder catheterization
Internal fetal/uterine pressure monitoring
Epidural anesthesia
Retained placental fragments
Postpartum hemorrhage
Episiotomy or lacerations
Hematomas

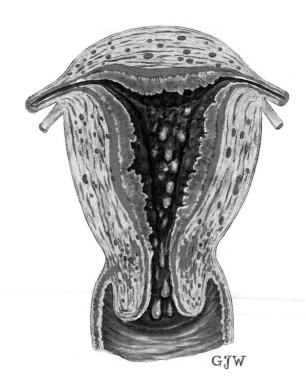

Fig. 26-3 Postpartum infection—endometritis.

(aerobic and anaerobic) should reveal the offending pathogens within 36 to 48 hours.

Wound Infections

Wound infections are also common postpartum infections, but these often develop after the woman is at home. Sites of infection include the cesarean incision and the episiotomy or repaired laceration site. Predisposing factors are similar to those for endometritis (see Box 26-4). Signs of wound infection include erythema, edema, warmth, tenderness, seropurulent drainage, and wound separation. Fever and pain may also be present.

Urinary Tract Infections

Urinary tract infections (UTIs) occur in 2% to 4% of postpartum women. Risk factors include urinary catheterization, frequent pelvic examinations, epidural anesthesia, genital tract injury, history of UTI, and cesarean birth (Clark, 1995). Signs and symptoms include dysuria, frequency and urgency, low-grade fever, urinary retention, hematuria, and pyuria. Costovertebral angle (CVA) tenderness or flank pain may indicate upper UTI. Urinalysis results may reveal *Escherichia coli*, although other gram-negative aerobic bacilli may also cause UTIs.

Mastitis

Mastitis, or breast infection, affects about 1% of women soon after childbirth, most of whom are first-time mothers who are breastfeeding. Mastitis almost always is unilateral and develops well after the flow of milk has been

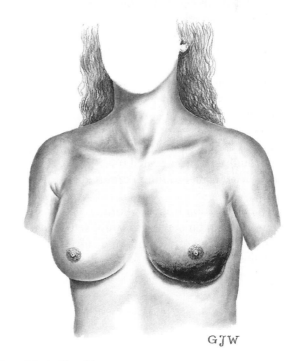

Fig. 26-4 Mastitis.

established (Fig. 26-4). The infecting organism generally is the hemolytic *S. aureus*. An infected nipple fissure usually is the initial lesion, but the ductal system is involved next. Inflammatory edema and engorgement of the breast soon obstruct the flow of milk in a lobe; regional, then generalized, mastitis follows. If treatment is not prompt, mastitis may progress to breast abscess.

Symptoms rarely appear before the end of the first postpartum week and are more common in the second to fourth weeks. Chills, fever, malaise, and local breast tenderness are noted first. Localized breast tenderness, pain, swelling, redness, and axillary adenopathy may also occur. Antibiotics are prescribed. Lactation is maintained (if desired) by emptying the breasts every 2 to 4 hours by breastfeeding, manual expression, or breast pump.

I CARE MANAGEMENT

Assessment and nursing diagnoses

A number of prenatal and intrapartum factors can predispose a woman to postpartum infection. These risk factors are listed in Box 26-4. Signs and symptoms and laboratory results associated with postpartum infection have been discussed with each infection. Suggested nursing diagnoses for women experiencing postpartum infection are listed in the Nursing Diagnoses box.

I Nursing Diagnoses_____

Women Experiencing Postpartum Infection
Knowledge deficit related to:
- Etiology, management, course of infection
- Transmission and prevention of infection
Impaired tissue integrity related to:
- Effects of infection process
Pain related to:
- Mastitis
- Puerperal infection
- Urinary tract infection
Altered family processes related to:
- Unexpected complication to expected postpartum recovery
- Possible separation from newborn
- Interruption in process of realigning relationships after the addition of the new family member
Risk of altered parenting related to:
- Fear of spread of infection to newborn

Expected Outcomes of Care

A plan of care is formulated that relates specifically to the needs of the woman and her family. Expected outcomes are determined in collaboration with the woman and her family and include that the woman will:
- State the etiology, management, and sequelae of infection; identify measures to prevent reinfection
- Describe a reduction or elimination of pain
- With her family, verbalize acceptance of the unexpected events; verbalize positive coping measures (e.g., arrangement for home health care)

HOME CARE *Patient Instructions for Self-Care*

Prevention of Genital Tract Infections
- Practice genital hygiene.
- Choose underwear or hosiery with a cotton crotch.
- Avoid tight-fitting clothing (especially tight jeans).
- Select cloth car seat covers instead of vinyl.
- Limit time spent in damp exercise clothes (especially swimsuits and leotards or tights).
- Limit exposure to bath salts or bubble bath.
- Avoid colored or scented toilet tissue.
- If sensitive, discontinue use of feminine hygiene deodorant sprays.
- Use condoms.
- Void before and after intercourse.
- Decrease dietary sugar.
- Drink yeast-active milk and eat yogurt (with lactobacilli).
- Avoid douching.

From Lowdermilk D, Perry S & Bobak I: *Maternity and women's health care,* ed 6, St Louis, 1997, Mosby.

Plan of Care and Interventions

The most effective and cheapest treatment of postpartum infection is prevention. Preventive measures include good prenatal nutrition to control anemia and intrapartal hemorrhage. Good maternal perineal hygiene is emphasized. Strict adherence by all health care personnel to aseptic techniques during childbirth and the postpartum period is very important.

Management of endometritis consists of IV broad-spectrum antibiotic therapy and supportive care, including hydration, rest, and pain relief. Assessments of lochia, vital signs, and changes in the woman's condition continue during treatment. Comfort measures depend on the symptoms and may include cool compresses, warm blankets, perineal care, and sitz baths. Teaching should include side effects of therapy, prevention of spread of infection (see Home Care box), signs and symptoms of a worsening condition, and adherence to the treatment plan and the need for follow-up care. Women may need to be encouraged or helped to maintain mother-infant interactions and breastfeeding (if allowed during treatment).

Postpartum women are usually discharged to home by 48 hours after birth. This is often before signs of infection are evident. Nurses in birth centers and hospital settings need to be able to identify women at risk for postpartum infection and to provide anticipatory teaching and counseling before discharge. After discharge, telephone follow-up, hot lines, support groups, lactation counselors, home visits by nurses, and teaching materials (videos, written materials) are all interventions that can be implemented to decrease the risk of postpartum infections. Home care nurses need to be able to recognize signs and symptoms of postpartum infection so that the woman can contact her primary health care provider. These nurses must also be able to provide the

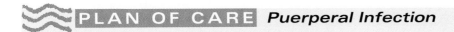

PLAN OF CARE   *Puerperal Infection*

NURSING DIAGNOSIS Infection of genital canal related to retained placental fragments

Expected Outcome *Infection is resolved with no adverse effects.*

Nursing Interventions/*Rationales*

Administer and monitor broad-spectrum antibiotics per physician order *to stem invading pathogens and prevent systemic infection until specific pathogen can be identified.*

Collect intrauterine cultures per physician order for laboratory analysis *to identify specific causative organism.*

Maintain Standard Precautions and use good handwashing technique when providing care *to prevent spread of infection.*

Monitor vital signs *to assess patient's response to treatment and status of infection.*

Monitor level of fatigue and lethargy, evidence of chills, loss of appetite, nausea and vomiting, and abdominal pain, *which are indicative of extent of infection and serve as indicators of status of infection.*

Monitor lochia for foul smell and profusion *as indicators of infection state.*

Monitor laboratory values (i.e., white blood cell [WBC] count, cultures) *for indicators of type and status of infection.*

Help patient to maintain good handwashing technique (particularly before handling her newborn) and to maintain scrupulous perineal care with frequent change and careful disposal of perineal pads *to avoid spread of infection.* Avoid use of communal sitz baths.

Ensure adequate fluid and nutritional intake *to fight infection;* administer antiemetics as needed per physician order.

Monitor intake and output and electrolyte laboratory values *to evaluate fluid and electrolyte balance.*

From Wong D & Perry S: *Maternal child nursing care,* St Louis, 1998, Mosby.

---

appropriate nursing care for women who need follow-up home care (see Plan of Care).

Treatment of wound infections may combine antibiotic therapy with wound debridement. Wounds may be opened and drained. Nursing care includes frequent wound and vital sign assessments and wound care. Comfort measures include sitz baths, warm compresses, and perineal care. Teaching includes good hygiene techniques (i.e., changing perineal pads front to back, handwashing before and after perineal care), self-care measures, and signs of worsening conditions to report to the health care provider. The woman is usually discharged to home for self-care or home nursing care after treatment is initiated in the inpatient setting.

Medical management for UTIs consists of antibiotic therapy, analgesia, and hydration. Postpartum women are usually treated on an outpatient basis; therefore teaching should include instructions on how to monitor temperature, bladder function, and appearance of urine. The woman should also be taught about signs of potential complications and the importance of taking all antibiotics as prescribed. Other suggestions for prevention of UTIs include proper perineal care, wiping from front to back after urinating or having a bowel movement, and increasing fluid intake (Clark, 1995).

Since mastitis rarely occurs before the postpartum woman is discharged, teaching should include warning signs of mastitis and counseling about prevention of cracked nipples. Management includes intensive antibiotic therapy (such as cephalosporins and vancomycin, which are particularly useful in staphylococcal infections), support of the breasts, local heat (or cold), adequate hydration, and analgesics.

Almost all instances of acute mastitis can be avoided by proper breastfeeding technique to prevent cracked nipples. Missed feedings, waiting too long between feedings, and abrupt weaning may lead to clogged nipples and mastitis. Cleanliness practiced by all who have contact with the newborn and new mother also reduces the incidence of mastitis (see Chapter 21).

Evaluation

Evaluation of the effectiveness of care of the woman with postpartum infection is based on the expected outcomes.

SEQUELAE OF CHILDBIRTH TRAUMA

Women are at risk for problems related to the reproductive system from the age of menarche through menopause and the older years. These problems include structural disorders of the uterus and vagina related to pelvic relaxation and urinary incontinence. They can be a delayed result of childbearing. For example, the structures and soft tissues of the vagina and bladder may be injured during a prolonged labor, a precipitous birth, or when cephalopelvic disproportion occurs.

Uterine Displacement and Prolapse

Normally, the round ligaments hold the uterus in anteversion, and the uterosacral ligaments pull the cervix backward and upward (see Fig. 5-2). **Uterine displacement** is a variation of this normal placement. The most common type of displacement is posterior displacement, or *retroversion*, in which the uterus is tilted posteriorly and the cervix rotates

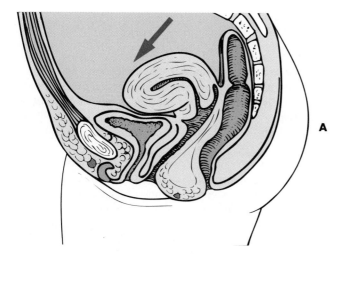

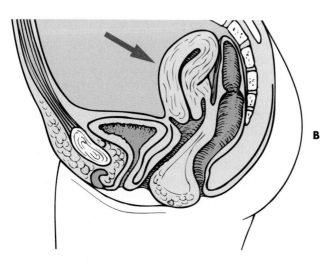

Fig. **26-5** Types of uterine displacement. **A,** Anterior displacement. **B,** Retroversion (backward displacement of uterus).

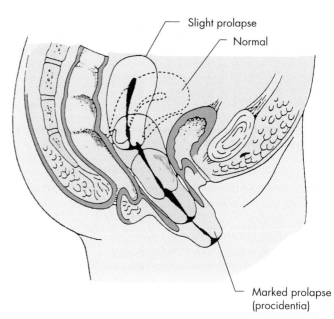

Fig. **26-6** Prolapse of uterus.

anteriorly. Other variations include retroflexion and anteflexion (Fig. 26-5).

By 2 months' postpartum, the ligaments should return to normal length, but in about one third of women the uterus remains retroverted. This condition is rarely symptomatic, but conception may be difficult because the cervix points toward the anterior vaginal wall and away from the posterior fornix, where seminal fluid pools after coitus. If symptoms occur, they may include pelvic and low back pain, dyspareunia, and exaggeration of premenstrual symptoms.

Uterine prolapse is a more serious type of displacement. The degree of prolapse can vary from mild to complete. In complete prolapse, the cervix and body of the uterus protrude through the vagina and the vagina is inverted (Fig. 26-6).

Uterine displacement and prolapse can be caused by congenital or acquired weakness of the pelvic support structures (often referred to as **pelvic relaxation**). In many cases problems can be related to a delayed but direct result of childbearing. Although extensive damage may be noted and repaired shortly after birth, symptoms related to pelvic relaxation most often appear during the perimenopausal period, when the effects of ovarian hormones on pelvic tissues are lost and atrophic changes begin. Pelvic trauma, stress and strain, and the aging process are also contributing causes. Other causes of pelvic relaxation include reproductive surgery and pelvic radiation.

Generally, symptoms of pelvic relaxation relate to the structure involved: urethra, bladder, uterus, vagina, cul-de-sac, or rectum. The most common complaints are pulling and dragging sensations, pressure, protrusions, fatigue, and low backache. Symptoms may be worse after prolonged standing or deep penile penetration during intercourse. Urinary incontinence may be present.

Cystocele and Rectocele

Cystocele and rectocele almost always accompany uterine prolapse, causing it to sag even further backward and downward into the vagina. *Cystocele* (Fig. 26-7) is the protrusion of the bladder downward into the vagina that develops when supporting structures in the vesicovaginal septum are injured. Anterior wall relaxation gradually develops over time as a result of congenital defects of supports, childbearing, obesity, or advanced age. When the woman stands, the weakened anterior vaginal wall cannot support the weight of the urine in the bladder; the vesicovaginal septum is forced downward, the bladder is stretched, and its capacity

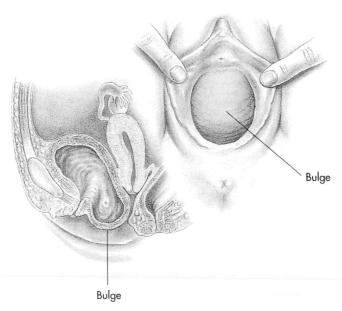

Fig. **26-7** Side and direct views of cystocele. (From Seidel H et al: *Mosby's guide to physical examination,* ed 4, St Louis, 1998, Mosby.)

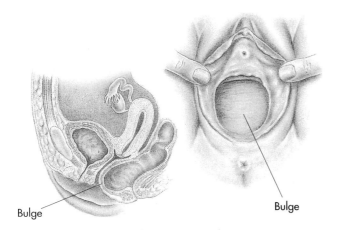

Fig. **26-8** Side and direct views of rectocele. (From Seidel H et al: *Mosby's guide to physical examination,* ed 4, St Louis, 1998, Mosby.)

is increased. With time the cystocele enlarges until it protrudes into the vagina. Complete emptying of the bladder is difficult because the cystocele sags below the bladder neck. *Rectocele* is the herniation of the anterior rectal wall through the relaxed or ruptured vaginal fascia and rectovaginal septum; it appears as a large bulge that may be seen through the relaxed introitus (Fig. 26-8).

Cystoceles and rectoceles often are asymptomatic. If symptoms of cystocele are present, they may include complaints of a bearing-down sensation or that "something is in my vagina." Other symptoms include urinary frequency, retention, and/or incontinence, and possible recurrent cystitis and UTIs. Pelvic examination will reveal a bulging of the anterior wall of the vagina when the woman is asked to

bear down. Unless the bladder neck and urethra are damaged, urinary continence is unaffected. Women with large cystoceles complain of having to push upward on the sagging anterior vaginal wall to be able to void.

Rectoceles may be small and produce few symptoms, but some are so large that they protrude outside of the vagina when the woman stands. Symptoms are absent when the woman is lying down. A rectocele causes a disturbance in bowel function, the sensation of "bearing down," or the sensation that the pelvic organs are falling out. With a very large rectocele, it may be difficult to have a bowel movement. Each time the woman strains during bowel evacuation, the feces are forced against the thinned rectovaginal wall, stretching it more. Some women facilitate evacuation by applying digital pressure vaginally to hold up the rectal pouch.

Urinary Incontinence

About 20% of women between the ages of 25 and 54 years have **urinary incontinence (UI)** (uncontrollable leakage of urine). Although nulliparous women can have UI, the incidence is higher in women who have given birth and also increases with parity (Sampselle et al., 1997). Conditions that disturb urinary control include *stress incontinence,* due to sudden increases in intraabdominal pressure (such as that due to sneezing or coughing); *urge incontinence,* caused by disorders of the bladder and urethra, such as urethritis and urethral stricture, trigonitis, and cystitis; neuropathies, such as multiple sclerosis, diabetic neuritis, and pathologic conditions of the spinal cord; and congenital and acquired urinary tract abnormalities (Skoner, Thompson & Caron, 1994).

Stress incontinence may follow injury to bladder neck structures. A sphincter mechanism at the bladder neck compresses the upper urethra, pulls it upward behind the symphysis, and forms an acute angle at the junction of the posterior urethral wall and the base of the bladder (Fig. 26-9). To empty the bladder, the sphincter complex relaxes and the trigone contracts to open the internal urethral orifice and pull the contracting bladder wall upward, forcing urine out. The angle between the urethra and the base of the bladder is lost or increased if the supporting pubococcygeus muscle is injured; this change, coupled with urethrocele, causes incontinence. Urine spurts out when the woman is asked to bear down or cough in the lithotomy position.

Genital Fistulas

Genital fistulas are perforations between genital tract organs. They can develop after a labor in which tissues of the genital tract are compressed between the fetal head and the bony pelvis. Most occur between the bladder and the genital tract (e.g., vesicovaginal); between the urethra and the vagina (urethrovaginal); and between the rectum or sigmoid colon and the vagina (rectovaginal) (Fig. 26-10). Genital fistulas may

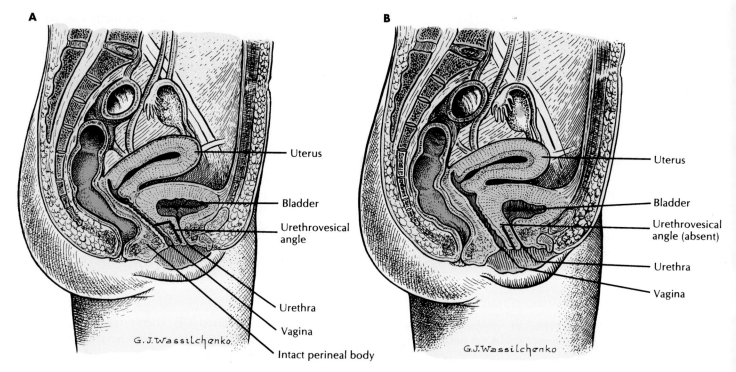

Fig. 26-9 Urethrovesical angle. **A,** Normal angle. **B,** Widening (absence) of angle.

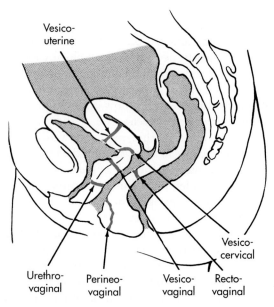

Fig. 26-10 Types of fistulas that may develop in vagina, uterus, and rectum. (From Phipps W et al: *Medical-surgical nursing: concepts and clinical practice,* ed 6, St Louis, 1999, Mosby.)

also be a result of a congenital anomaly, gynecologic surgery, obstetric trauma, cancer, radiation therapy, gynecologic trauma, or infection (e.g., in the episiotomy).

Signs and symptoms of vaginal fistulas depend on the site but may include presence of urine, flatus, or feces in the vagina; odors of urine or feces in the vagina; and irritation of vaginal tissues.

▌CARE MANAGEMENT

Assessment and Nursing Diagnoses

Assessment for problems related to structural disorders of the uterus and vagina focuses primarily on the genitourinary tract, the reproductive organs, bowel elimination, and psychosocial and sexual factors. A complete health history, physical examination, and laboratory tests are done to support the appropriate medical diagnosis. The nurse needs to assess the woman's knowledge of the disorder, its management, and possible prognosis. Suggested nursing diagnoses for structural problems of the uterus and vagina are listed in the Nursing Diagnoses box.

▌Nursing Diagnoses

Women Experiencing Structural Problems of the Uterus and Vagina

Knowledge deficit related to:
• Causes of structural disorders and treatment options

Constipation or diarrhea related to:
• Anatomic changes

Stress or urge (urinary) incontinence related to:
• Anatomic changes

Pain related to:
• Relaxation of pelvic support and/or elimination difficulties

Ineffective individual coping related to:
• Change in body image

Altered family processes or interpersonal relationships related to:
• Woman's anatomic and functional changes
Risk for injury related to:
• Lack of skill in self-care procedures
• Lack of understanding of the rationale for the need to comply with therapy
Social isolation, spiritual distress, body image disturbance, or self-esteem disturbance
Anxiety related to:
• Surgical procedure
• Prognosis

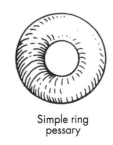

Simple ring pessary

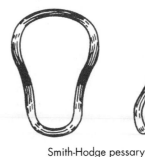

Smith-Hodge pessary

Fig. 26-11 Examples of pessaries: simple ring and Smith-Hodge.

Expected Outcomes of Care

Expected outcomes are mutually negotiated between the patient and the health care provider and stated in patient-centered terms. Possible expected outcomes may include that the woman will:
• Verbalize understanding of possible disorders related to alterations in pelvic support
• Use good hygiene and practice measures to prevent problems related to alterations in pelvic support
• Accept change in body functions (if they occur) without loss of positive body image, self-concept, and self-esteem
• Report less anxiety related to treatment and her prognosis

Plan of Care and Interventions

The health care team works together to treat the disorders related to alterations in pelvic support and to assist the woman in management of her symptoms. In general, nurses working with these women can provide information and self-care education to prevent problems before they occur, to manage or reduce symptoms and promote comfort and hygiene if symptoms are already present, and to recognize when further intervention is needed. This information can be part of all postpartum discharge teaching or can be provided at postpartum follow-up visits in clinics or physician/midwife offices, or during postpartum home visits. In addition, information on how to prevent or recognize structural problems of the uterus and vagina can be a topic for workshops for women for health fairs in community settings.

Interventions for specific problems depend on the problem and the severity of the symptoms. If discomfort related to uterine displacement is a problem, several interventions can be implemented to treat uterine displacement. Kegel exercises can be performed several times daily to increase muscular strength. A knee-chest position performed for a few minutes several times a day can correct a mildly

retroverted uterus. A fitted pessary to support the uterus and hold it in the correct position (Fig. 26-11) may be inserted in the vagina. Usually a pessary is used only for a short time because it can lead to pressure necrosis and vaginitis. Good hygiene is important; some women can be taught to remove the pessary at night, cleanse it, and replace it in the morning. If the pessary is always left in place, regular douching with commercially prepared solutions or weak vinegar solutions (1 tablespoon to 1 quart of water) to remove increased secretions and keep the vaginal pH at 4 to 4.5 are suggested. After a period of treatment, most women are free of symptoms and do not require the pessary. Surgical correction is rarely indicated.

Treatment for uterine prolapse depends on the degree of prolapse. Pessaries may be useful in mild prolapse. Estrogen therapy also may be used in the older woman to improve tissue tone. If these conservative treatments do not correct the problem, or if there is a significant degree of prolapse, abdominal or vaginal hysterectomy is usually recommended.

Treatment for a cystocele includes use of a vaginal pessary or surgical repair. Pessaries may not be effective. Anterior repair (colporrhaphy) is the usual surgical procedure and is usually done for large, symptomatic cystoceles. This involves a surgical shortening of pelvic muscles to provide better support for the bladder. An anterior repair is often combined with a vaginal hysterectomy.

Small rectoceles may not need treatment. The woman with mild symptoms may get relief from a high-fiber diet and adequate fluid intake, stool softeners, or mild laxatives.

Vaginal pessaries usually are not effective. Large rectoceles that are causing significant symptoms are usually repaired surgically. A posterior repair (colporrhaphy) is the usual procedure. This surgery is performed vaginally and involves shortening the pelvic muscles to provide better support for the rectum. Anterior and posterior repairs may be performed at the same time and with a vaginal hysterectomy.

Mild to moderate urinary incontinence can be significantly decreased or relieved in many women by bladder training and pelvic muscle (Kegel) exercises (Sampselle et al., 1997). Other management strategies include insertion of a bladder neck support prosthesis, estrogen therapy, and surgery (Mishell at al., 1997).

Nursing care of the woman with a cystocele, rectocele, or fistula requires great sensitivity, because the woman's reactions are often intense. She may become withdrawn or hostile because of embarrassment about odors and soiling of her clothing beyond her control. The nurse needs to be tactful in suggesting hygiene practices that reduce odor. Commercial deodorizing douches are available, or noncommercial solutions, such as chlorine solution (1 teaspoon of chlorine household bleach to 1 quart of water) may be used. The chlorine solution is also useful for external perineal irrigation. Sitz baths and thorough washing of the genitals with unscented, mild soap and warm water help. Sparse dusting with deodorizing powders can be useful. If a rectovaginal fistula is present, enemas given before leaving the house may provide temporary relief from oozing of fecal material until corrective surgery is performed. Irritated skin and tissues may benefit from use of the heat lamp or application of vitamin A&D ointment. Hygienic care is time consuming and may need to be repeated frequently throughout the day; protective pads or pants may need to be worn. All of these activities can be demoralizing to the woman and frustrating to her and her family.

Evaluation

Care of the woman with an alteration in pelvic support can be evaluated as effective if the problems are prevented or treated, or if the woman adapts positively to the change in body functions.

▌POSTPARTUM PSYCHOLOGIC COMPLICATIONS

Mental health disorders have implications for the mother, the newborn, and the entire family. Such conditions can interfere with attachment to the newborn and family integration, and some may threaten the safety and well-being of the mother, newborn, and other children. Because birth is usually thought to be a happy event, a new mother's emotional distress may puzzle and immobilize family and friends. At a time when she most needs the caring attention of loved ones, they may either criticize or withdraw because of their own anxiety.

Mood disorders are the predominant mental health disorder in the postpartum period, typically occurring within 4 weeks of childbirth (American Psychiatric Association [APA], 1994). The majority of women experience a mild depression or "baby blues" following the birth of a child. Others can have more serious depressions that can eventually incapacitate them to the point of being unable to care for themselves or their babies. Postpartum depression exerts a moderate to large effect on the interaction of mothers and infants (Beck, 1995b), and disturbances in early mother-infant interactions are found to be predictive of poorer infant cognitive outcome (Murray, Fiori-Crowley & Hooper, 1996). Male babies seem to be especially vulnerable. For example, in one study, 3-year-old boys with depressed mothers scored approximately 1 standard deviation lower on standardized tests of intellectual attainment than boys whose mothers were well (Sharp et al., 1995). In the rarest of cases, a disturbed mother may kill her infant, herself, and/or other family members. Nurses are strategically positioned to offer anticipatory guidance, to assess the mental health of new mothers, to offer therapeutic interventions, and to refer when necessary. Failure to do so may result in tragic consequences.

Clinical Manifestations

The Diagnostic and Statistical Manual of Mental Disorders contains the official guidelines for the assessment and diagnosis of psychiatric illness (APA, 1994). From less severe to most severe, the disorders are categorized as postpartum blues (discussed in Chapter 18), postpartum depression without psychotic features, and postpartum depression with psychotic features (postpartum psychosis).

Postpartum depression without psychotic features

Postpartum depression (PPD), an intense and pervasive sadness with severe and labile mood swings, is more serious and persistent than postpartum blues. The intense fears, anger, anxiety, and despondency that persist past the baby's first few weeks are not a normal part of postpartum blues (Shrock, 1994). Occurring in approximately 10% to 15% of new mothers, these symptoms rarely disappear without outside help. Wickberg and Hwang (1997) reported a prevalence of depression of 12.5% at 8 weeks and 8.3% at 12 weeks' postpartum in a Swedish population.

The symptoms of postpartum major depression do not differ from the symptoms of nonpostpartum mood disorders except that the mother's ruminations of guilt and inadequacy feed her worries about being an incompetent and inadequate parent (Kumar, 1990). To be diagnosed with major depression, at least five of the following must be present nearly every day: depressed mood—often with spontaneous crying; markedly diminished interest in all activities; insomnia or hypersomnia; weight changes (increases and decreases); psychomotor retardation or agitation; fatigue or loss of energy; feelings of worthlessness or inappropriate guilt; diminished ability to concentrate; and/or suicidal ideation with or without a suicidal plan (Fishel, 1995). In PPD, there may be odd food cravings (often sweet desserts) and binges with abnormal appetite and weight gain (Shrock, 1994). New mothers report an increased yearning for sleep, sleeping heavily, but awakening instantly with any infant noise, and an inability to go back to sleep after infant feedings (Herz, 1992).

A distinguishing feature of PPD is irritability (Shrock, 1994). These episodes of irritability may flare up with little provocation and may sometimes escalate to violent outbursts or dissolve into uncontrollable sobbing (Shrock, 1994). Many of these outbursts are directed against significant others ("He never helps me") or the baby ("She cries all the time, and I feel like hitting her"). Women with postpartum major depressive episodes often have severe anxiety, panic attacks, and spontaneous crying long after the usual duration of baby blues.

Many women feel especially guilty about having depressive feelings at a time when they believe they should be happy (APA, 1994). They may be reluctant to discuss their symptoms or their negative feelings toward the child. A prominent feature of PPD is rejection of the infant, often caused by abnormal jealousy. The mother may be obsessed by the notion that the offspring may take her place in her partner's affections. Attitudes toward the infant may include disinterest, annoyance with care demands, and blaming because of her lack of maternal feeling. When observed, she may appear awkward in her responses to the baby. Obsessive thoughts about harming the child are very frightening to her. Often she does not share these thoughts because of embarrassment, but when she does, other family members become very frightened.

Medical management. The natural course is one of gradual improvement over the 6 months after birth. Support treatment alone is not efficacious for major PPD. Pharmacologic intervention is needed in most instances. Treatment options include antidepressants, anxiolytic agents, and electroconvulsive therapy. Psychotherapy focuses on the mother's fears and concerns regarding her new responsibilities and roles, as well as monitoring for suicidal or homicidal thoughts. For some women, hospitalization is necessary.

Postpartum depression with psychotic features

Postpartum psychosis is a syndrome most often characterized by depression (as described in the preceding section), delusions, and thoughts by the mother of harming either the infant or herself (Kaplan, Sadock & Grebb, 1994).

A postpartum mood disorder with psychotic features occurs in 1 to 2 per 1,000 births (Kaplan, Sadock & Grebb, 1994). Once a woman has had one postpartum episode with psychotic features, there is a 35% to 60% likelihood of recurrence with each subsequent birth (APA, 1994). Recent research, however, reported that women with histories of PPD (both with and without psychotic features) who were treated with high-dose oral estrogen immediately following birth had a low relapse rate—9% (Sichel et al., 1995). The authors hypothesized that the low rate of relapse suggests that oral estrogen may stem the rapid rate of change in estrogen following birth, thereby preventing the potential impact of dopaminergic and serotonergic neuroreceptors, which trigger depression.

Symptoms often begin within days after the birth, although the mean time to onset is 2 to 3 weeks and almost always within 8 weeks of the birth (Kaplan, Sadock & Grebb, 1994). Characteristically, the woman begins to complain of fatigue, insomnia, and restlessness and may have episodes of tearfulness and emotional lability. Complaints regarding the inability to move, stand, or work are also common. Later, suspiciousness, confusion, incoherence, irrational statements, and obsessive concerns about the baby's health and welfare may be present (Kaplan, Sadock & Grebb, 1994). Delusions may be present in 50% of all women, and hallucinations may be present in about 25%. Auditory hallucinations that command the mother to kill the infant can also occur in severe cases. When delusions are present, they are often related to the infant. The mother may think the infant is possessed by the devil, has special powers, or is destined for a terrible fate (APA, 1994). Grossly disorganized behavior may be manifested as a disinterest in the infant or an inability to provide care. Some will insist that something is wrong with the baby or accuse nurses or family of hurting or poisoning their child (Shrock, 1994). Nurses are advised to be alert for mothers who are agitated, overactive, confused, complaining, or suspicious.

A specific illness included in depression with psychotic features is **bipolar disorder** (formerly called manic-depressive illness). This mood disorder is preceded or accompanied by manic episodes and is characterized by elevated, expansive, or irritable moods. Bipolar disorders occur in approximately 0.6% to 0.88% of the population (APA, 1994). Clinical manifestations of a manic episode include at least three of the following symptoms, which have been significantly present for at least 1 week: grandiosity, decreased need for sleep, pressured speech, flight of ideas, distractibility, psychomotor agitation, and excessive involvement in pleasurable activities without regard for negative consequences (APA, 1994). Because patients are hyperactive, they may not take the time to eat or sleep, which leads to inadequate nutrition, dehydration, and sleep deprivation. While in a manic state, mothers will need constant supervision when caring for their infant. Mostly they will be too preoccupied to provide child care.

Medical management. A favorable outcome is associated with a good premorbid adjustment (before the onset of the disorder) and a supportive family network (Kaplan, Sadock & Grebb, 1994). The course of the syndrome is similar to that seen in patients with mood disorders. Because mood disorders are usually episodic, patients may experience another episode of symptoms within a year or two of the birth. Postpartum psychosis is a psychiatric emergency. In one study, 5% of the patients committed suicide, and 4% committed infanticide (Kaplan, Sadock & Grebb, 1994). Antidepressants and lithium are the treatments of choice. If the mother is breastfeeding, some sources say no pharmacologic agents should be prescribed (Kaplan, Sadock & Grebb, 1994), but other sources advise caution while prescribing some agents (Schatzberg & Nemeroff, 1995) (see later discussion). The mother will probably need psychiatric hospitalization. It is usually advantageous for the mother to have contact with her baby if she so desires, but visits must be closely supervised. Psychotherapy is indicated after the period of acute psychosis is past.

Etiology

A multidisciplinary approach is needed to understand the causes of PPD, including biologic (hormonal, neurotransmitter, and genetic theories), psychologic (personality and attributional theories), and sociocultural (social support, life stress, culture, preparation for childbearing) factors (Boyer, 1990). In the following discussion, each of these theories is explained by at least one current research study illustrating the significance of that particular approach.

Biologic theories

Some factors unique to the reproductive process play a major role. Alterations in hypothalamic-pituitary-adrenal (HPA) axis function attributable to childbearing show remarkable similarity to those observed in depressed women (Wisner & Stowe, 1997). Postpartum women are also at increased risk for hypothalamic-pituitary-thyroidal (HPT) axis dysfunction that may increase affective disorder vulnerability. Women with a history of major depression who relapsed during the postpartum period were found to have a significantly greater growth hormone response to apomorphine than those who remained well. The development of increased sensitivity of hypothalamic dopamine D_2 receptors in the postpartum period appears to predict the onset of depression (McIvor et al., 1996).

Psychologic theories

Theories that predict risk factors for PPD include a poor marital relationship (Shrock, 1994), family stress (Gotlib, 1991), fewer support systems, more stressful life events, and fewer personal resources (Logsdon, McBride & Birkimer, 1994). One study of Portuguese women reported that, aside from a history of depression, the only other powerful predictor of PPD was the negative impact score of life events (Areias et al., 1996). Women who feel close to their husbands report fewer depressive symptoms; women with psychiatric histories who did not relapse in the postpartum period had partners who were more positive about them than were partners of high-risk women who relapsed (Marks et al., 1996). Postnatal depression in fathers was associated with PPD in their wives (Areias et al., 1996). Low self-esteem was found to be a reliable contributing factor to PPD in several studies (Chen, 1996; Fontaine & Jones, 1997). Mothers with low self-esteem were 39 times more likely to have high depressive symptoms than those with high self-esteem (Hall et al., 1996).

Sociocultural theories

Theories about contributing causes of PPD are also reported from sociology. Stress (Chen, 1996), labeling, and feminist models have been hypothesized to contribute to PPD (Thurtle, 1995). Leathers, Kelley, and Richman (1997) reported that low levels of self-reported social gratification, support, and control at work and in the parenting role were related to PPD.

I CARE MANAGEMENT

Even though the prevalence of PPD is fairly well established, only 2 or 3 out of 100 are referred to a mental health care provider; of the remainder, only about half are identified by family physicians, nurse-practitioners, or other persons (Kumar, 1990). Those identified are often treated inappropriately with benzodiazepines or subtherapeutic doses of antidepressants.

Assessment and Nursing Diagnoses

To recognize symptoms of PPD as early as possible, the nurse needs to be an active listener and demonstrate a caring attitude. In one research study (Whitton, Warner & Appleby, 1996), British women suffering from PPD were interviewed about their symptoms, help-seeking behavior, and treatment. Over 90% recognized that there was something wrong, but only one third believed they were suffering from PPD. Over 80% had not reported their symptoms to any health professional. Nurses cannot depend on women volunteering unsolicited information about their depression or asking for help. The nurse needs to observe for signs of depression and ask appropriate questions to determine moods, appetite, sleep, energy/fatigue levels, and ability to concentrate. Examples of ways to initiate conversation include: "How is your life going now that you have a baby (or another child)? . . . Have you changed much since having the baby?" (Shrock, 1994) "How much of the time do you spend crying?" If it appears that the

| BOX 26-5 | Suggested Questions to Elicit Responses from the Postpartum Depression Checklist |

LACK OF CONCENTRATION

Are you experiencing difficulty concentrating?
Does your mind seem to be filled with cobwebs?
Does it seem at times like fogginess sets in?

LOSS OF INTERESTS

Do you feel your life is empty of your previous interests and goals?
Have you lost interest in your hobbies that used to bring you pleasure and enjoyment?

LONELINESS

Are you experiencing feelings of loneliness?
Do you feel as though no one really understands what you are experiencing?
Do you feel uncomfortable around other people?
Have you been isolating yourself from other people?

INSECURITY

Have you been feeling insecure, fragile, or vulnerable?
Does the responsibility of motherhood seem overwhelming?

OBSESSIVE THINKING

Is your mind constantly filled with obsessive thinking, such as "What's wrong with me?" "Am I going crazy?" "Why can't I enjoy being with my baby?"
When trying to fall asleep at night, is your mind still racing with repetitive thoughts?

LACK OF POSITIVE EMOTIONS

Are you experiencing feelings of emptiness?
Do you feel like a robot just going through the motions?
When caring for your infant/child, do you feel any joy or love?

LOSS OF SELF

Do you feel as though you are not the same person you used to be?
Are you afraid that your life will never be normal again?

ANXIETY ATTACKS

Are you experiencing uncontrollable anxiety attacks?
Are you experiencing periods of palpitations, chest pains, sweating, or tingling hands?
When going through an anxiety attack, do you feel as though you're losing your mind?

LOSS OF CONTROL

Do you feel you are in control of your emotions and thoughts?
Are you experiencing loss of control in any aspects of your life?

GUILT

Are you feeling guilty because you believe you are not giving your infant/child the love and attention he or she needs?
Are you experiencing guilt over thoughts of harming your infant/child?
Do you feel you are a good mother?

CONTEMPLATING DEATH

Have you experienced thoughts of harming yourself?
Have you been feeling so low that the thought of leaving this world was appealing to you?

From Beck C: Screening methods for postpartum depression, *J Obstet Gynecol Neonatal Nurs* 4(4):308, 1995b.

new mother is depressed, the nurse must ask if the mother has thought about hurting herself or the baby. The patient may be more willing to answer honestly if she is told, "Lots of women feel depressed after having a baby, and some feel so badly that they think about hurting themselves or the baby. Have you had these thoughts?"

NURSE ALERT *Recalling risk factors for PPD can alert the nurse to identify those postpartum women at greatest risk. Such factors include a history of a mood disorder, meager or absent social support, stressful life events, low self-esteem, poor marital relationship, depressed father, unplanned pregnancy, not breastfeeding, unemployment in the mother (no job to return to following maternity leave), and unemployment in the head of the household (Warner et al., 1996).*

Nurses can use screening tools in assessing whether the depressive symptoms have progressed from postpartum blues to PPD. Examples are the Postpartum Depression Checklist developed by Beck (1995b) (Box 26-5) and the Edinburgh Postnatal Depression Scale (EPDS) (Cox, Holden & Sagovsky, 1989) (Box 26-6). The EPDS, with a cutoff point of 11.5, was found to identify all but two women with major depression, giving it a sensitivity of 96% (Wickberg & Hwang, 1996b). Particularly if the initial interaction reveals some question that the patient might be depressed, a formal screening is helpful in determining the urgency of the referral and the type of provider. Also important is the need to assess the woman's family because they may be able to offer valuable information, as well as have a need to express how they have been affected by the woman's emotional disorder.

BOX 26-6 *Edinburgh Postnatal Depression Scale (EPDS)*

Name:
Address:
Baby's age:

As you have recently had a baby, we would like to know how you are feeling. Please UNDERLINE the answer which comes closest to how you have felt IN THE PAST 7 DAYS, not just how you feel today.

Here is an example, already completed.
I have felt happy
     Yes, all the time
     <u>Yes, most of the time</u>
     No, not very often
     No, not at all
This would mean: "I have felt happy most of the time" during the past week. Please complete the other questions in the same way.

IN THE PAST 7 DAYS:

1. I have been able to laugh and see the funny side of things
     As much as I always could
     Not quite so much now
     Definitely not so much now
     Not at all
2. I have looked forward with enjoyment to things
     As much as I ever did
     Rather less than I used to
     Definitely less than I used to
     Hardly at all
* 3. I have blamed myself unnecessarily when things went wrong
     Yes, most of the time
     Yes, some of the time
     Not very often
     No, never
4. I have been anxious or worried for no good reason
     No, not at all
     Hardly ever
     Yes, sometimes
     Yes, very often

* 5. I have felt scared or panicky for no very good reason
     Yes, quite a lot
     Yes, sometimes
     No, not much
     No, not at all
* 6. Things have been getting on top of me
     Yes, most of the time I haven't been able to cope at all
     Yes, sometimes I haven't been coping as well as usual
     No, most of the time I have coped quite well
     No, I have been coping as well as ever
* 7. I have been so unhappy that I have had difficulty sleeping
     Yes, most of the time
     Yes, sometimes
     Not very often
     No, not at all
* 8. I have felt sad or miserable
     Yes, most of the time
     Yes, quite often
     Not very often
     No, not at all
* 9. I have been so unhappy that I have been crying
     Yes, most of the time
     Yes, quite often
     Only occasionally
     No, never
*10. The thought of harming myself has occurred to me
     Yes, quite often
     Sometimes
     Hardly ever
     Never

Scoring: Response categories are scored 0, 1, 2, and 3 according to increased severity of the symptom.
Items marked with an asterisk are reverse scored (i.e., 3, 2, 1 and 0). The total score is calculated by adding together the scores for each of the 10 items.

From Cox J, Holden J, & Sagovsky M: Edinburgh postnatal depression scale, *Br J Psych* 150:782, 1989.

Planning is based on the nursing diagnoses (see Nursing Diagnoses box) and is focused on meeting the individualized needs of the family to ensure safety, especially for the mother and infant and any other children, and to facilitate functional family coping.

▌ Nursing Diagnoses_____

Women Experiencing Postpartum Emotional Complications
Risk for injury to newborn related to:
• Mother's depression (inattention to infant's needs for hygiene, nutrition, safety) and psychotropic medications via breast milk

Ineffective family coping related to:
• Increased care needs of mother and infant
Risk for altered parenting related to:
• Inability of depressed mother to attach to infant
Risk for altered growth and development of infant related to:
• Lack of stimulation and inadequate loving care
Anxiety in the mother related to:
• Postpartum hormonal fluctuation
Self-esteem disturbance in the mother related to:
• Stresses associated with role changes
Risk for violence toward self (mother) or children related to:
• Postpartum depression

Expected Outcomes of Care

Specific measurable criteria can be developed based on the following general outcomes:

- The mother will no longer be depressed.
- The mother's and infant's physical well-being will be maintained.
- The family will cope effectively.
- Family members will demonstrate continued healthy growth and development.
- The infant will be fully integrated into the family.

Plan of Care and Interventions

On the postpartum unit

The postpartum nurse must observe the new mother carefully for any signs of teariness and conduct further assessments as necessary. Information about PPD must be discussed by nurses to prepare new parents for potential problems in the postpartum period. The family must be able to recognize the symptoms and know where to go for help. In addition, a teaching brochure that explains what the woman can do to prevent depression could be used as part of discharge planning (Boyer, 1990). This brochure might include an elaboration of the ideas listed in the Home Care box.

In these days of early discharge, postpartum mothers usually leave the hospital before the blues or depression hits (Shrock, 1994). If the postpartum nurse is concerned about the mother, a mental health consult should be requested before the mother leaves the hospital. All patients should be urged to maintain contact with the postpartum staff for urgent referrals or resources. A routine message to whoever comes to take the patient home should be, "If you notice that your wife (or daughter) is upset or crying a lot, please call the postpartum care provider immediately—don't wait for the routine postpartum appointment."

In the home and community

Postpartum home visits can reduce the incidence of or complications from depression. A brief home visit or phone call at least once a week until the new mother returns for her postpartum visit may save the life of a mother and her infant. In a Swedish research project, 41 postpartum depressed women were randomly allocated to a study and a control group (Wickberg & Hwang, 1996a). The women in the study group received six weekly counseling visits by the Child Health Clinic nurse, and the control group received routine primary care. Twelve (80%) postpartum women with major depression in the study group were fully recovered after the intervention compared with four (25%) in the control group. More research about the effectiveness of home visits as an intervention for PPD is needed.

Supervision of the mother with emotional complications may become a primary concern. Since depression can greatly interfere with her mothering functions, family and friends may need to participate in the infant's care. This

HOME CARE *Patient Instructions for Self-Care*

Activities to Prevent Postpartum Depression

- Share knowledge about postpartum emotional problems with close family and friends.
- Take care of yourself, including eating a balanced diet, getting exercise on a regular basis, and getting adequate sleep. Ask someone to take care of the baby so that you can get a full night's sleep.
- Share your feelings with someone close to you; don't isolate yourself at home.
- Don't overcommit yourself or feel like you need to be superwoman.
- Don't place unrealistic expectations on yourself.
- Don't be ashamed of having emotional problems after your baby is born—it happens to about 15% of women.

supervision can be planned by the collaborative efforts of the nurse and family members. This is a time for the extended family and friends to determine what they can do to help, and the nurse will work with them to ensure adequate supervision of the woman and their understanding of the woman's mental illness.

Caring is one of the nurses' most powerful tools. Using a phenomenologic research methodology, interviews with 10 mothers who had experienced PPD were analyzed. Seven themes emerged that illustrated nurses' caring for mothers experiencing PPD: having sufficient knowledge about PPD; using astute observation and intuition to make quick, correct diagnoses; providing hope that the mothers' living nightmares will come to an end; readily sharing their time; making appropriate referrals for the right path to recovery; providing continuity of care; and understanding what the mothers were experiencing (Beck, 1995a).

Facilitating relationship with partner. Women with PPD may not be able to attend to their partners' needs. The nurse can guide the woman and her partner in working together to cope with this stressful time. Depression can make a woman overly observant of a loved one's unhelpful behavior while failing to recognize loving, helpful gestures. The health care provider must not agree that the partner is nonsupportive, even when the postpartum woman is being critical. The nurse can say, "It seems right now that you feel he is not being supportive of you," or "You feel like your needs are not being met, even though he may be doing the best he knows how." The nurse can also encourage the postpartum woman to identify several specific requests for her partner, such as asking for a hug or asking him to watch the baby so that she can take a walk outside.

When the woman has PPD, a partner often reacts with confusion, shock, denial, and anger and feels neglected and blamed. The nurse can talk with the woman about how her condition is hard on her partner, too, and that he is probably very worried about her. Men often withdraw or criticize when they are deeply worried about their significant others. The nurse can provide nonjudgmental opportunities for the partner to verbalize feelings and concerns, help the partner identify positive coping strategies, and be a source of encouragement for the partner to continue supporting the woman. Both the woman and her partner need an opportunity to express their needs, fears, thoughts, and feelings in a nonjudgmental environment (Shrock, 1994).

Suggesting changes and resources. Even if the mother is severely depressed, if adequate resources can be mobilized to ensure safety for both mother and infant, hospitalization can be avoided. Whether the mother has private insurance or is referred to state-supported agencies, the home health care nurse will need to make frequent phone calls or home visits to do assessment and counseling. Some parents may need to reassess their daily routines, their expectations of parenthood, and the concept of "good mothering." Postpartum women may indeed need rest, household help, or a prescription for medication (Shrock, 1994). Other community resources that may be helpful are temporary child care or foster care, homemaker service, meals on wheels, parenting guidance centers, mother's-day-out programs, and telephone support groups. Mild cases of PPD can be referred to support groups (Berchtold & Burrough, 1990), such as Postpartum Support International Hotline ([206] 881-6580) or Depression after Delivery (DAD) (P.O. Box 1282, Morrisville, PA 19067; [908] 575-9121).

Providing safety. When depression is suspected, the nurse asks, "Have you thought about hurting yourself?" If delusional thinking about the baby is suspected, the nurse asks, "Have you thought about hurting your baby?" There are four criteria to measure in assessing the seriousness of a suicidal plan: method, availability, specificity, and lethality. Has the woman specified a method? Is the method of choice available? How specific is the plan? If the method is concrete and detailed, with access to it right at hand, the suicide risk increases. How lethal is the method? The most lethal method is shooting, with hanging a close second. The least lethal is slashing one's wrists.

| NURSE ALERT | *Suicidal thoughts or attempts are one of the most serious symptoms of PPD and require immediate assessment and intervention (Fishel, 1995).*

Referral. Women with moderate to severe cases of PPD should be referred to a mental health therapist, such as an advanced practice psychiatric nurse, for evaluation and therapy so as to avoid the effects that PPD can have on the woman and on her relationships with her partner, baby, and other children (Shrock, 1994). Inpatient psychiatric hospitalization may be necessary. This decision is made when the safety needs of the mother or children are threatened.

Psychiatric hospitalization

Women with postpartum psychosis are a psychiatric emergency and must be referred immediately to a psychia-

trist who can prescribe medication and other forms of therapy and assess the need for hospitalization.

| LEGAL TIP | **Legal Commitment for Treatment of PPD**
If a woman with PPD is experiencing active suicidal ideation or harmful delusions about the baby and is unwilling to seek treatment, legal intervention may be necessary to commit the woman to an inpatient setting for treatment.

To review the question of whether an infant should be admitted to psychiatric services when a severe psychiatric disorder necessitates admission of the mother, Barnett and Morgan (1996) reviewed all available literature on mother-infant admission. Early reports favored joint admission, then opinions changed, possibly for economic reasons. Recent research data report on longer-term adverse effects of postnatal depression on the children, and on the finding of psychologic and psychiatric morbidity in many of the fathers. Joint admission to designated special units can be valuable, but such facilities are only cost-efficient and effective if established as part of an appropriate broader plan for managing postpartum psychiatric disorder.

Within the hospital setting, the reintroduction of the baby to the mother can occur at the mother's own pace. A schedule is set for increasing the hours of the mother's caring for the baby over several days, culminating in the infant staying overnight in the mother's room. This allows the mother to experience meeting the infant's needs and giving up sleep for the baby, a situation difficult for new mothers even under ideal conditions. The mother's readiness for discharge and caring for the baby is assessed. Her interactions with her baby are also carefully supervised and guided.

Nurses should also observe the mother for signs of bonding with the baby. Attachment behaviors are defined as eye-to-eye contact; physical contact that involves holding, touching, cuddling, and talking to the baby and calling the baby by name; and the initiation of appropriate care. A staff member is assigned to keep the baby in sight at all times. Indirect teaching, praise, and encouragement are designed to bolster the mother's self-esteem and self-confidence. The Bethlem Mother-Infant Interaction Scale can be used by inpatient nurses to aid clinical decisions about the safety of parenting by individual mothers with severe mental illness in the postpartum period (Hipwell & Kumar, 1996).

Psychotropic medications

PPD is usually treated with antidepressant medications. If the woman with PPD is not breastfeeding, then antidepressants can be prescribed without special precautions. The commonly used antidepressant drugs are often divided into four groups: selective serotonin reuptake inhibitors (SSRIs), heterocyclics (including the tricyclics–TCAs), monoamine oxidase inhibitors (MAOIs), and other antidepressant agents not in the above classifications (Keltner & Folks, 1997) (Box 26-7). None of these medications is

---

BOX 26-7 *Antidepressant Medications*

SELECTIVE SEROTONIN REUPTAKE INHIBITORS
Fluoxetine (Prozac)
Fluvoxamine (Luvox)
Paroxetine (Paxil)
Sertraline (Zoloft)

HETEROCYCLICS/TRICYCLICS
Amitriptyline (Elavil)
Amoxapine (Asendin)
Clomipramine (Anafranil)
Desipramine (Norpramin)
Doxepin (Sinequan)
Imipramine (Tofranil)
Nortriptyline (Pamelor)
Maprotiline (Ludiomil)
Protriptyline (Vivactil)

MONOAMINE OXIDASE INHIBITORS
Phenelzine (Nardil)
Tranylcypromine (Parnate)

OTHER AGENTS
Bupropion (Wellbutrin)
Nefazodone (Serzone)
Trazadone (Desyrel)
Venlafaxine (Effexor)

BOX 26-8 *Mood Stabilizers*

Carbamazepine (Tegretol)
Clonazepam (Klonopin)
Divalproex (Depakote)
Lithium carbonate (Eskalith)

BOX 26-9 *Commonly Used Antipsychotic Medications*

PHENOTHIAZINES
Chlorpromazine (Thorazine)
Fluphenazine (Prolixin)
Perphenazine (Trilafon)
Thioridazine (Mellaril)
Trifluoperazine (Stelazine)

OTHER
Clozapine (Clozaril)
Haloperidol (Haldol)
Loxapine (Loxitane)
Olanzapine (Zyprexa)
Pimozide (Orap)
Risperidone (Resperdal)
Thiothixene (Navane)

---

rated for use in pregnancy as a Food and Drug Administration (FDA) category A drug (controlled studies show no risk to the fetus). The only ones classified as category B (no evidence of risk in humans) are maprotiline (Ludiomil), bupropion (Wellbutrin), fluoxetine (Prozac), fluvoxamine (Luvox), paroxetine (Paxil), and sertraline (Zoloft). The remaining antidepressant medications are rated as category C (risk cannot be ruled out, but potential benefits may justify potential risk) or D (positive evidence of risk to the fetus but potential benefits may outweigh risk).

The SSRIs are prescribed more frequently today than other groups of antidepressant medications. They are relatively safe and carry fewer side effects than the TCAs. However, if an SSRI is taken with dextromethorphan, an agent found in cough syrup, the combination could trigger the serotonin syndrome (mental status changes, agitation, hyperreflexia, shivering, diarrhea, etc.) (Keltner & Folks, 1997). The most frequent side effects with the SSRIs are GI disturbances (nausea, diarrhea), headache, and insomnia. In about one third of patients the SSRIs reduce libido, arousal, or orgasmic function. SSRIs can also inhibit specific P-450 isoenzymes, resulting in marked elevations in drug concentrations and reduction in drug clearance.

The TCAs cause many central nervous system (CNS) and peripheral nervous system (PNS) side effects. Although some are simply annoying, others are significant—even dangerous (Keltner & Folks, 1997). In overdose, these medications can cause death. A common CNS effect is sedation, and this could easily interfere with mothers caring for their babies. A mother could fall asleep while holding the baby and drop him or her, or she could have trouble getting fully awake during the night to care for the baby. Other side effects include weight gain, tremors, grand mal seizures, nightmares, agitation or mania, and extrapyramidal side effects. Anticholinergic side effects include dry mouth, blurred vision (usually temporary), difficulty voiding, constipation, sweating, and orgasm difficulty (Keltner & Folks, 1997).

Hypertensive crisis is the main reason why MAOIs are not prescribed more frequently, even though they are quite effective. The patient should be taught to watch for signs of hypertensive crisis—throbbing, occipital headache, stiff neck, chills, nausea, flushing, retroorbital pain, apprehension, pallor, sweating, chest pain, and palpitations (Keltner & Folks, 1997). This crisis is brought on by the patient taking a large variety of over-the-counter medications or eating foods that contain tyramine, a sympathomimetic pressor amine, which normally is broken down by the enzyme monoamine oxidase. The nurse would need to do extensive teaching about foods and medications to avoid those that contain tyramine.

The patient taking mood stabilizers (Box 26-8) needs to be taught about the many side effects and, especially for those taking lithium, the need to have serum lithium levels drawn every 6 months. Women with severe psychiatric syndromes such as schizophrenia, bipolar disorder, or psychotic depression will probably require antipsychotic medications (Box 26-9).

Patient education is especially important when caring for people who are taking antipsychotic drugs. The nurse should use discretion in selecting the content to be shared because patients may become anxious about the potential side effects. The nurse may choose to do more extensive education with a close family member. Most of these medications can cause sedation and orthostatic hypotension—both of which could interfere with the mother being able to safely care for her baby. In addition, they can cause PNS effects such as constipation, dry mouth, blurred vision, tachycardia, urinary retention, weight gain, and agranulocytosis, to name a few. CNS effects may include dystonias, parkinsonism-like symptoms, tardive dyskinesia (irreversible), and neuroleptic malignant syndrome (potentially fatal).

Psychotropic medications and lactation. About one half of all new mothers breastfeed. A major clinical dilemma is the antidepressant treatment of women suffering from PPD who want to breastfeed their infants. In the past, women were told to discontinue lactation. To date, the FDA has not approved any psychotropic medication for use during lactation. However, the American Academy of Pediatrics (AAP) (1994) published a report on excretion of drugs into human breast milk. Their classification includes drugs that are contraindicated during breastfeeding, drugs whose effects on nursing infants are unknown but may be of concern because they could alter CNS development, and drugs usually compatible with breastfeeding. Because all psychotropic medications pass through breast milk to the infant, the risks associated with the use of such medication must be weighed against the risks associated with maternal agitation and potentially self-destructive behavior.

In PPD with psychotic features, the mother may need to discontinue breastfeeding in order to take antipsychotic and antimanic medications without fear of harm to the baby. This loss, however, can intensify the mother's depression. It has been recommended that nonpharmacologic interventions be used before medications; however, in today's managed care climate, interventions such as frequent psychotherapy sessions, constant supervision by home health care nurses and family, and inpatient hospitalizations for mother and infant may not be readily available (Schatzberg & Nemeroff, 1995).

To date, breast milk excretion studies have demonstrated that antidepressants are present in breast milk, with a milk-serum ratio that is typically greater than 1:1 (Schatzberg & Nemeroff, 1995). For amitriptyline and desipramine, there is a peak increase in breast milk concentrations 4 to 6 hours after an oral dose. Adjusting both the schedule of dosing of the antidepressant and the infant's feeding schedule may considerably reduce the concentration of the drug to which the infant is exposed. The majority of investigators recommend using the secondary amine TCAs (nortriptyline and desipramine) (Schatzberg & Nemeroff, 1995). Typically, MAOIs are avoided; minimal data are available concerning the SSRIs. No human data have been published on the newer antidepressants. Most of the drugs listed in Boxes 26-7, 26-8, and 26-9 are rated 4—drug effects on infants are unknown but may be of concern (see Appendix C).

Wisner, Perel, and Findling (1996) reviewed 15 studies that systematically investigated the antidepressant effects during the postpartum period. The results revealed that sertraline and several tricyclics, including amitriptyline, nortriptyline, desipramine, and clomipramine, fail to exert significant adverse effects and do not increase infant antidepressant levels. In contrast, colic and increased blood levels have been reported in breastfed infants whose mothers took fluoxetine, and respiratory depression occurred in those whose mothers were treated with doxepin. The data to date suggest that no documented developmental delays are evident in 9- to 36-month-old infants of antidepressant-treated mothers (Wisner, Perel & Findling, 1996).

Antipsychotic drugs are excreted into breast milk. With the exception of clozapine (Clozaril), which is category B, all of the other antipsychotic medications are category C. The most widely studied is chlorpromazine; seven infants did not demonstrate any developmental deficits at 16-month and 5-year follow-ups. The breast milk concentrations of several other antipsychotics have been measured; the milk-serum ratio is less than or equal to 1.0 (Schatzberg & Nemeroff, 1995). The older antipsychotic medications have been widely used for three decades, and risks are minimal for nursing infants; their use should be avoided during the first trimester of pregnancy (Schatzberg & Nemeroff, 1995). None of these medications has been proved safe during lactation; the AAP does not rate any of the antipsychotic medications as compatible with breastfeeding.

Mood-stabilizing or antimanic medications are present in breast milk. Carbamazepine and clonazepam are category C, and lithium and divalproex are category D. Nursing infants can achieve serum lithium concentrations that are 40% to 50% of maternal levels (Schatzberg & Nemeroff, 1995); therefore lithium is contraindicated in breastfeeding. In contrast, both carbamazepine and divalproex appear in low concentrations in human milk, and both are considered compatible with breastfeeding; however, the benefits of breastfeeding and the potential risks need to be carefully considered (AAP, 1994).

Nursing implications. When breastfeeding women have emotional complications and need psychotropic medications, referral to a psychiatrist who specializes in postpartum disorders is preferred. Depressed women who are not breastfeeding will need the nurse to reinforce the need to take antidepressants as ordered. Because they do not exert any effect before about 2 weeks and usually do not reach full effect before 4 to 6 weeks, many women discontinue taking the medication on their own. Patients taking any of the antidepressants should be cautioned about combining alcohol or over-the-counter medications with the antidepressants. (For additional information, see Fishel, 1995.)

Evaluation

The nurse can be assured that care has been effective if the physical well-being of the mother and infant is maintained, the mother and family are able to cope effectively, and each family member continues to show a healthy adaptation to the presence of the new member of the family.

RESEARCH

Clinical Presentation of Women Readmitted with Severe Postpartum Preeclampsia or Eclampsia

Birth of an infant is described as the cure for pregnancy-induced hypertension. Although the majority of patients with preeclampsia or eclampsia have no symptoms after birth, manifestations of severe preeclampsia and/or eclampsia have been observed up to 3 weeks' postpartum. In this retrospective, case-controlled study, the participants were 53 women readmitted in the postpartum period (<6 weeks) with severe preeclampsia or eclampsia. The control group was matched 2 to 1 with an index study participant and consisted of 106 women who had intrapartum severe preeclampsia or who did not require readmission. The medical records of the study and control participants were reviewed for symptoms, laboratory changes, and physical findings associated with preeclampsia/eclampsia. Women readmitted for postpartum severe preeclampsia or eclampsia had a clinical presentation that differed from that of intrapartum preeclampsia. Neurologic complaints, malaise, and nausea and vomiting were reported more often in women who were readmitted than in mothers with intrapartum preeclampsia.

Clinical Application of the Study: Nurses should be aware that women requiring readmission for postpartum severe preeclampsia have a unique clinical presentation that is different from women who present with intrapartum preeclampsia. Postpartum assessments before hospital discharge should include checking for signs and symptoms relating to the unique presentation of postpartum preeclampsia/eclampsia. Women and their families need to be educated about the signs and symptoms of preeclampsia and instructed to report such signs and symptoms to their physician or certified nurse-midwife.

Source: Attenbury J et al: Clinical presentation of women readmitted with postpartum severe preeclampsia or eclampsia, *J Obstet Gynecol Neonatal Nurs* 27(2):134, 1998.

KEY POINTS

- Postpartum hemorrhage is the most common and most serious type of excessive obstetric blood loss.
- Hemorrhagic (hypovolemic) shock is an emergency situation in which the perfusion

KEY POINTS—cont'd

of body organs may become severely compromised, leading to significant morbidity or mortality rate for the mother.

- The potential hazards of the therapeutic interventions may further compromise the woman with a hemorrhagic disorder.
- Clotting disorders are associated with many obstetric complications.
- The first symptom of postpartum infection is usually fever greater than 38° C on 2 consecutive days in the first 10 postpartum days (after the first 24 hrs).
- Prevention is the most effective and inexpensive treatment of postpartum infection.
- Structural disorders of the uterus and vagina related to pelvic relaxation and urinary incontinence may be a delayed result of childbearing.
- Mood disorders account for most mental health disorders in the postpartum period.
- Identification of women at greatest risk for postpartum depression can be facilitated by use of various screening tools.
- Suicidal thoughts or attempts are one of the most serious symptoms of postpartum depression.
- Antidepressant medications are the usual treatment for postpartum depression; however, specific precautions are needed for breastfeeding women.

CRITICAL THINKING EXERCISES

1 *Two objectives of the Healthy People 2000: National Health Promotion and Disease Prevention Objectives are to reduce the maternal mortality rate to no more than 3.3 per 100,000 live births and to reduce severe complications of pregnancy to no more than 15 per 100 births. What is the maternal mortality rate in the state in which you live? Discuss the potential impact of current health care reform initiatives in achieving these goals in your state.*

2 *Identify resources in your community for women with postpartum depression. Develop criteria to evaluate these resources and compare these resources according to the criteria. Develop an informational packet that could be distributed to postpartum patients during discharge teaching on how to find a resource for postpartum depression and include the strengths and weaknesses (or pros and cons) of each.*

References

Akins S: Postpartum hemorrhage: a 90s approach to an age-old problem, *J Nurse Midwifery* 39(2 suppl):123s, 1994.

American Academy of Pediatrics, Committee on Drugs: The transfer of drugs and other chemicals into human milk, *Pediatrics* 93(1):137, 1994.

American College of Obstetricians and Gynecologists: *Diagnosis and management of postpartum hemorrhage*, vol 143, Washington, DC, 1990, The College.

American Psychiatric Association: *Diagnostic and statistical manual of mental disorders*, ed 4, Washington, DC, 1994, American Psychiatric Association Press.

Areias M et al.: Correlates of postnatal depression in mothers and fathers, *Br J Psychiatry* 169(1):36, 1996.

Barnett B & Morgan M: Postpartum psychiatric disorder: who should be admitted and to which hospital? *Aust NZ J Psychiatry* 30(6):709, 1996.

Beck C: Perceptions of nurses' caring by mothers experiencing postpartum depression, *J Obstet Gynecol Neonatal Nurs* 24(9):819, 1995a.

Beck C: Screening methods for postpartum depression, *J Obstet Gynecol Neonatal Nurs* 4(4):308, 1995b.

Berchtold N & Burrough M: Reaching out: depression after delivery support group network, *NAACOG Clin Issues Perinat Women Health Nurs* 1(3):385, 1990.

Berg C et al.: Pregnancy-related mortality in the United States—1987-1990, *Obstet Gynecol* 8(2):161, 1996.

Bowes W: Clinical aspects of normal and abnormal labor. In Creasy R & Resnick R, editors: *Maternal-fetal medicine: principles and practice*, Philadelphia, 1994, WB Saunders.

Boyer D: Prediction of postpartum depression, *NAACOG Clin Issues Perinat Women Health Nurs* 1(3):359, 1990.

Calhoun B & Brost B: Emergency management of sudden puerperal fever, *Obstet Gynecol Clin North Am* 22(2):357, 1995.

Chen C: Postpartum depression among adolescent mothers and adult mothers, *Kaohsiung J Med Sci* 12(2):104, 1996.

Clark R: Infection during the postpartum period, *J Obstet Gynecol Neonatal Nurs* 24(6):542, 1995.

Clark S et al., editors: *Handbook of critical care obstetrics*, Boston, 1994, Blackwell Scientific Publications.

Cox J, Holden J & Sagovsky R: Edinburgh Postnatal Depression Scale, *Br J Psychiatry* 150:782, 1989.

Cunningham F et al.: *Williams obstetrics*, ed 20, Stamford, Conn, 1997, Appleton & Lange.

Doan-Wiggins L: Drug therapy for obstetric emergencies, *Emerg Med Clin North Am* 12(1):257, 1994.

Druelinger L: Postpartum emergencies, *Emerg Med Clin North Am* 12(1):219, 1994.

Fishel A: Mental health. In Fogel C & Woods N, editors: *Women's health care*, Thousand Oaks, London, 1995, Sage Publications.

Fontaine K & Jones L: Self-esteem, optimism, and postpartum depression, *J Clin Psychiatry* 53(1):59, 1997.

Gotlib I et al.: Prospective investigation of postpartum depression: factors involved in onset and recovery, *J Abnorm Psychol* 100(2):122, 1991.

Grimes D: The morbidity and mortality of pregnancy: still risky business, *Am J Obstet Gynecol* 170(5 part 2):1489, 1994.

Hall L et al.: Self-esteem as a mediator of the effects of stressors and resources on depressive symptoms in postpartum mothers, *Nurs Res* 45(4):231, 1996.

Hamadeh G, Dedmon C & Mozley P: Postpartum fever, *Am Fam Physician* 52(2):531, 1995.

Herz E: Prediction, recognition, and prevention. In Hamilton F & Harberger P, editors: *Postpartum psychiatric illness: a picture puzzle*, Philadelphia, 1992, University of Pennsylvania Press.

Hipwell A & Kumar R: Maternal psychopathology and prediction of outcome based on mother-infant interaction ratings, *Br J Psychiatry* 169(5):655, 1996.

Hunter S & Weiner C: Obstetric hemorrhage. In Repke J, editor: *Intrapartum obstetrics*, New York, 1996, Churchill Livingstone.

Kaplan H, Sadock B & Grebb J: *Kaplan and Sadock's synopsis of psychiatry*, ed 7, Baltimore, 1994, Williams & Wilkins.

Keltner N & Folks D: *Psychotropic drugs*, St Louis, 1997, Mosby.

Kleinert D et al.: von Willebrand disease: a nursing perspective, *J Obstet Gynecol Neonatal Nurs* 26(3):271, 1997.

Knuppel R & Hatangadi S: Acute hypotension related to hemorrhage in the obstetric patient, *Obstet Gynecol Clin North Am* 22(1):111, 1995.

Kumar R: An overview of postpartum psychiatric disorders, *NAACOG Clin Issue Perinat Women Health Nurs* 1(3):351, 1990.

Leathers S, Kelley M & Richman J: Postpartum depressive symptomatology in new mothers and fathers: parenting, work, and support, *J Nerv Ment Disord* 185(3):129, 1997.

Logsdon M, McBride A & Birkimer J: Social support and postpartum depression, *Res Nurs Health* 17(6):449, 1994.

Marks M et al.: How does marriage protect women with histories of affective disorder from postpartum relapse? *Br J Med Psychol* 69(4):329, 1996.

McIvor R et al.: The growth hormone response to apormophine at 4 days postpartum in women with a history of major depression, *J Affect Disord* 40(3):131, 1996.

Mishell D et al.: *Comprehensive gynecology*, ed 3, St Louis, 1997, Mosby.

Murray L, Fiori-Crowley A & Hooper R: The impact of postnatal depression and associated adversity on early mother-infant interactions and later infant outcome, *Child Dev* 67(5):2512, 1996.

Norris T: Management of postpartum hemorrhage, *Am Fam Physician* 55(2):635, 1997.

Phipps W et al.: *Medical-surgical nursing: concepts and clinical practice*, ed 6, St Louis, 1999, Mosby.

Richey M, Gilstrap L & Ramin S: Management of disseminated intravascular coagulopathy, *Clin Obstet Gynecol* 38(3):514, 1995.

Ridgeway L: Puerperal emergency: vaginal and vulvar hematomas, *Obstet Gynecol Clin North Am* 22(2):275, 1995.

Roberts W: Emergent obstetric management of postpartum hemorrhage, *Obstet Gynecol Clin North Am* 22(2):283, 1995.

Sampselle C et al.: Continence for women: evidence-based practice, *J Obstet Gynecol Neonatal Nurs* 26(4):375, 1997.

Schatzberg A & Nemeroff C: *Textbook of psychopharmacology*, Washington, DC, 1995, American Psychiatric Press.

Sharp D et al.: The impact of postnatal depression on boys' intellectual development, *J Child Psychol Psychiatry* 36(8):1315, 1995.

Shrock P: More than baby blues, *Adv Nurse Pract* 2(6):24, 1994.

Sichel D et al.: Prophylactic estrogen in recurrent postpartum affective disorder, *Biol Psychiatry* 38(1):814, 1995.

Skoner M, Thompson W & Caron V: Factors associated with risk of stress urinary incontinence, *Nurs Res* 42(5):301, 1994.

Thurtle V: Post-natal depression: the relevance of sociological approaches, *J Adv Nurs* 22(3):416, 1995.

Warner R et al.: Demographic and obstetric risk factors for postnatal psychiatric morbidity, *Br J Psychiatry* 168(5):607, 1996.

Weed S: *Wise woman herbal for the childbearing year,* Woodstock NY, 1986, Ash Tree Publishing.

Wendel P & Cox S: Emergent obstetric management of uterine inversion, *Obstet Gynecol Clin North Am* 22(2):261, 1995.

White D & Poole J, editors: *Obstetrical emergencies for the perinatal nurse,* White Plains, NY, 1996, March of Dimes Birth Defects Foundation.

Whitton A, Warner R & Appleby L: The pathway to care in post-natal depression: women's attitudes to post-natal depression and its treatment, *Br J Gen Pract* 46(408):427, 1996.

Wickberg B & Hwang C: Counseling of postnatal depression: a controlled study on a population-based Swedish sample, *J Affect Disord* 39(3):209, 1996a.

Wickberg B & Hwang C: The Edinburgh Postnatal Depression Scale: validation on a Swedish community sample, *Acta Psychiatr Scand* 94(3):181, 1996b.

Wickberg B & Hwang C: Screening for postnatal depression in a population-based Swedish sample, *Acta Psychiatr Scand* 95(1):62, 1997.

Wisner K, Perel J & Findling R: Antidepressant treatment during breast-feeding, *Am J Psychiatry* 153(9):1132, 1996.

Wisner K & Stowe Z: Psychobiology of postpartum mood disorders, *Semin Reprod Endocrinol* 15(1):77, 1997.

Wong D & Perry S: *Maternal child nursing care,* St Louis, 1998, Mosby.

Zahn C & Yeomans E: Postpartum hemorrhage: placenta accreta, uterine inversion and puerperal hematomas, *Clin Obstet Gynecol* 33(3):422, 1990.

CHAPTER

27 The Newborn at Risk: Problems Related to Gestational Age

LISA B. FIKAC

LEARNING OBJECTIVES

- Define the key terms.
- Compare and contrast the characteristics of preterm, term, postterm, and postmature neonates.
- Review techniques for assessing the gestational age of newborns.
- Discuss respiratory distress syndrome and the approach to treatment.
- Review the topics of prematurity and oxygen therapy.
- Discuss the pathophysiology of retinopathy of prematurity and bronchopulmonary dysplasia, and identify risk factors that predispose preterm infants to these problems.
- List the signs and symptoms of perinatal asphyxia.
- Describe meconium aspiration syndrome.
- Examine the needs of parents of infants at risk because of their gestational age and birth weight.
- Identify appropriate responses and interventions the nurse can use in caring for families experiencing anticipatory grief or loss and grief in the neonatal period.

KEY TERMS

anticipatory grief
appropriate for gestational age (AGA)
bronchopulmonary dysplasia (BPD)
continuous positive airway pressure (CPAP)
corrected age
extracorporeal membrane oxygenation (ECMO)
hypoglycemia
insensible water loss (IWL)
intrauterine growth restriction (IUGR)
kangaroo care
large for gestational age (LGA)
low birth weight (LBW)
mechanical ventilation
meconium aspiration syndrome (MAS)
necrotizing enterocolitis (NEC)
neutral thermal environment (NTE)
nonnutritive sucking
patent ductus arteriosus (PDA)
periventricular-intraventricular hemorrhage (PV-IVH)
postmature
postterm
premature
preterm
respiratory distress syndrome (RDS)
retinopathy of prematurity (ROP)
small for gestational age (SGA)
term
very low birth weight (VLBW)

Accurate assessment of gestational age and birth weight is important because of the bearing these factors have on perinatal morbidity and mortality and long-term developmental outcome for the infant. Modern technology has made an important contribution to improving the health and overall survival of infants at risk because of their gestational age or birth weight. However, infants who are born considerably before term and survive are particularly susceptible to the development of sequelae related to their preterm birth. These conditions, which can also occur in term and near-term infants, but not as frequently, include necrotizing enterocolitis, bronchopulmonary dysplasia, intraventricular and periventricular hemorrhage, and retinopathy of prematurity.

Newborns are classified according to their gestational age in the following ways:

- **Preterm** or **premature:** Born before the completion of 37 weeks' gestation, regardless of birth weight.
- **Term:** Born between the beginning of week 38 and the end of week 42 of gestation.
- **Postterm:** Pregnancy that extends beyond the completion of 42 weeks' gestation.
- **Postmature:** Born after the completion of 42 weeks' gestation.

The causes of preterm and postterm birth are largely unknown. However, it is known that the incidence of preterm birth is highest among women from low socioeconomic groups. The lack of comprehensive prenatal health care in this population is a likely contributing factor. Other social factors associated with preterm birth include African-American race, single status, low maternal age, low prepregnancy weight, stress, standing for long periods, short stature, and less than 12 years of education. Obstetric events associated with preterm birth include previous fetal or neonatal death, previous preterm birth or spontaneous abortion, incompetent cervix, maternal genital abnormality, maternal in utero exposure to diethylstilbestrol (DES), short intervals between pregnancies, premature rupture of membranes, late and/or no prenatal care, preeclampsia or eclampsia, hyperemesis, placental complications, multifetal pregnancy, and fetal congenital anomalies (Cloherty & Stark, 1997; Witter & Keith, 1993).

There is a normal range of birth weights for each gestational week (Fig. 27-1), but the birth weights of preterm, term, or postmature newborns may also be outside these normal ranges. Birth weights are classified in the following ways:

- **Large for gestational age (LGA):** Weight is above the 90th percentile for gestational age.
- **Appropriate for gestational age (AGA):** Weight falls between the 10th and 90th percentiles for gestational age.
- **Small for gestational age (SGA):** Weight is below the 10th percentile for gestational age.
- **Low birth weight (LBW):** Weight of 2,500 gm or less at birth. These newborns have had either less than the expected rate of intrauterine growth or a shortened gestation period. Preterm birth and LBW commonly occur together (e.g., less than 32 weeks' gestation and less than 1,200 gm birth weight).
- **Very low birth weight (VLBW):** Weight of 1,500 g or less at birth.

Intrauterine growth restriction (IUGR) is the term applied to the fetus whose rate of growth does not meet the expected growth pattern.

Common causes of LGA newborns include glucose intolerance of pregnancy, maternal diabetes mellitus, maternal overnutrition, parity, heredity, and certain congenital anomalies. Causes of SGA newborns may be maternal smoking, hypertensive states, undernutrition, anemia, or nephritis. In addition, the birth of an SGA newborn may be associated with multifetal gestation, a discordant twin pregnancy, or congenital anomalies. Living at a high altitude, infection with the rubella virus, or other maternal infection may also predispose a woman to giving birth to an SGA newborn. Fetal malnutrition, IUGR, and chronic fetal stress are other conditions associated with the birth of SGA infants.

There is an array of maternal, fetal, and prenatal placental factors associated with IUGR. Maternal factors include socioeconomic factors, preeclampsia, advanced diabetes, malnutrition, cigarette smoking, alcohol consumption, drug addiction, and living at a high altitude. Fetal factors include multifetal pregnancy, chromosomal and nonchromosomal congenital anomalies, and chronic infection (rubella and cytomegalovirus). Placental factors include

placental insufficiency and abnormal vascular anastmoses, twin-to-twin transfusion, and abnormal cord insertion (Fanaroff & Martin, 1997).

INFANT MORBIDITY AND MORTALITY

Preterm birth is responsible for causing almost two thirds of infant deaths. Preterm infants are at higher risk for dying because they have not grown and developed enough to be able to make an uncomplicated transition to extrauterine life. As a result, the prospects for survival or good health in these infants may be severely diminished (Box 27-1). Infants weighing more than 2,500 gm and born after 37 weeks' gestation have the best prospects of survival. There is a dramatic reduction in the mortality rate of infants, regardless of weight, born after week 36 of gestation. The mortality rate is less than 5% if the pregnancy has progressed to 35 weeks and the fetus weighs more than 2,000 gm.

Children and adults who were LBW infants are more likely to have major problems such as cerebral palsy, mental retardation, and sensory and cognitive disabilities and are also more likely to have difficulty successfully adapting socially, psychologically, and physically to an increasingly complex environment (Fanaroff & Martin, 1997). In addition to the potential alterations in the lifestyles of such people and their families, the cost of the care required by LBW infants is estimated to be in the billions of dollars each year.

PRETERM INFANTS

Preterm infants are at risk because their organ systems are immature and they lack adequate reserves of bodily nutrients. The potential problems and care needs of the preterm infant weighing 2,000 gm differ from those of the term, postterm, or postmature infant of equal weight (Philip, 1987).

As mentioned, preterm infants are at a distinct disadvantage when trying to make the transition from intrauterine to extrauterine life, but the degree of this disadvantage depends primarily on their level of maturity. If these infants have physiologic disorders and anomalies as well, these affect the infant's response to treatment. In general, the closer infants are to term from the standpoint of both gestational age and birth weight, the easier their adjustment to the external environment.

CARE MANAGEMENT

Assessment and Nursing Diagnoses

Gestational age

Gestational age assessment, which incorporates physical and neurologic criteria, remains the standard approach for newborns in well-baby, as well as intensive care, nurseries.

Ballard and associates (1991) developed a gestational tool that is more accurate for determining the gestational ages of

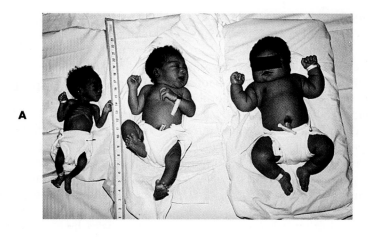

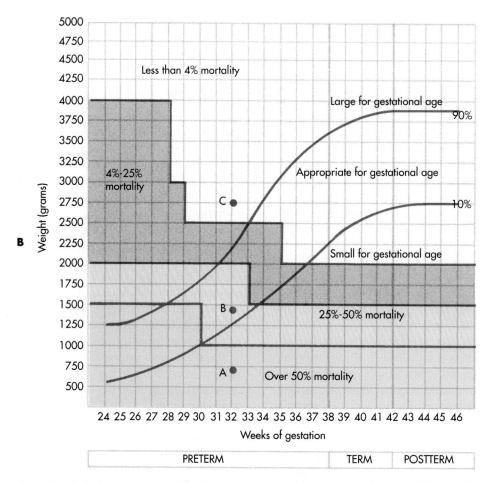

Fig. 27-1 **A,**Three babies of the same gestational age, with weights of 600, 1,400, and 2,750 gm, respectively, from left to right. Their weights are plotted in **B** at points *A, B,* and *C.* **B,** Intrauterine growth status for gestational age and according to appropriateness of growth. (**A** from *Perinatal assessment of maturation,* National Audiovisual Center, Washington, DC; **B** Courtesy Mead Johnson & Co, Evansville, Ind; modified from Battaglia F & Lubchenco L: *J Pediatr* 71:59, 1967.)

Resuscitation of Extremely Premature Infants

There are many different opinions about the resuscitation of extremely preterm infants weighing between 500 and 750 gm. Ethical issues that nurses caring for such infants are confronted with include:
- Whether to resuscitate?
- Who should decide?
- Is the cost of resuscitation justified?
- Do the benefits of technology outweigh the burdens in relation to the quality of life?

All people involved (health care providers and parents) should participate in the discussions in which these controversial issues are resolved.

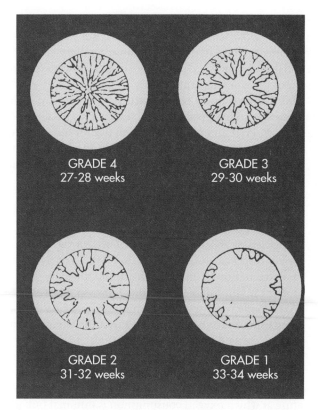

Fig. 27-2 Grading system for assessment of gestational age by examination of the anterior vascular capsule of the lens. (From Hittner H, Hirsch N & Rudolph A: Assessment of gestational age by examination of the anterior vascular capsule of the lens, *J Pediatr* 91[3]:456, 1977.)

extremely premature infants. This assessment tool has been adopted by many neonatal intensive care units (NICUs) in the United States (see Fig. 20-1, *A*).

Examination of the anterior vascular capsule of the lens has also been used to determine gestational age (Fig. 27-2). This method involves the use of direct ophthalmoscopy of the lens (Hittner, Hirsch & Rudolph, 1977) and uses as its basis the fact that the hyaloid system and the tunica vasculosa lentis are an embryologic vascular system that invade the eye beginning at approximately 27 weeks' gestation and atrophy after 34 weeks (Trotter, 1993). However, the corneas of infants at less than 27 weeks' gestation are too hazy to permit the lens vessels to be visualized, and the lens vessels in infants at greater than 34 weeks' gestation are minimal. Therefore the use of this assessment of the anterior vascular capsule of the lens to determine gestational age is applicable only to infants between 27 and 34 weeks' gestation and is limited by the capability of the examiner (Hittner, Hirsch & Rudolph, 1977).

Physiologic assessment

An accurate assessment of gestational age is critical in helping the nurse to identify the potential problems a preterm newborn is likely to experience. In further assessments of the preterm infant, the nurse follows a systematic approach similar to that used for the term infant. However, the response of the preterm infant to extrauterine life is different from that of the term infant. By understanding the physiologic basis of these differences, the nurse can assess these infants, determine the response of the preterm infant, and discern which potential problems are most likely to occur.

Respiratory function. Just as with the term infant, the initial assessment begins with an assessment of the infant's respiratory function, during which the nurse observes the infant's ability to make the pulmonary transition from intrauterine to extrauterine life. The preterm infant is likely to have difficulty making this transition

because of the numerous problems that affect the respiratory systems of such infants:
- Decreased number of functional alveoli
- Deficient surfactant levels
- Smaller lumen in the respiratory system
- Greater collapsibility or obstruction of respiratory passages
- Insufficient calcification of the bony thorax
- Weak or absent gag reflex
- Immature and friable capillaries in the lungs
- Greater distance between functional alveoli and the capillary bed

In combination, these deficits severely hinder the infant's respiratory efforts and can produce respiratory distress or apnea. The nurse needs to be prepared to provide oxygen and ventilation as necessary (Cloherty & Stark 1997).

Cardiovascular function. After the respiratory assessment, the nurse assesses the infant's cardiovascular system and its ability to adequately perfuse essential tissues and organs. Evaluation of heart rates and rhythm, skin color, blood pressure, perfusion, pulses, oxygen saturation, and acid-base status provides information on the cardiovascular status. The nurse must be prepared to intervene if symptoms of hypovolemia, shock, or both, are found. These symptoms include hypotension, slow capillary refill (>3 seconds), and continued respiratory distress despite the provision of oxygen and ventilation.

Maintaining body temperature. The preterm infant is susceptible to temperature instability as a result of numerous factors. Preterm infants are at high risk for heat loss due to the large body surface area in relation to weight. Other factors that place the preterm infant at risk for temperature instability include:

- Minimal insulating subcutaneous fat
- Limited stores of brown fat (an internal source for the generation of heat present in normal term infants)
- Decreased or absent reflex control of skin capillaries (shiver response)
- Inadequate muscle mass activity (rendering the preterm infant unable to produce its own heat)
- Poor muscle tone resulting in more body surface area being exposed to the cooling effects of the environment
- Friable (easily damaged) capillaries
- An immature temperature regulation center in the brain.

The goal of thermoregulation is to create a **neutral thermal environment (NTE),** which is the environmental temperature at which oxygen consumption is minimal but adequate to maintain the body temperature (Cloherty & Stark, 1997). Armed with the knowledge of the four mechanisms of heat transfer (convection, conduction, radiation, and evaporation), the nurse can then create an environment for the preterm infant that prevents temperature instability (see Chapter 19). The infant will be kept in a radiant warmer or isolette with control settings at a temperature to maintain the NTE.

Central nervous system function. The preterm infant's central nervous system (CNS) is susceptible to injury as a result of the following problems:

- Birth trauma that includes damage to immature structures
- Bleeding from fragile capillaries
- An impaired coagulation process, including prolonged prothrombin time
- Recurrent anoxic episodes
- Predisposition to hypoglycemia

Research data indicate that the developing nervous system has the ability to reorganize neural connection after injury, meaning that some injuries that would be permanent in adults are not so in infants. Certain neurologic signs appear to be predictive of later neurologic abnormalities. These signs include hypotonia, a decreased level of activity, weak cry for more than 24 hours, and an inability to coordinate suck and swallow (Fanaroff & Martin, 1997). Ongoing assessment and documentation of these neurologic signs is needed for the purpose of discharge teaching and making follow-up recommendations, as well as for their predictive value.

Maintaining adequate nutrition. The goal of neonatal nutrition is to promote normal growth and development (Cloherty & Stark, 1997). However, the maintenance of adequate nutrition in the preterm infant is complicated by problems with intake and metabolism. The preterm infant has the following disadvantages with regard to intake: weak or absent suck, swallow, and gag reflexes; a small stomach capacity; and weak abdominal muscles. The preterm infant's metabolic functions are compromised by a limited store of nutrients, a decreased ability to digest proteins or absorb nutrients, and immature enzyme systems.

The nurse must continuously assess the infant's ability to take in and digest nutrients. Some preterm infants require gavage or intravenous (IV) feedings instead of oral feedings.

Maintaining renal function. The preterm infant's immature renal system is unable to (1) adequately excrete metabolites and drugs, (2) concentrate urine, or (3) maintain acid-base, fluid, or electrolyte balance (Cloherty & Stark, 1997; Gomella, Cunningham & Eyal, 1994). Therefore intake and output, as well as specific gravity, must be assessed. Laboratory tests must be done to assess acid-base and electrolyte balance. Drug levels are also monitored in preterm infants because certain drugs can overwhelm the immature system's ability to excrete them.

Maintaining hematologic status. The preterm infant is also particularly predisposed to hematologic problems due to the following problems:

- Increased capillary friability
- Increased tendency to bleed (prolonged prothrombin time and partial thromboplastin time)
- Slowed production of red blood cells resulting from rapid decrease in erythropoiesis after birth
- Loss of blood due to frequent blood sampling for laboratory tests
- Decreased red blood cell survival related to the relatively larger size of the red blood cell and its increased permeability to sodium and potassium

The nurse assesses such infants for any evidence of bleeding from puncture sites and the gastrointestinal (GI) tract. Infants are also examined for signs of anemia (decreased hemoglobin and hematocrit levels, pale skin, increased apnea, lethargy, tachycardia, and poor weight gain) (Fanaroff & Martin, 1997).

Resisting infection. Preterm infants are at increased risk for infection because they have a shortage of stored maternal immunoglobulins, an impaired ability to make antibodies, and a compromised integumentary system (thin skin and fragile capillaries). Preterm infants exhibit various nonspecific signs and symptoms of infection (Box 27-2). The nurse must be diligent in assessing preterm infants so that sepsis can be identified and treated early. As with all aspects of care, strict handwashing is the single most important measure to prevent iatrogenic infections.

| BOX 27-2 | *Signs and Symptoms of Infection* |

- Temperature instability
  —Hypothermia
  —Hyperthermia
- CNS changes
  —Lethargy
  —Irritability
- Changes in color
  —Cyanosis, pallor
  —Jaundice
- Cardiovascular instability
  —Poor perfusion
  —Hypotension
- Respiratory distress
  —Apnea
- Gastrointestinal problems
  —Feeding intolerance
  —Vomiting
  —Diarrhea
  —Glucose instability
- Metabolic acidosis

Growth and development potential

Although it is impossible to predict with complete accuracy the growth and development potential of each preterm infant, some findings support an anticipated favorable outcome in the absence of ongoing medical sequelae that can affect growth, such as bronchopulmonary dysplasia, necrotizing enterocolitis, and CNS problems (Witter & Keith, 1993). The growth and development milestones (e.g., motor milestones, vocalization, growth) are corrected for gestational age until the child is approximately 2½ years of age (Avery, Fletcher & MacDonald, 1994).

The age of a preterm newborn is corrected by adding the gestational age and the postnatal age. For example, an infant born at 32 weeks' gestation 4 weeks ago would now be considered 36 weeks of age. The infant's **corrected age** at 6 months after the birth date is then 4 months, and the infant's responses are accordingly evaluated against the norm expected for a 4-month-old infant.

There are certain measurable factors that predict normal growth and development. The preterm infant experiences catch-up body growth during the first 2 to 3 years of life, with maximum growth occurring between 36 and 40 weeks' postconceptional age (Avery, Fletcher & MacDonald, 1994; Fanaroff & Martin, 1997). The head is the first to experience catch-up growth, followed by a gain in weight and height (Avery, Fletcher & MacDonald, 1994; Cloherty & Stark, 1997). At the infant's discharge from the hospital, which usually occurs between 37 and 40 weeks' postconceptional age, the infant should exhibit the following characteristics:

- An ability to raise the head when prone and to hold the head parallel with the body when tested for the head lag response
- An ability to cry with vigor when hungry
- An appropriate amount and pattern of weight gain according to a growth grid
- Neurologic responses appropriate for corrected age

At 39 to 40 weeks' corrected age, the infant should be able to focus on the examiner's or parent's face and to follow with his or her eyes.

At the corrected ages of 6 and 12 months, the infant is assessed again for age-appropriate responses. The infant who continues to be a poor eater; is irritable; displays sensory, perceptual, intellectual, or motor deviations in development; or displays hypertonia or hypotonia may be at risk for developmental delay. These behaviors must be interpreted with caution; such infants should be frequently reevaluated by an interdisciplinary team. Because of the increased potential for long-term developmental impairment, the parents need continued support and attention. Minor behavioral deviations also are identified for the parents to help them understand and accept their child, as well as provide the child with activities to help initiate learning. Deviations such as clumsiness, varying degrees of incoordination, slowness in reading and writing, and similar problems may be distressing to the child, parents, and other family members. Of the very low-birth-weight (VLBW) survivors, approximately 15% to 25% will have neurologic and/or cognitive disabilities in varying degrees of severity (Avery, Fletcher & MacDonald, 1994).

Parental adaptation to preterm infant

The experience of parents whose infant is born prematurely is different from the experience of parents whose infant is born at term (Shields-Poe & Pinelli, 1997; Wereszczak, Miles & Holditch-Davis, 1997). This may cause parental attachment and the adaptation to the parental role to differ as well. The key differences in the two experiences are summarized in Table 27-1.

Parental tasks. Parents of preterm infants must accomplish numerous psychologic tasks before effective relationships and parenting patterns can evolve. These tasks include the following:

- Experiencing **anticipatory grief** over the potential loss of an infant. The parent grieves in preparation for the infant's possible death, although the parent clings to the hope that the child will survive. This begins during labor and lasts until the infant dies or shows evidence of surviving. Anticipatory grief occurs when families have knowledge of an impending loss, such as when a baby is admitted to an NICU with problems or when a diagnosis of an anencephalic fetus is made by ultrasonography. The baby is still alive, but the prognosis is poor. Being able to anticipate the loss gives families an opportunity to plan, feel more in control of their situation, and say good-bye in a special way. However, some individuals or family members may distance or detach themselves from the experience or from their loved ones as a way of protecting themselves from the pain of loss and grief.
- The mother's acceptance of her failure to give birth to a healthy, full-term infant. Grief and depression typify this phase, which persists until the infant is out of danger and is expected to survive.

TABLE 27-1   *Differences in Parental Experiences with Term and Preterm Infants*

TERM BIRTH	PRETERM BIRTH
Parents have had a 38- to 40-week pregnancy in which to go through the emotional process of attachment and bonding.	Parents have not had a term gestation and may not be emotionally ready for attachment and bonding.
The parents are usually pleased with the first sight of the full-term infant; they may be joyous and show affectionate behaviors.	Parents may feel shock, panic, anxiety, and helplessness. They may be overwhelmed by the event.
The infant and parents participate actively in an acquaintance process; the infant cues the parents with eye contact.	Parents may not get the opportunity to see or touch the infant at birth if conditions warrant the start of immediate care for stabilization.
Parents progress from fingertip to palm to full enfolding (cuddling) of the infant, usually within a few minutes after the birth.	Parents may fear harming their small, fragile infant; progression from fingertip to palm touching may take hours, days, or several visits. Parents are not satisfied with just touching; they want to hold their baby.
Parents begin immediately to engage in caretaking activities—feeding, grooming, comforting, playing, etc.	Caretaking is often delayed until the baby's condition is stable, which can be days to several months.

- Resuming the process of relating to the infant. As the baby's condition begins to improve and the baby gains weight, feeds by nipple, and is weaned from the isolette, the parent can begin the process of developing an attachment to the infant that was interrupted by the infant's critical condition at birth.
- Learning about the ways in which this baby differs in terms of his or her special needs and growth patterns. Another parental task is to learn, understand, and accept the infant's caregiving needs and growth and development expectations (Sammons & Lewis, 1985).
- Adjusting the home environment to accommodate the needs of the new infant. Parents are encouraged to limit the number of visitors to minimize exposure of the infant to pathogens. The environmental temperature may need to be altered to optimize conditions for the infant. Grandparents and siblings also react to the birth of the preterm infant. Parents must deal with the grief of grandparents and the bewilderment and anger of the infant's siblings at the seemingly disproportionate amount of parental time spent on the newborn.

Parental responses. Newman (1980) noted two different approaches to the way in which parents cope with having a premature infant—coping through commitment and coping through distance. In the first approach, parents take each day as it comes, recognizing and accepting the lessened responses of their infant and noting the gradual progress in their child's condition. In the second approach, the parents pull away from becoming emotionally attached to the infant; they postpone becoming attached until the infant is in better health.

Parents have also been observed to progress through stages as they spend more time with their infants. In the first stage they maintain an *en face* position, stroking and touching their infant (Fig. 27-3). In the second stage they assume some child care activities, such as feeding, bathing,

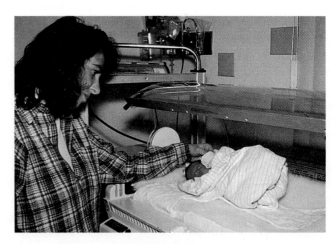

A

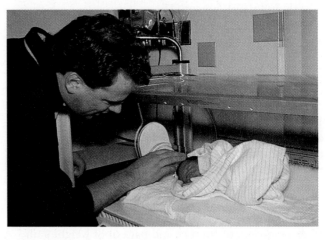

B

Fig. **27-3 A,** Mother interacts with her premature infant by touch. **B,** Father interacts with his baby by stroking and touching baby with fingertip. (Courtesy Michael S. Clement, MD, Mesa, Ariz.)

and changing the infant. In the third stage the infant becomes a person in their eyes and is seen as a whole child (Schraeder, 1980).

Infant responsiveness. The preterm infant's behavior is difficult to interpret because the infant is unable to provide positive reciprocal cues that encourage continued interaction with the parents (Lindsay et al., 1993). The quiet alert state is less evident and is unpredictable. Field (1979) noted that if a mother concentrated her interactions on imitating the infant's behavior, the preterm infant would become increasingly attentive and interested. Too active an involvement in child care tended to cause the infant to become disinterested and look away (gaze aversion). One young mother noted that "gentle stroking of her infant's head caused him to look at her." She also reported that even at age 7 years, gentle head stroking calmed her child. Oehler, Hannan, and Catlett (1993) reported eye opening or orienting as the most frequent way preterm infants respond to maternal interaction.

Parenting disorders. The incidence of physical and emotional abuse has been found to be greater in infants who, because of preterm birth or illness, are separated from their parents for a time after birth (Fanaroff & Martin, 1997). Physical abuse includes varying degrees of poor nutrition, poor hygiene, and battering. Emotional abuse ranges from subtle disinterest to outright dislike of the infant to abandonment. Parents may also show preferential treatment toward the brothers and sisters of the infant, nag the infant, have extremely high expectations of the infant, or show other types of overt or covert negative parental responses.

Factors surrounding the birth may predispose parents to treat their infant this way because subconsciously they have rejected the infant. These factors might include parental pain and anxiety, a heavy financial burden because of the cost of the infant's care, unresolved anticipatory grief, a threat to self-esteem, or the fact that the infant was the product of an unwanted pregnancy. The goal of health professionals is to identify abuse and neglect early so that further problems can be prevented and, in turn, the incidence of such abuse can be reduced.

Growth in the parental role. Parents go through numerous phases of adjustment as they become the "real" parents of their infant (Sammons & Lewis, 1985). These phases of adjustment, which include grieving and bereavement, bonding and attachment, and adapting to the role of parent, parallel the parental tasks already discussed. While parents are adapting to their new role, the preterm infant is achieving medical milestones and becoming progressively more accessible to the parents. As this occurs, the parents actively participate in caregiving, experience joy at the baby's increased awake time and responsiveness, and start to use the baby's name—not just "it," "he," or "she."

Nurses are in a unique position to assist parents during their infant's hospitalization. The iatrogenic complications parents suffer include confusion over the parental role, both in the unit and at home, a lack of self-confidence in their ability to care for their infant at home, lack of control, fear that the infant will become sick after discharge, and inability to discuss concerns with health care professionals before discharge (Kenner, 1990).

Potential nursing diagnoses for preterm infants and their parents are listed in the Nursing Diagnoses box.

I Nursing Diagnoses

Preterm Infants and Their Parents

Impaired gas exchange related to:
- Decreased number of functional alveoli
- Deficiency of surfactant

Ineffective breathing pattern related to:
- Inadequate chest expansion, secondary to infant position

Ineffective thermoregulation related to:
- Immature thermoregulation center

Risk for infection related to:
- Invasive procedures
- Decreased immune response

Anxiety (parental) related to:
- Lack of knowledge regarding infant condition
- Lack of knowledge regarding infant cues

Expected Outcomes of Care

The plan of nursing care for the preterm infant is directed by the physiologic needs of the infant's immature systems and often involves emergency treatments and procedures. Nursing care is a critical element in determining the infant's chances for survival, as well as normal development. In addition to meeting the infant's physical needs, nursing care is planned in conjunction with parents to promote parent-infant attachment and interaction. Expected outcomes are presented in patient-centered terms and include that the infant will:

- Maintain physiologic functioning
- Maintain adequate nutrition
- Experience no or minimal hematologic problems
- Remain free of infection
- Not develop retinal problems
- Not suffer trauma to the immature musculoskeletal system
- Experience attachment to parents

Expected outcomes for the parents include that they will:
- Perceive the infant as potentially normal (if this is medically substantiated)
- Provide care comfortably
- Experience pride and satisfaction in the care of their infant
- Organize their time and energies to meet the love, attention, and care needs of the other members of the family, as well as their own needs

Plan of Care and Interventions

The best environment for fetal growth and development is the uterus of a healthy, well-nourished woman. The goal of care for the preterm infant is to provide an extrauterine environment that approximates the healthy intrauterine environment in order to promote normal growth and development. Physicians, nurses, and respiratory therapists work together as a team to provide the intensive care needed. However, it is the nurse who is a constant presence in the infant's support system.

The admission of a preterm newborn to the intensive care nursery usually represents an emergency situation. Immediately after admission, a rapid initial evaluation is done to determine the infant's need for lifesaving treatment. Resuscitation is started in the birthing unit, and the newborn's need for warmth and oxygen is continued during transfer to the nursery.

A knowledge of the physiologic problems that typically arise in a preterm infant and of the infant's need to conserve energy for repair, maintenance, and growth serves as the basis for nursing actions. Nursing care is focused on the continuous assessment and analysis of the infant's physiologic status. In collaboration with the health care team, nurses make decisions and initiate therapies on the basis of their interpretation of these data. Nurses fulfill many roles in providing the intensive and extended care that these infants require. In addition, they are the support persons and teachers during the first phase of the parents' adjustment to the birth of their preterm infant.

The nurse-to-infant ratio is decided by the assessment and intervention needs of the particular infant and can vary from one infant per nurse, in the case of extremely critical infants, to as many as five infants per nurse, in the case of infants almost ready for transfer to a general care nursery. Hospitals not equipped to care for high-risk infants arrange for their immediate transfer to specialized centers.

The nurse uses many technologic support systems to monitor the body responses and maintain the body functions of the infant. Technical skill needs to be combined with a gentle touch and concern about the traumatic effects of harsh lighting and the volume of machinery noise.

Physical care

The environmental support measures for the preterm infant typically consist of the following equipment and procedures:

- An isolette or radiant warmer placed over the infant to control body temperature (NTE)
- Oxygen administration, depending on the infant's cardiopulmonary and circulatory status
- Electronic monitors as needed for the observation of respiratory and cardiac functions
- Assistive devices for positioning the infant in neutral flexion

- Clustering of care and minimization of stimulation

Various metabolic support measures that may be instituted consist of the following:

- Parenteral fluids to help support nutrition and maintain normal arterial blood gas (ABG) levels and acid-base balance
- IV access to facilitate the administration of antibiotic therapy if sepsis is a concern
- Blood work to monitor ABG levels, pH, blood glucose levels, electrolytes, and the status of blood cultures

Maintaining body temperature

The premature or otherwise compromised infant is even more susceptible to heat loss and its complications. In addition, LBW infants may be unable to increase their metabolic rate because of impaired gas exchange, caloric intake restrictions, or poor thermoregulation. Transepidermal water loss is greater because of skin immaturity in very premature infants (those at less than 28 weeks' gestation) (Endo & Nishioka, 1993) and can contribute to temperature instability.

Compromised infants are cared for in the thermoneutral environment created by use of an external heat source (Klaus, Martin & Fanaroff, 1993). The infant is attached by a probe to an external heat source supplied by a radiant warmer or a servocontrolled incubator. This idealized environment maintains an infant's normal body temperature between 36.5° and 37.2° C. Maintaining a thermoneutral condition in the youngest, most immature infants decreases the need for them to generate additional heat. As a result, excessive oxygen consumption is prevented in such compromised infants (Blake & Murray, 1998; Thomas, 1994).

Oxygen therapy

Clinical criteria for identifying the need for oxygen administration include increased respiratory effort, respiratory distress with apnea, tachycardia, bradycardia, and central cyanosis with or without hypotonia. In addition, the need for oxygen should be substantiated by biochemical data (arterial oxygen pressure [PaO_2] of less than 60 mm Hg or an oxygen saturation of less than 92%). Compromised infants often require saturations of more than 95% to maintain respiratory stability because their hemoglobin levels are frequently low. As the PaO_2 falls, less oxygen is released from the hemoglobin, which increases the risk for cellular hypoxia (Klaus, Martin & Fanaroff, 1993). Continuous monitoring can reveal significant oxygen level changes, and steps can be taken to improve oxygenation and saturation as soon as possible.

Oxygen administered to an infant is warmed and humidified to prevent cold stress and drying of the respiratory mucosa. During the administration of oxygen, the concentration, volume, temperature, and humidity of the gas are carefully controlled. Delivery of oxygen for more

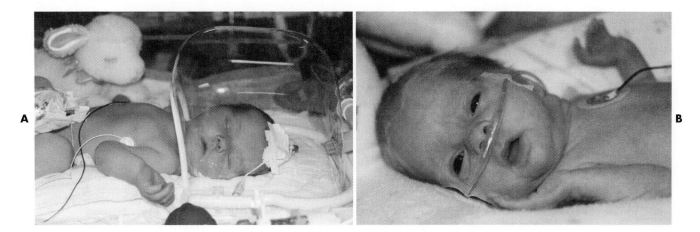

Fig. **27-4** **A,** Infant under hood. **B,** Infant with nasal cannula. (Courtesy Victoria Langer, RNC, MSN, NNP; from Dickason E, Silverman B & Kaplan J: *Maternal-infant nursing care,* ed 3, St Louis, 1998, Mosby.)

than a few minutes requires the use of special equipment (hood, nasal cannula, positive-pressure mask, or endotracheal tube) because the concentration of free-flow oxygen cannot be monitored accurately (Bloom & Cropley, 1994). In addition, free-flow oxygen into an incubator should not be used because the concentration would fluctuate dramatically every time the doors or portholes were opened. The indiscriminant use of oxygen may be hazardous. Possible complications of oxygen therapy include retinopathy of prematurity and bronchopulmonary dysplasia. It is important to remember that the administration of a therapeutic level of oxygen for a severely depressed infant could cause significant physiologic harm if given to an infant with mild respiratory disease (Hagedorn, Gardner & Abman, 1998).

Infants who need oxygen should have their respiratory status assessed accurately every 1 to 2 hours, and this should include a continuous pulse oximetry reading and at least one ABG measurement (Donovan & Spengler, 1993). The interventions implemented are then determined on the basis of the findings yielded by the clinical assessment, including telemetry (pulse oximetry or tcPO$_2$ monitoring) and laboratory tests (Hagedorn, Gardner & Abman, 1998; Wong, 1995). The interventions ordered are those that can directly manage the underlying disease process and range from hood oxygen administration to ventilator therapy.

Hood therapy. Oxygen can be administered by a hood to infants who do not require mechanical pressure support. The hood is a clear plastic cover that is sized to fit over the head and neck of the infant (Fig. 27-4, *A*). Inside the hood the infant receives the correct amount of oxygen. The infant is also protected from fluctuations in the ambient concentration of oxygen, such as occur when the portholes of the incubator are opened (Hagedorn, Gardner & Abman, 1998). The nurse checks the oxygen level every 1 to 2 hours because the concentration must be adjusted in response to the infant's condition.

Nasal cannula. Infants requiring low-flow amounts of oxygen can benefit from the use of a nasal cannula (Fig. 27-4, *B*). These are of particular value for older infants who are recuperating but still require supplemental oxygen. They are the preferred method for home oxygen administration (Hall, 1993). They permit the infant to receive an adequate, continuous flow of oxygen while allowing optimal vision, positioning, and parental holding. Infants can also breastfeed while receiving oxygen by this method. However, the nasal prongs must be inspected frequently to make sure they are not partially obstructed by milk or secretions (Hagedorn, Gardner & Abman, 1998). The use of nasal cannulas rather than hood therapy is encouraged because this allows easier feedings and psychosocial interactions (Ludington-Hoe et al., 1994). Nasal cannulas are preferred because the humidified oxygen delivered by a hood creates a fine mist that may alter the infant's vision.

Continuous positive airway pressure therapy. Infants who are unable to maintain an adequate PaO$_2$ despite the administration of oxygen by hood or nasal cannula may require the delivery of oxygen using **continuous positive airway pressure (CPAP).** CPAP infuses oxygen or air under a preset pressure (Fig. 27-5, *A*) by means of nasal prongs, a face mask, or an endotracheal tube. This pressure increases the alveolar volume by preventing the alveoli from collapsing on expiration (Wong, 1995). CPAP also increases the functional residual capacity, improves the diffusion time of pulmonary gases, including oxygen, and can decrease pulmonary shunting. If implemented early enough, CPAP may preclude the need for mechanical ventilation (Hagedorn, Gardner & Abman, 1998; Klaus, Martin & Fanaroff, 1993). One drawback to its use is that it can cause vascular shunting in the pulmonary beds, which can lead to persistent pulmonary hypertension and which can in turn cause severe respiratory distress.

Mechanical ventilation. Mechanical ventilation must be implemented if other methods of therapy cannot

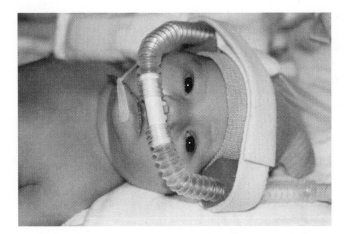

A

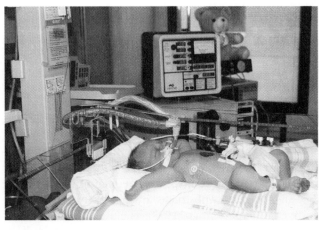

B

Fig. **27-5 A,** Infant receiving ventilatory assistance with continuous positive airway pressure (CPAP). **B,** Infant intubated and on ventilator. (*Courtesy Victoria Langer, RNC, MSN, NNP; from Dickason E, Silverman B & Kaplan J: Maternal-infant nursing care, ed 3, St Louis, 1998, Mosby.*)

---

provide adequate oxygenation (Bloom & Cropley, 1994). Its use is indicated whenever blood gas values reveal the existence of severe hypoxemia or severe hypercapnia (Fig. 27-5, *B*). The condition of the infant suffering from apnea with bradycardia, ineffective respiratory effort, shock, asphyxia, infection, meconium aspiration syndrome, respiratory distress syndrome, or congenital defects that affect ventilation may also deteriorate and require intubation to reverse the process (Donovan & Spengler, 1993; Klaus, Martin & Fanaroff, 1993; Wong, 1995).

The ventilator settings are determined by the infant's particular needs. The ventilator is set to provide a predetermined amount of oxygen to the infant during spontaneous respirations and also to provide mechanical ventilation in the absence of spontaneous respirations (Hagedorn, Gardner & Abman, 1998).

BOX 27-3	*Medications for Surfactant Replacement*

Bovine lung extract: beractant (Survanta)
Artificial surfactant: colfosceril (Exosurf)

INDICATIONS
Prevention and treatment of respiratory distress syndrome in premature infants
• For *prevention,* drug is administered within 15 minutes of birth to infants with clinical manifestations of surfactant deficiency or with birth weight less than 1,250 gm.
• For *treatment,* drug is administered to infant with confirmed diagnosis of respiratory distress syndrome, preferably within 8 hours of birth.

DOSAGE AND ROUTE
Depends on drug used. Administer via endotracheal tube.

SIDE EFFECTS AND ADVERSE EFFECTS
Bradycardia and oxygen desaturation after administration
Respiratory distress immediately after administration

NURSING CONSIDERATIONS
Observe infants' condition for changes. Diuresis may occur with improvement. Ventilator settings may need changing as the infant's ability to oxygenate increases.

Surfactant administration. Surfactant can be administered as an adjunct to oxygen and ventilation therapy. Before 34 weeks' gestation, most infants do not produce enough surfactant to survive extrauterine life (Hagedorn, Gardner & Abman, 1998). As a result, lung compliance is decreased, and not enough gas exchange occurs as the lungs become atelectatic and require greater pressures to expand. By administering artificial surfactant, respiratory compliance is improved until the infant can generate enough surfactant on his or her own. Exogenous surfactant is manufactured from human, porcine, or bovine amniotic fluid and is given in several doses through an endotracheal tube (Wong, 1995). As with any drug therapy, the infant must be monitored for the occurrence of potential side effects such as a patent ductus arteriosus and pulmonary hemorrhage. Use of this drug has been associated with a significantly reduced length of time on ventilators and oxygen therapy, and an increased survival rate in premature infants (Mauskopf et al., 1995) (Box 27-3).

Extracorporeal membrane oxygenation therapy. Infants with severe pulmonary dysfunction who are at more than 34 weeks' gestation may be candidates for **extracorporeal membrane oxygenation (ECMO)** therapy. ECMO makes use of cardiopulmonary bypass to oxygenate the infant's blood outside the body through a membrane oxygenator. The membrane oxygenator serves as an artificial

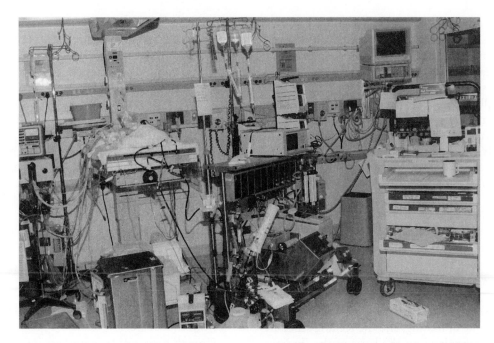

Fig. **27-6** Infant being treated with extracorporeal membrane oxygenation (ECMO) therapy. Note emergency supply cart next to oxygenator. (Courtesy Dale Ikuta, San Jose, Calif.)

lung while the infant's lungs heal (Fig. 27-6). Because of the massive systemic anticoagulation therapy required in the pump tubing and the increased risk for hemorrhage, the criteria for its use are very strict, and the use of this therapy is therefore limited (Donovan & Spengler, 1993). The risk for intraventricular hemorrhages in premature infants is particularly high, and for this reason ECMO therapy cannot be used in them. ECMO has been successful in the treatment of various acute and chronic lung diseases, including meconium aspiration syndrome and persistent pulmonary hypertension (Hagedorn, Gardner & Abman, 1998).

Other therapies. Other ventilator therapies that may reduce pulmonary tissue damage are currently either being used or studied. These include high-frequency oscillator ventilation, jet ventilation, flow interruption ventilation, and liquid ventilation (Donovan & Spengler, 1993). These methods of high-frequency ventilation work by providing smaller volumes of oxygen at a significantly more rapid rate (greater than 300 breaths/min) than traditional mechanical ventilators do. As a result, the intrathoracic pressure is decreased, and along with this, the risk of barotrauma. In liquid ventilation the surface tension is reduced while oxygenation is improved through the recreation of a fetal lung environment. Instead of air pressure, an experimental oxygenated lipid solution is pumped continuously through the lungs. Nitric oxide therapy used in conjunction with conventional ventilation is also being investigated as a substitute intervention for infants requiring ECMO.

Respiratory assistance is weaned slowly as the infant's status improves. The infant is ready to be weaned from respiratory assistance once the ABG and oxygen saturation levels are maintained within normal limits. A spontaneous, adequate respiratory effort must be present, and the infant must also show improved muscle tone during increased activity. Weaning is done in a stepwise and gradual manner. This may consist of the infant being extubated, placed on continuous positive airway pressure, and then weaned to oxygen by means of a hood or nasal cannula. Throughout the weaning process the infant's oxygen levels are monitored by pulse oximetry, $tcPO_2$ monitoring, and blood gas levels.

The goal of weaning is the withdrawal of all oxygen support. However, some infants do not achieve this before discharge from the hospital and may require home oxygen therapy for several months. Throughout the weaning period, health care providers assess the infant for signs and symptoms indicating poor tolerance of the process. These include an increased pulse, respiratory distress, or cyanosis, or a combination of these. If these occur, the amount of oxygen being delivered is increased, and weaning proceeds more slowly while further assessments are done. Underlying causes of intolerance of weaning may be bronchopulmonary dysplasia, a patent ductus arteriosus, or CNS damage (Hagedorn, Gardner & Abman, 1998).

The parents need to be given consistent information and to be reassured about the infant's respiratory progress. Decisions regarding the nature of continued interventions should be included in a multidisciplinary plan of care, and the therapy should be frequently reinforced to the family. Daily updates are imperative, especially if unexpected complications arise.

Nutritional care

It is not always possible to provide enteral (by the GI route) nourishment to a preterm infant. Such infants are often too ill or weak to breastfeed or bottle feed because of respiratory distress or sepsis (Blackburn & VandenBerg, 1993; Price & Kalhan, 1993). Early enteral feeding of the asphyxiated neonate with a low Apgar score is also avoided to prevent bowel necrosis. In such cases, nutrition is provided parenterally. Those infants who require parenteral nutrition may have one or more of the following problems (Schanler, Shulman & Prestridge, 1994; Townsend, Johnson & Hay, 1998):

- Lack of a coordinated suck-and-swallow reflex
- Inability to suck because of a congenital anomaly
- Respiratory distress requiring aggressive ventilator support
- Asphyxiation with a potential for necrotizing enterocolitis

Type of nourishment. The types of formulas used, the mode and volume of feeding, and the feeding schedule of the infant are determined on the basis of the findings yielded by assessment of the following variables:

- Initially, the birth weight, then the current weight of the preterm infant
- Pattern of weight gain or loss (infants weighing less than 1,500 gm require more energy for growth and thermoregulation and may gain weight poorly with either breastfeedings or bottle feedings)
- Presence or absence of suck-and-swallow reflex in all infants at less than 35 weeks' gestation (Lefrak-Okikawa & Meier, 1993)
- Demonstrated behavioral readiness to take oral feedings (Cagan, 1995)
- Physical condition, including presence or absence of bowel sounds, abdominal distention, or bloody stools, as well as presence and degree of respiratory distress or apneic episodes (Price & Kalhan, 1993)
- Residual from previous feeding, if being gavage fed
- Malformations (especially GI defects such as omphalocele or esophageal atresia) including the need for a gastrostomy feeding tube
- Renal function, including urinary output and laboratory values (nitrogen balance, electrolyte balance, glucose level); premature infants are especially susceptible to altered renal function (Schanler, Schulman & Prestridge, 1994).

The infant's ability to tolerate the solute and fluid load is also assessed. Complications, including feeding intolerance and metabolic imbalances, may arise from inappropriate nutritional intake, and the nurse should assess the infant for these (Price & Kalhan, 1993).

Weight and fluid loss or gain. For many reasons, the caloric, nutrient, and fluid requirements of compromised infants are greater than those of the term, normal newborn. One reason is that premature or dysmature (malnourished) newborns often have limited stores of nutrients and fluids. In addition, symptomatic or asymptomatic hypoglycemia, electrolyte imbalances, or other metabolic disturbances can develop in an infant whose nutritional intake is poor. Such hypoglycemia may cause serious damage to carbohydrate-dependent brain cells. Weight gain or loss in such infants is therefore monitored carefully to detect any need for a change in the therapy.

The infant's weight is measured and recorded daily, and the rate of weight loss or gain is calculated. Further depletion of weight and metabolic stores can occur as a result of one or a combination of the following factors:

- Birth asphyxia
- Increased respirations or respiratory effort
- Patent ductus arteriosus
- Hypothermic environment
- Insensible fluid loss caused by evaporation (with radiant heat or phototherapy)
- Vomiting, diarrhea, and dysfunctional absorption from the GI tract
- Growth demands (a premature infant's growth rate approximates that of fetal growth during the last trimester and is at least two times faster than a term infant's growth rate after birth)
- Inability of the renal system to concentrate urine and maintain an adequate rate of urea excretion, as well as infant's inadequate response to antidiuretic hormone

The compromised newborn is predisposed to have weight and fluid losses because of the greater amount of fluid needed to meet the demands of the increased cellular metabolic processes (resulting from stress, repair, or growth). The body weight of premature infants weighing less than 1,500 gm consists of 83% to 89% water, compared with the term infant's water content of 75% (Price & Kalhan, 1993). Most of this water is in the extracellular fluid compartment. Even with the early institution of fluid and nutrition intake, the premature infant's weight and fluid losses seem exaggerated. Inadequate fluid intake, resulting from either delayed administration or insufficient volume, can further cause weight and fluid losses in the premature infant.

Insensible water loss (IWL) is an evaporative loss that occurs largely through the skin. Approximately 30% of this IWL comes from the respiratory tract. The total IWL in a normal infant ranges anywhere from 30 to 60 ml/kg/24 hr (Blake & Murray, 1998). The effects of radiant warmers, incubators, phototherapy, and other factors can augment the IWL. Some of this loss can be prevented by humidifying the respiratory gases administered to such compromised infants.

During the first week of extrauterine life, the premature infant can lose up to 15% of his or her birth weight. In contrast, a weight loss of up to only 10% is acceptable in a term AGA infant (Price & Kalhan, 1993). After the initial week, a premature infant's loss or gain during each 24-hour period should not exceed 2% of the previous day's weight. The nurse assesses weight trends. (To calculate a weight loss or

---

BOX 27-4	*Calculation of a Weight Loss or Gain*

EXAMPLE 1

Day 4   1,750 gm

Day 5   1,730 gm

‾‾‾‾‾‾‾‾‾‾‾‾‾‾‾‾‾

      20-gm loss

$$\frac{20}{1,750} = \frac{X\%}{100\%}$$

$1,750X = 2,000$

$$\begin{array}{r} 1.1 \\ 1,750\overline{)2,000.0} \end{array}$$

$X = 1.1\%$ weight loss

EXAMPLE 2

Day 4   1,750 gm

Day 5   1,790 gm

‾‾‾‾‾‾‾‾‾‾‾‾‾‾‾‾‾

      40-gm gain

$$\frac{40}{1,750} = \frac{X\%}{100\%}$$

$1,750X = 4,000$

$$\begin{array}{r} 2.3 \\ 1,750\overline{)4,000.00} \end{array}$$

$X = 2.3\%$ weight gain

---

gain, see Box 27-4.) Weight loss may be caused by increased stooling or voiding, increased evaporative losses, inadequate volume or incorrect fluid administration, and problems with malabsorption. Implementation of interventions and frequent reassessment of the infant and its environment are necessary to correct the problems (Townsend, Johnson & Hay, 1998). Such interventions include adjusting the incubator temperature; monitoring and adjusting the volume and type of fluids being administered; assessing the urinary output, including the specific gravity; and assessing the blood glucose levels. The glucose determinations are used to assess urine osmolarity and hence renal function. High glucose levels (greater than 125 mg/dl) can stimulate an excessive osmotic diuresis (Wong, 1995). Weight gain may be due to overfeeding or fluid retention. The nurse reports and records her findings and continues to assess the infant's fluid status, urinary output, and blood glucose levels. The interventions implemented are determined by the infant's specific disorder and nutritional needs.

Elimination patterns. The infant's elimination patterns are also assessed. This includes the frequency of urination, as well as the amount, color, pH, and specific gravity of the urine. The assessment of the infant's bowel movements includes the frequency of stooling and the character of the stool, as well as whether there is constipation, diarrhea, or loss of fats (steatorrhea). All of these findings are documented. The nurse may request guaiac tests to assess for blood in the stool, tests to detect stool-reducing substances, and a pH determination to assess for malabsorption (Townsend, Johnson & Hay, 1998; Wong, 1995). Infants with unexplained abdominal distention are assessed carefully to rule out the presence of hypomotility or obstructions of the GI tract.

Oral feeding. Nourishment by the oral route is preferred for the infant who has adequate strength and GI function. Breast milk may be fed by breast or bottle. Formula may be fed by bottle or a supplementer (see Fig. 21-3). Throughout the feeding, the nurse assesses the newborn's tolerance of the procedure. When the infant breastfeeds, the nurse assists the mother by providing support and help, as necessary.

The needs of the compromised infant must be considered when determining the type and frequency of the feedings. Many compromised infants cannot suck well enough to breastfeed or bottle feed until they have recovered from their initial illness or matured physically (greater than 32 weeks' gestation). Mothers of compromised infants are encouraged to continue pumping breast milk, especially if theirs is a very premature infant who may not breastfeed for many weeks (Townsend, Johnson & Hay, 1998). Because of the significant breastfeeding attrition rates among these mothers, they need support and encouragement every few days to continue pumping while their infant is not yet able to nurse. If there is no available breast milk (from the mother or a milk bank), commercial formula is used. The calories, protein, and mineral content of commercial formulas vary (see Chapter 21). The type of nipple selected ("preemie," regular, orthodontic) depends on the infant's ability to suck from the specific type of nipple. The nurse also considers the energy the infant needs to expend in the process.

Overfeeding of the preterm infant should be avoided because this can lead to abdominal distention, with apnea, vomiting, and possibly aspiration of the feeding. The nurse monitors the infant's abdominal girth when distention is obvious.

Gavage feeding. Gavage feeding is a method of providing nourishment to the infant who is compromised by respiratory distress, the infant who is too immature to have a coordinated suck-and-swallow reflex, or the infant who is easily fatigued by sucking. In gavage feeding, breast milk or formula is given to the infant through a nasogastric or orogastric tube. This spares the infant the work of sucking.

Gavage feeding can be done either with an intermittently placed tube or continuously through an indwelling catheter. Infants who cannot tolerate large-bolus feedings (those on ventilators for more than a week) are given continuous feedings. Breast milk or formula can be supplied intermittently using a syringe with gravity-controlled flow or can be given continuously using an infusion pump. The type of fluid instilled is recorded with every syringe change. The volume of the continuous feedings is recorded hourly, and the residual gastric aspirate is measured every 4 hours. Residuals of less than a quarter of a feeding can be refed to the infant to prevent the loss of gastric electrolytes. Feeding is stopped if the residual is greater than a quarter of the feeding and is not resumed until the infant can be assessed for a possible feeding intolerance (Townsend, Johnson & Hay, 1998).

The orogastric route for gavage feedings is preferred because most infants are preferential nose breathers. However, some infants do not tolerate oral tube placement. A small nasogastric feeding tube can be placed in older infants who would otherwise gag or vomit or in ones who are learning to suck (Townsend, Johnson & Hay, 1998). To insert the tube, the nurse should follow the sequence given in the Procedure box.

To begin the feeding, the nurse connects the barrel of a syringe to the gavage tube. While crimping the feeding tube, the nurse pours the specified amount of breast milk or formula into the syringe. The nurse then releases the crimp in the tube and allows the feeding to flow down by gravity (Fig. 27-7). The infant usually tolerates the feeding better if the rate approximates that of an oral feeding (about 1 ml/min). The parent or nurse can swaddle or hold the infant to help the infant associate the feeding with positive interactions

PROCEDURE

Inserting a Gavage Feeding Tube

1. Measure the length of the gavage tube:
   a. From the tip of the nose,
   b. To the lobe of the ear, and
   c. Down to the upper abdomen (Fig. 27-7, *A*).
2. Mark the tube with a piece of tape on the centimeter mark (average 16 to 18 cm), then:
   a. Lubricate the tip of the tube with sterile water.
   b. Insert gently (to avoid tissue trauma) through the mouth or nare (Fig. 27-7, *B*).
   c. Guide the tube down the esophagus until the predetermined mark is reached.
3. Correct placement of the tube can be checked before instilling any fluid by either:
   a. Injecting a small amount of air (1 to 3 ml) into the tube while simultaneously listening for sounds of gurgling or by using a stethoscope placed over the stomach area.
   b. Pulling back on the plunger to aspirate stomach contents to check for previous feeding or mucus. Lack of fluid is not necessarily evidence of improper placement.
4. Tape the tube in place and also tape it to the cheek to prevent accidental dislodgment and incorrect positioning (Fig. 27-7, *C*).
   a. Assess the infant's skin integrity before taping the tube.
   b. Edematous or very premature infants need to have a pectin barrier placed under the tape to prevent abrasions (Kuller & Lund, 1993).
5. Tube placement must be assessed before each feeding.
   a. Placement of the tube in the trachea will cause the infant to gag, cough, or become cyanotic (Townsend, Johnson & Hay, 1998).
   b. Aspiration of respiratory secretions may be mistaken for stomach contents (Metheny et al., 1994).
   c. Check the length of the tube, because it is possible to hear air entering the stomach even if the tube is positioned above the gastroesophageal (cardiac) sphincter

●

From Wong D: *Whaley & Wong's nursing care of infants and children,* ed 5, St Louis, 1995, Mosby.

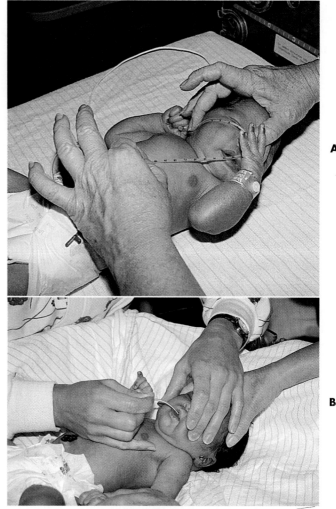

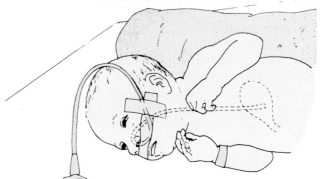

Fig. **27-7** Gavage feeding. **A,** Measurement of gavage feeding tube from tip of nose to earlobe and to midpoint between end of xyphoid process and umbilicus. Tape may be used to mark correct length on tube. **B,** Insertion of gavage tube using orogastric route. **C,** Indwelling gavage tube, nasogastric route. After feeding by orogastric or nasogastric tube, infant is propped on right side for 1 hour to facilitate emptying of stomach into small intestine. Note rolled towel for support. (**A** and **B** courtesy Marjorie Pyle, RNC, Lifecircle, Costa Mesa, Calif.)

(Lefrak-Okikawa & Meier, 1993). The parents are encouraged to talk to their infant during the feedings.

Once the prescribed volume has been delivered, the nurse crimps or pinches the tube and removes the syringe. The gavage tube is capped (or the nurse continues to pinch it) while removing it in one steady motion. Capping the tube (or pinching it off) prevents breast milk or formula from leaking from the tube and being aspirated during removal of the tube.

After the feeding, the infant is positioned to prevent aspiration. The documentation of the procedure includes the size of the feeding tube, the amount and quality of the residual from the previous feeding, the type and quantity of fluid instilled (sterile water, breast milk, or formula), and the infant's response to the procedure.

Gastrostomy feedings. Infants with certain congenital malformations require gastrostomy feedings. This involves the surgical placement of a tube through the skin of the abdomen into the stomach (Wong, 1995). The tube is then taped in an upright position to prevent trauma to the incision site. After the site heals, the nurse initiates small bolus feedings per the physician's orders (Fig. 27-8). Feedings by gravity are done slowly over 20 to 30 minutes. Special

care must be taken to prevent rapid bolusing of the fluid because this may lead to bloating, GI reflux into the esophagus, or respiratory compromise. Meticulous skin care at the tube insertion site is necessary to prevent skin breakdown or infections. In addition, intake and output are monitored scrupulously because these infants are initially prone to diarrhea until regular feedings are established.

Parenteral fluids. Feeding supplemental parenteral fluids is indicated for infants who are unable to obtain sufficient fluids or calories by enteral feeding (see Fig. 27-8). Some of these infants are dependent on total parenteral nutrition (TPN) for extensive periods. The nurse assesses and documents the following in infants receiving parenteral fluids or TPN:

- Type and infusion rate of the solution
- Functional status of the infusion equipment, including the tubing and infusion pump
- Infusion site for possible complications (phlebitis, infiltration, dislodgment)
- Caloric intake
- Infant's responses to therapy

The physician orders TPN per the hospital protocol. These orders must specify the electrolytes and nutrients

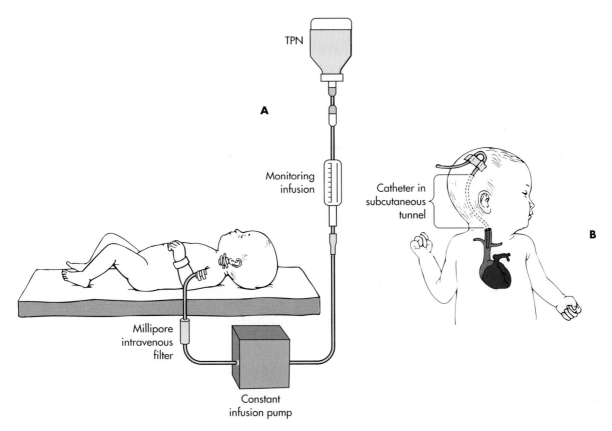

Fig. 27-8 A, Total parenteral nutrition (TPN). **B,** Close-up showing infusion site and internal placement of catheter into descending vena cava. Parenteral nutrition often is used in conjunction with other forms of feedings, particularly during weaning to oral feedings.

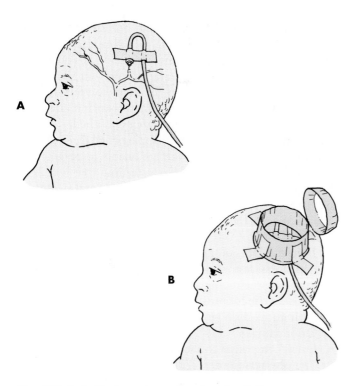

Fig. 27-9 **A,** Venipuncture of scalp vein. **B,** Paper cup protecting venipuncture site.

desired, as well as the volume and rate of infusion. The amounts of calories, protein, and fat are determined on the basis of the individual infant's energy needs (Price & Kalhan, 1993).

While caring for the infant receiving parenteral fluids or TPN, the nurse secures and protects the insertion site (Fig. 27-9). In addition to observing the principles of asepsis, the nurse must observe the principles of neonatal skin care (Kuller & Lund, 1993). The nurse should also inspect the infusion site for signs of infiltration and reposition the infant frequently to maintain body alignment and protect the site. Parents of infants need to be given explanations about TPN and the way in which the IV equipment and solutions affect their infant.

Advancing infant feedings. Feedings are advanced as assessment data and the infant's ability to tolerate the feedings warrant it. Documentation of a premature infant's sucking patterns can also be used to determine its readiness to nipple feed (Medoff-Cooper, Verklan & Carlson, 1993). Feedings are advanced from passive (parenteral and gavage) to active (nipple and breastfeeding). Infants with a cleft lip or palate who have a gastrostomy are often changed to nipple feedings once their deformity is repaired surgically. At each step, the nurse must carefully assess the infant's response to prevent overstressing the infant.

The infant receiving nutrition parenterally is gradually weaned off of this type of nutrition. To do this, the nourishment given by continuous or intermittent gavage feedings is increased while the parenteral fluids are decreased.

For all compromised infants, feedings are advanced slowly and cautiously because, if feedings are advanced too rapidly, the infant may experience vomiting (with an attendant risk of aspiration), diarrhea, abdominal distention, and apneic episodes. Rapid advancement of feedings may also cause fluid retention with cardiac compromise or a pronounced diuresis with hyponatremia.

If the infant needs additional calories, a commercial human milk fortifier can be added to the gavaged breast milk, or the number of calories per 30 ml of commercial formula can be increased. Soy and elemental formulas are used only for infants with very special dietary needs, such as allergies to cow's milk or chronic malabsorption (Townsend, Johnson & Hay, 1998). Calories in breast milk can be lost if the cream separates and adheres to the tubing during continuous infusion (Brennan-Brehm et al., 1994). This problem is decreased if microbore tubing is used for both continuous and intermittent gavage feedings.

The infant receiving gavage feedings progresses to bottle feeding or breast milk feedings. To do this, the gavage feedings are decreased as the infant's ability to suckle breast milk or formula improves. Often during this transition the infant is fed by both nipple and gavage feeding to ensure the intake of both the prescribed volume of food and nutrients. However, an increased respiratory effort is a documented problem in premature infants who have a gavage tube that is left in place during nipple feedings (Shiao et al., 1995), so nurses must watch for this. The parents need support during this transition because many families measure their parenting competence by how well they can feed their infant (Green, 1994).

As the time of discharge nears, the appropriate method of feeding, as well as the assessments pertaining to the method (e.g., tolerance of feedings, status of gavage tube placement), are reviewed with the parents. The parents should be encouraged to interact with the infant by talking and making eye contact with the infant during the feeding. This interaction is encouraged to stimulate the psychosocial development of the infant and to facilitate bonding and attachment (Haut, Peddicord & O'Brien, 1994; Oehler, Hannan & Catlett, 1993).

Nonnutritive sucking. If the infant is nourished by the gavage or the parenteral route, **nonnutritive sucking** is encouraged (Fig. 27-10) for several reasons. One is that allowing the infant to suckle on a pacifier during gavage or between oral feedings may improve oxygenation. In addition, such nonnutritive sucking may lead to a decreased energy expenditure with less restlessness and promote faster attachment to the nipple when oral feedings are initiated (Lefrak-Okikawa & Meier, 1993; Pickler & Terrell 1994). Mothers of premature infants should be encouraged to let their premature infants start sucking at the breast during kangaroo care because some infant's suck-and-swallow reflexes may be coordinated as early as 32 weeks' gestation.

Infants with IUGR may have an age-appropriate sucking reflex but require thermoregulatory support, making it

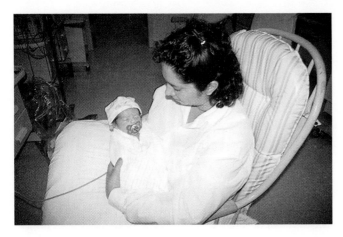

Fig. **27-10** Nonnutritive sucking by infant. (Courtesy Marjorie Pyle, RNC, Lifecircle, Costa Mesa, Calif.)

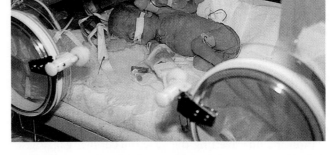

Fig. **27-11** Ventilator-dependent infant. (Courtesy Marjorie Pyle, RNC, Lifecircle, Costa Mesa, Calif.)

difficult to breastfeed. These infants may also benefit from nonnutritive sucking at the breast for short periods.

Developmental and emotional care

All infants and their families have developmental and emotional needs. However, the events in the compromised infant's life are distinctly different from those of the healthy term infant, and each challenge faced by the infant also affects the family. Whenever an infant shows increased physical distress (oxygen desaturations), the family members are affected in turn by such things as the resulting potential for more medical procedures or a longer hospital stay. The size of premature infants frequently distresses families, who cannot relate as well to other care issues of their infant, such as routine diaper changes, because they are focused on how tiny and fragile the infant appears.

Besides these factors, the infant's vision may be altered by respiratory equipment or a phototherapy mask, making it difficult for the infant to interact with caregivers and family members (Fig. 27-11). The infant may also be unable to establish diurnal and nocturnal rhythms because of the continuous exposure to overhead lighting. In addition, sedation or pain medications affect the way in which the infant perceives the environment.

Infants in NICUs are also exposed to high levels of auditory input from the various machine alarms, and this can have adverse effects (Fig. 27-12). In addition, continuous noise levels of 45 to 85 decibels (db) are common in NICUs. An incubator alone produces a constant noise level of 60 to 80 db (Haubrich, 1993), and each new piece of life-support equipment used adds another 20 db to the background noise (Strauch, Brandt & Edwards-Beckett, 1993). The infant's hearing may be damaged if it is exposed to a constant decibel level of 90 db or frequent decibel swings higher than 110 db.

An additional concern in the care of compromised infants is that environmental hazards can be potentiated

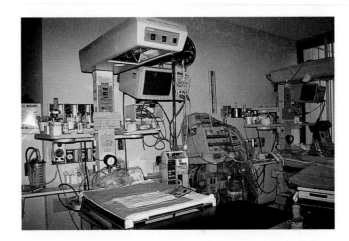

Fig. **27-12** Significant environmental stimulation. Note bed, wall oxygen attachments, monitor, ventilator, incubator, and pumps, all of which have alarm systems. (Courtesy Marjorie Pyle, RNC, Lifecircle, Costa Mesa, Calif.)

by some drugs used for infant therapy. Diuretics (especially furosemide [Lasix]), antibiotics (gentamicin), and antimalarial agents can potentiate noise-induced hearing loss (Haubrich, 1993). Therefore routine hearing screening should be performed in all infants before discharge, with universal screening completed by no later than the third month of life (National Institutes of Health, 1993).

Parents of compromised infants must learn their new infant's special characteristics and needs under the close supervision of the nursery staff while their infant copes with his or her illness or physical deformities. At times they may become confused or frustrated as their infant's condition improves one day and regresses the next. Other parents may have to cope with the death of their infant. Constant support from all staff members from admission through discharge can help families get through this highly stressful and emotional time.

Infant communication. Infants communicate their needs and ability to tolerate sensory stimulation through physiologic responses. The nurses and parents of these compromised infants must therefore be alert to such cues. Although full-term infants may thrive on stimulation, this same stimulation in compromised infants can instead provoke physical symptoms of stress and anxiety (Blackburn & VandenBerg, 1993; Gardner & Lubchenco, 1998). Armed with a knowledge of normal gestational age responses, and by frequently assessing such infants, the nurse can recognize the developmental and emotional needs of even the tiniest infant.

Problems with noxious stimuli and barriers to normal contact may cause anxiety and tension. Clues to overstimulation include averting the gaze, hiccuping, gagging, or regurgitating food. Term infants exhibit a startle reflex, and premature infants move all of their limbs in an uncoordinated fashion in response to noxious stimuli. An irregular respiratory rate or an increased heart rate may develop in severely distressed infants, and they may then be unable to regain a calm state.

A relaxed infant state is indicated by stabilization of vital signs, closed eyes, and a relaxed posture. Nonintubated infants may make soothing verbal sounds when they are relaxed. Infants requiring artificial ventilation cannot cry audibly and often show their distress through posturing; they then relax once their needs are met. Pinyard (1994) recommends evaluating an infant's cry as part of a developmental assessment, because specific cry sounds have been correlated with certain behavioral responses. As compromised infants heal and mature, they increasingly respond to stimuli in a self-regulated manner rather than with a dissociated response. Infants who do not show increased self-regulation should be evaluated for a neurologic problem.

Infant stimulation. A neonatal individualized developmental care and assessment program (NIDCAP) routinely integrates aspects of neurodevelopmental theory with caregivers' observations, environmental interventions, and parental support (Blackburn & VandenBerg, 1993; Gardner & Lubchenco, 1998). Routine reassessment is built into the program's design. Developmental stimuli may consist of such simple measures as placing a waterbed on the top of the infant's mattress or kangaroo (skin-to-skin) holding. The simplest calming technique is to contain the infant's extremities close to the body using both hands. The care of the infant is organized to allow extended periods of undisturbed rest and sleep. Pain medications or sedatives should be administered consistently, per the unit's protocol.

Data from studies examining the effects of high-intensity lighting suggest that there is a link between exposure to background nursery light and the occurrence of retinopathy of prematurity. More significantly, infants exposed to a diurnal light pattern show better neuromuscular integration (Blackburn & VandenBerg, 1993). For this reason, there should be routine periods of diminished

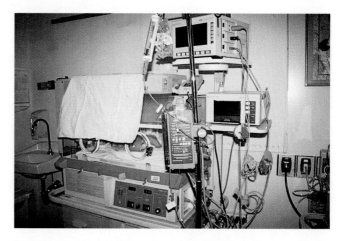

Fig. **27-13** Infant in doubled-walled incubator with a blanket for a light shield. (Courtesy Marjorie Pyle, RNC, Lifecircle, Costa Mesa, Calif.)

lighting in neonatal units to provide infants with a more normal environment. A folded blanket can also be arranged over the incubator to shield the infant from bright overhead lights (Fig. 27-13).

In the nursery, conversation and noise are minimized. This includes setting items gently on the incubator (such as formula bottles, charts, and other equipment) and not slamming the porthole doors. A "do not disturb" sign can be placed on the incubator as a reminder. The volume of mechanical alarms and overhead paging systems should also be monitored. The institution of a quiet hour is one way to reduce the amount of noise infants are exposed to on a busy unit.

Infants acquire a sense of trust as they learn the feel, sound, and smell of their parents (Gardner & Lubchenco, 1998). Compromised infants must also learn to trust their caregivers to obtain comfort. However, because caregivers in the nursery may also inflict pain as part of the care they must give, some compromised infants may not learn to trust as readily as a healthy infant. For this reason, it is important for both the parents and the caregivers of such infants to employ comforting interventions such as removing painful stimuli, stopping hunger, and changing wet or soiled clothing to foster trust (Green, 1994).

When the infant is ready for stimulation, the nurse has many options. All infants can tolerate being held, even if only for short periods. Additional ways for the nurse or parents to stimulate infants include cuddling, rocking, singing, and talking to the infant (Fig. 27-14). These activities are beneficial, especially during feedings. Stroking the infant's skin during medical therapy can provide tactile stimulation. The caregiver responds to the infant's cues by offering reassurance, providing for nonnutritive sucking, stroking the infant's back, and talking to the infant.

Mobiles and decals that can be changed frequently may also be placed within the infant's visual range to stimulate

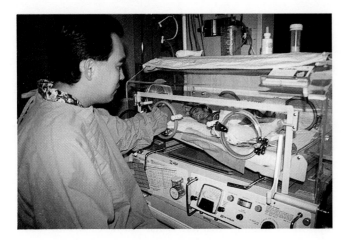

Fig. 27-14 A father caresses his tiny preterm infant in the NICU. (Courtesy Marjorie Pyle, RNC, Lifecircle, Costa Mesa, Calif.).

the infant visually. Wind-up musical toys provide rhythmic distractions as long as they are not too loud. If the infant is receiving phototherapy, the protective eye patches are removed periodically (e.g., during feeding) so that the infant can see the caregiver's face for short, comforting sessions.

Kangaroo care. Kangaroo care (skin-to-skin holding) helps premature infants to directly interact with their parents. In this technique the infant, dressed only in a diaper, is placed directly on the parent's bare chest and then covered with the parent's clothing or a warmed blanket (Fig. 27-15). In this way, the parent's body temperature also functions as an external heat source that enhances the infant's temperature regulation (Gale, Franck & Lund, 1993). Even ventilator-dependent infants weighing under 1 kg have been found to benefit from this measure, although they usually tolerate it for only 30 minutes or less at a time.

Kangaroo holding was originally developed in Bogota, Colombia, where radiant warmers and incubators were in severely short supply. Although such care has its roots in severe economic hardships, it stems from a deep respect for natural processes. Infants and parents who participate in such kangaroo care have been observed to have dramatically better outcomes (Affonso et al., 1993). The mothers report increased breast milk output and fewer feelings of helplessness related to their experiences in the NICU. The infants have been found to maintain their temperatures and oxygenation levels better and to experience fewer episodes of crying, apnea, and periodic respirations. They have also been observed to be alert and quiet longer and to have slightly higher heart rates. Kangaroo care also meets developmental needs by fostering neurobehavioral development (Ludington-Hoe & Swinth, 1996).

Positioning. The positioning of infants plays an important role in the effectiveness of care. For instance, positioning an infant in a nest or with rolls is very beneficial in

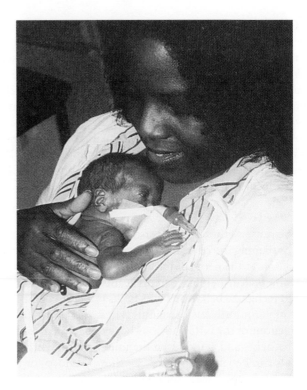

Fig. 27-15 Kangaroo care. Parent wraps her shirt around the infant. (From Gale G et al.: Skin-to-skin holding of the intubated premature infant, *Neonatal Netw* 12[6]:51, 1993.)

reducing stress. It does so by providing defined boundaries, which helps the infant acquire organizational skills (Oehler et al., 1996). In addition, it promotes the proper body alignment that is necessary to prevent developmental problems that may prevent walking as the child matures. Positioning the infant in a side-lying fetal position or prone with both legs tucked up close to the abdomen gives the infant a sense of security. Teaching parents the various ways to position the infant and to do so in an organized and composed manner supports their sense of autonomy and provides them with the skills necessary for assessing their infant's cues after discharge (Oehler, Hannan & Catlett, 1993).

Parents are often concerned about the head molding that occurs in premature infants. Chan, Kelley, and Khan (1993) investigated the effectiveness of a water mattress placed under the infant's head in preventing this phenomenon but concluded that such relief of pressure on the baby's head would not completely alter the outcome. There needs to be further research on the effectiveness of positioning in alleviating this problem.

Parent education

Cardiopulmonary resuscitation. Sudden infant death syndrome (SIDS) is 8 to 10 times more likely to develop in preterm infants than in term infants. Furthermore, it has been found that infants discharged from an

NICU are about twice as likely to die unexpectedly during the first year of life as infants in the general population. Instruction in cardiopulmonary resuscitation (CPR) is essential for parents of all infants but especially for those of infants at risk for life-threatening events (see Chapter 20). Infants considered at risk include those who are premature, have apnea or bradycardia spells, or have a tendency to choke (Wright, Norton & Kesten, 1989). Before taking their infant home, parents must be able to administer CPR. All parents should be encouraged to obtain instruction in CPR at their local Red Cross or other community agency.

Parental support

The nurse as the support person and teacher is responsible for shaping the environment and making the caregiving responsive to the needs of the parents and infant. Nurses are instrumental in helping parents learn who their infant is and to recognize behavioral cues in his or her development.

If preterm birth has been anticipated, the family can be given a tour of the NICU or shown a video to prepare them for the sights and activities of the unit. After the birth, the parents can be given a booklet, be shown a video, or have someone describe what they will see when they go to the unit to see their infant. As soon as possible, the parents should see and touch their infant so that they can begin to acknowledge the reality of the birth and the infant's true appearance and condition. They will need encouragement as they begin to accomplish the psychologic tasks imposed by the preterm birth. For the following reasons, a nurse or physician should be present during the parents' first visit to see the infant:

- To help them "see" the infant rather than focus on the equipment. The importance and purpose of the apparatus that surrounds their infant should also be explained to them
- To explain the characteristics normal for an infant of their baby's gestational age. In this way parents do not compare their child with a full-term, healthy infant
- To encourage the parents to express their feelings about the pregnancy, labor, and birth and the experience of having a preterm infant
- To assess the parents' perceptions of the infant to determine the appropriate time for them to become actively involved in care

Parents who have negative feelings about the pregnancy or the infant need support and may benefit from participation in groups or from counseling. Their feelings should be acknowledged as valid, including the financial and emotional burden they are experiencing and their understandable feelings toward the infant.

As soon as possible after the birth, the parents are given the opportunity to meet the infant in the *en face* position, to touch the infant, and to see his or her favorable characteristics. As soon as possible, depending primarily on her physical condition, the mother is encouraged to visit the nursery as desired and help with the infant's care. When the family cannot be present physically, staff members devise appropriate methods to keep them in almost constant touch with the newborn, such as with daily phone calls, notes written as if by the infant, or photographs of the infant.

Some hospitals have support groups for the parents of infants in NICUs. These groups help parents experiencing anxiety and grief by encouraging them to share their feelings. Hospitals also often arrange to have an experienced NICU parent make contact with a new group member to provide additional support. The volunteer parents provide support by making hospital visits, phone calls, and home visits (Lindsay et al., 1993).

Many NICUs use volunteers in varying capacities. After they have gone through the orientation program, volunteers can perform tasks such as holding the infants, stocking bedside cabinets, assembling parent packets, and, in some nurseries, feeding the infants.

Some preterm infants can be discharged earlier than the expected time. The criteria showing an infant's readiness for early discharge are that the infant's physiologic condition is stable, the infant is receiving adequate nutrition, and the infant's body temperature is stable. The parents, or other caregivers, also need to exhibit a physical, emotional, and educational readiness to assume responsibility for the care of the infant. Ideally, the home environment is adequate for meeting the needs of the infant. The parents also need to show that they know the way to take the infant's temperature, know the signs and symptoms to report, and understand the dietary needs of the infant (Brooten, 1995). The nurse's assessment, counseling, and teaching skills are invaluable for ensuring the success of the home care of infants after early hospital discharge.

Anticipatory grief. Families experience anticipatory grief when they are told of the impending death of their infant (Nichols, 1993). Parents who have an infant with a debilitating disease (with or without a congenital deformity), but one that may not necessarily threaten the life of the child, may also experience anticipatory grief. An alteration in relationships, a change in lifestyle, and a very real threat to their hopes and dreams for the future may affect the day-to-day interaction of the family with their infant and the staff (Loizeaux, 1993; Mehren, 1991). Nurses should help facilitate the family's grieving process. If the nurse observes that a family member's day-to-day interactions with the infant change, the nurse should assess the situation and request psychosocial support or intervention by a chaplain or social worker, if necessary.

Loss of an infant. Parents who know their infant is going to die experience a very difficult time. Before the infant's death, the parents need to direct their attention, energy, and caregiving activities toward the dying infant.

However, some parents find it difficult to visit their infant even for short periods once a terminal diagnosis has been made. Grandparents also grieve but often are unsure how to comfort their own child (the infant's parent) during the period of impending death. Health care professionals can help by involving the family in the infant's care, providing privacy, answering questions, and preparing them for the inevitability of the death.

Intensive care nurseries consist of multiple-bed rooms, making a family's grief a very public event. A designated private family room with technical support available allows the entire grieving family to have time to make their initial farewells out of the public eye. The staff must be prepared for the expression of a variety of grief reactions ranging from anger to copious weeping.

There may not be time for parents to anticipate the loss. Such parents may experience a delayed grief response. Contributing to this is the fact that at the time of death parents are being asked to make decisions immediately regarding organ donation, autopsy, and funeral arrangements—things they might never have had to think of before. Because of their unpreparedness, they may react by simply refusing to discuss these issues.

Certain special circumstances also affect the parents' responses (Harrigan et al., 1993). For instance, if one or more of the infants of a multifetal pregnancy die, even if at least one is expected to live, parents may act as if all of the infants are alive or dead. One reason for their denial of the infant's death may be that it causes them to lose the special status society accords the parents of twins or triplets. For weeks such parents may continue to speak of all of their children in the present tense to family and friends who have not seen the babies. Parents of infants who die during transport to another facility may also find it difficult to accept the event as a reality. The nursing staff must therefore provide every opportunity for the parents to see their infant and grieve for it (see Chapter 25).

The physical and emotional trauma felt by the families of infants who have died may have a debilitating effect and prolong their grief (Klaus & Kennell, 1993). They may desire to avoid the terrible acknowledgment that their infant is dead. This can cause them to suffer a low-level clinical depression that can be more pronounced if the mother has endured additional crises related to the pregnancy and postpartum period. The death of an infant is also made more difficult to accept by the fact that it violates one of the basic laws of nature—that parents should precede their children in death. Follow-up of the family after any death is therefore important to determine the family's well-being and their need for referral and support.

Parents of infants who have died face other issues as well, such as how to continue to function in the role of parent. Coping with one's grief while parenting and explaining the death to surviving children can be extremely difficult for bereaved parents (Loizeaux, 1993; Mehren, 1991). However, the physical, emotional, and social responses to grief that parents experience gradually diminish as they begin to reenter and become more involved in the events of everyday life.

The nursing staff also experiences grief (Downey et al., 1993). Many primary staff nurses find themselves grieving as if the infant were their own because they often have been the primary caregiver for weeks, or even months. Managers and other staff members must acknowledge this grief. Talking about the infant or attending the funeral may help the affected staff members resolve their feelings about the infant's death.

Evaluation

The nurse uses the previously stated expected outcomes of care to evaluate the effectiveness of the physical and psychosocial aspects of care (see Plan of Care).

COMPLICATIONS COMMON TO PRETERM INFANTS

Respiratory Distress Syndrome

Respiratory distress syndrome (RDS) refers to a lung disorder usually affecting premature infants. Maternal and fetal conditions associated with a decreased severity of RDS include female infant, African-American race, maternal pregnancy-induced hypertension, maternal drug abuse, maternal steroid therapy (betamethasone), chronic retroplacental abruption, prolonged rupture of membranes, and IUGR (Korones & Bada-Ellzey, 1993). The incidence and severity of RDS increase with a decrease in the gestational age. Perinatal asphyxia, hypovolemia, male infant, white race, maternal diabetes (types 1 and 2), second-born twin, familial predisposition, maternal hypotension, cesarean birth without labor, hydrops fetalis, and third-trimester bleeding are all factors that place an infant at increased risk for RDS (Avery, Fletcher & Macdonald, 1994; Goetzman & Wennberg, 1991; Korones & Bada-Ellzey, 1993). The incidence of RDS in infants born between 26 and 28 weeks' gestation is approximately 50%, whereas the incidence in infants born at 30 to 31 weeks' gestation is approximately 25% (Avery, Fletcher & MacDonald, 1994; Gomella, Cunningham & Eyal, 1994).

RDS is caused by a lack of pulmonary surfactant, which leads to progressive atelectasis, loss of functional residual capacity, and a ventilation-perfusion imbalance with an uneven distribution of ventilation. This surfactant deficiency may be caused by insufficient surfactant production, abnormal composition and function, disruption of surfactant production, or a combination of these factors. The sequence of events that occurs is further compromised by the weak respiratory muscles and an overly compliant chest wall common to premature infants. Lung capacity is further compromised by the presence of proteinaceous material and

PLAN OF CARE *High-Risk Premature Newborn*

NURSING DIAGNOSIS Ineffective breathing pattern related to pulmonary and neuromuscular immaturity, decreased energy, fatigue

Expected Outcome *Infant exhibits adequate oxygenation (i.e., ABGs and acid-base within normal limits [WNL], oxygen saturations 92% or greater, respiratory rate and pattern WNL, breath sounds clear, absence of grunting, nasal flaring, minimal retractions, skin color WNL).*

Nursing Interventions/*Rationales*

Position neonate prone or supine, avoiding neck hyperextension *to promote optimum air exchange.* Use a side-lying position after feeding or in cases of excessive mucus production *to avoid aspiration.* Avoid Trendelenburg's position *as it can cause increased intracranial pressure and reduce lung capacity.*

Suction nasopharynx, trachea, and endotracheal tube as indicated *to remove mucus.* Avoid oversuctioning *as it can cause bronchospasm, bradycardia, hypoxia, and predispose neonate to intraventricular hemorrhage.*

Administer percussion, vibration, and postural drainage as prescribed *to facilitate drainage of secretions.*

Administer oxygen and monitor neonatal response *to maintain oxygen saturation.*

Maintain a neutral thermal environment *to conserve oxygen use.*

Monitor arterial blood gases, acid-base balance, oxygen saturation, respiratory rate and pattern, breath sounds, airway patency; observe for grunting, nasal flaring, retractions, cyanosis *to detect signs of respiratory distress.*

NURSING DIAGNOSIS Ineffective thermoregulation related to immature temperature regulation and minimal subcutaneous fat stores

Expected Outcome *Infant exhibits maintenance of stable body temperature within normal range for postconceptional age (36.5° to 37.2° C).*

Nursing Interventions/*Rationales*

Place neonate in a prewarmed radiant warmer *to maintain stable temperature.*

Place temperature probe on neonatal abdomen *to control heat levels in radiant warmer.*

Take axillary temperature periodically *to monitor temperature and cross-check functioning of warmer unit.*

Avoid infant exposure to cool air and drafts, cold scales, cold stethoscopes, cold examination tables, prolonged bathing *that predispose the infant to heat loss.*

Monitor probe frequently *as detachment can cause overheating or warmer-induced hyperthermia.*

Transfer infant to a servocontrolled open warmer bed or incubator *when temperature has stabilized.*

NURSING DIAGNOSIS Risk for infection related to immature immune system

Expected Outcome *Infant exhibits no evidence of nosocomial infection.*

Nursing Interventions/*Rationales*

Institute scrupulous handwashing techniques before and after handling neonate, ensure all supplies and/or equipment are clean before use, ensure strict aseptic technique with invasive procedures *to minimize exposure to infective organisms.*

Prevent contact with persons who have communicable infections and instruct parents in infection control procedures *to minimize infection risk.*

Administer prescribed antibiotics *to provide coverage for infection during sepsis workup.*

Continuously monitor vital signs for stability *as instability, hypothermia, or prolonged temperature elevations serve as indicators for infection.*

NURSING DIAGNOSIS Risk for nutrition alteration less than body requirements related to inability to ingest nutrients secondary to immaturity

Expected Outcome *Infant receives adequate amount of nutrients with sufficient caloric intake to maintain positive nitrogen balance; demonstrates steady weight gain.*

Nursing Interventions/*Rationales*

Administer parenteral fluid/total parenteral nutrition (TPN) as prescribed to provide adequate nutrition and fluid intake.

Monitor for signs of intolerance to TPN, *which can interfere with effective replenishment of nutrients.*

Periodically assess readiness to orally feed (i.e., strong suck, swallow, and gag reflexes) *to provide appropriate transition for TPN to oral feeding as soon as neonate is ready.*

Advance volume and concentration of formula when orally feeding per unit protocol *to avoid overfeeding and feeding intolerance.*

If mother desires to breastfeed when neonate is stable, demonstrate how to express milk *to establish and maintain lactation until infant can breastfeed.*

PLAN OF CARE *High-Risk Premature Newborn—cont'd*

> **NURSING DIAGNOSIS** Risk for fluid volume deficit/excess related to immature physiology

Expected Outcome *Infant exhibits evidence of fluid hemostasis.*

Nursing Interventions/*Rationales*

Administer parenteral fluids as prescribed and regulate carefully *to maintain fluid balance.* Avoid hypertonic fluids such as undiluted medications, concentrated glucose, *as they can cause excess solute load on immature kidneys.*

Implement strategies (use of plastic covers and increase of ambient humidity) *that minimize insensible water loss.*

Monitor hydration status (i.e., skin turgor, blood pressure, edema, weight, mucous membranes, fontanels, urine specific gravity, electrolytes) and intake and output *to evaluate for evidence of dehydration or overhydration.*

> **NURSING DIAGNOSIS** Risk for impaired skin integrity related to immature skin structure, immobility, invasive procedures

Expected Outcome *Infant's skin remains intact with no evidence of irritation or injury.*

Nursing Interventions/*Rationales*

Cleanse skin as needed with plain warm water and apply moisturizing agents to skin *to prevent dryness and reduce friction across skin surface.*

When performing procedures: minimize use of tape and apply a skin barrier between tape and skin; use transparent elastic film for securing central and peripheral lines; use limb electrodes for monitoring or attach with hydrogel and rotate electrodes frequently; remove adhesives with soap and water rather than alcohol or acetone-based adhesive removers *to minimize skin damage.*

Monitor use of thermal devices such as warmers or heating pads carefully *to prevent burns.*

Monitor skin closely for evidence of redness, rash, irritation, bruising, breakdown, ischemia, infiltration *to detect and treat potential complications early.*

> **NURSING DIAGNOSIS** Risk for injury related to increased intracranial pressure and intraventricular hemorrhage secondary to immature central nervous system

Expected Outcome *Infant will exhibit normal intracranial pressure (ICP) with no evidence of intraventricular hemorrhage.*

Nursing Interventions/*Rationales*

Institute minimum stimulation protocol (i.e., minimal handling, clustering care techniques, avoidance of sudden head movements to one side, undisturbed sleep periods, light variations to simulate day and night, limiting personnel and equipment noise in environment) *to decrease stress responses, which can increase ICP.*

Institute ordered pharmacologic and nonpharmacologic pain control methods *to manage pain and reduce physical stress.*

Avoid hypertonic solutions and medications *as they increase cerebral blood flow.*

Elevate head of bed 15 to 20 degrees *to decrease ICP.*

Monitor vital signs *for evidence of ICP.*

Recognize signs of overstimulation (i.e., flaccidity, yawning, irritability, crying, staring, active averting) *so stimulation can be stopped to allow rest.*

> **NURSING DIAGNOSIS** Altered parenting related to separation and interruption of parent/infant attachment secondary to premature birth

Expected Outcome *Parents establish contact with neonate; demonstrate competent parenting skills and willingness to care for neonate.*

Nursing Interventions/*Rationales*

Before parents' first visit to the NICU, prepare them by explaining what the neonate will look like, what the equipment will look like and its function *to diminish fear and decrease sense of shock.*

Keep parents informed about infant's condition (improvements and setbacks) and important aspects of infant's care; encourage and answer parental questions; actively listen to parent concerns *to establish trust, open communication, and caring atmosphere to aid in coping.*

Encourage parents to visit the NICU often; to name infant; to touch, hold, or caress infant as physical condition permits; to be actively involved in infant's care; to bring personal items (i.e., clothing, stuffed animals, or pictures of family) *to allow for formation of emotional bond.*

Reinforce parent involvement and praise care endeavors *to increase self-confidence in their contribution.*

Encourage parents to bring other siblings to visit; explain to siblings what they are seeing; encourage siblings to draw pictures or write letters for infant and place in or near infant's crib *to promote family involvement, help ease sibling fears, and let them contribute to infant's care.*

Refer parents to social services as needed *to ensure comprehensive care.*

From Wong D & Perry S: *Maternal child nursing care,* St Louis, 1998, Mosby.

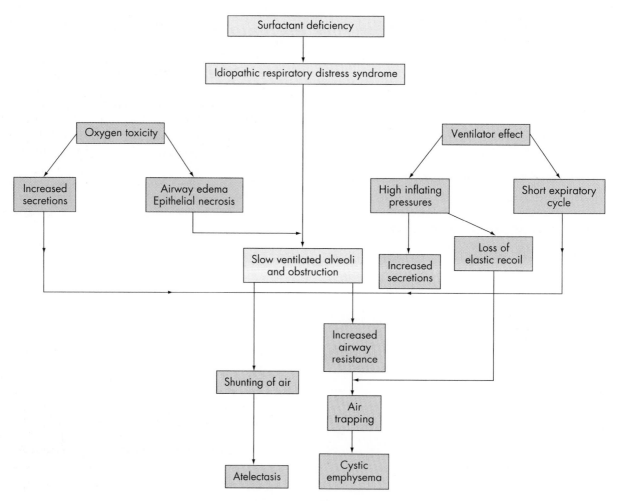

Fig. **27-16** Pathogenesis of respiratory distress syndrome (RDS). (From Merenstein G & Gardner S: *Handbook of neonatal intensive care,* ed 4, St Louis, 1998, Mosby.)

epithelial debris in the airways. The resulting decreased oxygenation, cyanosis, and metabolic or respiratory acidosis can cause the pulmonary vascular resistance (PVR) to be increased. This increased PVR can lead to right-to-left shunting and a reopening of the ductus arteriosus and foramen ovale (Avery, Fletcher & MacDonald, 1994; Gomella, Cunningham & Eyal, 1994) (Fig. 27-16).

Clinical symptoms of RDS are listed in Box 27-5. These respiratory symptoms usually appear immediately after birth or within 6 hours of birth. Physical examination reveals crackles, poor air exchange, pallor, the use of accessory muscles (retractions), and occasionally apnea. Radiographic findings include a uniform reticulogranular appearance and air bronchograms (Avery, Fletcher & MacDonald, 1994; Fanaroff & Martin, 1997; Gomella, Cunningham & Eyal, 1994). The infant's clinical course typically is variable. There is usually an increased oxygen requirement and increased respiratory effort as atelectasis, a loss of functional residual capacity, and ventilation-perfusion imbalance worsen.

However, RDS is a self-limiting disease, with the respiratory symptoms abating after 72 hours. This disappearance of respiratory symptoms coincides with the production of surfactant in the type 2 cells of the alveoli.

The treatment for RDS is supportive. Adequate ventilation and oxygenation must be established and maintained in an attempt to prevent ventilation-perfusion mismatch and atelectasis. Exogenous surfactant may be administered at birth or shortly after birth, and this has the effect of altering the typical course of RDS. Positive-pressure ventilation, CPAP, and oxygen therapy may be needed during the respiratory illness. However, the prevention of complications associated with mechanical ventilation is also critical. These complications include pulmonary interstitial emphysema, pneumothorax, pneumomediastinum, and pneumopericardium. The mortality and morbidity rates associated with RDS are attributed to the immature organ systems of the infant and the complications associated with the treatment of the disease (Avery, Fletcher & MacDonald, 1994; Fanaroff & Martin, 1997; Gomella, Cunningham & Eyal, 1994).

BOX 27-5	Clinical Signs of Respiratory Distress Syndrome

Tachypnea
Grunting
Flaring
Retractions
Cyanosis
Increased work of breathing
Hypercapnia
Respiratory or mixed acidosis
Hypotension and shock

TABLE 27-2	Normal Arterial Blood Gas Values for Neonates

VALUE	RANGE
pH	7.33-7.42
Arterial oxen pressure (PaO_2)	50-80 mm Hg
Carbon dioxide pressure ($PaCO_2$)	38-48 mm Hg
Bicarbonate (HCO_3)	20-24 mEq/L
Oxygen saturation	>90%

From Dickason E, Silverman B & Kaplan J: *Maternal-infant nursing care,* ed 3, St Louis, 1998, Mosby.

Acid-base balance is evaluated by monitoring the ABG values (Table 27-2). Frequent blood sampling requires arterial access accomplished either by umbilical artery catheterization or by a peripheral arterial line. Pulse oximetry and transcutaneous carbon dioxide and oxygen monitors document trends in ventilation and oxygenation. Capillary blood gas values indicate the pH and PCO_2 status in infants who are in a more stable condition (Cloherty & Stark, 1997).

The maintenance of an NTE continues to be of critical importance in infants with RDS because infants suffering from hypoxemia are unable to increase their metabolic rate when cold stressed (Fanaroff & Martin, 1997).

The clinical and radiographic presentation (radiodense lung fields and air bronchograms) of neonatal pneumonia may be similar to that of RDS. Fluid in the minor tissue may also be noted in infants with neonatal pneumonia. Therefore sepsis evaluation, including blood culture, complete blood count (CBC) with differential, and occasionally a lumbar puncture, is done in infants with RDS to rule out neonatal pneumonia. Broad-spectrum antibiotics are begun while the results of cultures are awaited (Avery, Fletcher & Macdonald, 1994; Cloherty & Stark, 1997).

Fluid and nutrition need to be maintained in the critically ill infant with RDS. Parenteral nutrition can be implemented to provide protein and fats to promote a positive nitrogen balance. Daily monitoring of the electrolyte values, urinary output, specific gravity, and weight help evaluate the infant's hydration status (Cloherty & Stark, 1997; Fanaroff & Martin, 1997).

The need for frequent blood sampling may make blood transfusions necessary. The critically ill infant usually needs to have a venous hematocrit level of more than 40% to maintain adequate oxygen-carrying capacity (Fanaroff & Martin, 1997).

NURSE ALERT *Directed-donor blood has become more frequently requested. This is donor blood usually obtained from a family member or close friend of the family who has the same blood type as the infant or a compatible blood type. It may be necessary to notify the infant's family of the potential need for blood transfusion on admission to allow for the processing of directed-donor blood.*

Reassuring the family that stringent testing of all blood products is done may alleviate some of their anxiety about the transmission of blood-borne pathogens. Because some religions prohibit the use of blood transfusions, it is critical to obtain a complete history from the family, including their religious preference. Alternative strategies for maintaining the hematocrit may need to be employed in these instances.

Complications Associated with Oxygen Therapy

Retinopathy of prematurity

Retinopathy of prematurity (ROP) is a complex multi-causal disorder that affects the developing retinal vessels of premature infants. The normal retinal vessels begin to form in utero at approximately 16 weeks in response to an unknown stimulus. These vessels continue to develop until they reach maturity at approximately 42 to 43 weeks' post-conception. Once the retina is completely vascularized, the retinal vessels are not susceptible to ROP. The mechanism of injury in ROP is unclear. Oxygen tensions that are too high for the level of retinal maturity initially result in vasoconstriction. After oxygen therapy is discontinued, neovascularization occurs in the retina and vitreous, with capillary hemorrhages, fibrotic resolution, and possible retinal detachment. Cicatricial (scar) tissue formation and consequent visual impairment may be mild or severe. The entire disease process in severe cases may take as long as 5 months to evolve. Examination by an ophthalmologist before discharge and a schedule for repeat examinations thereafter are recommended for the parents' guidance.

The key to the management of ROP is prevention and early detection of premature birth. Circumferential cryopexy, laser photocoagulation, vitamin E therapy, and decreasing the intensity of ambient light are used in the treatment of ROP, with varying results (Fanaroff & Martin, 1997; Gomella, Cunningham & Eyal, 1994).

Bronchopulmonary dysplasia

Bronchopulmonary dysplasia (BPD) is a chronic pulmonary condition affecting infants who have experienced respiratory failure; been oxygen dependent for more than

28 days, with therapy continued beyond 36 weeks of post-conceptional age; show abnormal radiographic findings with areas of overinflation and areas of atelectasis; or exhibit respiratory symptoms (Avery, Fletcher & MacDonald, 1994; Lund, 1990). The etiology of BDP is multifactorial and includes pulmonary immaturity, surfactant deficiency, lung injury and stretch, barotrauma, inflammation caused by oxygen exposure, and a genetic predisposition (Gomella, Cunningham & Eyal, 1994; Knoppert & Mackanjee, 1994; Lund, 1990).

Clinical symptoms of BPD include tachypnea, retractions, nasal flaring, increased work of breathing, and tachycardia. Auscultation of the lung fields in affected infants typically reveals crackles, decreased air movement, and occasionally expiratory wheezing (Gomella, Cunningham & Eyal, 1994). The treatment for BPD includes oxygen therapy, nutrition, fluid restriction, and medications (diuretics, corticosteroids, bronchodilators). However, the key to the management of BPD is prevention by preventing prematurity and RDS and by using less toxic therapies.

The prognosis for infants with BPD depends on the degree of pulmonary dysfunction. Most deaths occur within the first year of life as a result of cardiorespiratory failure, sepsis, or respiratory infection; in some infants the deaths are sudden and unexplained (Gomella, Cunningham & Eyal, 1994).

Patent ductus arteriosus

The ductus arteriosus is a normal muscular contractile structure in the fetus connecting the left pulmonary artery and the dorsal aorta. The duct constricts after birth as oxygenation, the levels of circulating prostaglandins, and the muscle mass increase. Other factors that promote ductal closure include catecholamines, low pH, bradykinin, and acetylcholine (Korones & Bada-Ellzey, 1993). When the fetal ductus arteriosus fails to close after birth, **patent ductus arteriosus (PDA)** occurs. The incidence of PDA in premature infants weighing less than 1,500 gm is 40% to 60%, with an increased percentage of cases occurring in premature infants weighing less than 1,000 gm (Gomella, Cunningham & Eyal, 1994).

The clinical presentation in an infant with a PDA includes systolic murmur, active precordium, bounding peripheral pulses, tachycardia, tachypnea, crackles, and hepatomegaly. The systolic murmur is heard best at the second or third intercostal space at the upper left sternal border. An active precordium is caused by an increased left ventricular stroke volume. In addition, a widened pulse pressure may result in an increase in peripheral pulses (Gomella, Cunningham & Eyal, 1994).

Radiographic studies in infants with PDA typically show cardiac enlargement and pulmonary edema. ABG findings reveal hypercapnia and metabolic acidosis. Echocardiography can demonstrate a PDA and can quantitate the amount of blood shunting across the PDA (Avery, Fletcher & MacDonald, 1994; Gomella, Cunningham & Eyal, 1994).

The PDA can be managed medically or surgically. Medical management consists of ventilatory support, fluid restriction, and the administration of diuretics and indomethacin. Indomethacin is a prostaglandin synthetase inhibitor that blocks the effect of the arachidonic acid products on the ductus and causes the PDA to constrict in approximately 85% of infants (Avery, Fletcher & MacDonald, 1994). Ventilatory support is adjusted based on the ABG values. Fluid restriction is implemented to decrease cardiovascular volume overload in association with the diuretic therapy (Gomella, Cunningham & Eyal, 1994). Surgical ligation is done when a PDA is clinically significant and medical management has failed (Gomella, Cunningham & Eyal, 1994).

The nursing care of the infant with PDA focuses on supportive care. The infant needs an NTE, adequate oxygenation, meticulous fluid balance, and parental support.

Periventricular-intraventricular hemorrhage. Periventricular-intraventricular hemorrhage (PV-IVH) is one of the most common types of brain injury that occurs in neonates and is among the most severe from the standpoint of both the short- and long-term outcomes. The incidence of PV-IVH in infants weighing less than 1,000 gm is 50% to 70%. Use of prenatal corticosteroids can reduce the incidence to about 25% (Dietch, 1993; Fanaroff & Martin, 1997).

The pathogenesis of PV-IVH includes intravascular factors (fluctuating or increasing cerebral blood flow, increases in cerebral venous pressures, and coagulopathy), vascular factors, extravascular factors, and nursery care (Dietch, 1993). PV-IVH events typically occur within the first week of life, with 50% occurring in the first 24 hours, 90% occurring in the first 72 hours, and 95% occurring in the first week (Gomella, Cunningham & Eyal, 1994; Volpe, 1992).

PV-IVH is classified according to a grading system of I to IV, with grade I being the least severe and grade IV the most severe. The hemorrhage is further categorized as small, moderate, or severe (Fanaroff & Martin, 1997) (Box 27-6).

The long-term neurodevelopmental outcome is determined by the severity of the PV-IVH. In studies comparing infants with PV-IVH with similar infants without PV-IVH, the incidence of handicaps in infants with moderate PV-IVH was found to be threefold and in those with severe PV-IVH sevenfold greater than that in infants without PV-IVH (Fanaroff & Martin, 1997).

Nursing care focuses on recognition of factors that increase the risk of PV-IVH, interventions to decrease the risk of bleeding, and supportive care to infants who have bleeding episodes. The infant is positioned with the head in midline and the head of the bed elevated slightly to prevent or minimize fluctuations in intracranial blood pressure. NTE is maintained, as well as oxygenation. Rapid infusions of fluids should be avoided. Blood pressure is monitored closely for fluctuations. The infant is monitored for signs of pneumothorax, since it often precedes PV-IVH.

<table>
<tr><td>

BOX 27-6   *Classification for the Spectrum of Periventricular-Intraventicular Hemorrhage*

SMALL HEMORRHAGE

Grade I

Isolated germinal matrix hemorrhage

Grade II

Intraventricular hemorrhage with normal ventricular size

MODERATE HEMORRHAGE

Grade III

Intraventricular hemorrhage with acute ventricular dilatation

SEVERE HEMORRHAGE

Grade IV

Intraventricular hemorrhage with parenchymal hemorrhage

From Fanaroff A & Martin R: *Neonatal-perinatal medicine: disease of the fetus and infant,* ed 6, St Louis, 1997, Mosby.

</td></tr>
</table>

BOX 27-7   *Proposed Risk Factors for Necrotizing Enterocolitis*

Asphyxia
Respiratory distress syndrome
Umbilical artery catheter
Exchange transfusion
Early enteral feedings
Patent ductus arteriosus
Congenital heart disease
Polycythemia
Anemia
Shock

Necrotizing enterocolitis

Necrotizing enterocolitis (NEC) is an acute inflammatory disease of the GI mucosa, commonly complicated by perforation. This often fatal disease occurs in about 2% to 5% of newborns in NICUs. Although the cause is unknown, the factors listed in Box 27-7 are known to contribute to its development.

Reversal of perinatal asphyxia within 30 minutes may prevent GI tract insult and thus prevent the pathophysiologic events that trigger NEC. After 30 minutes the distribution of cardiac output tends to be directed more toward the heart and brain and away from the abdominal organs. Therefore prompt birth of the intrauterine-asphyxiated fetus or ventilation of the asphyxiated newborn may be beneficial to the GI tract, as well as to other organs.

The onset of NEC in the full-term infant usually occurs between 4 and 10 days after birth. In the preterm infant the onset may be delayed for up to 30 days. The signs of developing NEC are nonspecific, which is characteristic of many neonatal diseases. Some generalized signs include decreased activity, hypotonia, pallor, recurrent apnea and bradycardia, decreased oxygen saturation values, respiratory distress, metabolic acidosis, oliguria, hypotension, decreased perfusion, temperature instability, and cyanosis. GI symptoms include abdominal distention, increasing or bile-stained residual gastric aspirates, vomiting (bile or blood), grossly bloody stools, abdominal tenderness, and erythema of the abdominal wall (Korones & Bada-Ellzey, 1993).

A diagnosis of NEC is confirmed by a radiographic examination that reveals bowel loop distention, pneumatosis intestinalis, pneumoperitoneum, portal air, or a combination of these findings. The abnormal radiographic findings are caused by the bacterial colonization of the GI tract associated with NEC, resulting in ileus. Pneumatosis intestinalis, pneumoperitoneum, and portal air are caused by gas produced by the bacteria that invade the wall of the intestines and escape into the peritoneum and portal system when perforation occurs. The laboratory evaluation in such infants consists of a CBC with differential coagulation studies, ABG analysis, measurement of serum electrolyte levels, and blood culture (Korones & Bada-Ellzey, 1993). The white blood cell count on the CBC may be either increased or decreased. The platelet count and coagulation study findings may be abnormal, showing thrombocytopenia and DIC. Electrolyte levels may be abnormal with leaking capillary beds and fluid shifts with the infection.

Treatment in such infants is supportive. Oral or tube feedings are discontinued to rest the GI tract. An orogastric tube is placed and attached to low wall suction to provide gastric decompression. Parenteral therapy (often TPN) is begun. Because NEC is an infectious disease, control of the infection is imperative, with an emphasis on careful handwashing before and after infant contact. Antibiotic therapy may be instituted, and surgical resection is performed if perforation or clinical deterioration occurs. Therapy is usually prolonged, and recovery may be delayed by the formation of adhesions, the development of the complications associated with bowel resection, the occurrence of short gut syndrome (especially if the ileocecal valve is removed), or the development of intolerance to oral feedings.

Research findings indicate that a decrease in the incidence of NEC correlates with the use of nonnutritive sucking during gavage feedings (Pickler & Terrell, 1994). The authors hypothesize that nonnutritive sucking has this effect because it makes the GI tract less susceptible to the factors that precipitate NEC by promoting gastric motility and thus increasing the release of gastric enzymes. The improvement in the infant's behavioral organization brought about by nonnutritive sucking also appears to play a role in this.

PAIN IN NEONATES

Pain has been defined physiologically and psychologically. The psychologic component of pain and the diffuse total body response to pain exhibited by the neonate led many health care providers to believe that infants, especially premature infants, do not experience pain (Franck & Gregory, 1993). It is now known, however, that the CNS of fetuses is well developed as early as 24 weeks. The peripheral and spinal structure that transmits pain information is present and functional between the first and second trimester. Synaptic development begins in the cortex and achieves functional maturity by 20 to 24 weeks' gestation. The pituitary-adrenal axis is also well developed at this time, and a fight-or-flight reaction is observed in response to the catecholamines released in response to stress (Franck, 1993; Lawrence et al., 1993).

The physiologic response to pain in neonates can be life threatening because it can involve a decrease in the tidal volume, an increase in the demands on the cardiovascular system, an increase in metabolism, and neuroendocrine imbalance. The hormonal-metabolic response to pain in a term infant is also of a greater magnitude and shorter duration than that of adults. In addition, the newborn's sympathetic response to pain is less mature and thus less predictable than an adult's (Franck & Gregory, 1993). Besides these factors, the decreased lipid stores and immature enzyme activity characteristic of premature infants result in an increase in tissue breakdown in response to pain.

Assessment

There are three components to the response to pain that must be considered in the pain assessment of newborns: behavioral, physiologic and autonomic, and metabolic (Franck & Gregory, 1993). Each component is reviewed separately.

Behavioral responses

The most common behavioral sign of pain is a vocalization or cry. Through acoustical analysis the pain cry has been found to be distinctive (Craig & Grunau, 1993). It has been described as being high pitched and shrill (Lynam, 1995). A cry face is also characteristic of an infant experiencing pain. Such infants also flex and adduct their upper body and lower limbs in an attempt to withdraw from the painful stimulus. The premature infant's threshold for the initiation of this flexor response is lower than the term infant's, but it may increase with repeated stimulation. However, critically ill infants may become flaccid in response to a pain stimulus (Franck & Gregory, 1993). Other facial features exhibited during pain include eye squeeze, brow contraction, deepened nasolabial furrows, a taut and quivering tongue, and open mouth. The extremities and body will exhibit withdrawal, thrashing, jerking, and rigid posture (Craig & Grunau, 1993).

Physiologic and autonomic responses

Significant changes in heart rate, blood pressure (increased or decreased), intracranial pressure, vagal tone, respiratory rate, and oxygen saturation occur during noxious stimuli (Franck & Gregory, 1993; Lynam, 1995).

Metabolic responses

Epinephrine, norepinephrine, glucagon, corticosterone, cortisol, 11-deoxycorticosterone, lactate, pyruvate, and glucose are released in infants in response to pain (Franck & Gregory, 1993; Lynam, 1995).

Management

The goals of the management of neonatal pain are (1) to minimize the intensity, duration, and physiologic cost of the pain and (2) to maximize the neonate's ability to cope and recover from the pain (Franck & Gregory, 1993). Nonpharmacologic and pharmacologic strategies are used.

Nonpharmacologic management

Containment, also known as *swaddling*, is effective in reducing excessive immature motor responses. This may also provide comfort through other senses, such as the thermal, tactile, and proprioceptive senses (Franck & Gregory, 1993; Lynam, 1995). Nonnutritive sucking is the most common comfort measure used. However, the effectiveness of nonnutritive sucking in reducing the pain response has been found to be limited and confined to the pain caused by certain procedures (Lynam, 1995). Distraction with visual, oral, auditory, or tactile stimulation may be helpful in term or older infants (Franck & Gregory, 1993).

Pharmacologic management

Pharmacologic agents are routinely used for adults during painful procedures. These same agents are also now becoming routinely used in neonates to alleviate such pain. Local anesthesia may be used for circumcision and has also become a routine measure during certain invasive procedures such as chest tube insertion. Topical anesthesia has been used for lumbar puncture, venipuncture, and heel sticks (Franck, 1993). Opioids have been used as preprocedural analgesia. However, if the infant is not ventilated, the use of opioids is of concern because of the potential for these agents to cause respiratory depression (Franck, 1993; Franck & Gregory, 1993).

Anesthesia is used for prolonged surgical procedures. The American Academy of Pediatrics recommends the same guidelines for the safe administration of anesthesia to critically ill infants as those used for adult patients in unstable conditions (Franck, 1993). Pain control is also crucial during the immediate postoperative period. A low-dose continuous infusion or an intermittent bolus of narcotic analgesia is given to infants. The pharmacokinetic properties of morphine in premature infants are different from those in adults. That is, this drug has a longer half-life and a delayed clearance in premature infants. Other effects of morphine and meperidine observed in premature infants include decreased intestinal motility, abdominal distention, and hypotension, which is seen in dehydrated infants. Fentanyl has effects similar to those of morphine and meperidine, including an ability to cause significant respiratory depression (Franck & Gregory, 1993). Sufentanil is 10 times more potent than fentanyl and is used for neonates undergoing cardiac surgical procedures. Alfentanil is short acting and has been used for short procedures (Franck & Gregory, 1993). Methadone has been used for the relief of postoperative pain and treatment of the neonatal abstinence syndrome. A 50- to 100-mg/kg dose of methadone relieves pain in neonates for 6 to 10 hours (Franck & Gregory, 1993).

POSTMATURE INFANTS

A pregnancy that is prolonged beyond 42 weeks is a post-term pregnancy, and the infant who is born is called postmature. Postmaturity can be associated with placental insufficiency, resulting in a fetus who has a wasted appearance (dysmaturity) at birth due to loss of subcutaneous fat and muscle mass. However, not all postmature infants will show signs of dysmaturity; some will continue to grow in utero and be large at birth.

The perinatal mortality rate is significantly higher in the postmature fetus and neonate. One reason for this is that during labor and birth the increased oxygen demands of the postmature fetus may not be met. Insufficient gas exchange in the postmature placenta also increases the likelihood of intrauterine hypoxia, which may result in the passage of meconium in utero, thereby increasing the risk for meconium aspiration syndrome. Of all the deaths that occur in postmature newborns, one half occur during labor and birth, about one third occur before the onset of labor, and one sixth occur during the postpartum period.

Meconium Aspiration Syndrome

Meconium staining of the amniotic fluid can be indicative of nonreassuring fetal status, especially in a vertex presentation. It appears in about 8% to 20% of all births. Many infants with meconium staining exhibit no signs of depression at birth; however, the presence of meconium in the amniotic fluid necessitates careful supervision of labor and close monitoring of fetal well-being. The presence of a team skilled at neonatal resuscitation is required at the birth of any infant with meconium-stained amniotic fluid. The mouth and nares of the infant should be suctioned on the perineum before the infant's first breath. In the event of thick or particulate meconium the standard of care is to intubate the infant at birth and suction any meconium visualized below the vocal cords. Appropriate management of the airway at birth can largely prevent **meconium aspiration syndrome (MAS).**

If meconium is not removed from the airway at birth, it can migrate down to the terminal airways, causing mechanical obstruction. It is also possible that the fetus aspirated meconium in utero. Such meconium aspiration can cause a chemical pneumonitis. These infants may develop persistent pulmonary hypertension of the newborn (PPHN), further complicating their management.

> **LEGAL TIP** Standard of Care—Meconium Aspiration
>
> *When there are particles of meconium in the amniotic fluid, the standard of care is that the infant should be suctioned below the vocal cords immediately after birth. The nurse's responsibility is to notify the appropriate personnel to be at the birth and have suctioning equipment available.*

Persistent Pulmonary Hypertension of the Newborn

The term *persistent pulmonary hypertension of the newborn (PPHN)* is applied to the combined findings of pulmonary hypertension, right-to-left shunting, and a structurally normal heart. PPHN may present either as a single entity or as the main component of MAS, congenital diaphragmatic hernia, RDS, hyperviscosity syndrome, or neonatal pneumonia or sepsis. PPHN is also called *persistent fetal circulation (PFC)* because the syndrome includes a reversion to fetal pathways for blood flow.

A brief review of the characteristics of fetal blood flow can help in the visualization of the problems with PPHN (see Fig. 8-9). In utero, oxygen-rich blood leaves the placenta via the umbilical vein, goes through the ductus venosus, and enters the inferior vena cava. From there it empties into the right atrium and is mostly shunted across the foramen ovale to the left atrium, effectively bypassing the lungs. This blood enters the left ventricle, leaves via the aorta, and preferentially perfuses the carotid and coronary arteries. Thus the heart and brain receive the most oxygenated blood. Blood drains from the brain into the superior vena cava, reenters the right atrium, proceeds to the right ventricle, and exits via the main pulmonary artery. The lungs are a high-pressure circuit, needing only enough perfusion for growth and nutrition. The ductus arteriosus (connecting the main pulmonary artery and the aorta) is the path of least resistance for the blood leaving the right side of the fetal heart, shunting most of the cardiac output away from the lungs and toward the systemic system. This *right-to-left shunting* is the key to fetal circulation.

After birth, both the foramen ovale and the ductus arteriosus close in response to various biochemical processes, pressure changes within the heart, and dilatation of the pulmonary vessels. This dilatation allows virtually all of the cardiac output to enter the lungs, become oxygenated, and provide oxygen-rich blood to the tissues for normal metabolism. Any process that interferes with this transition from fetal to neonatal circulation may precipate PPHN. PPHN characteristically proceeds into a downward spiral of exacerbating hypoxia and pulmonary vasoconstriction. Prompt recognition and aggressive intervention are required to reverse this process.

The infant with PPHN is typically born at term or post-term and presents with tachycardia and cyanosis. Management depends on the underlying cause of the persistent pulmonary hypertension. The use of ECMO has improved the chances of survival in these infants (see earlier discussion).

Another mode of treatment for PPHN and other respiratory disorders of the newborn is high-frequency ventilation, a group of assisted-ventilation methods that deliver small volumes of gas at high frequencies and limit the development of high airway pressure, thus reducing barotrauma (Fanaroff & Martin, 1997).

I CARE MANAGEMENT

To ensure the safe birth of the fetus, it becomes important to determine whether the pregnancy is actually prolonged and also whether there is any evidence of fetal jeopardy as a result.

Most postmature infants are oversized but otherwise normal, with advanced development and bone age. A postmature infant will have some, but not necessarily all, of the following physical characteristics:

*   Generally a normal skull, but the reduced dimensions of the rest of the body make the skull look inordinately large
*   Dry, cracked (desquamating), parchmentlike skin at birth
*   Hard nails extending beyond the fingertips
*   Profuse scalp hair
*   Depleted subcutaneous fat layers, leaving the skin loose and giving the infant an "old person" appearance
*   Long and thin body
*   Absent vernix
*   Often meconium staining (golden yellow to green) of skin, nails, and cord, indicative of a hypoxic episode in utero
*   May have an alert, wide-eyed appearance symptomatic of chronic intrauterine hypoxia

Possible nursing diagnoses for the postmature infant are listed in the Nursing Diagnoses box.

I Nursing Diagnoses

Postmature Infant
Impaired airway clearance related to:
*   Meconium aspiration syndrome
Ineffective thermoregulation related to:
*   Immature thermoregulation center
Risk for injury related to:
*   Birth trauma
Risk for injury secondary to hypoglycemia related to:
*   Depleted glycogen stores

Immediate outcomes of care are that the postmature newborn will:
*   Initiate and maintain respirations
*   Experience no CNS trauma or infection
*   Have any birth trauma identified and treated promptly without sequelae

The long-term expected outcome is that the infant will not experience adverse effects of postmaturity.

The immediate care rendered in postmature infants is similar to that given to preterm infants. Potential complications experienced by postmature infants include polycythemia, hypothermia, hypoglycemia, and meconium aspiration (Avery, Fletcher & MacDonald, 1994). See other sections for the management and care of these complications.

The nurse can be assured that care was effective when the short-term outcomes for care have been achieved. Long-term follow-up will be needed to evaluate whether there are any adverse effects as a result of postmaturity.

I OTHER PROBLEMS RELATED TO GESTATION

Small for Gestational Age and Intrauterine Growth Restriction

Infants whose birth weight falls below the 10th percentile expected at term or who fall two standard deviations below the mean for gestational age, for reasons other than heredity, are considered at high risk, with the perinatal mortality rate four to eight times greater than that for the normal term infant (Gomella, Cunningham & Eyal, 1994).

Various conditions can affect and impede growth in the developing fetus. The cause, severity, and gestational age at which the insult occurs determine the way in which fetal growth is affected and what problems affect the newborn. Conditions occurring in the first trimester that affect all aspects of fetal growth (infections, teratogens, and chromosomal abnormalities) or extrinsic conditions occurring early in pregnancy result in a symmetric IUGR (head circumference, length, and weight all fall below the 10th percentile). Conditions causing symmetric IUGR will result in a short SGA infant, usually with a smaller head circumference and reduced brain capacity (Gomella, Cunningham & Eyal, 1994).

Growth restriction in the later stages of pregnancy results in asymmetric IUGR (with respect to gestational age, weight falls below the 10th percentile, whereas length and head circumference fall above the 10th percentile). Asymmetric IUGR occurs as a result of maternal, fetal, and placental conditions (Korones & Bada-Ellzey, 1993). Such infants can grow and develop normally. Abnormal fetal size may also indicate an adaptive response with diminished fetal weight–sparing brain growth (Fanaroff & Martin, 1997).

Common problems that affect SGA, IUGR, and dysmature infants are perinatal asphyxia, meconium aspiration, hypoglycemia, and heat loss.

Perinatal asphyxia

Commonly, IUGR infants have been exposed to chronic hypoxia for varying periods before labor and birth. Labor is a stressor to the normal fetus, but it is an even greater stressor for the growth-restricted fetus. The chronically hypoxic infant is severely compromised even by a normal labor and has difficulty compensating after birth. The alert, wide-eyed appearance of such newborns is attributed to the prolonged fetal hypoxia. Appropriate management and resuscitation are essential for these depressed infants.

The birth of SGA babies with perinatal asphyxia may be associated with a maternal history of heavy cigarette smoking; preeclampsia; low socioeconomic status; multifetal gestation; gestational infections such as rubella, cytomegalovirus, and toxoplasmosis; advanced diabetes mellitus; and cardiac problems. The nursing staff must be alert to and prepared for possible perinatal asphyxia during the birth of an infant in a woman with such a history. Sequelae to perinatal asphyxia include MAS and hypoglycemia.

Hypoglycemia

All stressed infants are at risk for the development of hypoglycemia (Merenstein & Gardner, 1998). Such stress may include perinatal asphyxia and IUGR. The definition of **hypoglycemia** differs for the term and the preterm infant. Hypoglycemia occurring within the first 3 days of life in the term infant is defined as a blood glucose level of less than 40 mg/dl; that occurring in the preterm infant within the same time frame is defined as a blood glucose level of less than 25 mg/dl. Symptoms of hypoglycemia include poor feeding, hypothermia, and diaphoresis. CNS symptoms can include tremors and jitteriness, weak cry, lethargy, floppy posture, convulsions, or coma. Diagnosis is confirmed by blood glucose determinations performed by the laboratory when suspected or by unit visual methods using reagent strips such as Chemstrip-BG or Dextrostix (Merenstein & Gardner, 1998).

Heat loss

For numerous reasons, SGA infants are particularly susceptible to temperature instability, and close attention must be paid to them to maintain thermoneutrality. These reasons include the fact that they have less muscle mass, less brown fat, less heat-preserving subcutaneous fat, and little ability to control skin capillaries. Nursing considerations in these infants focus on the maintenance of thermoneutrality to promote recovery from perinatal asphyxia, because cold stress jeopardizes such recovery (Merenstein & Gardner, 1998).

I CARE MANAGEMENT

Several physical findings are characteristic of the SGA neonate:

- Generally a normal skull, but the reduced dimensions of the rest of the body make the skull look inordinately large
- Reduced subcutaneous fat stores
- Loose and dry skin
- Diminished muscle mass, especially over buttocks and cheeks
- Sunken abdomen (scaphoid) as opposed to the well-rounded abdomen seen in normal infants
- Thin, yellowish, dry, and dull umbilical cord (normal cord is gray, glistening, round, and moist)
- Sparse scalp hair
- Wide skull sutures (inadequate bone growth)

SGA infants are also likely to suffer perinatal asphyxia, MAS, hypoglycemia, and heat loss.

The nursing care given to the SGA infant is determined by the nature of the clinical problems and is the same as that given to the preterm infant with the same problems. Gas exchange is supported by maintaining a clear airway and preventing cold stress. Hypoglycemia is treated with oral feedings (e.g., breast milk, formula, dextrose solution) per the hospital protocol. Parenteral infusions may be necessary. An external heat source is used until the infant's temperature is stabilized (radiant warmer or isolette). The nursing support given to parents is also similar to that given to parents of preterm infants.

Large for Gestational Age

The LGA, or oversized, infant traditionally has been regarded as one weighing 4,000 gm or more at birth. An infant is considered LGA despite gestation when the weight falls above the 90th percentile on growth charts or two standard deviations above the mean weight for gestational age (Gomella, Cunningham & Eyal, 1994; Korones & Bada-Ellzey, 1993). About 10% of newborns weigh this much, and about 0.4% to 0.9% weigh 4,500 gm or more (Korones & Bada-Ellzey, 1993). Most of these newborns also have other proportionately larger measurements. Many are born well after the estimated date of birth. Better maternal health and nutrition probably are responsible for such greater growth in the recent past; genetic disposition is another factor—large mothers have large babies. Certain fetal disorders can also result in LGA infants. These include transposition of the great vessels and Beckwith-Wiedemann syndrome (Korones & Bada-Ellzey, 1993).

Maternal pelvic diameters have not kept pace with the better maternal health and nutrition resulting in larger babies. As a result, fetopelvic disproportion often occurs with LGA babies, particularly in obese women, women who gain 16 kg or more during gestation, and women with undiagnosed or uncontrolled diabetes, who are prone to having large babies. Birth trauma, especially in infants with a breech or shoulder presentation, is a serious hazard for the oversized neonate. Asphyxia or CNS injury, or both, may occur.

A biparietal diameter greater than 10 cm verified by fetometry (ultrasound or x-ray examination), a uterine fundal measurement greater than 42 cm in the absence of hydramnios, and only average or smaller interior pelvic diameters are frequent findings. All pregnancies of more than 42 weeks' gestation need to be carefully evaluated. All large fetuses are monitored during a trial of labor, and preparation is made for cesarean birth if a nonreassuring fetal status or poor progress of labor occurs. LGA newborns may be preterm, term, or postterm; they may be the infants of diabetic (or prediabetic) mothers; and they may be postmature. Each of these problems carries special concerns. Regardless of any coexisting potential problems, the oversized infant is at risk just by virtue of its size.

I CARE MANAGEMENT

The nurse assesses the LGA infant for gestational age, hypoglycemia, and trauma resulting from vaginal or cesarean birth. The blood glucose levels of LGA infants are monitored, and any hypoglycemia is corrected. Any specific birth injuries are identified and treated appropriately. Care depends on the LGA infant's condition.

RESEARCH

Breastfeeding Patterns of Low-Birth-Weight Infants after Discharge

Although human milk is recognized as the best source of nutrition for most infants and especially for low-birth-weight (LBW) infants, many mothers who initiate breastfeeding with LBW infants are unsuccessful at sustaining lactation until their infants are discharged. The feeding patterns of LBW infants on the day of hospital discharge and 4 weeks after birth were examined. The convenience sample consisted of 110 mothers who intended to breastfeed their LBW infants. Maternal and infant data were collected using a three-part breastfeeding questionnaire and a hospital data form. The first part of the questionnaire included maternal demographics, previous experiences with breastfeeding, and breastfeeding goals. The second part included an infant feeding diary; the third part included the breastfeeding pattern and feeding mode and the reasons for a decrease or cessation in breastfeeding. Part 1 was completed 72 hours after birth. The feeding diary was initiated at the first feeding and continued for the next 7 days. The mothers completed part 3 of the questionnaire by telephone 4 and 8 weeks after birth. The researchers found that at hospital discharge, 38% of the infants were fed exclusively at the breast. Only 52% of the full-term LBW infants and 52% of the preterm LBW infants had effective vigorous feedings at the breast at hospital discharge as rated by the mothers. At 4 weeks, 40% of the infants were fed exclusively at the breast and 19% were weaned to formula.

RESEARCH—cont'd

CLINICAL APPLICATION OF THE STUDY

The ability to group infants into a category to determine feeding patterns is very difficult. Specifically, the feeding patterns of the LBW or preterm infant differ from those of the full-term infant. Data from this study suggest cautious use of breastfeeding assessment tools, since each individual infant must be assessed for feeding needs. In addition, the definition of breastfeeding that is widely accepted for full-term infants does not fit breastfeeding patterns for this population.

Source: Hill P et al.: Breastfeeding patterns of low-birth-weight infants after hospital discharge, *J Obstet Gynecol Neonatal Nurs* 26(2):189, 1997.

KEY POINTS

- Preterm infants are at risk for problems stemming from the immaturity of their organ systems.
- Nurses who work with preterm infants observe them for respiratory distress and other early symptoms of physiologic disorders.
- The adaptation of parents to preterm infants differs from that of parents to full-term infants.
- Nurses can facilitate the development of a positive parent-child relationship.
- Nurses' skills in interpreting data, making decisions, and initiating therapy in newborn intensive care units are crucial to ensuring infants' survival.
- Parents need special instruction (e.g., cardiopulmonary resuscitation, oxygen therapy, suctioning, developmental care) before they take a high-risk infant home.
- SGA infants are considered at risk because of fetal growth restriction.
- The high incidence of nonreassuring fetal status among postmature infants is related to the progressive placental insufficiency that can occur in a postterm pregnancy.
- Parents need assistance with coping with anticipated grief or loss and grief.

CRITICAL THINKING EXERCISES

1 *A single, unemployed woman has a preterm infant who was born at 31 weeks' gestation. The woman does not live in the city where the hospital is located, and she is to be discharged tomorrow. It is anticipated that the infant will require a stay in the hospital for at least 6 more weeks*

CRITICAL THINKING EXERCISES—cont'd

and will likely require oxygen therapy at home after discharge. What kinds of assistance will this mother need now and after the infant goes home? Identify resources in the community that may have services she can use and investigate the eligibility requirements for these services.

2 Identify an infant who is SGA. Review the prenatal and postnatal history. Identify reasons for an infant being SGA. Identify problems that may occur in this SGA infant.

3 Identify an infant who is LGA. Review the prenatal and postnatal history. Identify reasons for an infant being LGA. Identify problems that may occur in this LGA infant.

4 During a scheduled clinical experience in the NICU or a special care nursery:

a Identify problems affecting a premature infant and observe the technique used by the NICU staff for managing each problem identified. Discuss interventions that were based on nursing research or suggest what could have been done.

b Observe and compare parental interactions with a premature infant during the acute and chronic stages.

References

Affonso D et al.: Reconciliation and healing for mothers through skin-to-skin contact provided in an American tertiary level intensive care nursery, *Neonatal Netw* 12(3):25, 1993.

Avery G, Fletcher M & MacDonald M: *Neonatology: pathophysiology and management of the newborn*, ed 4, Philadelphia, 1994, JB Lippincott.

Ballard J et al.: New Ballard score, expanded to include extremely premature infants, *J Pediatr* 119(3):417, 1991.

Blackburn S & VandenBerg K: Assessment and management of neonatal neurobehavioral development. In Kenner C, Bruggemeyer A & Gunderson L, editors: *Comprehensive neonatal nursing: a physiologic perspective*, Philadelphia, 1993, WB Saunders.

Blake W & Murray J: Heat balance. In Merenstein G & Gardner S, editors: *Handbook of neonatal intensive care*, ed 4, St Louis, 1998, Mosby.

Bloom R & Cropley C: *Textbook of neonatal resuscitation*, Elk Grove, Ill, 1994, American Heart Association.

Brennan-Brehm M et al.: Calorie loss from expressed mother's milk during continuous gavage infusion, *Neonatal Netw* 13(2):27, 1994.

Brooten D: Perinatal care across the continuum: early discharge and nursing home follow-up, *J Perinat Neonat Nurs* 9(1):38, 1995.

Cagan J: Feeding behavior in preterm infants, *Neonatal Netw* 14(2):82, 1995 (abstract).

Chan J, Kelley M & Kahn J: The effects of a pressure relief mattress on postnatal head molding in very low birth weight infants, *Neonatal Netw* 12(5):19, 1993.

Cloherty J & Stark A: *Manual of neonatal care*, ed 4, Boston, 1997, Little, Brown.

Craig K & Grunau R: Neonatal pain perception and behavioral measurement. In Anand K & McGrath P, editors: *Pain in neonates*, Amsterdam, 1993, Elsevier.

Dickason E, Silverman B & Kaplan J: *Maternal-infant nursing care*, ed 3, St Louis, 1998, Mosby.

Dietch J: Periventricular-intraventricular hemorrhage in the very low birth weight infant, *Neonatal Netw* 12(1):7, 1993.

Donovan E & Spengler L: New technologies applied to the management of respiratory dysfunction. In Kenner C, Brueggemeyer A & Gunderson L, editors: *Comprehensive neonatal nursing: a physiologic perspective*, Philadelphia, 1993, WB Saunders.

Downey V et al.: Dying babies and associated stress in NICU nurses, *Neonatal Netw* 12(6):49, 1993.

Endo A & Nishioka E: Neonatal assessment. In Kenner C, Brueggemeyer A & Gunderson L, editors: *Comprehensive neonatal nursing: a physiologic perspective*, Philadelphia, 1993, WB Saunders.

Fanaroff A & Martin R: *Neonatal-perinatal medicine: disease of the fetus and infant*, ed 6, St Louis, 1997, Mosby.

Field T: Interaction patterns of preterm and term infants. In Field T, editor: *Infants born at risk*, Jamacia, NY, 1979, Spectrum Publications.

Franck L: Identification, management, and prevention of pain in the neonate. In Kenner C, Brueggemeyer A & Gunderson L, editors: *Comprehensive neonatal nursing: a physiologic perspective*, Philadelphia, 1993, WB Saunders.

Franck L & Gregory G: Clinical evaluation and treatment of infant pain in the neonatal intensive care unit. In Schechter M, Berde C & Yaster M, editors: *Pain in infants, children, and adolescents*, Baltimore, 1993, Williams & Wilkins.

Gale G, Franck L & Lund C: Skin-to-skin (kangaroo) holding of the intubated premature infant, *Neonatal Netw* 12(6):49, 1993.

Gardner S & Lubchenco L: The neonate and the environment: impact on development. In Merenstein G & Gardner S, editors: *Handbook of neonatal intensive care*, ed 4, St Louis, 1998, Mosby.

Goetzman B & Wennberg R: *Neonatal intensive care handbook*, ed 8, St Louis, 1991, Mosby.

Gomella T, Cunningham M & Eyal F: *Neonatology: management, procedure, on-call problems, diseases and drugs*, ed 3, Norwalk, Conn, 1994, Appleton & Lange.

Green M, editor: *Bright futures, guidelines for health supervision of infants, children and adolescents*, Arlington, Va, 1994, National Center for Education in Maternal and Child Health.

Hagedorn M, Gardner S & Abman S: Respiratory distress. In Merenstein G & Gardner S, editors: *Handbook of neonatal intensive care*, ed 4, St Louis, 1998, Mosby.

Hall L: Home care. In Kenner, C, Brueggemeyer A & Gunderson L (eds): *Comprehensive neonatal nursing: A physiologic perspective*, Philadelphia, 1993, WB Saunders.

Harrigan R et al.: Perinatal grief: response to the loss of an infant, *Neonatal Netw* 12(5):25, 1993.

Haubrich K: Assessment and management of auditory dysfunction. In Kenner C, Bruggemeyer A & Gunderson L, editors: *Comprehensive neonatal nursing: a physiologic perspective*, Philadelphia, 1993, WB Saunders.

Haut G, Peddicord K & O'Brien E: Supporting parental bonding in the NICU: a care plan for nurses, *Neonatal Netw* 13(8):19, 1994.

Hittner H, Hirsch N & Rudolph A: Assessment of gestational age by examination of the anterior vascular capsule of the lens, *J Pediatr* 91(3):455, 1977.

Kenner C: Caring for the NICU parent, *J Perinat Neonatal Nurs* 4(2):78, 1990.

Klaus M & Kennell J: Care of the parents. In Klaus M & Fanaroff A, editors: *Care of the high-risk neonate*, ed 4, Philadelphia, 1993, WB Saunders.

Klaus M, Martin R & Fanaroff A: The physical environment. In Klaus M & Fanaroff A, editors: *Care of the high-risk neonate*, ed 4, Philadelphia, 1993, WB Saunders.

Knoppert D & Mackanjee H: Current strategies in the management of bronchopulmonary dysplasia: the role of corticosteroids, *Neonatal Netw* 13(3):53, 1994.

Korones A & Bada-Ellzey H: *Neonatal decision making,* St Louis, 1993, Mosby.

Kuller J & Lund C: Assessment and management of integumentary dysfunction. In Kenner C, Brueggemeyer A & Gunderson L, editors: *Comprehensive neonatal nursing: a physiologic perspective,* Philadelphia, 1993, WB Saunders.

Lawrence J et al.: The development of a tool to assess neonatal pain, *Neonatal Netw* 12(6):59, 1993.

Lefrak-Okikawa L & Meier P: Nutrition: physiologic basis of metabolism and management of enteral and parenteral nutrition. In Kenner C, Brueggemeyer A & Gunderson L, editors: *Comprehensive neonatal nursing: a physiologic perspective,* Philadelphia, 1993, WB Saunders.

Lindsay J et al.: Creative caring in the NICU: parent-to-parent support, *Neonatal Netw* 12(4):37, 1993.

Loizeaux W: *Anna, a daughter's life,* New York, 1993, Arcade Publishing.

Ludington-Hoe S & Swinth J: Developmental aspects of kangaroo care, *J Obstet Gynecol Neonatal Nurs* 25(8):691, 1996.

Ludington-Hoe S et al.: Kangaroo care: research results, practice implications and guidelines, *Neonatal Netw* 13(1):19, 1994.

Lund C, editor: *Bronchopulmonary dysplasia: strategies for total patient care,* Petaluma, Calif, 1990, NICU INK.

Lynam L: Research utilization: nonpharmacological management of pain in neonates, *Neonatal Netw* 14(5):59, 1995.

Martin R, Faranoff A & Klaus M: Respirating problems. In Klaus M & Faranoff A, editors: *Care of the high-risk neonate,* ed 4, Philadelphia, 1993, WB Saunders.

Mauskopf J et al.: Synthetic surfactant for rescue treatment of respiratory distress syndrome in premature infants weighing from 700 to 1350 grams: impact on hospital resource use and charges, *J Pediatr* 126(1):94, 1995.

Medoff-Cooper B, Verklan T & Carlson S: The development of sucking patterns and physiologic correlates in very-low-birth-weight infants, *Nurs Res* 42(2):100, 1993.

Mehren E: *Born too soon,* New York, 1991, Doubleday.

Merenstein G & Gardner S: *Handbook of neonatal intensive care,* ed 4, St Louis, 1998, Mosby.

Metheny N et al.: Characteristics of aspirates from feeding tubes as a method for predicting tube location, *Nurs Res* 43(5): 282, 1994.

National Institutes of Health: Early identification of hearing impairment in infants and young children, *NIH Consensus Statement* 11(1), 1993.

Nichols J: Bereavement: a state of having suffered a loss. In Kenner C, Brueggemeyer A & Gunderson L, editors: *Comprehensive neonatal nursing: a physiologic perspective,* Philadelphia, 1993, WB Saunders.

Newman L: Parents' perception of their low birth weight infants, *Paediatrician* 9(3-4):182, 1980.

Oehler J, Hannan T & Catlett A: Maternal views of preterm infants' responsiveness to social interaction, *Neonatal Netw* 12(6):67, 1993.

Oehler J et al: Behavioral characteristics of very low-birth-weight infants of varying biologic risk at 6, 15, and 24 months of age, *J Obstet Gynecol Neonatal Nurs* 25(3):233, 1996.

Philip A: *Neonatology: a practical guide,* ed 3, Philadelphia, 1987, WB Saunders.

Pickler R & Terrell B: Nonnutritive sucking and necrotizing enterocolitis, *Neonatal Netw* 13(8):15, 1994.

Pinyard B: Infant cries: physiology and assessment, *Neonatal Netw* 13(4):15, 1994.

Price P & Kalhan S: Nutrition and selected disorders of the gastrointestinal tract. In Klaus M & Fanaroff A, editors: *Care of the high-risk neonate,* ed 4, Philadelphia, 1993, WB Saunders.

Sammons W & Lewis J: *Premature babies: a different beginning,* St Louis, 1985, Mosby.

Schanler R, Schulman R & Prestridge L: Parenteral nutrient needs of very low birth weight infants, *J Pediatr* 125(6):961, 1994.

Schraeder B: Attachment and parenting despite lengthy intensive care, *MCN Am J Matern Child Nurs* 5(1):37, 1980.

Shiao S et al.: Nasogastric tube placement: effects of breathing and sucking in very-low-birth-weight infants, *Nurs Res* 44(2):82, 1995.

Shields-Poe D & Pinelli J: Variables associated with parental stress in neonatal intensive care units, *Neonatal Netw* 16(1):29, 1997.

Strauch C, Brandt S & Edwards-Beckett J: Implementation of a quiet hour: effect on noise level and infant sleep state, *Neonatal Netw* 12(2):31, 1993.

Thomas K: Back to basics: thermoregulation in neonates, *Neonatal Netw* 13(2):15, 1994.

Townsend S, Johnson C & Hay W: Enteral nutrition. In Merenstein G & Gardner S, editors: *Handbook of neonatal intensive care,* ed 4, St Louis, 1998, Mosby.

Trotter C: Gestational age assessment. In Tappero E & Honeyfield M, editors: *Physical assessment of the newborn,* Petaluma, Calif, 1993, NICU INK.

Volpe J: Intraventricular hemorrhage in the premature infant: morphologic characteristics. In Polin R & Fox W, editors: *Fetal and neonatal physiology,* vol 2, Philadelphia, 1992, WB Saunders.

Wereszczak J, Miles M & Holditch-Davis D: Maternal recall of the neonatal intensive care unit, *Neonatal Netw* 16(4):33, 1997.

Witter F & Keith L: *Textbook of prematurity: antecedents, treatment, and outcome,* Boston, 1993, Little, Brown.

Wong D: *Whaley and Wong's nursing care of infants and children,* ed 5, St Louis, 1995, Mosby.

Wong D & Perry S: *Maternal child nursing care,* St Louis, 1998, Mosby.

Wright S, Norton C & Kesten K: Retention of infant CPR instruction by parents, *Pediatr Nurs* 15(1):37, 1989.

CHAPTER

28

The Newborn at Risk: Acquired and Congenital Conditions

DEBBIE ASKIN

LEARNING OBJECTIVES

- *Define the key terms.*
- *Discuss the assessment of the newborn with hyperbilirubinemia.*
- *Compare Rh and ABO incompatibility.*
- *Develop a nursing care plan that addresses the prevention, identification and management of hyperbilirubinemia in a newborn.*
- *Describe common congenital anomalies and identify nursing care priorities for each anomaly.*
- *Develop a nursing care plan that focuses on the parents of a newborn with a defect or disorder.*
- *Describe the assessment of infants for birth trauma and for sequelae of a diabetic pregnancy.*
- *Develop nursing care plans for complications typically seen in infants of diabetic mothers.*
- *Describe in detail the assessment of a newborn for infection.*
- *Outline the assessment of a newborn experiencing drug withdrawal.*
- *Assess the effects of maternal use of alcohol, heroin, methadone, marijuana, cocaine, and smoking on the fetus and newborn.*
- *Discuss discharge planning and home care for high risk newborns and their families.*

KEY TERMS

ABO incompatibility
anencephaly
caput succedaneum
cephalhematoma
choanal atresia
cleft lip and palate
clubfoot
congenital
congenital hip dysplasia
Coomb's test
diaphragmatic hernia
epispadias
erythroblastosis fetalis
esophageal atresia
exchange transfusion
fetal alcohol effects (FAE)
fetal alcohol syndrome (FAS)
gastroschisis
hydrocephalus
hydrops fetalis
hyperbilirubinemia
hypospadias
imperforate anus
isoimmunization
jaundice
kernicterus
macrosomia
microcephaly
myelomeningocele
neonatal abstinence syndrome
neural tube defects
omphalocele
spina bifida
thrush
TORCH

Nurses must always be prepared to provide immediate and emergency care to newborns who are born with or develop problems during the newborn period. Nurses assist in the stabilization of the infant before transporting the infant to a regional intensive care nursery. Nurses detect deviations from normal and participate in the care of infants with acquired or congenital problems. They deal with parents who are trying to cope with the birth of a baby who does not meet their expected ideal. In this chapter some of the problems encountered during the newborn period are discussed, and nursing care of compromised infants is described.

HYPERBILIRUBINEMIA

Hyperbilirubinemia is the name for the condition in which the bilirubin level in the blood is increased. It is characterized by a yellow discoloration of the skin, mucous membranes, sclera, and various organs. This yellow discoloration is referred to as **jaundice,** or *icterus*. Jaundice is caused primarily by the accumulation in the skin of unconjugated bilirubin, a breakdown product of hemoglobin formed after its release from hemolyzed red blood cells (RBCs). Physiologic jaundice, discussed in Chapter 19 is the most common abonormal finding in newborns and is usually benign. The challenge in the care of neonates with hyperbilirubinemia is to distinguish physiologic jaundice from a serious clinical pathologic condition.

Physiologic Jaundice

Physiologic jaundice occurs in about half of all healthy full-term newborns and typically arises more than 24 hours after birth. In both Caucasian and African-American infants it is manifested by a progressive increase in the unconjugated bilirubin level in cord blood of from 2 mg/dl to a mean peak of 5 to 6 mg/dl between 60 to 72 hours of age. In Asian and Native American infants the level may increase to 10 to 14 mg/dl between 72 and 120 hours of age. Resolution in Caucasian and African-American newborns is evidenced by a rapid decline in the unconjugated bilirubin level to 2 mg/dl by 5 days after birth; in Asian and Native American infants this takes 7 to 10 days.

Physiologic jaundice is more common and typically more severe in preterm infants, in whom the serum bilirubin level typically reaches a mean peak of 10 to 12 mg/dl by the fifth day of life. The primary reason why it takes longer for the maximum concentration to be reached in preterm than in full-term infants is that the livers of preterm infants are immature, and hence liver function is not fully developed.

Pathologic Jaundice

Pathologic jaundice, or hyperbilirubinemia, is not defined solely in terms of the serum concentrations of unconjugated bilirubin. It also refers to that level of serum bilirubin which, if left untreated, can result in kernicterus, or the deposition of bilirubin in the brain and in other body cells. Following are the findings that support a diagnosis of pathologic jaundice and that, if encountered in an infant, warrant further investigation (Fanaroff & Martin, 1997):

- Serum bilirubin concentrations of greater than 4 mg/dl in cord blood
- Clinical jaundice evident within 24 hours of birth
- Total serum bilirubin levels increasing by more than 5 mg/dl in 24 hours or increasing at a rate of 0.5 mg/dl or greater over a 4- to 8-hour period
- A serum bilirubin level in a full-term newborn that exceeds 15 mg/dl at any time or clinical jaundice lasting more than 10 days
- A serum bilirubin level in a preterm newborn that exceeds 10 mg/dl at any time

- Any case of visible jaundice that persists more than 10 days of life in a full-term infant or 21 days in a preterm infant, unless they are receiving breast milk

There are many potential causes of pathologic hyperbilirubinemia in neonates. The most common is incompatibility between the maternal and fetal blood, specifically Rh and ABO incompatibility, and these are discussed later in this chapter. Other less common conditions that may be associated with pathologic jaundice in the neonate are bacterial or nonbacterial maternal infections and maternal medical conditions such as diabetes. In addition, both oxytocin administration and the maternal ingestion of sulfonamides, diazepam, or salicylates near the time of birth can affect the neonate's ability to excrete bilirubin.

There are also neonatal conditions that can predispose to the development of pathologic hyperbilirubinemia. One of these is the decreased ability of preterm or low-birth-weight (LBW) neonates to conjugate bilirubin because of an ineffective glucuronyl transferase enzyme system. Hepatic cell damage caused by infection or drugs also interferes with the functioning of this enzyme system. Other conditions that can result in pathologic jaundice include neonatal hypothyroidism or other metabolic abnormalities; polycythemia resulting from twin-to-twin transfusion or the transfusion of a large volume of blood by means of the placenta; and an intestinal obstruction such as meconium ileus (the most common presentation of cystic fibrosis in the neonate) or pyloric stenosis or that results from such disorders as Hirschsprung's disease. Biliary atresia may also cause jaundice, but such jaundice usually occurs after the neonatal period.

Sequestered blood can also be responsible for causing pathologic jaundice. Such an increase in the serum bilirubin level occurs when the blood in cephalhematomas, ecchymosis, or hemangiomas or the blood that becomes trapped during bleeding into internal organs is hemolyzed. Maternal blood swallowed by the neonate during birth may also be responsible for causing the bilirubin levels to increase as the blood is absorbed and broken down in the neonate's intestinal mucosa.

Kernicterus

The goal of the care given the infant with hyperbilirubinemia is the prevention of kernicterus. **Kernicterus,** or bilirubin encephalopathy, is caused by the deposition of bilirubin in the brain, especially within the basal ganglia, cerebellum, and hippocampus. This deposition can occur because unconjugated bilirubin is highly lipid soluble, making it capable of crossing the blood-brain barrier if it is not bound to protein. It results in the yellowish staining of the brain tissue and the necrosis of neurons and occurs if the concentration of unconjugated bilirubin reaches toxic levels. Kernicterus, which can develop in newborns who show no apparent signs of clinical jaundice, is generally considered to be directly related to the total serum bilirubin level, although these levels alone do not predict the risk of brain injury. In a healthy full-term infant, a total serum bilirubin level of 25 mg/dl is considered the upper limit beyond which the risk for kernicterus increases, although the condition may occur at much lower levels in premature infants or infants with other complications (Fanaroff & Martin, 1997). Some of the perinatal events that increase the likelihood of kernicterus developing, even at lower bilirubin levels, include hypoxia, asphyxia, acidosis, hypothermia, hypoglycemia, sepsis, treatment with certain medications, and hypoalbuminemia. These conditions cause kernicterus by interfering with the conjugation of bilirubin or by competing for albumin-binding sites. The resulting unconjugated bilirubin can then pass through the blood-brain barrier and enter the brain, resulting in kernicterus.

Kernicterus has been associated with acute and long-term symptoms of neurologic damage; it is never present at birth. The clinical manifestations typically appear between 2 and 6 days after birth and go through several phases as the disease progresses, generally beginning after the bilirubin level has peaked. During the first phase, the newborn is hypotonic and lethargic and shows a poor suck and depressed or absent Moro's reflex. These more subtle signs are followed by the appearance of a high-pitched cry, opisthotonos (severe muscle spasm that causes the back to arch acutely), spasticity, hyperreflexia, and often by fever and seizures. All of this occurs over a period of approximately 24 hours. About half of the affected infants survive, although they often suffer permanent neurologic sequelae, such as choreoathetoid cerebral palsy or ataxia, sensorineural hearing loss, perceptual problems, mental retardation, or an attention deficit disorder.

Choreoathetoid cerebral palsy is a chronic condition characterized by both choreiform (jerky, tick-like twitching) and athetoid (slow, writhing) movements. Fortunately, because it is now possible to identify the problem early and institute timely treatment with phototherapy and exchange transfusions, the classic bilirubin encephalopathy just described is not as prevalent as it once was.

> **NURSE ALERT** | *There have been reports of several cases of kernicterus in infants of mothers who were discharged early after birth. The discharge teaching for and follow-up of infants who are discharged early is therefore imperative.*

Hemolytic disorders in the newborn

The most common causes of pathologic hyperbilirubinemia are hemolytic disorders in the newborn. These occur most often if the blood groups of the mother and baby are different, and the most frequent of these are ABO and Rh factor incompatibilities.

The four major blood groups in the ABO system are A, B, AB, and O. People with type A blood have A antigen, those with type B have B antigen, those with type AB have both A and B antigens, and those with type O have no antigen. In turn, people with type A blood have plasma antibodies to type B blood, those with type B blood have antibodies to type A blood, those with type AB blood have no antibodies, and those with type O blood have antibodies to type A and B blood. If a person is administered or exposed to an incompatible blood type, he or she will form antibodies against the antigen in that blood, with an agglutination, or clumping, occurring as the antibodies in the plasma mix with the antigens of the different blood group.

The Rh factor, which is a genetically determined factor present on RBCs, can be a major source of incompatibility. There are several forms of the Rh antigen, with the D antigen the most significant one because it causes the most antibody production in a person who is Rh negative. Rh positivity is a dominant trait, so one must inherit the recessive gene from both parents to be Rh negative. A person who has the Rh factor is considered Rh positive; a person without it is considered Rh negative. As an illustration of the foregoing discussion, a mother who has A negative blood, has the A antigen, plasma antibodies to the B antigen, and no Rh factor on her RBCs.

Hemolytic disorders occur because maternal antibodies are present naturally or form in response to an antigen from the fetal blood crossing the placenta and entering the maternal circulation. The maternal antibodies of the IgG class in turn cross the placenta, causing the neonate's RBCs to lyse, with hyperbilirubinemia and jaundice the result.

ABO incompatibility. **ABO incompatibility** is more common than Rh incompatibility but causes less severe problems in the affected infant. It occurs if the fetal blood type is A, B, or AB and the maternal type is O. It rarely occurs in infants with type B blood born to mothers with type A blood. The incompatibility arises because naturally occurring anti-A and anti-B antibodies are transferred across the placenta to the fetus. Unlike the situation that pertains to Rh incompatibility (discussed in next section), first-born infants may be affected, because mothers with type O blood already have anti-A and anti-B antibodies in their blood. Such a newborn may show a weakly positive result to a direct Coombs' test. The cord bilirubin level usually is less than 4 mg/dl, and any resulting hyperbilirubinemia usually can be treated with phototherapy. Exchange transfusions are required only occasionally. Although ABO incompatibility is a common cause of hyperbilirubinemia, it rarely precipitates significant anemia resulting from the hemolysis of RBCs.

Rh incompatibility. Rh incompatibility, or **isoimmunization,** occurs when an Rh-negative mother has an Rh-positive fetus who inherits the dominant Rh-positive gene from the father. If the mother is Rh negative and the father is Rh positive and homozygous for the Rh factor, all the offspring will be Rh positive. If the father is heterozygous for the factor, there is a 50% chance that each infant born of the union will be Rh positive and a 50% chance that each will be born Rh negative (see Fig. 8-13). An Rh-negative fetus is in no danger because it has the same Rh factor as the mother. An Rh-negative fetus with an Rh-positive mother is also in no danger. It is only the Rh-positive offspring of an Rh-negative mother who is at risk. The incidence of Rh sensitization and resulting hemolytic disease of the newborn has decreased dramatically since the development of Rh$_0$ (D) immune globulin in 1968. However, hemolytic disease of the fetus or newborn resulting from isoimmunization still occurs in 1.5% of all pregnancies (Vomund & Witter, 1994).

The pathogenesis of Rh incompatibility is as follows. Hematopoiesis in the fetus, or the formation of blood cells, begins as early as the eighth week of gestation and, in up to 40% of pregnancies, some of these cells may pass through the placenta into the maternal circulation. When the fetus is Rh positive and the mother Rh negative, the mother may form antibodies against the fetal blood cells—first IgM antibodies that are too large to pass through the placenta, and then later, IgG antibodies that can cross the placenta. The process of antibody formation is called *maternal sensitization*. Sensitization may occur during pregnancy, birth, abortion, or amniocentesis. Usually women become sensitized in their first pregnancy with an Rh-positive fetus but do not produce enough antibodies to cause lysis of fetal blood cells. During subsequent pregnancies, antibodies form in response to repeated contact with the antigen from the fetal blood, resulting in lysis or destruction of fetal RBCs.

Severe Rh incompatibility results in marked fetal hemolytic anemia because the fetal erythrocytes are destroyed by maternal Rh-positive antibodies. Although the placenta usually clears the bilirubin generated by the red blood cell breakdown, in extreme cases fetal bilirubin levels increase. This results in fetal jaundice, also known as *icterus gravis*.

The fetus compensates for the anemia by producing large numbers of immature erythrocytes to replace those hemolyzed, thus the name for this condition—**erythroblastosis fetalis.** In the most severe form of this disease, **hydrops fetalis,** the fetus has marked anemia, together with cardiac decompensation, cardiomegaly, and hepatosplenomegaly. Hypoxia results from the severe anemia. In addition, because of the decreased intravascular oncotic pressure involved, fluid leaks out of the intravascular space, resulting in generalized edema, as well as effusions into the peritoneal (ascites), pericardial, and pleural (effusion) spaces. The placenta is often edematous, which, along with the edematous fetus, can cause the uterus to rupture.

Intrauterine or early neonatal death may occur as a result of hydrops fetalis, although intrauterine exchange transfusions and early delivery of the fetus may avert this. Intrauterine transfusion involves the infusion of Rh-negative, type O blood into the umbilical vein or the peritoneal cavity of the fetus, where it is absorbed by the lymphatics and enters the fetal circulation. Such transfusions are administered as needed until birth. This is a risky procedure, however, and is reserved for use in seriously affected fetuses in which the hazards of transfusion are judged to be less than the complications of prematurity, should premature birth occur (Fanaroff & Martin, 1997).

CARE MANAGEMENT

Assessment and Nursing Diagnoses

It is important to determine the blood type and Rh factor of the pregnant woman prenatally. A thorough history must then be obtained in the Rh-negative pregnant woman to assess for the existence of events that could have caused her to develop antibodies to the Rh factor. Such events include (1) previous pregnancy with an Rh-positive fetus, (2) transfusion with Rh-positive blood, which causes immediate sensitization, (3) spontaneous or elective abortions after 8 or more gestational weeks, (4) amniocentesis performed for any reason, (5) premature separation of the placenta, and (6) trauma.

Because hematopoiesis begins in the fetus during the eighth gestational week, a woman who has experienced an abortion after this time or has previously given birth to a child may have been inoculated with fetal blood at the time of placental separation. During amniocentesis, the needle may cause localized damage to the single layer of cells that separates the maternal and fetal circulation in the placenta, thereby also allowing fetal RBCs to enter the maternal circulation.

If any of these events have occurred, the woman's record is checked to determine whether she has received Rh$_0$ (D) immune globulin, such as Rhogam, which is a commercial preparation of passive antibodies against the Rh factor. This injection of anti-Rh antibodies binds with any fetal red blood cell antigens that are in the maternal circulation causing the cells to be phagocytosed before the woman's immune system is activated to produce antibodies.

An indirect **Coombs' test** should be done at the first prenatal visit of an Rh-negative woman to determine whether she has antibodies to the Rh antigen. In this test the maternal blood serum is mixed with Rh-positive RBCs. If the Rh-positive RBCs agglutinate or clump, this indicates that maternal antibodies are present. The dilution of the specimen of blood at which clumping occurs determines the titer, or level, of maternal antibodies. This titer indicates the degree of maternal sensitization. A level of 1:8 rarely results in fetal jeopardy. If the titer reaches 1:16, amniocentesis is performed to determine optical density (ΔOD) to estimate the fetal hemolytic process (see Chapter 22). Rising bilirubin levels may indicate the need for an intrauterine transfusion or the termination of the pregnancy by labor induction.

The indirect Coombs' test is repeated at 28 weeks and, if the result remains negative, indicating that sensitization has not occurred, the woman is given an intramuscular injection of Rh_o (D) immune globulin. If the test result is positive, showing that sensitization has occurred, it is repeated every 4 to 6 weeks to monitor the maternal antibody titer, as just described.

Nursing diagnoses pertinent to newborns at risk because of hyperbilirubinemia are listed in the accompanying box.

▌ Nursing Diagnoses

Newborns with Hyperbilirubinemia

Risk for injury to neurons and cells in the kidney, pancreas, and intestine related to:
- Hyperbilirubinemia

Impaired gas exchange related to:
- Hemolytic anemia

Risk for fluid volume deficit related to:
- Phototherapy

Risk for parental anxiety related to:
- Hyperbilirubinemia, its management, and potential sequelae

Risk for impaired skin integrity related to:
- Increased stooling while undergoing phototherapy

Risk for ineffective thermoregulation (increased or decreased) related to:
- Phototherapy

Expected Outcomes of Care

Hospital protocols for the care of infants with hyperbilirubinemia are developed as a collaborative effort of the health care team. These protocols are then used in individualizing care for the infant and parents. Expected outcomes for care are stated in patient-centered terms, as in the following:

- The infant's prenatal and perinatal risk factors will be identified, and intervention will be implemented when appropriate.
- The infant will not develop hyperbilirubinemia or its sequela, kernicterus.
- The infant will have minimal or no sequelae from hyperbilirubinemia and its treatment.
- The infant will tolerate the treatment for hyperbilirubinemia without complications.
- The infant's serum bilirubin levels will return to normal.
- The infant's parents will demonstrate an understanding of the infant's condition, the therapies, and the possible sequelae of the condition.

Plan of Care and Interventions

Prenatally the prevention of hyperbilirubinemia is the primary focus of care. The implementation of interventions focused on the care of the woman whose fetus is considered at risk for hyperbilirubinemia is essential to prevent problems in the newborn. Prenatal control of diabetes mellitus, prevention of maternal infection, avoidance of drugs such as diazepam and salicylates near the time of birth, and prevention of preterm birth reduce the risk.

There must be early identification of the Rh-negative woman, and care must be taken to prevent sensitization. The Rh-negative woman should be asked about any blood transfusion or any of the other factors already cited that would predispose her to sensitization. Rh_o (D) immune globulin is administered in the following amounts to Rh-negative women whose Coombs' tests are negative (Fanaroff & Martin, 1997; Wandstrat, 1997):

- 50 µg after
  —chorionic villus sampling, ectopic pregnancy or abortion before 13 weeks' gestation
- 300 µg after
  —spontaneous or elective abortion after 13 weeks' gestation
  —percutaneous umbilical sampling
  —amniocentesis
  —abruptio placentae/placenta previa
  —trauma
  —at 28 weeks' gestation
  —within 72 hours of the preterm or term birth of an Rh-positive infant
- More than 300 µg after
  —large transplacental hemorrhage
  —mismatched blood transfusion

The fetus and maternal antibody titers are monitored prenatally. If amniocentesis reveals that the ΔOD is high and ultrasound reveals the fetus is in jeopardy, intrauterine transfusion may be done every 1 to 2 weeks between 26 and 32 weeks. If the endangered fetus is at more than 32 weeks' gestation, a preterm delivery may be performed, usually by cesarean.

Postpartum interventions focus on preventing sensitization in the mother, if it has not occurred already, and treating any complications in the neonate resulting from the hemolysis of RBCs. The unsensitized Rh-negative mother whose baby is Rh positive should receive 300 µg of Rh_o (D) immune globulin within 72 hours of birth. This should prevent her from producing antibodies to the fetal blood cells that entered her bloodstream during the birth.

The neonate's cord blood is sent to the laboratory to determine the infant's blood type and Rh status. A direct Coombs' test is performed on this cord blood to determine whether there are maternal antibodies in the fetal blood. If antibodies are found to be present, the titer, indicating the degree of maternal sensitization, is measured. If the titer is 1:64, an exchange transfusion is indicated. In addition, the prevention of or prompt therapy for perinatal asphyxia, acidosis, cold stress, sepsis, and hypoglycemia will decrease the newborn's risk for severe hemolytic disease and his or her susceptibility to kernicterus. Early frequent feedings are also initiated to stimulate the gastrocolic reflex and thus to facilitate the removal of bilirubin through stooling.

If pathologic jaundice is present, the cause is determined and therapeutic management begun. This includes monitoring and reducing the raised bilirubin level. The bilirubin level can also be measured noninvasively using transcutaneous bilirubinometry. This is a screening test for neonatal jaundice that uses as its basis the relationship between the yellow color of the skin and the total serum bilirubin level.

Phototherapy is used to reduce the serum bilirubin levels, particularly if the jaundice is physiologic rather than pathologic, occurs past the 24-hour period after birth, and the bilirubin levels are generally less than 15 mg/dl. Phototherapy using bili-lights or a phototherapy blanket is carried out in the normal newborn nursery (see Chapter 20 and Fig. 20-9).

Exchange transfusions are needed less frequently today because of the decrease in the incidence of hemolytic disease in newborns resulting from isoimmunization. However, it is still the treatment of choice for some infants, including full-term infants with bilirubin levels of 20 mg/dl or greater after intensive phototherapy has failed to lower the bilirubin level by 1 to 2 mg/dl within 4 to 6 hours of therapy or show a steady decrease in total bilirubin to levels below the exchange transfusion level (Provisional Committee AAP, 1994). A positive result to a direct Coombs' test performed on cord blood and a hemoglobin concentration of less than 12 gm/dl, indicating hemolytic disease in the newborn, are also indications for transfusion. However, other factors must always be considered as well, particularly the clinical condition of the infant, because the risks of treatment must be weighed against the risks of the outcome if the infant is not treated (Peterec, 1995).

An exchange transfusion reduces the serum bilirubin level in infants who have severe hyperbilirubinemia resulting from any cause. In infants with Rh incompatibility, it removes the RBCs that would otherwise be hemolyzed by circulating maternal antibodies, removes the antibodies responsible for hemolysis, and corrects the anemia caused by hemolysis of the infant's sensitized RBCs. It also reduces the serum bilirubin level in infants who have severe hyperbilirubinemia resulting from any cause.

Exchange transfusion is accomplished by alternately removing a small amount of the infant's blood and replacing it with an equal amount of donor blood. If the infant has Rh incompatibility, type O Rh-negative blood is used for transfusion, so the maternal antibodies still present in the infant do not hemolyze the transfused blood. Depending on the infant's size, maturity, and condition, amounts of from 5 to 20 ml of the infant's blood are removed at one time and replaced with donor blood. The total amount of blood exchanged approximates 170 ml/kg of body weight, or 75% to 85% of the infant's total blood volume. During the procedure the health care team members observe the infection control precautions for invasive procedures. The infant is monitored closely during and after the procedure, including the heart rate and rhythm, respirations, blood pressure,

temperature, pedal pulses, and the presence of edema. Hypervolemia or hypovolemia, as well as air emboli, may be a complication of the procedure. Symptoms of hypocalcemia, such as jitteriness, irritability, convulsions, tachycardia, and electrocardiogram changes, may be triggered by preservatives in the donor blood that lower the infant's serum calcium level. This may necessitate an infusion of calcium gluconate to correct the deficit. The nurse also monitors the infusion site for hemorrhage and is constantly alert for any other complications of blood transfusion that may occur, such as heart failure, hypercalcemia, hyperkalemia, hypernatremia, hypoglycemia, acidosis, sepsis, shock, thrombus formation, and a transfusion mismatch reaction (Wise & Lawrence-Nolan, 1990).

Planning for rehabilitative measures is necessary if kernicterus occurs. The family will need the services of many community resources to care for the affected child. An interdisciplinary approach that includes social services must be taken.

Home care

In cases in which the infant is discharged from the hospital before 48 hours of age, the parents should receive teaching regarding adequate hydration and assessment of the infant for the appearance of jaundice. Appropriate testing and follow-up of the infant should be available. A program of home phototherapy, where available, allows infants to receive treatment of uncomplicated hyperbilirubinemia following discharge from the hospital. For these infants, nurses provide monitoring of treatment and of serum bilirubin levels as outlined by hospital or agency policy.

Evaluation

On a short-term basis, the nurse can consider nursing care to be effective to the degree that the outcomes for care were achieved (Plan of Care).

❙ BIRTH TRAUMA

Birth trauma (injury) is physical injury sustained by a neonate during labor and birth. The significance of birth injuries is assessed most accurately by review of mortality data. These data show a steady decline in fatal birth injuries. In 1981, birth injuries ranked sixth in major causes of neonatal mortality, resulting in 23.8 deaths per 100,000 live births. As of 1993, birth injuries ranked eleventh and caused 3.7 deaths per 100,000 live births. This ongoing improvement has been attributed to refinements in obstetric techniques, increased use of cesarean birth for births that would be difficult vaginally, and decreased use of vacuum extraction and version and extraction. Despite this decrease, birth injuries still represent an important source of neonatal morbidity. Therefore the clinician should consider the broad range of birth injuries in the differential diagnosis of neonatal clinical disorders (Fanaroff & Martin, 1997).

PLAN OF CARE *Infant with Hyperbilirubinemia*

> **NURSING DIAGNOSIS** Risk for injury related to hemolytic disease and treatment effects

Expected Outcomes *Bilirubin levels decrease with treatment, there is no evidence of harmful effects from phototherapy (i.e., no eye irritation, dehydration, temperature instability, or skin breakdown), and there are no complications from exchange transfusions.*

Nursing Interventions/*Rationales*

Initiate early feedings *to enhance excretion of bilirubin in stools.*

Observe skin and mucous membranes for signs of jaundice, *indicative of rising bilirubin levels;* monitor serum bilirubin levels *to determine rate of rise and treatment response.*

Note time of jaundice onset *to help distinguish physiologic from other causes of jaundice.*

Observe for signs of hypoxia, hypothermia, hypoglycemia, and metabolic acidosis, *which occur as a result of hyperbilirubinemia and increase the risk of brain damage.*

Initiate phototherapy per physician order *to decrease bilirubin levels.*

During phototherapy, shield infant's eyes *to prevent damage to corneas and retinas:* keep infant nude and change positions frequently *for maximum body surface exposure:* cleanse skin frequently *to prevent irritation;* maintain adequate fluid intake *to prevent dehydration;* monitor body temperature *to prevent hyperthermia.*

Before exchange transfusion, keep infant NPO (2 to 4 hours) *to prevent aspiration;* check donor blood for compatibility *to prevent transfusion reaction;* have resuscitation equipment (oxygen, Ambu bag, endotracheal tubes, laryngoscope) at bedside *in preparation for emergency action.*

Assist physician with exchange transfusion procedure; track amounts of blood withdrawn and transfused *to maintain balanced blood volume;* maintain body temperature *to avoid hypothermia and cold stress;* monitor vital signs and observe for rash *for indicators of transfusion reaction.*

After transfusion, continue to monitor vital signs *for transfusion reaction or other complications;* check umbilical cord *for bleeding or signs of infection.*

> **NURSING DIAGNOSIS** Risk for knowledge deficit related to administration of home phototherapy

Expected Outcome *Family demonstrates ability to provide home therapy.*

Nursing Interventions/*Rationales*

Explore family's willingness to try home phototherapy *to evaluate feasibility of home therapy option.*

Explore family's understanding of jaundice and proposed therapy *to establish baseline for teaching.*

Teach family with demonstration-return demonstration, allowing for several practice sessions and supplement with written materials with pictorial representations *to ensure safe and optimum results.*

Include the following in your instructions: placement of lamp or fiberoptic unit; proper eye care and patching; proper skin care; proper positioning under lamp; provision of increased fluid intake; monitoring of time under lamp; monitoring of vital signs, skin, eyes, feeding patterns, stooling and voiding patterns; observation for complications.

Stress importance of obtaining the prescribed bilirubin tests on schedule *as a way of tracking success of therapy.*

Give parents a contact if they have any questions while carrying out therapy *to offer ongoing support and increase parent comfort.*

From Wong D & Perry S: *Maternal child nursing care,* St Louis, 1998, Mosby.

In theory, most birth injuries may be avoidable, especially if careful assessment of risk factors and appropriate planning of birth occur. The use of ultrasonography allows antepartum diagnosis of macrosomia, hydrocephalus, and unusual presentations. Elective cesarean birth can be chosen for some pregnancies to prevent significant birth injury. A small percentage of significant birth injuries are unavoidable despite skilled and competent obstetric care, as in especially difficult or prolonged labor or when the infant is in an abnormal presentation (Fanaroff & Martin, 1997). Some injuries cannot be anticipated until the specific circumstances are encountered during childbirth. Emergency cesarean birth may provide a last-minute salvage, but in these circumstances the injury may be truly unavoidable. The same injury might be caused in several ways. For example, a cephalhematoma could result from an obstetric technique such as forceps or vacuum-assisted birth or from pressure of the fetal skull against the maternal pelvis.

Many injuries are minor and resolve readily in the neonatal period without treatment. Other traumas require some degree of intervention. A few are serious enough to be fatal. The nurse's contributions to the welfare of the newborn begin with early observation and accurate recording. The prompt reporting of signs that indicate deviations from normal permits early initiation of appropriate therapy. Table 28-1 provides an overview of neurologic birth injuries and the sites in which they occur.

TABLE 28-1 *Types of Birth Injuries*

SITE OF INJURY	TYPE OF INJURY
Scalp	Caput succedaneum
	Subgaleal hemorrhage
	Cephalhematoma
Skull	Linear fracture
	Depressed fracture
	Occipital osteodiastasis
Intracranial	Epidural hematoma
	Subdural hematoma (laceration of
	falx, tentorium, or superficial veins)
	Subarachnoid hemorrhage
	Cerebral contusion
	Cerebellar contusion
	Intracerebellar hematoma
Spinal cord	Vertebral artery injury
(cervical)	Intraspinal hemorrhage
	Spinal cord transection or injury
Plexus	Erb's palsy
	Klumpke's paralysis
	Total (mixed) brachial plexus injury
	Horner's syndrome
	Diaphragmatic paralysis
	Lumbosacral plexus injury
Cranial and	Radial nerve palsy
peripheral	Medial nerve palsy
nerve	Sciatic nerve palsy
	Laryngeal nerve palsy
	Diaphragmatic paralysis
	Facial nerve palsy

From Moe P & Paige P: Neurologic disorders. In Merenstein G & Gardner S, editors: *Handbook of neonatal intensive care,* ed 4, St Louis, 1998, Mosby.

I CARE MANAGEMENT

Assessment and Nursing Diagnoses

Several factors predispose an infant to birth injuries (Fanaroff & Martin, 1997; Merenstein & Gardner, 1998). Maternal factors include uterine dysfunction that leads to prolonged or precipitous labor, preterm or postterm labor, and cephalopelvic disproportion. Injury may result from dystocia caused by fetal macrosomia, multifetal gestation, abnormal or difficult presentation (not caused by maternal uterine or pelvic conditions), and congenital anomalies. Intrapartum events that can result in scalp injury include the use of intrapartum monitoring of fetal heart rate (FHR) and collection of fetal scalp blood for acid-base assessment. Obstetric birth techniques can cause injury. Forceps- and vacuum-assisted birth, version and extraction, and cesarean birth are potential contributory factors. Often more than one factor is present, and multiple predisposing factors may be related to a single maternal disease.

The Apgar score may alert the caregiver to birth injuries and help in identifying infants in need of immediate resuscitation. Flaccid muscle tone, regardless of cause, increases the risk of joint dislocations and separation during the birth process. Flaccid tone in extremities may be traced to nerve plexus injuries or long-bone fractures. A weak or hoarse cry is characteristic of laryngeal nerve palsy as a result of excessive traction on the neck during birth. Pronounced bruising of the skin may preclude accurate assessment for color.

A complete physical assessment of the newborn is performed soon after birth. Because evidence of birth injury may not be apparent at the initial examination, assessment continues during each contact with the neonate.

Nursing diagnoses depend on the type of injury. Examples are listed in the accompanying box.

I Nursing Diagnoses

Infants with Birth Injuries
Infant
Impaired physical mobility related to:
• Brachial plexus injury
Impaired gas exchange related to:
• Diaphragmatic paralysis (partial or complete)
Pain related to:
• Injury
Injury related to:
• Bruising, cephalhematoma, hyperbilirubinemia
Parents and family
Anxiety related to knowledge deficit regarding:
• Injury
• Cause of injury
• Management and therapy
• Prognosis
Anticipatory grieving related to:
• Possible sequelae of the birth injury

Expected Outcomes of Care

Meeting the unique needs of the birth-injured newborn requires constant vigilance. Expected outcomes are established and prioritized. Nursing actions are selected in terms of the particular disorder and individual needs of the infant and family. The overall outcomes for care of infants with birth trauma include the following:
• The newborn will suffer minimal or no sequelae of trauma
• The infant will receive prompt and appropriate treatment
• The parents will initiate and maintain a positive parent-child relationship
• The parents' and family's educational needs regarding the injury and its management will be met

Plan of Care and Interventions

Soft tissue injuries

Caput succedaneum is a localized edematous swelling of the scalp that crosses the suture lines of the skull. The swelling persists for a few days after birth and then disappears without treatment. It is most often seen after vertex vaginal births and has no pathologic significance (Fig. 19-4, *A*).

Cephalhematoma is a collection of blood from ruptured blood vessels between the periosteum and the surface of the skull. Because blood collects beneath the periosteum, it does not cross the cranial suture lines (see Fig. 19-4, *B*). The swelling may appear unilaterally or bilaterally, usually is minimal or absent at birth, increases over the first 3 days of life, and disappears gradually in 2 to 3 weeks. Occasionally, hyperbilirubinemia may result from breakdown of the accumulated blood.

Subconjunctival (scleral) and retinal hemorrhages result from rupture of capillaries caused by increased intracranial pressure during birth. They clear within 5 days after birth and usually present no problems. However, parents need reassurance about their presence.

Erythema, ecchymoses, petechiae, abrasions, lacerations, and edema of buttocks and extremities may be present. Localized discoloration may appear over presenting or dependent parts. Ecchymoses and edema may appear anywhere on the body and on the presenting body part from the application of forceps. They also may result from manipulation of the infant's body during birth.

Bruises over the face may be the result of face presentation (Fig. 28-1). In a breech presentation, bruising and swelling may be seen over the buttocks or genitalia (Fig. 28-2). The skin over the entire head may be ecchymotic and covered with petechiae caused by a tight nuchal cord. Petechiae, or pinpoint hemorrhagic areas, acquired during birth may extend over the upper portion of the trunk and face. These lesions are benign if they disappear within 2 days of birth and no new lesions appear. Ecchymoses and petechiae may be signs of a more serious disorder, such as thrombocytopenic purpura. If they do not disappear spontaneously in 2 days, the physician is notified. To differentiate hemorrhagic areas from skin rashes and discolorations such as mongolian spots, the nurse blanches the skin with two fingers. Because extravasated blood remains within the tissues, petechiae and ecchymoses do not blanch.

Forceps injury occurs at the site of application of the instrument. Forceps injury typically has a linear configuration across both sides of the face, outlining the placement of the forceps. The affected areas are kept clean to minimize the risk of secondary infection. These injuries usually resolve spontaneously within several days with no specific therapy. The increased use of padded forceps blades and vacuum assisted birth may reduce the incidence of these lesions (Fanaroff & Martin, 1997).

Accidental lacerations may be inflicted with a scalpel during cesarean birth or with scissors during an episiotomy. These cuts may occur on any part of the body but most often are found on the scalp, buttocks, and thighs. Usually they are superficial, needing only to be kept clean. Butterfly adhesive strips will hold the edges of more serious lacerations together. Rarely, sutures are needed.

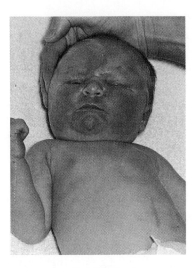

Fig. **28-1** Marked bruising of the entire face of an infant born vaginally after face presentation. Less severe ecchymoses were present on the extremities. Phototherapy was required for treatment of jaundice resulting from the breakdown of accumulated blood. (From O'Doherty N: *Neonatology: micro atlas of the newborn,* Nutley, NJ, 1986, Hoffmann-LaRoche.)

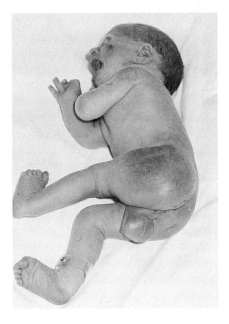

Fig. **28-2** Swelling of the genitals and bruising of the buttocks after a breech delivery. (From O'Doherty N: *Neonatology: micro atlas of the newborn,* Nutley, NJ, 1986, Hoffmann-LaRoche.)

Skeletal injuries

The newborn's immature, flexible skull can withstand a great degree of molding before fracture results. Considerable force is required to fracture the newborn's skull. Two types of skull fractures typically are identified in the newborn: linear fractures and depressed fractures. The location of the fracture and involvement of underlying structures determine its significance.

If an artery lying in a groove on the undersurface of the skull is torn as a result of the fracture, increased intracranial pressure will ensue. Unless a blood vessel is involved, linear fractures (which account for 70% of all fractures for this age group) heal without special treatment. The soft skull may become indented without laceration of either the skin or the dural membrane. These depressed fractures, or "ping-pong ball" indentations, may occur during difficult births from pressure of the head on the bony pelvis (Fig. 28-3). They also can occur as a result of injudicious application of forceps. Spontaneous or nonsurgical elevation of the indentation using a hand breast pump or vacuum extractor has been reported (Fanaroff & Martin, 1997).

Fracture of the *clavicle,* or collarbone, is the most common birth injury. It is often associated with difficult vertex or breech birth of infants of greater than average size. *Crepitus* (the crackling sound produced by the rubbing together of fractured bone fragments) is often heard and/or felt (especially if the infant is in a prone position), and radiographs usually reveal a complete fracture with overriding of the fragments (Fig. 28-4).

A newborn with a fractured clavicle may have no symptoms, but suspect a fracture if the infant has limited use of the affected arm, malposition of the arm, an asymmetric Moro's reflex, or focal swelling or tenderness or if the infant cries in pain when the arm is moved. Eliciting the scarf sign (extending arm across chest toward opposite shoulder) for assessment of gestational age is contraindicated if a fractured clavicle is suspected. Often no intervention may be prescribed other than proper body alignment, careful dressing and undressing of the infant, and handling and carrying that support the affected bone. For example, if the infant has a fractured clavicle, it is important to support the upper and lower back rather than pull the infant up from under the arms. Occasionally, for immobilization and relief of pain, the arm on the side of the fractured clavicle may be fixed on the body by pinning the sleeve to the shirt or by application of a triangular sling.

The humerus and femur are other bones that may be fractured during a difficult birth. Fractures in newborns generally heal rapidly. Immobilization is accomplished with slings, splints, swaddling, and other devices.

The parents need support in handling these infants because they often are fearful of hurting them. Parents are encouraged to practice handling, changing, and feeding the affected neonate under the guidance of nursery personnel. This increases their confidence and knowledge and facilitates attachment. A plan for follow-up therapy is developed with the parents so that the times and arrangements for therapy are acceptable to them.

Peripheral nervous system injuries

Erb-Duchenne paralysis (brachial paralysis of the upper portion of the arm) is the most common type of paralysis associated with a difficult birth, occurring at rates of 0.5 to

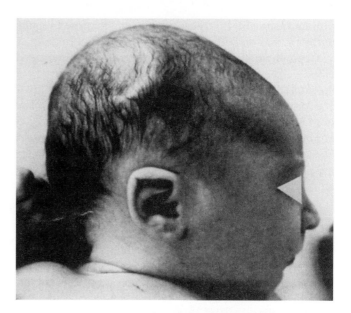

Fig. 28-3 Depressed skull fracture in a full-term male after rapid (1-hour) labor. The infant was delivered by occiput-anterior presentation after rotation from occiput-posterior position. (From Fanaroff A & Martin R, editors: *Neonatal-perinatal medicine: diseases of the fetus and infant,* ed 6, St Louis, 1997, Mosby.)

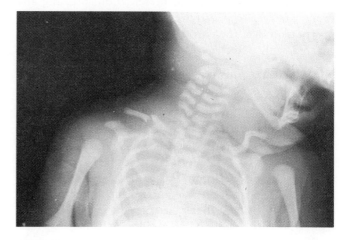

Fig. 28-4 Fractured clavicle after shoulder dystocia. (From O'Doherty N: *Neonatology: micro atlas of the newborn,* Nutley, NJ, 1986, Hoffmann-LaRoche.)

1.9 per 1,000 live births (Merenstein & Gardner, 1998) (Fig. 28-5). Injury to the upper plexus results from stretching or pulling the head away from the shoulder during the difficult birth. Typical symptoms are a flaccid arm with the elbow extended and the hand rotated inward, absence of Moro's reflex on the affected side, sensory loss over the lateral aspect of the arm, and an intact grasp reflex.

Treatment is by intermittent immobilization, proper positioning, and range of motion (ROM) exercises. Gentle manipulation and ROM exercises are delayed until

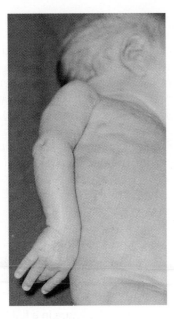

Fig. 28-5 Erb-Duchenne paralysis in newborn infant. Moro's reflex was absent in right upper extremity. Recovery was complete. (From O'Doherty N: *Neonatology: micro atlas of the newborn*, Nutley, NJ, 1986, Hoffmann-LaRoche.)

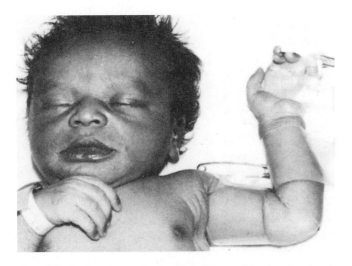

Fig. 28-6 Recommended corrective positioning for treatment of Erb-Duchenne paralysis. Notice abduction and external rotation at shoulder, flexion at elbow, supination of forearm and slight dorsiflexion at wrist. (From Behrmann R, editor: *Neonatology: diseases of the fetus and infant*, St Louis, 1973, Mosby.)

about the tenth day to prevent additional injury to the brachial plexus.

Immobilization may be accomplished with a brace or splint or by pinning the infant's sleeve to the mattress. The infant should be positioned for 2 or 3 hours at a time as follows (Fig. 28-6):

• Abduct the arm 90 degrees
• Externally rotate the shoulder

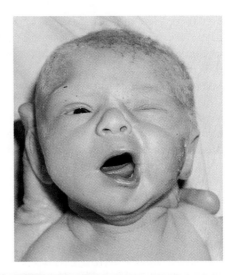

Fig. 28-7 Facial paralysis 15 minutes after forceps birth. Absence of movement on affected side is especially noticeable when infant cries. (From O'Doherty N: *Neonatology: micro atlas of the newborn*, Nutley, NJ, 1986, Hoffmann-LaRoche.)

• Flex the elbow 90 degrees
• Supinate the wrist with the palm directed slightly toward the face.

Damage to the lower plexus, *Klumpke's palsy*, is less common. With lower arm paralysis, the wrist and hand are flaccid, the grasp reflex is absent, deep tendon reflexes are present, and dependent edema and cyanosis may be apparent (in the affected hand). Treatment consists of placing the hand in a neutral position, padding the fist, and gently exercising the wrist and fingers.

Parents are taught to position and immobilize the arm or wrist or both. They can gently massage and manipulate the muscles to prevent contractures while the arm is healing. If edema or hemorrhage is responsible for the paralysis, the prognosis is good and recovery may be expected in a few weeks. If laceration of the nerves has occurred and healing does not result in return of function within a few months (3 to 6 months or 2 years at the most), surgery may be indicated; however, little or no function will develop. Full recovery is expected in 85% to 95% of infants (Merenstein & Gardner, 1998).

Facial palsy or paralysis (Fig. 28-7) generally is caused by pressure on the facial nerve during birth. The face on the affected side is flattened and unresponsive to the grimace that accompanies crying or stimulation, and the eye will remain open. Moreover, the forehead will not wrinkle. Often the condition is transitory, resolving within hours or days of birth. Permanent paralysis is rare.

Treatment involves assistance with feeding, prevention of damage to the cornea of the open eye, and supportive care of the parents. Usually the infant's face appears distorted, especially when crying. Feeding may be prolonged, with the milk flowing out the newborn's mouth around the nipple on the affected side. The mother will need understanding and sympathetic encouragement while learning how to feed and care for the infant, as well as how to hold and cuddle the baby.

Phrenic nerve injury almost always occurs as a component of brachial plexus injury rather than as an isolated problem. Injury to the phrenic nerve results in diaphragmatic paralysis. Cyanosis and irregular thoracic respirations, with no abdominal movement on inspiration, are characteristic of paralysis of the diaphragm. Babies with diaphragmatic paralysis usually require mechanical ventilatory support, at least for the first few days after birth. Other treatments include diaphragmatic pacing or surgical correction.

Central nervous system injuries

All types of intracranial hemorrhage (ICH) occur in newborns. ICH as a result of birth trauma is more likely to occur in the full-term, large infant. The frequency and severity of ICH are different in the newborn than in older children or adults. In the newborn more than one type of hemorrhage can and does frequently occur (Fanaroff & Martin, 1997; Wong, 1995).

Subdural hemorrhages (hematomas), life-threatening collections of blood in the subdural space, most often are produced by the stretching and tearing of the large veins in the tentorium of the cerebellum, the dural membrane that separates the cerebrum from the cerebellum. When this type of bleeding occurs, the typical history includes a nulliparous mother, with the total labor and birth occurring in less than 2 or 3 hours, a difficult birth involving high or midforceps application, or a large-for-gestational age (LGA) infant. Subdural hematoma occurs infrequently today because of improvements in obstetric care. However, it is especially serious because of its inaccessibility to aspiration by subdural tap (Fanaroff & Martin, 1997; Wong, 1995).

Subarachnoid hemorrhage, the most common type of ICH, occurs in term infants as a result of trauma and in preterm infants as a result of hypoxia. Small hemorrhages are the most common. Bleeding is of venous origin, and underlying contusion also may occur (Wong, 1995).

The clinical presentation of hemorrhage in the full-term infant can vary considerably. In many infants, signs are absent, and hemorrhaging is diagnosed only because of abnormal findings on lumbar puncture, for example, RBCs in the cerebrospinal fluid (CSF). The initial clinical manifestations of neonatal subarachnoid hemorrhage may be the early onset of alternating depression and irritability, with refractory seizures (Fanaroff & Martin, 1997). Occasionally the infant appears normal initially and then has seizures on the second or third day of life, followed by no apparent sequelae.

Intracerebellar hemorrhage, although infrequent, may occur in LBW infants in association with perinatal trauma and asphyxia. At present the exact causes are not fully understood. The clinical picture is characterized by severe progressive apnea, a falling hematocrit level, and death (Fanaroff & Martin, 1997).

In general, nursing care of an infant with ICH is supportive and includes monitoring of ventilatory and intravenous therapy, observation and management of seizures, and prevention of increased ICP. Minimal handling to promote rest and reduce stress should guide nursing care (Wong, 1995).

Spinal cord injuries almost always result from breech births, especially difficult ones in which version and extraction are used. Brow and face presentations, dystocia, preterm birth, maternal nulliparity, and precipitous birth have also been identified as predisposing factors in these types of injuries. Stretching of the spinal cord, usually by forceful longitudinal traction on the trunk while the head is still firmly engaged in the pelvis, is the most common mechanism of injury. This injury is rarely seen today because cesarean birth is often used for breech presentation (Fanaroff & Martin, 1997).

Clinical manifestations depend on the severity and location of the injury. High cervical cord injuries are more likely to cause stillbirths or rapid death of the neonate (Menitocoglou, Perlman & Manning, 1995). Lower lesions cause an acute spinal cord syndrome. Common signs of spinal shock include flaccid extremities, diaphragmatic breathing, paralyzed abdominal movements, atonic anal sphincter, and distended bladder. Therapy is supportive and usually unsatisfactory. Infants who survive present a therapeutic challenge that requires combined treatment from many health care providers, including the nurse, pediatrician, neurologist, neurosurgeon, urologist, orthopedist, physical therapist, and occupational therapist. Parents need to understand fully the implications of severe injury to the spinal cord and the overwhelming implications it presents for the family (Fanaroff & Martin, 1997; Merenstein & Gardner, 1998).

Evaluation

The nurse can be assured that care has been effective if the previously stated outcomes for care have been achieved.

CONGENITAL ANOMALIES

The desired and expected outcome of every wanted pregnancy is a normal, functioning infant with a good intellectual potential. Fulfillment of this hope depends on numerous hereditary and environmental factors. Probably all human characteristics have a genetic component, including those that produce symptoms or physical abnormalities that impair the fitness of the person. Some disorders or diseases occur through the influence of a single gene or the combined action of many genes inherited from the parents; others result from the action of the intrauterine environment. Many defects appear to occur as the result of multifactorial inheritance, which is the interaction of multiple genes with environmental factors that affect the embryonic development of the affected system. Examples of these include neural tube defects, congenital heart defects, congenital hip dysplasia, and cleft lip or palate. A disease or disorder that is transmitted from generation to generation is termed *genetic* or *hereditary*. A **congenital** disorder is one that is present at birth and can be caused by genetic or environmental factors, or both.

Congenital defects occur in 3% to 4% of all live births (Wardinsky, 1994), but this number increases if one includes the congenital defects that are diagnosed later in childhood. In addition, the incidence of congenital malformations in fetuses that are aborted is higher than that in infants who are born alive, thus also adding to the overall incidence. Major congenital defects are the leading cause of death in infants younger than 1 year of age in the United States and account for 20% of neonatal deaths. Although there has been a decrease in the incidences of other causes of neonatal mortality, the death rate associated with most congenital anomalies has essentially remained stable since 1932. For example, although the incidence of congenital heart defects has increased, probably because of better diagnostic capabilities, the death rate in such children has remained at approximately 1.5 per 10,000 children (Hoekelman et al., 1996).

The most common major congenital anomalies that cause serious problems in the neonate are congenital heart disease, neural tube defects, cleft lip or palate, clubfoot, and congenital hip dysplasia. These are thought to result from the interaction of multiple genetic and environmental factors. Minor anomalies are less apparent but are important to identify because they may be a part of a characteristic pattern of malformations. That is, they may point to the presence of a more serious major anomaly and aid in its diagnosis. Minor malformations are more common in areas of the body that have variable features, such as the face and distal extremities. Some of the most common malformations include the lack of a helical fold of the pinna, complete or incomplete simian creases, and a capillary hemangioma other than on the face or posterior aspect of the neck.

The seriousness of congenital anomalies in terms of their effect on society is reflected in the more than 6 million hospital days and $200 billion a year required for the care and treatment of these neonates. Ways of preventing and detecting these anomalies are being improved continuously, as are the techniques for the care of the fetus with certain anomalies. Promoting the availability of these services to populations at risk challenges the community health care systems. An interdisciplinary team approach is vital for providing holistic care: the surgical treatment, rehabilitation, and education of the child, as well as psychosocial and financial assistance for the parents. Parental disappointment and disillusion add to the complexity of the nursing care needed for these infants.

Cardiovascular System Anomalies

During fetal development there are periods when cell division and differentiation of the organs and tissues of a particular body system are occurring rapidly. During these various sensitive, or critical, periods, particular body systems are more susceptible to environmental influences than they are later in gestation. For example, the critical period for the cardiovascular system is from week 3 of embryonic development to week 8, a time when many women may not be aware that they are pregnant.

Congenital heart defects (CHDs) are anatomic abnormalities in the heart that are present at birth, although they may not be diagnosed immediately. Some type of cardiologic problem is present in 10 of every 1,000 live births (Hoffman, 1995). Ventricular septal defects, constituting more than 20% of all CHDs, are the most common type of acyanotic lesion. Tetralogy of Fallot, constituting 10% of all CHDs, is the most common type resulting in cyanosis. After prematurity, CHDs are the next major cause of death in the first year of life.

The etiology of CHDs is unknown in more than 90% of the cases. This is an important fact for parents to know, because they often feel guilt that they have done something to cause the defect. Maternal factors that are associated with a higher incidence of CHD include maternal rubella, alcoholism, diabetes, poor nutrition, or age over 40. The maternal ingestion of folic acid antagonists, anticonvulsants, progesterone, estrogen, lithium, or coumadin, or use of the acne medication Accutane (isotretinoin) are thought to be involved in the cause of heart defects, as is radiation exposure. There is also an increased likelihood of cardiac disease in LBW infants, especially those small for gestational age, as well as in premature infants and those with congenital infections. In addition, CHDs may be associated with other extracardiac defects such as renal agenesis, tracheoesophageal fistula, and diaphragmatic hernias.

Genetic factors are implicated in the pathogenesis of CHD. As a general rule, these defects are thought to be multifactorial in origin, involving both genetic and environmental influences; however, a familial occurrence of virtually all forms of CHD has been noted. If a family has one affected child, the risk for them having a second child with CHD has been thought to be 1% to 3%, but the risk for the acquisition of some defects is greater than this. For example, the risk for the acquisition of left-sided lesions such as hypoplastic left heart syndrome is 14%; that for coarctation of the aorta is 8% (Fyler, 1992). The risk of an affected mother having a child with a CHD ranges from 8% to 16%. This number will become more important as children with CHDs live longer and reproduce; therefore continuing epidemiologic studies are needed in this area.

Chromosomal abnormalities may also be associated with CHDs. For example, 40% of children with trisomy 21, or Down syndrome, have a cardiac defect. All children who have trisomy 18, the second most common

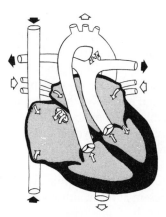

Complete transposition of great vessels

The anomaly is an embryologic defect caused by a straight division of the bulbar trunk without normal spiraling. As a result, the aorta originates from the right ventricle, and the pulmonary artery from the left ventricle. An abnormal communication between the two circulations must be present to sustain life.

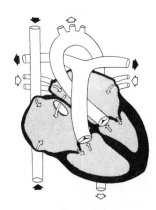

Atrial septal defects

An atrial septal defect is an abnormal opening between the right and left atria. Basically, three types of abnormalities result from incorrect development of the atrial septum. An incompetent foramen ovale is the most common defect. The high ostium secundum defect results from abnormal development of the septum secundum. Improper development of the septum primum produces a basal opening known as an ostium primum defect, frequently involving the atrioventricular valves. In general, left to right shunting of blood occurs in all atrial septal defects.

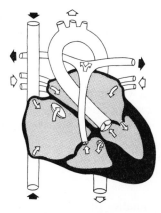

Tricuspid atresia

Tricuspid valvular atresia is characterized by a small right ventricle, large left ventricle, and usually a diminished pulmonary circulation. Blood from the right atrium passes through an atrial septal defect into the left atrium, mixes with oxygenated blood returning from the lungs, flows into the left ventricle, and is propelled into the systemic circulation. The lungs may receive blood through one of three routes: (1) a small ventricular septal defect, (2) patent ductus arteriosus, (3) bronchial vessels.

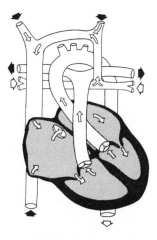

Anomalous venous return

Oxygenated blood returning from the lungs is carried abnormally to the right heart by one or more pulmonary veins emptying directly, or indirectly, through venous channels into the right atrium. Partial anomalous return of the pulmonary veins to the right atrium functions the same as an atrial septal defect. In complete anomalous return of the pulmonary veins, an interatrial communication is necessary for survival.

Fig. 28-8 Congenital heart abnormalities. (Used with permission of Ross Products Division, Abbott Laboratories, Inc., Columbus, Ohio 43216. From Clinical Education Aid #7, copyright 1976, Ross Products Division, Abbott Laboratories, Inc.)

chromosomal abnormality, have cardiac anomalies, and most die within a week of birth.

Although traditionally CHD has been classified as either cyanotic or acyanotic, a classification that categorizes cardiac defects physiologically is now considered more descriptive. The first of the four categories in this classification includes defects that result in increased pulmonary blood flow, often with congestive heart failure. Examples of the CHDs in this category are atrial and ventricular septal defects and patent ductus arteriosus (Fig. 28-8). The second category includes defects that involve decreased pulmonary blood flow and typically result in cyanosis. The most common example of this type of defect is tetralogy of

Fallot; tricuspid atresia is a less common defect in this category. The third category includes those defects that cause obstruction to blood flow out of the heart. Pulmonary stenosis is an example of an obstruction to the flow of blood out of the right side of the heart that causes cyanosis. Coarctation of the aorta and subaortic stenosis are examples of obstructions to the flow of blood out of the left side of the heart that can result in congestive heart failure but not cyanosis. The fourth category comprises those complex cardiac anomalies that involve a flow of mixed saturated and desaturated blood in the heart or great vessels. These include such defects as transposition of the great vessels and total anomalous venous return.

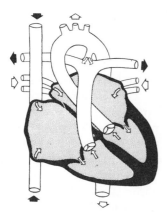

Patent ductus arteriosus

The patent ductus arteriosus is a vascular connection that, during fetal life, bypasses the pulmonary vascular bed and directs blood from the pulmonary artery to the aorta. Functional closure of the ductus normally occurs soon after birth. If the ductus remains patent after birth, the direction of blood flow in the ductus is reversed by the higher pressure in the aorta.

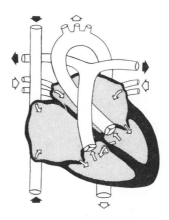

Ventricular septal defects

A ventricular septal defect is an abnormal opening between the right and left ventricle. Ventricular septal defects vary in size and may occur in either the membranous or muscular portion of the ventricular septum. Due to higher pressure in the left ventricle, a shunting of blood from the left to right ventricle occurs during systole. If pulmonary vascular resistance produces pulmonary hypertension, the shunt of blood is then reversed from the right to the left ventricle, with cyanosis resulting.

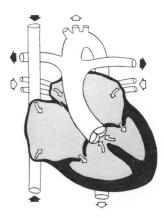

Truncus arteriosus

Truncus arteriosus is a retention of the embryologic bulbar trunk. It results from the failure of normal septation and division of this trunk into an aorta and pulmonary artery. This single arterial trunk overrides the ventricles and receives blood from them through a ventricular septal defect. The entire pulmonary and systemic circulation is supplied from this common arterial trunk.

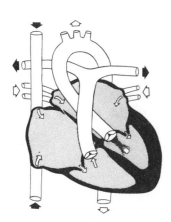

Subaortic stenosis

In many instances, the stenosis is valvular with thickening and fusion of the cusps. Subaortic stenosis is caused by a fibrous ring below the aortic valve in the outflow tract of the left ventricle. At times, both valvular and subaortic stenosis exist in combination. The obstruction presents an increased work load for the normal output of the left ventricular enlargement.

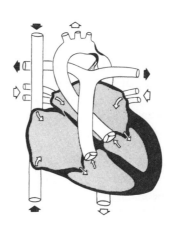

Coarctation of the aorta

Coarctation of the aorta is characterized by a narrowed aortic lumen. It exists as a preductal or postductal obstruction, depending on the position of the obstruction in relation to the ductus arteriosus. Coarctations exist with great variation in anatomic features. The lesion produces an obstruction to the flow of blood through the aorta causing an increased left ventricular pressure and work load.

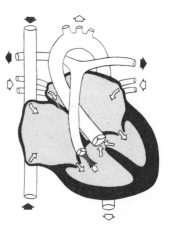

Tetralogy of Fallot

Tetralogy of Fallot is characterized by the combination of four defects: (1) pulmonary stenosis, (2) ventricular septal defect, (3) overriding aorta, (4) hypertrophy of right ventricle. It is the most common defect causing cyanosis in patients surviving beyond 2 years of age. The severity of symptoms depends on the degree of pulmonary stenosis, the size of the ventricular septal defect, and the degree to which the aorta overrides the septal defect.

Fig. 28-8—cont'd Congenital heart abnormalities.

Severe CHDs often are evident immediately after birth, especially defects that cause cyanosis such as transposition of the great vessels. Infants with these anomalies are transferred directly to special care nurseries or pediatric units. Even though the structural or functional anomalies are always present at birth, some affected newborns may be asymptomatic. Some of these CHDs, such as a small coarctation of the aorta, become apparent only as the infant or child is exposed to stresses such as growth demands or infection.

If symptoms are present at birth, they may be obvious with the first cry, which may be weak and muffled or loud and breathless. Affected newborns may be cyanotic and unrelieved by oxygen treatment, with the cyanosis increasing whenever the child is in the supine position or cries. The bluish-gray, dusky color of cyanotic infants may be mild, moderate, or severe. Other infants may be acyanotic and pale, with or without mottling on exertion, which includes crying, feeding, or stooling.

The affected newborn's activity level varies from restlessness to lethargy, and possibly unresponsiveness, except to pain. Persistent bradycardia (resting heart rate of less than 80 to 100 beats/min) or tachycardia (rate exceeding 160 to 180 beats/min) may be noted (Wong, 1995). The cardiac rhythm may be abnormal, and murmurs may be heard. Signs of congestive heart failure, diminished cardiac output, and decreased tissue perfusion may be evident.

Because the cardiac and respiratory systems function together, cardiac disease may be manifested by respiratory signs and symptoms. The respiratory rate should be determined when the newborn is in a resting state. Abnormal findings may include tachypnea, which is a rate of 60 breaths/min or more; retractions with nasal flaring; grunting occurring with or without exertion; and dyspnea, which may worsen when the infant is supine or exerting itself.

A major role of the nurse is to assess infants for abnormal findings, which, if observed, must be reported immediately. Newborns exhibiting these symptoms require prompt diagnosis and appropriate therapy in a neonatal or pediatric intensive care unit. Interventions planned if a nursing diagnosis of decreased cardiac output is made include administering oxygen as ordered, as well as cardiotonic and other medications such as diuretics that rid the body of accumulated fluid; decreasing the workload of the heart by maintaining a thermoneutral environment; feeding using the gavage method if necessary; and preventing crying if this precipitates cyanosis. Various diagnostic tests such as echocardiography and cardiac catheterization are performed to obtain specific information about the defect and the need for surgical intervention.

Central Nervous System Anomalies

Most congenital anomalies of the central nervous system (CNS) result from defects in the closure of the neural tube during fetal development. Although the cause of **neural tube defects** is unknown, they are thought to stem from the interaction of many genes that in turn are influenced by factors in the fetal environment. Environmental influences such as exposure to potato blight or organic solvents, treatment with valproic acid (an anticonvulsant), and alcohol consumption have been implicated. There is growing evidence that a maternal folic acid deficit has a direct bearing on failure of the neural tube to close, therefore, in 1993 the American Academy of Pediatrics issued recommendations that folic acid be administered to women of childbearing-age (Rowe et al., 1995). Although myelomeningocele is usually an isolated defect, it can occur with some syndromes and also with other defects such as cleft palate, ventricular septal defect, tracheoesophageal fistula, diaphragmatic hernia, imperforate anus, and renal anomalies. Some neural tube defects can be diagnosed prenatally by ultrasound studies and the finding of elevated levels of alpha-fetoprotein in the amniotic fluid and maternal serum.

Spina bifida

Spina bifida, the most common defect of the CNS, results from failure of the neural tube to close at some point. There are two categories of spina bifida: spina bifida occulta and spina bifida cystica. Spina bifida occulta is a malformation in which the posterior portion of the laminas fails to close but the spinal cord or meninges do not herniate or protrude through the defect (Fig. 28-9, *A*). Spina bifida is usually asymptomatic and may not be diagnosed unless there are associated problems. Spina bifida cystica includes meningocele and myelomeningocele. A meningocele is an external sac that contains meninges and CSF and that protrudes through a defect in the vertebral column. A **myelomeningocele** is similar, except that it also contains nerves; therefore the infant has motor and sensory deficits below the lesion. In the United States, myelomeningocele occurs in approximately 1 in 1,000 live births (Romanczuk & Brown, 1994).

A myelomeningocele, which is visible at birth and most often in the lumbosacral area, is usually covered with a very fragile, thin membrane (Fig. 28-9, *B*). The sac can tear easily, allowing CSF to leak out, as well as providing an entry for infectious agents into the CNS. Myelomeningocele usually is associated with an Arnold-Chiari malformation, which results from the improper development and downward displacement of part of the brain into the cervical spinal canal. This in turn results in the development of hydrocephalus, which affects approximately 90% of children with myelomeningocele, although it may not be present at birth. The long-term prognosis in an affected infant can be determined to a large extent at birth, with the degree of neurologic dysfunction related to the level of the lesion, which determines the nerves involved. Although decisions regarding closure of the sac and treatment traditionally have been a matter of controversy, many physicians now recommend that treatment be instituted regardless of the

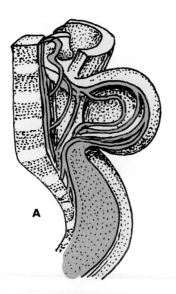

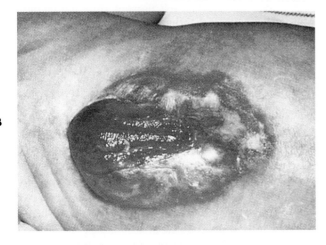

Fig. **28-9** **A,** Myelomeningocele. Note absence of vertebral arches. **B,** Myelomeningocele (spina bifida). (From Zitelli B & Davis H: *Atlas of pediatric diagnosis,* ed 3, St Louis, 1997, Mosby-Wolfe.)

level of the lesion, unless there is a severe CNS anomaly, advanced hydrocephalus at birth, severe anoxic brain damage, active CNS infection, or a congenital malformation or syndromes incompatible with long-term survival (Rowe et al., 1995).

A major preoperative nursing intervention for a neonate with a myelomeningocele is to protect the protruding sac from injury to prevent its rupture and resultant risk of CNS infection. Such infants should be positioned in a side-lying or prone position to prevent pressure on the sac until surgical repair is done. If the infant is allowed to be held, the nurse or parent must be careful to keep the defect from being injured. The sac should be covered with a sterile, moist, nonadherent dressing and sterile techniques used in its care. The skin around the defect must be cleansed and dried carefully to prevent breakdown, which would establish a portal of entry for infectious agents.

Because a lack of normal innervation may prevent the bladder from emptying completely, the nurse should use Credé's method at regular intervals to express urine from the bladder.

Other nursing care involves an assessment of the infant's neurologic function that includes the status of the following: apparent paralysis of lower extremities; the flaccidity and spasticity of muscles below the defect; and sphincter control, as evidenced by the number and character of voidings and stools, as well as the leakage of urine and stool. The infant's head circumference is measured and other neurologic assessments are performed to determine the presence and degree of hydrocephalus.

A major nursing intervention is providing support and needed information to parents as they begin to learn to cope with an infant who has immediate needs for intensive care and likely will have long-term needs as well. Surgical repair is often done in the neonatal period, preferably within the first 24 hours. Very early closure can prevent CNS infection and trauma to the exposed nerves. It can also prevent stretching of other nerve roots, which can occur as the sac continues to enlarge after birth. Surgical shunt procedures to prevent increasing hydrocephalus may be needed. Other problems, such as infection, are treated as they occur.

Encephalocele and anencephaly

Encephalocele and anencephaly are abnormalities resulting from failure of the anterior end of the neural tube to close. An encephalocele is a herniation of the brain and meninges through a skull defect. Treatment consists of surgical repair and shunting to relieve hydrocephalus, unless a major brain malformation is present. Most of these infants will have some degree of cognitive deficit. **Anencephaly** is the absence of both cerebral hemispheres and of the overlying skull. It is a condition that is incompatible with life; many of the infants are stillborn or die within a few days of birth. Warmth, fluids, and comfort measures are supplied until the infant eventually dies of respiratory failure.

Hydrocephalus

Hydrocephalus refers to a condition in which the ventricles of the brain are enlarged as a result of an imbalance between the production and absorption of the CSF. It is almost always caused by interference with the circulation and absorption of CSF. Congenital hydrocephalus usually arises as a result of a malformation in the brain or an intrauterine infection. It occurs in approximately 3 to 4 per 1,000 live births (Shiminski-Maher & Disabato, 1994). About one third of all cases of congenital hydrocephalus result from stenosis of the aqueduct of Sylvius in the brain. Hydrocephalus frequently occurs in conjunction with a myelomeningocele, which blocks the flow of CSF.

An infant with congenital hydrocephalus will initially have a bulging anterior fontanel and a head circumference that increases at an abnormal rate, resulting from the increase in

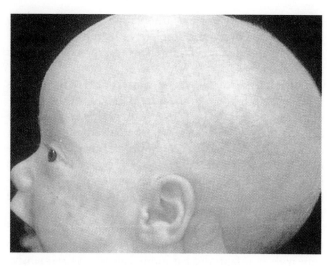

Fig. 28-10 Infantile hydrocephalus. The characteristic appearance is an enlarged head, thinning of the scalp, distended scalp veins, and a full fontanel. (From Booth I & Wozniak E: *Pediatrics*, Baltimore, 1984, Williams & Wilkins.)

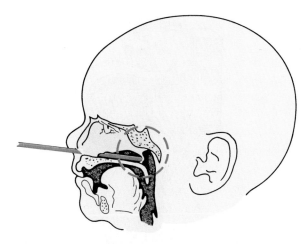

Fig. 28-11 Choanal atresia. Posterior nares are obstructed by membrane or bone either bilaterally or unilaterally. Infant becomes cyanotic at rest. With crying, newborn's color improves. Nasal discharge is present. Snorting respirations often are observed with increased respiratory effort. Newborn may be unable to breathe and eat at the same time. Diagnosis is made by noting inability to pass small feeding tube through one or both nares. (Used with permission of Ross Products Division, Abbott Laboratories, Inc., Columbus, Ohio 43216. From Clinical Education Aid #6, Copyright 1963, Ross Products Division, Abbott Laboratories, Inc.)

CSF pressure (Fig. 28-10). Enlargement of the forehead with depressed eyes that are rotated downward, causing a "setting sun" sign, occurs as the condition worsens. If the surgical shunting of excess CSF from the brain is not done soon after birth, the resulting increasing intracranial pressure will lead to irreversible neurologic damage, as evidenced by palpably widening sutures and fontanels, lethargy, poor feeding, vomiting, irritability, opisthotonos, and a high-pitched, shrill cry.

Nursing actions appropriate to the needs of a newborn with hydrocephalus include careful documentation of the ongoing observations. Measurement of the head circumference and other neurologic assessments are done frequently. If the infant's head is large, the placement of sheepskin or a flotation mattress under the infant and frequent position changes are necessary to prevent skin breakdown resulting from the pressure.

The infant's heavy head should be supported carefully during holding or turning, and positioning in the crib should be done in such a way that a patent airway is maintained. The method, amount, and frequency of feeding are determined by the infant's tolerance and energy level. The nurse should be alert to the possibility of projectile vomiting, which is a frequent occurrence in the presence of increased intracranial pressure, and maintain aspiration precautions. Nonnutritive sucking, touching, and cuddling needs should be met.

The surgical correction of hydrocephalus involves the placement of a shunt that goes from the ventricles of the brain usually to the peritoneum to allow the drainage of excess CSF. Damaged or destroyed brain tissue cannot be restored; the long-term prognosis in affected infants depends on the presence and extent of such tissue damage, along with the cause of the hydrocephalus, the presence of concurrent neurologic problems, and the long-term success of the shunt procedure.

Microcephaly

Microcephaly refers to a small brain in a generally normally formed head. It can be an autosomal-recessive disorder or caused by a chromosomal abnormality; exposure of the woman to x-rays; or rubella, cytomegalovirus, or other maternal infections. Microcephalic infants require supportive nursing care and medical observation to determine the extent of the psychomotor retardation that almost always accompanies this abnormality. There is no treatment. Parents need support to learn to care for a child with such cognitive impairment.

Respiratory System Anomalies

Screening for congenital anomalies of the respiratory system is necessary even in infants who are apparently normal at birth. Respiratory distress at birth or shortly thereafter may be the result of lung immaturity or anomalous development. Congenital laryngeal web and bilateral choanal atresia are readily apparent at birth. Respiratory distress caused by diaphragmatic hernia and tracheoesophageal fistula may appear immediately or be delayed, depending on the severity of the defect.

Laryngeal web and choanal atresia

A laryngeal web, which is uncommon, results from the incomplete separation of the two sides of the larynx and is most often between the vocal cords. **Choanal atresia** (Fig. 28-11) is the most common congenital anomaly of the nose; it is a bony or membranous septum located between the nose and the pharynx. Inability to pass a suction catheter

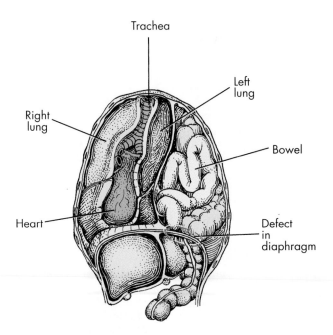

Fig. 28-12 Diaphragmatic hernia. (Used with permission of Ross Products Division, Abbott Laboratories, Inc., Columbus, Ohio 43216. From Clinical Education Aid #6, Copyright 1963, Ross Products Division, Abbott Laboratories, Inc.)

through the nose into the pharynx usually leads to its detection. Nearly half of the infants with choanal atresia have other anomalies. Infants with either a laryngeal web or choanal atresia require emergency surgery.

Diaphragmatic hernia

Diaphragmatic hernia results from a defect in the formation of the diaphragm, allowing the abdominal organs to be displaced into the thoracic cavity. It occurs in approximately 1 in 3,000 live births (Guzzetta et al., 1994); however, if stillbirths resulting from this defect are included, the incidence increases to 1 in 2,000. Herniation of the abdominal viscera into the thoracic cavity may cause severe respiratory distress and represent a neonatal emergency (Fig. 28-12). The defect and herniation may be minimal and easily repaired, or the defect may be so extensive that the viscera present in the thoracic cavity during embryonic life have prevented the normal development of pulmonary tissue. The defect is usually on the left because that is the side of the diaphragm that fuses last.

Most congenital diaphragmatic hernias are discovered prenatally on ultrasound studies and in some research institutions may be repaired by fetal surgery. At birth most affected infants have severe respiratory distress, and respiratory assessment reveals worsening distress as the bowels fill with air. Typically the breath sounds are diminished and bowel sounds are heard in the chest. Heart sounds may be heard on the right side of the chest because the heart has been displaced there by the abdominal contents. Physical examination reveals a flat or scaphoid abdomen and a prominent ipsilateral chest. Diagnosis can be made on the basis of the x-ray study finding of loops of intestine in the thoracic cavity and the absence of intestine in the abdominal cavity.

Preoperative nursing interventions include participating in the stabilization of the infant's condition until surgical repair can be done. The infant should be positioned with the head and chest elevated and the affected side downward to allow the normal lung to expand. Gastric contents are aspirated and suction applied to decompress the gastrointestinal tract and prevent further cardiothoracic compromise. Oxygen therapy, mechanical ventilation, and the correction of acidosis are necessary in infants with large defects. Extracorporeal membrane oxygenation (ECMO) may be used preoperatively or postoperatively (see Chapter 27) in infants with severe circulatory and respiratory complications who do not respond to conventional medical therapy (Nugent & Matranga, 1997). The prognosis depends largely on the degree of pulmonary development and the success of diaphragmatic closure, but the prognosis in severe cases is guarded. The overall survival for infants who are symptomatic within the first few hours of life is approximately 50%, although it has improved with the advent of ECMO.

Gastrointestinal System Anomalies

Anomalies in the gastrointestinal system can occur anywhere along the gastrointestinal tract, from the mouth to the anus. Some anomalies, such as cleft lip, omphalocele, and gastroschisis, are apparent at birth. Others, including cleft palate, esophageal atresia, pyloric stenosis, intestinal obstructions, and imperforate anus become apparent as the infant is further assessed or becomes symptomatic. These anomalies arise as a result of the interrupted development of that particular organ at a crucial point during organogenesis.

Cleft lip and palate

Cleft lip or **palate** is a commonly occurring congenital midline fissure, or opening, in the lip or palate resulting from failure of the primary palate to fuse (Fig. 28-13, *A-D*). One or both deformities may occur. Multiple genetic and, to a lesser extent, environmental factors, such as maternal infection, radiation exposure, alcohol ingestion, and treatment with medications such as corticosteroids, some tranquilizers, and anticonvulsants, appear to be involved in their development.

Cleft lip with or without cleft palate occurs in approximately 1 in 1,000 live births (Rowe et al., 1995); the incidence is greatest for Native Americans and Asians and lowest for African-Americans. It is more common in males. The defect can range from a simple notch in the lip to complete separation of the lip that extends to the floor of the nose. The treatment for a cleft lip is surgical repair, which usually is done between 6 and 12 weeks of age, if the infant is healthy and free of infection. Advances in surgical techniques have made it possible for some infants, particularly

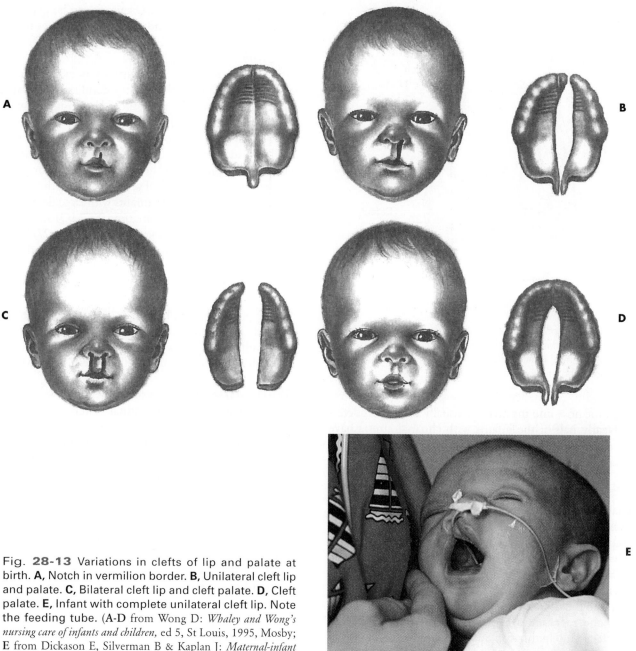

Fig. **28-13** Variations in clefts of lip and palate at birth. **A,** Notch in vermilion border. **B,** Unilateral cleft lip and palate. **C,** Bilateral cleft lip and cleft palate. **D,** Cleft palate. **E,** Infant with complete unilateral cleft lip. Note the feeding tube. (A-D from Wong D: *Whaley and Wong's nursing care of infants and children,* ed 5, St Louis, 1995, Mosby; E from Dickason E, Silverman B & Kaplan J: *Maternal-infant nursing care,* ed 3, St Louis, 1998, Mosby.)

those with unilateral cleft lip, to have a near-normal appearance (see Fig. 28-13). The results of the repair depend on the severity of the defect, with more severe bilateral cleft lip requiring surgical repair done in stages.

Anomalies of the palate often occur in association with cleft lip. A cleft palate alone occurs half as frequently as cleft lip. It is more common in females and occurs more frequently as a constituent of certain syndromes. This defect can range from a cleft in the uvula to a complete cleft of the hard and soft palates that may be unilateral, bilateral, or midline. Feeding is difficult because the cleft

lip renders the newborn unable to maintain a seal around a nipple; the cleft palate renders the infant unable to form a vacuum to maintain suction when feeding. In addition, the inability to suck and swallow normally allows milk to pool in the nasopharynx, which increases the likelihood of aspiration. Furthermore, as the infant attempts to suck, milk often comes out through the cleft and out of the nares. Although the degree of difficulty depends on the size of the cleft, feeding problems are greater in infants with a cleft palate than in those with a cleft lip. Regardless of the extent and type of defect, feeding may become a

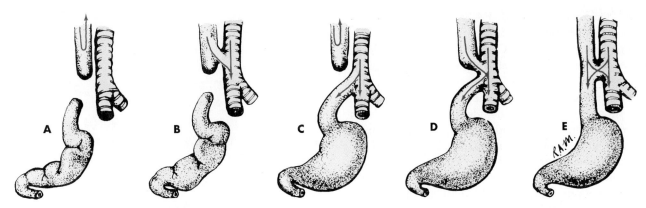

Fig. **28-14** Congenital atresia of esophagus and tracheoesophageal fistula. **A,** Upper and lower segments of esophagus end in blind sac, occurring in approximately 8% of such infants. **B,** Upper segment of esophagus ends in atresia and connects to trachea by fistulous tract, occurring in less than 1% of such infants. Infant may drown with first feeding. **C,** Upper segment of esophagus ends in blind pouch; lower segment connects with trachea by small fistulous tract, occurring in approximately 87% of such infants. **D,** Both segments of esophagus connect by fistulous tracts to trachea, occurring in less than 1% of such infants. Infant may drown with first feeding. **E,** Esophagus is continuous but connects by fistulous tract to trachea; know as *H-type.* (From Wong D: *Whaley and Wong's nursing care of infants and children,* ed 5, St Louis, 1995, Mosby.)

very frustrating experience for parents. Breastfeeding can be successful in some infants (Danner, 1992). There are also special nipples, bottles, and appliances available to aid in feeding (Fig. 28-13, *E*). In general, parents of infants with these defects need a great deal of education and support as they learn to feed their baby, to prevent what should be a normal part of infant care from becoming a very frustrating experience.

The type of surgical repair done to close the cleft palate is based on the degree of the cleft and, as with a cleft lip, if severe, may necessitate repair done in stages. Repair is begun at 6 to 18 months, after some development of the affected area has occurred. Early repair helps avert some of the speech problems that may occur in people with palate defects. Long-term care is often necessary for children with a cleft palate and involves the combined efforts of a health care team comprising acute care and community nurses, social workers, ear, nose, and throat and plastic surgeons, speech therapists, and orthodontists.

Parents of infants with a cleft lip or palate need much support, particularly in the case of a cleft lip because this is both a cosmetic and functional defect. Recognizing that this may interfere with normal parent-infant bonding in the neonatal period, the nurse must assess for this and intervene appropriately.

Esophageal atresia and tracheoesophageal fistula

Esophageal atresia (EA) and tracheoesophageal fistula (TEF), the most life-threatening anomalies of the esophagus, often occur together, although they can also occur singly.

Esophageal atresia is a congenital anomaly in which the esophagus ends in a blind pouch or narrows into a thin cord, thus failing to form a continuous passageway to the stomach. TEF is an abnormal connection between the esophagus and trachea. Hydramnios is a common finding in pregnancy, particularly if the fetus has an EA without TEF. More than half of the infants have associated anomalies, most often cardiac and gastrointestinal tract ones. Variations of the anomalies are possible, depending on the presence or absence of a TEF, the site of the fistula, and the location and degree of the esophageal obstruction. The most common variant is the combination of a proximal EA, in which the esophagus ends in a blind pouch, with a distal TEF, in which the lower esophagus exits the stomach and joins the trachea rather than forming a continuous tube to the upper esophagus (Fig. 28-14, *C*). This defect occurs in approximately 1 in 3,000 live births (Stapleton, 1996).

Infants with the life-threatening anomaly EA with TEF show significant respiratory difficulty immediately after birth. EA with or without TEF results in excessive oral secretions, drooling, and feeding intolerance. Soon after the first feeding is begun in such infants, there is regurgitation of unaltered formula, that is, formula that has not mixed with gastric secretions, since it could not enter the stomach because of the EA. Respiratory distress can result from aspiration or from the acute gastric distention produced by the TEF. Choking, coughing, and cyanosis occur after even a small amount of fluid is taken by mouth.

Nursing interventions are supportive until surgery is performed. Any infant with excessive oral secretions and respiratory distress should not be fed orally until a physician is consulted. The infant with EA and TEF is placed in a semi-Fowler's position, which facilitates respiratory efforts and diminishes the reflux of gastric contents into the trachea. A double-lumen catheter is placed in the proximal esophageal pouch and attached to continuous suction to remove secretions and decrease the possibility of aspiration. Other supportive measures include maintaining fluid and electrolyte balance by IV and thermoregulation. Surgical correction, done in one stage if possible, consists of ligating the fistula and anastomosing the two segments of the esophagus. Prematurity and the presence of significant pneumonia or severe associated congenital anomalies may increase the risk of poor outcome. The prognosis for a normal life is good, however, with an overall survival rate of 85% to 90%; the chances for survival in those infants in a good-risk category exceed 95%.

Omphalocele and gastroschisis

Omphalocele and gastroschisis are two of the more common congenital defects that occur in the abdominal wall. They are rare, however, with omphalocele occurring in approximately 1 in 5,000 live births and the incidence of gastroschisis much less than that of omphalocele (Rowe et al., 1995). An **omphalocele** is a covered defect of the umbilical ring into which varying amounts of the abdominal organs may herniate (Fig. 28-15, *A*). Although it is covered with a peritoneal sac, the sac may rupture during or after birth. Many infants born with an omphalocele are premature, and more than half have other serious syndromes or anomalies involving the gastrointestinal, cardiac, genitourinary, musculoskeletal, and nervous systems.

Gastroschisis is the herniation of the bowel through a defect in the abdominal wall to the right of the umbilical cord. No membrane covers the contents, as occurs with an omphalocele (Fig. 28-15, *B*). Unlike infants with omphalocele, these infants rarely have associated anomalies.

The preoperative nursing care is similar for infants with either defect. Exposure of the viscera causes problems with thermoregulation and fluid and electrolyte balance. Before closure is performed, the exposed viscera are covered with moistened saline gauze and plastic wrap. Antibiotics, fluid and electrolyte replacement, gastric decompression, and thermoregulation are needed for physiologic support. If complete closure is impossible because of the small size of the defect and the large amount of viscera to be replaced, a Silastic (Dow Corning, Midland, Mich.) silo pouch is created to protect the contents as they are gradually placed back into the abdominal cavity. The defect is closed surgically after the reduction of contents is complete. Gastric decompression is necessary preoperatively to prevent aspiration pneumonia and to allow as much bowel as possible to be placed into the abdomen during surgery. Surgery is usually performed soon after birth. With surgical treatment and nutritional support, the survival rate is greater than 90% in such infants (Rowe et al., 1995).

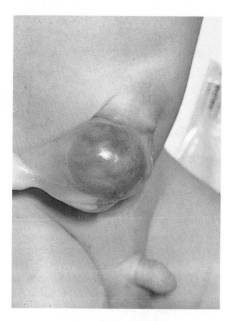

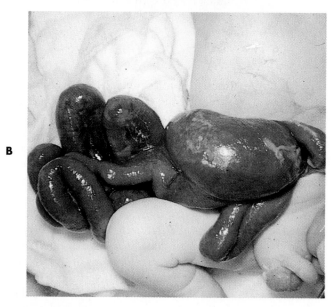

Fig. 28-15 A, Omphalocele. **B,** Gastroschisis of bowel and stomach. (**A** from O'Doherty N: *Neonatology microatlas of the newborn,* Nutley, NJ, 1986, Hoffmann-LaRoche; **B** Courtesy Wyeth International.)

Parental support is essential because the infant has an obvious disfiguring anomaly that can be quite shocking and repulsive in appearance. Depending on the size of the defect, the infant may also be critically ill preoperatively. The nurse must be aware of the effect this may have on parental bonding and intervene appropriately as the parents cope with this crisis.

Gastrointestinal obstruction

Congenital intestinal obstruction occurs in from 1 in 400 to 1 in 5,000 live births (Rowe et al., 1995). Such an obstruction can occur anywhere in the gastrointestinal track and occur in the form of atresia, which is a complete obliteration of the passage; partial obstruction, in which the symptoms may vary in severity and sometimes not be detected in the neonatal period; or malrotation of the intestine, which leads to twisting of the intestine (volvulus) and obstruction. Meconium ileus is an obstruction caused by impacted meconium and is the earliest sign of cystic fibrosis, a life-threatening chronic illness. Infants presenting with this type of obstruction should be tested for cystic fibrosis.

In addition to hydramnios in the pregnant woman, the infant shows the following cardinal signs and symptoms: bilious vomiting, abdominal distention, and failure to pass normal amounts of meconium in the first 24 hours. High intestinal obstruction is characterized by vomiting, even if the infant is not being fed orally. A low obstruction is characterized primarily by distention, with vomiting occurring later. Abdominal distention can elevate the diaphragm, which causes respiratory difficulties. Careful evaluation must be done to make a correct diagnosis.

Nursing care is aimed at supporting the infant until surgical intervention can be carried out to eliminate the obstruction. Oral feedings are discontinued, a nasogastric tube is placed for suction, and intravenous therapy is initiated to provide needed fluid and electrolytes. In infants with an intestinal obstruction, surgery consists of resecting the obstructed area of bowel and anastomosing the non-affected bowel. In recent years the survival rate for these infants has risen to 85% to 90% as a result of better treatments, better neonatal intensive care, and a better understanding of the total problem.

Imperforate anus

Imperforate anus is a term used to describe a wide range of congenital disorders involving the anus and rectum (Fig. 28-16). These anomalies are relatively common, with an incidence of approximately 1 in 500 live births (Wong, 1995). Occurring more in male than in female infants, they result from the failure of anorectal development in week 7 and 8 of gestational life. Such infants have no anal opening (Fig. 28-17), and frequently there is also a fistula from the rectum to the peritoneum or genitourinary system. They can be further classified according to the location of the defect into a "high" or "low" type, which determines the treatments necessary, as well as the prognosis. Infants with high anomalies, which occur primarily in males, require a colostomy in the neonatal period, with corrective surgery done in stages over time. Low anomalies may involve stenotic areas or there may be a thin translucent membrane covering the anal opening. Treatment for such a membrane is excision followed by daily dilatation, which parents are taught to do. Other low lesions are surgically corrected by anoplasty. The preoperative nursing care is similar to that described for other gastrointestinal obstructions.

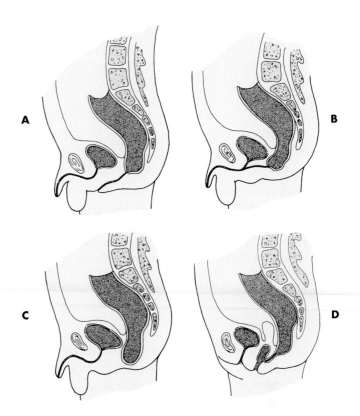

Fig. **28-16** Types of imperforate anus. Anal sphincter muscle may be present and intact. **A,** High lesion opening onto perineum through narrow fistulous tract. **B,** High lesion ending in fistulous tract to urinary tract. **C,** Low lesion in bowel passes through puborectal muscle. **D,** High lesion ending in fistulous tract to vagina.

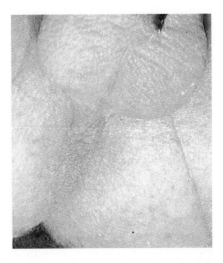

Fig. **28-17** Imperforate anus. (From Chessell G et al.: *Diagnostic picture tests in clinical medicine,* vol 2, 1984, Mosby-Wolfe.)

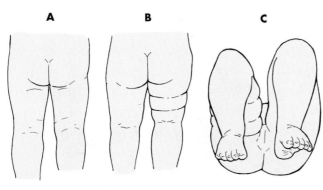

A   B   C

Fig. **28-18** Congenital dysplasia of hip. **A,** Normal gluteal and popliteal skin creases. **B,** Abnormal skin creases and asymmetry of skin folds. **C,** Apparent shortening of femur. Femoral head is displaced. (Used with permission of Ross Products Division, Abbott Laboratories, Inc., Columbus, Ohio 43216. From Clinical Education Aid #15, Copyright 1965, Ross Products Division, Abbott Laboratories, Inc.)

Musculoskeletal System Anomalies

The two most common musculoskeletal system anomalies seen in neonates are congenital hip dysplasia and congenital clubfoot. Both of these conditions must be detected and treated early for them to be successfully corrected.

Congenital hip dysplasia

Congenital hip dysplasia consists of disorders that result from the abnormal development of one or all of the components of the hip joint, resulting in instability of the hip. This causes one or both of the femoral heads to be displaced from the hip socket, or acetabulum. The dislocated femoral head does not exert pressure on the acetabulum, causing delayed development of the femoral head and failure of the acetabulum to form normally. The etiology is considered to be multifactorial, with genetic factors involved, and females are more often affected than males. Risk factors for the defect include breech presentation, a positive family history, the birth order (firstborn), and prenatal maternal oligohydramnios with fetal compression and deformation. The effect of maternal hormones during pregnancy may foster hip joint capsule laxity, especially in the female. The defect occurs in approximately 1.5 to 2 per 1,000 live births (Speers & Speers, 1992). The examiner tests for an unstable or actually dislocated femoral head by abducting the hips and feeling for a click when the femoral head passes back into the acetabulum (see Table 20-1 and Fig. 28-18).

Early detection, often by the nurse during a routine newborn assessment, allows for early treatment, which is more effective than later treatment and can prevent complications. The use of double or triple diapering to maintain the hip in an abducted position, which keeps the head of the femur in the acetabulum, may be recommended as a temporary measure until definitive treatment can begin. Treatment often involves the use of a Pavlik harness, a device that keeps the

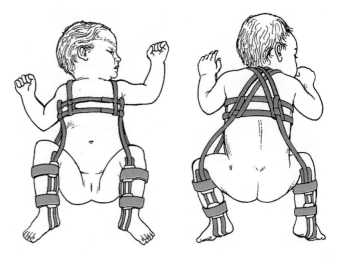

Fig. **28-19** Treatment for congenital hip dislocation by application of the Pavlik harness. 1. Position the infant in a relaxed supine position. 2. The shoulder straps on the chest halter should cross in the back to prevent slippage down the shoulders. 3. The buckles for the anterior (flexor) stirrup-straps should be placed at the anterior line. 4. The buckles for the posterior (abduction) stirrup-straps should be placed over the scapula. 5. The Velcro straps for the proximal part of the leg should be placed just below the popliteal fossa. 6. Place the feet into the stirrups and secure the straps. 7. The posterior straps should already be attached and should not need to be unfastened when the harness is removed. 8. Secure the straps attached to the stirrups to the anterior buckles positioning the hips at 70-degree abduction. (From Lowdermilk D, Perry S & Bobak I: *Maternity and women's health care,* ed 6, St Louis, 1997, Mosby.)

hips and knees flexed, the hips abducted, and the femoral head in the acetabulum (Fig. 28-19). Worn continuously for 3 to 6 months, it promotes the development of muscle and cartilage, resulting in a stable hip. Although the harness is effective up to 90% of the time, traction, casting, and even surgery may be necessary to stabilize the hip.

In addition to the major intervention of assessing and helping identify the disorder, another key nursing intervention is teaching the parents about the care of the infant, who will remain in the harness continuously during the treatment. Because this occurs during a time of maximum growth, it will be necessary for them to adjust the infant's care to accommodate the infant's changing needs. Continuing thorough follow-up care is necessary, as well as psychosocial support for the family.

Clubfoot

Clubfoot is a congenital deformity in which portions of the foot and ankle are twisted out of a normal position. These can be of varying degrees of severity and assume a variety of combinations of abnormal positions. The most common, seen in approximately 95% of infants with clubfoot, is talipes equinovarus. In this abnormality, the foot points downward and inward; the ankle is inverted, and the

Achilles tendon is shortened. Unless treated, further stiffening occurs, and bony changes will result.

Clubfoot is one of the most common congenital anomalies, occurring in approximately 1 per 700 to 1 per 1,000 live births, with two times more males than females affected (Wong, 1995). The exact cause is unknown, but possibilities include a genetic predisposition, in utero compression, and abnormal embryonic development. Treatment begins soon after birth. This consists of manipulation and frequent serial casting, which is necessary because of the rapid growth of the infant. If this is ineffective, surgical correction is necessary. Although a controversial issue, the optimal age for surgery is generally acknowledged to be between 4 to 12 months. Treatment, which may continue into adolescence, often results in good function of the foot, although the feet may differ in size. The deformity may recur, and repeat surgery may then be necessary.

Because these infants are often placed in a cast before they are discharged, the nurse must teach the parents the way to care for an infant in a cast, including protecting the cast and assessing the toes for neurovascular compromise. This is particularly important because of the growth of the child, which could cause the child to outgrow the cast. As is true with the birth of any child with any anomaly, the nurse should be supportive of the parents as they learn the ways in which to meet the infant's normal needs, as well as those brought about by the infant's physical problem.

Genitourinary System Anomalies

Anomalies involving the genitourinary system can be distressing to parents because they may be readily apparent and, in the case of some conditions, because of the concern about sexuality and reproductive functioning. These anomalies range from obvious anomalies of the external genitalia, such as hypospadias, to those involving internal organs that may not be detected but may cause damage to the urinary tract. An example of the latter is an obstruction in the urinary tract that can cause hydronephrosis, which is the abnormal collection of urine in the renal pelvis that can eventually destroy the kidney.

Hypospadias and epispadias

Hypospadias constitutes a range of penile anomalies associated with an abnormally located urinary meatus. The meatus can open below the glans penis or anywhere along the ventral surface of the penis, the scrotum, or the perineum. It is the most common anomaly of the penis, affecting approximately 1 in 300 to 500 male infants (Rowe et al., 1995). It is classified according to the location of the meatus and the presence or absence of chordee, which is a ventral curvature of the penis. The cause is unknown, although it is thought to be of multifactorial inheritance.

Mild cases of hypospadias are often repaired for cosmetic reasons and involve a single surgical procedure. In more

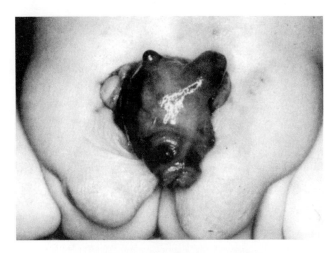

Fig. 28-20 Exstrophy of bladder. (Courtesy Edward S. Tank, MD, Division of Urology, Oregon Health Sciences University, Portland, Ore.)

severe cases, several operations are required to reconstruct the urethral opening and correct the chordee, thereby straightening the penis. The goals are to improve the appearance of the genitalia and make it possible for the child to be able to urinate in a standing position and have a sexually adequate organ. It is vital that these infants not be circumcised, because the foreskin may be needed during surgical repair. Repair is done early, often during or soon after the first year of life, so that the child's body image is not impaired.

Epispadias is rare, occurring in approximately 1 in 100,000 live births (Kaplan, 1994). The urethral opening is located along the dorsal surface of the penis, and the severity ranges from a mild to a severe anomaly that is associated with exstrophy of the bladder. Surgical correction is necessary, and affected infants should not be circumcised.

Exstrophy of the bladder

The most common bladder anomaly is exstrophy (Fig. 28-20), which often occurs in conjunction with epispadias. It is rare, occurring only in approximately 1 in 25,000 live births and twice as frequently in females (Kaplan, 1994). It results from the abnormal development of the bladder, abdominal wall, and the symphisis pubis that causes the bladder, urethra, and ureteral orifices to all be exposed. The bladder is visible in the suprapubic area as a red mass with numerous folds, with urine draining from it onto the infant's skin. Surgical reconstruction is accomplished in several steps, beginning in infancy with closure of the bladder. Repair is completed before school age, if possible, although some children never attain normal voiding patterns and later may be considered for surgery for urinary diversion.

Immediately after birth the exposed bladder is covered with a sterile, nonadherent dressing to protect it until closure can be performed. It is recommended that reconstructive surgery be started in the neonatal period, although it

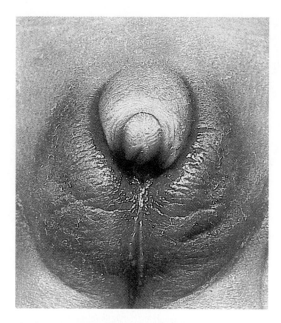

Fig. 28-21 Ambiguous external genitals (i.e., structure can be enlarged clitoral hood and clitoris or malformed penis). (Courtesy Edward S. Tank, MD, Division of Urology, Oregon Health Sciences University, Portland, Ore.)

may be delayed. If the bladder is left open, an ongoing need is the prevention of infection and excoriation of the surrounding skin caused by the draining urine. Parents will need much support as they deal with caring for an infant who has such an obvious defect.

Sexual ambiguity

Sexual ambiguity in the newborn (Fig. 28-21) often is discovered by the nurse during a physical assessment. Erroneous or abnormal sexual differentiation may be a genetic aberration, such as congenital adrenal hypoplasia, which can be life threatening because of the deficiency of all adrenal cortical hormones involved. Other possible causes of sexual ambiguity include chromosomal abnormalities, defective sex hormone synthesis in males, and the placental transfer of masculinizing agents to female fetuses. Gender assignment should be done as quickly as possible after birth. The data on which this is based may be gathered from the following sources: maternal and family history, including the ingestion of steroids during pregnancy and relatives with ambiguous genitalia or who died during the neonatal period; physical examination; chromosomal analysis (results are available in 2 to 3 days); endoscopy, ultrasonography, and radiographic contrast studies; biochemical tests, such as analysis of urinary steroid excretion, which helps detect several of the adrenal cortical syndromes; and, in some instances, laparotomy or gonad biopsy (Wong, 1995). Therapeutic intervention, including any surgery, should be started as soon as possible to prevent long-term psychoso-

cial problems. Parents need much support as they learn to deal with this very challenging situation.

Teratoma

A teratoma is an embryonal tumor that may be solid, cystic, or mixed. It is composed of at least two and usually three types of embryonal tissue: ectoderm, mesoderm, and endoderm. A teratoma in the newborn may occur in the skull, mediastinum, abdomen, or sacral area, with more than half located in the sacrococcygeal area; 80% of all teratomas are benign. They are uncommon, occurring in approximately 1 in 35,000 live births (Rowe et al., 1995). The treatment of choice for such neonates is complete surgical resection. Most such sacrococcygeal tumors are benign, and no additional therapy is needed after complete resection done in the neonatal period. If the tumor is not surgically resected before the infant is 1 to 2 months old, the likelihood of the teratoma becoming malignant increases rapidly.

▌ CARE MANAGEMENT

Perinatal diagnosis

Many congenital anomalies require intervention soon after birth. By careful observations in the birth room or nursery, the nurse can identify most of these conditions. An excessive amount of amniotic fluid, hydramnios, is commonly associated with congenital anomalies in the newborn, and such infants should be examined closely at the earliest possible time.

Oligohydramnios, which is an insufficient amount of amniotic fluid, is associated primarily with anomalies of the urinary tract that prevent normal micturition in utero. It is most often associated with renal agenesis or dysplasia and obstructive lesions in the lower urinary tract. Anomalies of the ears sometimes occur with renal abnormalities. Bilateral renal agenesis, resulting in oligohydramnios, commonly presents as Potter's syndrome, which is characterized by atypical facial appearance consisting of a flat nose, recessed chin, epicanthal folds, and low-set abnormal ears; limb abnormalities; pulmonary hypoplasia; and fetal growth restriction. These conditions may be diagnosed prenatally.

Postnatal diagnosis

Apgar scoring and a brief assessment are completed for all neonates after birth. Any deviations from normal are reported to the physician or midwife immediately. A thorough assessment of all body systems follows, with identification of both visible anomalies and those that might not be visible.

Some infants have multiple congenital anomalies. A recognized pattern of malformations is referred to as a *syndrome.* The most common is Down syndrome (Table 28-2, Fig. 28-22), with diagnosis confirmed early in the neonatal period.

Diagnostic procedures for the detection of genetic disorders are performed after birth at any time from the

TABLE 28-2 *Common Autosomal Aberrations*

SYNDROME	CHROMOSOMAL ABNORMALITY AND NOMENCLATURE	AVERAGE INCIDENCE* (LIVE BIRTHS)	MAJOR CLINICAL MANIFESTATIONS
Cri-du-chat	Deletion of short arm of a B (no. 5) chromosome—46,XY	1:50,000	Distinctive weak, high-pitched mewlike cry resembling the cry of a cat; small head; hypertelorism; failure to thrive; severe mental retardation
Trisomy 13 (Patau's)	Trisomy of a group D (no. 13) chromosome—47,XY,13+	1:4,000 to 1:15,000	Multiple anomalies, including cleft lip and palate (frequently bilateral); ear malformations; microphthalmia; polydactyly; eye defects; mental retardation; early death
Trisomy 18 (Edwards')	Trisomy of a group E (no. 18) chromosome—47,XY,18+	1:3,500-8,000	Deformed and low-set ears; micrognathia; rocker-bottom feet; overlapping (index over third) fingers; prominent occiput; hypertelorism; failure to thrive and early death; mental retardation
Trisomy 21 (Down)	Trisomy of a group G (no. 21) chromosome—47,XY,21+ (trisomy; 46,XY,D—G- (Dq-Gq)+ (translocation); 46,XY/47,XY,21+ (mosaic)	1:70[†]	Brachycephaly with flat occiput; inner epicanthal folds; small ears, nose, and mouth with protruding tongue; muscular hypotonia; broad, short hands with stubby fingers and simian palmar crease; broad, stubby feet with wide space between big and second toes; mental retardation; variable life expectancy

Modified from Wong D: *Whaley and Wong's nursing care of infants and children,* ed 5, St Louis, 1995, Mosby.
*Data from Nora J & Fraser F: *Medical genetics: principles and practice,* ed 3, Philadelphia, 1989, Lea & Febiger; D'Alton M & DeCherney A: Prenatal diagnosis, *N Engl J Med* 322:114, 1993.
[†]Risk related to maternal age: 30 years, 1/952; 35 years, 1/385; 40 years, 1/106; 45 years, 1/30; 49 years 1/11.

postnatal period through adulthood. There are many tests for various disorders; only the most frequently used ones are discussed here.

Biochemical tests. The most widespread use of postnatal testing for genetic disease is the routine screening of newborns for inborn errors of metabolism such as phenylketonuria (PKU), which is mandatory in most states in the United States. An inborn error of metabolism is the term applied to a large group of disorders caused by a metabolic defect that results from the absence of or change in a protein, usually an enzyme, and mediated by the action of a certain gene. These defects can involve any substrate produced from protein, carbohydrate, or fat metabolism. Inborn errors of metabolism are recessive disorders, and, for this reason, for them to occur, a person must receive a defective gene from each parent. The parents usually are unaffected because their normal dominant gene directs the synthesis of sufficient protein to meet their metabolic needs under normal circumstances. With the advent of new biochemical techniques,

it is now possible to detect the abnormal gene responsible for causing an increasing number of these disorders.

PKU results from a deficiency of the enzyme phenylalanine dehydrogenase (see Chapter 8). The test for PKU is not reliable, however, until the newborn has ingested an ample amount of the amino acid phenylalanine, a constituent of both human and cow milk.

NURSE ALERT | *The nurse must document the initial ingestion of milk and perform the test at least 24 hours after that time.*

If the infant is found to have PKU, a diet low in phenylalanine is begun soon after birth. Breastfeeding or partial breastfeeding may be possible for some infants if the phenylalanine levels are monitored carefully and remain within acceptable limits (Lawrence, 1994). Although severe mental retardation is seen less in affected children living in countries where there is neonatal screening for PKU, many affected children have some intellectual impairment.

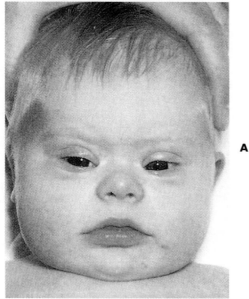

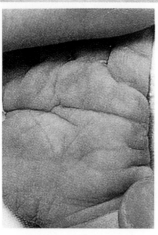

Fig. 28-22 **A,** Clinical features of Down syndrome. **B,** Simian crease. (From Zitelli B & Davis H: *Atlas of pediatric diagnosis,* ed 3, St Louis, 1997, Mosby-Wolfe.)

Galactosemia, caused by a deficiency of the enzyme galactose 1-phosphate uridyltransferase, results in the inability to convert galactose to glucose. Galactosemia can be detected by measuring the blood levels of galactose in the urine of newborns suspected of having the disease who have ingested formula containing galactose. Early symptoms are vomiting, weight loss, and CNS symptoms, including poor feeding, drowsiness, and seizures. If the disorder goes untreated, the galactose levels will continue to increase and the affected infant will show failure to thrive, mental retardation, cataracts, jaundice, hepatomegaly, and cirrhosis of the liver, with death possibly occurring in the first month of life. Therapy consists of eliminating galactose from the diet.

Many states in the United States mandate routine screening for hypothyroidism. This involves the measurement of thyroxine (T_4) in a drop of blood obtained from a heel stick at 2 to 5 days of age. At this time the normally expected increase in T_4 is lacking in newborns with hypothyroidism. Cretinism develops in untreated affected people. The same blood sample can be used to test for all three of these metabolic disorders—PKU, galactosemia, and hypothyroidism.

Cytologic studies. Abnormalities can occur in either the autosomes or the sex chromosomes. Chromosomal disorders often can be diagnosed on the basis of the clinical manifestations alone. However, an infant may have a clinical appearance that is only suggestive of a problem. Cytologic studies then need to be done to confirm or rule out a suspected diagnosis (see Chapter 8).

Dermatoglyphics. Dermatoglyphics is the study of the patterns formed by the ridges in the skin on the hands and feet. Characteristic dermatoglyphic patterns have been noted for almost all the chromosomal abnormalities, such as Down syndrome (see *simian crease* in Fig. 28-22, *B*).

The nursing diagnoses formulated for an infant born with a congenital anomaly depend on the anomaly the infant has. For example, the diagnoses in an infant born with a CHD causing cyanosis will relate to inadequate oxygenation of body tissues, such as "activity intolerance related to imbalance between oxygen supply and demand." General nursing diagnoses pertaining to the care of neonates with congenital abnormalities are listed in the box.

▌Nursing Diagnoses

Infants with Congenital Abnormalities
Newborn
Risk for injury or death related to:
• Presence of a congenital disorder
Risk for infection related to:
• Anomaly or its treatment
Risk for impaired gas exchange, nutrition, or mobility related to:
• Congenital anomaly
Risk for altered growth and development related to:
• Inborn error of metabolism
Parents and Family
Dysfunctional grieving or spiritual distress related to:
• Birth of a child with a defect
Risk for ineffective individual or family coping related to:
• Birth of a child with a defect
Knowledge deficit related to:
• Cause of disorder, its management, alternative courses of action, community resources, prognosis, and the care needed by the child after discharge
Anxiety related to:
• Uncertainty regarding prognosis or ability to care for child
Risk for altered parenting related to:
• Birth of a child with a disorder or defect

Interventions: newborn

A collaborative health team approach that includes specialists (e.g., orthodontists, physical therapists, geneticists) and community service representatives is needed in the care of infants with some disorders. Surgical intervention in the neonatal period may be necessary for the infant requiring either immediate correction or a palliative procedure to relieve the symptoms of the anomaly until definitive correction can be done. However, the complications induced by the stress of surgery may upset the delicate metabolic balance in a neonate already attempting to adapt to its extrauterine environment. This is compounded by the fact that there is only a limited amount of nutrient reserves normally present in the neonate and these reserves are already being drawn on by the energy-expending processes involved in rapid growth. Any surgical procedures performed during this time of growth place additional demands on these reserves. There is also a higher morbidity and mortality in neonates than in older children or adults undergoing similar procedures (Rowe et al., 1995). However, despite these problems unique to neonates, advances in surgical techniques, anesthesia, and the nursing care given in intensive care nurseries have together been responsible for lessening the risk of surgery in neonates.

The health care team must be highly skilled to meet the needs of these infants. In addition to stabilization of the infant's condition, other preoperative interventions such as orogastric tube placement for abdominal decompression, the management of open lesions, and the maintenance of fluid and electrolyte balance, are implemented to manage specific anomalies.

Postoperatively the infant is returned to the intensive care nursery, where close monitoring is maintained. The infant's respiratory efforts are supported; this often requires suctioning and usually mechanical ventilation. Constant surveillance is necessary to detect any respiratory complications resulting from the anesthesia. A pulse oximeter is attached to measure the oxygen saturation in hemoglobin, which closely correlates with arterial oxygen saturation. Oxygen is provided as needed. An indwelling gastric catheter attached to intermittent suction is placed to remove gastric secretions, thereby preventing aspiration and the abdomen from becoming distended. The infant's fluid, electrolyte, and acid-base status are monitored and adjusted as needed. Urinary output is monitored and should equal 1 to 2 ml/kg/hr. Other nursing interventions are focused on caring for the surgical site, maintaining thermoregulation, and promoting comfort.

Interventions: parents and family

While the infant is receiving optimal care, the parents also have needs that must be met as they deal with the crisis of having an infant with an abnormal condition. Their reactions are carefully assessed and are likely to be those typical of a grief response. Facilitating their understanding of the information given them about their infant's condition is a vital nursing intervention. A newly diagnosed disorder often implies the need for the implementation of a therapeutic regimen. For example, the disorder may be an inborn error of metabolism, such as PKU, which requires consistent and rigid adherence to a diet. The family of such an infant may need help with securing the required formula and receiving counseling from the clinical dietitian. The importance of maintaining the diet, keeping an adequate supply of special preparations, and avoiding the use of unauthorized substitutions must be impressed on the family.

Referral to appropriate agencies is another essential component of the follow-up management, and the nurse should make the parents aware of all possible sources of aid, including pertinent literature, parent groups, and national organizations. Many organizations and foundations, such as the Cystic Fibrosis Foundation and the Muscular Dystrophy Association, provide services and equipment for affected children. There are also numerous parent groups the family can join where they can share experiences and derive mutual support in coping with problems similar to those of other group members. Nurses need to be familiar with the services available in their community that provide assistance and education to families with these special problems (see Appendix D).

A major nursing function is providing emotional support to the family during all aspects of the care of the child born with a defect or disorder. The feelings stemming from the real or imagined threat posed by a congenital anomaly are as varied as the people being counseled. Responses may include apathy, denial, anger, hostility, fear, embarrassment, grief, and loss of self-esteem.

Parents benefit from seeing before-and-after pictures of other babies born with the same defect. Coupled with other verbal and nonverbal supportive care, this visual reassurance may be effective in allaying their concerns.

Families need much information, guidance, and support as they make decisions regarding the care of their infant. Once they have been given the facts and possible consequences and all the assistance they need in problem solving, the final decision regarding a course of action must be their own. It is then incumbent on health care providers to support the decision of the family.

INFANTS OF DIABETIC MOTHERS

No single physiologic or biochemical event can explain the diverse clinical manifestations seen in the infants of diabetic mothers (IDMs) or infants of gestational diabetic mothers (IGDMs). A better understanding of maternal and fetal metabolism, resulting in stricter control of maternal diabetes and improved obstetric and neonatal intensive care, has led to a decrease in perinatal mortality in diabetic pregnancy. However, maternal diabetes continues to play a significant role in neonatal morbidity and mortality.

All infants born to mothers with diabetes are at some risk for complications. The degree of risk is affected by the severity and duration of maternal disease. Problems seen in

IDMs include congenital anomalies, macrosomia, birth trauma and perinatal asphyxia, respiratory distress syndrome (RDS), hypoglycemia, hypocalcemia and hypomagnesemia, cardiomyopathy, and hyperbilirubinemia and polycythemia.

Pathophysiology

The mechanisms responsible for the problems seen in IDMs are not fully understood. In early pregnancy, fluctuations in blood glucose levels and episodes of ketoacidosis are believed to cause congenital anomalies. Later in pregnancy, when the mother's pancreas cannot release sufficient insulin to meet increased demands, maternal hyperglycemia results. The high levels of glucose cross the placenta and stimulate the fetal pancreas to release insulin. The combination of the increased supply of maternal glucose and other nutrients and increased fetal insulin results in excessive fetal growth called macrosomia (see later discussion).

Hyperinsulinemia accounts for many of the problems the fetus or infant develops. In addition to fluctuating glucose levels, maternal vascular involvement or superimposed maternal infection adversely affects the fetus. Normally, maternal blood has a more alkaline pH than carbon dioxide–rich fetal blood does. This phenomenon encourages the exchange of oxygen and carbon dioxide across the placental membrane. When the maternal blood is more acidotic than the fetal blood, such as during ketoacidosis, little carbon dioxide or oxygen exchange occurs at the level of the placenta. The mortality for the unborn baby resulting from an episode of maternal ketoacidosis may be as high as 50% or more (Fanaroff & Martin, 1997).

There are indications that some neonatal conditions— macrosomia, hypoglycemia, hypocalcemia, hyperbilirubinemia, and perhaps fetal lung immaturity—may be eliminated or the incidence decreased by maintaining control over maternal glucose levels within narrow limits (Creasy & Resnik, 1994).

Neonatal Complications

Congenital anomalies

Congenital anomalies occur in approximately 7% to 10% of IDMs. Their incidence is two to four times that for infants born to mothers without diabetes (Ogata, 1994). The incidence is greatest among small-for-gestational-age (SGA) newborns. Intrauterine growth restriction (IUGR) leading to SGA infants is seen in IDMs with severe vascular disease. The most frequently occurring anomalies involve the cardiac, musculoskeletal, and central nervous systems. In most defects associated with diabetic pregnancies, the structural abnormality occurs before the eighth week after conception. This reinforces the importance of control of blood glucose both before conception and in the early stages of pregnancy.

The incidence of congenital heart lesions in these infants is five times higher than that in the general population. Coarctation of the aorta, transposition of the great vessels, and atrial or ventricular septal defects are the most common lesions encountered in the IDM. Maternal diabetic

control is negatively correlated with the incidence of lesions; that is, the better the control, the fewer the lesions.

Central nervous system anomalies include anencephaly, encephalocele, meningomyelocele, and hydrocephalus. The musculoskeletal system may be affected by *caudal regression syndrome* (*sacral agenesis,* with weakness or deformities of the lower extremities, malformation and fixation of the hip joints, and shortening or deformity of the femurs). Hypertrichosis on the pinnae (excessive hair growth on the external ear) has been added to the list of characteristic clinical features (Fanaroff & Martin, 1997). Other defects noted in this population include gastrointestinal atresia and urinary tract malformations.

Neonatal small left colon syndrome, also called *lazy colon syndrome,* occurs in some IDMs and IGDMs. This syndrome is suspected when failure to pass meconium, abdominal distention, and bile-stained vomitus are noted. Contrast enemas show a greatly diminished caliber of the left colon from the splenic flexure. The syndrome is transient, with normal bowel function developing early in infancy (Fanaroff & Martin, 1997).

Macrosomia

Despite improvements in the control of maternal blood sugar levels, the incidence of **macrosomia** in the insulin-dependent diabetic is 20% to 30% (Ogata, 1994). At birth the typical LGA infant has a round, cherubic ("tomato" or cushingoid) face, chubby body, and a plethoric or flushed complexion (Fig. 28-23). These are the characteristics of macrosomia. The infant has enlarged internal organs (hepatosplenomegaly, splanchnomegaly, cardiomegaly) and increased body fat, especially around the shoulders. The placenta and umbilical cord are larger than average. The

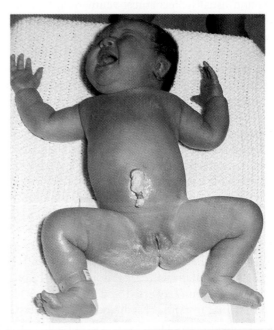

Fig. **28-23** Macrosomia. (From O'Doherty N: *Neonatology: micro atlas of the newborn,* Nutley, NJ, 1986, Hoffmann-LaRoche.)

brain is the only organ that is not enlarged. IDMs may be LGA but physiologically immature.

Insulin has been implicated as the primary growth hormone for intrauterine development. Uncontrolled maternal diabetes results in elevated maternal levels of amino acids and free fatty acids along with hyperglycemia. As the nutrients cross the placenta, the fetal pancreas responds by producing insulin to match the fuel supply. The resulting accelerated protein synthesis, together with a deposition of excessive glycogen and fat stores, is responsible for the typical macrosomic infant. This is the infant most at risk for the neonatal complications of hypoglycemia, hypocalcemia, hyperviscosity, and hyperbilirubinemia. The excessive amounts of metabolic fuels presented to the fetus from the mother and the consequent fetal hyperinsulinism are now understood to represent the basic pathologic mechanism in the diabetic pregnancy (Fanaroff & Martin, 1997).

Birth trauma and perinatal asphyxia

The excessive shoulder size in these infants often leads to dystocia, particularly because the head may be smaller in proportion to the shoulders than in a nonmacrosomic infant. Macrosomic infants, who may be born vaginally or by cesarean birth after a trial of labor, may incur birth trauma.

Birth injury (resulting from macrosomia or method of birth) and perinatal asphyxia occur in 20% of IGDMs and 35% of IDMs. Examples of birth trauma include cephalhematoma; paralysis of the facial nerve (seventh cranial nerve) (see Fig. 28-7); fracture of the clavicle or humerus; brachial plexus paralysis, usually Erb-Duchenne (right upper arm) palsy (see Fig. 28-5); and phrenic nerve paralysis, invariably associated with diaphragmatic paralysis.

Respiratory distress syndrome

IDMs or IGDMs are four to six times more likely than normal infants to develop RDS. With improved maternal glucose control, this risk has been substantially reduced. Some recent studies have found no increased risk of RDS in matched controlled studies of IDM and non-IDM infants (Mimouni et al., 1987), whereas others have shown a continued delay in lung maturation in the presence of maternal diabetes (Piper & Langer, 1993).

In the fetus exposed to high levels of maternal glucose, synthesis of surfactant may be delayed because of the high fetal serum level of insulin (Philip, 1996). Fetal lung maturity, as evidenced by a lecithin/sphingomyelin (L/S) ratio of 2:1, is not reassuring if the mother has diabetes mellitus or gestation-induced diabetes mellitus. For the infants of such mothers, an L/S ratio of 3:1 or more or the presence of phosphatidylglycerol in the amniotic fluid is more indicative of adequate lung maturity.

Hypoglycemia

Hypoglycemia (blood glucose levels less than 40 mg/dl in term infants) affects many IDMs. After constant exposure to high circulating levels of glucose, hyperplasia of the fetal pancreas occurs, resulting in hyperinsulinemia. Disruption of the fetal glucose supply occurs with the clamping of the umbilical cord, and the neonate's blood glucose level falls rapidly in the presence of fetal hyperinsulinism. Hypoglycemia is most common in the macrosomic infant but blood glucose levels should be monitored in all infants of known or suspected diabetic mothers.

Asymptomatic or symptomatic hypoglycemia most frequently presents within the first 1 to 3 hours after birth. Signs of hypoglycemia include jitteriness, apnea, tachypnea, and cyanosis. Significant hypoglycemia may result in seizures. Hypoglycemia is worsened by the presence of hypothermia or respiratory distress.

Hypocalcemia and hypomagnesemia

Hypocalcemia occurs in 10% to 20% of IDMs and is believed to be related to decreased levels of parathormone (Ogata, 1994). Hypomagnesemia is believed to develop because of maternal renal losses that occur in diabetes. Hypocalcemia is associated with preterm birth, birth trauma, and perinatal asphyxia. Signs of hypocalcemia, a prevalent finding in IDMs and IGDMs, are similar to those of hypoglycemia, but they occur between 24 and 36 hours of age. Hypocalcemia must be considered if therapy for hypoglycemia is ineffective.

Cardiomyopathy

All IDMs need careful observation for cardiomyopathy. Two types of cardiomyopathy can occur. Clinicians must be alert to identify correctly the type of lesion so that appropriate therapy is instituted. Both types of lesions are associated with respiratory symptoms and congestive heart failure.

Hypertrophic cardiomyopathy (HCM) is characterized by a hypercontractile and thickened myocardium. The ventricular walls are thickened, as is the septum, which in severe cases results in outflow tract obstructions. The mitral valve is poorly functioning. In nonhypertrophic cardiomyopathy (non-HCM) the myocardium is poorly contractile and overstretched. The ventricles are increased in size, and there is no outflow obstruction. Most infants are asymptomatic, but severe outflow obstruction may cause left ventricular heart failure. HCM may be treated with a β-adrenergic blocker (such as propranolol to decrease contractility and heart rate). A cardiotonic agent is used to treat non-HCM (such as digoxin to increase contractility and decrease heart rate). The abnormality usually resolves in 3 to 12 months (Fanaroff & Martin, 1997).

Hyperbilirubinemia and polycythemia

Hyperbilirubinemia develops in 20% to 25% of IDMs (Ogata, 1994). Many IDMs are also polycythemic. Polycythemia increases blood viscosity, thereby impairing circulation. In addition this increased number of RBCs to be hemolyzed increases the potential bilirubin load that the neonate must clear. The excessive RBCs are produced in extramedullary foci (liver and spleen) in addition to the usual sites in bone marrow. Therefore both liver function and bilirubin clearance may be adversely affected. Bruising associated with birth of a macrosomic infant will contribute further to high bilirubin levels.

Nursing Care

Nursing care depends on the neonate's particular problems. If the maternal blood glucose level was well controlled throughout the pregnancy, the infant may require only monitoring. Because euglycemia (normal blood glucose levels) is not always possible, the nurse must promptly recognize and treat any consequences of maternal diabetes that arise. The most common problems IDMs experience that require intervention include birth trauma and perinatal asphyxia; RDS; difficult metabolic transition, including hypoglycemia and hypocalcemia; and congenital anomalies (Plan of Care).

PLAN OF CARE *Infant of Mother with Gestational Diabetes*

NURSING DIAGNOSIS Risk for injury related to hypoglycemia, hypocalcemia, polycythemia, hyperbilirubinemia secondary to maternal gestational diabetes

Expected Outcomes *Infant will exhibit blood glucose, serum calcium, hematocrit, and serum bilirubin levels that are within normal limits.*

Nursing Interventions/*Rationales*

Monitor blood glucose levels (less than 40 mg/dl indicative of hypoglycemia); serum calcium levels (less than 7 mg/dl indicative of hypocalcemia); serum bilirubin levels (over 15 mg/dl indicative of hyperbilirubinemia) *to assess and detect early onset to prevent complications.*

Observe for signs of hypoglycemia (i.e., jitteriness, twitching, lethargy, apathy, convulsions, cyanosis, sweating, eye rolling, refusal to eat); hypocalcemia (i.e., jitters, apnea, high-pitched cry, abdominal distention); polycythemia (plethora); and hyperbilirubinemia (i.e., jaundice) *to assess and detect signs of onset to prevent complications.*

Early feeding of infant, glucose supplements as prescribed *to prevent or treat early hypoglycemia;* increased milk feedings/calcium supplements per physician order *to prevent or treat early hypocalcemia;* early and frequent feedings *to reduce hematocrit and enhance excretion of bilirubin in stool;* phototherapy *for bilirubin over 12 to 15 mg/dl.*

Reduce environmental factors (i.e., stimuli such as jarring or shaking, cold stress, and respiratory distress), *which can predispose infant to hypoglycemia or precipitate a seizure.*

NURSING DIAGNOSIS Risk for impaired gas exchange related to lung immaturity/cardiomyopathy secondary to maternal gestational diabetes

Expected Outcomes *Infant will exhibit signs of adequate oxygen supply (respiratory rate, rhythm, and amplitude, blood gas levels within normal limits).*

Nursing Interventions/*Rationales*

Monitor infant vital signs, blood gas levels per order, patency of airway *to evaluate pulmonary and circulatory status.*

Avoid activities that may lower body temperature and lead to cold stress, *which can induce respiratory distress.*

Suction as needed *to keep airway patent and prevent aspiration.*

Position infant on side *to facilitate mucous drainage.*

Have resuscitation equipment and oxygen available *for quick treatment of respiratory distress.*

NURSING DIAGNOSIS Risk for ineffective thermoregulation related to physiologic immaturity; potential for infection related to immature immunologic defenses/environmental exposure

See the Nursing Care Plan for the normal newborn in Chapter 20.

NURSING DIAGNOSIS Anxiety (risk for powerlessness, situational low self-esteem, ineffective coping) related to neonate's condition, management, and prognosis

Expected Outcome *Parents demonstrate understanding of prognosis and therapy for infant.*

Nursing Interventions/*Rationales*

Explain potential effects of maternal diabetic condition on newborn *to relieve fear of unknown and support ability to cope.*

Encourage open communication (i.e., inform parents of ongoing condition, procedures, and treatment; answer questions; correct misperceptions; actively listen to parental concerns) *to provide support and help provide sense of control.*

Encourage parents to interact with infant and to become involved in care routines *to foster emotional connection.*

From Wong D & Perry S: *Maternal child nursing care,* St Louis, 1998, Mosby.

NEONATAL INFECTIONS

Sepsis

Sepsis (presence of microorganisms or their toxins in blood or other tissues) continues to be one of the most significant causes of neonatal morbidity and mortality. The newborn infant is susceptible to infection. Maternal immunoglobulin (IgM) does not cross the placenta. IgA and IgM require time to reach optimum levels after birth. Phagocytosis is less efficient. Serum complement levels are inadequate; serum complement (C1 through C6) is involved in immunologic reactions, some of which kill or lyse bacteria and enhance phagocytosis. Dysmaturity seen with IUGR and preterm and postterm birth further compromises the neonate's immune system.

Table 28-3 outlines risk factors for neonatal sepsis. Special precautions for preventing infection, as well as prompt recognition when it occurs, are necessary for optimum newborn care. Neonatal infections may be acquired in utero, during birth, during resuscitation, and nosocomially (Fanaroff & Martin, 1997).

Prenatal acquisition of infection occurs by organisms placentally transferred directly into the fetal circulatory system and from infected amniotic fluid, such as with herpes simplex virus (HSV), cytomegalovirus (CMV), and rubella.

TABLE 28-3	Risk Factors for Neonatal Sepsis
SOURCE	**RISK FACTORS**
Maternal	Low socioeconomic status
	Poor prenatal care
	Poor nutrition
	Substance abuse
Intrapartum	Premature rupture of fetal membranes
	Maternal fever
	Chorioamnionitis
	Prolonged labor
	Preterm labor
	Maternal urinary tract infection
Neonatal	Twin gestation
	Male
	Birth asphyxia
	Meconium aspiration
	Congenital anomalies of skin or mucous membranes
	Galactosemia
	Absence of spleen
	Low birth weight or prematurity
	Malnourishment
	Prolonged hospitalization

From Askin D: Bacterial and fungal sepsis in the neonate, *J Obstet Gynecol Neonatal Nurs* 24(7):635, 1995.

Microorganisms ascend from the vagina and pass through the cervix. The membranes become infected and may rupture. Infection of the fetal skin and respiratory or gastrointestinal tract may result.

During birth, contact with an infected birth canal can result in generalized or local infection. The upper airway and gastrointestinal tract are again the principal pathways for generalized infections. The conjunctiva and oral cavity are the usual sites of local infection.

Postnatal infection may be acquired during resuscitation or through the introduction of foreign objects such as indwelling catheters or endotracheal tubes. Nursery-acquired infections may be transferred to the infant by the hands of the parents or health care personnel or spread from contaminated equipment. The umbilicus is a receptive site for cutaneous infection leading to sepsis (Fanaroff & Martin, 1997).

Neonatal bacterial infection is classified into two patterns according to the time of presentation. Early-onset or congenital sepsis usually presents within 24 hours of birth, progresses more rapidly than later-onset infection, and carries a mortality of 15% to 50% (Klein & Marcy, 1995). Early-onset infection is usually caused by microorganisms from the normal flora of the maternal vaginal tract, including group B streptococcus, *Haemophilus influenzae*, *Listeria monocytogenes*, *Escherichia coli*, and *Streptococcus pneumoniae*. It is associated with a history of obstetric complications, such as preterm labor, premature rupture of membranes, maternal fever during labor, and chorioamnionitis (Klein & Marcy, 1995).

Acquired infection is most frequently seen after 1 week of age and is slower in progression. Bacteria responsible for *late-onset sepsis* are varied, may be acquired from the birth canal or from the external environment, and include *Staphylococcus aureus*, *Staphylococcus epidermidis*, *Pseudomonas* organisms, and group B streptococci. *S. aureus* is most common, accounting for 40% of all late-onset sepsis (Lott & Kilb, 1992).

Viral infections may cause abortion, stillbirth, intrauterine infection, congenital malformations, and acute disease. These pathogens also may cause chronic infection, with subtle manifestations that may be recognized only after a prolonged period. It is important to recognize the manifestations of infections in the neonatal period to treat the acute infection and to prevent nosocomial infections in other infants, and to anticipate effects on the infant's subsequent growth and development.

Fungal infections are of greatest concern in the immunocompromised or premature infant. Occasionally, fungal infections such as thrush are found in otherwise healthy term infants.

Septicemia refers to a generalized infection in the bloodstream. Pneumonia, the most common form of neonatal infection, is one of the leading causes of perinatal death (Fanaroff & Martin, 1997). Bacterial meningitis affects 1 in 2,500 live-born infants. Gastroenteritis is sporadic, depending on epidemic outbreaks. Local infections such as conjunctivitis and omphalitis occur frequently, but incidence rates are unavailable. Infection continues to be a significant factor in fetal and neonatal morbidity and mortality.

CARE MANAGEMENT

Assessment and Nursing Diagnoses

The prenatal record is reviewed for risk factors associated with infection and signs and symptoms suggestive of it. Maternal vaginal or perineal infection may be transmitted directly to the infant during passage through the birth canal. Psychosocial history and history of sexually transmitted diseases (STDs) may indicate possible human immunodeficiency virus (HIV), hepatitis B virus (HBV), or CMV infection.

The perinatal events also are reviewed. Premature rupture of membranes (PROM) may be caused by maternal or intrauterine infection. Ascending infection may occur after prolonged PROM, prolonged labor, or intrauterine fetal monitoring. A maternal history of fever during labor or the presence of foul-smelling amniotic fluid may also indicate the presence of infection. Antibiotic therapy initiated during labor should be noted. Resuscitation that requires intubation and deep suctioning may result in infection. The neonate's gestational age, maturity, birth weight, and gender all affect the incidence of infection. Sepsis occurs about twice as often and results in a higher mortality in male than in female infants. The neonate is assessed for respiratory distress, skin abscesses, rashes, and other indications of infection.

During the postnatal period the time of onset of suspicious signs is noted. Onset within the first 48 hours of life is more often associated with prenatal or perinatal predisposing factors. Onset after 2 or 3 days more frequently reflects disease acquired at or subsequent to birth (Fanaroff & Martin, 1997).

The earliest clinical signs of neonatal sepsis are characterized by a lack of specificity. The nonspecific signs include lethargy, poor feeding, poor weight gain, or irritability. The nurse or parent may simply note that the infant is just not doing as well as before. Differential diagnosis may be difficult because signs of sepsis are similar to signs of noninfectious neonatal problems such as anemia or hypoglycemia. Additional clinical and laboratory information and appropriate cultures supplement the findings described. Table 28-4 outlines signs of sepsis.

Laboratory studies are performed. Specimens for cultures include blood, nasopharyngeal or oropharyngeal, CSF,

TABLE 28-4	*Signs of Sepsis**
SYSTEM	**SIGNS**
Respiratory	Apnea, bradycardia
	Tachypnea
	Grunting, nasal flaring
	Retractions
	Decreased oxygen saturation
	Acidosis
Cardiovascular	Decreased cardiac output
	Tachycardia
	Hypotension
	Decreased perfusion
Central nervous	Temperature instability
	Lethargy
	Hypotonia
	Irritability, seizures
Gastrointestinal	Feeding intolerance
	Abdominal distention
	Vomiting, diarrhea
Integumentary	Jaundice
	Pallor
	Petechiae

From Askin D: Bacterial and fungal sepsis in the neonate, *J Obstet Gynecol Neonatal Nurs* 24(7):635, 1995.
*Laboratory findings include neutropenia, increased bands, hypoglycemia or hyperglycemia, metabolic acidosis, and thrombocytopenia.

stool, and urine. Increased direct (conjugated) bilirubin levels may be found, especially if the infecting microorganism is gram negative. Complete blood cell count with differential is performed to determine the presence of anemia, increased white blood cell count, or decreased white blood cell count (an ominous sign). C-reactive protein may or may not be elevated.

Vigilant assessment continues during and after treatment. The newborn continues to be assessed for sequelae to septicemia. Before the advent of antibiotics, 90% of newborns with sepsis died. Antibiotic therapy decreased mortality to between 13% and 45% depending on the causative organism. Sequelae to septicemia include meningitis, disseminated intravascular coagulation (DIC), and septic shock.

Septic shock results from the toxins released into the bloodstream. The most common sign is a drop in blood pressure, a vital sign often overlooked in the care of the neonate. Other signs are rapid, irregular respirations and pulse (similar to septicemia in general).

Any number of nursing diagnoses are possible, depending on the infant's gestational age and birth weight, the organ systems involved, and the nature of the infection. Examples of nursing diagnoses related to neonatal infections are listed in the accompanying box.

Nursing Diagnoses

Newborns with Infections

Newborn

Risk for infection related to:
- Maternal vaginal (or other) infection
- Need for resuscitation or ventilation therapy
- Need for indwelling umbilical catheters, total parenteral nutrition (TPN), parenteral fluids
- Intrauterine electronic fetal monitoring
- Male gender
- Dysmaturity, IUGR, gestational age

Ineffective thermoregulation related to:
- Infection

Impaired tissue integrity related to:
- Need for multiple supportive measures (e.g., biometric monitoring, TPN, inhalation therapy)

Pain related to:
- Need for multiple supportive measures

Parents and family

Anxiety, fear, or anticipatory grieving related to:
- Uncertainty about infant's prognosis
- Poor prognosis

Risk for altered parent-infant attachment related to:
- Separation of parent and newborn
- Feelings of inadequacy in caring for infant
- Inability to breastfeed

Powerlessness or spiritual distress related to:
- Perinatal events or newborn's condition

Anxiety related to knowledge deficit regarding:
- Newborn's condition, its course, and its management

Expected Outcomes of Care

Planning begins with the development of standards for preventive measures in nurseries and protocols for diagnosis and treatment of infections. Individual assessment findings are used to plan care for each infant. Parents and family are encouraged to participate in planning. Expected outcomes include the following:

- The newborn will remain free of sepsis
- The newborn's early signs of sepsis will be recognized, and appropriate therapy will be instituted
- If therapy is necessary, the newborn will suffer no harmful sequelae
- Parents will begin bonding and attachment to newborn
- Parents will maintain self-esteem
- Staff members will establish caring relationship with parents to foster their trust and to encourage continuing, active, positive interactions of family with members of health care system.

Plan of Care and Interventions

Preventive measures

Virtually all controlled clinical trials have demonstrated that effective handwashing is responsible for the prevention of nosocomial infection in nursery units (Fanaroff & Martin, 1997). Nurses are directly or indirectly responsible for minimizing or eliminating environmental sources of infectious agents in the nursery. Measures to be taken include Standard Precautions (see Chapter 6), careful and thorough cleaning, frequent replacement of used equipment (e.g., changing intravenous tubing per hospital protocol, cleaning resuscitation and ventilation equipment), and disposal of excrement and linens in an appropriate manner. Overcrowding must be avoided in nurseries.

Instillation of antibiotic in newborns' eyes 1 to 2 hours after birth is done to prevent infection, such as gonorrhea and chlamydia. The skin, its secretions, and normal flora are natural defenses that protect against invading pathogens. Warm water may be used to remove blood and meconium from the neonate's face, head, and body. A mild nonmedicated soap (in single-use container or in a small bar reserved for a single newborn) can be used with careful water rinsing. The vernix caseosa is left in place. No single method of cord care has been shown to prevent colonization and subsequent disease. Alcohol, triple dye, or an antimicrobial agent are agents typically used. Nurses need to follow agency protocols for cord care.

Curative measures

Breastfeeding or feeding the newborn breast milk from the mother is encouraged. Protective mechanisms exist in breast milk. Colostrum contains immunoglobulin A (IgA), which offers protection against infection in the gastrointestinal tract. Human milk contains iron-binding protein that exerts a bacteriostatic effect on *E. coli*. Human milk also contains macrophages and lymphocytes. The vulnerability of infants to common mucosal pathogens such as respiratory syncytial virus (RSV) may be reduced by passive transfer of maternal immunity in the colostrum and breast milk.

Administering medications, taking precautions when performing treatments, and following isolation procedures are also interventions to be considered when a newborn has an infection.

Monitoring the intravenous infusion rate and administering antibiotics are the nurse's responsibility. It is important to administer the prescribed dose of antibiotic within 1 hour after it is prepared to avoid loss of drug stability. If the intravenous fluid the infant is receiving contains electrolytes, vitamins, or other medications, the nurse should check with the hospital pharmacy before adding antibiotics. The antibiotic (or other medication) may be deactivated or may form a precipitate when combined with other substances. In that case a piggyback solution of the prescribed fluid is attached with a three-way stopcock at the infusion site.

Care must be taken in suctioning secretions from any newborn's oropharynx or trachea. These secretions may be infected.

Isolation procedures are implemented according to hospital policy as indicated. Isolation protocols are changing rapidly, and the nurse is urged to participate in continuing education and in-service programs to remain up to date.

In some jurisdictions, medically stable infants may be discharged home to complete a course of intravenous or intramuscular antibiotics. The home care nurse provides daily assessments of the infant's condition, parent teaching and support, and administration of the antibiotic dose.

Rehabilitative measures

Rehabilitative measures vary with the individual needs of the neonate. Some neonates will need to be weaned from ventilatory support systems. Those who suffer sequelae such as mental retardation and epilepsy will require a knowledgeable family and supportive community resources. Some children will require corrective care for problems with dentition, vision, and hearing.

Evaluation

The nurse can be reasonably assured that care was effective if the previously stated outcomes for care are achieved.

TORCH Infections

The occurrence of certain maternal infections during early pregnancy is known to be associated with various congenital malformations and disorders. The most common and best understood infections are represented by the acronym **TORCH**, for *T*oxoplasmosis, *o*ther (gonorrhea, syphilis, varicella, HBV, and HIV), *r*ubella, *c*ytomegalovirus, and *h*erpes simplex virus (Box 28-1). HSV may result in a severe, often fatal systemic illness in neonates. Survivors of herpetic infection may have residual neurologic defects and chorioretinitis. The other congenital infections also may result in encephalopathy with various anomalies, including microcephaly, chorioretinitis intracranial calcifications, microphthalmos, and cataracts. To a certain extent the varied clinical manifestations of these infections overlap, but a specific diagnosis can be made by the clustering of clinical findings, as well as by specific antibody studies collectively referred to as a TORCH screen (Fanaroff & Martin, 1997).

Toxoplasmosis

Toxoplasmosis is a multisystem disease caused by the protozoan *Toxoplasma gondii*. Approximately 30% of

---

| **BOX 28-1** | **TORCH Infections Affecting Newborns** |

T Toxoplasmosis
O Other: gonorrhea, syphilis, varicella, hepatitis B virus (HBV), human immunodeficiency virus (HIV)
R Rubella
C Cytomegalovirus (CMV) infections or cytomegalic inclusion disease (CMID)
H Herpes simplex virus (HSV) infection

---

women who contract toxoplasmosis during gestation transmit the disease to their offspring. Fetal infection rates vary according to geographic location. Reported rates vary from 0.12 to 3.5 per 1,000 births (Remington, McLeod & Desmonts, 1995). The diagnosis of toxoplasmosis in the neonate is supported by elevated levels of cord blood serum IgM.

More than 70% of affected infants are free of symptoms. The clinical features of toxoplasmosis resemble cytomegalic inclusion disease (CMID) in the infant. Both diseases are responsible for serious perinatal mortality and morbidity: 10% to 15% die, 85% have severe psychomotor problems or mental retardation by 2 to 4 years, and 50% have visual problems by 1 year.

Severe toxoplasmosis is associated with preterm birth, growth restriction, microcephaly or hydrocephaly, microphthalmos, chorioretinitis, central nervous system (CNS) calcification, thrombocytopenia, jaundice, and fever. Petechiae or a maculopapular rash may also be evident. Some clinical manifestations do not develop until later in life. The affected infant may be treated with pyrimethamine, as well as oral sulfadiazine; folic acid supplement is needed to prevent leukopenia and anemia, side effects of pyrimethamine.

Gonorrhea

Neonatal infection with *Neisseria gonorrhoeae* occurs in 30% to 50% of newborns of women who have gonococcal infections (Ament & Whalen, 1996). After rupture of membranes, ascending infection can result in orogastric contamination of the fetus. The organism also may invade mucosal surfaces such as the conjunctiva (ophthalmia neonatorum), rectal mucosa, and pharynx. Contamination may occur as the infant passes through the birth canal, or it may occur postnatally from an infected adult. Neonatal gonococcal arthritis, septicemia, meningitis, vaginitis, and scalp abscesses also can develop.

Eye prophylaxis (e.g., with 0.5% erythromycin ointment or 1% silver nitrate) is administrated at or shortly after birth to prevent ophthalmia neonatorum. The infant with a mild infection often recovers completely with appropriate treatment, such as neonatal ceftriazone. Occasionally, infants die of overwhelming infection in the early neonatal period.

Syphilis

Congenital and neonatal syphilis have reemerged in recent years as significant health problems. It is estimated that for every 100 women diagnosed with primary or secondary disease, 2 to 5 infants will contract congenital syphilis. If syphilis during pregnancy is untreated, 40% to 50% of neonates born to these women will have symptomatic congenital syphilis (Cohen & Goldstein, 1996). Treatment failure can occur, particularly when treatment is given in the third trimester; therefore infants born to women treated after 20 weeks of gestation should be investigated for congenital syphilis.

Fetal infestation with the spirochete *Treponema pallidum* is blocked by Langhans' layer in the chorion until this layer begins to atrophy between 16 and 18 weeks of gestation. If spirochetemia is untreated, it will result in fetal death by midtrimester abortion or stillbirth in one in four cases. All neonates in whom the infection occurs before 7 months of gestation are affected. Only 60% are affected if the infection occurs late in pregnancy. If maternal infection is treated adequately before the eighteenth week, neonates seldom demonstrate signs of the disease unless reinfection occurs.

Because the fetus becomes infected after the period of organogenesis (first trimester), maldevelopment of organs does not result. Congenital syphilis may stimulate preterm labor, but no evidence indicates that it causes IUGR. Signs of congenital syphilis may include inflammatory and destructive changes in the placenta; in organs such as the liver, spleen, kidneys, adrenal glands; and in bone covering and marrow. Disorders of the CNS, teeth, and cornea may not become evident until several months after birth.

Clinical manifestations. The most severely affected infants may be hydropic (edematous) and anemic, with enlarged liver and spleen. Hepatosplenomegaly probably is the result of extramedullary hematopoietic activity stimulated by the severe anemia.

In some infants, signs of congenital syphilis do not appear until late in the neonatal period. In these newborns, early signs, such as poor feeding, slight hyperthermia, and snuffles, may be nonspecific. *Snuffles* refers to the copious, clear, serosanguineous mucous discharge from the obstructed nose. A mucopurulent discharge indicates secondary infection, usually by streptococci or staphylococci.

By the end of the first week of life, a copper-colored maculopapular dermal rash appears in untreated newborn cases. The rash is characteristically first noticeable on the palms of the hands, soles of the feet, the diaper area, and around the mouth and anus. Rough, cracked, mucocutaneous lesions of the lips heal to form circumoral radiating scars known as *rhagades.*

Other involvement results in exfoliation (separation, flaking) of nails and loss of hair. Iritis and choroiditis are characteristic of infection of the eyes. Nephrotic syndrome secondary to renal infection; hepatitis with jaundice, lymphadenopathy, and inflammation of the pancreas, testes, and colon; and a pseudoparalysis of the extremities may be noted. If syphilis is suspected, the neonate undergoes a lumbar puncture for CSF analysis.

Medical management. If the mother was adequately treated before giving birth and serologic testing of the infant does not show syphilis, generally the infant is not treated with antibiotics. In this case the infant is checked for antibody titer (received from the mother via the placenta) every 2 weeks for 3 months, at which time the test result should be negative. Some physicians recommend antibiotic therapy for asymptomatic or inconclusive cases.

For antibiotic treatment to be effective, an "adequate" blood level must be maintained for an "adequate" period. The suggested medication protocol in the presence of symptomatic systemic disease differs from author to author and from physician to physician. Penicillin is the usual treatment (Paryani et al., 1994). After 12 hours of antibiotic therapy, the infant's condition is not considered contagious. It generally is accepted that erythromycin is the substitute antibiotic of choice for infants sensitive to penicillin.

Prognosis. In general, treatment of syphilis is more effective if it is begun early rather than late in the course of the disease. However, a recurrence rate of 5% can be expected. Even adequate treatment of congenital syphilis after birth does not always prevent late (5 to 15 years after initial infection) complications. Potential complications include neurosyphilis, deafness, Hutchinson's teeth (notched incisors), saber shins, joint involvement, saddle nose (depressed bridge), gummas (soft, gummy tumors) over the skin and other organs, and interstitial keratitis (inflammation of the cornea). The failure of therapy with the persistence of spirochetes in the eyes is not unusual because antibiotics penetrate ocular tissue poorly. Congenital syphilis during early childhood rarely causes death.

Varicella-zoster

The varicella-zoster virus responsible for chickenpox and shingles is a member of the herpes family. Approximately 95% of women in the childbearing years are immune; therefore, the risk of infection in pregnancy is low (1 to 7 cases per 10,000 pregnancies) (Freij & Sever, 1994).

Varicella transmission to the fetus may occur across the placenta when the disease is contracted in the first half of pregnancy, but this is relatively infrequent. When transmission to the fetus does occur in the early part of pregnancy, the effects on the fetus include limb atrophy, neurologic abnormalities, eye abnormalities, and IUGR.

When maternal infection occurs in the last 3 weeks of pregnancy, 25% of infants born to these mothers develop clinical varicella (Freij & Sever, 1994). The severity of the infant's illness increases greatly if maternal infection occurred within 5 days before or 2 days after birth. The mortality in severe illness is 30% (Freij & Sever, 1994).

Seroimmune pregnant women exposed to active chickenpox can be given varicella-zoster immune globulin (VZIG), which does not reduce the incidence of infection but should decrease the effects of the virus on the fetus. The immunoglobulin must be given within 72 hours of exposure to be effective.

Infants born to mothers who develop chickenpox between 5 days before birth and 48 hours after should be given VZIG at birth because of the risk of severe disease. Vidarabine or acyclovir can be used to treat infants with generalized involvement and pneumonia (Strodtbeck, 1995).

Term infants exposed to chickenpox after birth will have a mild or no infection if they are born to immune mothers. Those born to nonimmune mothers may develop chickenpox, but the course is not usually severe. Experts are divided as to whether this group of infants should receive VZIG. Infants less than 28 weeks are at risk regardless of their mother's status and likely benefit from VZIG if exposed to chickenpox.

Hepatitis B virus

Hepatitis B virus (HBV) infection during pregnancy is not associated with an increase in malformations, stillbirths, or IUGR; however, about a 32% increase in risk exists for preterm birth (Fanaroff & Martin, 1997). The transmission rate of HBV to the newborn is dependent upon the timing of the infection (Cowles & Gonik, 1997). Transmission occurs transplacentally, serum to serum, and by contact with contaminated urine, feces, saliva, semen, or vaginal secretions during birth. Infants are more frequently infected during birth or in the first few days of life. The rate of transmission is highest when the mother contracts the virus immediately before birth. These mothers will be positive for hepatitis B surface antigen (HBsAg). Transmission may possibly occur through breast milk, but antigens also develop in formula-fed infants at the same or higher rate. Diagnosis is made by viral culture of amniotic fluid and the presence of HBsAg and IgM in the cord or baby's serum.

Neonatal and fetal effects are serious. Preterm birth exposes the neonate to the problems of prematurity. Infants may be symptom free at birth or show evidence of acute hepatitis with changes in liver function. The mortality for full-blown hepatitis is 75%. Infants who become carriers are at high risk for chronic hepatitis, cirrhosis of the liver, or liver cancer even years later (Fanaroff & Martin, 1997).

Infants whose mothers have antibodies for HBsAg or who have developed hepatitis during pregnancy or the postpartum period should be treated with hepatitis B immunoglobulin (HBIG), 0.5 ml intramuscularly, as soon as possible after birth—within the first 12 hours of life. Concurrently, but at a different site, the vaccine also should be given (Fanaroff & Martin, 1997). The second dose of vaccine is given at 1 month and the third dose at 6 months. The vaccine should protect the child for up to 9 years. After the infant has been cleansed thoroughly and has received the vaccine, breastfeeding may be initiated. Vaccination for infants not exposed to HBV is recommended before discharge; breastfeeding for these infants may begin before the vaccine is given.

Human immunodeficiency virus and acquired immunodeficiency syndrome

Although the transmission rate of HIV infections has been reported by some authors to be as high as 50% to 60% in infants born to mothers infected with HIV, most researchers cite a transmission rate of 20% to 35% (Bastin et al., 1992; Lindberg, 1995; Merenstein & Gardner, 1998). Pediatric acquired immunodeficiency syndrome (AIDS) accounts for 1.5% of reported AIDS cases in the United States, and 89% of these children are the offspring of HIV-infected mothers (Shannon, 1995). The incidence is likely to increase. The blood supply in the United States and Canada is now screened for HIV, thus decreasing the chance of transmission by this route. However, the number of women of childbearing age infected with HIV is increasing.

Transmission of HIV from the mother to the infant occurs transplacentally at various gestational ages, perinatally through maternal blood and secretions, and postnatally through breast milk (Fanaroff & Martin, 1997; Shannon, 1995).

Routine screening and counseling of all pregnant women have been a source of controversy but have been recommended by several groups, including the American Academy of Pediatrics (Frenkel & Gaur, 1994; Provisional Committee on Pediatric AIDS, 1995). This has become especially important in light of findings that indicate administration of zidovudine to HIV-infected pregnant women and their infants significantly reduces the perinatal transmission of HIV (Kline, 1996).

Diagnosis. Diagnosis of HIV infection in the neonate is problematic (Chadwick & Yogev, 1995). Pregnant women infected with HIV produce IgG antibodies, which cross the placenta to the fetus. Therefore cord blood is positive for antibody when tested by enzyme-linked immunosorbent assay (ELISA) or Western blot techniques. Because of their physiologically depressed immune response, infants generally produce a less vigorous and more limited antibody response to HIV infection.

Virtually every baby born to a mother who is seropositive for HIV will have HIV antibody at birth; however only 13% to 40% are actually infected (Connor & McSherry, 1994). Uninfected infants lose this maternal antibody during the first 8 to 15 months of life. Most infected infants begin to develop their own antibody and remain seropositive (Fanaroff & Martin, 1997). Many tests are used to diagnose HIV infection in infants and children, but improvements in sensitivity and reliability of tests are needed (Chadwick & Yoger, 1995; Lindberg, 1995). It may be possible to identify infected infants earlier (3 to 6 months) using a combination of tests, including viral cultures, polymerase chain reaction (PCR) and p24 antigen (Merenstein, Adams & Weisman, 1998).

Typically the HIV-infected neonate is asymptomatic at birth and bears no obvious physical signs. The occurrence of an opportunistic infection (caused by an organism that does not usually cause disease) in the neonate may alert the caregiver to the presence of HIV infection or assist in the confirmation of the diagnosis of HIV infection. The average age of onset for an opportunistic infection is 3 to 6 months of age (Provisional Committee on Pediatric AIDS, 1995). In pediatrics the presence of lymphoid interstitial pneumonitis is now considered a criterion for diagnosis (Fanaroff & Martin, 1997). During the first year of life the presence of failure to thrive, developmental delay and oral candidiasis (thrush) that does not respond to treatment with topical antifungal agents carries a high index of suspicion for HIV infection (Kline, 1996).

Before 1 year of age, infected infants usually manifest some symptoms similar to those seen in adults, including lymphadenopathy, hepatosplenomegaly, chronic diarrhea, interstitial pneumonitis, and persistent thrush. In addition, infants fail to thrive and have developmental delays, recurrent severe bacterial infections, and occasionally recurrent enlargement of the parotid glands. *Pneumocystis carinii* pneumonia (PCP) has occurred in 62% and Kaposi's sarcoma in 5% of affected infants. Viral infection caused by CMV and Epstein-Barr virus is commonly observed in children with AIDS. Bacterial sepsis also may be an initial manifestation (Fanaroff & Martin, 1997).

The average survival time between testing positive for HIV infection and death for infants is 9 months, with a 70% to 85% death rate by 2 years of age (Shannon, 1995). The disease progression has been slower and the mortality lower in infants with a later onset than with those diagnosed at birth.

Management. Although it is rare for an infant to be born with symptoms of HIV, all infants born to HIV-positive mothers should be presumed to be HIV positive. Management begins by implementing Standard Precautions and precautions for invasive procedures to prevent further transmission of HIV (Craven et al., 1994; Fanaroff & Martin, 1997). Measures should also be undertaken to protect the infant from further exposure to maternal blood and body fluids. The infant's skin should be cleansed with soap and water and alcohol before invasive procedures such as vitamin K administration or heel punctures. Umbilical cord stumps are cleaned meticulously every day until healing is complete. Isolation is not required, and the infant can usually be cared for in the normal nursery. The use of gloves is not required for care activities such as dressing or feeding the infant (Benson, 1994).

Therapy for the symptomatic infant includes antimicrobial medications specific for the infections encountered and corticosteroids in the presence of lymphoid interstitial pneumonitis. Prophylaxis for PCP should be administered according to the guidelines established by the U.S. Public Health Service (Centers for Disease Control and Prevention, 1998). Pediatric data are not available, but it has been recommended that asymptomatic infants receive zidovudine (ZDV; formerly Azidothymidine, AZT) according to their lymphocyte counts (Connor & McSherry, 1994).

Counseling regarding the care of the mothers themselves, the family's care of the infant, and future pregnancies challenges the caregiver. In industrialized countries it is generally recommended that mothers with HIV infections not breastfeed; however, the World Health Organization (WHO) does not discourage women with HIV in developing countries from breastfeeding although this advice may be changing.

Some parents opt to place the infected infants in foster homes despite the low risk for transmission among members of the same household. Social services are required in these cases. If the parent chooses to keep the infant, home health care is arranged. For more information and updated information, parents are offered the following resource: the National AIDS hotline, 1-800-342-AIDS.

The family must be counseled about vaccinations. Children with symptomatic or asymptomatic HIV infection should receive all routine vaccines except oral poliovirus vaccine. The family should be advised that household contacts should not receive oral polio vaccine because the virus can be transmitted to the immunocompromised child. Inactivated poliomyelitis vaccine can be given (Wong, 1995).

Rubella infection

Congenital rubella infection is a major concern. Since vaccination was begun in 1969, congenital rubella cases have been reduced drastically.

The risk of a congenitally infected infant varies with the gestational age of the fetus when maternal infection occurs. Anomalies are most severe if the mother contracts the virus during the first trimester.

More than two thirds of infected infants show no apparent involvement at birth, but consequences develop years later. Central and peripheral hearing defects, the most common result, appear to be progressive after birth. The major teratogenic effects of rubella involve the cardiovascular system (pulmonary artery hypoplasia, patent ductus arteriosus, and coarctation of the aortic isthmus) and cataract formation. Multiple other abnormalities typically occur, including intrauterine and postnatal growth restriction, thrombocytopenic purpura (Fig. 28-24), dermal erythropoiesis, interstitial pneumonia, bony radiolucencies, retinopathy, and hepatosplenomegaly. Severe infections may result in fetal death. Delayed effects of infection manifest as thyroid dysfunction, diabetes mellitus, growth hormone deficiency, and progressive rubella panencephalopathy (Fanaroff & Martin, 1997).

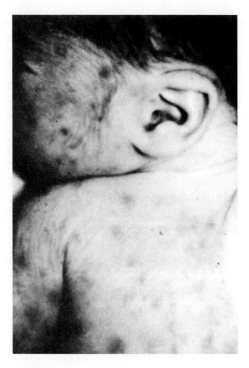

Fig. **28-24** Newborn with congenital rubella syndrome, showing multiple purpuric lesions over face and trunk. (Courtesy Donald C. Anderson, Baylor College of Medicine, Houston, Tex.)

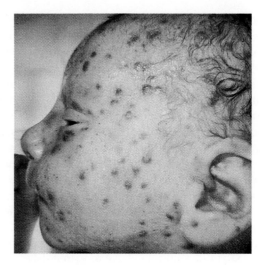

Fig. **28-25** Neonatal cytomegalovirus (CMV) infection. Typical rash seen in a severely affected infant. Note the small head size. (Courtesy David A. Clarke, Philadelphia.)

The rubella virus has been cultured in infants for up to 18 months after their birth. These infants are a serious source of infection to susceptible individuals, particularly women in the childbearing years. Extended pediatric isolation is mandatory until the noncontagious stage of rubella has been reached. (The infant should be isolated until pharyngeal mucus and urine are free of virus).

Cytomegalovirus infection

Cytomegalovirus infection (CMV) during pregnancy may result in abortion, stillbirth, or congenital or neonatal cytomegalic inclusion disease (CMID). It is the most common cause of congenital viral infections in humans, occurring in 1% of all newborns (Fanaroff & Martin, 1997). Most (90% to 95%) of the affected infants are asymptomatic at birth; however, hearing loss and learning disabilities have been reported in previously asymptomatic infants (Strodtbeck, 1995).

The neonate with classic, full-blown CMID displays IUGR and has microcephaly. The neonate also has a rash, jaundice, and hepatosplenomegaly (Fig. 28-25). Anemia, thrombocytopenia, and hyperbilirubinemia are to be expected. Intracranial, periventricular calcification often is noted on x-ray films. Inclusion bodies ("owl's eye" figures) in cells sedimented from freshly voided urine or in liver biopsy specimens are typical.

Elevated levels of cord blood IgM are suggestive of disease. The virus may be isolated from urine or saliva of the newborn. Differential diagnosis includes other causes of jaundice, syphilis (positive Venereal Disease Research Laboratory [VDRL] findings), toxoplasmosis (positive Sabin-Feldman dye test result), hemolytic disease of the newborn (positive Coombs' test reaction), or coxsackievirus infection (positive culture).

Despite the extensive, endemic nature of the disease in women and men and its potential for havoc in perinatal life, critically affected newborns are born only occasionally. Milder forms of the disease often may result when the fetus is affected late in pregnancy. CMV can be transmitted through breast milk while the mother is experiencing acute CMV syndrome. CMV infections acquired after birth are often asymptomatic and have no sequelae. Exceptions to this occur in preterm infants in whom postnatal acquisition of CMV can result in pneumonia, hepatitis, thrombocytopenia, and long-term neurologic sequelae.

Antenatally infected infants who are asymptomatic at birth are at risk for late sequelae. Hearing loss may not be apparent until after the first year of life. Chorioretinitis, microcephaly, mental retardation, and neuromuscular deficits may occur by 2 years of age. Some children are at risk for a defect in tooth enamel, resulting in severe caries.

Herpes simplex virus

Herpes simplex virus (HSV) infection among newborns is being diagnosed more frequently. HSV infection is estimated to occur in as many as 1 in 2,000 to 1 in 5,000 births (Fanaroff & Martin, 1997).

The neonate may acquire the virus by any of four modes of transmission:
- Transplacental infection
- Ascending infection by way of the birth canal

- Direct contamination during passage through an infected birth canal
- Direct transmission from infected personnel or family

Transplacental transmission of HSV infection to the neonate may occur during maternal viremia. However, an ascending transcervical infection first involves the intact fetal membranes, causing chorioamnionitis. This infection then is likely to be the cause of rupture of membranes rather than the sequela to their rupture. Ascending transcervical infection of intact membranes occurs in approximately 5% of HSV-infected neonates (Kohl, 1997). Transcervical infection can be accelerated by fetal monitoring scalp electrodes. The electrodes break the fetal skin barrier and increase the risk of infection; however, most infants show no evidence of infection in utero.

Congenital infection is rare and characterized by in utero destruction of normally formed organs. Affected infants are growth restricted. They have severe psychomotor restriction, with intracranial calcifications, microcephaly, hypertonicity, and seizures. They suffer eye involvement, including microphthalmos, cataracts, chorioretinitis, blindness, and retinal dysplasia. Some infants have patent ductus arteriosus, limb anomalies, and recurrent skin vesicles, with a short life expectancy.

Most infants are infected directly during passage through the birth canal. The risk of infection during vaginal birth in the presence of genital herpes has not been clearly delineated. It may be as high as 40% to 60%, with active primary infection at term. Primary maternal infections after 32 weeks of gestation carry a higher risk for the fetus and newborn than do recurrent infections (Fanaroff & Martin, 1997). The transmission rate of chronic vaginal herpes from the pregnant woman to her newborn is low, 5% or less (Cohen & Goldstein, 1996). Passive intrauterine immunity to herpes may be responsible.

Postnatal acquisition of the virus and spread within a nursery have been documented by DNA analysis. Both mother and father, as well as maternal breast lesions, have been implicated in neonatal infections. There also is concern regarding symptomatic and asymptomatic shedding among hospital personnel. Nursery personnel with cold sores should practice strict handwashing and follow hospital policy, but no evidence indicates that they should be removed from the nursery unless they have a herpetic whitlow (primary HSV infection of the terminal segment of a finger) (Fanaroff & Martin, 1997).

Clinically, neonatal HSV infections are classified as disseminated infection, encephalitis, or localized infection of the skin, eye, or mouth.

Disseminated infections may involve virtually every organ system, but the liver, adrenal glands, and lungs are primarily involved. Affected infants exhibit initial symptoms usually in the first week of life but sometimes in the second week, with signs of bacterial sepsis or shock. Clinical manifestations include skin vesicles in approximately 50% of

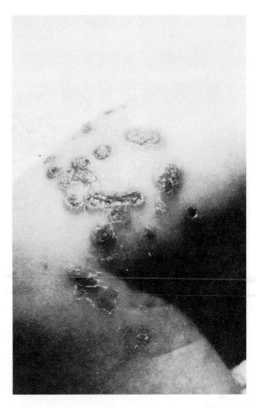

Fig. 28-26 Neonatal herpes simplex virus (HSV) skin infection. (From Fanaroff A & Martin R: *Neonatal-perinatal medicine: diseases of the fetus and infant,* ed 5, St Louis, 1995, Mosby.)

infants (Fig. 28-26). Death results from progression of CNS involvement, respiratory distress and pneumonitis, shock, DIC, and bleeding. Overall, the mortality without antiviral therapy is 82%.

Encephalitis may occur as a component of disseminated disease. Blood-borne seeding of the brain results in multiple lesions of cortical hemorrhagic necrosis. It also can occur alone or in association with oral, eye, or skin lesions. In the second to fourth week of life, brain involvement usually manifests. Only 60% of the infants have skin lesions, and the CSF of fewer than 50% will reveal the virus. Lethargy, poor feeding, irritability, and local or generalized seizures may be the presenting manifestations. Almost half the infants die of neurologic deterioration as late as 6 months after onset, and virtually all survivors have severe sequelae, including microcephaly and blindness (Fanaroff & Martin, 1997).

Localized HSV infections most often occur with skin findings or rarely with isolated oral cavity lesions (Fig. 28-27). CNS or disseminated disease will develop in 70% of the infants with skin vesicles. Ocular involvement, which can occur alone, may be secondary to either HSV-1 or HSV-2. Ocular disease may not be discovered for months. Microphthalmos, cataracts, optic atrophy, and corneal scarring may result from chorioretinitis, keratitis, and retinal hemorrhage (Fanaroff & Martin, 1997).

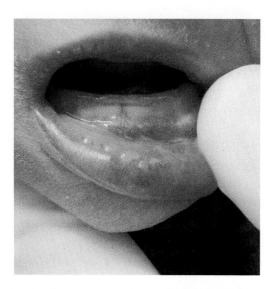

Fig. **28-27** Neonatal HSV oral lesions. (Courtesy David A. Clarke, Philadelphia.)

Management. Gloves should be worn when caregivers are in contact with these infants. The neonate's eyes, oral cavity, and skin are inspected carefully for the presence of any lesions. Cultures are obtained from the mouth, the eyes, and any possible lesions. Circumcision, if performed, is delayed until the infant is ready to be discharged. The infant may be discharged with the mother if the infant's cultures are negative for the virus. As long as no suspicious lesions are on the mother's breasts, breastfeeding is allowed. For the infant at risk, prophylactic topical eye ointment (vidarabine) is administered for 5 days for prevention of keratoconjunctivitis. No current recommendations exist for prophylactic systemic therapy; each case should be considered individually. Blood, urine, and CSF specimens should be cultured when indicated clinically. If herpetic lesions first occur after 6 weeks of life, the risk of dissemination and severe illness is very low (Fanaroff & Martin, 1997).

Therapy includes general supportive measures, as well as treatment with vidarabine or acyclovir. Acyclovir is the most frequently used drug. It is considered safe because only viral replication is inhibited, although long-term sequelae are not yet known. Acyclovir is easier to administer and is more effective than vidarabine for herpes encephalitis. The current recommended dose of acyclovir is 10 mg/kg/day intravenously every 8 hours for at least 14 days. Continuing therapy may be required in case of recurrence. Ophthalmic ointment should be administered simultaneously (Fanaroff & Martin, 1997).

Bacterial Infections

Group B streptococcus

The most common cause of neonatal sepsis and meningitis in the United States is the group B streptococcus (GBS) (Greatrex, 1997). Early-onset GBS infection in the neonate most often presents within 24 hours of birth and is most common in premature infants (Lott et al., 1994). Transplacental or vertical transmission to the fetus results in a respiratory illness that initially mimics the symptoms of severe respiratory distress. The infant rapidly deteriorates and often develops septic shock, which has a mortality rate of 30% to 50% (Fuller, 1992). Risk factors for GBS infection include preterm birth, maternal chorioamnionitis, and rupture of membranes longer than 18 hours before birth (Baker, 1997).

Late-onset GBS infection presents between 1 week and 3 months of age with an average age of onset of 24 days. Eighty-five percent of infants with late-onset GBS have meningitis, which has a mortality rate of 25% (Fuller, 1992).

If the mother is positive for GBS and is treated with antibiotics during labor, the infant is usually not treated. If the mother is not given antibiotics or her GBS status is unknown, the infant may be observed for 48 hours and a CBC may be done. Antibiotic therapy is usually not given unless the infant is symptomatic; however, there is no set procedure (Alkalay et al., 1996).

Escherichia coli

Escherichia. coli is the second most common cause of neonatal sepsis and meningitis in the United States. *E. coli* is found in the gastrointestinal tract soon after birth and makes up the bulk of human fecal flora. In addition to meningitis, *E. coli* can also cause infections in other body systems, including the urinary tract.

Tuberculosis

The incidence of tuberculosis (TB), caused by *Mycobacterium tuberculosis,* is increasing in Canada and the United States. Congenitally acquired TB can present with otitis media, pneumonia, hepatosplenomegaly, enlarged lymph glands, or abdominal distention (Starke, 1997). After birth, exposed infants contract TB through droplets expelled by infected individuals, which results in pneumonia and necrosis of lung tissue. Treatment is with antituberculosis drugs. Untreated TB of the neonate is almost always fatal (Smith & Teele, 1995).

Listeriosis

Neonatal infection is the most common clinical form of listeriosis in humans. Meconium-stained fluid is a common feature; pneumonia is also common. A granulomatous rash occurs in severe cases. Listeriosis can also present as meningitis in a late-onset infection. Ampicillin is the preferred treatment in combination with an aminoglycoside (Bortolussi & Schlech, 1995).

Chlamydia infection

Chlamydia trachomatis is an intracellular bacterium that causes neonatal conjunctivitis and pneumonia. The conjunctivitis (congestion and edema), with minimal discharge, develops 5 days to 2 weeks after birth. Inclusion conjunctivitis is usually self-limiting, but if untreated, chronic follicular conjunctivitis, with conjunctival scarring and corneal neovascularization, has been reported (Hess, 1993).

The neonate also is treated with oral erythromycin for 2 to 3 weeks. Silver nitrate is not effective against *C. trachomatis*, but erythromycin or tetracycline ointment may prevent ophthalmic infection (Fanaroff & Martin, 1997). Eye prophylaxis is not sufficient to prevent the development of chlamydial pneumonia; therefore infants at risk should also be treated with systemic antibiotics such as oral erythromycin syrup.

Fungal Infections

Candidiasis

Candida infections, formerly known as moniliasis, may occur in the newborn. *Candida albicans,* the organism usually responsible, may cause disease in any organ system. It is a yeastlike fungus (producing yeast cells and spores) that can be acquired from a maternal vaginal infection during birth, by person-to-person transmission, or from contaminated hands, bottles, nipples, or other articles. It usually is a benign disorder in the neonate, often confined to the oral and diaper regions (Wong, 1995).

Candidal diaper dermatitis appears on the perianal area, inguinal folds, and lower portion of the abdomen. The affected area is intensely erythematous, with a sharply demarcated, scalloped edge, frequently with numerous satellite lesions that extend beyond the larger lesion. The source of the infection is through the gastrointestinal tract. Treatment is with applications of an anticandidal ointment, such as nystatin (Mycostatin) or miconazole 2% (Monistat), with each diaper change. The infant also may be given an oral antifungal preparation to eliminate any gastrointestinal source of infection (Wong, 1995).

Oral candidiasis (**thrush,** or mycotic stomatitis) is characterized by the appearance of white plaques on the oral mucosa, gums, and tongue. The white patches are easily differentiated from milk curds; the patches cannot be removed and tend to bleed when touched. In most cases the infant does not seem to be in discomfort from the infection. A few infants seem to have some difficulty swallowing.

Infants who are sick, debilitated, or receiving antibiotic therapy are more susceptible to thrush. Those with conditions such as cleft lip or palate, neoplasms, and hyperparathyroidism seem to be more vulnerable to mycotic infection.

The objectives of management are to eradicate the causative organism, to control exposure to *C. albicans,* and to improve the infant's resistance. Interventions include maintenance of scrupulous cleanliness to prevent reinfection (nursing personnel, parents, others). Good handwashing technique is always essential. Clean surfaces should be provided for neonates. Proper cleanliness of the equipment and environment is ensured. If the infant is breastfeeding, the mother's breasts are treated with topical nystatin.

Medications are administered as ordered. Nystatin is instilled into the newborn's mouth with a medicine dropper after the infant is given sterile water to wash out any residual milk. Nystatin also may be swabbed over mucosa, gums, or tongue. Less frequently, an aqueous solution of gentian violet (1% to 2%) is applied with a swab to oral mucosa, gums, and tongue. The nurse should guard against staining the skin, clothes, and equipment and should inform parents about the purple staining of the baby's mouth.

INFANTS OF SUBSTANCE-ABUSING MOTHERS

Certain maternal behaviors result in perinatal risk. Maternal habits hazardous to the fetus and neonate include drug addiction, smoking, and alcohol abuse. Occasional withdrawal reactions have been reported in neonates of mothers who use to excess such drugs as barbiturates, alcohol, or amphetamines. Serious reactions are seen in neonates whose mothers abuse psychoactive drugs or are treated with methadone. Almost 50% of pregnancies of women addicted to opioids result in LBW infants who are not necessarily preterm. Alcohol is a teratogen. Maternal ethanol abuse during gestation creates a readily identifiable fetal alcohol syndrome.

The adverse effects of exposure of the fetus to drugs are varied. They include transient behavioral changes such as fetal breathing movements or irreversible effects such as IUGR, structural malformations, or mental retardation or fetal death. Critical determinants of the effect of the drug on the fetus include the specific drug, the dosage, the route of administration, the genotype of the mother or fetus, and the timing of the drug exposure. Fig. 28-28 shows critical periods of human embryogenesis and the teratogenic effects of drugs. Table 28-5 summarizes the effects of commonly abused substances on the fetus and neonate.

Alcohol

Documentation of the **fetal alcohol syndrome (FAS)** can be found in the literature since the early part of the eighteenth century. The incidence of FAS in the United States is approximately 2 per 10,000 live births (Centers for Disease Control and Prevention, 1993).

FAS is based on a minimum criteria of signs in each of three categories: prenatal and postnatal growth restriction; CNS malfunctions, including mental retardation; and facial features such as microcephaly, small eyes or short palpebral fissures, and a thin upper lip (Bartram, Joffe & Perry, 1988). Infants exposed prenatally to alcohol who are affected but do not meet the criteria for FAS may be said to have **fetal alcohol effects (FAEs)** or alcohol-related birth defects (ARBDs) (Coles, 1993). These effects run the gamut from learning disabilities and behavioral problems to speech or language problems and hyperactivity. Often these problems are not detected until the child goes to school and learning

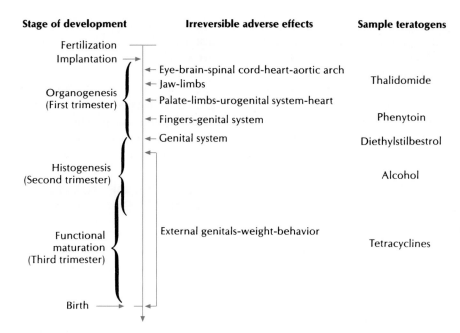

Stage of development   **Irreversible adverse effects**   **Sample teratogens**

Fig. **28-28** Critical periods in human embryogenesis. (From Fanaroff A & Martin R: *Neonatal-perinatal medicine: diseases of the fetus and infant,* ed 6, St Louis, 1997, Mosby.)

TABLE 28-5   *Summary of Neonatal Effects of Commonly Abused Substances*

SUBSTANCE	NEONATAL EFFECTS
Alcohol	*Fetal alcohol syndrome* (FAS): craniofacial anomalies, including short eyelid opening, flat midface, flat upper lip groove, thin upper lip; microcephaly, hyperactivity, developmental delays, attention deficits *Fetal alcohol effects:* milder forms of FAS; cardiac anomalies
Cocaine	Prematurity, small for gestational age, microcephaly, poor feeding, irregular sleep pattern, diarrhea, visual attention problems, hyperactivity, difficult to console, hypersensitivity to noise and external stimuli, irritability, developmental delays, congenital anomalies such as prune belly syndrome (distended, flabby, wrinkled abdomen caused by lack of abdominal muscles)
Heroin	Low birth weight, small for gestational age, neonatal abstinence syndrome (see Table 28-7)
Amphetamines	Small for gestational age, prematurity, poor weight gain, lethargy
Tobacco	Prematurity, low birth weight, increased risk for sudden infant death syndrome, increased risk for bronchitis, pneumonia, developmental delays
Marijuana	Possible neonatal tremors, possible low birth weight

---

problems become evident. FAEs can be seen with other disorders, such as fetal hydantoin syndrome; therefore a careful history is needed.

Predictable abnormal patterns of fetal and neonatal morphogenesis are attributed to severe, chronic alcoholism in women who continue to drink heavily during pregnancy. The pattern of growth deficiency begun in prenatal life persists after birth, especially in the linear growth rate, rate of weight gain, and growth of head circumferences.

Ocular structural anomalies are common findings (Fig. 28-29). Limb anomalies and a variety of cardiocirculatory anomalies, especially ventricular septal defects, pose problems for the child. Table 28-6 outlines physical findings in FAS. Mental retardation (IQ of 79 or below at 7 years of age), hyperactivity and fine motor dysfunction (poor hand-to-mouth coordination, weak grasp) add to the handicapping problems that maternal alcoholism can impose. Genital abnormalities are seen in daughters of alcohol-addicted mothers. Two thirds of newborns with FAS are girls; the cause of this altered fetal sex ratio is unknown. Severe and chronic alcoholism (ethanol toxicity), not maternal malnutrition is responsible for the severity and consistency

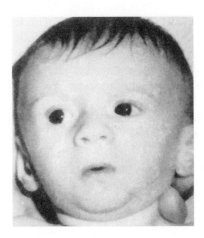

Fig. 28-29 Fetal alcohol anomaly. (Courtesy Dr. Charles Linder, Medical College of Georgia. From Goodman R & Gorlin R: *Atlas of the face in genetic disorders*, ed 2, St Louis, 1977, Mosby.)

TABLE 28-6	*Features of Fetal Alcohol Syndrome (FAS)*

AFFECTED PART	CHARACTERISTICS
Eyes	Epicanthal folds, strabismus, ptosis, hypoplastic retinal vessels
Mouth	Poor suck, cleft lip, cleft palate, small teeth
Ears	Deafness
Skeleton	Radioulnar synostosis, fusion of cervical vertebrae, restricted bone growth
Heart	Atrial and ventricular septal defects, tetralogy of Fallot, patent ductus arteriosus
Kidney	Renal hypoplasia, hydronephrosis, urogenital sinus
Liver	Extrahepatic biliary atresia, hepatic fibrosis
Immune system	Increased infections: otitis media, upper respiratory infections, immune deficiencies
Tumors	Nonspecific neoplasms
Skin	Abnormal palmar creases, irregular hair, whorls

From Weiner L & Morse B: FAS: clinical perspectives and prevention. In Chasnoff I, editor: *Drugs, alcohol, pregnancy and parenting,* Boston, 1991, Kluwer Academic Publishers.

of postnatal performance problems (Fanaroff & Martin, 1997). High alcohol levels are lethal to the developing embryo. Lower levels cause brain and other malformations. Long-term prognosis (no studies are available as yet) is discouraging even in an optimum psychosocial environment, when one considers the combination of growth failure and mental retardation.

Alcohol effects, however, depend not only on the amount of alcohol consumed but also on the interaction of quantity, frequency, type of alcohol, and other drug abuse. Other drugs, such as cigarettes, caffeine, and marijuana, may potentiate the fetal effects of alcohol consumption during gestation (Fanaroff & Martin, 1997).

The infant of a mother who abuses alcohol is faced with many clinical problems. Identification of the problems leads to the medical diagnosis of FAS. The infant may suffer respiratory distress related to preterm birth, neurologic damage, and a "floppy" epiglottis and small trachea. Tracheoepiglottal anomalies may cause cardiopulmonary arrest. Other disorders include recurrent otitis media and hearing loss. Craniofacial features may be important in diagnosing craniofacial and oral anomalies, dental development abnormalities, and long-term body growth patterns (Lewis & Woods, 1994). Feeding difficulties are related to preterm birth, poor sucking ability, and possible cleft palate. The infant may exhibit brain dysfunction, microcephaly, and grand mal seizures.

Long-term effects into childhood may include poor attention span; disciplinary problems; autism; learning disabilities; and motor, mental, and social delays (Bell & Lau, 1995). FAS is now recognized as one of the leading causes of mental retardation in the United States. Although the distinctive facial features of the infant tend to become less evident, the mental capacities never become normal (Budd, 1995).

Nursing care involves many of the same strategies used for the care of preterm infants (see Chapter 27). Special efforts are made to involve the parents in their child's care and to encourage opportunities for parent-child attachment.

Infants placed in a warm, caring environment with understanding caregivers who can deal with the infant's hyperirritability can be helped to lead a more normal existence than their condition might warrant. These caregivers provide human contact and can deal with the eating problems that typically lead to a diagnosis of failure to thrive. However, these infants may not go home to such an environment. Often the family is dysfunctional.

Heroin

Heroin crosses the placenta and frequently results in IUGR. Heroin may have a direct growth-inhibiting effect on the fetus, but the exact mechanisms of growth inhibition are not clear. There is an increased rate of stillbirths but not of congenital anomalies. Most medical complications attributed to heroin ingestion result from prematurity (Finnegan, 1991).

Maternal detoxification in the first trimester carries an increased risk of spontaneous abortion. Detoxification is not recommended after the thirty-second week because of possible withdrawal-induced fetal distress (Glantz & Woods, 1993).

Heroin withdrawal occurs in 50% to 75% of infants born to addicted mothers, usually within the first 24 to 48 hours of life. The signs depend on the length of maternal addiction, the amount of drug taken, and the time of injection before birth. The infant whose mother is taking methadone may not demonstrate signs of withdrawal until a week or so after birth. The symptoms of infants whose mothers used heroin or methadone are similar in nature. Initially the infant may be depressed. The withdrawal syndrome may manifest as a combination of any of the following signs. The infant may be jittery and hyperactive. Usually the infant's cry is shrill and persistent. The infant may yawn or sneeze frequently. The tendon reflexes are increased, but Moro's reflex is decreased. The neonate may exhibit poor feeding and sucking, tachypnea, vomiting, diarrhea, hypothermia or hyperthermia, and sweating. In addition, an abnormal sleep cycle, with absence of quiet sleep and disturbance of active sleep, has been described in these infants (Fanaroff & Martin, 1997).

If withdrawal is not treated, vomiting, diarrhea, dehydration, apnea, and convulsions may develop. Death may follow. Therapy is individualized. Dehydration and electrolyte imbalance are prevented or treated. Usually one of the following drugs is ordered: phenobarbital, paregoric (compound tincture of opium), or diazepam, singly or in combination.

NURSE ALERT *The use of naloxone (Narcan) is contraindicated in infants born to narcotic addicts because it may cause severe signs and symptoms of narcotic abstinence syndrome and seizures.*

The long-term effect on these infants is now being studied. The risk of sudden infant death syndrome (SIDS) is 5 to 10 times higher for infants with significant withdrawal problems than for infants in the general population.

Methadone

Methadone, a synthetic opiate, has been the therapy of choice for heroin addiction since 1965. It does cross the placenta. An increasing number of infants have been born to methadone-maintained mothers, who seem to have better prenatal care and a somewhat better lifestyle than those taking heroin (Fanaroff & Martin, 1997).

Some question exists concerning the benefits of methadone therapy during pregnancy because of its effect on the fetus. In one study (Levine & Rebarber, 1995), nonstress tests performed on women receiving methadone were found to be significantly less reactive than nonstress tests reported in the general population of pregnant women. These findings question the benefits of methadone treatment for pregnant heroin abusers and the related ethical issues. Methadone withdrawal occurs in approximately 80% to 95% of infants born to these women.

Methadone withdrawal resembles heroin withdrawal but tends to be more severe and prolonged. In addition, the incidence of seizures is higher. Seizures usually occur between days 7 and 10. The infants exhibit a disturbed sleep pattern similar to that seen in heroin withdrawal. The infants have a higher birth weight than that in heroin withdrawal, usually appropriate for gestational age. No increased incidence of congenital anomalies is seen.

Late-onset withdrawal occurs at 2 to 4 weeks and may continue for weeks or months. A higher incidence of SIDS also has been reported in these infants. This factor is important for perinatal nurses who coordinate follow-up care for the infant and education for the mother or other caregiver. Community health nurses need to know about the potential for withdrawal symptoms to occur.

Therapy for methadone withdrawal is similar to that for heroin withdrawal. The few available follow-up studies of these infants reveal a high incidence of hyperactivity, learning and behavior disorders, and poor social adjustment (Fanaroff & Martin, 1997).

Marijuana

Marijuana crosses the placenta. Its use during pregnancy may result in a shortened gestation and a higher incidence of IUGR (Day, Cottreau & Richardson, 1993). Some investigators have found a higher incidence of meconium staining (Fanaroff & Martin, 1997). Some association has been reported between the use of marijuana and a decrease in infant birth weight and length and the occurrence of congenital anomalies; however, the findings have been inconsistent (Zuckerman, 1991). A longitudinal study by Fried (1993) followed infants of marijuana users for 2 years and found no association between marijuana use and cognitive abilities at 12, 24, or 36 months but at 48 months found memory and verbal measures of cognitive ability affected in the infants of heavy marijuana users. Compounding the issue of the effects of marijuana is multidrug use, especially among adolescents, thus combining the harmful effects of marijuana, tobacco, alcohol, and cocaine. Long-term follow-up studies on exposed infants are needed.

Cocaine

Cocaine crosses the placenta and is found in breast milk. Antenatal effects of maternal cocaine ingestion are not common but include infarctions to developing organs, resulting in defects such as hydronephrosis, hypospadias, prune belly syndrome (distended flabby abdomen and renal anomalies), congenital heart disease, skull defects, ileal atresia, and limb reduction. Infants born to cocaine-abusing mothers show a high rate of perinatal morbidity, IUGR, preterm birth, and cerebral hemorrhage or infarction and are at risk for intellectual and developmental problems (Bell & Lau, 1995; Fanaroff & Martin, 1997).

Cocaine-dependent neonates do not experience a process of withdrawal seen in narcotic-exposed infants but rather suffer from neurotoxic effects of the drug. Signs of exposure have some of the same characteristics as heroin withdrawal but can be quite varied. There may be an increased risk for SIDS (Mays et al., 1996). Box 28-2 summarizes neonatal effects of maternal cocaine use.

Phencyclidine

Phencyclidine (PCP) (Angel Dust) increases the risk of injury to the pregnant woman and therefore also to her passively dependent fetus. The user may be unaware that

BOX 28-2	*Neonatal Effects of Maternal Cocaine Use*

PHYSICAL	BEHAVIORAL
Preterm birth	Irritability
Decreased length	Tremors
Decreased head circumference	Poor feeding
	Abnormal sleep patterns
Intrauterine growth restriction	Increased startles
	Disorganized behavior
Ileal atresia	Lability
Prune belly syndrome	Poor visual processing
Cryptorchidism	Difficult to console
Hypospadias	
Hydronephrosis	
Seizures	
Fever	
Congenital heart disease	
Skull defects	
Hypertension	
Cerebral infarction	
Vomiting	
Diarrhea	
SIDS	
Tachypnea	

she is ingesting PCP because it frequently is misrepresented as another drug of abuse or mixed with other drugs (Carroll, 1990).

PCP crosses the placenta and is found in breast milk. Literature about the effects on infants is limited. The infants exposed to PCP may exhibit abnormal motor behavior such as irritability, jitteriness, and hypertonicity (Glantz & Woods, 1993).

Miscellaneous Substances

The fetal and neonatal effects of maternal use of methamphetamines in pregnancy are not well known. The effects appear to be dose related. LBW, preterm birth, and perinatal mortality may be consequences of higher doses used throughout pregnancy. Infants may be drowsy and jittery and hypertonic with a high pitched cry and poor feeding (Bell & Lau, 1995). Lethargy may continue for several months, along with frequent infections and poor weight gain. Emotional disturbances and delays in gross and fine motor coordination may be seen during early childhood.

Phenobarbital crosses the placenta readily and is subsequently found in high levels in the fetal liver and brain. Because of its slow metabolic rate, when withdrawal does occur, onset is generally at 2 to 14 days after birth and duration is approximately 2 to 4 months. Irritability, crying, hiccoughs, and sleepiness mark the initial response. During the second stage the infant is extremely hungry, regurgitates and gags frequently, and demonstrates episodic irritability, sweating, and a disturbed sleep pattern.

Treatment consists of swaddling, frequent feedings, and protection from noxious external stimuli. If no improvement occurs, the neonate should be given phenobarbital and then slowly withdrawn from this drug after control of symptoms (Fanaroff & Martin, 1997).

Caffeine has not been implicated as a teratogen in humans. Fenster, Eskenazi, and Windham (1991) reported that caffeine consumption of greater than 300 mg a day was associated with IUGR and LBW. Mills, Holmes, and Aarons (1993) reported no adverse effects in the fetus with consumption of less than 300 mg of caffeine a day.

Tobacco

Cigarette smoking in pregnancy has been found to be associated with birth weight deficits of up to 250 gm for a full-term neonate (Fanaroff & Martin, 1997). Maternal cigarette smoking is implicated in 21% to 39% of LBW infants. Passive exposure to second-hand smoke by a pregnant woman may also result in the birth of an LBW infant. Also, if pregnant smokers drink five or more cups of coffee and one or more drinks of alcohol per day, the risk of IUGR is increased considerably (Fried, 1993).

The rate of spontaneous abortion and preterm birth is increased in the smoking population. When other variables have been controlled for, no association has been found between maternal smoking and congenital anomalies (Fried, 1993). Nicotine and cotinine, the two pharmacologically active substances in tobacco, are found in higher concentrations in infants whose mothers smoke. These substances can be secreted in breast milk for up to 2 hours after the mother has smoked. Cigarette smoke contains more than 2,000 compounds, including carbon monoxide, dioxin, cyanide, and cadmium. Long-term studies show residual effects beyond the neonatal period (Floyd et al., 1993). Deficits in growth, in intellectual and emotional development, and in behavior have been documented. These include poor auditory responsiveness, increased fine motor tremors, hypertonicity, and decreased verbal comprehension.

Pregnant women need to be aware of the harmful effects of smoking on their unborn baby's health. These include IUGR, spontaneous abortions, PROM, placenta previa, and SIDS (Blair, 1996). Increasing concern surrounds second-hand smoke and its potential effects on infants and siblings. Mothers and all others need to refrain from smoking near the infant. It is not clear whether the association between SIDS and maternal smoking reflects in utero exposure or passive exposure postnatally, or both.

I CARE MANAGEMENT

Assessment of the newborn requires a review of the mothers prenatal record. A medical and social history of drug abuse and detoxification is noted. The infant may have IUGR or be preterm with LBW.

The woman who is addicted to narcotics may have infections that compound the risk to the infant, including hepatitis, septicemia, and STDs, including AIDS.

The nurse often is the first to observe the signs of drug dependence in the infant. The nurse's observations help the physician differentiate between drug dependence and other conditions, such as tracheoesophageal fistula, CNS disorder, sepsis, hypoglycemia, and electrolyte imbalance.

The infant is assessed by means of the guidelines discussed in Chapter 20. The infant's gestational age and maturity are noted. In utero exposure to some drugs results in observable malformations or dysmorphism (abnormality of shape). Neonatal behavior may arouse suspicion. **Neonatal abstinence syndrome** is the term given to the group of signs and symptoms associated with drug withdrawal in the neonate (Table 28-7). Fig. 28-30 provides an example of a scoring system for assessing withdrawal symptoms. Because many women are multidrug users, the newborn initially may exhibit a confusing complex of signs.

Urine or meconium screening may be used to identify substances abused by the mother. Initially costly and of limited availability, tests of meconium collected on day 1 or 2 of life have been shown to be both sensitive and reliable in detecting the metabolites of several street drugs, including cocaine (Bibb et al., 1995) (Box 28-3).

Nursing diagnoses, which depend on the assessment findings, are tailored to the individual needs of the neonate and the family. Examples of nursing diagnoses are listed in the accompanying box.

Nursing Diagnoses

Infants of Substance-Abusing Mothers

Neonate

Risk for infection related to:
- Maternal risk behaviors
- PROM

Altered growth and development related to:
- Effects of maternal substance abuse

Sleep pattern disturbance related to:
- Drug withdrawal

Disorganized infant behavior related to:
- Effects of maternal substance abuse

Parents

Altered parenting related to:
- Continuation of substance abuse or detoxification program
- Guilt about infant's condition
- Inability to cope with care needs of a special infant

Anxiety related to knowledge deficit regarding:
- Care needs of an affected infant

Violence: self-directed or directed toward infant related to:
- Drug-dependent lifestyle

TABLE 28-7	*Signs of Neonatal Abstinence Syndrome*
SYSTEM	**SIGNS**
Gastrointestinal	Poor feeding, vomiting, regurgitation, diarrhea, excessive sucking
Central nervous	Irritability, tremors, shrill crying, incessant crying, hyperactivity, little sleep, excoriations on knees and face, convulsions
Metabolic, vasomotor, respiratory	Nasal congestion, tachypnea, sweating, frequent yawning, increased respiratory rate >60/min, fever >37.2° C

BOX 28-3	*Neonatal Drug Screening: Ethical Consideration*

Testing of neonatal urine or meconium for the presence of drug metabolites is a sensitive and reliable means of identifying neonates at risk for withdrawal symptoms. Controversy arises over whether universal drug screening should be instituted and whether informed consent is needed for screening neonates. Ethical issues include the cost versus benefit of universal testing and the rights of parents versus the medical need to diagnose withdrawal.

Nursing care

Planning for care of the infant born to a substance-abusing mother presents a challenge to the health care team. Parents are included in the planning for the newborn's care and also are encouraged to plan for their own care. A multidisciplinary approach is needed that includes home health or community resource personnel (e.g., regulatory agencies such as child protective services).

Education and social support to prevent the abuse of drugs provide the ideal approach. However, given the scope of the drug abuse problem, total prevention is unrealistic.

Nursing care of the drug-dependent neonate involves supportive therapy for fluid and electrolyte balance, nutrition, infection control, and respiratory care. Swaddling, holding, reducing stimuli, and feeding as necessary may be helpful in easing withdrawal (Plan of Care). Specific suggestions for providing care to infants experiencing withdrawal are listed in Box 28-4.

Pharmacologic treatment is usually based on the severity of withdrawal symptoms, as determined by an assessment tool such as the one shown in Fig. 28-30. When indicated, medications are given as ordered. Common medications to control symptoms are phenobarbital and paregoric.

Drug dependence in the neonate is physiologic, not psychologic. Thus a predisposition to dependence later in life is not believed to exist. However, the psychosocial

NEONATAL ABSTINENCE SCORING SYSTEM

SYSTEM	SIGNS AND SYMPTOMS	SCORE	AM				PM						COMMENTS
CENTRAL NERVOUS SYSTEM DISTURBANCES	Excessive High Pitched (Or Other) Cry	2											Daily Weight:
	Continuous High Pitched (Or Other) Cry	3											
	Sleeps < 1 Hour After Feeding	3											
	Sleeps < 2 Hours After Feeding	2											
	Sleeps < 3 Hours After Feeding	1											
	Hyperactive Moro's Reflex	2											
	Markedly Hyperactive Moro's Reflex	3											
	Mild Tremors Disturbed	1											
	Moderate-Severe Tremors Disturbed	2											
	Mild Tremors Undisturbed	3											
	Moderate-Severe Tremors Undisturbed	4											
	Increased Muscle Tone	2											
	Excoriation (Specific Area)	1											
	Myoclonic Jerks	3											
	Generalized Convulsions	5											
METABOLIC/VASOMOTOR/RESPIRATORY DISTURBANCES	Sweating	1											
	Fever <101°F (99-100.8°F./37.2-38.2°C.)	1											
	Fever >101°F (38.4°C. and Higher)	2											
	Frequent Yawning (> 3-4 Times/Interval)	1											
	Mottling	1											
	Nasal Stuffiness	1											
	Sneezing (> 3-4 Times/Interval)	1											
	Nasal Flaring	2											
	Respiratory Rate > 60/min	1											
	Respiratory Rate > 60/min with Retractions	2											
GASTROINTESTINAL DISTURBANCES	Excessive Sucking	1											
	Poor Feeding	2											
	Regurgitation	2											
	Projectile Vomiting	3											
	Loose Stools	2											
	Watery Stools	3											
	TOTAL SCORE												
	INITIALS OF SCORER												

Fig. **28-30** Neonatal Abstinence Scoring (NAS) System, developed by L. Finnegan. (From Nelson N: *Current therapy in neonatal-perinatal medicine,* ed 2, St Louis, 1990, Mosby.)

PLAN OF CARE *Infant Undergoing Drug Withdrawal*

NURSING DIAGNOSIS Risk for injury related to hyperactivity, seizures secondary to passive narcotic addiction resulting from maternal substance abuse during pregnancy

Expected Outcome *Infant exhibits no signs of seizure activity.*

Nursing Interventions/*Rationales*

Administer phenobarbital, diazepam per physician order *to decrease CNS irritability and control seizure activity.*

Decrease environmental stimuli *that may trigger irritability and hyperactive behaviors.*

Plan care activities carefully *to allow for minimum stimulation.*

Wrap infant snugly and hold infant tightly *to reduce self-stimulation behaviors and protect skin from abrasions.*

If infant is cocaine addicted, position to avoid eye contact, swaddle infant, use vertical rocking techniques, use a pacifier *to counter poor organizational response to stimuli and depressed interactive behaviors.*

Monitor activity level, note the relationship between activity level and external stimulation, and stop external stimulation *if it causes activity increase.*

NURSING DIAGNOSIS Altered nutrition, less than body requirements related to CNS irritability, poor suck reflex, vomiting, and diarrhea

Expected Outcome *Infant exhibits ingestion and retention of adequate nutrients and appropriate weight gain.*

Nursing Interventions/*Rationales*

Feed in frequent small amounts, elevate head during and after feeding, burp well *to diminish vomiting and aspiration.*

Experiment with various nipples *to find one most effective in compensating for poor suck reflex.*

Monitor weight daily and maintain strict intake and output *to evaluate success of feeding.*

If intake is insufficient, feed by oral gavage per physician order *to ensure ingestion of needed nutrients.*

Have suction available as required *to reduce chances of aspiration.*

NURSING DIAGNOSIS Risk for fluid volume deficit related to diarrhea and vomiting

Expected Outcome *Infant exhibits evidence of fluid homeostasis.*

Nursing Interventions/*Rationales*

Administer oral and parenteral fluids per physician order and regulate *to maintain fluid balance.*

Monitor hydration status (i.e., skin turgor, weight, mucous membranes, fontanels, urine specific gravity, electrolytes) and intake and output *to evaluate for evidence of dehydration.*

NURSING DIAGNOSIS Ineffective maternal coping, anxiety, powerlessness related to drug use, infant distress during withdrawal, and single-parent status

Expected Outcome *Woman will accept newborn's condition and participate in care activities, showing evidence of maternal-infant bonding process.*

Nursing Interventions/*Rationales*

Explain effects of maternal drug use on newborn and the withdrawal process *to provide understanding and reality concerning effects of drug use.*

Encourage open communication (i.e., inform mother of ongoing condition, procedures, and treatment; answer questions; correct misperceptions; actively listen to her concerns) *to provide a sense of respect, support, and encourage a sense of control.*

Encourage mother to interact with infant and to become involved in care routines *to foster emotional connection.*

Explain how to do care procedures, how to avoid excess stimulation, how to hold and rock infant *to enhance mother's care abilities and her sense of confidence and control.*

If the mother is addicted to cocaine, explain infant's inability to interact, gaze aversion, arching back, and lack of response to cuddling *to enhance understanding of infant behaviors.*

Make appropriate referrals to social agencies for treatment of maternal drug addiction, infant development programs, and other needed support services *to ensure adequate resources for care of self and infant.*

From Wong D & Perry S: *Maternal child nursing care,* St Louis, 1998, Mosby.

environment in which the infant may be raised may create a tendency to addiction.

The mother requires considerable support. Her need for and her abuse of drugs result in a decreased capacity to cope. The infant's withdrawal signs and decreased consolability stress her coping abilities even further. Home health

care, treatment for addiction, and education are important considerations. Sensitive exploration of the woman's options for the care of her infant and herself and for future fertility management may help her see that she has choices. This approach helps communicate respect for the new mother as a person who can make responsible decisions.

BOX 28-4 *Care of the Infant Experiencing Withdrawal*

- Place the infant in a side-lying position with the spine and legs flexed.
- Position the infant's hands in midline with the arms at the side.
- Carry the infant in a flexed position.
- When interacting with the infant, introduce one stimulus at a time when the infant is in a quiet, alert state. Watch for time-out or distress signals (gaze aversion, yawning, sneezing, hiccoughs, arching, mottled color).
- When the infant is distressed, swaddle in a flexed position and rock in a slow, rhythmic fashion.
- Put the infant in a sitting position with chin tucked down for feeding.

TABLE 28-8 *Drugs of Abuse Contraindicated during Breastfeeding**

DRUG	REPORTED EFFECT OR REASONS FOR CONCERN
Amphetamine[†]	Irritability, poor sleeping pattern
Cocaine	Cocaine intoxication
Heroin	Tremors, restlessness, vomiting, poor feeding
Marijuana	Only one report in literature; no effect mentioned; at risk for inhaling smoke
Nicotine (smoking)	Shock, vomiting, diarrhea, rapid heart rate, restlessness; decreased milk production
Phencyclidine	Potent hallucinogen

Modified from American Academy of Pediatrics Committee on Drugs: The transfer of drugs and other chemicals into human milk, *Pediatrics* 93(1):137, 1994; Lawrence R: *Breastfeeding,* ed 4, St Louis, 1994, Mosby.
*The Committee on Drugs strongly believes that nursing mothers should not ingest any compounds listed here. Not only are they hazardous to the unborn infant, but they are also detrimental to the physical and emotional health of the mother. This list is obviously not complete; no drug of abuse should be ingested by nursing mothers even though adverse reports are not in the literature.
[†]Drug is concentrated in human milk.

The issue of breastfeeding in this population is a difficult one. Although breast milk remains the optimum source of nutrition for these infants, care must be taken to avoid exposing the infant to additional drugs through the breast milk. The American Academy of Pediatrics has compiled a list of drugs contraindicated in breastfeeding (Table 28-8).

DISCHARGE PLANNING FOR THE HIGH RISK INFANT

Discharge planning for the high risk infant begins on admission. The admission history should include important information regarding the family of the infant that can affect discharge. Who makes up the immediate family? Does the mother have others who depend on her for support? How are they being taken care of during this period?

Questions about the home environment should be asked as soon as possible. Is there gas or electric heating in the home, or is the family dependent on a fireplace or wood-burning stove? Is there access to a telephone for emergencies? Is there a home at all, or is the family living in a shelter? Problems posed by answers to these questions require the intervention of social services and can take a long time to resolve.

Successful discharge of the high risk infants to their home or community hospital requires a multidisciplinary approach. Medical, nursing, and social services are crucial to the smooth transition of these infants and their families to the community and home. If the infant is transported back to the community hospital that referred either the mother before birth or the infant after birth, interfacility communication is essential to continuity of care.

Discharge to home, whether from the regional center or community hospital setting, requires parental competence. Discharge teaching begins as soon as the infant is stable and the parents wish to become involved in the care. Discharge teaching must include normal newborn care as well as

TEACHING GUIDELINES

Discharge Teaching for Parents of High Risk Infants

Discharge teaching includes (but is not limited to) the following:
- Helping parents understand their baby's condition
- Infant/child car safety
- Safety measures in the home
- Feeding
- Elimination
- Bathing
- Cord care
- Taking the baby's temperature
- Medication administration
- CPR for infants
- Impact of environmental factors (maintaining thermoregulation at home)
- Teaching related to the infant's specific condition (signs and symptoms of deterioration, etc.)
- Developmental concerns related to their infant
- Follow-up appointments/consultations

specific information pertinent to the medical condition of the infant. Discharge teaching is extensive, requires time, and cannot be adequately accomplished on the day of discharge. Important considerations in the discharge teaching of the parents of high risk infants are listed in the Teaching Guidelines box.

Discharge to home does not mean the infants can be treated like normal newborns. Follow-up by a pediatrician or nurse practitioner familiar with the complications common to the high risk newborn is essential. Further follow-up of specific complications by qualified specialists and referral to high-risk centers for developmental interventions can help ensure the best outcome possible for these fragile infants.

KEY POINTS

- Hyperbilirubinemia is caused by a variety of factors, including maternal-fetal Rh and ABO incompatibility.
- Erythroblastosis fetalis leads to anemia, edema, and the cytotoxic effects of unconjugated bilirubin.
- Perinatal events such as hypoxia and cold stress increase the infant's susceptibility to the neurotoxic effects of bilirubin.
- Major congenital defects are the leading cause of death in infants younger than 1 year of age in the United States and account for 20% of neonatal deaths.
- Hydramnios and oligohydramnios are associated with the occurrence of many congenital anomalies.
- The curative and rehabilitative problems of an infant with a congenital disorder are often complex and require a multidisciplinary approach to care.
- The supportive care given to the parents of infants with an abnormal condition must begin at birth or at the time of diagnosis and continue for years.
- A small percentage of significant birth injuries may occur despite skilled and competent obstetric care.
- Metabolic abnormalities of diabetes mellitus in pregnancy adversely affect embryonic and fetal development.
- Infection in the neonate may be acquired in utero, during birth, during resuscitation, and from within the nursery.
- The most common maternal infections during early pregnancy that are associated with various congenital malformations are represented by the acronym TORCH.
- HIV transmission from mother to infant occurs transplacentally at various gestational ages, perinatally by maternal blood and secretions, and by breast milk.
- Signs and symptoms of infant withdrawal vary in time of onset depending on the drug involved.

CRITICAL THINKING EXERCISES

1 *Discuss the ethical implications of routinely screening the urine of all infants for the presence of drug metabolites, including possible punitive measures taken against the mother.*

2 *Mary is HIV positive and has just given birth to Joshua. She is being discharged tomorrow and says she has no place to go. (She was living at the homeless shelter before she delivered.) In planning for Mary and Joshua's discharge, what community social and health services need to be considered? If Mary lived in your area, what services would be available? How could the nurse make a difference in this family's situation?*

3 *Dianna has just given birth to Ben who has a cleft lip and palate.*

   a *How do you think any parent might respond to having an infant with a congenital defect? What do you think Dianna may be feeling at this time?*

   b *As you go with Dianna to the nursery to see Ben, what do you anticipate her reaction might be, and how might you respond?*

   c *What are your priority nursing diagnoses at this time?*

   d *Why might Ben have feeding problems? Describe the feeding related interventions that would be most appropriate. Dianna wishes to breastfeed Ben. What is your response?*

   e *What community resources and home care supports can be put in place to support this family?*

References

Alkalay A et al.: Management of neonates born to mothers with group B streptococcus colonization, *J Perinatal* 16(6):470, 1996.

Ament L & Whalen E: Sexually transmitted diseases in pregnancy: diagnosis, impact and interventions, *J Obstet Gynecol Neonatal Nurs* 25(8):657, 1996.

American Academy of Pediatrics, Committee on Drugs: The transfer of drugs and other chemicals into human milk, *Pediatrics* 93(1):137, 1994.

American Academy of Pediatrics, Committee on Genetics: Folic acid for the prevention of neural tube defects, *Pediatrics* 92(3):493, 1993.

Askin D: Bacterial and fungal sepsis in the neonate, *J Obstet Gynecol Neonatal Nurs* 24(7):635, 1995.

Baker C: Group B streptococcal infections, *Clin Perinatol* 24(1):59, 1997.

Bartram J, Joffe G & Perry L: Prenatal environment: effect on neonatal outcome. In Merenstein G & Gardner S: *Handbook of neonatal intensive care*, ed 4, St Louis, 1998, Mosby.

Bastin N et al.: HIV disease and pregnancy, postpartum care of the HIV positive woman and her newborn, *J Obstet Gynecol Neonatal Nurs* 21(2):105, 1992.

Bell G & Lau K: Perinatal and neonatal issues of substance abuse, *Pediatr Clin North Am* 42(2):261, 1995.

Benson M: Management of infants born to women infected with human immunodeficiency virus, *J Perinatal Neonatal Nurs* 7(4):79, 1994.

Bibb K et al.: Drug screening in mothers using meconium samples, paired urine samples and interviews, *J Perinatol* 15(3):199, 1995.

Blair T: Smoking and the sudden infant death syndrome, *Br Med J* 313(7051):195, 1996.

Bortolussi R & Schlech W: Listeriosis. In Remington J & Klein J: *Infectious diseases of the fetus and newborn infant*, ed 4, Philadelphia, 1995, WB Saunders.

Budd K: Perinatal substance use: promoting abstinence in acute care settings, *AACN Clin Issues* 6(1):70, 1995.

Carroll M: PCP and hallucinogens, *Adv Alcohol Substance Abuse* 9(1-2):167, 1990.

Centers for Disease Control and Prevention: Fetal alcohol syndrome in the United States–1979-1992, *MMWR* 42(17):339, 1993.

Centers for Disease Control and Prevention: 1998 Guidelines for treatment of sexually transmitted diseases, *MMWR* 47(RR-1):1 1998.

Chadwick E & Yogev R: Pediatric AIDS, *Pediatr Clin North Am* 42(4):969, 1995.

Cohen S & Goldstein E: Infectious disease complications. In Niswander K & Evan A, editors: *Manual of obstetrics*, Boston, 1996, Little, Brown.

Coles C: Impact of prenatal alcohol exposure on the newborn and the child, *Clin Obstet Gynecol* 36(2):255, 1993.

Connor E & McSherry G: Treatment of HIV infection in infancy, *Clin Perinatol* 21(1):163, 1994.

Cowles T & Gonik B: Perinatal infections. In Fanaroff A & Martin R: *Neonatal-perinatal medicine: diseases of the fetus and newborn*, ed 6, St Louis, 1997, Mosby.

Craven D et al.: Human immunodeficiency virus infection in pregnancy: epidemiology and prevention of vertical transmission, *Infect Control Hosp Epidemiol* 15(1):36, 1994.

Creasy R & Resnik R: *Maternal-fetal medicine: principles and practice*, ed 3, Philadelphia, 1994, WB Saunders.

D'Alton M & DeCherney A: Prenatal diagnosis, *N Engl J Med* 328(2):114, 1993.

Danner S: Breastfeeding the infant with a cleft palate, *NAACOG's Clin Issues Perinatol Women Health Nurs* 3(4):634, 1992.

Day N, Cottreau C & Richardson G: Epidemiology of alcohol, marijuana and cocaine use, *Clin Obstet Gynecol* 36(2):232, 1993.

Fanaroff A & Martin R: *Neonatal-perinatal medicine: diseases of the fetus and infant*, ed 6, St Louis, 1997, Mosby.

Fenster L, et al.: Caffeine consumption during pregnancy and fetal growth, *Am J Public Health* 81(4):458, 1991.

Finnegan L: Drug addiction and pregnancy: the newborn. In Chasnoff I, editor: *Drugs, alcohol, pregnancy and parenting*, Boston, 1991, Kluwer Academic Publishers.

Floyd R et al.: A review of smoking in pregnancy: effect on pregnancy outcome and cessation efforts, *Annu Rev Public Health* 14:379, 1993.

Freij B & Sever J: Chronic infection. In Avery G, Fletcher M & MacDonald M, editors: *Neonatology: pathophysiology and management of the newborn*, ed 4, Philadelphia, 1994, JB Lippincott.

Frenkel L & Gaur S: Perinatal HIV infection and AIDS, *Clin Perinatol* 21(1):95, 1994.

Fried P: Prenatal exposure to tobacco and marijuana: effects during pregnancy, infancy and early childhood, *Clin Obstet Gynecol* 36(2):319, 1993.

Fuller R: Group B streptococcal infection in the newborn, *Crit Care Clin North Am* 4(3):487, 1992.

Fyler D, editor: *Nardas pediatric cardiology*, St Louis, 1992, Mosby.

Glantz J & Woods J: Cocaine, heroin and phencyclidine: obstetric perspectives, *Clin Obstet Gynecol* 36(2):279, 1993.

Greatrex B: A review of beta-haemolytic streptococcal infections in babies, *Br J Nurs* 6(9):8, 1997.

Guzzetta P et al.: General surgery. In Avery G et al., editors: *Neonatology: pathophysiology and management of newborns*, Philadelphia, 1994, Lippincott.

Hess D: Chlamydia in the neonate, *Neonat Netw* 12(3):9, 1993.

Hoekelman R et al.: *Primary pediatric care*, St Louis, 1996, Mosby.

Hoffman J: Incidence of congenital heart disease: I. Postnatal incidence, *Pediatr Cardiol* 16(4):103, 1995.

Kaplan G: Structural abnormalities of the genitourinary system. In Avery G et al., editors: *Neonatology: pathophysiology and management of the newborn*, Philadelphia, 1994, Lippincott.

Klein J & Marcy S: Bacterial sepsis and meningitis. In Remington J & Klein J, editors: *Infectious diseases of the fetus and newborn infant*, ed 4, Philadelphia, 1995, WB Saunders.

Kline M: Vertical human immunodeficiency virus infection. In Hansen T & McIntosh N, editors: *Current topics in neonatology*, Philadelphia, 1996, WB Saunders.

Kohl S: Neonatal herpes simplex infection, *Clin Perinatol* 24(1):129, 1997.

Lawrence R: *Breastfeeding: a guide for the medical profession*, ed 4, St Louis, 1994, Mosby.

Levine A & Rebarber A: Methadone maintenance, treatment and the nonstress test, *J Perinatol* 15(3):229, 1995.

Lewis D & Woods S: Fetal alcohol syndrome, *Am Fam Phys* 50(1):1025, 1994.

Lindberg C: Perinatal transmission of HIV: how to counsel women, *MCN Am J Matern Child Nurs* 20(4):207, 1995.

Lott J & Kilb J: The selection of antibacterial agents for treatment of neonatal sepsis or which drug kills which bug? *Neonat Pharmacol Q*, 1(1):19, 1992.

Lott J et al.: Assessment and management of immunologic dysfunction. In Kenner C, Brueggemeyer A & Gunderson L, editors: *Comprehensive neonatal nursing*, Philadelphia, 1994, WB Saunders.

Mays L et al.: Neurobehavioural profiles of neonates exposed to cocaine prenatally, *Pediatrics* 91(4):778, 1996.

Menticoglou S, Perlman M & Manning F: High cervical spinal cord injury in neonates delivered with forceps: report of 15 cases, *Obstet Gynecol* 86(4):589, 1995.

Merenstein G, Adams K & Weisman L: Infections in the neonate. In Merenstein G & Gardner S, editors: *Handbook of neonatal intensive care*, ed 4, St Louis, 1998, Mosby.

Merenstein G & Gardner S: *Handbook of neonatal intensive care*, ed 4, St Louis, 1998, Mosby.

Mills J et al.: Moderate caffeine use and the rash of spontaneous abortion and intrauterine growth retardation, *JAMA* 269(5):593, 1993.

Mimouni F et al.: Respiratory distress syndrome in infants of diabetic mothers in the 1980's: no direct adverse effect of maternal diabetes with modern management, *Obstet Gynecol* 69(2):191, 1987.

Moe P & Paige P: Neurologic disorders. In Merenstein G & Gardner S, editors: *Handbook of neonatal intensive care,* ed 4, St Louis, 1998, Mosby.

Nelson N: *Current therapy in neonatal-perinatal medicine,* ed 2, St Louis, 1990, Mosby.

Nora J & Fraser F: *Medical genetics: principles and practice,* ed 3, Philadelphia, 1989, Lea & Febiger.

Nugent J & Matranga G: Extra corporeal membrane oxygenation in the newborn. In Askin D, editor: *Acute respiratory care of the neonate,* ed 2, Petaluma, Calif, 1997, NICU INK.

O'Doherty N: *Neonatology: microatlas of the newborn,* Nutley, NJ, 1986, Hoffman-LaRoche.

Ogata E: Carbohydrate homeostasis. In Avery G, Fletcher M & MacDonald M, editors: *Pathophysiology and management of the newborn,* Philadelphia, 1994, JB Lippincott.

Paryani S et al.: Treatment of asymptomatic congenital syphilis: benzathine versus procaine penicillin G therapy, *J Pediatr* 125(3):471, 1994.

Peterec S: Management of neonatal Rh disease, *Clin Perinatol* 22(3):561, 1995.

Philip A: *Neonatology: a practical guide,* ed 4, Philadelphia, 1996, WB Saunders.

Piper J & Langer O: Does maternal diabetes delay fetal pulmonary maturity? *Am J Obstet Gynecol* 168(3):783, 1993.

Provisional Committee on Pediatric AIDS, AAP: Perinatal human immunodeficiency virus testing, *Pediatrics* 95(2):303, 1995.

Provisional Committee for Quality Improvement and Subcommittee on Hyperbilirubinemia, AAP: Practice parameter: management of hyperbilirubinemia in the healthy term newborn, *Pediatrics* 94(4):558, 1994.

Remington J, McLeod R & Desmonts G: Toxoplasmosis. In Remington J & Klein J, editors: *Infectious diseases of the fetus & newborn infant,* ed 4, Philadelphia, 1995, WB Saunders.

Romanczuk A & Brown J: Folic acid will reduce the risk of neural tube defects, *MCN Am J Matern Child Nurs* 19(6):331, 1994.

Rowe M et al.: *Essentials of pediatric surgery,* St Louis, 1995, Mosby.

Shannon L: Clinical perspectives and future trends of HIV infection in the newborn and child, *Neonatal Netw* 14(3):21, 1995.

Shiminski-Maher T & Disabato J: Current trends in the diagnosis and management of hydrocephalus in children, *J Pediat Nurs* 9(2):74, 1994.

Smith M & Teele D: Tuberculosis. In Remington J & Klein J, editors: *Infectious diseases of the fetus and newborn infant,* ed 4, Philadelphia, 1995, WB Saunders.

Speers A & Speers M: Care of the infant in a Pavlik harness, *Pediatr Nurs* 18(3):229, 1992.

Stapleton S: The infant with tracheoesophageal fistula and esophageal atresia, *Mother Baby J* 1(5):13, 1996.

Starke J: Tuberculosis: an old disease but a new threat to mother, fetus and neonate, *Clin Perinatol* 24(1):107, 1997.

Strodtbeck F: Viral infection of the newborn, *J Obstet Gynecol Neonatal Nurs* 24(7):659, 1995.

Vomund S & Witter S: Advanced techniques for the treatment of severe isoimmunization, *MCN Am J Matern Child Nurs* 19(1):18, 1994.

Wandstrat T: Rho (D) immune globulin, *Mother Baby J* 2(5):45, 1997.

Wardinsky T: Visual clues to the diagnosis of birth defects and genetic disease, *J Pediatr Health Care* 8(2):63, 1994.

Weiner L & Morse B: FAS: clinical perspectives and prevention. In Chasnoff I, editor: *Drugs, alcohol, pregnancy and parenting,* Boston, 1991, Kluwer Academic Publishers.

Wise B & Lawrence-Nolan L: A risk of blood transfusions for premature infants, *MCN Am J Matern Child Nurs* 15(2):96, 1990.

Wong D: *Whaley and Wong's nursing care of infants and children,* ed 5, St Louis, 1995, Mosby.

Wong D & Perry S: *Maternal child nursing care,* St Louis, 1998, Mosby.

Zitelli B & Davis H: *Atlas of pediatric diagnosis,* ed 3, St Louis, 1997, Mosby-Wolfe.

Zuckerman B: Marijuana and cigarette smoke. In Chasnoff I, editor: *Drugs, alcohol, pregnancy and parenting,* Boston, 1991, Kluwer Academic Publishers.

Glossary

abdominal Belonging or relating to the abdomen and its functions and disorders.

  a. birth Birth of a child through a surgical incision made into the abdominal wall and uterus; cesarean birth.

  a. gestation Implantation of a fertilized ovum outside the uterus but inside the peritoneal cavity.

ABO incompatibility Hemolytic disease that occurs when the mother's blood type is O and the newborn's is A, B, or AB.

abortion Termination of pregnancy before the fetus is viable and capable of extrauterine existence, usually less than 20 weeks of gestation (or when the fetus weighs less than 500 gm).

  complete a. Abortion in which fetus and all related tissue have been expelled from the uterus.

  elective a. Termination of pregnancy chosen by the woman that is not required for her physical safety.

  habitual (recurrent) a. Loss of three or more successive pregnancies for no known cause.

  incomplete a. Loss of pregnancy in which some but not all the products of conception have been expelled from the uterus.

  induced a. Intentionally produced loss of pregnancy by woman or others.

  inevitable a. Threatened loss of pregnancy that cannot be prevented or stopped and is imminent.

  missed a. Loss of pregnancy in which the products of conception remain in the uterus after the fetus dies.

  septic a. Loss of pregnancy in which there is an infection of the products of conception and the uterine endometrial lining, usually resulting from attempted termination of early pregnancy.

  spontaneous a. Loss of pregnancy that occurs naturally without interference or known cause.

  therapeutic a. Pregnancy that has been intentionally terminated for medical reasons.

  threatened a. Possible loss of a pregnancy; early symptoms are present (e.g., the cervix begins to dilate).

abruptio placentae Partial or complete premature separation of a normally implanted placenta.

abstinence Refraining from sexual intercourse periodically or permanently.

access to care Opportunity to receive health care services.

accreta, placenta See *placenta accreta.*

acid mantle Covering of skin formed by uppermost horny layer of epidermis, sweat, superficial fat, metabolic products, and external substances.

acidosis Increase in hydrogen ion concentration resulting in a lowering of blood pH below 7.35.

acini cells Milk-producing cells in the breast.

acme Highest point (e.g., of a contraction).

acoustic stimulation test Antepartum test to elicit fetal heart rate response to sound; performed by applying sound source (laryngeal stimulator) to maternal abdomen over the fetal head.

acquaintance Process used by parents to get to know or become familiar with their new infant; an important step in attachment.

acrocyanosis Peripheral cyanosis; blue color of hands and feet in most infants at birth that may persist for 7 to 10 days.

acromion Projection of the spine of the scapula (forming the point of the shoulder); used to explain the presentation of the fetus.

active phase Phase in first stage of labor from 4 to 7 cm dilatation.

adnexa Adjacent or accessory parts of a structure.

  uterine a. Ovaries and uterine (fallopian) tubes.

adolescence That period of an individual's transformation from a child to an adult.

adult respiratory distress syndrome (ARDS) Set of symptoms including decreased compliance of lung tissue, pulmonary edema, and acute hypoxemia. The condition is similar to respiratory distress syndrome of the newborn.

afibrinogenemia Absence or decrease of fibrinogen in the blood such that the blood will not coagulate. In obstetrics, this condition occurs from complications of abruptio placentae or retention of a dead fetus.

afterbirth Lay term for the placenta and membranes expelled after the birth of the child.

afterbirth pains (afterpains) Painful uterine cramps that occur intermittently for approximately 2 or 3 days after birth and that result from contractile efforts of the uterus to return to its normal involuted condition.

AGA Appropriate (growth) for gestational age.

agenesis Failure of an organ to develop.

agonist-antagonist compounds An agonist is an agent that activates something; an antagonist is an agent that blocks something.

albuminuria Presence of readily detectable amounts of albumin in the urine.

alkalosis Abnormal condition of body fluids characterized by a tendency toward an increased pH, as from an excess of alkaline bicarbonate or a deficiency of acid.

amenorrhea Absence or suppression of menstruation.

amniocentesis Procedure in which a needle is inserted through the abdominal and uterine walls into the amniotic fluid; used for assessment of fetal health and maturity.

amnioinfusion Infusion of normal saline warmed to body temperature through an intrauterine catheter into the uterine cavity in an attempt to increase the fluid around the umbilical cord and prevent compression during uterine contractions.

amnion Inner membrane of two fetal membranes that form the sac and contain the fetus and the fluid that surrounds it in utero.

amnionitis Inflammation of the amnion, occurring most frequently after early rupture of membranes.

amniotic Pertaining or relating to the amnion.
   a. fluid Fluid surrounding fetus derived primarily from maternal serum and fetal urine.
   a. fluid embolism Embolism resulting from amniotic fluid entering the maternal bloodstream during labor and birth after rupture of membranes; this is often fatal to the woman if it is a pulmonary embolism.
   a. fluid index (AFI) Estimation of amount of amniotic fluid by means of ultrasound to determine excess or decrease.
   a. sac Membrane "bag" that contains the fetus and fluid before birth.

amniotomy Artificial rupture of the fetal membranes (AROM), using a plastic amnihook or surgical clamp.

analgesia Absence of pain without loss of consciousness.

analgesic Any medication or agent that will relieve pain.

anaphylaxis Immediate hypersensitivity reaction characterized by local reactions such as urticaria or by systemic reactions; may be fatal.

android pelvis Male type of pelvis; heart-shaped inlet.

anencephaly Congenital deformity characterized by the absence of cerebrum, cerebellum, and flat bones of skull.

anesthesia Partial or complete absence of sensation with or without loss of consciousness.

aneuploidy Having an abnormal number of chromosomes.

announcement phase The first developmental task experienced by expectant fathers as identified by May. During this phase the expectant father accepts the biologic fact of pregnancy.

anomaly Organ or structure that is malformed or in some way abnormal with reference to form, structure, or position.

anovulatory Failure of the ovaries to produce, mature, or release eggs.

anoxia Absence of oxygen.

antenatal Occurring before or formed before birth (newborn).

antepartal Before labor (maternal).

anthropoid pelvis Pelvis in which the anteroposterior diameter is equal to or greater than the transverse diameter; oval inlet.

antibody Specific protein substance made by the body that exerts restrictive or destructive action on specific antigens, such as bacteria, toxins, or Rh factor.

anticipatory grief Grief that predates the loss of a beloved object.

antigen Protein foreign to the body that causes the body to develop antibodies (e.g., bacteria, dust, Rh factor).

Apgar score Numeric expression of the condition of a newborn obtained by rapid assessment at 1 and 5 minutes of age; developed by Dr. Virginia Apgar.

apnea Cessation of respirations for more than 15 seconds associated with generalized cyanosis.

Apt test Differentiation of maternal and fetal blood when there is vaginal bleeding. It is performed as follows: Add 0.5 ml of blood to 4.5 ml of distilled water. Shake. Add 1 ml of 0.25 N sodium hydroxide. Fetal and cord blood remain pink for 1 or 2 minutes. Maternal blood becomes brown in 30 seconds.

areola Pigmented ring of tissue surrounding the nipple.
   secondary a. During the fifth month of pregnancy, a second faint ring of pigmentation seen around the original areola.

asphyxia Decreased oxygen with or without excess of carbon dioxide in the body.
   perinatal a. Condition occurring in utero with the following biochemical changes: hypoxemia (lowering of Po_2), hypercapnia (increase in Pco_2), and respiratory and metabolic acidosis (reduction of blood pH).

aspiration pneumonia Inflammatory condition of the lungs and bronchi caused by the inhalation of vomitus containing acid gastric contents.

assisted reproductive therapies (ARTs) Treatments for infertility, including in vitro fertilization procedures, embryo adoption, embryo hosting, and therapeutic insemination.

asynclitism Oblique presentation of the fetal head at the superior strait of the pelvis; the pelvic planes and those of the fetal head are not parallel.

ataractics Drugs capable of promoting tranquility; a tranquilizer.

atelectasis Pulmonary pathosis involving alveolar collapse.

atony Absence of muscle tone.

atresia Absence of a normally present passageway.
   biliary a. Absence of the bile duct.
   choanal a. Complete obstruction of the posterior nares, which open into the nasopharynx, with membranous or bony tissue.
   esophageal a. Congenital anomaly in which the esophagus ends in a blind pouch or narrows into a thin cord, thus failing to form a continuous passageway to the stomach.

attachment A specific and enduring affective tie to another person.

attitude Body posture or position.
   fetal a. Relation of fetal parts to each other in the uterus (e.g., all parts flexed, all parts flexed except neck is extended).

augmentation of labor Artificial stimulation of uterine contractions after labor has started spontaneously but is not progressing satisfactorily.

autoimmune disorders Body produces antibodies against itself, causing tissue damage.

autoimmunization Development of antibodies against constituents of one's own tissues (e.g., a man may develop antibodies against his own sperm).

autolysis "Self-digestive" process by which the uterus returns to a nonpregnant state after childbirth. The decrease in estrogen and progesterone levels after childbirth results in this destruction of excess hypertrophied uterine tissue.

autosomal inheritance Characteristics transmitted by genes on the autosomes, not the sex chromosomes.

autosomes Any of the paired chromosomes other than the sex (X and Y) chromosomes.

azoospermia Absence of sperm in the semen.

bacteremic shock Shock that occurs in septicemia when endotoxins are released from certain bacteria into the bloodstream.

bag of waters Lay term for the sac containing amniotic fluid and fetus.

ballottement (1) Movability of a floating object, such as a fetus. (2) Diagnostic technique using palpation: a floating object, when tapped or pushed, moves away and then returns to touch the examiner's hand.

Bandl's ring Abnormally thickened ridge of uterine musculature between the upper and lower segments that occurs after a mechanically obstructed labor, with the lower segment thinning abnormally.

barotrauma Tissue damage caused by pressure, often applied to the lungs.

Bartholin's glands Two small glands situated on either side of the vaginal orifice that secrete small amounts of mucus during coitus and that are homologous to the bulbourethral glands in the male.

basal body temperature Lowest body temperature of a healthy person taken immediately after awakening and before getting out of bed.

basalis, decidua See *decidua basalis.*

bearing-down effort "Secondary powers"; energy exerted by the woman during contractions to push out the baby.

behavioral assessment Assessment of activity, feeding and sleeping patterns, and responsiveness.

behavioral repertoire A set of behaviors (actions and reactions) that both parent and infant use to facilitate interactions.

Bell's palsy See *palsy, Bell's.*

bereavement The feelings of loss, pain, desolation, and sadness that occur after the death of a loved one.

bicornuate uterus Anomalous uterus that may be either a double or single organ with two horns.

biliary atresia See *atresia, biliary.*

bilirubin Yellow or orange pigment that is a breakdown product of hemoglobin. It is carried by the blood to the liver, where it is chemically changed and excreted into the bile or is conjugated and excreted by the kidneys.

Billings method See *ovulation method.*

bimanual Performed with both hands.
    b. palpation Examination of a woman's pelvic organs done by placement of one hand on the abdomen and one or two fingers of the other hand into the vagina.

biophysical profile (BPP) Noninvasive assessment of the fetus and its environment using ultrasonography and uterine fetal monitoring; includes fetal breathing movements, gross body movements, fetal tone, reactive fetal heart rate, and qualitative amniotic fluid volume.

biopsy Removal of a small piece of tissue for microscopic examination and diagnosis.

biorhythmicity Cyclic changes that occur with established regularity, such as sleeping and eating patterns.

biparietal diameter Largest transverse diameter of the fetal head; extends from one parietal bone to the other.

bipolar disorders Depression with previous or current manic episodes.

birth plan A tool by which parents can explore their childbirth options and choose those that are most important to them.

birth rate Number of live births per 1,000 population per year. See also *fertility.*

Bishop score Rating system to evaluate inducibility of the cervix; a higher score increases the rate of successful induction of labor.

blastocyst Stage in the development of a mammalian embryo, occurring after the morula stage, that consists of an outer layer, or trophoblast, and a hollow sphere of cells enclosing a cavity.

blended family Family form that includes stepparents and stepchildren.

bloody show Vaginal discharge that originates in the cervix and consists of blood and mucus; increases as cervix dilates during labor.

body boundaries Boundaries that serve to separate the self from the nonself and provide a feeling of safety.

body image Person's subjective concept of his or her physical appearance.

bonding A process by which parents, over time, form an emotional relationship with their infant.

Bradley method Husband-coached childbirth using labor breathing techniques.

Braxton Hicks sign Mild, intermittent, painless uterine contractions that occur during pregnancy. These contractions occur more frequently as pregnancy advances but do not represent true labor.

Brazelton assessment Method for assessing the interactional behavior of a newborn.

breakthrough bleeding Escape of blood occurring between menstrual periods; may be noted by women using chemical contraception (birth control pills).

breast self-examination (BSE) Self-examination of the breasts.

breast shells Rigid plastic cups that are worn inside a bra to put pressure on the areola to help a nipple protrude or to protect sore nipples from the pressure of clothing.

breech presentation Presentation in which buttocks or feet are nearest the cervical opening and are born first; occurs in approximately 3% of all births.
    complete b.p. Simultaneous presentation of buttocks, legs, and feet.
    footling (incomplete) b.p. Presentation of one or both feet.
    frank b.p. Presentation of buttocks, with hips flexed so that thighs are against abdomen.

bregma Point of junction of the coronal and sagittal sutures of the skull; the area of the anterior fontanel of the fetus.

brim Edge of the superior strait of the true pelvis; the inlet.

bronchopulmonary dysplasia (BPD) Pulmonary condition affecting preterm infants who have experienced respiratory failure and have been oxygen dependent for more than 28 days.

brown fat Source of heat unique to neonates that is capable of greater thermogenic activity than ordinary fat. Deposits are found around the adrenals, kidneys, and neck, between the scapulas, and behind the sternum for several weeks after birth.

bruit, uterine See *uterine bruit.*

calendar method See *rhythm method.*

***Candida* vaginitis** Vaginal, fungal infection; formerly moniliasis.

candidiasis Infection of the skin or mucous membrane by a yeastlike fungus, *Candida albicans;* see *thrush.*

capacitation Enzymatic process resulting in removal of plasma protein over acrosome of sperm; prerequisite for sperm to fertilize an ovum.

capsularis, decidua See *decidua capsularis.*

caput Occiput of fetal head appearing at the vaginal introitus preceding birth of the head.

    c. succedaneum Swelling of the tissue over the presenting part of the fetal head caused by pressure during labor.

carcinoma Malignant, often metastatic epithelial neoplasm; cancer.

cardiac decompensation A condition of heart failure in which the heart is unable to maintain a sufficient cardiac output.

cardiac output (CO) Volume of blood ejected from the left ventricle in 1 minute, measured in liters per minute. Cardiac output is the product of stroke volume and heart rate (CO = HR × SV).

cardinal movements of labor The mechanism of labor in a vertex presentation; includes engagement, descent, flexion, internal rotation, extension, external rotation (restitution), and expulsion.

carpal tunnel syndrome Pressure on the median nerve at the point at which it goes through the carpal tunnel of the wrist. It causes soreness, tenderness, and weakness of the muscles of the thumb.

carrier Individual who carries a gene that does not exhibit itself in physical or chemical characteristics but that can be transmitted to children (e.g., a female carrying the trait for hemophilia, which is expressed in male offspring).

caul Hood of fetal membranes covering fetal head during birth.

cephalhematoma NOTE: This is spelled cephalohematoma in some sources. Extravasation of blood from ruptured vessels between a skull bone and its external covering, the periosteum. Swelling is limited by the margins of the cranial bone affected (usually parietals).

cephalic Pertaining to the head.

    c. presentation Presentation of the fetal head.

cephalocaudal development Principle of maturation that development progresses from the head to tail (rump).

cephalopelvic disproportion (CPD) Condition in which the infant's head is of such a shape, size, or position that it cannot pass through the mother's pelvis.

cerclage Use of nonabsorbable suture to keep a premature dilating cervix closed; released when pregnancy is at term to allow labor to begin.

cervical cap Individually fitted contraceptive barrier for the cervix.

cervical intraepithelial neoplasm (CIN) Uncontrolled and progressive abnormal growth of cervical epithelial cells.

cervical mucus method See *ovulation method.*

cervical os "Mouth" or opening to the cervix.

cervicitis Cervical infection.

cervix Lowest and narrow end of the uterus; the "neck." The cervix is situated between the external os and the body, or corpus, of the uterus, and its lower end extends into the vagina.

cesarean birth Birth of a fetus by an incision through the abdominal wall and uterus.

cesarean hysterectomy Removal of the uterus immediately after the cesarean birth of an infant.

Chadwick's sign Violet color of vaginal mucous membrane that is visible from about the fourth week of pregnancy; caused by increased vascularity.

chloasma Increased pigmentation over bridge of nose and cheeks of pregnant women and some women taking oral contraceptives; also known as *mask of pregnancy.*

choanal atresia See *atresia, choanal.*

cholecystitis Acute or chronic inflammation of the gallbladder

cholelithiasis Presence of gallstones in the gallbladder.

choreoathetoid cerebral palsy Condition characterized by both choreiform (jerky, ticklike twitching) and athetoid (slow, writhing) movements.

chorioamnionitis Inflammatory reaction in fetal membranes to bacteria or viruses in the amniotic fluid, which then become infiltrated with polymorphonuclear leukocytes.

chorion Fetal membrane closest to the intrauterine wall that gives rise to the placenta and continues as the outer membrane surrounding the amnion.

chorionic villus (villi) Tiny vascular protrusions on the chorionic surface that project into the maternal blood sinuses of the uterus and that help to form the placenta and secrete hCG.

chorionic villus sampling (CVS) Removal of fetal tissue from placenta for genetic diagnostic studies.

chromosome Element within the cell nucleus carrying genes and composed of DNA and proteins.

circumcision

    female c. Religious or cultural removal of a portion of the clitoris and labia; practiced in some Third World countries but illegal in the United States. Mutilating procedure that can cause problems in childbirth.

    male c. Excision of the prepuce (foreskin) of the penis, exposing the glans; may be done for religious or cultural reasons.

claiming process Process by which the parents identify their new baby in terms of likeness to other family members, differences, and uniqueness.

cleft lip Incomplete closure of the lip. Lay term used is harelip.

cleft palate Incomplete closure of the palate or roof of mouth; a congenital fissure.

climacteric The period of a woman's life when she is passing from a reproductive to a nonreproductive state, with regression of ovarian function. The cycle of endocrine, physical, and psychosocial changes that occurs during the termination of the reproductive years. Also called *climacterium.*

clitoris Female organ analogous to male penis; a small, ovid body of erectile tissue situated at the anterior junction of the vulva.

clonus (ankle) Spasmodic alternation of muscular contraction and relaxation; counted in beats.

clubfoot Congenital deformity in which portions of the foot and ankle are twisted out of a normal position.

coitus Penile-vaginal intercourse.

    c. interruptus Intercourse during which penis is withdrawn from vagina before ejaculation.

cold stress Excessive loss of heat that results in increased respirations and nonshivering thermogenesis to maintain core body temperature.

colostrum The fluid in the breast from pregnancy into the early postpartal period. It is rich in antibodies, which provide protection from many diseases; high in protein, which binds bilirubin; and laxative acting, which speeds the elimination of meconium and helps to loosen mucus.

colposcopy Examination of vagina and cervix with a colposcope to identify neoplastic or other changes.

complete abortion See *abortion, complete.*

complete breech presentation See *breech presentation, complete.*

conception Union of the sperm and ovum resulting in fertilization; formation of the one-celled zygote.

conceptional age In fetal development the number of completed weeks since the moment of conception. Because the moment of conception is almost impossible to determine, conceptional age is estimated at 2 weeks less than gestational age.

conceptus Embryo or fetus, fetal membranes, amniotic fluid, and the fetal portion of the placenta.

condom Mechanical barrier worn on the penis for contraception or to protect against STDs; a "rubber."

condyloma acuminatum (*plural* condylomata acuminata) Wartlike growth on the skin usually seen near the anus or external genitals caused by human papillomavirus (HPV); genital warts. (Must be differentiated from condyloma latum seen in secondary syphilis.)

congenital Present or existing before birth as a result of either hereditary or prenatal environmental factors.

congenital rubella syndrome Complex of problems including hearing defects, cardiovascular abnormalities, and cataracts caused by maternal rubella in the first trimester of pregnancy.

conjoined twins See *twins, conjoined.*

conjugate

    diagonal c. Radiographic measurement of distance from inferior border of symphysis pubis (SP) to sacral promontory; may be obtained by vaginal examination; 12.5 to 13 cm.

    true c. (conjugata vera) Radiographic measurement of distance from upper margin of symphysis pubis (SP) to sacral promontory; 1.5 to 2 cm less than diagonal conjugate.

conjuctivitis Inflammation of the mucous membrane that lines the eyelids and is reflected onto the eyeball.

conscious relaxation Technique used to release the mind and body from tension through conscious effort and practice.

contraception Prevention of impregnation or conception.

contractions

    contraction stress test (CST) Test to stimulate uterine contractions for the purpose of assessing fetal response; a healthy fetus does not react to contractions, whereas a compromised fetus demonstrates late decelerations in the fetal heart rate that are indicative of uteroplacental insufficiency.

    duration Period from the beginning of the contraction to the end.

    frequency How often the contractions occur—the period from the beginning of one contraction to the beginning of the next.

    intensity Strength of the contraction at its peak.

    interval Period between uterine contractions, timed from the end of one contraction to the beginning of the next.

    resting tone The tension in the uterine muscle between contractions.

contraction ring See *Bandl's ring.*

Coombs' test *Indirect:* determination of Rh-positive antibodies in maternal blood; *direct:* determination of maternal Rh-positive antibodies in fetal cord blood. A positive test result indicates the presence of antibodies or titer.

coping mechanism Any effort directed at stress management. It can be task oriented and involve direct problem-solving efforts to cope with the threat itself or be intrapsychic or ego-defense oriented with the goal of regulating one's emotional distress.

copulation Coitus; sexual intercourse.

corpus luteum Yellow body. After rupture of the graafian follicle at ovulation, the follicle develops into a yellow structure that secretes progesterone and some estrogen in the second half of the menstrual cycle, atrophying about 3 days before sloughing of the endometrium in menstrual flow. If impregnation occurs, it continues to produce the hormones until the placenta can take over this function.

cotyledon One of the 15 to 28 visible segments of the placenta on the maternal surface, each made up of fetal vessels, chorionic villi, and an intervillous space.

counterpressure Pressure to sacral area of back during uterine contractions.

couplet care One nurse, educated in both mother and infant care, functions as the primary nurse for both mother and infant (also known as mother-baby care or single-room maternity care).

couvade Custom whereby the father behaves in specific ways during the pregnancy and labor.

Couvelaire uterus See *uterus, Couvelaire.*

cradle cap Common seborrheic dermatitis of infants consisting of thick, yellow, greasy scales on the scalp.

craniotabes Localized softening of cranial bones.

creatinine Substance found in blood and muscle; measurement of levels in maternal urine correlates with amount of fetal muscle mass and therefore fetal size.

crib death Unexpected and sudden death of an apparently normal and healthy infant that occurs during sleep and with no physical or autopsic evidence of disease. Also referred to as *sudden infant death syndrome* (SIDS).

cri-du-chat syndrome Rare congenital disorder recognized at birth by a kittenlike cry, which may prevail for weeks and then disappear. Other characteristics include low birth weight, microcephaly, "moon face," wide-set eyes, strabismus, and low-set misshapen ears. Infants are hypotonic; heart defects and mental and physical retardation are common. Also called *cat-cry syndrome.*

critical path The exact timing of all key incidents that must occur to achieve the standard outcomes within the diagnosis related group (DRG)–specific length of stay.

crowning Stage of birth when the top of the fetal head can be seen at the vaginal orifice as the widest part of the head distends the vulva.

cryosurgery Local freezing and removal of tissue without injury to adjacent tissue and with minimum blood loss, done with special equipment.

cryptorchidism Failure of one or both of the testicles to descend into the scrotum. Also called *undescended testis.*

cul-de-sac of Douglas Pouch formed by a fold of the peritoneum dipping down between the anterior wall of the rectum and the posterior wall of the uterus; also called *Douglas's cul-de-sac, pouch of Douglas,* and *rectouterine pouch.*

culdocentesis Puncture of Douglas's cul-de-sac through the vagina for aspiration of fluid.

Cullen's sign Faint, irregularly formed, hemorrhagic patches on the skin around the umbilicus. The discolored skin is blue black and becomes greenish brown or yellow. Cullen's sign may appear 1 to 2 days after the onset of anorexia and the severe, poorly localized abdominal pains characteristic of acute pancreatitis. Cullen's sign is also present in massive upper gastrointestinal hemorrhage and ruptured ectopic pregnancy.

cultural context Setting in which one considers the individual's and the family's beliefs and practices (culture).

curettage Scraping of the endometrium lining of the uterus with a curet to remove the contents of the uterus (as is done after an inevitable or incomplete abortion) or to obtain specimens for diagnostic purposes.

cycle of violence Pattern of three phases: period of increasing tension, the abusive episode, and a period of contrition and kindness.

cystocele Bladder hernia: injury to the vesicovaginal fascia during labor and birth may allow herniation of the bladder into the vagina.

cytology Study of cells, including their formation, origin, structure, function, biochemical activities, and pathology.

daily fetal movement counts (DFMCs) Maternal assessment of fetal activity; the number of fetal movements within a specific time are counted.

death Cessation of life.
    fetal d. Intrauterine death; death of a fetus weighing 500 gm or more of 20 weeks of gestation or more.
    infant d. Death during the first year of life.
    maternal d. Death of a woman as a result of a pregnancy or birth-related problem.
    neonatal d. Death of a newborn within the first 28 days after birth.
    perinatal d. Death of a fetus of 20 weeks of gestation or older or death of a neonate 28 days old or younger.

decidua Mucous membrane, lining of uterus, or endometrium of pregnancy that is shed after giving birth.
    d. basalis Maternal aspect of the placenta made up of uterine blood vessels, endometrial stroma, and glands. It is shed in lochial discharge after delivery.
    d. capsularis That part of the decidual membranes surrounding the chorionic sac.
    d. vera Nonplacental decidual lining of the uterus.

decrement Decrease or stage of decline, as of a contraction.

deep tendon reflexes (DTRs) Reflex caused by stimulation of tendons, such as elbow, wrist, knee, triceps, and ankle jerk reflexes.

delivery (birth) Expulsion of the child with placenta and membranes by the mother or their extraction by the obstetric practitioner.
    abdominal d. See *abdominal birth.*

ΔOD$_{450}$ (*read delta OD$_{450}$*) Delta optical density (or absorbance) at 450 nm, obtained by spectral analysis of amniotic fluid. This prenatal test is used to measure the degree of hemolytic activity in the fetus and to evaluate fetal status in women sensitized to the Rh factor.

demand feeding Feeding a newborn every third hour or when the baby cries to be fed, whichever comes first.

deoxyribonucleic acid (DNA) Intracellular complex protein that carries genetic information, consisting of two purines (adenine and guanine) and two pyrimidines (thymine and cytosine).

depression An intense and pervasive sadness with severe and labile mood swings.

depressive reactions Depression related to the postpartum period including postpartum blues, postpartum nonpsychotic depression, and postpartum psychosis.

DES Diethylstilbestrol; female fetus is predisposed to reproductive tract malformations and (later) dysplasia if her mother ingested this medication during pregnancy.

desquamation Shedding of epithelial cells of the skin and mucous membranes.

developmental crisis Severe, usually transient, stress that occurs when a person is unable to complete the tasks of a psychosocial stage of development and is therefore unable to move on to the next stage.

developmental task Physical or cognitive skill that a person must accomplish during a particular age period to continue developing, such as walking, which precedes the development of the sense of autonomy in the toddler period.

developmental theory Theoretic approach for viewing the family. The developmental perspective sees family members pass through phases of growth from dependence through active independence to interdependence.

diabetes mellitus Systemic disorder of carbohydrate, protein, and fat metabolism; caused by deficient insulin production or ineffective use of insulin at the cellular level.

diaphragmatic hernia Congenital malformation of diaphragm that allows displacement of the abdominal organs into the thoracic cavity.

diastasis recti abdominis Separation of the two rectus muscles along the median line of the abdominal wall. This is often seen in women with repeated childbirths or with a multiple gestation (e.g., triplets). In the newborn it is usually attributable to incomplete development.

Dick-Read method An approach to childbirth based on the premise that fear of pain produces muscular tension, producing pain and greater fear. The method includes teaching physiologic processes of labor, exercise to improve muscle tone, and techniques to assist in relaxation and prevent the fear-tension-pain mechanism.

dilatation of cervix Stretching of the external os from an opening a few millimeters in size to an opening large enough to allow the passage of the infant.

dilatation and curettage (D&C) Vaginal procedure in which the cervical canal is stretched enough to admit passage of an instrument called a *curet* (or *curette*). The endometrium of the uterus is scraped with the curet to empty the uterine contents or to obtain tissue for examination.

diploid number Having two sets of chromosomes; found normally in somatic (body) cells; 23 sets or 46 chromosomes.

discordance Discrepancy in size (or other indicator) between twins.

disorganization A dimension of bereavement characterized by depression, anorexia, difficulty in concentration, and a generalized feeling of not feeling good about oneself physically and emotionally.

disparate twins See *twins, disparate.*

disseminated intravascular coagulation (DIC) Pathologic form of coagulation in which clotting factors are consumed to such an extent that generalized bleeding can occur; associated with abruptio placentae, eclampsia, intrauterine fetal demise, amniotic fluid embolism, and hemorrhage.

dizygotic Related to or proceeding from two zygotes (fertilized ova).

dizygotic twins See *twins, dizygotic.*

Döderlein's bacillus Gram-positive bacterium occurring in normal vaginal secretions.

dominant trait Gene that is expressed whenever it is present in the heterozygous gene state (e.g., brown eyes are dominant over blue).

Doppler blood flow analysis Device for measuring blood flow noninvasively in the fetus and placenta to detect intrauterine growth restriction.

Douglas's cul-de-sac See *cul-de-sac of Douglas.*

doula Experienced assistant hired to give the woman support during labor and birth.

Down syndrome Abnormality involving the occurrence of a third chromosome, rather than the normal pair (trisomy 21), that characteristically results in a typical picture of mental retardation and altered physical appearance. This condition was formerly called *mongolism.*

drug dependence (addiction) Physical or psychologic dependence or both on a substance.

dry labor Lay term referring to labor in which amniotic fluid has already escaped. A "dry birth" does not exist.

Dubowitz assessment Estimation of gestational age of a newborn based on criteria developed for that purpose.

ductus arteriosus In fetal circulation an anatomic shunt between the pulmonary artery and arch of the aorta. It is obliterated after birth by a rising PO_2 and a change in intravascular pressures in the presence of normal pulmonary function. It normally becomes a ligament after birth but in some instances remains patent.

ductus venosus In fetal circulation, a blood vessel carrying oxygenated blood between the umbilical vein and the inferior vena cava, bypassing the liver. It is obliterated and becomes a ligament after birth.

Duncan's mechanism Delivery of placenta with the maternal surface presenting, rather than the shiny fetal surface.

dys- Prefix meaning abnormal, difficult, painful, faulty.

dysfunctional labor Abnormal uterine contractions that prevent normal progress of cervical dilatation and effacement.

dysfunctional uterine bleeding (DUB) Abnormal bleeding from the uterus for reasons that are not readily established.

dysmaturity See *intrauterine growth restriction (IUGR).*

dysmenorrhea
primary d. Painful menstruation beginning 2 to 6 months after menarche, related to ovulation.
secondary d. Painful menstruation related to organic disease such as endometriosis, pelvic inflammatory disease, uterine neoplasm.

dyspareunia Painful sexual intercourse, for either sex.

dysplasia Any abnormal development of tissues or organs.

dystocia Prolonged, painful, or otherwise difficult birth because of mechanical factors produced by the passenger (the fetus) or the passage (the pelvis and soft tissues of the birth canal of the mother), inadequate powers (uterine and other muscular activity), or maternal position.

ecchymosis Bruise; bleeding into tissue caused by direct trauma, serious infection, or bleeding diathesis.

eclampsia Severe complication of pregnancy of unknown cause and occurring more often in the primigravida; characterized by tonic and clonic convulsions, coma, high blood pressure, albuminuria, and oliguria occurring during pregnancy or shortly after birth.

ectoderm Outer layer of embryonic tissue giving rise to skin, nails, and hair.

ectopic Out of normal place.
e. pregnancy Implantation of the fertilized ovum outside of its normal place in the uterine cavity. Locations include the abdomen, uterine tubes, and ovaries.

edema Generalized accumulation of interstitial fluid.
dependent e. Edema of lower or most dependent parts of body where hydrostatic pressure is greater.
pitting e. Edema that leaves a small depression or pit when pressure is applied to a swollen area.

effacement Thinning and shortening or obliteration of the cervix that occurs during late pregnancy or labor or both.

effleurage Gentle stroking used in massage.

ejaculation Sudden expulsion of semen from the male urethra.

elective abortion See *abortion, elective.*

electronic fetal monitoring (EFM) Electronic surveillance of fetal heart rate by external and internal methods.

embolus Any undissolved matter (solid, liquid, or gaseous) that is carried by the blood to another part of the body and obstructs a blood vessel.

embryo Conceptus from the second or third week of development until about the eighth week after conception, when mineralization (ossification) of the skeleton begins. This period is characterized by cellular differentiation and predominantly hyperplastic growth.

emotional lability Rapid mood changes from irritability to anger or sadness to joy and cheerfulness; often seen in the first trimester of pregnancy.

endocarditis Inflammation of the inner layer of the heart muscle (endocardium).

endocervical Pertaining to the interior of the canal of the cervix of the uterus.

endocrine glands Ductless glands that secrete hormones into the blood or lymph.

endometriosis Tissue closely resembling endometrial tissue but located outside the uterus in the pelvic cavity. Symptoms may include pelvic pain or pressure, dysmenorrhea, dyspareunia, abnormal bleeding from the uterus or rectum, and sterility.

endometritis Postpartum uterine infection, often beginning at the site of the placental implantation.

endometrium Inner lining of the uterus that undergoes changes caused by hormones during the menstrual cycle and pregnancy; decidua.

endorphins Endogenous opioids secreted by the pituitary gland that act on the central and peripheral nervous systems to reduce pain.

en face Face-to-face position in which the parent's and infant's faces are approximately 20 cm apart and on the same plane.

engagement In obstetrics, the entrance of the fetal presenting part into the superior pelvic strait and the beginning of the descent through the pelvic canal.

engorgement Distention or vascular congestion. In obstetrics, the process of swelling of the breast tissue brought about by an increase in blood and lymph supply to the breast, which precedes true lactation. It lasts about 48 hours and usually reaches a peak between the third and fifth postbirth days.

engrossment A parent's absorption, preoccupation, and interest in his or her infant; term typically used to describe the father's intense involvement with his newborn.

enterocele Herniation of the peritoneum of the posterior cul-de-sac between the uterosacral ligaments into the rectovaginal septum.

entoderm Inner layer of embryonic tissue giving rise to internal organs such as the intestine.

entrainment Phenomenon observed in the microanalysis of sound films in which the speaker moves several parts of the body and the listener responds to the sounds by moving in ways that are coordinated with the rhythm of the sounds. Infants have been observed to move in time to the rhythms of adult speech but not to random noises or disconnected words or vowels. Entrainment is believed to be an essential factor in the process of maternal-infant bonding.

epicanthus Fold of skin covering the inner canthus and caruncle that extends from the root of the nose to the median end of the eyebrow; characteristically found in certain races but may occur as a congenital anomaly.

epidural block Type of regional anesthesia produced by injection of a local anesthetic into the epidural (peridural) space.

epidural blood patch A patch formed by a few millimeters of the mother's blood occluding a tear or hole in the dura mater around the spinal cord.

episiotomy Surgical incision of the perineum at the end of the second stage of labor to facilitate birth and to avoid laceration of the perineum.

epispadias Defect in which the urethral canal terminates on the dorsum of the penis or above the clitoris (rare).

Epstein's pearls Small, white blebs found along the gum margins and at the junction of the soft and hard palates. They are a normal manifestation and are typically seen in the newborn. Similar to Bohn's nodules.

epulis Tumorlike benign lesion of the gingiva seen in pregnant women.

equilibrium State of balance or rest resulting from the equal action of opposing forces, as with calcium and phosphorus in the body. In psychiatry, a state of mental or emotional balance.

Erb-Duchenne paralysis Paralysis caused by physical injury to the upper brachial plexus, occurring most often in childbirth from forcible traction during birth. The signs of Erb's paralysis include loss of sensation in the arm and paralysis and atrophy of the deltoid, the biceps, and the branchialis muscles. Also called *Erb's palsy.*

ergot Drug obtained from *Claviceps purpurea,* a fungus, which stimulates the smooth muscles of blood vessels and the uterus, causing vasoconstriction and uterine contractions.

erythema toxicum Innocuous pink papular neonatal rash of unknown cause, with superimposed vesicles appearing within 24 to 48 hours after birth and resolving spontaneously within a few days.

erythroblastosis fetalis Hemolytic disease of the newborn usually caused by isoimmunization resulting from Rh incompatibility or ABO incompatibility.

esophageal atresia See *atresia, esophageal.*

estimated date of birth (EDB) Approximate date of birth. Usually determined by calculation using Nägele's rule; "due date."

estradiol An estrogen.

estriol Major metabolite of estrogen that increases during the second half of pregnancy with an intact fetoplacental unit (normal placenta, normal fetal liver and adrenals) and normal maternal renal function.

estrogen Female sex hormone produced by the ovaries and placenta.

estrogen replacement therapy (ERT) Exogenous estrogen given to women during and after menopause to prevent hot flashes, mood changes, osteoporosis, and genitourinary symptoms.

ethics Systematic inquiry into the principles of right and wrong conduct, of virtue and vice, and of good and evil as they relate to conduct.

eutocia Normal or natural labor or birth.

evidence-based practice Practice based on analysis of research findings.

exchange transfusion Replacement of 75% to 85% of circulating blood by withdrawal of the recipient's blood and injection of a donor's blood in equal amounts, the purposes of which are to prevent an accumulation of bilirubin in the blood above a dangerous level, to prevent the accumulation of other by-products of hemolysis in hemolytic disease, and to correct anemia and acidosis.

expressive style Expectant father's strong emotional response to partner's pregnancy.

expulsive Having the tendency to drive out or expel.

   e. contractions Labor contractions that are characteristic of the second stage of labor.

extended family Family form that includes the nuclear family and other blood-related persons.

external cephalic version (ECV) Turning the fetus to a vertex position by exertion of pressure on the fetus externally through the maternal abdomen.

extracorporeal membrane oxygenation (ECMO) Oxygenation of blood external to body using cardiopulmonary by-pass and a membrane oxygenator. Used primarily for newborns with refractory respiratory failure or meconium aspiration syndrome.

extrauterine Occurring outside the uterus.

   e. pregnancy Pregnancy in which the fertilized ovum implants itself outside the uterus.

extrusion reflex Infant automatically extends tongue when it is stimulated.

facies Pertaining to the appearance or expression of the face; certain congenital syndromes typically present with a specific facial appearance.

FAD Fetal activity determination; also called *fetal activity test* (FAT).

failure to thrive Condition in which neonate's or infant's growth and development patterns are below the norms for age.

fallopian tubes Two canals or oviducts extending laterally from each side of the uterus through which the ovum travels, after ovulation, to the uterus; also called uterine tubes.

false labor Uterine contractions that do not result in cervical dilatation, are irregular, are felt more in front, often do not last more than 20 seconds, and do not become longer or stronger.

false pelvis Part of the pelvis superior to a plane passing through the linea terminalis (brim or outlet).

family dynamics Process by which family members assume varying social roles.

family functions Activities carried out within families for the well-being of family members; including biologic, economic, educational, psychologic, and sociocultural aspects.

family stress theory Theory that explains how families react and adapt to stressors that they experience.

family systems theory Theory that conceptualizes the family as a unit and focuses on observing interactions among family members.

family violence Interpersonal violence including child, elder, sibling, and spouse.

fantasy child The imagined dream child; the "ideal" unborn child.

fantasy mom A composite of the ideal mother ("supermom") whom a woman envisions in her mind's eye but who may have enviable but totally unrealistic accomplishments to her credit.

feeding readiness cues Infant responses that indicate optimal times to begin a feeding. The baby may make mouthing motions, suck a fist, or awaken and cry.

Ferguson's reflex Reflex contractions of the uterus after stimulation of the cervix.

ferning (arborization) test The appearance of a fernlike pattern found on slides of certain fluids.

   ovulation f.t. Test in which cervical mucus, placed on a slide, dries in a branching pattern in the presence of high estrogen levels at the time of ovulation.

fertile period Period before and after ovulation during which the human ovum can be fertilized; usually 3 days before and 4 days after ovulation.

fertility Quality of being able to reproduce; also number of births per 1,000 women aged 15 through 44 years. See also *birth rate.*

fertilization Union of an ovum and a sperm

fetal Pertaining or relating to the fetus

   f. alcohol effect (FAE) Lesser set of the same symptoms that make up fetal alcohol syndrome.

   f. alcohol syndrome (FAS) Congenital abnormality or anomaly resulting from excessive maternal alcohol intake during pregnancy. It is characterized by typical craniofacial and limb defects, cardiovascular defects, intrauterine growth restriction, and developmental delay.

   f. asphyxia See *asphyxia, fetal.*

   f. attitude See *attitude, fetal.*

   f. compromise Evidence such as a nonreassuring fetal heart rate pattern that indicates the fetus may be in jeopardy.

   f. death See *death, fetal.*

   f. lie Relation of the fetal spine to the maternal spine; that is, in vertical lie, maternal and fetal spines are parallel and the fetal head or breech presents; in transverse lie, fetal spine is perpendicular to the maternal spine and the fetal shoulder presents.

   f. membrane See *membrane.*

   f. presentation The part of the fetus that enters the pelvic inlet first.

   f. heart rate (FHR) Beats per minute (bpm) of the fetal heart. Normal range is 120 to 160 bpm.

      acceleration Increase in fetal heart rate, usually seen as a reassuring sign.

      baseline Average fetal heart rate between uterine contractions.

      bradycardia Baseline fetal heart rate below 110 bpm.

      deceleration Slowing of fetal heart rate attributed to a parasympathetic response and described in relation to uterine contractions.

         early d. Onset corresponding to onset of uterine contraction, related to fetal head compression.

         late d. Onset after peak of contraction, continuing into interval after contraction; caused by uteroplacental insufficiency.

         variable d. Onset at any time unrelated to contraction; caused by cord compression.

         prolonged d. Slowing of fetal heart rate lasting longer than 2 minutes.

   f. scalp spiral electrode Internal signal source for electronically monitoring the fetal heart rate.

   f. tobacco syndrome Diagnostic term applicable to infants who fit criteria: mother who smoked more than 5 cigarettes a day during pregnancy and had no prenatal evidence of hypertension; infant has symmetric growth restriction, weighs less than 2,500 gm, and has no other cause of intrauterine growth restriction.

α-fetoprotein (AFP) Fetal antigen; elevated levels in amniotic fluid associated with neural tube defects.

fetotoxic Poisonous or destructive to the fetus.

fetus Child in utero from about the eighth week after conception, until birth.

fibroid Fibrous, encapsulated connective tissue tumor, especially of the uterus.

fimbria Structure resembling a fringe, particularly the fringelike end of the uterine tube.

first stage Stage of labor from the onset of regular uterine contractions to full dilatation of the cervix.

fissure Groove or open crack in tissue.

fistula Abnormal tubelike passage that forms between two normal cavities, possibly congenital or caused by trauma, abscesses, or inflammatory processes.

flaccid Having relaxed, limp, or absent muscle tone.

flaring of nostrils Widening of nostrils (alae nasi) during inspiration in the presence of air hunger; sign of respiratory distress.

flexion Opposite of extension. In obstetrics, resistance to the descent of the baby down the birth canal causes the head to flex, or bend, so that the chin approaches the chest. Thus the smallest diameter (suboccipitobregmatic) of the vertex presents.

focusing phase Third developmental task experienced by expectant fathers as identified by May. This phase is characterized by the father's active involvement in both the pregnancy and his relationship with his infant.

follicle Small secretory cavity or sac.

> **graafian f.** Mature, fully developed ovarian cyst containing the ripe ovum. The follicle secretes estrogens, and after ovulation the corpus luteum develops within the ruptured graafian follicle and secretes estrogen and progesterone.

follicle-stimulating hormone (FSH) Hormone produced by the anterior pituitary during the first half of the menstrual cycle. Stimulates development of the graafian follicle.

fomites Nonliving material on which disease-producing organisms may be conveyed (e.g., bed linen).

fontanel Broad area, or soft spot, consisting of a strong band of connective tissue contiguous with cranial bones and located at the junctions of the bones.

> **anterior f.** Diamond-shaped area between the frontal and two parietal bones just above the baby's forehead at the junction of the coronal and sagittal sutures.

> **mastoid f.** Posterolateral fontanel usually not palpable.

> **posterior f.** Small, triangular area between the occipital and parietal bones at the junction of the lambdoidal and sagittal sutures.

> **sagittal f.** Soft area located in the sagittal suture, halfway between the anterior and posterior fontanels; may be palpated in normal newborns and in some neonates with Down syndrome.

> **sphenoid f.** Anterolateral fontanel usually not palpable.

footling (incomplete) breech presentation See *breech presentation, footling.*

foramen ovale Septal opening between the atria of the fetal heart. The opening normally closes shortly after birth, but if it remains patent, surgical repair usually is necessary.

forceps Curved-bladed instruments used to protect head of fetus during birth and to apply traction to assist birth.

forceps-assisted birth Birth in which forceps are used to assist in delivery of the fetal head.

foreskin Prepuce, or loose fold of skin covering the glans penis.

fornix Any structure with an arched or vaultlike shape.

> **f. of the vagina** Anterior and posterior spaces, formed by the protrusion of the cervix into the vagina, into which the upper vagina is divided.

fourth stage of labor Initial period of recovery from childbirth. It is usually considered to last for the first 1 to 2 hours after the expulsion of the placenta.

fourth trimester Another term for the puerperium; the 3-month interval after the birth of the newborn that includes return of the reproductive organs to their nonpregnant state and psychologic adaptation to parenthood.

frank breech presentation See *breech presentation, frank.*

fraternal twins Nonidentical twins that come from two separate fertilized ova.

free-standing birth center A center that provides prenatal care, labor and birth, and postbirth care outside of a hospital setting.

frenulum Thin ridge of tissue in midline of undersurface of tongue extending from its base to varying distances from the tip of the tongue.

friability Easily broken. May refer to a fragile condition of the cervix, especially during pregnancy, that causes the cervix to bleed easily when touched.

Friedman's curve Labor curve; pattern of descent of presenting part and of dilatation of cervix; partogram.

FSH See *follicle-stimulating hormone.*

fundus Dome-shaped upper portion of the uterus between the points of insertion of the uterine tubes.

funic souffle See *souffle, funic.*

funis Cordlike structure, especially the umbilical cord.

galactosemia Inherited, autosomal recessive disorder of galactose metabolism, characterized by a deficiency of the enzyme galactose-1-phosphate uridyltransferase.

gamete Mature male or female germ cell; the mature sperm or ovum.

gastroschisis Abdominal wall defect at base of umbilical stalk.

gastrostomy Surgical creation of an artificial opening into the stomach through the abdominal wall, performed to feed a patient when oral feeding is not possible.

gate control theory Proposed in 1965 by Melzack and Wall, this theory explains the neurophysical mechanism underlying the perception of pain: the capacity of nerve pathways to transmit pain is reduced or completely blocked by using distraction techniques.

gavage Feeding by means of a tube passed through the nose or mouth to the stomach.

gender identity Sense or awareness of knowing to which sex one belongs. The process begins in infancy, continues throughout childhood, and is reinforced during adolescence.

gene Factor on a chromosome responsible for hereditary characteristics of offspring.

genetic Dependent on the genes. A genetic disorder may or may not be apparent at birth.

genetic counseling Process of determining the occurrence or risk of occurrence of a genetic disorder within a family and of providing appropriate information and advice about the courses of action that are available, whether care of a child already affected, prenatal diagnosis, termination of a pregnancy, sterilization, or artificial insemination is involved.

genitalia Organs of reproduction.

genome Complete copy of genetic material in an organism.

genotype Hereditary combinations in an individual determining physical and chemical characteristics. Some genotypes are not expressed until later in life (e.g., Huntington's chorea); some hide recessive genes, which can be expressed in offspring; and others are expressed only under the proper environmental conditions (e.g., diabetes mellitus appearing under the stress of obesity or pregnancy).

gestation Period of intrauterine fetal development from conception through birth; the period of pregnancy.

gestational age In fetal development, the number of completed weeks counting from the first day of the last normal menstrual cycle.

gestational diabetes Glucose intolerance first recognized during pregnancy.

gestational trophoblastic neoplasia (GTN) Persistent trophoblastic tissue that is presumed to be malignant.

GIFT Gamete intrafallopian transfer of ova and washed sperm into uterine tubes.

gingivitis Inflammation of the gums characterized by redness, swelling, and tendency to bleed.

glans penis Smooth, round head of the penis, analogous to the female glans clitoris.

glomerulonephritis Noninfectious disease of the glomerulus of the kidney, characterized by proteinuria, hematuria, decreased urine production, and edema.

glucose tolerance test A test of the body's ability to use carbohydrates; used as a screening measure for gestational diabetes.

glycosuria Presence of glucose (a sugar) in the urine.

glycosylated hemoglobin (Ghb) Glycohemoglobin, a minor hemoglobin with glucose attached. Ghb concentration represents the average blood glucose level over the previous several weeks and is a measurement for glycemic control in diabetic therapy.

gonad Gamete-producing, or sex, gland; the ovary or testis.

gonadotropic hormone Hormone that stimulates the gonads.

gonadotropin-releasing hormone (GnRH) Hormone released from hypothalamus that stimulates pituitary gland to produce FSH and LH.

Goodell's sign Softening of the cervix, a probable sign of pregnancy, occurring during the second month.

graafian follicle (vesicle) See *follicle, graafian.*

gravida Pregnant woman.

gravidity Number of times a woman has been pregnant.

grief responses The physical, emotional, social, and cognitive responses to the death of a loved one.

grieving process A complex of somatic and psychologic symptoms associated with some extreme sorrow or loss, specifically the death of a loved one.

growth spurts Times of increased neonatal growth that usually occur at approximately 6 to 10 days, 6 weeks, 3 months, and 4 to 5 months. The increased caloric needs necessitate more frequent feedings to increase the amount of milk needed.

grunt, expiratory Sign of respiratory distress (hyaline membrane disease [respiratory distress syndrome, or RDS] or advanced pneumonia) indicative of the body's attempt to hold air in the alveoli for better gaseous exchange.

gynecoid pelvis Pelvis in which the inlet is round instead of oval or blunt; typical female pelvis.

gynecology Study of the diseases of the female, especially of the genital, urinary, and rectal organs.

habitual (recurrent) abortion See *abortion, habitual.*

habituation An acquired tolerance from repeated exposure to a particular stimulus. Also called *negative adaptation;* a decline and eventual elimination of a conditioned response by repetition of the conditioned stimulus.

haploid number Having half the normal number of chromosomes found in somatic (body) cells; 23 chromosomes.

harlequin sign Rare color change of no pathologic significance occurring between the longitudinal halves of the neonate's body. When infant is placed on one side, the dependent half is noticeably pinker than the superior half.

Hegar's sign Softening of the lower uterine segment that is classified as a probable sign of pregnancy and that may be present during the second and third months of pregnancy and is palpated during bimanual examination.

HELLP syndrome Condition characterized by hemolysis, elevated liver enzymes, and low platelet count; is a form of severe preeclampsia.

hematocrit Volume of red blood cells per deciliter (dl) of circulating blood; packed cell volume (PCV).

hematoma Collection of blood in a tissue; a bruise or blood tumor.

hematopoiesis Production of blood cells.

hemoconcentration Increase in the number of red blood cells in proportion to the volume, resulting from either a decrease in plasma volume or increased erythropoiesis.

hemodilution An increase in fluid content of blood, resulting in diminution of the proportion of formed elements.

hemoglobin Component of red blood cells consisting of globin, a protein, and hematin, an organic iron compound.

   h. electrophoresis Test to diagnose sickle cell disease in newborns. Cord blood is used.

hemolytic disease of the newborn Breakdown of fetal red blood cells by maternal antibodies, usually from an Rh-negative mother.

hemorrhagic disease of newborn Bleeding disorder during first few days of life based on a deficiency of vitamin K.

hemorrhagic shock Clinical condition in which the peripheral blood flow is inadequate to return sufficient blood to the heart for normal function, particularly oxygen transport to the organs or tissue.

hereditary Pertaining to a trait or characteristic transmitted from parent to offspring by way of the genes; used synonymously with *genetic.*

hermaphrodite Person having genital and sexual characteristics of both sexes.

heterozygous Having two dissimilar genes at the same site, or locus, on paired chromosomes (e.g., at the sites for eye color, one chromosome carrying the gene for brown, the other for blue).

high risk Increased possibility of suffering harm, damage, loss, or death. See also *risk factor.*

hirsutism Condition characterized by the excessive growth of hair.

Homan's sign Early sign of phlebothrombosis of the deep veins of the calf in which there are complaints of pain when the leg is in extension and the foot is dorsiflexed.

home birth Planned birth of the child at home, usually done under the supervision of a midwife.

homologous Similar in structure or origin but not necessarily in function.

homologous insemination Insemination in which the semen specimen is provided by the husband. The procedure is used primarily in cases of impotence or when the husband is incapable of sexual intercourse because of some physical disability.

homosexual family Family in which parents form a homosexual union. Children may be the offspring of a previous heterosexual union or may be conceived by one or both members of a homosexual couple through artificial insemination or by adoption.

homozygous Having two similar genes at the same locus, or site, on paired chromosomes.

hormone Chemical substance produced in an organ or gland that is conveyed through the blood to another organ or part of the body, stimulating it to increased functional activity or secretion. See also *specific hormones.*

hormone replacement therapy (HRT) Progestin and estrogen given for menopausal symptoms. See *estrogen replacement therapy.*

hot flash (flush) Transient sensation of warmth experienced by some women during or after menopause, resulting from autonomic vasomotor disturbances that accompany changes in the neurohormonal activity of the ovaries, hypothalamus, and pituitary gland.

human chorionic gonadotropin (hCG) Hormone that is produced by chorionic villi; the biologic marker in pregnancy tests.

hyaline membrane disease (HMD) See *respiratory distress syndrome (RDS).*

hydatidiform mole (molar pregnancy) Gestational trophoblastic neoplasm usually resulting from fertilization of egg that has no nucleus or an inactivated nucleus.

hydramnios (polyhydramnios) Amniotic fluid in excess of 1.5 liters; often indicative of fetal anomaly and frequently seen in poorly controlled, insulin-dependent, diabetic pregnant women even if there is no coexisting fetal anomaly.

hydrocele Collection of fluid in a saclike cavity, especially in the sac that surrounds the testis, causing the scrotum to swell.

hydrocephalus Accumulation of fluid in the subdural or subarachnoid spaces.

hydrops fetalis Most severe expression of fetal hemolytic disorder, a possible sequela to maternal Rh isoimmunization; infants exhibit gross edema (anasarca), cardiac decompensation, and profound pallor from anemia, and seldom survive.

hymen Membranous fold that normally partially covers the entrance to the vagina.

hymenal tag Normally occurring redundant hymenal tissue protruding from the floor of the vagina of a newborn female that disappears spontaneously in a few weeks after birth.

hyperbilirubinemia Elevation of unconjugated serum bilirubin concentrations.

hyperemesis gravidarum Abnormal condition of pregnancy characterized by protracted vomiting, weight loss, and fluid and electrolyte imbalance.

hyperesthesia Unusual sensibility to sensory stimuli, such as pain or touch.

hyperglycemia Excess glucose in the blood.

hyperplasia Increase in number of cells; formation of new tissue.

hyperreflexia Increased action of the reflexes.

hyperthyroidism Excessive functional activity of the thyroid gland.

hypertonic uterine dysfunction Uncoordinated, painful, frequent uterine contractions that do not cause dilatation and effacement; primary dysfunctional labor.

hypertrophic cardiomyopathy Enlargement and loss of elasticity of the heart muscle, that is, the septum and the left ventricle, causing impaired filling during diastole resulting in decreased cardiac output.

hypertrophy Enlargement, or increase in size, of existing cells.

hyperventilation Rapid, shallow (or prolonged, deep) respirations resulting in respiratory alkalosis: a decrease in H^+ concentration and PCO_2 and an increase in the blood pH and the ratio of $NaHCO_3$ to H_2CO_3. Symptoms may include faintness, palpitations, and carpopedal (hands and feet) muscular spasms.

hypocalcemia Deficiency in calcium often seen in preterm infants, in infants of diabetic mothers, or after long stressful labor in full-term infants.

hypofibrinogenemia Deficient level of a blood-clotting factor, fibrinogen, in the blood; in obstetrics, it occurs after complications of abruptio placentae or retention of a dead fetus.

hypogastric arteries Branches of the right and left iliac arteries carrying deoxygenated blood from the fetus through the umbilical cord, where they are known as *umbilical arteries,* to the placenta.

hypoglycemia Less than normal amount of glucose in the blood, usually caused by administration of too much insulin, excessive secretion of insulin by the islet cells of the pancreas, or dietary deficiency.

hypospadias Anomalous positioning of urinary meatus on undersurface of penis or close to or just inside the vagina.

hypothalamus Portion of the diencephalon of the brain forming the floor and part of the lateral wall of the third ventricle. It activates, controls, and integrates the peripheral autonomic nervous system, endocrine processes, and many somatic functions, such as body temperature, sleep, and appetite.

hypothermia Temperature that falls below normal range, that is, below 35° C, usually caused by exposure to cold.

hypothyroidism Deficiency of thyroid gland activity with underproduction of thyroxine.

hypotonic uterine dysfunction Weak, ineffective uterine contractions usually occurring in the active phase of labor; often related to cephalopelvic disproportion (CPD) or malposition of the fetus.

hypoxemia Reduction in arterial PO_2 resulting in metabolic acidosis by forcing anaerobic glycolysis, pulmonary vasoconstriction, and direct cellular damage.

hypoxia Insufficient availability of oxygen to meet the metabolic needs of body tissue.

hysterectomy Surgical removal of the uterus.

    TAH-BSO Total abdominal hysterectomy and bilateral salpingo-oophorectomy; removal of uterus, both tubes, and both ovaries.

    TVH Total vaginal hysterectomy.

hysterosalpingography Recording by x-rays of the uterus and uterine tubes after they are injected with radiopaque material.

hysterotomy Surgical incision into the uterus.

iatrogenic Caused by a health care provider's words, actions, or treatment.

icterus neonatorum Jaundice in the newborn.

idiopathic peripartum cardiomyopathy. A primary disease of the heart muscle with no apparent cause, occurring during the peripartum period.

IDM Infant of a diabetic mother.

Immunity

    acquired i. Protection against microorganisms that develops in response to actual infection or transfer of antibody from an immune donor.

    active i. Protection against specific microorganisms that develops in response to actual infection or vaccination.

    natural i. Nonspecific protection against microorganisms. Natural immunity is the first line of defense and includes skin and phagocytic cells.

    passive i. Protection against specific microorganisms that develops in response to the transfer of antibody or lymphocytes from an immune donor.

immunocompetent Ability of the immune system to respond appropriately to foreign antigens and to develop antigen-specific antibodies.

immunoglobin

    IgA Primary immunoglobulin in colostrum.

    IgG Transplacentally acquired immunoglobulin that confers passive immunity to the fetus against the infections to which the mother is immune.

    IgM Immunoglobulin neonate can manufacture soon after birth. Fetus produces it in the presence of amnionitis.

immunology The study of the components essential to the recognition and disposal of foreign (nonself or antigenic) material and maintenance of body defenses.

impaired fertility Inability to conceive or to carry fetus to live birth at a time a couple chooses to do so.

implantation Embedding of the fertilized ovum in the uterine mucosa; nidation.

impotence Term designating a man's inability, partial or complete, to perform sexual intercourse or to achieve orgasm; erectile dysfunction.

inborn error of metabolism Hereditary deficiency of a specific enzyme needed for normal metabolism of specific chemicals (e.g., deficiency of phenylalanine hydroxylase results in phenylketonuria [PKU]; a deficiency of hexosaminidase results in Tay-Sachs disease).

incompetent cervix Cervix that is unable to remain closed until a pregnancy reaches term because of a mechanical defect in the cervix resulting in dilatation and effacement usually during the second or early third trimester of pregnancy. Premature dilatation of the cervix is the preferred term.

incomplete abortion See *abortion, incomplete.*

increment Increase, or buildup, as of a contraction.

induced abortion See *abortion, induced.*

induction Artificial stimulation of labor.

inertia Sluggishness or inactivity; in obstetrics, refers to the absence or weakness of uterine contractions during labor.

inevitable abortion See *abortion, inevitable.*

infant Child who is under 1 year of age.

infective endocarditis Inflammation of the inner layer of the heart muscle (endocardium), caused by a bacterial infection.

infertility Decreased capacity to conceive.

informed consent Choice based on full comprehension of relevant information.

inhalation analgesia Reduction of pain by administration of anesthetic gas. Occasionally given during the second stage of labor. Consciousness is retained to allow the woman to follow instructions and to avoid the adverse effects of general anesthesia.

inlet Passage leading into a cavity.

    pelvic i. Upper brim of the pelvic cavity.

insemination Introduction of semen into the vagina or uterus for impregnation.

    therapeutic i. Introduction of semen by instrument injection into the vagina or uterus for impregnation.

instrumental style Characteristic style displayed by expectant fathers that emphasizes tasks to be accomplished.

insulin Hormone produced by the beta cells of the pancreatic islets of Langerhans; promotes glucose transport into the cells; aids in protein and lipid synthesis.

internal os Inside mouth or opening.

intertuberous diameter Distance between ischial tuberosities. Measured to determine dimension of pelvic outlet.

intervillous space Irregular space in the maternal portion of the placenta, filled with maternal blood and serving as the site of maternal-fetal gas, nutrient, and waste exchange.

intoxication Development of a reversible substance-specific syndrome caused by the recent ingestion of or exposure to a substance. The symptoms of intoxication are attributable to the direct physiologic effects of the substance on the central nervous system.

intrapartum During labor and birth.

intrathecal Within the subarachnoid space.

intrauterine device (IUD) Small plastic or metal form placed in the uterus to prevent implantation of a fertilized ovum.

intrauterine growth restriction (IUGR) Fetal undergrowth of any cause, such as deficient nutrient supply or intrauterine infection, or associated with congenital malformation.

intrauterine pressure catheter (IUPC) Catheter inserted into uterine cavity to assess uterine activity and pressure by electronic means.

intrauterine resuscitation Interventions initiated when nonreassuring fetal heart rate patterns are noted and are directed at improving intrauterine blood flow.

introitus Entrance into a canal or cavity such as the vagina.

intussusception Prolapse of one segment of bowel into the lumen of the adjacent segment.

in utero Within or inside the uterus.

in vitro fertilization Fertilization in a culture dish or test tube.

inversion Turning end for end, upside down, or inside out.
> **i. of uterus** Condition in which the uterus is turned inside out so that the fundus intrudes into the cervix or vagina, caused by a too vigorous removal of the placenta before it is detached by the natural process of labor.

involution (1) Rolling or turning inward. (2) Reduction in size of the uterus after birth and its return to its nonpregnant condition.

isoimmune hemolytic disease Breakdown (hemolysis) of fetal/neonatal Rh-positive red blood cells because of Rh antibodies formed by an Rh-negative mother who had been previously exposed to Rh-positive RBCs.

isoimmunization Development of antibodies in a species of animal with antigens from the same species (e.g., development of anti-Rh antibodies in an Rh-negative person).

ITP Abbreviation for idiopathic thrombocytopenic purpura.

jaundice Yellow discoloration of the body tissues caused by the deposit of bile pigments (unconjugated bilirubin); icterus.
> **breast milk j.** Term used by some clinicians to describe late-onset (after day 5) jaundice in the breastfed infant. A cause for this phenomenon has not been conclusively identified. See *physiologic j.*
> **pathologic j.** Jaundice usually first noticeable within 24 hours after birth; caused by some abnormal condition such as an Rh or ABO incompatibility and resulting in bilirubin toxicity (e.g., kernicterus).
> **physiologic j.** Yellow tinge to skin and mucous membranes in response to increased serum levels of unconjugated bilirubin; not usually apparent until after 24 hours; also called *neonatal jaundice, physiologic hyperbilirubinemia.*

kangaroo care Skin-to-skin infant care, especially for preterm infants, which provides warmth to infant. Infant is placed naked or diapered against mother's or father's bare chest and is covered with parent's shirt or a warm blanket.

karyotype Schematic arrangement of the chromosomes within a cell to demonstrate their numbers and morphology.

Kegel exercises Pelvic muscle exercises to strengthen the pubococcygeal muscles.

kernicterus Bilirubin encephalopathy involving the deposit of unconjugated bilirubin in brain cells, resulting in death or impaired intellectual, perceptive, or motor function and adaptive behavior.

ketoacidosis The accumulation of ketone bodies in the blood as a consequence of hyperglycemia; leads to metabolic acidosis.

Kleihauer-Betke test Laboratory test that detects the presence of fetal blood cells in the maternal circulation.

labia majora Two folds of skin containing fat and covered with hair that lie on either side of the vaginal opening and form each side of the vulva. (Singular, *labium majus.*)

labia minora Two thin folds of delicate, hairless skin inside the labia majora. (Singular, *labium minus.*)

labor Series of processes by which the fetus is expelled from the uterus; parturition; childbirth.
> **active phase** Phase in first stage of labor from 4 to 7 cm in dilatation.
> **first stage** Stage of labor from the onset of regular uterine contractions to full dilatation of the cervix.
> **latent phase** Phase in first stage of labor from none to 3 cm in dilatation.
> **second stage** Stage of labor from full dilatation of the cervix to the birth of the baby.
> **third stage** Stage of labor from the birth of the baby to the expulsion of the placenta.
> **transition phase** Phase in first stage of labor from 8 to 10 cm in dilatation.

labor, delivery, recovery (LDR) A single room where all steps of the birth process occur. Avoids having to move the woman to different rooms for each phase of the birth process. The woman is moved to a postpartum room after recovery.

labor, delivery, recovery, postpartum (LDRP) A single room where all steps of the birth process and hospitalization occur. The woman stays in the same room throughout her hospitalization.

laceration Irregular tear of wound tissue; in obstetrics, it usually refers to a tear in the perineum, vagina, or cervix caused by childbirth.

lactase Enzyme necessary for the digestion of lactose.

lactation Function of secreting milk or period during which milk is secreted.
> **l. consultant** A health care professional who has specialized training in breastfeeding.
> **l. suppression** Stopping the production of breast milk through the use of medication (rare) or nonpharmacologic interventions.

lactogenesis stage I Initial synthesis of milk components (colostrum) that begins during pregnancy.

lactogenesis stage II Beginning of milk production 2 to 5 days' postpartum.

lactogen Medication or other substance that enhances the production and secretion of milk.

lactose intolerance Inherited absence of the enzyme lactose.

lactosuria Presence of lactose in the urine during late pregnancy and during lactation. Must be differentiated from glycosuria.

Lamaze (psychoprophylaxis) method Method of preparation for childbirth developed in the 1950s by a French obstetrician, Fernand Lamaze, that gained popularity in the United States in the 1960s. It requires practice at home and coaching during labor and birth. The goals are to minimize fear and the perception of pain and to promote positive family relationships by using both mental and physical preparation.

lambdoid suture Suture line extending across the posterior third of the skull, separating the occipital bone from the two parietal bones, and forming the base of the triangular posterior fontanel.

***Laminaria* tent** Cone of dried seaweed that swells as it absorbs moisture. Used to dilate the cervix nontraumatically in preparation for an induced abortion or in preparation for induction of labor.

lanugo Downy, fine hair characteristic of the fetus between 20 weeks of gestation and birth that is most noticeable over the shoulder, forehead, and cheeks but is found on nearly all parts of the body except the palms of the hands, soles of the feet, and the scalp.

laparoscopy Examination of the interior of the abdomen by insertion of a small telescope through the anterior abdominal wall.

large for gestational age (LGA) Exhibiting excessive growth for gestational age.

last menstrual period (LMP) Date of the first day of the last menstrual bleeding.

latch-on Attachment of the infant to the breast for feeding.

latent phase Phase in first stage of labor from none to 3 cm in dilatation.

lecithin A phospholipid that decreases surface tension; surfactant.

lecithin/sphingomyelin ratio Ratio of lecithin to sphingomyelin in the amniotic fluid. It is used to assess maturity of the fetal lung.

leiomyoma Benign smooth muscle tumor.

Leopold's maneuver Four maneuvers for diagnosing the fetal position by external palpation of the mother's abdomen.

letdown or letdown reflex See *milk ejection reflex.*

letting-go phase Interdependent phase after birth in which the mother and family move forward as a system with interacting members.

leukorrhea White or yellowish mucous discharge from the cervical canal or the vagina that may be normal physiologically or caused by pathologic states of the vagina and endocervix (e.g., *Trichomonas vaginalis* infections).

LH See *luteinizing hormone (LH).*

libido Sexual drive.

lie Relationship existing between the long axis of the fetus and the long axis of the mother. In a longitudinal lie, the fetus is lying lengthwise or vertically, whereas in a transverse lie, the fetus is lying crosswise or horizontally in the uterus.

lightening Sensation of decreased abdominal distention produced by uterine descent into the pelvic cavity as the fetal presenting part settles into the pelvis. It usually occurs 2 weeks before the onset of labor in nulliparas.

linea nigra Line of darker pigmentation seen in some women during the latter part of pregnancy that appears on the middle of the abdomen and extends from the symphysis pubis toward the umbilicus.

linea terminalis Line dividing the upper (false) pelvis from the lower (true) pelvis.

lithotomy position Position in which the woman lies on her back with her knees flexed and with abducted thighs drawn up toward her chest.

live birth Birth in which the neonate, regardless of gestational age, manifests any heartbeat, breathes, or displays voluntary movement.

living ligature Configuration of smooth muscle fibers of the uterus that gives them the capacity to ligate blood vessels and control blood loss after abortion and childbirth.

local infiltration anesthesia Process by which a substance such as a local anesthetic drug is deposited within the tissue to anesthetize a limited region.

lochia Vaginal discharge during the puerperium consisting of blood, tissue, and mucus.

   l. alba Thin, yellowish to white, vaginal discharge that follows lochia serosa on about the tenth day after birth and that may last from 2 to 6 weeks' postpartum.

   l. rubra Red, distinctly blood-tinged vaginal flow that follows birth and lasts 2 to 4 days.

   l. serosa Serous, pinkish brown, watery vaginal discharge that follows lochia rubra until about the tenth day after birth.

low birth weight (LBW) An infant birth weight of less than 2,500 gm.

low spinal (saddle) block anesthesia Type of regional anesthesia produced by injection of a local anesthetic solution into the cerebrospinal fluid intrathecal (subarachnoid) space in the spinal canal.

L/S ratio See *lecithin/sphingomyelin ratio.*

lunar month Four weeks (28 days).

luteinizing hormone (LH) Hormone produced by the anterior pituitary that stimulates ovulation and the development of the corpus luteum.

luteotropin (LTH) Lactogenic hormone; prolactin; an adenohypophyseal hormone.

lysozyme Enzyme with antiseptic qualities that destroys foreign organisms and that is found in blood cells of the granulocytic and monocytic series and is also normally present in saliva, sweat, tears, and breast milk.

maceration (1) Process of softening a solid by soaking it in a fluid. (2) Softening and breaking down of fetal skin from prolonged exposure to amniotic fluid as seen in a postterm infant. Also seen in a dead fetus.

macroglossia Hypertrophy of tongue or tongue large for oral cavity; seen in some preterm neonates and in neonates with Down syndrome.

macrophage Any phagocytic cell of the reticuloendothelial system, including Kupffer cells in the liver, splenocytes in the spleen, and histocytes in the loose connective tissue.

macrosomia Large body size as seen in neonates of diabetic or prediabetic mothers.

magnetic resonance imaging (MRI) Noninvasive nuclear procedure for imaging tissues with high fat and water content; in obstetrics, uses include evaluation of fetal structures, placenta, amniotic fluid volume.

malpractice Professional negligence that is the proximate cause of injury or harm to a client, resulting from a lack of professional knowledge, experience, or skill that can be expected in others in the profession or from a failure to exercise reasonable care or judgment in the application of professional knowledge, experience, or skill.

mammary gland Compound gland of the female breast that is made up of lobes and lobules that secrete milk for nourishment of the young. Rudimentary mammary glands exist in the male.

mammography X-ray examination technique used to screen for and evaluate breast lesions.

managed care System of guiding care to promote efficiency and cost effectiveness.

Marfan syndrome An inherited disorder that is an autosomal dominant trait resulting in an abnormal condition characterized by elongation of the bones, causing significant musculoskeletal disturbances. Also usually associated with cardiovascular and eye abnormalities.

mask of pregnancy See *chloasma*.

mastectomy Excision, or removal, of the mammary gland.
> **modified radical m.** Removal of breast tissue, skin, and axillary nodes.

mastitis Infection in a breast, usually confined to a milk duct, characterized by influenza-like symptoms and redness and tenderness in the affected breast.

maternal adaptation Process that a woman goes through in adjusting to her version of the maternal role; includes three phases: taking in, taking hold, and letting go.

maternal mortality Death of a woman related to childbearing.

maturation (1) Process of attaining maximum development. (2) In biology, a process of cell division during which the number of chromosomes in the germ cells (sperm or ova) is reduced to one half the number (haploid) characteristic of the species.

maturational crisis Crisis that arises during normal growth and development, such as puberty.

McDonald's sign Easy flexion of the fundus on the cervix.

mean arterial pressure (MAP) Average of systolic and diastolic blood pressures. A MAP of greater than 90 mm Hg in the second trimester is associated with an increase in the incidence of pregnancy-induced hypertension in the third trimester.

meatus Opening from an internal structure to the outside (e.g., urethral meatus).

mechanical ventilation Technique used to provide predetermined amount of oxygen; requires intubation.

meconium First stools of infant: viscid, sticky; dark greenish brown, almost black; sterile; odorless.
> **m. aspiration syndrome (MAS)** Function of fetal hypoxia: with hypoxia, the anal sphincter relaxes and meconium is released; reflex gasping movements draw meconium and other particulate matter in the amniotic fluid into the infant's bronchial tree, obstructing the airflow after birth.
> **m. ileus** Lower intestinal obstruction by thick, puttylike, inspissated (dried) meconium that may be the result of deficiency of trypsin production in the newborn with cystic fibrosis.
> **m.-stained fluid** In response to hypoxia, fetal intestinal activity increases and anal sphincter relaxes, resulting in the passage of meconium, which imparts a greenish coloration.

meiosis Process by which germ cells divide and decrease their chromosomal number by one half.

membrane(s) Thin, pliable layer of tissue that lines a cavity or tube, separates structures, or covers an organ or structure; in obstetrics, the amnion and chorion surrounding the fetus.
> **artificial rupture of m. (AROM)** Rupture of membranes using a plastic amnihook or surgical clamp.
> **preterm rupture of m. (PROM)** Spontaneous rupture of membranes before 37 weeks of gestation.
> **spontaneous rupture of m. (SROM)** Rupture of membranes by natural means.

menarche Onset, or beginning, of menstrual function.

meningomyelocele Saclike protrusion of the spinal cord through a congenital defect in the vertebral column.

menopausal hormone therapy (MHT) Hormonal therapy for menopausal symptoms, usually estrogen and progestin.

menopause From the Greek word *mēn* (month) and Greek word *pausis* (cessation), the actual permanent cessation of menstrual cycles; so diagnosed after 1 year without menses.

menorrhagia Abnormally profuse or excessive menstrual flow.

menses (menstruation) (Latin plural of *mensis* "month.") Periodic vaginal discharge of bloody fluid from the nonpregnant uterus that occurs from the age of puberty to menopause.

mentum Chin, a fetal reference point in designating position (e.g., "left mentoanterior" [LMA], meaning that the fetal chin is presenting in the left anterior quadrant of the maternal pelvis).

mesoderm Embryonic middle layer of germ cells giving rise to all types of muscles, connective tissue, bone marrow, blood, lymphoid tissue, and urogenital system.

metastasis Process by which tumor cells spread from site of origin to distant parts of the body.

metrorrhagia Abnormal bleeding from the uterus, particularly when it occurs at any time other than the menstrual period.

microcephaly Congenital anomaly characterized by abnormal smallness of the head in relation to the rest of the body and by underdevelopment of the brain, resulting in some degree of mental retardation.

midwife One who practices the art of helping and aiding a woman to give birth.
> **certified nurse m.** Registered nurse with advanced education in midwifery.
> **lay m.** Midwife who learned skills through practice; has no formal education in midwifery

milia Unopened sebaceous glands appearing as tiny, white, pinpoint papules on forehead, nose, cheeks, and chin of a neonate that disappear spontaneously in a few days or weeks.

milk ejection reflex (MER) Release of milk caused by the contraction of the myoepithelial cells within the milk glands in response to oxytocin; also called *letdown*.

milk-leg Thrombophlebitis of femoral vein resulting in edema of leg and pain; may occur after difficult vaginal birth.

milk transfer Infant's removal of milk from the breast, which is dependent on correct latch-on and the efficiency of the baby's suck, as well as the mother's milk ejection reflex.

miscarriage Spontaneous abortion; lay term usually referring to the loss of the fetus.

missed abortion See *abortion, missed*.

mitleiden "Suffering along," or the psychosomatic symptoms of fathers-to-be.

mitosis Process of somatic cell division in which a single cell divides, but both of the new cells have the same number of chromosomes as the first.

mitral valve prolapse (MVP) A disorder in which one or both of the cusp(s) of the mitral valve protrude backward into the left atrium during ventricular systole, resulting in incomplete closure of the valve. A midsystolic click or a late systolic murmur may be heard.

mitral valve stenosis Narrowing of the opening of the mitral valve caused by stiffening of value leaflets, obstructing the blood flow from the atrium to the ventricle.

mittelschmerz Abdominal pain in the region of an ovary during ovulation that usually occurs midway through the menstrual cycle. Present in many women, mittelschmerz is useful for identifying ovulation, thus pinpointing the fertile period of the cycle.

molding Overlapping of cranial bones or shaping of the fetal head to accommodate and conform to the bony and soft parts of the mother's birth canal during labor.

mongolian spot Bluish gray or dark nonelevated pigmented area usually found over the lower back and buttocks present at birth in some infants, primarily nonwhite. The spot usually fades by school age.

mongolism See *Down syndrome*.

moniliasis See *candidiasis*.

monitrice One trained in psychoprophylactic methods and who supports women during labor.

monosomy Chromosomal aberration characterized by the absence of one chromosome from the normal diploid complement.

monozygotic Originating or coming from a single fertilized ovum, such as identical twins.

monozygotic twins See *twins, monozygotic*.

mons veneris Pad of fatty tissue and coarse skin that overlies the symphysis pubis in the woman and that, after puberty, is covered with hair.

Montgomery's glands (tubercles) Small, nodular prominences (sebaceous glands) on the areolas around the nipples of the breasts that enlarge during pregnancy and lactation.

mood disorders Disorders that have a disturbance in the prevailing emotional state as the dominant feature. Cause is unknown.

moratorium phase The second developmental task experienced by expectant fathers as identified by May. During this phase the expectant father adjusts to the reality of pregnancy.

morbidity (1) Condition of being diseased. (2) Number of cases of disease or of sick persons in relationship to a specific population; incidence.

morning sickness Nausea and vomiting that affect some women during the first few months of their pregnancy; may occur at any time of day.

Moro's reflex Normal, generalized reflex in a young infant elicited by a sudden loud noise or by striking the table next to the child, resulting in flexion of the legs, an embracing posture of the arms, and usually a brief cry. Also called *startle reflex*.

mortality (1) Quality or state of being subject to death. (2) Number of deaths in relation to a specific population; incidence.

　fetal m. Number of fetal deaths per 1,000 births (or per live births). See also *death, fetal*.

　infant m. Number of deaths per 1,000 children 1 year of age or younger.

　maternal m. Number of maternal deaths per 100,000 births.

　neonatal m. Number of neonatal deaths per 1,000 births (or per live births). See also *neonatal mortality*.

　perinatal m. Combined fetal and neonatal mortality. See also *death, perinatal*.

morula Developmental stage of the fertilized ovum in which there is a solid mass of cells resembling a mulberry.

mosaicism Condition in which some somatic cells are normal, whereas others show chromosomal aberrations.

mourning The process of finding the answers to the questions surrounding the loss, coping with grief responses, and determining how to live again.

multigravida Woman who has been pregnant two or more times.

multipara Woman who has carried two or more pregnancies to viability, whether they ended in live infants or stillbirths.

multifetal pregnancy Pregnancy in which there is more than one fetus in the uterus at the same time; multiple pregnancy.

mutation Change in a gene or chromosome in gametes that may be transmitted to offspring.

mutuality Component of parent-infant attachment; infant behaviors and characteristics call forth corresponding parent behaviors and characteristics.

myelomeningocele External sac containing meninges, spinal fluid, and nerves that protrudes through defect in vertebral column.

Nägele's (or Naegele's) rule Method for calculating the estimated date of birth (EDB) or "due date."

narcotic antagonist A compound such as naloxone (Narcan) that promptly reverses the effects of narcotics such as meperidine (Demerol).

natal Relating or pertaining to birth.

navel Depression in the center of the abdomen, where the umbilical cord was attached to the fetus; umbilicus.

necrotizing enterocolitis (NEC) Acute inflammatory bowel disorder that occurs primarily in preterm or low-birth-weight neonates. It is characterized by ischemic necrosis (death) of the gastrointestinal mucosa, which may lead to perforation and peritonitis; formula-fed infants are at higher risk for this disease.

negligence Commission of an act that a prudent person would not have done or the omission of a duty that a prudent person would have fulfilled, resulting in injury or harm to another person. In particular, in a malpractice suit a professional person is negligent if harm to a patient results from such an act or such a failure to act, but it must be proved that other prudent persons of the same profession would ordinarily have acted differently under the same circumstances.

neonatal abstinence syndrome Signs and symptoms associated with drug withdrawal in the neonate.

neonatal mortality Statistical rate of infant death during the first 28 days after live birth, expressed as the number of such deaths per 1,000 live births in a specific geographic area or institution in a given period of time.

neonatal narcosis Central nervous system (CNS) depression in the newborn caused by a narcotic; may be exhibited by respiratory depression, hypertonia, lethargy, and delay in temperature regulation.

neonatology Branch of medicine that studies care of the neonate.

neoplasia Growth of new tissue; tumor that serves no physiologic function; may be benign or malignant.

neural tube Tube formed from fusion of the neural folds from which develop the brain and spinal cord.

   n. t. defect Improper development of tube resulting in malformation of brain or spinal cord; see α-*fetoprotein*.

neutral thermal environment (NTE) Environment that enables the neonate to maintain a body temperature of at least 36.6° C with minimum use of oxygen and energy.

nevus Natural blemish or mark; a congenital circumscribed deposit of pigmentation in the skin; mole.

   n. flammeus Port-wine stain; reddish, usually flat, discoloration of the face or neck. Because of its large size and color, it is considered a serious deformity.

   n. vasculosus (strawberry hemangioma) Elevated lesion of immature capillaries and endothelial cells that regresses over a period of years.

nidation Implantation of the fertilized ovum in the endometrium, or lining, of the uterus.

nipple confusion Difficulty experienced by some infants in mastering breastfeeding after having been given a pacifier or bottle. This problem appears to be more related to tactile sensation than flow of liquid.

nipple cup A device used to make inverted nipples erectile.

nonmaleficence The principle in bioethics directing us to act so as to avoid causing harm.

nonnutritive sucking Use of a pacifier by infants.

nonreassuring fetal heart rate pattern Fetal heart rate pattern that indicates the fetus is not well oxygenated and requires intervention.

nonshivering thermogenesis Infant's method of producing heat from brown fat by increasing metabolic rate.

nonstress test (NST) Evaluation of fetal response (fetal heart rate) to natural contractile uterine activity or to an increase in fetal activity.

normoglycemia Blood glucose level within normal limits; glycemic control.

nosocomial Pertaining to a hospital.

nuchal cord Encircling of fetal neck by one or more loops of umbilical cord.

nuclear family Family form consisting of parents and their dependent children.

nulligravida Woman who has never been pregnant.

nullipara Woman who has not yet carried a pregnancy to viability.

nurse practitioner Registered nurse who has additional education to practice nursing in an expanded role.

observer style Characteristic style described by May that is displayed by expectant fathers who show a detached approach to involvement in his partner's pregnancy.

occipitobregmatic Pertaining to the occiput (the back part of the skull) and the bregma (junction of the coronal and sagittal sutures) or anterior fontanel.

occiput Back part of the head or skull.

oligohydramnios Abnormally small amount or absence of amniotic fluid; often indicative of fetal urinary tract defect.

oliguria Urine output below 25 to 30 ml by the kidneys for 2 consecutive hours.

omphalitis Inflammation of the umbilical stump characterized by redness, edema, and purulent exudate in severe infections.

omphalocele Congenital defect resulting from failure of closure of the abdominal wall or muscles and leading to hernia of abdominal contents through the navel.

oocyte Primordial or incompletely developed ovum.

oogenesis Formation and development of the ovum.

operculum Plug of mucus that fills the cervical canal during pregnancy.

ophthalmia neonatorum Infection in the neonate's eyes usually resulting from gonorrheal or other infection contracted when the fetus passes through the birth canal (vagina).

opisthotonos Tetanic spasm resulting in an arched, hyperextended position of the body.

oral GTT (glucose tolerance test) Test for blood glucose after oral ingestion of a concentrated sugar solution.

orchitis Inflammation of one or both of the testes, characterized by swelling and pain, often caused by mumps, syphilis, or tuberculosis.

orifice Normal mouth, entrance, or opening, to any aperture.

os Mouth, or opening.

   external o. (o. externum) External opening of the cervical canal.

   internal o. (o. internum) Internal opening of the cervical canal.

   o. uteri Mouth, or opening, of the uterus.

ossification Mineralization of fetal bones.

osteoporosis Deossification of bone tissue resulting in structural weakness; decreased bone mass increasing risk of fractures, especially after menopause.

outlet Opening by which something can leave.

   pelvic o. Lower aperture, or opening, of the true pelvis.

ovary One of two glands in the female situated on either side of the pelvic cavity that produces the female reproductive cell, the ovum, and two known hormones, estrogen and progesterone.

ovulation Periodic ripening and discharge of the ovum from the ovary, usually 14 days before the onset of menstrual flow.

   o. method Control of fertility using evaluation of cervical mucus throughout the menstrual cycle; ovulation occurs just after the appearance of the peak mucus sign; Billings method.

ovum Female germ, or reproductive cell, produced by the ovary; egg.

oxygen toxicity Oxygen overdosage that results in pathologic tissue changes (e.g., retinopathy of prematurity, bronchopulmonary dysplasia).

oxytocics Drugs that stimulate uterine contractions, thus accelerating childbirth and preventing postbirth hemorrhage. They may be used to increase the letdown reflex during lactation.

oxytocin Hormone produced by the posterior pituitary that stimulates uterine contractions and the release of milk in the mammary gland (letdown reflex).

    o. challenge test (OCT) Evaluation of fetal response (fetal heart rate) to contractile activity of the uterus stimulated by exogenous oxytocin (Pitocin).

Paco$_2$ Partial pressure of carbon dioxide in arterial blood.

palmar erythema Rash on the surface of the palms sometimes seen in pregnancy.

palsy Permanent or temporary loss of sensation or ability to move and control movement; paralysis.

    Bell's p. Peripheral facial paralysis of the facial nerve (cranial nerve VII), causing the muscles of the unaffected side of the face to pull the face into a distorted position.

    Erb's p. See *Erb-Duchenne paralysis.*

Pao$_2$ Partial pressure of oxygen in arterial blood.

Papanicolaou (Pap) smear Microscopic examination using scrapings from the cervix, endocervix, or other mucous membranes that will reveal, with a high degree of accuracy, the presence of premalignant or malignant cells.

para Usually expressed as a number that refers to parity. See *parity.*

paracervical block Type of regional anesthesia produced by injection of a local anesthetic into the lower uterine segment just beneath the mucosa adjacent to the outer rim of the cervix (3 and 9 o'clock positions).

parental adjustment Process that a person goes through in adapting to the parental role; includes three stages: expectations, reality, and transition to mastery.

parity Number of past pregnancies that have reached viability, regardless of whether the infant or infants were alive or stillborn. See *para.*

parturient Woman giving birth.

parturition Process or act of giving birth.

patent Open.

pathogen Substance or organism capable of producing disease.

pathologic jaundice See *jaundice, pathologic.*

peau d'orange Orange peel–like skin secondary to cancerous lesions and seen over edematous breasts.

pedigree Shorthand method of depicting family lines of individuals that is usually used for tracing manifestations of a physical or chemical disorder.

pelvic Pertaining or relating to the pelvis.

    p. inflammatory disease (PID) Infection of internal reproductive structures and adjacent tissues usually secondary to sexually transmitted infections.

    p. inlet See *inlet, pelvic.*

    p. outlet See *outlet, pelvic.*

    p. relaxation Refers to the lengthening and weakening of the fascial supports of pelvic structures.

    p. tilt (rock) Exercise used to help relieve low back discomfort during menstruation and pregnancy.

pelvimetry Measurement of dimensions and proportions of the pelvis to determine its capacity and ability to allow the passage of the fetus through the birth canal.

pelvis Bony structure formed by the sacrum, coccyx, innominate bones, and symphysis pubis and the ligaments that unite them.

    android p. See *android pelvis.*

    anthropoid p. See *anthropoid pelvis.*

    gynecoid p. See *gynecoid pelvis.*

    platypelloid p. See *platypelloid pelvis.*

    true p. Pelvis below the linea terminalis.

penis Male organ used for urination and copulation.

percutaneous umbilical blood sampling (PUBS) Procedure during which the fetal umbilical vessel is accessed for blood sampling or for transfusions.

perimenopause Period of transition of changing ovarian activity before menopause and through first few years of amenorrhea.

perinatal Of or pertaining to the time and process of giving birth or being born.

perinatal period Period extending from the twentieth or twenty-eighth week of gestation through the end of the twenty-eighth day after birth.

perinatologist Physician who specializes in fetal and neonatal care.

perineum Area between the vagina and rectum in the female and between the scrotum and rectum in the male.

periodic breathing Sporadic episodes of cessation of respirations for periods of 10 seconds or less not associated with cyanosis typically noted in preterm infants.

periods of reactivity (newborn infant) *First period* (within 30 minutes after birth): brief cyanosis, flushing with crying; crackles, nasal flaring, grunting, retractions; heart sounds loud, forceful, irregular; alert; mucus; no bowel sounds; followed by period of sleep. *Second period* (4 to 8 hours after birth): swift color changes; irregular respiratory and heart rates; mucus with gagging; meconium passage; temperature stabilizing.

peripartum heart failure Inability of the heart to maintain an adequate cardiac output. Heart failure occurring during pregnancy.

periventricular Intraventricular hemorrhage, a common type of brain injury in preterm infants; prognosis depends on severity of hemorrhage.

pessary Device placed inside the vagina to function as a supportive structure for the uterus.

petechiae Pinpoint hemorrhagic areas caused by numerous disease states involving infection and thrombocytopenia and occasionally found over the face and trunk of the newborn because of increased intravascular pressure in the capillaries during birth.

pH Hydrogen ion concentration.

phenotype Expression of certain physical or chemical characteristics in an individual resulting from interaction between genotype and environmental factors.

phenylketonuria (PKU) Recessive hereditary disease that results in a defect in the metabolism of the amino acid phenylalanine caused by the lack of an enzyme, phenylalanine hydroxylase, that is necessary for the conversion of the amino acid phenylalanine into tyrosine. If PKU is not treated, brain damage may occur, causing severe mental retardation.

phimosis Tightness of the prepuce, or foreskin, of the penis.

phlebitis Inflammation of a vein with symptoms of pain and tenderness along the course of the vein, inflammatory swelling and acute edema below the obstruction, and discoloration of the skin because of injury or bruise to the vein, possibly occurring in acute or chronic infections or after procedures or childbirth.

phlebothrombosis Formation of a clot or thrombus in the vein; inflammation of the vein with secondary clotting.

phocomelia Developmental anomaly characterized by the absence of the upper portion of one or more limbs so that the feet or hands or both are attached to the trunk of the body by short, irregularly shaped stumps, resembling the fins of a seal.

phosphatidylglycerol A phospholipid, a component of pulmonary surfactant; its presence in amniotic fluid is considered a sign of fetal lung maturity when the pregnancy is complicated by maternal diabetes.

phototherapy Utilization of lights to reduce serum bilirubin levels by oxidation of bilirubin into water-soluble compounds that are then processed in the liver and excreted into bile and urine.

physiologic jaundice See *jaundice, physiologic.*

pica Unusual craving during pregnancy (e.g., of laundry starch, dirt, red clay).

pinch test Determines if nipples are everted or inverted by placing thumb and forefinger on areola and pressing inward. The nipple will stand erect or invert.

placenta Latin, flat cake; afterbirth, specialized vascular disc-shaped organ for maternal-fetal gas and nutrient exchange. Normally it implants in the thick muscular wall of the upper uterine segment.
>   **abruptio p.** See *abruptio placentae.*
>   **battledore p.** Umbilical cord insertion into the margin of the placenta.
>   **circumvallate p.** Placenta having a raised white ring at its edge.
>   **p. accreta** Invasion of the uterine muscle by the placenta, thus making separation from the muscle difficult if not impossible.
>   **p. increta** Deep penetration in myometrium by placenta.
>   **p. percreta** Perforation of uterus by placenta.
>   **p. previa** Placenta that is abnormally implanted in the thin, lower uterine segment and that is typed according to proximity to cervical os: total—completely occludes os; partial—does not occlude os completely; and marginal—placenta encroaches on margin of internal cervical os.
>   **p. succenturiata** Accessory placenta.

placental Pertaining or relating to the placenta.
>   **p. infarct** Localized, ischemic, hard area on the fetal or maternal side of the placenta.
>   **p. souffle** See *souffle, placental.*

platypelloid pelvis Broad pelvis with a shortened anteroposterior diameter and a flattened, oval, transverse shape.

plethora Deep, beefy-red coloration of a newborn caused by an increased number of blood cells (polycythemia) per volume of blood.

plugged ducts Milk ducts blocked by small curds of dried milk.

podalic Concerning or pertaining to the feet.
>   **p. version** Shifting of the position of the fetus so as to bring the feet to the outlet during labor.

polycythemia Increased number of erythrocytes per volume of blood, which may be caused by large placental transfusion, fetus transfusion, or maternal-fetal transfusion, or it may be attributable to hypovolemia resulting from movement of fluid out of vascular into interstitial compartment.

polydactyly Excessive number of digits (fingers or toes).

polyhydramnios See *hydramnios.*

polyp Small tumorlike growth that projects from a mucous membrane surface.

polyuria Excessive secretion and discharge of urine by the kidneys.

position Relationship of an arbitrarily chosen fetal reference point, such as the occiput, sacrum, chin, or scapula on the presenting part of the fetus to its location in the front, back, or sides of the maternal pelvis.

positive signs of pregnancy Definite indication of pregnancy (e.g., hearing the fetal heartbeat, visualization and palpation of fetal movement by the examiner, sonographic examination).

posterior Pertaining to the back.
>   **p. fontanel** See *fontanel, posterior.*

postmature infant Infant born at or after the beginning of week 43 of gestation or later and exhibiting signs of dysmaturity.

postnatal Happening or occurring after birth (newborn).

postpartum Happening or occurring after birth (mother).

postpartum blues A letdown feeling, accompanied by irritability and anxiety, which usually begins 2 to 3 days after giving birth and disappears within a week or two. Sometimes called the "baby blues."

postpartum depression Depression occurring within 6 months of childbirth, lasting longer than postpartum blues and characterized by a variety of symptoms that interfere with activities of daily living and care of the baby.

postpartum psychosis Symptoms begin as postpartum blues or depression but are characterized by a break with reality. Delusions, hallucinations, confusion, delirium, and panic can occur.

postterm pregnancy Pregnancy prolonged past 42 weeks of gestation (also called postdate pregnancy).

precipitous labor Rapid or sudden labor of less than 3 hours beginning from onset of cervical changes to completed birth of neonate.

preconception care Care designed for health maintenance before pregnancy.

preeclampsia Disease encountered after 20 weeks of gestation or early in the puerperium; a vasospastic disease process characterized by increasing hypertension, proteinuria, and hemoconcentration.

pregestational diabetes Diabetes mellitus type 1 or type 2 that exists before pregnancy.

pregnancy Period between conception through complete birth of the products of conception. The usual duration of pregnancy in the human is 280 days, 9 calendar months, or 10 lunar months.
>   **abdominal p.** See *abdominal gestation.*

ectopic p. See *ectopic pregnancy.*

extrauterine p. See *extrauterine pregnancy.*

pregnancy-induced hypertension (PIH) Hypertensive disorders of pregnancy including preeclampsia, eclampsia, and transient hypertension.

premature infant Infant born before completing week 37 of gestation, irrespective of birth weight; preterm infant.

premenstrual syndrome Syndrome of nervous tension, irritability, weight gain, edema, headache, mastalgia, dysphoria, and lack of coordination occurring during the last few days of the menstrual cycle preceding the onset of menstruation.

premonitory Serving as an early symptom or warning.

prenatal Occurring or happening before birth.

prepartum Before birth; before giving birth.

prepuce Fold of skin, or foreskin, covering the glans penis of the male.

    p. of the clitoris Fold of the labia minora that covers the glans clitoris.

presentation That part of the fetus that first enters the pelvis and lies over the inlet: may be head, face, breech, or shoulder.

    breech p. See *breech presentation.*

    cephalic p. See *cephalic presentation.*

presenting part That part of the fetus that lies closest to the internal os of the cervix.

pressure edema Edema of the lower extremities caused by pressure of the heavy pregnant uterus against the large veins; edema of fetal scalp after cephalic presentation (caput succedaneum).

presumptive signs of pregnancy Manifestations that are suggestive of pregnancy but are not absolutely positive. These include the cessation of menses, Chadwick's sign, morning sickness, and quickening.

preterm birth Birth occurring before 37 weeks of gestation.

preterm or premature rupture of membranes (PROM) Spontaneous rupture of membranes before 37 weeks of gestation.

previa, placenta See *placenta previa.*

primigravida Woman who is pregnant for the first time.

primipara Woman who has carried a pregnancy to viability whether the child is dead or alive at the time of birth.

primordial Existing first or existing in the simplest or most primitive form.

probable signs of pregnancy Manifestations or evidence that indicates that there is a definite likelihood of pregnancy. Among the probable signs are enlargement of abdomen, Goodell's sign, Hegar's sign, Braxton Hicks sign, and positive hormonal tests for pregnancy.

prodromal Serving as an early symptom or warning of the approach of a disease or condition (e.g., prodromal labor).

progesterone Hormone produced by the corpus luteum and placenta whose function is to prepare the endometrium of the uterus for implantation of the fertilized ovum, develop the mammary glands, and maintain the pregnancy.

prolactin A pituitary hormone that triggers milk production.

prolapsed cord Protrusion of the umbilical cord in advance of the presenting part.

proliferative phase of menstrual cycle Preovulatory, follicular, or estrogen phase of the menstrual cycle.

promontory of the sacrum Superior projecting portion of the sacrum at the junction of the sacrum and L5.

prophylactic (1) Pertaining to prevention or warding off of disease or certain conditions. (2) Condom, or "rubber."

proscription Forbidden; taboos.

prostaglandin (PG) Substance present in many body tissues; has a role in many reproductive tract functions; used to induce abortions, cervical ripening for labor induction.

proteinuria Presence of protein in urine.

pruritus Itching.

pseudocyesis Condition in which the woman has all the usual signs of pregnancy, such as enlargement of the abdomen, cessation of menses, weight gain, and morning sickness, but is not pregnant; phantom or false pregnancy.

pseudopregnancy See *pseudocyesis.*

psychoprophylaxis Mental and physical education of the parents in preparation for childbirth, with the goal of minimizing the fear and pain and promoting positive family relationships.

ptyalism Excessive salivation.

puberty Period in life in which the reproductive organs mature and one becomes functionally capable of reproduction.

pubic Pertaining to the pubis.

pubis Pubic bone forming the front of the pelvis.

pudendal block Injection of a local anesthetizing drug at the pudendal nerve root to produce numbness of the genital and perianal region.

puerperal infection Infection of the pelvic organs during the postbirth period; childbed fever.

puerperium Period after the third stage of labor and lasting until involution of the uterus takes place, usually about 3 to 6 weeks.

pulse oximetry Noninvasive method of monitoring oxygen levels by detecting the amount of light absorbed by oxygen-carrying hemoglobin.

pyrosis A burning sensation in the epigastric and sternal region from stomach acid (heartburn).

quickening Maternal perception of fetal movement; usually occurs between weeks 16 and 20 of gestation.

radioimmunoassay Pregnancy test that tests for the beta subunit of human chorionic gonadotropin using radioactively labeled markers.

rape-trauma syndrome Characteristic symptoms seen in victims of rape and consisting of several phases; similar to posttraumatic stress syndrome.

recessive trait Genetically determined characteristic that is expressed only when present in the homozygotic state.

reciprocity Type of body movement or behavior that provides the observer with cues, such as the behavioral cues infants provide to parents and parents' responses to cues.

reconstituted family See *blended family.*

rectocele Herniation or protrusion of the rectum into the posterior vaginal wall.

referred pain Discomfort originating in a local area such as cervix, vagina, or perineal tissues but felt in the back, flanks, or thighs.

reflex Automatic response built into the nervous system that does not need the intervention of conscious thought (e.g., in the newborn, rooting, gagging, grasp).

reflex bradycardia Slowing of the heart in response to a particular stimuli.

regional anesthesia Anesthesia of an area of the body by injection of a local anesthetic to block a group of sensory nerve fibers.

regurgitate Vomiting or spitting up of solids or fluids.

residual urine Urine that remains in the bladder after urination.

respiratory distress syndrome (RDS) Condition resulting from decreased pulmonary gas exchange, leading to retention of carbon dioxide (increase in arterial PCO_2). Most common neonatal causes are prematurity, perinatal asphyxia, and maternal diabetes mellitus; hyaline membrane disease (HMD).

restitution In obstetrics, the turning of the fetal head to the left or right after it has completely emerged from the introitus as it assumes a normal alignment with the infant's shoulders.

resuscitation Restoration of consciousness or life in one who is apparently dead or whose respirations or cardiac function or both have ceased.

retained placenta Retention of all or part of the placenta in the uterus after birth.

retinopathy of prematurity (ROP) Associated with hyperoxemia, resulting in eye injury and blindness in premature infants.

retraction (1) Drawing in or sucking in of soft tissues of chest, indicative of an obstruction at any level of the respiratory tract from the oropharynx to the alveoli. (2) Retraction of uterine muscle fiber. After contracting, the muscle fiber does not return to its original length but remains slightly shortened, a unique attribute of uterine muscle that aids in preventing postdelivery hemorrhage and results in involution.

retroflexion Bending backward.

    r. of uterus Condition in which the body of the uterus is bent backward at an angle with the cervix, the position of which usually remains unchanged.

retrolental fibroplasia (RLF) See *retinopathy of prematurity*.

retroversion Turning or a state of being turned back.

    r. of uterus Displacement of the uterus; the body of the uterus is tipped backward with the cervix pointing forward toward the symphysis pubis.

Rh factor Inherited antigen present on erythrocytes. The individual with the factor is known as *positive* for the factor.

Rh immune globulin (RhIG) Solution of gamma globulin that contains Rh antibodies. Intramuscular (IM) administration of Rh immune globulin (trade name RhoGAM) prevents sensitization in Rh-negative women who have been exposed to Rh-positive red blood cells.

rheumatic heart disease Permanent damage of the heart muscle and valves secondary to an autoimmune reaction in the heart tissue precipitated by rheumatic fever.

rhythm method Contraceptive method in which a woman abstains from sexual intercourse during the ovulatory phase of her menstrual cycle; calendar method.

ribonucleic acid (RNA) Element responsible for transferring genetic information within a cell; a template, or pattern.

ring of fire Burning sensation as vagina stretches and fetal head crowns.

risk factors Factors that cause a person or a group of people to be particularly vulnerable to an unwanted, unpleasant, or unhealthful event.

risk taking Intentional behaviors with uncertain outcomes.

rite of passage Significant life event indicating movement from one maturational level to another.

Ritgen maneuver Procedure used to control the birth of the head.

rooming-in unit Maternity unit designed so that the newborn's crib is at the mother's bedside or in a nursery adjacent to the mother's room.

rooting reflex Normal response of the newborn to move toward whatever touches the area around the mouth and to attempt to suck. This reflex usually disappears by 3 to 4 months of age.

rotation In obstetrics, the turning of the fetal head as it follows the curves of the birth canal downward.

rubella vaccine Live attenuated rubella virus given to clients who have not had rubella or who are serologically negative. Exposure to the rubella virus through vaccination causes the client to form antibodies, producing active immunity.

Rubin's test Transuterine insufflation of the uterine tubes with carbon dioxide to test their patency; infrequently used.

rugae Folds in the vaginal mucosa and scrotum.

sac, amniotic See *amniotic sac*.

sacroiliac Of or pertaining to the sacrum and ilium.

sacrum Triangular bone composed of five united vertebrae and situated between L5 and the coccyx; forms the posterior boundary of the true pelvis.

safe passage Normal uneventful birth process for mother and child.

safe period The days in the menstrual cycle that are not designated as fertile days, that is, before and after ovulation.

sagittal suture Band of connective tissue separating the parietal bones, extending from the anterior to the posterior fontanel.

salpingo-oophorectomy Removal of a uterine tube and an ovary.

Schultze's mechanism Delivery of the placenta with the fetal surfaces (shiny in appearance) presenting.

scrotum Pouch of skin containing the testes and parts of the spermatic cords.

second stage Stage of labor from full dilatation of the cervix to the birth of the baby.

secondary areola See *areola, secondary*.

secretory phase of menstrual cycle Postovulatory, luteal, progestational, premenstrual phase of menstrual cycle; 14 days in length.

secundines Fetal membranes and placenta expelled after childbirth; afterbirth.

self-care Patient provides care for self as part of plan of care.

semen Thick, white, viscid secretion discharged from the urethra of the male at orgasm; the transporting medium of the sperm.

semen analysis Examination of semen specimen to determine liquefaction, volume, pH, sperm density, and normal morphology.

sensitization Development of antibodies to a specific antigen.

sensory behavior Responses of the five senses; indicate a readiness for social interaction.

septic abortion See *abortion, septic.*

sepsis Bacterial infections of the bloodstream.

sex chromosome Chromosome associated with determination of gender: the X (female) and Y (male) chromosomes. The normal female has two X chromosomes, and the normal male has one X and one Y chromosome.

sexual decision making Selection of choices concerned with intimate and sexual behavior.

sexual history Past and present health conditions, lifestyle behaviors, knowledge, and attitudes related to sex and sexuality.

sexual response cycle The phases of physical changes that occur in response to sexual stimulation and sexual tension release.

sexuality The part of life that has to do with being male or female.

sexually transmitted diseases (STDs) Disease acquired as a result of sexual activity with an infected individual.

shake test "Foam" test for lung maturity of fetus; more rapid than determination of lecithin/sphingomyelin ratio.

Sheehan syndrome Postpartum necrosis of the pituitary gland resulting from hypovolemic shock and disseminated intravascular coagulation.

sibling rivalry Negative behaviors exhibited by siblings in response to the addition of a new baby in the family.

sickle cell hemoglobinopathy Abnormal crescent-shaped red blood corpuscles in the blood.

Sims' position Position in which the client lies on the left side with the right knee and thigh drawn upward toward the chest.

single-parent family Family form characterized by one parent (male or female) in the household. This may result from loss of spouse by death, divorce, separation, desertion, birth of a child to a single woman, or adoption.

single-room maternity care (SRMC) Variation of care sites where one nurse provides care to a mother and infant, that is, mother-baby units, LDRPs.

singleton A single fetus.

situational crisis Crisis that arises suddenly in response to an external event or a conflict concerning a specific circumstance. The symptoms are transient, and the episode is usually brief.

sitz bath Application of moist heat or cold to the perineum by sitting in a tub or basin filled with warm or cold water.

sleep-wake cycles Variations in states of newborn consciousness.

Small for gestational age (SGA) Refers to inadequate growth for gestational age.

smegma Whitish secretion around labia minora and under foreskin of penis.

somatic pain Perineal discomfort resulting from stretching of perineal tissues.

souffle Soft, blowing sound or murmur heard by auscultation.

   funic s. Soft, muffled, blowing sound produced by blood rushing through the umbilical vessels and synchronous with the fetal heart sounds.

   placental s. Soft, blowing murmur caused by the blood current in the placenta and synchronous with the maternal pulse.

   uterine s. Soft, blowing sound made by the blood in the arteries of the pregnant uterus and synchronous with the maternal pulse.

sperm Male sex cell. Also called *spermatozoon, spermatozoa.*

spermatogenesis Process by which mature spermatozoa are formed, during which the diploid chromosome number (46) is reduced by half (haploid, 23).

spermicide Chemical substance that kills sperm by reducing their surface tension, causing the cell wall to break down by a bactericidal effect or by creating a highly acidic environment. Also called *spermatocide.*

spina bifida occulta Congenital malformation of the spine in which the posterior portion of laminas of the vertebrae fails to close but there is no herniation or protrusion of the spinal cord or meninges through the defect. The newborn may have a dimple in the skin or growth of hair over the malformed vertebrae.

spinnbarkeit Formation of a stretchable thread of cervical mucus under estrogen influence at time of ovulation.

splanchnic engorgement Excessive filling or pooling of blood within the visceral vasculature that occurs after the removal of pressure from the abdomen, such as birth of an infant, removal of an excess of urine from bladder, removal of large tumor.

spontaneous abortion See *abortion, spontaneous.*

spontaneous rupture of membranes (SROM) Rupture of membranes by natural means.

squamocolumnar junction Site in the endocervical canal where columnar epithelium and squamous epithelium meet; also called *transformation zone.*

square window Angle of wrist between hypothenar prominence and forearm; one criterion for estimating gestational age of neonate.

standard body weight An appropriate weight for height; a body mass index (BMI) within the normal range.

state-related behavior Behavioral responses dependent on current state of infant.

station Relationship of the presenting fetal part to an imaginary line drawn between the ischial spines of the pelvis.

sterility (1) State of being free from living microorganisms. (2) Complete inability to reproduce offspring.

sterilization Process or act that renders a person unable to produce children.

stillbirth The birth of a baby after 20 weeks of gestation and 1 day or weighing ≤350 gm (depending on the state code) that does not show any signs of life.

stress urinary incontinence (SUI) Loss of urine occurring with increased abdominal pressure (e.g., with coughing or sneezing).

striae gravidarum ("stretch marks") Shining reddish lines caused by stretching of the skin, often found on the abdomen, thighs, and breasts during pregnancy. These streaks turn to a fine pinkish white or silver tone in time in fair-skinned women and brownish in darker-skinned women.

subinvolution Failure of a part (e.g., the uterus) to reduce to its normal size and condition after enlargement from functional activity (e.g., pregnancy).

suboccipitobregmatic diameter Smallest diameter of the fetal head—follows a line drawn from the middle of the anterior fontanel to the undersurface of the occipital bone.

supine hypotension Shock; fall in blood pressure caused by impaired venous return when gravid uterus presses on ascending vena cava, when woman is lying flat on her back; vena cava syndrome.

support systems Network from which people receive help in times of crisis.

surfactant Phosphoprotein necessary for normal respiratory function that prevents the alveolar collapse (atelectasis). See also *lecithin* and *L/S ratio*.

suture (1) Junction of the adjoining bones of the skull. (2) Procedure uniting parts by their being sewn together.

symphysis pubis Fibrocartilaginous union of the bodies of the pubic bones in the midline.

synchrony Fit between an infant's cues and the parent's response.

syndactyly Malformation of digits, often seen as a fusion of two or more toes to form one structure.

systemic analgesia Analgesics administered either intramuscularly (IM) or intravenously (IV) that cross the blood-brain barrier and provide central analgesic effects.

systemic lupus erythematosus (SLE) A chronic inflammatory connective tissue disease affecting many systems, that is, the integumentary, renal, and nervous systems.

tachypnea Excessively rapid respiratory rate (e.g., in neonates, respiratory rate of 60 breaths/min or more).

taking-hold phase Period after birth characterized by a woman becoming more independent and more interested in learning infant care skills; learning to be a competent mother is an important task.

taking-in phase Period after birth characterized by the woman's dependency; maternal needs are dominant, and talking about the birth is an important task.

talipes equinovarus Deformity in which the foot is extended and the person walks on the toes.

telangiectasia Permanent dilatation of groups of superficial capillaries and venules.

telangiectatic nevi ("stork bites") Clusters of small, red, localized areas of capillary dilatation frequently seen in neonates at the nape of the neck or lower occiput, upper eyelids, and nasal bridge that can be blanched with pressure of a finger.

teratogenic agent Any drug, virus, or irradiation, the exposure to which can cause malformation of the fetus.

teratogens Nongenetic factors that cause malformations and disorders in utero.

teratoma Tumor composed of different kinds of tissue, none of which normally occurs together or at the site of the tumor.

term infant Live infant born between weeks 38 and 42 of completed gestation.

testis One of the glands contained in the male scrotum that produces the male reproductive cell, or sperm, and the male hormone, testosterone; testicle.

tetany, uterine Extremely prolonged uterine contractions.

thalassemia An anemia affecting Mediterranean and Southeast Asian populations in which there is an insufficient amount of globin produced to fill the red blood cells.

therapeutic abortion See *abortion, therapeutic*.

therapeutic insemination See *insemination, therapeutic*.

therapeutic rest Administration of analgesics to decrease pain and induce rest for management of hypertonic uterine dysfunction.

thermal shift Drop and subsequent rise in basal body temperature around the time of ovulation.

thermistor probe Automatic sensor used to monitor skin temperature of infant under radiant warmer.

themogenesis Creation or production of heat, especially in the body.

thermoregulation Control of temperature.

third stage Stage of labor from the birth of the baby to the expulsion of the placenta.

threatened abortion See *abortion, threatened*.

thrombocytopenia Abnormal hematologic condition in which the number of platelets is reduced, usually by destruction of erythroid tissue in bone marrow because of certain neoplastic diseases or an immune response to a drug.

thrombocytopenic purpura Hematologic disorder characterized by prolonged bleeding time, decreased number of platelets, increased cell fragility, and purpura, which result in hemorrhages into the skin, mucous membranes, organs, and other tissue.

thromboembolism Obstruction of a blood vessel by a clot that has become detached from its site of formation.

thrombophlebitis Inflammation of a vein with secondary clot formation.

thrombus Blood clot obstructing a blood vessel that remains at the place it was formed.

thrush Fungal infection of the mouth or throat that is characterized by the formation of white patches on a red, moist, inflamed mucous membrane and is caused by *Candida albicans*.

toco- (toko-) Combining form that means childbirth or labor.

tocolytic drug Drug used to relax the uterus, to suppress preterm labor, or for version.

tocotransducer Electronic device for measuring uterine contractions.

TORCH infections Infections caused by organisms that damage the embryo or fetus; acronym for *t*oxoplasmosis, *o*ther (e.g., syphilis), *r*ubella, *c*ytomegalovirus, and *h*erpes simplex.

toxemia Term previously used for hypertensive states of pregnancy.

toxicology screen Laboratory analysis of blood or urine to test for alcohol or drug content. Urine drug screening is the most common because it is noninvasive.

tracheoesophageal fistula Congenital malformation in which there is an abnormal tubelike passage between the trachea and esophagus.

transformation zone See *squamocolumnar junction.*

transition—labor See *transition phase.*

transition period—newborn Period from birth to 4 to 6 hours later; infant passes through period of reactivity, sleep, and second period of reactivity.

transition to parenthood Period of time from the preconception parenthood decision through the first months after birth of the baby during which parents define their parental roles and adjust to parenthood.

transition phase Phase in first stage of labor from a cervical dilatation of 8 to 10 cm.

translocation Condition in which a chromosome breaks and all or part of that chromosome is transferred to a different part of the same chromosome or to another chromosome.

trial of labor (TOL) Period of observation to determine if a laboring woman is likely to be successful in progressing to a vaginal birth.

Trichomonas **vaginitis** Inflammation of the vagina caused by *Trichomonas vaginalis,* a parasitic protozoon, and characterized by persistent burning and itching of the vulvar tissue and a profuse, frothy, white discharge.

trimester One of 3 periods of about 3 months each into which pregnancy is divided.

trisomy Condition whereby any given chromosome exists in triplicate instead of the normal duplicate pattern.

trophoblast Outer layer of cells of the developing blastodermic vesicle that develops the trophoderm or feeding layer, which will establish the nutrient relationships with the uterine endometrium.

trophoblastic disease A condition in which trophoblastic cells covering the chorionic villi proliferate and undergo cystic changes, which may be malignant.

tubal ligation Abdominal procedure in which the uterine tubes are tied off and a section is removed to interrupt tubal continuity and thus sterilize the woman.

tubercles of Montgomery Small papillae on surface of nipples and areolae that secrete a fatty substance that lubricates the nipples.

twins Two neonates from the same impregnation developed within the same uterus at the same time.

   conjoined t. Twins who are physically united; Siamese twins.

   disparate t. Twins who are different (e.g., in weight) and distinct from one another.

   dizygotic t. Twins developed from two separate ova fertilized by two separate sperm at the same time; fraternal twins.

   monozygotic t. Twins developed from a single fertilized ovum; identical twins.

ultrasonography Use of high-frequency sound waves for a variety of obstetric diagnoses and for fetal surveillance.

ultrasound transducer External signal source for monitoring fetal heart rate electronically.

umbilical cord (funis) Structure connecting the placenta and fetus and containing two arteries and one vein encased in a tissue called *Wharton's jelly.* The cord is ligated at birth and severed; the stump falls off in 4 to 10 days.

umbilicus Navel, or depressed point in the middle of the abdomen that marks the attachment of the umbilical cord during fetal life.

urethra Small tubular structure that drains urine from the bladder.

urinary frequency Need to void often or at close intervals.

urinary meatus Opening, or mouth, of the urethra.

uterine Referring or pertaining to the uterus.

   u. adnexa See *adnexa, uterine.*

   u. atony Relaxation of uterus; leads to postpartum hemorrhage.

   u. bruit Abnormal sound or murmur heard while auscultating the uterus.

   u. ischemia Decreased blood supply to the uterus.

   u. prolapse Falling, sinking, or sliding of the uterus from its normal location in the body.

   u. souffle See *souffle, uterine.*

uteroplacental insufficiency (UPI) Decline in placental function—exchange of gases, nutrients, and wastes—leading to fetal hypoxia and acidosis; evidenced by late fetal heart rate decelerations in response to uterine contractions.

uterus Hollow muscular organ in the female designed for the implantation, containment, nourishment of the fetus during its development, and expulsion of fetus during labor and birth; also organ of menstruation.

   Couvelaire u. Interstitial myometrial hemorrhage after premature separation (abruptio) of placenta. A purplish-bluish discoloration of the uterus and boardlike rigidity of the uterus are noted.

   inversion of u. See *inversion of uterus.*

   retroflexion of u. See *retroflexion of uterus.*

   retroversion of u. See *retroversion of uterus.*

vaccination Intentional injection of antigenic material given to stimulate antibody production in the recipient.

vacuum curettage Uterine aspiration method of early abortion.

vacuum-assisted birth Birth involving attachment of vacuum cup to fetal head and using negative pressure to assist in birth of the fetus.

vagina Normally collapsed musculomembranous tube that forms the passageway between the uterus and the entrance to the vagina.

vaginal birth after cesarean (VBAC) Giving birth vaginally after having had a previous cesarean birth.

vaginismus Intense, painful spasm of the muscles surrounding the vagina.

Valsalva maneuver Any forced expiratory effort against a closed airway such as holding one's breath and tightening the abdominal muscles (i.e. pushing during the second stage of labor).

variability Normal irregularity of fetal cardiac rhythm; short term—beat-to-beat changes; long term—rhythmic changes (waves) from the baseline value.

varicocele Enlargement of veins of the spermatic cord.

varicosity (varicose veins) Swollen, distended, and twisted veins that may develop in almost any part of the body but are most commonly seen in the legs, caused by pregnancy, obesity, congenital defective venous valves, and occupations requiring much standing.

vasectomy Ligation or removal of a segment of the vas deferens, usually done bilaterally to produce sterility in the male.

VDRL test Abbreviation for Venereal Disease Research Laboratories test, a serologic flocculation test for syphilis.

vernix caseosa Protective gray-white fatty substance of cheesy consistency covering the fetal skin.

version Act of turning the fetus in the uterus to change the presenting part and facilitate birth.

    external cephalic v. See *external cephalic version*.

    podalic v. Shifting of the fetus's position so as to bring the feet to the outlet during birth.

vertex Crown or top of the head.

    v. presentation Presentation in which the fetal head is nearest the cervical opening and is born first.

very low birth weight (VLBW) Refers to infant weighing 1,500 gm or less at birth.

viable, viability Capable, capability of living, as in a fetus that has reached a stage of development, usually 22 menstrual weeks (20 weeks of gestation), which will permit it to live outside the uterus.

visceral pain Discomfort from cervical changes and uterine ischemia located over the lower portion of the abdomen and radiating to the lumbar area of the back and down the thighs.

vulva External genitalia of the female that consist of the labia majora, labia minora, clitoris, urinary meatus, and vaginal introitus.

vulvar self-examination (VSE) Systematic examination of the vulva by the patient.

vulvectomy Surgical removal of all or parts of the vulva.

warm line A help line, or consultation service, for families to access; most often for support of newborn care and postpartum care after hospital discharge.

weaning Process of changing from breastfeeding or bottle feeding to drinking from a cup.

Wharton's jelly White, gelatinous material surrounding the umbilical vessels within the cord.

witch's milk Secretion of a whitish fluid for about a week after birth from enlarged mammary tissue in the neonate, presumably resulting from maternal hormonal influences.

withdrawal (1) Physiologic or cognitive changes that occur after removal of the substance in the substance-dependent person; (2) removing penis from vagina before ejaculation (coitus interruptus).

womb See *uterus*.

X chromosome Sex chromosome in humans existing in duplicate in the normal female and singly in the normal male.

X linkage Genes located on the X chromosome.

Y chromosome Sex chromosome in the human male necessary for the development of the male gonads.

zona pellucida Inner, thick, membranous envelope of the ovum.

zygote Cell formed by the union of two reproductive cells or gametes; the fertilized ovum resulting from the union of a sperm and an ovum.

Standard Laboratory Values: Pregnant and Nonpregnant Women

	NONPREGNANT	PREGNANT
HEMATOLOGIC VALUES		
Complete Blood Count (CBC)		
Hemoglobin, g/dl	12 to 16*	>11*
Hematocrit, PCV, %	37 to 47	>33*
Red blood cell (RBC) volume, per ml	1,600	1,500 to 1,900
Plasma volume, per ml	2,400	3,700
RBC count, million/mm^3	4.2 to 5.4	5 to 6.25
White blood cells, total per mm^3	5,000 to 10,000	5,000 to 15,000
Polymorphonuclear cells, %	55 to 70	60 to 85
Lymphocytes, %	20 to 40	15 to 40
Erythrocyte sedimentation rate, mm/hr	20/hr	Elevated second and third trimesters
MCHC, g/dl packed RBCs (mean corpuscular hemoglobin concentration)	32 to 36	No change
MCH/(mean corpuscular hemoglobin) per picogram (less than a nanogram)	27 to 31	No change
MCV/μm^3 (mean corpuscular volume) per cubic micrometer	80 to 95	No change
Blood Coagulation and Fibrinolytic Activity†		
Factors VII, VIII, IX, X		Increase in pregnancy, return to normal in early puerperium; factor VIII increases during and immediately after birth
Factors XI, XIII		Decrease in pregnancy
Prothrombin time (PT)	11 to 12.5 sec	Slight decrease in pregnancy
Partial thromboplastin time (PTT)	60 to 70 sec	Slight decrease in pregnancy and again decrease during second and third stage of labor (indicates clotting at placental site)
Bleeding time	1 to 9 min (Ivy)	No appreciable change
Coagulation time	6 to 10 min (Lee/White)	No appreciable change
Platelets	150,000 to 400,000/mm^3	No significant change until 3 to 5 days after birth and then a rapid increase (may predispose woman to thrombosis) and gradual return to normal
Fibrinolytic activity		Decreases in pregnancy and then abrupt return to normal (protection against thromboembolism)
Fibrinogen	200 to 400 mg/dl	Increased levels late in pregnancy
Mineral/Vitamin Concentrations		
Vitamin B$_{12}$, folic acid, ascorbic acid	Normal	Moderate decrease
Serum proteins		
Total, g/dl	6.4 to 8.3	5.5 to 7.5
Albumin, g/dl	3.5 to 5.0	Slight increase
Globulin, total, g/dl	2.3 to 3.4	3 to 4
Blood glucose		
Fasting, mg/dl	70 to 105	Decreases
2-hour postprandial, mg/dl	<140	Under 140 after a 100-gm carbohydrate meal is considered normal

	NONPREGNANT	PREGNANT
HEPATIC VALUES		
Bilirubin total	Not more than 1 mg/dl	Unchanged
Serum cholesterol	120 to 200 mg/dl	Increases from 16 to 32 weeks of pregnancy; remains at this level until after birth
Serum alkaline phosphatase	42 to 128 U/L	Increases from week 12 of pregnancy to 6 weeks after birth
Serum globulin albumin	2.3 to 3.4 g/dl	Slight increase
RENAL VALUES		
Bladder capacity	1,300 ml	1,500 ml
Renal plasma flow (RPF), ml/min	490 to 700	Increase by 25%
Glomerular filtration rate (GFR), ml/min	88 to 128	Increase by 50%
Nonprotein nitrogen (NPN), mg/dl	25 to 40	Decreases
Blood urea nitrogen (BUN), mg/dl	10 to 20	Decreases
Serum creatinine, mg/dl	0.5 to 1.1	Decreases
Serum uric acid, mg/dl	2.0 to 6.6	Decreases
Urine glucose	Negative	Present in 20% of pregnant women
Intravenous pyelogram (IVP)	Normal	Slight-to-moderate hydroureter and hydronephrosis; right kidney larger than left kidney

From Pagana K & Pagana T: *Mosby's diagnostic and laboratory test reference,* ed 3, St Louis, 1997, Mosby.
*At sea level. Permanent residents of higher levels (e.g., Denver) require higher levels of hemoglobin.
†Pregnancy represents a hypercoagulable state.

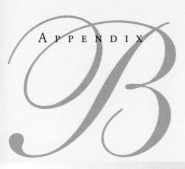

APPENDIX

Standard Laboratory Values in the Neonatal Period

	NEONATAL

1. HEMATOLOGIC VALUES

Clotting factors

Activated clotting time (ACT)	2 min
Bleeding time (Ivy)	2 to 7 min
Clot retraction	Complete 1 to 4 hr
Fibrinogen	125 to 300 mg/dl*

	TERM	PRETERM
Hemoglobin (g/dl)	14.5 to 22.5	15 to 17
Hematocrit (%)	44 to 72	45 to 55
Reticulocytes (%)	0.4 to 6	Up to 10
Fetal hemoglobin (% of total)	40 to 70	80 to 90
Red blood cells (RBCs)/mm^3	4.0^6-6.0^6	
Platelet count/mm^3	84,000 to 478,000	120,000 to 180,000
White blood cells (WBCs)/mm^3	9,000 to 30,000	10,000 to 20,000
Neutrophils (%)	54 to 62	47
Eosinophils and basophils (%)	1 to 3	
Lymphocytes (%)	25 to 33	33
Monocytes (%)	3 to 7	4
Immature WBC (%)	10	16

*dl refers to deciliter (1 dl = 100 ml); this conforms to the SI system (standardized international measurements).

	NEONATAL

2. BIOCHEMICAL VALUES

Bilirubin, direct			0 to 1 mg/dl
Bilirubin, total	Cord:		<2 mg/dl
	Peripheral blood:	0 to 1 day	6 mg/dl
		1 to 2 day	8 mg/dl
		3 to 5 day	12 mg/dl
Blood gases	Arterial:		pH 7.31 to 7.45
			Pco_2 33 to 48 mm Hg
			Po_2 50 to 70 mm Hg
	Venous:		pH 7.28 to 7.42
			Pco_2 38 to 52 mm Hg
			Po_2 20 to 49 mm Hg
α_1-Fetoprotein			0
Fibrinogen			150 to 300 mg/dl
Serum glucose			40 to 60 mg/dl

NORMAL RANGES
NEONATAL

3. URINALYSIS

Color	Clear, straw
Specific gravity	1.001 to 1.018
pH	5 to 7
Protein	Negative
Glucose	Negative
Ketones	Negative
RBCs	Rare
WBCs	0 to 4
Casts	Rare
17-Ketosteroids	Under 1
17-Hydroxycorticosteroids	Same
Urinary calcium	5 mg/kg of body weight
Urinary sodium	20% of adult values
Urinary vanillylmandelic acid (VMA)	<1.0 mg/24 hrs

Volume: 20 to 40 ml excreted daily in the first few days; by week 1, 24-hour urine volume close to 200 ml
Protein: may be present in first 2 to 4 days
Osmolarity (mOsm/L): 100 to 600

4. URINE SCREENING TESTS FOR INBORN ERRORS OF METABOLISM

Benedict's test: for reducing substances in the urine—glucose, galactose, fructose, lactose; phenylketonuria (PKU), alkaptonuria, tyrosyluria, and tyrosinosis may give a positive Benedict's test result.
Ferric chloride test: an immediate green color for PKU, histidinemia, and tyrosinuria; a gray to green color for presence of phenothiazines, isoniazid; red to purple color for presence of salicylates or ketone bodies.
Dinitrophenylhydrazine test: for PKU, maple syrup urine disease, Lowe's syndrome.
Cetyltrimethylammonium bromide test: for mucopolysaccharides: immediate positive reaction in gargoylism (Hurler's syndrome); delayed, moderately positive reaction for Marfan's, Morquio-Ullrich, and Murdoch syndromes.
Metachromatic stain (or urine sediment): granules (free or as inclusion bodies in cells) are seen in metachromatic leukodystrophy; may also be seen rarely in Tay-Sachs and other lipid diseases of central nervous system.
Amino acid chromatography: aminoaciduria may be normal in newborns; chromatography may be helpful to detect hypophosphatasia and argininosuccinicaciduria.
Diaper test, Phenistix test, and *Dinitrophenylhydrazine (DNPH) test:* simple, inexpensive tests for PKU; used for screening; most useful when infant is at least 6 weeks of age.

5. BLOOD SERUM PHENYLALANINE TESTS

Guthrie inhibition assay methods: drops of blood placed on filter paper; laboratory uses bacterial growth inhibition test; phenylalanine level above 8 mg/dl blood: diagnostic of PKU. Effective in newborn period; used also to monitor PKU diet; blood easily obtained by heel or finger puncture; inexpensive; used for wide-scale screening.

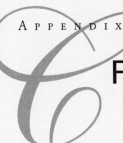

Relationship of Drugs to Breast Milk and Effect on Infant

The drugs listed in this appendix have been categorized by their major use. The ratings given are those published by the American Academy of Pediatrics (AAP) Committee on Drugs. These ratings label drugs that transfer into human milk. Drugs without a rating were not included in the AAP list. The ratings are described as the following:

1. Drugs that are contraindicated during breastfeeding
2. Drugs of abuse that are contraindicated during breastfeeding
3. Radioactive compounds that require temporary cessation of breastfeeding
4. Drugs with unknown effects on breastfeeding but may be of concern
5. Drugs that have been associated with significant effects on some nursing infants and should be given to breastfeeding mothers with caution
6. Maternal medication usually compatible with breastfeeding
7. Food and environmental agents: effect on breastfeeding

DRUG	EXCRETED IN MILK	% ADULT DOSE IN MILK	AAP RATING	COMMENTS
ANALGESICS AND ANTIINFLAMMATORY DRUGS (NONNARCOTIC)				
Acetaminophen (Datril, Tylenol)	Yes	0.04 to 1.85	6	Detoxified in liver. Avoid in immediate postbirth period; otherwise no problems with therapeutic dose.
Aspirin (Bayer, Anacin, Bufferin, Excedrin, etc.)	Yes	10.55 ± 10.45	6	Long history of experience shows complications rare. Can cause interference with platelet aggregation and diminished factor XII (Hageman factor) at birth. When mother requires high, continuing level of medication for arthritis, aspirin is drug of choice. Observe infant for bruisability. Platelet aggregation can be evaluated. Salicylism seen only in maternal overdosing. Mother should increase vitamin C and vitamin K intake.
Ibuprofen (Advil, Nuprin, Motrin, etc.)	Yes	<0.8	6	No apparent effects in therapeutic doses.
Indomethacin (Indocin)	Yes	0.11 to 0.98	6	Convulsions in breastfed neonate (case report). Used to close patent ductus arteriosus. Insufficient data as to effect on other vessels. May be nephrotoxic.

DRUG	EXCRETED IN MILK	% ADULT DOSE IN MILK	AAP RATING	COMMENTS
ANALGESICS AND ANTIINFLAMMATORY DRUGS (NONNARCOTIC)—cont'd				
Mefenamic acid (Ponstel)	Yes	0.036 to 0.8	6	No apparent effect on infant at therapeutic doses; infant able to excrete via urine.
Naproxen (Naproxyn, Anaprox, Naprosyn, Aleve)	Yes	1.1		Less toxic in adults than some other organic derivatives.
Propoxyphene (Darvon)	Yes	Trace amounts	6	Only symptoms detectable would be failure to feed and drowsiness. On daily, around-the-clock dosage, infant could consume 1 mg/day.
ANTIINFECTIVES (May change intestinal flora of infant and sensitize for later allergic reaction)				
Acyclovir (Zovirax)	Yes	5.6 ± 4.4	6	Minimal absorption through maternal skin.
Ampicillin (Polycillin, Amcill, Omnipen, Penbritin)	Yes	0.05 to 0.04		Sensitivity resulting from repeated exposure; diarrhea or secondary candidiasis.
Carbenicillin (Pyopen, Geopen)	Yes	0.001		Levels not significant. Drug is given to neonate. Not well absorbed from gastrointestinal (GI) tract.
Cefazolin (Ancef, Kefzol)	Yes	0.075	6	Probably not significant. Detected in milk if given intravenously (IV).
Cephalexin (Keflex)	Yes	0.86 ± 0.35		Completely gone by 8 hours; absorption less in first few months.
Cephalothin (Keflin)	Yes	0.4		Negligible.
Chloramphenicol (Chloromycetin)	Yes	1.6	4	Gray syndrome. Infant does not excrete drug well, and small amounts may accumulate. Contraindicated. May be tolerated in older infant with mature glycuronide system.
Colistin (Colymycin)	Yes	0.07		Not absorbed orally.
Demeclocycline (Declomycin)	Yes	Trace		Not significant in therapeutic doses. Can be given to infants. Drug remains in milk 3 days after dose.
Erythromycin (Ilosone, E-Mycin, Erythrocin)	Yes	0.1 to 2.1	6	Higher concentrations have been reported in milk than in plasma. Should not be given under 1 month of age because of risk of jaundice. Dose in milk higher when given IV to mother.
Gentamicin	Yes			Not absorbed from GI tract, may change gut flora. Drug is given to newborns directly.
Isoniazid (Nydrazid)	Yes	2.3		Infant at risk for toxicity, but need for breast milk may outweigh risk.
Kanamycin (Kantrex)	Yes	0.95	6	Infant absorbs little from GI tract. Infants can be given drug.
Metronidazole (Flagyl)	Yes	0.13 to 36	4	Caution should be exercised because of its high milk concentrations. Contraindicated when infant under 6 months; may cause neurologic disorders and blood dyscrasia. AAP says to discard milk for 12 hours if mother takes 2-gm dose.
Nitrofurantoin (Furadantin, Macrodantin)	Yes	0.6	6	No significant effect in therapeutic doses except in infant with G6PD deficiency.

DRUG	EXCRETED IN MILK	% ADULT DOSE IN MILK	AAP RATING	COMMENTS
ANTIINFECTIVES —cont'd				
Novobiocin (Albamycin, Cathomycin)	Yes	0.15		Infant can be given drug directly.
Nystatin (Mycostatin)	No	Not absorbed orally		Can be given to infant directly.
Oxacillin (Prostaphlin)	No	Trace		
Penicillin G, benzathine (Bicillin)	Yes	0.8		Clinical need should supersede possible allergic responses.
Penicillin G, potassium	Yes	0.8		Infant can be given penicillin directly. Parents should be told to inform physician that infant has been exposed to penicillin because of potential sensitivity.
Streptomycin	Yes	0.5	6	Not to be given more than 2 weeks. Ototoxic and nephrotoxic with long use. Is given to infants directly.
Sulfisoxazole (Gantrisin)	Yes	0.45	6	To be avoided during first month after birth; may cause kernicterus.
Tetracycline HCl (Achromycin, Panmycin, Sumycin)	Yes	0.3 to 4.8	6	Not enough to treat an infection in an infant. May cause discoloration of the teeth in the infant; the antibiotic, however, may be largely bound to the milk calcium. Do not give longer than 10 days or repeatedly.
ANTICOAGULANTS				
Coumarin derivatives Dicumarol (bishydroxy-coumarin), warfarin (Panwarfin)	Yes	6.5	6	Monitor prothrombin time. Give vitamin K to infant. Discontinue if surgery or trauma occurs. Drug of choice if mother to continue breastfeeding. May cause bleeding.
Heparin	No			Heparin ineffective orally.
ANTICONVULSANTS AND SEDATIVES (Barbiturates may pass into milk but do not sedate infant)				
Magnesium sulfate	Yes	0.5	6	May produce sedation in infant.
Pentobarbital (Nembutal)	Yes	Traces		Depends on liver for detoxification so may accumulate in first week of life until infant is able to detoxify. No problem for older infant in usual doses.
Phenytoin (Dilantin)	Yes	1.4 to 7.2	6	No problem if mother's dose is in therapeutic range.
Phenobarbital (Luminal)	Yes	1.5 5		Sleepiness and decreased sucking possible. On usual analeptic doses, infants alert and feed well. On hypnotic doses, infants depressed and difficult to rouse.
Sodium bromide (Bromo-Seltzer and over-the-counter sleeping aids)	Yes	6, 7		Drowsy, decreased crying, rash, decreased feeding. No longer available in the United States.
ANTIHISTAMINES (May suppress lactation; administer after nursing; all pass into breast milk)				
Brompheniramine (Dimetane)	Yes	Unknown		Drugs used in neonates. May cause sedation, decreased feeding, or may produce stimulation and tachycardia. Should avoid long-acting preparations, which may accumulate in infant.

DRUG	EXCRETED IN MILK	% ADULT DOSE IN MILK	AAP RATING	COMMENTS
ANTIHISTAMINES—cont'd				
Diphenhydramine (Benadryl)	Yes	Unknown		When combined with decongestants, may cause decrease in milk.
Promethazine (Phenergan)	Yes	Unknown	6	Passage into breast is expected; increases serum prolactin levels.
AUTONOMIC DRUGS				
Atrophine sulfate*	Yes	Traces	6	Hyperthermia, atropine toxicity, infants especially sensitive; also inhibits lactation. Infant dose 0.01 mg/kg.
Ergotamine	Yes	Unknown	1	May inhibit lactation.
Neostigmine	No	No known harm to infant.		
Propantheline bromide (Pro-Banthine)	No	Uncontrolled data indicate no measurable levels		Drug rapidly metabolized in maternal system to inactive metabolite. Mother should avoid long-acting preparations, however.
CARDIOVASCULAR DRUGS				
Diazoxide (Hyperstat)				Arteriolar dilators and antihypertensive, given only IV, not active orally.
Digoxin	Yes	0.07 to 14	6	Not detected in infant's plasma.
Hydralazine (Apresoline)	Yes	0.8	6	Jaundice, thrombocytopenia, electrolyte disturbances possible.
Methyldopa (Aldomet)	Yes	0.02 to 0.09		Galactorrhea. No specific data except as affects mother's milk production.
Propranolol (Inderal)	Yes	Traces		Risk of effect almost nonexistent.
Quinidine	Yes	4.1	6	Arrhythmia may occur.
CATHARTICS				
Cascara	Yes	Low	6	Caused colic and diarrhea in infant.
Milk of magnesia	No	None	6	No effect.
Mineral oil	No	None	6	No effect.
Phenolphthalein	Unknown	Unknown	6	Reported to cause symptoms in some.
Rhubarb	Unknown	None	6	None in syrup form. Fresh rhubarb may give symptoms of colic and diarrhea.
Saline cathartics	No	None	6	No effect.
Senna	No	None	6	None
Stool softeners and bulk-forming laxatives	No	None	6	No effect.
Suppositories (for constipation)	No	None	6	Not absorbed.
DIURETICS				
Furosemide (sulfamoylan-thranilic acid) (Lasix)	Possible	Not found in all samples		Drug is given to children under medical management.
Spironolactone (Aldactone)	Yes	Canrenone, a metabolite, appears	6	Acts as antagonist of aldosterone; causes sodium excretion and potassium retention. The metabolite apparently has some activity.
Thiazides (Diuril, Enduron, Esidrix, HydroDiuril, Oretic, Thiuretic tablets)	Yes	0.25 to 0.43	6	Risk of dehydration and electrolyte imbalance, especially sodium loss, which would require monitoring. Watch weight and wet diapers and take an occasional specific gravity reading of urine and serum sodium to indicate status of infant. Risk, however, is extremely low. May suppress lactation because of dehydration in mother.

*An ingredient in many prescription and nonprescription drugs.

DRUG	EXCRETED IN MILK	% ADULT DOSE IN MILK	AAP RATING	COMMENTS
HORMONES AND CONTRACEPTIVES				
Contraceptives (oral) Ethinyl estradiol, mestranol, 19-nortestosterone, norethindrone (Norlutin)	Yes	0.16 ±0.14	6	May diminish milk supply. May decrease vitamins, protein, and fat in milk. Most significant concern is long-range influences of hormone on young infant, which is not certain. Reports of feminization of infant.
Corticotropin	Yes	1.1	6	May decrease quantity and quality of milk.
Cortisone	Yes	Significant amounts		May affect infant in therapeutic doses.
Epinephrine (Adrenalin)	Yes			Destroyed in GI tract of infant.
Estrogen	Yes	0.1	6	Risks as with oral contraceptives. May alter quality and quantity of milk.
Insulin	No			Destroyed in intestinal tract.
Medroxyprogesterone acetate (Provera)	Yes	0.86 to 5	6	6-month injection may affect milk supply; 3-month injection should not decrease supply.
Prednisone	Yes	0.06 to 3.6	6	Minimum amount not likely to cause effect on infant in short course.
Tolbutamide (Orinase)	Yes	18	6	Watch for jaundice.
NARCOTICS				
Cocaine	Yes	Significant levels in milk	1, 2	No metabolites or drug found in milk after 36 hours or in infant's urine after 60 hours.
Codeine	Yes	5 ±2	6	No effect in therapeutic level and transient use. Can accumulate. Individual variation. Watch for neonatal depression. Asians metabolize drug less than Caucasians do.
Heroin	Yes		2	Level in milk enough to cause addiction in infant.
Marijuana (*Cannabis sativa L.*)	Yes		2	Shown in laboratory animals to produce structural changes in nursling's brain cells; impairs DNA and RNA formation. Infant at risk of inhaling smoke during feeding or when held by person who is smoking.
Meperidine (Demerol)	Yes	Trace		Trace amounts may accumulate if drug taken around the clock when infant is neonate. Watch for drowsiness and poor feeding.
Methadone	Yes	2.2	6	When dosage not excessive, infant can be breastfed if monitored for evidence of depression and failure to thrive. Suggest mother take daily dose after evening feeding and supplement formula at next feeding.
Morphine	Yes	0.8 to 1.2	6	Single doses have minimum effect. Potential for accumulation. May be addicting to neonate. Amounts in breast milk too variable to consider breastfeeding as means of treating withdrawal symptoms.
Percodan (oxycodone [derived from opiate thebaine], aspirin, phenacetin, caffeine)	Yes	Unknown		Consider for its component parts. In neonatal period, sleepiness and failure to feed, which increase maternal engorgement and neonatal weight loss, have been observed, probably caused by oxycodone.

DRUG	EXCRETED IN MILK	% ADULT DOSE IN MILK	AAP RATING	COMMENTS
PSYCHOTROPIC AND MOOD-CHANGING DRUGS				
Alcohol (Ethanol)	Yes	1 to 19.5	6	Milk may smell like alcohol. Ethanol in doses of 1 to 2 g/kg to mother causes depression of milk-ejection reflex (dose dependent). No acetaldehyde found because infant cannot metabolize ethanol.
Amphetamine	Yes	6.1 ±0.1	2	Has caused stimulation in infants with jitteriness, irritability, sleeplessness. Long-acting preparations cumulative.
Benzodiazepines* Chlordiazepoxide (Librium)	Yes			Not sufficient to affect infant first week when glucuronyl system needed for detoxification. May accumulate. May cause jaundice. Older infant, no apparent problem.
Diazepam (Valium)	Yes	2 to 4.7	4	Detoxified in glucuronyl system. In first weeks of life may contribute to jaundice. Metabolite active. Effect on infant: hypoventilation, drowsiness, lethargy, weight loss. Single doses over 10 mg contraindicated during breastfeeding. Accumulation in infant possible.
Haloperidol (Haldol)	Yes	0.15 to 2	4	An antipsychotic: animal studies in nurslings show behavior abnormalities.
Lithium carbonate (Eskalith, Lithane, Lithonate)	Yes	1.8		Measurable lithium in infant's serum. Infant kidney can clear lithium; however, lithium inhibits adenosine 3′, 5′-cyclic monophosphate, significant for brain growth. Also affects amine metabolism. Report of cyanosis and poor muscle tone and ECG changes in nursing infant.
Meprobamate (Miltown, Equanil)	Yes	2 to 4 times maternal plasma level		If therapy continued, infant should be followed closely.
Phencyclidine (PCP)	Yes		1	Animal studies show PCP in milk even after drug has been discontinued for 40 days.
Phenothiazines Chlorpromazine (Thorazine)	Yes	0.07 to 0.2		Drowsiness and lethargy in infants.
Thioridazine (Mellaril)	Yes	No information		Thioridazine is less potent in general than other phenothiazines. Probably safe.
Trifluoperazine (Stelazine)	Yes	Minimum		
Tricyclic antidepressants				Apparently no accumulation. No infants who have been observed showed symptoms.
Amitriptyline (Elavil)	Yes	0.8 ±0.2	4	Watch for depression or failure to feed; increases maternal prolactin secretion.
Desipramine (Norpramin, Pertofrane)		1	4	
Imipramine (Tofranil)	Yes	0.1	4	

DRUG	EXCRETED IN MILK	% ADULT DOSE IN MILK	AAP RATING	COMMENTS
STIMULANTS				
Caffeine	Yes	0.66 to 10	6	Accumulates when intake moderate and continual. Causes jitteriness, wakefulness, and irritability. Caffeine present in many hot and cold drinks. Consider if infant very wakeful.
Theobromine	Yes	20	7	No adverse symptoms observed in the infants. Chocolate the most common cause of exposure.
Theophylline	Yes	<1 to 15	6	Irritability, fretfulness.
THYROID AND ANTITHYROID MEDICATIONS				
Thiouracil	Yes	0.3 to 2.6	6	Get baseline levels of T_3, T_4, and TSH before and 6 weeks after mother starts medication.
Thyroid and thyroxine	Yes	0.3 to 2.6	6	Does not produce adverse symptoms on long-range follow-up study. Noted to improve milk supply of hypothyroid mothers. No contraindication.
MISCELLANEOUS				
DPT	Yes	Minimum		Does not interfere with immunization schedule.
Methotrexate	Yes	0.93	1	Antimetabolite. Infant would receive 0.26 μg/dl, which researchers consider nontoxic for infant.
Nicotine	Yes		2	Decreases milk production. Smoking may interfere with let-down reflex if smoking started before onset of a feeding. Smoke exposure may be a concern.
Poliovirus vaccine	No			Live vaccine taken orally. Not necessary to withhold nursing 30 minutes before and after dose. Provide booster after infant no longer nursing.
Rh antibodies	Yes			Destroyed in GI tract; not effective orally.
Rubella virus vaccine	Yes	Minimum		Will not confer passive immunity. Mother should not be given vaccine when at risk for pregnancy.
Tuberculin test	No			Tuberculin-sensitive mothers can adaptively immunize their infants through breast milk, and that immunity may last several years.
Chest x-rays				No effect.

*Alcohol enhances the effects of these drugs.
Compiled from Lawrence RA: *Breastfeeding: a guide for the medical profession,* ed 4, St Louis, 1994, Mosby; The Committee on Drugs, American Academy of Pediatrics: The transfer of drugs and other chemicals into human breast milk, *Pediatrics,* 93:(1):137, 1994.

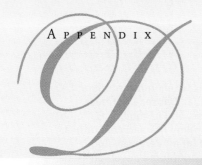

APPENDIX

Resources

This Appendix includes community and national resources, national clearinghouses, journals, and nursing organizations of interest to maternity and women's health nurses.

Community and National Resources

AIDS Network Hotline

(800) 342-2437 (AIDS)

AIDS Resource List

http://www.hivnet.org/aidsres.html

American Academy of Husband-Coached Childbirth

P.O. Box 5224
Sherman Oaks, CA 91413
(800) 42-Birth (in California)
(800) 423-2397 (outside California)

American Academy of Pediatrics

http://www.aap.org

American Association of Acupuncturists and Oriental Medicine

4104 Lake Boone Trail, Suite 201
Raleigh, NC 27607-6518
(919) 787-5181

American Cancer Society, Inc.

1599 Clifton Rd., NE
Atlanta, GA 30329
(800) ACS-2345
http://www.cancer.org

American Cleft Palate Association

1218 Grandview Ave.
Pittsburgh, PA 15211
(412) 681-1376
(800) 24-CLEFT

American College of Obstetricians and Gynecologists

409 12th St. SW
Washington, DC 20024
(800) 762-2264
http://www.acog.com

American Diabetes Association

Diabetes Information Service Center
1660 Duke St.
Alexandria, VA 22314
1-800-ADA-DISC
http://www.diabetes.org

American Fertility Foundation

2131 Magnolia Ave., Suite 201
Birmingham, AL 35256
(205) 251-9764

American Red Cross

430 17th St. NW
Washington, DC 20006
(202) 737-8300
http://www.redcross.org

American Society for Psychoprophylaxis in Obstetrics (ASPO)

1200 19th St. NW, Suite 300
Washington, DC 20036-2412
(800) 368-4404

Association for Childbirth at Home, International

P.O. Box 39498
Los Angeles, CA 90039
(213) 667-0839

Association of Maternal and Child Health Programs

1220 19th St. NW, Suite 801
Washington, DC 20036
(202) 775-0436
http://www.amchp.org

Centers for Disease Control and Prevention

1600 Clifton Rd., NE
Atlanta, GA 30333
(404) 329-1819
(404) 329-3286
http://www.cdc.gov

Center for Sickle Cell Disease
2121 Georgia Ave. NW
Washington, DC 20059
(202) 636-7930

Childbirth Graphics
P.O. Box 21207
Waco, TX 76702
(800) 229-3366

Compassionate Friends
(*Following death of an infant*)
P.O. Box 1347
Oak Brook, IL 60521
(312) 990-0010

COPE (Coping with the Overall Pregnancy/Parenting Experience)
37 Clarendon St.
Boston, MA 02116
(617) 357-5588

C/SEC, Inc. (Cesarean/Support Education and Concern)
22 Forest Rd.
Framingham, MA 01701
(508) 877-8266

Endometriosis Association
8585 North 76th Place
Milwaukee, WI 53223
(414) 355-2200
(800) 992-3636

Environmental Protection Agency (EPA)
Public Information Center
Room PM 211-B
401 M St. SW
Washington, DC 20460
(202) 382-7550
http://www.epa.gov

Equal Rights for Fathers
P.O. Box 90042
San Jose, CA 95109-3042
(408) 848-2323

Florence Crittenton Association of America
(*Assists in bringing about a greater understanding of factors relating to unmarried mothers and adolescent girls with other problems in adjustment*)
608 South Dearborn St.
Chicago, IL 60605

Healthy Mothers, Healthy Babies Coalition
409 12th St. SW
Washington, DC 20024
(202) 863-2458

Institute for Women's Policy Research
1400 20th St. NW
Washington, DC 20036
(202) 785-5100
http://www.iwpr.org

International Childbirth Education Association (ICEA)
P.O. Box 20048
Minneapolis, MN 55420
(612) 854-8660
http://www.icea.org

International Lactation Consultant Association
201 Brown Ave.
Evanston, IL 60202-3601
(708) 260-8874

Lact-Aid
(*Provides information and services to promote breastfeeding*)
P.O. Box 1066
Athens, TN 37303
(614) 744-9090

La Leche League
1400 N. Meacham Rd.
Shaumburg, IL 60173
(800) 525-3243 (24-hour line)
http://www.lalecheleague.org

March of Dimes Birth Defects Foundation
National Foundation/March of Dimes
1275 Mamaroneck Ave.
White Plains, NY 10605
(914) 428-7100
http://www.modimes.org

Maternity Center Association, Inc.
281 Park Ave. South, 5th Floor
New York, NY 10010
(212) 777-5000

National Abortion Federation Consumer Hotline
1156 15th St. NW, Suite 700
Washington, DC 20005
(800) 772-9100

National Association for Sickle Cell Disease
3345 Wilshire Blvd., Suite 1106
Los Angeles, CA 90010-1880
(213) 736-5455
(800) 421-8453

National Association of Childbearing Centers
3123 Gottschall Rd.
Perkiomenville, PA 18074
(215) 234-8068

**National Association of Parents and Professionals
for Safe Alternatives in Childbirth (NAPSAC)**
P.O. Box 267
Marble Hill, MO 63764
(314) 238-2010

National Breast Cancer Coalition
P.O. Box 66373
Washington, DC 20035
(202) 296-7477
(800) 935-0434

**National Cancer Institute Cancer Information
Service**
(800) 4-CANCER
http://www.nci.nih.gov

National Child Abuse Hotline
(800) 422-4453

National Coalition Against Domestic Violence
P.O. Box 34103
Washington, DC 20043-4301
(202) 638-8638

Hotline: (800) 333-SAFE (7233)
(*Many states have local coalitions against domestic violence.*)

National Coalition Against Sexual Assault
912 North 2nd St.
Harrisburg, PA 17102
(717) 232-6771

**National Coalition of Feminist
and Lesbian Cancer Projects**
P.O. Box 90437
Washington, DC 20090
(202) 332-5536

**The National Coalition of Hispanic Health and
Human Services Organizations (COSSMHO)**
1030 15th St. NW, Suite 1053
Washington, DC 20005
(202) 387-5000
http://www.cossmho.org

National Down Syndrome Congress
1800 Dempster St.
Park Ridge, IL 60068-1146
(708) 823-7550
(800) 232-6372

National Down Syndrome Society Hotline
666 Broadway
New York, NY 10012
(800) 221-4602

National Foundation for Jewish Genetic Diseases, Inc.
250 Park Ave., Suite 1000
New York, NY 10177
(212) 371-1030

**National Institute of Child Health and Human
Development (NICHD)**
National Institutes of Health
9000 Rockville Pike
Bldg 31, Room 2A32
Bethesda, MD 20892
(301) 496-4000
http://www.nih.gov

**National Organization of Mothers
of Twins Clubs, Inc.**
P.O. Box 23188
Albuquerque, NM 87192
(505) 275-0955

**National Organization for Women (NOW) Legal
Defense and Education Fund**
99 Hudson St.
New York, NY 10013-2871
(212) 925-6635

**National Organization on Adolescent Pregnancy,
Parenting, and Prevention**
4421A East-West Hwy.
Bethesda, MD 20814
(301) 913-0378
http://www.noappp.org

National Perinatal Association
101 ½ South Union St.
Alexandria, VA 22314-3323
(703) 549-5523

National Resource Center for Domestic Violence
(800) 537-2238

National Right to Life Committee
419 7th St. NW, Suite 500
Washington, DC 20004
(202) 626-8800

National Sudden Infant Death Syndrome Foundation

10500 Little Patuxent Parkway, Suite 420
Columbia, MD 21044
(301) 964-8000
(800) 221-7437

National Women's Health Resource Center

5255 Loughboro Rd, NW
Washington, DC 20016
(202) 537-4015
http://www.healthywomen.org

Office of Minority Health Resource Center

P.O. Box 37337
Washington, DC 20013-7337
(301) 587-1938

Parent Care, Inc.

(*Neonatal intensive care unit family support*)
101½ South Union
Alexandria, VA 22314-3323
(703) 836-4678

Parenthood After Thirty

451 Vermont
Berkeley, CA 94707
(415) 524-6635

Parents of Prematures

13613 NE 26th Place
Bellevue, WA 98005
(206) 883-6040

Parents Without Partners

8807 Colesville Rd.
Silver Spring, MD 20910
(301) 588-9354
(800) 637-7974

Planned Parenthood Federation of America, Inc.

810 Seventh Ave.
New York, NY 10019
(800) 230-PLAN
http://www.ppfa.org/ppfa

Pregnancy and Infant Loss

1421 East Wayzata Blvd., Suite 40
Wayzata, MN 55391
(614) 473-9372

Premenstrual Syndrome Action

P.O. Box 16292
Irving, CA 92713
(714) 854-4407

Reach to Recovery
(*see* American Cancer Society)
(*breast cancer*)

Read Natural Childbirth Foundation

P.O. Box 956
San Rafael, CA 94915
(415) 456-8462

Resolve, Inc.

(*Impaired fertility*)
1310 Broadway, Dept. GM
Summerville, MA 02144-1713
(617) 623-0744

RTS Bereavement Services

Lutheran Hospital–La Crosse
1910 South Ave.
La Crosse, WI 54601
(608) 791-4747
(800) 362-9567

Sex Information & Education Council of the United States

(*Provides publications [e.g., "Sexual relations in pregnancy and postpartum"] and teaching aids*)
130 W. 42nd St., Suite 350
New York, NY 10036
http://www.siecus.org

Special Supplemental Nutrition Program for Women, Infants, and Children (WIC)

Food and Consumer Service
3101 Park Center Dr., Rm 819
Alexandria, VA 22302
(703) 305-2286
http://www.usda.gov/fcs/wic.htm

Spina Bifida Association of America

4590 McArthur Blvd. NW, Suite 250
Washington, DC 20007-4226
(800) 621-3141

Twins Magazine

P.O. Box 12045
Overland Park, KS 66212
(800) 821-5533

National Clearinghouses

American Foundation for Maternal and Child Health

(*Research on the perinatal period*)
300 Beekman Place
New York, NY 10022
(212) 759-5510

Breastfeeding Resources

http://www.parentsplace.com/readroom/bf.html

CDC National Clearinghouse in AIDS

http://www.cdcnac/org

Food and Drug Administration (FDA)

Office of Consumer Affairs
Public Inquiries
5600 Fishers Lane (HFE-88)
Rockville, MD 20857
(301) 443-3170
http://www.fda.gov

Infertility Resources

http://www/ihr.com/infertility/index.html

National AIDS Information Clearinghouse

P.O. Box 6003
Rockville, MD 20849-6003
1-800-458-5231 (English and Spanish)

National Clearinghouse for Drug Abuse Information

P.O. Box 426
Dept DQ
Kensington, MD 20795
1-800-637-2045; 1-800-492-6605 (in Maryland only)
http://www.health.org

National Clearinghouse for Family Planning Information

P.O. Box 10716
Rockville, MD 20850
(703) 558-4990

National Clearinghouse for Human Genetic Disease

(Provides information about inherited diseases.)
National Center for Education in Maternal and Child Health
38th and R Sts., NW
Washington, DC 20057

Sudden Infant Death Syndrome Clearinghouse

8201 Greensboro Dr., Suite 600
McLean, VA 22102
(723) 821-8955

Nursing Journals

AWHONN's Lifelines

2000 L St. NW, Suite 740
Washington, DC 20036
(202) 261-2400
http://www.awhonn.org

Birth: Issues in Prenatal Care and Education

(Formerly Birth and Family Journal)
Blackwell Scientific Publications, Inc.
3 Cambridge Center, Suite 208
Cambridge, MA 02142
(617) 876-7000

Bookmarks

(Complimentary annotated catalog of book reviews)
ICEA Supplies Center
P.O. Box 20048
Minneapolis, MN 55420

Canadian Nurse

The Canadian Nurses Association
50 The Driveway
Ottawa, Canada K2P1E2

The Female Patient

Division Excerpta Medica
301 Gibraltar Dr.
P.O. Box 528
Morris Plains, NJ 07950

Journal of Nurse-Midwifery

Elsevier Science, Inc.
655 Avenue of the Americas
New York, NY 10010
(212) 989-5800

Journal of Obstetric, Gynecologic and Neonatal Nursing (JOGNN)

J.B. Lippincott Co.
12107 Insurance Way
Hagerstown, MD 21740

Journal of Perinatal and Neonatal Nursing

Aspen Publishers, Inc.
7201 McKinney Circle
Frederick, MD 21701
(800) 234-1660

Maternal/Newborn Advocate

The National Foundation/March of Dimes
P.O. Box 2000
White Plains, NY 10602

MCN The American Journal of Maternal Child Nursing

555 W. 57th St.
New York, NY 10019

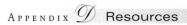

Mother-Baby Journal
1304 Southpoint Blvd., Suite 280
Petaluma, CA 95954
(707) 762-2646

Neonatal Network
1304 Southpoint Blvd., Suite 280
Petaluma, CA 95954
(707) 762-2646

Nurse Practitioner: A Journal of Primary Nursing Care
3845 42nd Ave. NE
Seattle, WA 98105

Nursing Research
555 W. 57th St.
New York, NY 10019

Loss and Grief
"Bereavement" Magazine
8133 Telegraph Dr.
Colorado Springs, CO 80920
(719) 282-1948

Women's Health Issues
The Jacob's Institute for Women's Health
409 12th St. SW
Washington, DC 20024
(888) 4ES-INFO

Nursing Organizations

American College of Nurse Midwives
818 Connecticut Ave. NW, Suite 900
Washington, DC 20006
(202) 728-9860
http://www.midwife.org

American Nurses Association
600 Maryland Ave. SW
Washington, DC
(202) 651-7000
http://www.nursingworld.org or www.ana.org

The Association of Women's Health, Obstetric, and Neonatal Nurses (AWHONN)
2000 L St. NW, Suite 740
Washington, DC 20036
(800) 673-8499 (US)
(800) 245-0231 (Canada)
http://www.awhonn.org

Canadian Nurses Association
50 The Driveway
Ottawa, Ont. K2P 1E2
(613) 237-2133

Midwives Alliance of North America
United States and Canada
c/o Concord Midwifery Service
30 South Main St.
Concord, NH 03301
(603) 225-9586

National Association of Neonatal Nurses (NANN)
1304 Southpoint Blvd., Suite 280
Petaluma, CA 94954
(800) 451-3785
http://www.ajn.org/ajnnet/nsorgs/nann/

National League for Nursing (NLN)
61 Broadway
New York, NY 10006
(800) 669-1656
http://www.nln.org

Human Milk Banking Association of North America (HMBANA) Member Banks

HMBANA Executive Office
P.O. Box 370464
West Hartford, CT 06137-0464
(860) 232-8809

Regional Milk Bank
The Medical Center of Central Massachusetts
Worcester, MA 01605
(508) 793-6005

Mothers' Milk Bank
Medical Center of Delaware
Wilmington, DE 19579
(302) 733-2340

Community Human Milk Bank
Georgetown University Hospital
Washington, DC 20007
(202) 784-2177

Triangle Mothers' Milk Bank
Wake Medical Center
Raleigh, NC 27610
(919) 250-8599

Mothers' Milk Bank

Central Baptist Hospital
Lexington, KY 40503
(606) 275-6502

Mothers' Milk Bank

Presbyterian/St. Luke's Medical Center
Denver, CO 80218
(303) 869-1888

Mothers' Milk Bank

Valley Medical Center
San Jose, CA 95128
(408) 998-4550

Lactation Support Service

British Columbia Children's Hospital
Vancouver, British Columbia, Canada V6H 3V4
(604) 875-2345, ext. 7607

Page numbers followed by "b" indicate boxes; "f" indicates figures; "t" indicates tables.

To help us publish the most useful materials for students, we would appreciate your comments on this book. Please take a few moments to complete the form below, then tear it out and mail it back to us. Thank you in advance for your input!

Book Title: _____

Author Name: _____

1. Did the content of this textbook help you meet the requirements for passing this course? Explain: _____

_____

2. What do you like most about this product? _____

_____

What do you like least? _____

_____

3. Which chapters were most helpful? Which were least helpful? _____

_____

4. If you could change one thing about this book, what would it be? _____

_____

5. If applicable, did you purchase/use the student learning guide accompanying the text? If so, did you purchase the student learning guide on your own or at the direction of the instructor? _____

_____

6. Was the book a good value for the price? _____

_____

7. Are you planning to keep this text? Why or why not? _____

_____

Are you interested in doing in-depth reviews of our nursing textbooks? If so, please fill out the information below:

Name: _____ Telephone: _____

Address: _____

Thank you!

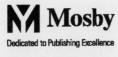

Mosby

Dedicated to Publishing Excellence

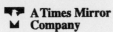

A Times Mirror Company

tape shut here

**NO POSTAGE
NECESSARY
IF MAILED
IN THE
UNITED STATES**

BUSINESS REPLY MAIL
FIRST-CLASS MAIL   PERMIT NO. 135   SAINT LOUIS MO

POSTAGE WILL BE PAID BY ADDRESSEE

**JANET BLANNER
NURSING MARKETING
MOSBY INC
11830 WESTLINE INDUSTRIAL DR
SAINT LOUIS MO 63146-9987**

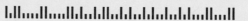

tape shut here